Anesthesia
and Neurosurgery

Anesthesia
and Neurosurgery

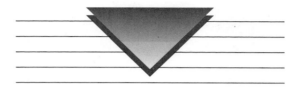

JAMES E. COTTRELL, M.D.

Senior Associate Dean for Clinical Practice
Professor and Chairman
Department of Anesthesiology
State University of New York
Health Science Center at Brooklyn
Brooklyn, New York

DAVID S. SMITH, M.D., PH.D.

Associate Professor
Department of Anesthesia
University of Pennsylvania
School of Medicine
Director
Division of Neuroanesthesia
Hospital of the University of Pennsylvania
Philadelphia, Pennsylvania

THIRD EDITION
with 285 illustrations

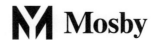 **Mosby**

St. Louis Baltimore Boston Chicago London Madrid Philadelphia Sydney Toronto

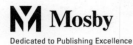

Executive Editor: Susan M. Gay
Developmental Editor: Sandra Clark Brown
Project Supervisor: John Rogers
Senior Production Editor: Helen Hudlin
Manufacturing Supervisor: Theresa Fuchs
Designer: Jeanne Wolfgeher
Cover Design: Renée Duenow

THIRD EDITION

Printed in the United States of America
Composition by the Clarinda Company
Printing/binding by Walsworth Publishing Company

Mosby–Year Book, Inc.
11830 Westline Industrial Drive
St. Louis, MO 63146

Library of Congress Cataloging in Publication Data

Anesthesia and neurosurgery / [edited by] James E. Cottrell, David S.
   Smith.— 3rd ed.
        p.   cm.
   Includes bibliographical references and index.
   ISBN 0-8016-6573-6
   1. Nervous system—Surgery.   2. Anesthesia in neurology.
   I. Cottrell, James E.   II. Smith, David S. (David Stuart), 1946-
   [DNLM: 1. Anesthesia.   2. Nervous System—surgery.   WO 200 A578
   1994]
   RD593.A5   1994
   617.9′6748—dc20
DNLM/DLC
for Library of Congress   94-3103
                                                                          CIP

94 95 96 97 98 / 9 8 7 6 5 4 3 2 1

Contributors

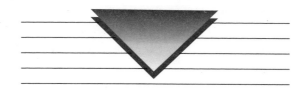

MAURICE S. ALBIN, M.D., M.SC. (ANES.)

Professor
Departments of Anesthesia and Surgery (Neurosurgery)
The University of Texas Health Science Center
San Antonio, Texas

ALAN A. ARTRU, M.D.

Professor and Head of Research
Department of Anesthesiology
University of Washington
School of Medicine
Seattle, Washington

DONALD P. BECKER, M.D.

W. Eugene Stern Former Professor and Chief
Division of Neurosurgery
UCLA Medical Center
Los Angeles, California

ROBERT BEDFORD, M.D.

Professor
Department of Anesthesia
University of Virginia
School of Medicine
Charlottesville, Virginia

MARVIN BERGSNEIDER, M.D.

Chief Resident
Division of Neurosurgery
UCLA Medical Center
Los Angeles, California

JAMES E. COTTRELL, M.D.

Senior Associate Dean for Clinical Practice
Professor and Chairman
Department of Anesthesiology
State University of New York
Health Science Center at Brooklyn
Brooklyn, New York

RICHARD M. DASHEIFF, M.D.

Director
University of Pittsburgh Epilepsy Center
Pittsburgh, Pennsylvania

BARBARA A. DODSON, M.D.

Assistant Professor
Department of Anesthesia
University of California
San Francisco, California

KAREN B. DOMINO, M.D.

Associate Professor
Departments of Anesthesiology and Neurosurgery
University of Washington
Harborview Medical Center
Seattle, Washington

CALVIN C. ENG, M.D.

Acting Professor
Department of Anesthesiology
University of Washington
Harborview Medical Center
Seattle, Washington

PROFESSOR WILLIAM FITCH, M.D.

Professor and Head
University Department of Anaesthesia
University of Glasgow
Glasgow Royal Infirmary
Glasgow, Scotland

EUGENE S. FLAMM, M.D.

Charles Harrison Frazier Professor
   and Chairman
Division of Neurosurgery
University of Pennsylvania
School of Medicine
Philadelphia, Pennsylvania

HUGH A. GELABERT, M.D.

Assistant Professor of Surgery in Residence
Section of Vascular Surgery
Center for Health Sciences
University of California
Los Angeles, California

ADRIAN W. GELB, M.D., M.B., CH.B., F.R.C.P.C.

Professor and Chairman
Department of Anesthesia
University of Western Ontario
University Hospital
London, Ontario, Canada

SHANKAR P. GOPINATH, M.D.

Research Associate
Department of Neurosurgery
Baylor College of Medicine
Houston, Texas

STEPHEN J. HAINES, M.D.

Professor of Neurosurgery, Otolaryngology, and Pediatrics
Department of Neurosurgery
University of Minnesota
Minneapolis, Minnesota

JOHN HARTUNG, PH.D.

Research Associate Professor
Department of Anesthesiology
State University of New York
Health Science Center at Brooklyn
Brooklyn, New York

IAN A. HERRICK, B.SC., M.D., F.R.C.P.C.

Assistant Professor
Department of Anaesthesia
University of Western Ontario
University Hospital
London, Ontario, Canada

W. ANDREW KOFKE, M.D.

Associate Professor
Department of Anesthesiology
Director, Neurologic Anesthesia and Supportive Care Program
University of Pittsburgh
School of Medicine
Pittsburgh, Pennsylvania

MARK J. KOTAPKA, M.D.

Assistant Professor
Division of Neurosurgery
University of Pennsylvania
School of Medicine
Philadelphia, Pennsylvania

FRED J. LAINE, M.D.

Assistant Professor
Department of Radiology
Medical College of Virginia
Richmond, Virginia

ARTHUR M. LAM, M.D., F.R.C.P.C.

Professor
Departments of Anesthesiology and Neurosurgery
University of Washington
Harborview Medical Center
Seattle, Washington

WARREN J. LEVY, M.D.

Associate Professor
Department of Anesthesia
University of Pennsylvania
School of Medicine
Philadelphia, Pennsylvania

WAYNE K. MARSHALL, M.D.

Associate Professor
Department of Anesthesia
M.S. Hershey Medical Center
Hershey, Pennsylvania

M. JANE MATJASKO, M.D.

Martin Helrich Professor and Chairman
Department of Anesthesiology
University of Maryland
Baltimore, Maryland

ROBERT W. MCPHERSON, M.D.

Director
Division of Neuroanesthesia
Johns Hopkins Medical Institution
Baltimore, Maryland

LESLIE NEWBERG MILDE, M.D.

Professor and Vice Chair
Department of Anesthesiology
Mayo Clinic
Rochester, Minnesota

THOMAS H. MILHORAT, M.D.

Professor and Chairman
Department of Neurosurgery
State University of New York
Health Science Center at Brooklyn
Director of Neurosurgery
Kings County Hospital Center
Brooklyn, New York

JOHN I. MILLER, M.D., F.A.C.S.

Director
Division of Pediatric Neurosurgery
State University of New York
Health Science Center at Brooklyn
Brooklyn, New York

WESLEY S. MOORE, M.D.

Professor of Surgery
Director, Section of Vascular Surgery
Center for Health Sciences
University of California
Los Angeles, California

JONATHAN D. MORENO, PH.D.

Professor of Pediatrics and of Medicine
Director, Division of Humanities in Medicine
State University of New York
Health Science Center at Brooklyn
Brooklyn, New York

JAMES L. MOSTROM, M.D.

Assistant Professor
Department of Anesthesia
M.S. Hershey Medical Center
Hershey, Pennsylvania

KAZUHIKO NAKAKIMURA, M.D.

Staff Anesthesiologist
Department of Anesthesiology-Resuscitology
Yamaguchi University
School of Medicine
Yamaguchi, Japan

EDWARD A. NEUWELT, M.D.

Professor
Department of Neurology
Oregon Health Sciences University
Portland, Oregon

PHILIPPA NEWFIELD, M.D.

Attending Anesthesiologist
California Pacific Medical Center
Assistant Clinical Professor
Departments of Anesthesia and Neurosurgery
University of California
San Francisco, California

EDWARD H. OLDFIELD, M.D.

Chief
Surgical Neurology Branch
National Institute of Neurological Disorders and Stroke
National Institutes of Health
Bethesda, Maryland

EUGENE ORNSTEIN, PH.D., M.D.

Associate Professor
Department of Anesthesiology
College of Physicians & Surgeons
Columbia University
New York, New York

DANIEL K. O'ROURKE, M.D.

Resident
Department of Neurosurgery
University of Pittsburgh
Pittsburgh, Pennsylvania

ANDREW T. PARSA, B.S.

Medical Scientist Training Program
Department of Neurosurgery
Department of Anatomy and Cell Biology
State University of New York
Health Science Center at Brooklyn
Brooklyn, New York

WILLIAM J. PERKINS, M.D.

Assistant Professor
Department of Anesthesiology
Mayo Clinic
Rochester, Minnesota

PATRICIA H. PETROZZA, M.D.

Associate Professor
Department of Anesthesia
Bowman Gray School of Medicine
Head, Neurosurgical Anesthesia
Wake Forest University Medical Center
Winston-Salem, North Carolina

DONALD S. PROUGH, M.D.

Professor and Chairman
Rebecca Terry White Distinguished Chair
Department of Anesthesiology
The University of Texas Medical Branch
Galveston, Texas

CLAUDIA S. ROBERTSON, M.D.
Professor
Department of Neurosurgery
Baylor College of Medicine
Houston, Texas

TAKEFUMI SAKABE, M.D.
Professor and Chairman
Department of Anesthesiology-Resuscitology
Yamaguchi University
School of Medicine
Yamaguchi, Japan

MARK S. SCHELLER, M.D.
Associate Professor
Department of Anesthesiology
Neuroanesthesia Research Laboratory
University of California
San Diego, California

JEFFREY S. SCHWEITZER, M.D., PH.D.
Fellow
Section of Neurological Surgery
Yale University
School of Medicine
New Haven, Connecticut

DAVID S. SMITH, M.D., PH.D.
Associate Professor
Department of Anesthesia
University of Pennsylvania
School of Medicine
Director, Division of Neuroanesthesia
Hospital of the University of Pennsylvania
Philadelphia, Pennsylvania

WENDY R.K. SMOKER, M.D.
Professor
Department of Radiology
Director ENT/Neuroradiology
Medical College of Virginia
Richmond, Virginia

RENÉ TEMPELHOFF, M.D.
Associate Professor
Department of Anesthesiology
Director of Neuroanesthesia
Washington University School of Medicine
St. Louis, Missouri

MITCHELL TOBIAS, M.D.
Assistant Professor
Department of Anesthesia
University of Pennsylvania
School of Medicine
Philadelphia, Pennsylvania

MARGARET R. WEGLINSKI, M.D.
Assistant Professor
Department of Anesthesiology
Mayo Clinic
Rochester, Minnesota

DENNIS Y. WEN, M.D.
Assistant Professor
Department of Neurosurgery
University of Minnesota
Minneapolis, Minnesota

MARIE L. YOUNG, M.D.
Associate Professor
Department of Anesthesia
University of Pennsylvania
School of Medicine
Philadelphia, Pennsylvania

WILLIAM L. YOUNG, M.D.
Associate Professor
Departments of Anesthesiology and Neurological Surgery
College of Physicians & Surgeons
Columbia University
New York, New York

MARK H. ZORNOW, M.D.
Associate Professor
Department of Anesthesiology
Neuroanesthesia Research Laboratory
University of California
San Diego, California

CONNIE ZUCKERMAN, J.D.
Assistant Professor of Humanities in Medicine
and of Family Medicine
Division of Humanities in Medicine
State University of New York
Health Science Center at Brooklyn
Brooklyn, New York

Foreword to the Third Edition

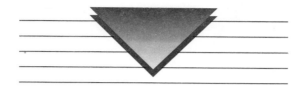

Since publication of the second edition of *Anesthesia and Neurosurgery*, the field of anesthesiology has been significantly enhanced by advances in technology, the manufacture and clinical validation of new equipment, and the development of new pharmacological agents. In combination with advances in electrophysiologic monitoring, these tools have expanded the research base upon which neuroanesthesiology is built. That enriched foundation has, in turn, resulted in a greater understanding of neuropharmacology and neuropathology.

Advances in neuroanesthesiology have also enabled neurosurgeons to expand their own field while anesthesiologists provide more appropriate perioperative management, superior postoperative care, and improved management of acute and chronic pain. Indeed, as our expanding abilities become applicable to a larger and more diversified patient population, neuroanesthesiologists are now faced with new challenges in providing assistance to colleagues in radiology, neonatology, critical care, and other specialities.

Subspecialities emerge as a result of an expansion of knowledge. The Oxford English Dictionary defines a "specialist" as an "authority who particularly or exclusively studies a single branch of his profession or subject." The editors of this volume have certainly devoted their lives to becoming masters in the subspecialty of neuroanesthesiology. Jim Cottrell was a founder and subsequent President of the Society of Neurosurgical Anesthesia and Critical Care. In addition, he initiated the *Journal of Neurosurgical Anesthesiology*, recognizing the need to bring the subspecialty's literature, previously fragmented across many journals, under one cover. David Smith, the new co-editor of this volume, has worked for many years in one of the leading research centers in neuroanesthesiology and is also a past President of the Society of Neurosurgical Anesthesia and Critical Care.

Outcome is the most important attribute of any anesthetic intervention of critical care experience. Brain damage can cause severe emotional and financial consequences—consequences which we can most fully appreciate when the damage affects someone close to us—a colleague, a friend, or, in particular, a member of our own family. I am certain that this third edition of *Anesthesia and Neurosurgery* will be an indispensable source of up-to-date knowledge and practical clinical advice for all anesthesiologists who strive to provide neurosurgical patients with the most appropriate care and the best possible outcome.

PROFESSOR DR. HUGO VAN AKEN
CHAIR, DEPARTMENT OF ANESTHESIOLOGY
UNIVERSITY HOSPITAL
CATHOLIC UNIVERSITY OF LEUVEN, BELGIUM

Preface

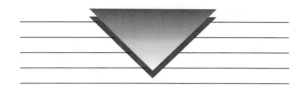

The nineties have been declared "The Decade of the Brain" and the third edition of *Anesthesia and Neurosurgery* will serve this decade well. When a subspecialty advances as rapidly as neuroanesthesiology, most material that was current just eight years ago must be left behind. Accordingly, with a preponderance of new chapters, new authors, and even a new co-editor, this edition of a once familiar text is essentially a new book with a 14-year legacy. That legacy has paralleled the development of the field itself, and we owe a debt of gratitude to Dr. Herman Turndorf for the contributions he made to previous editions of this text and to the foundations on which modern neuroanesthesiology has been built.

Putting first things first, Part I covers relevant biochemistry and physiology, including brain metabolism, cerebral and spinal cord blood flow, metabolically induced brain injury, cerebrospinal fluid, intracranial pressure monitoring, the blood-brain barrier and cerebral edema, and the effects of anesthetics on ICP and CBF. Part II reviews basic aspects of neuroradiology and neurophysiologic brain monitoring.

Part III focuses on the perioperative period, including fluid management; care of the acutely unstable patient; surgical and anesthetic management of supratentorial masses, the posterior fossa, aneurysms, and arteriovenous malformations; interventional neuroradiology; induced hypotension; blood-brain barrier disruption; occlusive cerebrovascular disease; seizure surgery; pediatric neurosurgery; neurologic diseases of the spine and spinal cord; and neuroendocrine disease.

Finally, Part IV takes us to the postoperative period and intensive care management of the neurosurgical patient. It covers management of severe head injury, spinal cord injury, and includes an innovative discussion of ethical considerations.

The new format of *Anesthesia and Neurosurgery* provides quick orientation, focused reading, and an index that facilitates comprehensive access to specific subjects. There is liberal use of color for emphasis. The international group of authors has been chosen for their ability to communicate and for their expertise. They have generously lived up to their reputations, and we, the editors, are grateful for their contribution.

Everyone involved hopes this book will serve its readers by helping them to better serve their patients.

JAMES E. COTTRELL
DAVID S. SMITH

ACKNOWLEDGMENTS

The editors would like to acknowledge the efforts of many individuals who, in addition to the authors of each chapter, spent hours in helping prepare this book for publication. These include Iris Karafin who was central to manuscript revision; Kathleen Grugan, R.N., M.S.N., David Bowden, B.A., and Cara Grugan who spent many hours reading chapters for flow and content; and Anne Miniadis, Dr. Cottrell's administrative assistant, and several associates, including Cynthia Cohen, Ph.D., J.D., Theodore Cheek, M.D., Ira Kass, Ph.D., John Hartung, Ph.D., and Audrée Bendo, M.D., who reviewed various chapters. The editors would also like to thank Susan Gay of Mosby–Year Book for her guidance and patience during the production of this text.

Contents

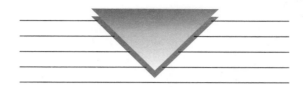

1

Brain Metabolism

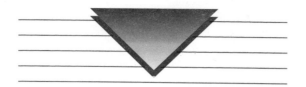

WILLIAM FITCH

The brain is a *converter* of energy: It converts substrates supplied as metabolic fuel (mainly D-glucose and oxygen) into the usable forms of energy with which it supports and regulates its many synaptic connections, voltage-dependent and agonist-operated ion channels, and the synthesis, transportation, and packaging of neurotransmitters. The brain is also a substantial *consumer* of energy. In humans, the central nervous system receives about 15% of the resting cardiac output (750 ml/min) and consumes about 20% (170 µmol/100 g/min) of the oxygen required by the body at rest (on average, the weight of the brain is only 2% to 3% of the total body weight). Moreover, one quarter (31 µmol/100 g/min) of the glucose consumed by the body is used by the brain. Fortunately, the brain is also a *conserver* of energy. Under physiologic conditions, the expenditure of energy is controlled by the activity of the cells: The consumption of fuel is related to the work done and not the reverse.

This chapter describes how the brain obtains energy from its supply of metabolic substrates, details why the brain consumes energy, and discusses briefly the clinical importance of its ability to conserve energy. In addition, the chapter considers those means by which the metabolic activity of the brain may be assessed, either relatively or absolutely, and their clinical applicability.

THE BRAIN AS A CONVERTER OF ENERGY

The brain's energy requirement is substantial; paradoxically, its store of energy-generating substrates (glycogen, glucose, oxygen) is small—so small, in fact, that at normal rates of ATP production the available stores of glycogen would be exhausted in less than 3 minutes. Thus the normal functioning of the central nervous system depends on the continuous provision of appropriate energy substrates and the adequate removal of the waste products of metabolism.

The requirement of the central nervous system for metabolic fuel is provided almost exclusively, at least under physiologic conditions, by the glycogenolysis of the glycogen stored in the liver (mainly), muscle, and, to a limited extent, other organs (per unit mass, muscle stores 10 times as much glycogen and liver 100 times as much as the brain), and the complete oxidation of the released glucose to carbon dioxide and water. In the absence of ketosis (such as may occur in association with starvation or diabetes), the adult brain uses glucose as its sole metabolic substrate. Although glucose may be formed from noncarbohydrate sources (certain amino acids, the glycerol portion of fat molecules), gluconeogenesis does not contribute much to the brain's energy supply. With starvation (perhaps also during the fast prior to anesthesia), gluconeogenesis—a process requiring the expenditure of significant quantities of energy in its own right[20]—is essential because the ability of the brain to metabolize ketone bodies depends on a basal input of glucose with which to regenerate certain of the intermediary substrates required by the citric acid cycle.[43] Under certain circumstances, the energy released by the oxidation of ketone bodies by the brain is important, such as under physiologic conditions in the neonate and during starvation in the adult. It has been recognized for some time that, with prolonged starvation, ketone bodies, acetoacetate, and beta-hydroxybuterate will replace glucose as the predominant metabolic substrate in the brain. More recent studies have shown an increase in the uptake of ketones by the brain (in proportion to their concentration in blood) in *healthy* individuals who have fasted for as little as 12 to 16 hours. However, even when ketone bodies are the predominant source of metabolic fuel, the brain cannot tolerate hypoglycemia; a supply of glucose, albeit small, is necessary.

Glucose is transported via facilitated diffusion from the blood into the brain by membrane-based carrier mechanisms specific for D-glucose, which exhibit the properties of saturability and competition.[22] At rest, the brain extracts from the blood around 10% of the glucose delivered to it. Obviously, there is some reserve, and more will be ex-

tracted if the blood flow decreases. However, because the concentration of glucose in the brain is lower than that in the blood, there is no "safety device" with which the brain can supplement its supply in the presence of systemic hypoglycemia.[22] The properties of the intact blood-brain barrier (as well as those of the membrane-based transporters) restrict the substrates used by the brain to the few mentioned previously. However, when blood-brain barrier function is absent or impaired, compounds such as various intermediaries of the citric acid cycle and dicarboxylic acids may be able to enter brain tissue and be metabolized.[3]

The oxidation of glucose occurs in every cell in the body with the exception of red blood cells, which lack mitochondria, and provides the cell's major source of energy. It occurs in three successive stages: glycolysis, the citric acid cycle, and the electron transport chain (Fig. 1-1).

Glycolysis is the term given to a series of 10 chemical reactions that occur in the cytoplasm of the cell and convert the six-carbon molecule of glucose into two three-carbon molecules of pyruvic acid (Fig. 1-2). Because two molecules of adenosine triphosphate (ATP) are required to initiate the glycolytic reactions and four molecules of ATP are generated to complete the process, there is a net gain of two molecules of ATP for each molecule of glucose oxidized (Table 1-1). The fate of the pyruvic acid depends on the availability of oxygen. Under anaerobic conditions, the pyruvic acid is reduced by the addition of two hydrogen atoms to form lactic acid. This may be transported back to the liver, where it is reconverted to pyruvic acid, or it may remain in the cell until aerobic conditions are restored.

In the presence of adequate amounts of oxygen, the complete oxidation of glucose continues in the mitochondria, where, in a cyclic series of reactions, the pyruvic acid (now as acetyl co-enzyme A) is oxidized to form carbon dioxide

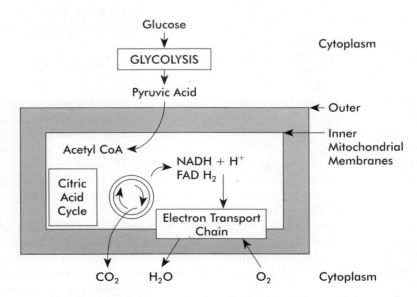

FIG. 1-1   Schematic representation of complete oxidation of glucose.

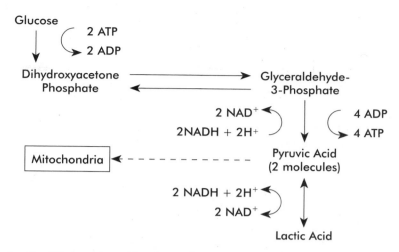

FIG. 1-2 Simplified version of biochemical reactions involved in glycolysis. *(Modified from Siesjo BK*: Brain energy metabolism, *New York, 1978, Wiley.)*

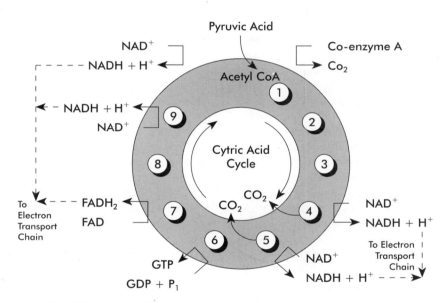

FIG. 1-3 Simplified version of biochemical reactions involved in the citric acid cycle. *(Modified from Siesjo BK*: Brain energy metabolism, *New York, 1978, Wiley.)*

TABLE 1-1
Summary of ATP Production (Aerobic Metabolism) from One Molecule of Glucose

Source	Yield of ATP
Glycolysis	
Oxidation of glucose to pyruvic acid	2
Krebs cycle	
Oxidation of succinyl CoA to succinic acid	2 (GTP)
Electron transport chain	
1. 2 Nicotinamide adenine dinucleotide (NADH) + 2 H$^+$ (glycolysis)	6
2. 2 NADH + 2 H$^+$ (acetyl CoA)	6
3. 6 NADH + 6 H$^+$ (Krebs cycle)	18
4. 2 Flavin adenine dinucleotide (FADH$_2$)	4
Total	38

and water. The citric acid (Krebs) cycle is a series of biochemical reactions in which the large amount of potential energy, stored in the intermediate substances derived from the pyruvic acid, is released in a stepwise manner (Fig. 1-3). A series of oxidations (pyruvic acid derivatives) and reductions (coenzymes) transfers the potential energy, in the form of electrons, to a number of coenzymes. The net result of the citric acid cycle is that for every two molecules of acetyl CoA that enter the cycle there is the liberation of four molecules of carbon dioxide, which are excreted via the lungs, the production of reduced coenzymes (six nicotinamide adenine dinucleotide (NADH) + 6H$^+$ and two flavin adenine dinucleotide (FADH$_2$)), which contain stored energy, and the generation of two molecules of GTP, a high-energy compound that is used to produce ATP. The reduced coenzymes (NADH, H^+, and $FADH_2$) are the most important end-products because they contain most of the energy stored originally in the glucose and subsequently in the pyruvic acid (Table 1-1).

During the third component of aerobic metabolism, the energy stored in the coenzymes is transferred to adenosine diphosphate (ADP) and inorganic phosphate to form ATP, a high-energy molecule that releases large amounts of *usable* energy (E) when it is hydrolyzed:

$$ATP + H_2O \rightarrow ADP + Pi + E \qquad (1)$$

Because the supply of ATP is limited and the energy released by the breakdown of ATP is being used by the cell constantly, the ATP is replenished as a phosphate group and is added to ADP:

$$ADP + Pi + E \rightarrow ATP + H_2O \qquad (2)$$

The carriers of the electron transport chain are organized into three complexes within the cristae of the inner membrane of the mitochondrion (Fig. 1-4): the NADH complex (which contains flavin mononucleotide [FMN]), the cytochrome b-c complex (which contains cytochromes b and c), and the cytochrome oxidase complex (which contains cytochromes a and a_3). Coenzyme Q transfers electrons between the first and second complexes and cytochrome c between the second and third. The NADH dehydrogenase complex, coenzyme Q, and the cytochrome b-c_1 complex are the three components of the system that pump (actively transport) hydrogen ions from one side of the membrane to the other and, as a result, establish a hydrogen ion gradient across the membrane and a "store" of potential energy. As the hydrogen ions on the side of the membrane with the higher hydrogen ion concentration diffuse back across the membrane with the help of ATPase, the energy is released and used by the enzyme to synthesize ATP from ADP and Pi. The various transfers of electrons in the electron trans-

port chain generate 34 molecules of ATP from each molecule of glucose oxidized, 3 from each of the 10 molecules of NADH + H^+ and 2 from each of the two molecules of $FADH_2$. Thus, theoretically, 38 molecules of ATP (usable energy) can be generated by aerobic metabolism (Table 1-1) from each molecule of glucose supplied as metabolic fuel:

$$C_6H_{12}O_6 + 6\ O_2 + 38\ ADP + 38\ Pi \qquad (3)$$
$$\downarrow$$
$$6\ CO_2 + 6\ H_2O + 38\ ATP$$

However, in reality, one molecule of glucose probably yields no more than 30 to 35 molecules of ATP. There are other (alternative) pathways by which small amounts of glucose and pyruvate are metabolized. Some of the glucose is required for the synthesis of nucleotides and is diverted into the pentose phosphate pathway,[38] some is used to sustain the store (albeit small) of glycogen in the brain, and 5% to 8% is metabolized to lactate.

The ATP generated by these reactions in the mitochondria next must be transported into the cytoplasm for use elsewhere in the cell. This is achieved by transport proteins in the inner membrane of the mitochondria that couple the outward movement of ATP with the passage of ADP (formed from metabolic reactions in the cytoplasm) into the mitochondria.

Glycolysis, the citric-acid cycle, and the electron transport chain normally provide all of the ATP required by cellular activities. Because the citric acid cycle and the electron transport chain are *aerobic* processes (and yield 17 to 18 times as much ATP as glycolysis alone), *anaerobic* metabolism clearly cannot satisfy the energy requirements of the brain (Table 1-1). Hence the central nervous system depends fundamentally on the continuous provision of oxygen.

The brain is an obligate aerobe; it cannot store oxygen, and its high metabolic requirements *(vide infra)* consume 40 to 70 ml O_2/min. Fortunately, under normal circum-

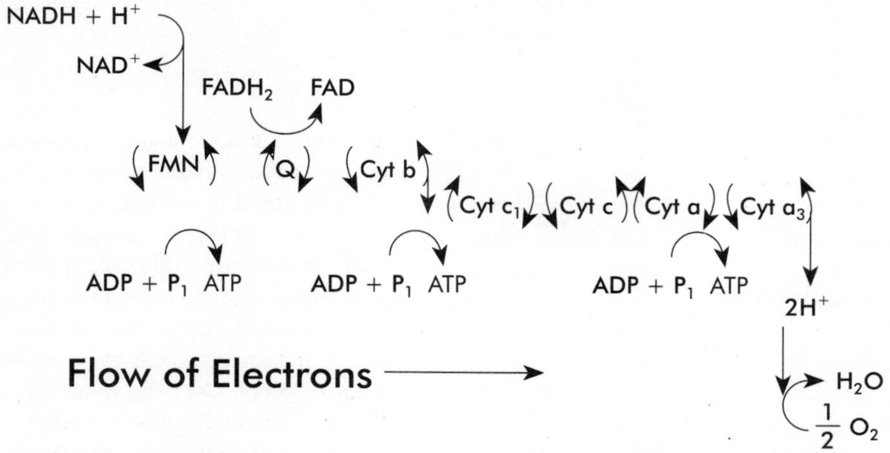

Flow of Electrons ⟶

FIG. 1-4 Simplified version of reactions involved in the electron transport chain. (*Modified from Siesjo BK*: Brain energy metabolism, *New York, 1978, Wiley, and* J Neurosurg 60:883-908, 1984.)

BOX 1-1
SUMMARY OF BALANCE BETWEEN DEMAND FOR
AND DELIVERY OF OXYGEN UNDER PHYSIOLOGIC
CONDITIONS

Demand for Oxygen
3-5 ml per 100 g brain tissue per minute (i.e., 40-70 ml
   per min)

Delivery of Oxygen
20 ml per 100 ml blood
50 ml blood per 100 g brain tissue per min (i.e., 150 ml
   per min)

---

stances, there is a substantial safety margin and the delivery of oxygen ($CaO_2 \times CBF$) is considerably greater than demand (Box 1-1). As a result, any decrease in delivery (unaccompanied by any decrease in demand) will be counteracted, at least initially, by an increase in the amount of oxygen extracted from the blood, with the preservation of aerobic metabolism and normal clinical function. If necessary, certain emergency reactions that delay the depletion of ATP or increase glycolysis can be brought into play. Ultimately, however, after the supply of oxygen at cellular level has become insufficient to support the continuing synthesis of adequate amounts of ATP, there is failure of those energy-requiring processes that sustain the normal function of the cell and its integrity.

It was conventionally taught that mitochondrial oxidations involve the acceptance by oxygen of a package of four electrons (with the formation of water) and that the production of ATP is coupled to the flow of electrons. On balance, it is now accepted that other reactions exist in which the univalent reduction of oxygen occurs with the subsequent formation of superoxide radicals, hydrogen peroxide, and hydroxyl radicals.[39] Fortunately, this liberation of free radicals does not appear to disadvantage the normal cell. However, this may not be the case under pathologic conditions in which the increase in the concentrations of these free radicals may threaten the survival of the cell.

THE BRAIN AS A CONSUMER OF ENERGY

Unlike muscle, the brain does no mechanical work. Nevertheless, as has been discussed previously, its consumption of energy is substantial. In this section, we will consider some anatomic and biochemical reasons for this.

Neurons are the basic information processors of the central nervous system. They are also responsible for the conduction of nerve impulses from one part of the body to another in a nondecremental manner. Most neurons consist of a cell body, dendrites, and an axon. The cell body contains a well-defined nucleus and a nucleolus surrounded by the cytoplasm, in which there are typical or-

ganelles (the Golgi apparatus, endoplasmic reticulum, mitochondria, Nissl bodies, and lysosomes). Dendrites are branched extensions of the cytoplasm that conduct nerve impulses toward the cell body. The axon is usually a single, long, thin, specially adapted process that conducts the nerve impulses away from the cell body to other neurons, muscles, or glands. The specialized terminals of the axon (synaptic terminals) contain unique structures that are usually vesicular in nature. These are believed to contain thousands of molecules of a transmitter substance that has been synthesized in the whole neuron and then packaged in remarkably regular amounts (quanta) within the vesicles. In most instances, a neuron synthesizes, stores, and releases only one neurotransmitter. Recently, some neurons have been identified that apparently produce two. However, as a general rule, it is possible to define a neuron by the type of transmitter released from its terminal(s) (acetylcholine, norepinephrine, dopamine, 5-hydroxytryptamine, gamma-aminohydroxybutyric acid, glutamate, and others). Until recently, it was believed that all neurotransmitters were small molecules; however, it is now clear that many neurons secrete peptides (e.g., substance P, enkephalins).

Macromolecules and macromolecular assemblies are being synthesized constantly in the cell body and transported peripherally to replace those lost or degraded. Although the rate at which this "wear and tear" occurs is not known with any degree of accuracy, it has been estimated that the cell body may reproduce up to 2000 mitochondria and renew its population of macromolecules in 1 day.[48] Moreover, it has been suggested that synaptic vesicles are used on only a few occasions before being degraded. Clearly such estimates are uncertain; nevertheless, they do highlight the fact that synthetic tasks must consume a significant proportion of the energy generated.[39]

Every living cell has a potential difference across its membrane because of the fact that charged particles are separated by a semipermeable membrane that prevents the charged particles from redistributing themselves randomly. The special feature of the so-called "excitable cells" (nerve, muscle) is that membrane permeability can be changed by processes that either increase (hyperpolarize) or decrease (depolarize) the potential difference. The cell membrane is formed of a double layer of phospholipid molecules (polar heads outside, hydrophobic fatty-acid tails inside) into which cholesterol molecules and specialized protein molecules (e.g., ATPases, adenylate cyclases, cytochrome oxidases) are inserted. Some of the proteins penetrate the membrane completely and are structured to form channels that permit the passage of water and ions. In addition to these specialized channels, there is an active pumping mechanism that transports sodium ions out of and potassium ions into the cell. Although the structural basis of the pump is unknown, the actions of certain metabolic inhibitors indicate that its carrier molecules are driven by energy derived from the metabolic processes within the cell, most likely by energy released when ATP is hydrolyzed by Na-K-ATPase.

The imbalance of positive charges across the cell membrane is due mostly to differences in permeability. This creates an electric potential across the membrane known as the resting potential and reflects mostly the potassium equilibrium potential (-97 mV). There is likely a constant leakage of ions through membrane gates that must be counteracted by ATP-driven transport. Thus, even when a neuron is not conducting an impulse, it is actively transporting ions across its membrane. If the membrane of an excitable cell is depolarized beyond a critical value, voltage-dependent sodium channels open and allow sodium ions to enter the cell until the sodium equilibrium potential ($+66$ mV) is reached. The passage of these positive ions into the cell depolarizes it further, the gate is opened wider, and the permeability of the membrane increases dramatically. It is likely that a similar voltage-dependent gate is opened at the internal end of the potassium channel such that potassium ions leave the cell (although on a slightly different time course) as the sodium enters. These fluxes activate the membrane-bound Na-K-ATPase. As a result, sodium is pumped out of the cell at the expense of ATP and restoration of the resting potential. Calcium is another ion that requires considerable amounts of ATP for its regulation. It is widely accepted that the influx of calcium into presynaptic terminals is a prerequisite for the release of transmitter and that calcium ions will enter the cell (along with sodium ions) when the membrane depolarizes. The restoration of normal calcium gradients and the maintenance of low intracellular calcium concentrations require energy (extracellular concentrations of calcium are much greater than intracellular). In all probability, the efflux of calcium ions is brought about mainly by a sodium/calcium exchange mechanism that utilizes the energy stored in the sodium gradient created by ATPase activity. However, there may be several other energy-dependent mechanisms (membrane pump, endoplasmic reticulum, calcium pump, mitochondrial calcium pump) both to export calcium ions from the cell and to ensure their sequestration in appropriate storage sites within the cell. The membrane-based calcium pump, although present in the general plasma membrane, is especially important in synaptic areas. It is activated by calmodulin and appears to exchange calcium ions for hydrogen ions.[5] About 3% of the total ATP consumption in the cell can be attributed to the activity of this pump.[14]

The phospholipid bilayer of the cell membrane is a dynamic structure. Phospholipid molecules can move sideways and exchange places with others in their own row. Moreover, there are enzymes (phosphatidyl methyltransferases) that can convert one phospholipid into another. This gives considerable fluidity to the membrane, a fluidity that is augmented by the normal turnover of the phospholipids. Several of the steps involved in these processes[39,50] require energy and may lead to the formation of compounds such as free fatty acids and prostaglandins that have either established or putative effects on metabolism and circulation.[39]

Glial tissue is of three main types: astroglia, oligodendroglia (responsible for laying down the spiral sheaths of myelin around axons), and microglia (immunologic function). Astroglia are not only supporting structures; they also play an important role in the metabolism of the neurons. They function as an intermediary between the blood vessels and the nerve cells, actively transferring material to and from the neurons, and act as a buffer of the internal milieu, especially in regard to ionic flow. Indeed, it seems likely that a major proportion of the glycogen stored in the brain is held in glial cells from which, presumably, the glycogen could be delivered rapidly to neighboring neurons in an emergency.[18] Glial cells may act as buffers of potassium ions by helping in their removal from the area surrounding the neuronal membranes and as buffers of neurotransmitters released from the neurons. Some of these neurotransmitters, notably the excitatory and inhibitory amino acids, are not broken down after release; thus their inactivation depends on reuptake, either into the presynaptic nerve terminals or into glial cells, a process that requires metabolic energy because the reaccumulation of, for example, glutamate within the cell occurs against a concentration gradient.

The contribution the glial cells make to the overall cerebral metabolic rate is controversial. On balance they appear to be less metabolically active than the neurons because they have a lower mitochondrial density and so should have a lower metabolic rate. This conclusion is in keeping with the fact that whereas neurons succcumb to hypoxia or hypoglycemia, glial cells do not.[39]

Three factors are involved in the control of the volume of a cell that does not have a rigid surrounding membrane: the quality of the fixed intracellular material, the external concentration of permeable material, and the ratio of the "leak" rate constant to the "pump" rate constant.[37] Energy is required for these processes; energy failure allows an influx of sodium and chloride ions in excess of any loss of potassium ions and as a result causes swelling of cells, both glial and neuronal.

In summary, the usable energy generated by the brain (as ATP) is consumed in the maintenance of the transmembrane electrical and ionic gradients (both in the resting state and after depolarization), the support of the structure of the membrane per se, the driving of axonal flow, and the synthesis, packaging, release, and reuptake of neurotransmitters. By far the most costly in terms of energy expenditure is ion transport. About 70% of the ATP produced is consumed in maintaining the nonequilibrium distribution of ions across the cell membrane.[14] Therefore any critical imbalance between the availability of energy and the demand for energy will result in a loss of activity in the membrane pump, the accumulation of sodium within the cell, and an increase in extracellular potassium concentration. These events lead to the depolarization of the membrane, the opening of voltage-dependent and agonist-operated calcium channels, and an increase in intracellular calcium concentration. The control of cell volume is lost, as are electrical excitability, synaptic function, and the regulation of acid-base balance.

THE BRAIN AS A CONSERVER OF ENERGY

As with any other energy converter, the brain must be efficient in its use of substrate; as an energy consumer, it should not squander the energy it has available. In 1890, Roy and Sherrington[35] proposed that ". . . the brain possesses an intrinsic mechanism by which its vascular supply can be varied locally in correspondence with local variations in functional activity." Much recent evidence supports this proposal, and it is accepted that, in conscious humans under physiologic conditions, the supply of substrate (as evidenced by the blood flow) parallels the expenditure of energy (as reflected in the oxygen consumption and glucose utilization). When cerebral function is depressed, as in coma, and the requirement for energy is decreased, total cerebral blood flow, oxygen consumption, and glucose use are much lower than in the normal fully conscious state. In contrast, during seizures (the most severe form of functional activation of the brain) the demand for energy substrates increases and must be met by a concomitant increase in supply. Moreover, the coupling between the processes that supply energy substrates and those that consume energy has been demonstrated in all the functional subunits of the central nervous system. Thus, under physiologic conditions, the heterogeneity of blood flow is mirrored by a heterogeneity of glucose utilization such that blood flow (substrate delivery) is greater to those areas in which the expenditure of energy is greatest (primary auditory cortex, neocortex) and least in those regions with the lowest demand for energy substrates (globus pallidus, white matter). Further evidence of this coupling between delivery and demand is available from studies in which neural pathways have been deliberately activated. For example, tactile stimulation has been shown to increase glucose utilization in the postcentral gyrus.[17] Likewise, stimulation of the visual and auditory pathways results in increases in glucose metabolism in the visual association cortex and the temporal lobe, respectively.[30] Thus it seems fair to conclude that the expenditure of energy by the brain is controlled tightly by the output of work, and that the amount of substrate delivered is coupled closely to the required expenditure of energy.[23]

It is clear from some of the descriptions presented earlier in the chapter that, at the cellular level, metabolism is normally a *balance* between the utilization of ATP during the performance of work and its resynthesis in sequences that themselves provide the energy (via phosphocreatine) to rephosphorylate the ADP.

In addition to glycolosis and oxidative phosphorylation, the brain has two other mechanisms that can help maintain a stable ATP concentration—the creatine phosphokinase and adenylate kinase reactions.[14] Creatine phosphokinase catalyzes the reversible transfer of phosphate between phos-

phocreatine and ATP:

$$PCr + ADP + H^+ \rightleftharpoons ATP + Cr \qquad (4)$$

The concentration of phosphocreatine, a high-energy compound found in excitable tissues, is about three times that of ATP (in brain), and it has been shown that a decrease in phosphocreatine concentration precedes a decrease in ATP concentration in those situations in which the synthesis of ATP is restricted (ischemia) or the demand for ATP is increased (seizures). Adenylate kinase makes available the energy contained in the terminal phosphate groups of the ADP molecule, particularly when the utilization of ATP outstrips the supply (ischemia):

$$ADP + ADP \rightleftharpoons ATP + AMP \qquad (5)$$

In the second place, adenylate kinase allows a "recharging" of the accumulated adenosine monophosphate (AMP) to ATP after the oxidative processes catch up with the deficit.[38]

Of the carbohydrate consumed by the brain, 95% undergoes oxidative metabolism;[3] 43% of the energy originally held in an unusable form in glucose is captured by the ATP. The remainder is given off as heat.

Finally, the neurons can conserve energy by "switching off" much of their expenditure of energy (before they have completely exhausted their reserves) when the delivery of substrate decreases to critical levels. In essence, function is sacrificed to conserve fuel. If we accept the concept proposed by Michenfelder and Theye (Fig. 1-5)[27] it is clear that by "switching off" 60% of its work, the brain can save 60% of its expenditure of energy and thus support its fundamental processes on a lessened supply of fuel. In other words, the brain has the capacity to "idle" and use less fuel. As long as damage has not been done to the "engine" of the cell itself, function can be restored when more fuel becomes available.

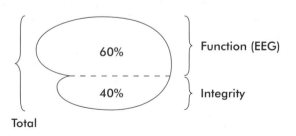

$$CMR_{O_2} = 5.5\ ml \cdot 100g^{-1} \cdot min^{-1}$$
$$Function = 3.3\ ml \cdot 100g^{-1} \cdot min^{-1}$$
$$Integrity = 2.2\ ml \cdot 100g^{-1} \cdot min^{-1}$$

FIG. 1-5 Oxygen requirements of the normal brain. Values are those obtained in the canine. *(From Michenfelder JD: The hypothermic brain. In Michenfelder JD: Anesthesia and the brain, New York, 1988, Churchill-Livingstone.)*

Effect of Temperature on Metabolic Processes

Now that the concept of "heat production" has been discussed, we should consider the effects of temperature (essentially hypothermia) on cerebral metabolic processes.

Hypothermia decreases the rate of all of the biochemical reactions that subserve metabolism, that is, those that support synaptic activity (as evidenced by spontaneous electrical activity) and those required to sustain the integrity of the cell (as reflected in ion fluxes and the activity of membrane-based ion pumps). As a result, the brain consumes less energy, is required to convert less substrate, and can therefore be more tolerant of any decrease in the supply of oxygen and, to a lesser extent, glucose.

The intrinsic velocity of a chemical reaction can be related to a defined rate constant K, the temperature dependence of which is given by:

$$K = Ae^{-E/RT} \qquad (6)$$

where

- T = The absolute temperature in degrees Kelvin
- A = A constant
- E = Another constant expressing the "activation energy" of the reaction

Thus temperature affects reaction rate by influencing the activation energy of the reaction. In essence, the relationship between temperature and the rate constant (metabolic rate) is exponential (logarithm of the rate constant is linearly related to $1/T$ with a slope equal to $-E/R$), and the magnitude of the relationship can be characterized by the temperature coefficient (Q_{10}), the ratio of the metabolic rates associated with two temperatures that differ by $10°$ C. The Q_{10} of the majority of chemical reactions is about 2; that is, a $10°$ C decrease in the temperature of a reaction will decrease the rate of the reaction by approximately 50%. For example, when the temperature decreases from 38 to $28°$ C, the cerebral metabolic rate for oxygen (CMR_{O_2}) decreases by about 55% and it decreases further to 20% of the normothermic value if the temperature is decreased by a further $10°$ C to $18°$ C (the Q_{10} for the CMR_{O_2} between 38 and $28°$ C is approximately 2.2[26]).

Classically, the Arrhenuis equation relates only to the kinetics of single reactions. As we have seen, the reactions by which the brain converts and consumes energy are complex. Thus it is not surprising to find that there has been some dispute about the exponential nature of the relationship between temperature and metabolism and about the absolute values of Q_{10}.[1,26,34] These issues were clarified by Steen et al.[45] in a study that examined the effects of hypothermia on functioning brain (active electroencephalogram [EEG]) and on brain in which electrical function had been suppressed by the administration of barbiturates (isoelectric EEG). They demonstrated that, in functioning brain, a simple exponential could not be used to describe the relationship between temperature and metabolic rate; between 37 and $28°$ C the calculated Q_{10} was 2.4, between 28 and $18°$ C it was 5.0, and below $18°$ C it was 2.3 (Table 1-2). The

TABLE 1-2

Interrelationships Between Temperature, CMR_{O_2} and Q_{10} Values

Temperature in Degrees Celsius	Functioning Brain CMR_{O_2}	Q_{10}	Nonfunctioning Brain CMR_{O_2}	Q_{10}
37	4.95	—	2.70	—
28	2.23	2.5	1.38	2.1
18	0.45	5.0	0.54	2.5

Modified from Michenfelder JD: *Anesthesia and the brain*, New York, 1988, Churchill-Livingstone, pp 23-34.

marked increase in Q_{10} between 28 and $18°$ C was accounted for by the cessation of electrical function (the onset of an isoelectric EEG), which tends to occur between 21 and $18°$ C. This abolition of the functional component of the energy-consuming reactions presumably caused a step decrease in metabolism and an increase in Q_{10}. The clinical significance of these concepts relates to the use of hypothermia as a means of protecting the brain. Thus, if the Q_{10} is 2 and if the normothermic brain can withstand complete ischemia for a period of 5 minutes, the brain should be able to withstand 10 minutes at $27°$ C and 20 minutes at $17°$ C. If the Q_{10} is 3 to 3.5, the values would be 15 to 18 minutes at $27°$ C and 45 to 63 minutes at $17°$ C, or if Q_{10} is 5, between $27°$ and $17°$ C for 75 to 90 min.[25] Table 1-2 also shows that the demand for oxygen (as reflected in the CMR_{O_2}) decreases progressively as temperature is decreased. Other studies have shown that the cerebral metabolic rate for glucose parallels that for oxygen[26,46] and that the breakdown of the available usable high-energy compounds (e.g., ATP) is decreased.[21,47] Thus it seems clear that hypothermia can decrease the demand by the brain for metabolic fuel and so, at least theoretically, make the brain more tolerant of any decrease in substrate delivery.

In humans, temperature can be decreased by 7 to $8°$ C and in other homeothermic animals such as the rat to $20°$ C before failure of the cardiovascular system begins to threaten the survival of the brain regardless of the decrease in the consumption of energy. If the circulation is supported artificially by cardiopulmonary bypass, neurons can withstand very low temperatures. A much narrower temperature range is tolerable in association with hyperthermia. Cardiovascular dysfunction is evident around $42°$ C; however, even the absence of overt circulatory failure, a similar (or slightly greater) increase in temperature appears to damage neurons directly because of inactivation of enzyme proteins. Thus, although initially the effects of hyperthermia on the brain must be the opposite of those produced by hypothermia, the range is small, and ultimately (around $43°$ C) the pathophysiology differs. There are very few studies of the effect of hyperthermia on cerebral metabolic rate; nevertheless, those that have been undertaken support the view that metabolism does increase as temperature increases to 40 and $42°$ C (CMR_{O_2} increases by 5% per degree C) and that oxygen uptake decreases at temperatures of around $43°$ C.

MEASUREMENT OF CEREBRAL METABOLIC ACTIVITY

The brain obtains usable energy principally through the *oxidative* phosphorylation of glucose. As we have seen, it converts metabolic fuel into energy in strict accordance with its consumption of energy such that, at steady state, the amount of ATP produced is equal to the amount used. In other words, there is a tight coupling between the production of ATP and the consumption of oxygen. Because this is so, the overall metabolic activity of the brain can be deduced from the measurement of the amount of oxygen consumed. It is true that similar information could be obtained from measurements of the utilization of glucose. However, substrates other than glucose may be used under certain circumstances and the tissue stores of glucose, although limited, are constantly varying. Thus measurements of oxygen consumption provide the most reliable information on metabolic activity.[38]

The law of the conservation of matter predicts that the amount of substrate *(Q)* (which, like oxygen, is consumed by a tissue) carried to the tissue in unit time *(At)* by the arterial blood *(Qa/At)* must be equal to the sum of the amount leaving the tissue in the venous blood *(Qv/At)*, the amount metabolized by the tissue *(Qm/At)*, and the amount that has accumulated in the tissue *(Qi/At)*:

$$\frac{Qa}{At} = \frac{Qv}{At} + \frac{Qm}{At} + \frac{Qi}{At} \qquad (7)$$

If the change in the amount of the substance accumulating in the tissue is small in comparison to the amount metabolized (as is the case for oxygen), *Qi* can be neglected and the equation written:

$$\frac{Qa - Qv}{At} = \frac{Qm}{At} \qquad (8)$$

That is, the amount of the substance metabolized (consumed) by the tissue is equal to the difference between the amount carried to and removed from the tissue within the stipulated period of time. The amount carried to the tissue during this time interval is equal to the product of the arterial blood flow *(Fa)* and the arterial concentration of the substance *(Ca)*, that is, Fa × Ca. Likewise, the amount leaving the tissue in the venous blood can be expressed as Fv × Cv. If the arterial inflow is equal to venous outflow, then:

$$\frac{Qm}{At} = F (Ca - Cv) \qquad (9)$$

where

F = The volume of nutrient blood flow to the tissue
Ca = The mean concentration of the substance in the arterial blood
Cv = The mean concentration in the venous blood draining the tissue (the Fick equation)

The application of the Fick principle to the measurement of metabolic activity requires, first, that the blood being sampled truly reflects the arterial inflow to the tissue under study and its venous outflow. Second, it must be possible to measure the flow to the tissue (in the context of this discussion, the cerebral blood flow) reliably and quantitatively. As far as the brain is concerned, we can make the reasonable assumption that the concentration of the substance (in this case the oxygen content) in arterial blood *(Ca)* sampled peripherally will be the same as that in the arterial blood supplying the brain. Unfortunately, the other two indices in equation 9 *(F* and *Cv)* cannot be dealt with so easily. The requirement to obtain samples of the venous blood that drains the tissue under investigation introduces the problem of what is and what is not the venous drainage of the brain itself. Although there is no doubt that the major portion of the blood leaving the brain will do so via the internal jugular veins, it is also acknowledged that there are numerous communications (emissary veins) between the intracranial venous sinuses and the extracranial veins that drain muscle, subcutaneous tissue, and skin, and between the facial veins and the internal jugular veins. In the experimental animal, this particular problem can be circumvented if blood is sampled from the superior sagittal sinus. Clinically, the jugular bulb is the only easily accessible site from which blood can be sampled, either by direct percutaneous puncture or by retrograde cannulation of the internal jugular vein. However, it is necessary to ensure that the tip of the cannula or catheter is placed as close as possible to the base of the skull (at least above the level of the second cervical vertebra) because a percentage of the blood in the more proximal part of the jugular bulb has drained from extracerebral tissues, that its position is confirmed radiologically, and that the samples of blood are withdrawn relatively slowly (particularly if flow is low) so as not to contaminate the sample with blood from extracerebral tissues. I have sought to emphasize these points because the actual source of the venous blood sample(s) is also a critically important determinant of the validity of the measurement of other variables, such as the cerebral metabolic rate for glucose, the cerebral venous lactate concentration, the arterial-jugular venous oxygen content difference, and the jugular venous oxygen saturation.

The means by which the flow of blood to the tissue in unit time *(F,* cerebral blood flow, CBF) may be measured and their applicability are described in detail elsewhere in this text. Nonetheless, several points are of particular relevance to the measurement of cerebral metabolic activity and are addressed here. First, although the Kety-Schmidt technique has been used extensively to measure CBF and, thus permits the calculation of cerebral metabolic rate, the actual value of metabolic rate obtained is an average of the metabolic rates in all of the tissues (gray matter and white matter), which have drained into the one jugular bulb from which the blood samples have been drawn; that is, most but not necessarily all of the ipsilateral hemisphere. A more extensive, although not more detailed, assessment of cerebral metabolic activity would require the cannulation of the jugular bulb bilaterally. The Kety-Schmidt technique can be used for the assessment of overall cerebral metabolism, but it cannot detect regional variations. However, application of the Kety-Schmidt technique (or one of its more appropriate modifications) in the experimental animal makes it possible to relate energy flux (CMR_{O_2}) to energy charge (e.g., tissue concentrations of ATP, inorganic phosphates, phosphocreatine).[14,38]

Radioactive Inert-Gas Clearance Technique

In the original application of the technique, the clearance of 85-Kr (beta emissions) from the surface of the cortex was monitored by a detector placed over the *exposed* cortex. Venous blood could be obtained easily from the superior sagittal sinus (after the elimination of extracranial anastomoses) and the CMR_{O_2} calculated. However, because the values obtained were higher than expected (and higher than those obtained using the Kety-Schmidt technique), it was concluded that this particular technique overestimated cortical oxygen consumption, most probably because the blood in the superior sagittal sinus was not representative of the venous blood from the actual tissue in which flow was measured, the superficial tissue layer (1 mm thick) of the cortex. The subsequent introduction of gamma-emitting isotopes facilitated the measurement of CBF and made possible the determination of regional blood flow. However, similar advantages did not accrue to the derivation of CMR_{O_2}. In animals, the sagittal sinus could be cannulated via a burr hole and metabolic rate calculated using the "fast" component of the clearance curve. However, a number of assumptions have to be made: that blood in the superior sagittal sinus drains only cortical tissue; that the "fast" component measures flow in cortical tissue; and that any recirculation or build-up of tracer in extracerebral tissues does not influence the results.[38] These assumptions are far from proven valid. In humans, there are no sampling sites from which one may obtain venous blood that would be a reflection of the tissue volume associated with these regional CBF techniques. Thus a measurement of cerebral metabolic rate can be obtained only by the derivation of mean flow, the measurement of the oxygen contents in arterial and jugular bulb blood, and the incorporation of these values into Equation 9. The measurement of CBF using the stochastic method is based on a quantitative principle, the law of the conservation of matter, and is the most valid measurement of flow in humans with which to derive cerebral metabolic rates. However, cannulation of a jugular bulb and a peripheral artery are necessary to obtain true cerebral venous and arterial blood. In addition, it is necessary to cannulate (or at least puncture) the internal carotid artery to permit the bolus administration of the tracer. Moreover, whether the venous blood sampled is representative of the particular tissue in which flow has been measured becomes a matter of speculation. The great advantage of the method is its ability to measure *regional* cerebral blood flow. Similar constraints apply to the inhalation and intravenous techniques (with the exception of puncture of the carotid artery). Therefore it is not surprising that the measurement of cere-

bral metabolic rates(s) has not achieved much prominence in clinical practice or that clinicians have examined other methods to assess the balance between the demand for energy by the brain and its supply.

Arterial-Jugular Venous Oxygen Content Difference; Jugular Venous Oxygen Saturation

It is clear from the previous discussion that Equation 9 could be just as correctly written:

$$CMR_{O_2} = CBF \times (Ca_{O_2} - Cjv_{O_2}) \qquad (10)$$

However, because of the difficulties described earlier, the relationship is expressed more commonly, clinically, as:

$$AjvD_{O_2} = CMR_{O_2}/CBF \qquad (11)$$

where $AjvD_{O_2}$ is the difference in oxygen content measured in simultaneously drawn samples of arterial and jugular venous (jugular bulb) blood. In this form, the equation indicates that measurements of $AjvD_{O_2}$ are indicative of the coupling (or lack of coupling) between metabolism and flow. $AjvD_{O_2}$ will remain constant (normal value 7 ml O_2/ 100 ml blood in adults) as long as the ratio between the demand for oxygen and its supply does not change. Of course, the absolute values of each may change, for example, with pyrexia, hypothermia, or the administration of anaesthetic agents. In certain pathophysiologic situations, the normal coupling between demand and supply can be abolished. For example, in patients with a head injury, the CMR_{O_2} is correlated closely with the Glasgow Coma Scale score and CBF can vary independently of metabolic rate.[29] In this situation the ratio between demand and supply will vary and the $AjvD_{O_2}$ will reflect the adequacy of the supply of oxygen for a given level of demand.[33] For example, if the $AjvD_{O_2}$ is less than 4 ml O_2/100 ml blood, it can be assumed that the supply of oxygen is excessive relative to the demand for oxygen (a hyperemic state). Conversely, an $AjvD_{O_2}$ value of greater than 8 to 9 ml O_2/100 ml blood indicates that the brain is extracting more oxygen from the blood, almost certainly because the supply is too low to meet its metabolic requirements (state of compensated hypoperfusion). Values of $AjvD_{O_2}$ greater than 9 ml O_2/100 ml blood are believed by many investigators to indicate impending or actual global ischemia.[8,29] Any further decrease in the supply of oxygen caused by a decrease in flow or in the oxygen content of arterial blood will exhaust the capacity of the brain to compensate for the hypoperfusion; metabolic rate will decrease, become delivery-dependent, and the relationship between $AjvD_{O_2}$ and CBF will become unpredictable. Finally, after infarction has occurred the $AjvD_{O_2}$ will decrease, infarcted tissue does not need to extract oxygen because it is not consuming energy.

The oxygen content of blood depends on the hemoglobin concentration, the amount of oxygen that will combine with 1 g hemoglobin, the percentage saturation of oxygen in the hemoglobin, and the amount of oxygen dissolved in the plasma (the Huffner factor, range 1.34 to 1.39) such that:

$$Co_2 = (Hb \times 1.39 \times So_2) + [0.003 \times Po_2 \text{ (mm Hg)}] \quad \textbf{(12)}$$

If, in the calculation of the $AjvDo_2$, the Huffner factor remains constant, the hemoglobin concentration does not change materially, the saturation of hemoglobin in arterial blood remains stable at around 100%, and the amount of oxygen dissolved in plasma is unimportant under normal circumstances, then one can argue that the $AjvDo_2$ is determined primarily by the oxygen saturation of jugular venous blood (Svo_2), that is:

$$AjvDo_2 \propto (1-Sjvo_2) \quad \textbf{(13)}$$

If we combine Equations 11 and 13, we can see that the balance between demand and supply is reflected in the changes in $Sjvo_2$ such that:

$$Sjvo_2 \propto CBF/CMRo_2 \quad \textbf{(14)}$$

It is now possible to measure $Sjvo_2$ continuously using intravascular catheters with embedded optical fibers and the technique of percutaneous retrograde cannulation of the internal jugular vein.[6] In the absence of anemia and any change in Sao_2, increases in $Sjvo_2$ to above a value of 75% (normal value is 69% to 70%) suggest either that there are large areas of brain in which supply is in excess of metabolic requirement or that there is global cerebral infarction. A decrease in value to less than 54% is said to be indicative of "compensated cerebral hypoperfusion" (increasing oxygen extraction but no frank ischemia), a situation that, in certain institutions, initiates a management protocol based on the work of Sheinberg et al.[36] A value of $Sjvo_2$ of less than 40% is usually associated with global cerebral ischemia, and this may be characterized further by the measurement of the concentration of lactic acid in the jugular venous blood and/or the calculation of the lactate oxygen index (LOI):

$$LOI = AjvDL/AjvDo_2 \quad \textbf{(15)}$$

where AjvDL is the difference in lactate concentration between arterial and jugular venous blood.[32]

Changes in the oxygenation of systemic blood will influence also the saturation of the blood in the jugular bulb. The continuous monitoring of Sao_2 in combination with $Sjvo_2$ allows the measurement of the arterial-jugular venous oxygen saturation difference, the calculation of the $AjvDo_2$ (by incorporating the hemoglobin concentration), and the derivation of the cerebral oxygen extraction ratio (OER)[7]; that is:

$$OER = Sao_2 - Sjvo_2/Sao_2 \quad \textbf{(16)}$$

The $AjvDo_2$ and the $Sjvo_2$ reflect the interactions between Cao_2, CBF, and $CMRo_2$. Even if Cao_2 is constant, $AjvDo_2$ and/or $Sjvo_2$ can provide only relative information about the consumption of energy by the brain and the delivery of metabolic fuel. Nevertheless, the monitoring of these variables complements the measurement of cerebral perfusion pressure and can be used clinically as a prognostic tool, as a means of detecting incipient cerebral ischemia, and as an identifier of different subgroups of patients with intracranial hypertension in an effort to target therapy more appropriately.

Near-Infrared Spectroscopy

Transmission spectroscopy using light in the visible spectrum has been employed by physiologists for many years and has become used widely in clinical practice with the introduction of pulse oximetry. However, because visible light is absorbed significantly by hemoglobin and other pigmented compounds (chromophores) present in biological tissues, the depth of penetration is limited to about 1 cm. In contrast, the absorption of light in the near-infrared region (700 to 1000 nm) is much less, and as a result, infrared light can penetrate tissue to up to 8 cm.[19]

In the near-infrared region of the spectrum there are only three chromophores of significance in brain tissue: oxyhemoglobin, deoxyhemoglobin, and oxidized cytochrome aa_3. Consequently, ability of the tissue to absorb near-infrared light provides information on the presence of these compounds within brain tissue. The initial investigations in newborn infants[4] and in adults during anesthesia[16] proved that such information could be acquired qualitatively. However, quantification was not possible until the relationship between the concentration of the chromophore and the optical absorption could be characterized[9,24,51,52] such that changes in optical attenuation could be converted into changes in concentration within the tissue. If several different wavelengths are used, it is possible to measure the changes in absorption caused by and thus changes in, the concentrations of oxyhemoglobin, deoxyhemoglobin, and cytochrome aa_3 simultaneously and continuously. The ability to measure the redox state of cytochrome aa_3 is, for the reasons given earlier, relevant in any assessment of metabolic state because it reflects directly the intracellular oxygen availability within the mitochondrion. The hemoglobin data can be processed to give values for cerebral blood volume and CBF,[12,13] the latter variable providing information on the supply of oxygen to the area of brain being examined.

In addition to an assessment of the concentrations of the individual chromophores, the equations used to quantify the data can be resolved into a final form that allows the determination of a "field value" for the "regional saturation of hemoglobin" ($rSHbo_2$).[24] This is the ratio of oxygenated hemoglobin to total hemoglobin in the "field" sampled by the detector. The spectrum obtained includes measurement of hemoglobin in three distinct compartments: arterial, venous, and microcirculatory. The value for $rSHbo_2$ is the weighted average of these three compartments but is dominated in the brain by the pools of relatively desaturated hemoglobin in the venous and microcirculatory compartments.

Although the physical principles underlying near-infrared spectroscopy have been known for some time, there have been a number of practical difficulties in its development as a clinically useful means of monitoring aspects of cerebral metabolic state. However, apparatus is now available that may permit the noninvasive measurement of intracellular oxygen availability and regional hemoglobin saturation. Clinical validation is awaited with interest.

^{14}C-2-Deoxyglucose Autoradiography

The ^{14}C-2-deoxyglucose technique is one of the most powerful tools with which to quantitatively investigate and measure regional cerebral metabolic activity. Three premises, all of which have been highlighted earlier in this chapter, provide the conceptual basis for the technique. First, the energy requirements of brain tissue are obtained, almost exclusively, from the oxidative catabolism of glucose. Second, the consumption of energy within a defined area of brain is intimately and directly related to the functional activity in that area. Third, these function-related requirements for energy must be met by the continuous supply of glucose as the metabolic fuel because of the limited stores of the substrate in the brain. The technique is designed to take advantage of the biochemical characteristics that differentiate glucose and 2-deoxyglucose. The entry of both D-glucose and 2-deoxyglucose into the brain is mediated via the same carrier mechanism; both are substrates for hexokinase and both are metabolized into their respective hexose-6-phosphates. Glucose-6-phosphate is metabolized further; 2-deoxyglucose-6-phosphate is not. Its catabolism ceases at this point (at least within the normal experimental period) and if the original 2-deoxyglucose is labeled with a suitable radioisotope (^{14}C), the trapped, radiolabeled metabolite can be quantified by the autoradiographic densitometry of slices of brain tissue prepared after sacrificing the animal and freezing the brain in situ. For a more detailed description of the theoretic basis and practical details, see the original description by Sokoloff[44] and subsequent reviews.[10,41,42]

The spatial resolution of quantitative autoradiography is one of the most obvious advantages of the 2-deoxyglucose technique. With the use of radiolabeled 2-deoxyglucose, isotope concentration and thus glucose use can be assessed readily in the individual layers of the cortex or hippocampus and in small hypothalamic or brainstem nuclei. Quantitative autoradiography also allows a nonprejudicial assessment of functional events.[10] Areas of interest can be identified on the autoradiograms after the study has been completed. As a result, the technique can be used to detect the involvement of areas of the brain in a response that could not have been predicted at the outset of the study. Not surprisingly, general anesthesia results in substantial disturbances in synaptic transmission, changes in the structure and function of cellular membranes, and alterations in most cerebral metabolic processes such as the level and turnover of neurotransmitters, the oxidative catabolism of glucose, and regeneration of energy. As such, general anesthesia could be considered a major confounding influence on investigations of cerebral metabolic activity. Thus the capac-

ity of the 2-deoxyglucose technique to assess function in fully conscious animals as readily as in anesthetized ones is a major advantage.

As with any technique, the 2-deoxyglucose technique has a number of constraints. Some of these relate to the theoretic basis of the technique (for more information see reviews mentioned earlier); others are more practical. For example, it has been noted previously that glucose is not the only energy-generating substrate that the brain may utilize. Under certain circumstances, ketone bodies or glycogen may be utilized. Thus the adequate nutrition of the animal is an important consideration, as is the avoidance of any unintentional hypoxemia, because this would stimulate anerobic glycolysis. However, the most obvious practical constraint on the technique is the requirement for the animal to be sacrificed. Thus, although a large amount of information may be generated, the profile obtained is relevant only to that one point in time. The manipulation of a variable or the administration of a drug requires that a further investigation be undertaken in another animal.

Positron Emission Tomography

The 2-deoxyglucose technique can be applied in vivo; the positron-emitting radionuclide ^{18}F-2-deoxyglucose can be administered to a patient, and three-dimensional representations of glucose utilization in the various regions of the brain can be constructed. Positron-emission tomography (PET) systems rely on the detection of the high-energy, gamma-ray photons (which result from the collisions between the positrons, which are released as isotope decays) and electrons. Because the two protons travel away from the collision at approximately 180 degrees to one another, PET systems involve the placing of a number of gamma-ray detectors around the body to detect and measure the emissions from an injected or inhaled positron-labeled tracer. Computer reconstruction techniques are then used to produce an image of the distribution of the tracer throughout the volume of the part of the patient under study.[15]

Over 95% of the human body is made up of oxygen, carbon, nitrogen, and hydrogen. Of these, oxygen, carbon, and nitrogen have positron-emitting isotopes with half-lives of less than 30 minutes (Table 1-3). Much of the power of PET lies in its use of organic molecules, which can be labeled with natural radiotracers. In addition, the short half-lives mean that the radiation dose to the patient is kept to a minimum; however, this requires a cyclotron placed close to the site of use to generate the short-lived radionuclides.

Regional cerebral metabolism can be quantified using either radiolabeled metabolic substrates (^{11}C glucose) or radiolabeled, metabolically inert analogues of the substrates (^{18}F-2-deoxy-2-fluoro-D-glucose [FDG]). As described for the 2-deoxyglucose technique, the FDG is taken up by actively metabolizing cells as if it were glucose. The FDG is phosphorylated; however, because FDG-6-phosphate is not a substrate for subsequent metabolism, it accumulates in the cell and the amount of accumulated radioactivity is an indication of the glucose utilization of that cell or that region

TABLE 1-3
Tracers Used in PET Scanning*

Radioisotope	Half-life (min)	Tracer	Application
^{18}F	109.8	^{18}F-FDG	Glucose metabolism
		^{18}F-Dopa	Dopamine storage
^{15}O	2.03	$C^{15}O_2$	Blood flow
		$H_2{}^{15}O_2$	Blood flow
		$^{15}O_2$	Oxygen metabolism
		$C^{15}O$	Blood volume
^{11}C	20.4	$^{11}CO_2$	pH

*Only tracers relevant to this chapter have been included.

of brain. If oxygen labeled with ^{15}O is inhaled, the tracer will become attached to hemoglobin. On reaching the brain, a fraction of the ^{15}O will be extracted from the blood to participate in aerobic metabolism. The oxygen extraction ratio (OER) can be calculated, and if CBF and the arterial oxygen content are known, the regional cerebral metabolic rate for oxygen can be derived:

$$OER \times Ca_{O_2} = CMR_{O_2}/CBF \qquad (17)$$

In contrast to some of our earlier discussions, however, CBF can be measured noninvasively and in absolute units using positron emission tomography and appropriate tracers (Table 1-3). In this way, it would be possible to insert appropriate values of CBF into the above equation and derive the CMR_{O_2}, which could, of course, be compared with the OER and the glucose utilization in the same regions of the brain. Such comparisons can increase our understanding of the basic physiologic interactions between functional activity, the demand for and utilization of substrate, and the delivery of metabolic fuel. Interrelationships that previously could only be assessed globally can now be examined regionally. The primary role of PET scanning, however, is to aid the understanding of disease processes, considerations that are outside the scope of this chapter. Thus we will only highlight one or two points.

PET is capable of looking at three areas of function that may be of interest to the anesthesiologist. First, it becomes possible to examine the functional effects of extracranial arterial stenosis on CBF, blood volume, and oxygen delivery. For example, in situations in which the blood supply to the brain is decreased, it is possible to note the increase in the extraction of oxygen and determine whether the hypoperfusion is compensated.

Second, it is possible to follow the development and resolution of ischemic lesions. However, one must take care in this context because, as has been emphasized previously, if insufficient oxygen is available to permit oxidative phosphorylation, glucose can still be metabolized anerobically. As noted earlier in the chapter, under these circumstances, the rate of anerobic glycolysis may be increased significantly yet be unable to supply the demand for energy. However, because glucose is actually being delivered to the

brain, PET scanning (as, indeed, autoradiography) may suggest that the production of energy is high when in reality it is not. This phenomenon may be particularly evident in the penumbra region around an infarct.

Third, the interrelationships between techniques of anesthesia, the administration of anesthetic agents, and the various indices of cerebral function (including receptor kinetics) can be compared readily using PET under both physiologic and pathophysiologic conditions.[28] To have this information on a regional basis would provide fascinating data. Unfortunately, however, the financial investment necessary, in both hardware and human resources, means that PET scanning is available in very few centers.

Magnetic Resonance Spectroscopy

Customarily, imaging of anatomic structures within the body has been achieved by measuring the differential absorption of x-rays. Magnetic resonance (MR) imaging makes possible not only the display of morphology (normal and pathologic) but also information on physiologic and biochemical changes in vivo without the use of ionizing radiation. The physical basis of the method was described initially by Bloch et al.[2] and Purcell et al.[31] in 1946. However, its use to generate cross-sectional images and study the metabolism of tissue were not available for another 25 years or so.

MR is a technique that involves the interaction of radiofrequency radiation and matter.[11,40] It relies on the fact that certain atomic nuclei such as hydrogen (^1H), phosphorous (^{31}P), and fluorine (^{19}F) have intrinsic magnetic properties such that when a sample containing such nuclei is placed in a magnetic field, the nuclei tend to align themselves along the direction of the field (as happens with a compass needle). This magnetic interaction between the nuclei and the applied field can be detected by applying pulses of radio-frequency radiation to the sample and observing the frequencies at which radiation is absorbed and subsequently reemitted. The frequencies of the various emitted signals are proportional to the field experienced by the nuclei. In MR spectroscopy, these frequencies provide chemical information; in MR imaging they provide spatial information.

MR spectroscopy is now established as a method by which the metabolism of living systems ranging from cellular suspensions to humans can be studied noninvasively. Initially used on excised tissues, It became feasible in the study of aspects of cerebral metabolism in small animals with the development of the surface coil, a type of detecting coil that could be placed adjacent to a superficial region of interest. With the construction of larger magnets, it was possible to extend the studies to humans (first of limbs and then of the neonatal brain). Currently, whole-body spectroscopy systems are available, and studies of the adult brain are possible. The nucleus that has been used most extensively for metabolic studies is ^{31}P, the naturally occurring phosphorus nucleus. MR can be used to measure the concentrations in brain tissue of those phosphorous metabolites that are important in the conversion and consumption of energy, ATP, PCr, Pi, phosphodiesters (PDE), and phosphomonoesters (PME). The relative areas of the signals provide information about the relative concentrations of the metabolites while the frequency of the Pi is sensitive to pH and therefore provides a monitor of the intracellular pH (Fig. 1-6, *A*). Thus in situations where oxidative phosphorylation is impaired, either because the oxygen supplied to the brain is decreased or because the mechanisms for consuming oxygen are damaged, the concentration of ATP will decrease (as discussed previously). However, because of the buffering effect of the creatine kinase reaction, the decrease in ATP will, at least initially, be small. ATP itself becomes appreciably depleted only after the PCr has decreased to a very low level (Fig. 1-6, *B*). These are the sort of changes that can be demonstrated using MR.[53] The phosphorylation potential of the tissue (ATP/ADP × Pi) can be assessed and may be used as a measure of energy reserve.

Although the ^{31}P nucleus has been studied most extensively, several other nuclei can be utilized for MR studies of metabolism, including ^{1}H, ^{19}F, ^{13}C, and ^{23}Na. ^{1}H MR is more sensitive than ^{31}P MR; unfortunately, it is technically more difficult to use because of the need to suppress the large signals that come from water. However, the use of this nucleus is of particular interest because it permits the monitoring of several metabolites such as lactate, alanine, glutamine, glutamate, and total creatine (Fig. 1-6, *C*). The spatial resolution for metabolic studies is considerably less precise than that for imaging. This is primarily because the metabolites of interest are present in relatively low concentrations compared with water (clinical imaging is based on the detection of ^{1}H signals from body water). As a result, the metabolites generate relatively weak signals such that for ^{31}P studies in humans, the linear resolution is in the range of 3 to 6 cm. However, it seems clear that ^{1}H spectroscopy provides better resolution than ^{31}P spectroscopy and may be better in the clinical situation.

As with PET scanning, the clinical impetus with MR has been the ability to understand disease processes rather than physiologic function. ^{31}Phosphorous MR has been used particularly in attempts to understand some of the mechanisms involved in hypoxic-ischemic injury in the newborn.[53] Although it has been used in adults in association with ischemic disease,[49] it seems likely that the ^{31}P spectroscopy is better suited to investigating acute rather than more longstanding effects of ischemia. It may be that ^{1}H spectroscopy will prove more useful as a means of investigating the more chronic effects. Indeed, ^{1}H MR may have an extensive role in the investigation of many disorders of the brain,[11] including cerebral neoplasms, cerebrovascular disease, and other disorders involving selective loss of neurons. It is now possible to integrate ^{1}H MR imaging and MR spectroscopy into a single examination, a combination of techniques that could prove to be very valuable, particularly in the investigation of disease states, because it would enable abnormalities of metabolic profile to be related very closely to the normal or abnormal structure of the central nervous system.

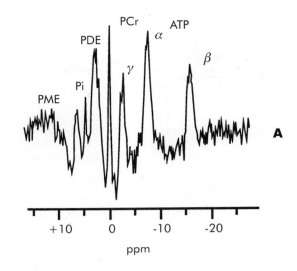

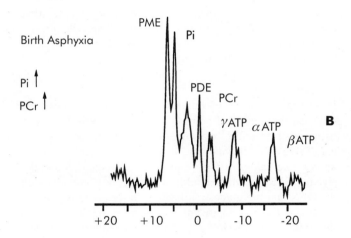

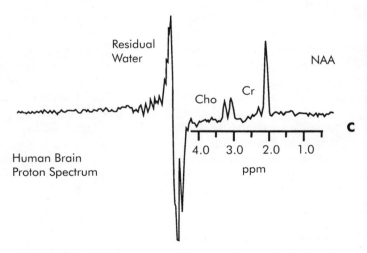

FIG. 1-6 Phosphorus and proton magnetic resonance spectroscopy of brain. **A,** ^{31}P spectrum from the normal human infant. **B,** ^{31}P spectrum from human infant with birth asphyxia. **C,** ^{1}H spectrum from human brain. The abscissa is frequency in parts per million (ppm); the ordinate is relative concentration. Compound abbreviations are defined in the text. (*Courtesy R.S. Hamid.*)

SUMMARY

One of the most amazing phenomena of modern medicine is the ability to temporarily and reversibly inhibit the normal physiologic functioning of the brain without subsequent alteration in neurologic function or psychologic performance. Our understanding of how this is achieved is imperfect, but we know it involves alterations in membrane function, synaptic transmission, and cerebral energy state. The brain has ongoing, substantial energy requirements and minimal stores of energy-generating substrates, so it is dependent on a continuous, uninterrupted substrate supply as well as waste product removal. Energy is used to maintain transmembrane electrical and ionic gradients as well as to support metabolic activities. In situations of substrate inadequacy, the brain has adaptive mechanisms, but the degree of adaptation is limited. The underlying metabolic requirements of the brain form the basis of the approach to patient care described in other chapters of this book and also provide an approach to diagnosis of brain function and disease.

References

1. Bering EA Jr: Effect of body temperature change on cerebral oxygen consumption of the intact monkey, *Am J Physiol* 200:417-419, 1961.
2. Bloch F, Hansen WW, Packard M: The nuclear induction experiment, *Phys Rev* 70:474-485, 1946.
3. Bickler PE: Energetics of cerebral metabolism and ion transport, *Anesth Clin North Am* 10:563-573, 1992.
4. Brazy JE, Lewis DV, Mitnick MH et al: Noninvasive monitoring of cerebral oxygenation in preterm infants: preliminary observations, *Pediatrics* 75:217-225, 1985.
5. Carafoli E: Intracellular calcium homeostasis, *Ann Rev Biochem* 56:395-433, 1987.
6. Cruz J: Continuous versus serial global cerebral haemometabolic monitoring: applications in acute brain trauma, *Acta Neurochir Scand Suppl* 42:35-39, 1988.
7. Cruz J, Miner ME, Allen SJ et al: Continuous monitoring of cerebral oxygenation in acute brain injury: assessment of cerebral haemodynamic reserve, *Neurosurgery* 29:743-749, 1991.
8. Deardon NM: Jugular bulb venous oxygen saturation in the management of severe head injury, *Curr Opinion Anaesthesiol* 4:279-286, 1991.
9. Delpy DT, Cope M, van der Zee P, et al: Estimation of optical pathlength through tissue from direct time of flight measurement, *Phys Med Biol* 33:1433-1442, 1988.
10. Dewar D, McCulloch J: Mapping functional events in the CNS with 2-deoxyglucose autoradiography. In Stewart MG, editor: *Quantitative methods in neuroanatomy,* Chichester, 1992, Wiley, pp 57-84.
11. Doran M, Gadian DG: Magnetic resonance imaging and spectroscopy of the brain. In Steward MG, editor: *Quantitative methods in neuroanatomy,* Chichester, 1992, Wiley, pp 163-179.
12. Edwards AD, Reynolds EOR, Richardson CE et al: Estimation of blood flow using near infra-red spectroscopy, *J Physiol* 410:50P.
13. Edwards AD, Wyatt JS, Richardson C et al: Cotside measurements of cerebral blood flow in ill newborn infants by near infra-red spectroscopy, *Lancet* ii:770-771, 1988.
14. Erecinska M, Silver IA: ATP and brain function, *J Cereb Blood Flow Metab* 9:2-19, 1989.
15. Eriksson L, Dahlbom M, Widen L: Positron emission tomography—a new technique for studies of the central nervous system, *J Microscopy* 157:305-333, 1990.
16. Fox E, Jobsis FF, Mitnick MH: Monitoring cerebral oxygen sufficiency in anaesthesia and surgery, *Adv Exp Med Biol* 191:849-854, 1985.
17. Greenberg JH, Reivich M, Alavi A et al: Metabolic mapping of functional activity in human subjects with the (18-F) fluorodeoxyglucose technique, *Science* 212:678-680, 1981.
18. Hertz L: Features of astrocytic function apparently involved in the response of central nervous tissue to ischemia-hypoxia, *J Cereb Blood Flow Metab* 1:143-153, 1981.
19. Jobsis FF: Noninvasive infrared monitoring of cerebral and myocardial oxygen sufficiency and circulatory parameters, *Science* 198:1264-1267, 1977.
20. Kinter D, Fitzpatrick JH, Louie JA et al: Cerebral oxygen and energy metabolism during and after 30 minutes of moderate hypoxia, *Am J Physiol* 247:E475-E482, 1984.
21. Kramer RS, Sanders AP, Lesage AM et al: The effect of profound hypothermia on preservation of cerebral ATP content during circulatory arrest, *J Thorac Cardiovasc Surg* 56:699-709, 1968.
22. Lajtha AL, Maker HS, Clark DD: Metabolism and transport of carbohydrates and amino acids. In Siegel GJ, Albers RW, Agranoff BW et al, editors: *Basic neurochemistry,* ed 3, Boston, 1981, Little, Brown, pp 329-353.
23. Lowry OH: Energy metabolism in brain and its control. In Inguar DH, Lassen NA, editors: *Brain work. The coupling of function, metabolism and blood flow in the brain,* Copenhagen, 1975, Munksgaard, pp 48-64.
24. McCormick PW, Stewart M, Dujovnj M et al: Clinical application of diffuse near infrared transmission spectroscopy to measure cerebral oxygen metabolism, *Hospimedica* 8:39-47, 1990.
25. Michenfelder JD: The hypothermic brain. In Michenfelder JD, editor: *Anesthesia and the brain,* New York, 1988, Churchill-Livingstone, pp 23-34.
26. Michenfelder JD, Theye RA: Hypothermia: effect on canine brain and whole-body metabolism, *Anesthesiology* 29:1107-1112, 1968.
27. Michenfelder JD, Theye RA: Cerebral protection by thiopental during hypoxia, *Anesthesiology* 39:510-517, 1973.
28. Myers R, Spinks TJ, Luthra SK et al: Positron emission tomography. In Stewart MG, editor: *Quantitative methods in neuroanatomy,* Chichester, 1992, Wiley, pp 117-161.

29. Obrist WD, Langfitt TW, Jaggi JL et al: Cerebral blood flow and metabolism in comatose patients with acute head injury, *J Neurosurg* 61:241-253, 1984.

30. Phelps ME, Kuhl DE, Mazziotta JC: Metabolic mapping of the brain's response to visual stimulation: studies in humans, *Science* 211:1445-1448, 1981.

31. Purcell EM, Torrey HC, Pound RV: Resonance moments by nuclear magnetic moments in a solid, *Phys Rev* 60:37-38, 1946.

32. Robertson CS, Grossman RG, Goodman JC et al: The predictive value of cerebral anaerobic metabolism with cerebral infarction after head injury, *J Neurosurg* 67:361-368, 1987.

33. Robertson CS, Narayan RK, Gokaslan ZL et al: Cerebral arteriovenous oxygen difference as an estimate of cerebral blood flow in comatose patients, *J Neurosurg* 70:222-230, 1989.

34. Rosomoff HL, Holiday DA: Cerebral blood flow and cerebral oxygen consumption during hypothermia, *Am J Physiol* 179:85-88, 1954.

35. Roy CS, Sherrington CS: On the regulation of the blood-supply of the brain, *J Physiol* (Lond) 11:85-109, 1890.

36. Sheinberg M, Kanter MJ, Robertson CS et al: Continuous monitoring of jugular venous oxygen saturation in head-injured patients, *J Neurosurg* 77:55-61, 1992.

37. Siegel GJ, Stahl WL, Swanson DD: Ion transport. In Siegel GJ, Albers RW, Agranoff BW et al, editors: *Basic neurochemistry,* ed 3, Boston, 1981, Little, Brown, pp 107-143.

38. Siesjo BK: *Brain energy metabolism,* New York, 1978, Wiley.

39. Siesjo BK: Cerebral circulation and metabolism, *J Neurosurg* 60:883-908, 1984.

40. Smith FW: Nuclear magnetic resonance in the investigation of cerebral disorder, *J Cereb Blood Flow Metab* 3:263-269, 1983.

41. Sokoloff L: Local cerebral energy metabolism: its relationships to local functional activity and blood flow. In *Ciba Foundation Symposium 56 (new series) cerebral vascular smooth muscle and its control,* Amsterdam, 1978, Elsevier, pp 171-196.

42. Sokoloff L: The (14-C)-deoxyglucose method: four years later, *Acta Neurol Scand* 60:640-649, 1979.

43. Sokoloff L: Circulation and energy metabolism of the brain. In Siegel GJ, Albers RW, Agranoff BW et al, editors: *Basic neurochemistry,* ed 3, Boston, 1981, Little, Brown, pp 471-495.

44. Sokoloff L, Reivich M, Kennedy C et al: The (14-C)-deoxyglucose method for the measurement of local cerebral glucose utilization: theory, procedure and normal values in the conscious and anesthetized albino rat, *J Neurochem* 28:897-916, 1977.

45. Steen PA, Newberg LA, Milde JH et al: Hypothermia and barbiturates: individual and combined effects on canine cerebral oxygen consumption, *Anesthesiology* 58:527-532, 1983.

46. Stephan H, Sonntag H, Lange H et al: Cerebral effects of anaesthesia and hypothermia, *Anaesthesia* 44:310-316, 1989.

47. Stocker F, Herschkowitz N, Bossi E et al: Cerebral metabolic studies in situ by 31-P nuclear magnetic resonance after hypothermic circulatory arrest, *Pediatr Res* 20:867-871, 1986.

48. Weiss PA: Neuronal dynamics and neuroplasmic ("axonal") flow. In Barondes SH, editor: *Cellular dynamics of the neuron,* New York, London, 1969, Academic Press, pp 3-34.

49. Welch KMA, Gross B, Licht J: Magnetic resonance spectroscopy of neurological diseases, *Curr Neurol* 8:295-331, 1988.

50. Wieloch T, Siesjo BK: Ischemic brain injury: the importance of calcium, lipolytic activities and free fatty acids, *Pathol Biol* 30:269-277, 1982.

51. Wray S, Cope M, Delpy DT et al: Characterisation of near infrared absorption spectra of cytochrome aa3 and haemoglobin for the non-invasive monitoring of cerebral oxygenation, *Biochem Biophys Acta* 933:184-192, 1988.

52. Wyatt JS, Cope M, Delpy DT et al: Quantitation of cerebral oxygenation and haemodynamics in sick newborn infants by near infrared spectrophotometry, *Lancet* ii:1063-1066, 1986.

53. Wyatt JS, Edwards AD, Azzopardi D et al: Magnetic resonance and near infrared spectroscopy for investigation of perinatal hypoxic-ischaemic brain injury, *Arch Dis Child* 64:953-963, 1989.

2

Cerebral and Spinal Cord Blood Flow

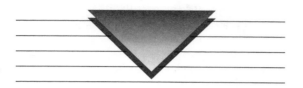

WILLIAM L. YOUNG
EUGENE ORNSTEIN

Studies of cerebral circulation have improved the understanding of the function and pathophysiology of the central nervous system (CNS).[26] This chapter will discuss aspects of the cerebral circulation and its regulation. The chapter begins with a discussion of circulatory regulation and its failure and proceeds to the methodology for measuring cerebral blood flow (CBF). A discussion of spinal cord blood flow follows, and the chapter ends with a discussion of monitoring CBF in the clinical setting. The purpose of this chapter is to review the basic mechanisms of CNS circulatory behavior and the tools used to understand them.

PHYSIOLOGY OF THE CEREBRAL CIRCULATION
Cerebral Metabolism

During most circumstances, neuronal function totally depends on oxidative metabolism of glucose to provide adenosine triphosphate (ATP), which ultimately fuels all cellular processes. Although only 2% of body weight, the brain accounts for 20% of resting oxygen consumption. Lack of substrate storage in the brain and high metabolic rate account for the relative sensitivity of the brain to oxygen deprivation.

17

Brain metabolism can be split into two parts. The portion that drives the "work" of the brain, that is, synaptic transmission (*activation metabolism*), and the portion necessary for cellular integrity (*basal metabolism*). A large part of the basal metabolism is devoted to the maintenance of the normal transmembrane ionic gradients (i.e., keeping K^+ inside and Na^+ and Ca^{++} outside the cell). The remainder of basal metabolism is concerned with protein and neurotransmitter synthesis and other basic cellular functions.

Regional CBF Requirements

The CNS is a most complex and structurally diverse organ and comprises multiple functional subdivisions. Neurons account for approximately half of the brain volume; the remainder consists of glial and vascular elements. In addition to mechanical support of neurons, the glia has important regulatory functions (e.g., neurotransmitter handling and maintenance of the metabolic milieu of the neuropile) that, at present, are imperfectly understood.

A wide range of metabolic rates exist in the brain (e.g., there is an approximately fourfold difference in CMR_{O_2} and CBF between cortical gray and white matter). Flow and metabolism are said to be *coupled,* and under physiologic circumstances, including during general anesthesia, this coupling is preserved (Figs. 2-1 and 2-2). In humans, this coupling is evident during anesthetic burst-suppression on the EEG as demonstrated by transcranial Doppler (TCD) studies during normothermia (W. Young, unpublished data) and during hypothermic cardiopulmonary bypass.[267]

Regulation of Cerebral Blood Flow

A rapid and precise regulatory system has evolved in the CNS whereby instantaneous increases in metabolic demand

can be rapidly met by a local increase in CBF and substrate delivery. It has been known for a long time and demonstrated with multiple imaging modalities that the time course of this regulatory process is rapid. Contralateral cortical areas "light up," demonstrating increased flow with hand movement,[187] and a variety of motor and cognitive tasks can be mapped using CBF techniques.[143] Visual stimulation results in almost immediate increases in flow velocity through the posterior cerebral arteries.[2,3,5] PET studies are beginning to unravel the interrelated functions of various cortical areas in such complex phenomena as language and visual processing.[199,241] As in most specialized vascular beds, this flow-metabolism coupling is critical during times of stress or extreme physiologic conditions such as hypotension or hypoxia. These pathologic processes engage regulatory mechanisms to maintain flow at physiologic levels.

The term *autoregulation* is used by some to describe the hemodynamic response of flow to changes in perfusion pressure independent of flow-to-metabolism coupling. The problem with this approach is that the precise mechanisms responsible for maintenance of cerebral blood flow are poorly understood.[148] We argue for the general case, that is, autoregulation implies a general matching of flow to metabolism, irrespective of mechanism. For example, the ability of the cerebral vasculature to dilate in response to tissue hypoxia certainly qualifies as an autoregulatory phenomenon, and it may be an oxygen-sensitive mechanism that regulates vascular resistance in the normoxic or hyperoxic range.[272] Perhaps when we know more precisely the mediators of these "autoregulatory" events we can devise better terminology. "Autoregulatory" responses are those that maintain the internal milieu of the CNS. Those that endanger CNS well-being are dysregulatory. Semantics aside, a clinical distinction can be made between two dis-

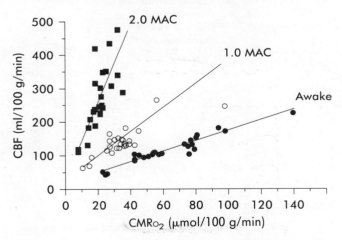

FIG. 2-1   CBF as a function of CMR_{O_2} in different brain regions of the rat determined by autoradiography during isoflurane anesthesia. Three groups are included: awake, 1.0 MAC, and 2.0 MAC. Note that the volatile anesthetic does not uncouple flow and metabolism, rather it is "reset" along a different line. (*Modified from Maekawa T, Tommasino C, Shapiro HM et al:* Anesthesiology 65:144, 1986. *Figure courtesy Dr. David S. Warner, University of Iowa.*)

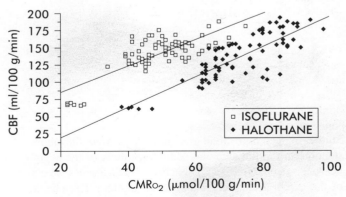

FIG. 2-2   CBF as a function of CMR_{O_2} in different brain regions of the rat determined by autoradiography during halothane and isoflurane anesthesia. As in Fig. 2-1, flow and metabolism remained coupled for both anesthetics. Note that for a given CMR_{O_2}, flow is actually higher for isoflurane than for halothane. (*From Hansen TD, Warner DS, Todd MM et al:* J Cereb Blood Flow Metab 9:323, 1989.)

tinct processes that may or may not be mechanistically related—flow-metabolism coupling and active vasomotion in response to circulatory perturbation.

Since Roy and Sherrington put forth their hypothesis more than 100 years ago,[219] the prevailing paradigm has been that local metabolic factors are involved in flow-metabolism coupling. However, pure changes in perfusion pressure undoubtedly involve a myogenic response in vascular smooth muscle as well (Bayliss effect).[194] This myogenic response actually may consist of two separate mechanisms, one responding to mean blood pressure changes and another sensitive to pulsatile pressure.[251] There is even evidence that flow, irrespective of pressure, may affect vascular resistance.[79] An overwhelming number of metabolic mediators for CBF regulation have been proposed, including hydrogen ion, potassium, adenosine, glycolytic intermediates, and phospholipid metabolites.[148,194] In a newer twist on the local metabolic hypothesis, the latest mediators are endothelium-derived factors,[101,102] nitric oxide being the subject of intense scrutiny at present.[147] Therefore the endothelium might be the "transducer" of hemodynamic responses to changes in perfusion pressure (see the following discussion).

Perivascular innervation in the brain has been recognized since Willis first described the cerebral circulation in 1664. Nevertheless, the precise function of this innervation remains obscure. The current paradigm holds that autonomic nerves are not necessary for regulatory responses but may modify them in several important ways. Nonetheless, this view may change as increasing attention is being paid to neural control mechanisms.[148,149] A major deficiency in the "local metabolic" theory is that the necessary temporal relationship between accumulation of vasoactive metabolites and flow increases has not been adequately demonstrated. In addition, there are many examples where CBF and CMR_{O_2} change in the same direction, but CBF increases out of proportion to metabolic rate, such as during seizure activity. Lou et al.[148] proposed that flow and metabolism level may be maintained after they have been set in place by a "rapid initiator" that involves a neurogenic mechanism.

Although unlikely to be directly involved in pressure autoregulation itself,[54] nitric oxide (NO) is the subject of intense scrutiny as a mediator of vascular tone[147] and as a neurotransmitter.[36] This area of research is rapidly expanding, and controversy prevails.[126]

The explosion of interest in NO is due to the identification of the multiple biologic roles it plays as a messenger molecule,[36] although, until recently, there was no evidence for it having any biologic function at all in vertebrates. However, it now appears that NO plays a major role in at least three systems: (1) bactericidal and tumoricidal effects in white blood cells, (2) as a neurotransmitter, and (3) as a moderator/mediator of vascular tone, functioning as an "endothelium-derived relaxing factor" or EDRF.

Nitric oxide is synthesized from L-arginine in the endothelial cell by the action of the enzyme nitric oxide syn-

thase (NOS). Calcium is intimately involved in this process. NO diffuses into the vascular myocyte and activates guanylate cyclase, forming cGMP. A protein kinase is stimulated by cGMP, resulting in phosphorylation of the light chain of myosin, and thus vascular relaxation.[36] NO appears to be formed on demand and is not stored in vesicles, as is the traditional fate of neurotransmitters.

Nitric oxide action has been studied by using arginine analogues such as L-N^G-nitroarginine methyl ester (L-NAME), which can be used as a specific antagonist of NO activity. NO appears to influence basal tone,[252] including the endothelium-dependent response to acetylcholine in cerebral arteries[65] and vasogenic dilation from stimulation of nonadrenergic, noncholinergic nerves.[83] Vascular abnormalities in disease states that significantly predispose the brain to damage, such as diabetes mellitus, also may be related to a NO-mediated mechanism.[198]

Although NO appears to play a role in dilation in response to CO_2,[123,198,268] in other experiments, participation in hypocapnia-induced vasoconstriction could not be demonstrated.[65] The site of action for CO_2-induced NO production may not be in the endothelium but rather in perivascular structures such as astroctyes[123] (Pelligrino, personal communication). The participation of NO in hypoxia-induced vasodilation does not appear to be physiologically important.[138,197,198] Regarding anesthetic effects on CBF, NO appears to interact with the cerebral vasodilatory effects of both halothane[135] and isoflurane.[168]

The role of NO as a neurotransmitter undoubtedly will prove to be significant for care of the patient with neurologic disease by its interactions with anesthetic depth[127] and cerebral ischemic states,[233] in particular the pathogenesis of vasospasm after subarachnoid hemorrhage.[127]

Anatomic Considerations

The primary arterial supply to the brain consists of the *anterior* circulation, which comprises the two carotid arteries and their derivations, and the *posterior* circulation, consisting of the two vertebral arteries, which join to form the basilar artery.

Collateral arterial inflow channels are a cornerstone of CBF compensation during ischemia. The principal pathways are embodied in the Circle of Willis. This hexagonal ring of vessels lies in the subarachnoid space and circles the pituitary gland (Fig. 2-3). In many patients the Circle of Willis is incomplete. The primary "collateral" pathways are the anterior communicating artery, which joins the two carotid circulations, and the posterior communicating arteries, which join the vertebral and carotid circulations bilaterally. In a normal individual there is probably no net flow through these communicating vessels, but rather a to-and-fro movement of blood that maintains patency by preventing thrombosis or atresia. These vessels allow flow when a pressure differential develops.

When the normal arterial supply is compromised and the Circle of Willis does not supply the remedy, other mecha-

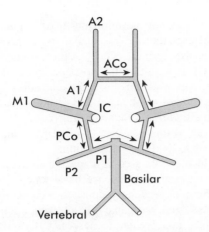

FIG. 2-3 Circle of Willis with collateral pathways. The principal pathways for collateral flow are marked by arrows. Not shown are potential pathways from the extracranial circulation, (e.g., via retrograde flow through the ophthalmic artery). *(From Young W: Clinical neuroscience lectures, Munster, Ind, 1991, Cathenart Publishing.)*

nisms may be activated. Deep, intraparenchymal collateral pathways are usually not present between arterial irrigation territories. Between major arterial distributions, however, there is the potential for leptomeningeal communications that bridge "watershed" areas. These are typified by surface connections between the anterior and middle cerebral arteries and middle and posterior cerebral arteries. This leptomeningeal circulation may compensate for reduced flow at the periphery of an arterial distribution. However, if perfusion pressure is reduced globally, these watershed areas are the furthest from the arterial input pressure and are the most vulnerable to ischemic damage.[154]

In addition, the external and internal carotid arteries have the potential for communication, which is most commonly manifested as flow from the external carotid artery, via facial pathways, to the ophthalmic artery. Thus retrograde flow is provided to the Circle of Willis. Several other pathways may develop between the carotid and vertebrobasilar system.[53] In rare situations meningeal collaterals may develop into the intracranial circulation (e.g., arteriovenous malformations and Moya Moya disease).

In summary, an elegant microcirculatory arrangement is provided for recruiting accessory inflow channels to the end-arterial perfusion territories of the brain. During normal circumstances these channels either lie dormant or are underutilized, becoming functional (critical) only when a pathologic stress is imposed on the circulation. In general, it is the Circle of Willis and the leptomeningeal communications that compensate for an acute interruption of the circulation; other pathways described previously are more likely to compensate for chronic cerebral insufficiency.

Regulation of cerebrovascular resistance takes place primarily in the smaller arteries and arterioles (muscular or resistance vessels) and not the larger arteries that are visible on an angiogram (elastic or conductance vessels). However,

the contribution of both venules and capillaries[177] and larger conductance arteries to regulatory activity is a subject of controversy.[108,137] There is probably a continuum of varying participation in autoregulatory function as one proceeds distally on the arterial tree.[137,228]

In humans the venous drainage of the brain is complex and considerably more variable than drainage of the arterial tree. The typically thin-walled and valveless intracerebral conduits terminate into thicker-walled venous sinuses, which are rigid by virtue of bony attachments. Because there is confluence of the larger venous sinuses, a considerable admixture of venous blood draining the cerebral hemispheres takes place, and it is not uncommon to note in the later venous phase of an angiogram that one side of the venous drainage appears to be dominant. This may be of interest in deciding which internal jugular vein to choose for cannulation.

A controversial topic is whether the capillary bed of the brain is fully perfused at all times, that is, whether capillary recruitment takes place.[74,75,81,82] There are probably mechanical influences on local flow by sphincter mechanisms at the microcirculatory level.[98,177] Based on current data, it is reasonable to assume that capillary recruitment is not a *major* control mechanism for recruitment of collateral flow, but it may be operative in flow-metabolism coupling or under certain pathologic conditions.

Hemodynamic Factors

Pressure Regulation.   Conceptually, a convenient way to model the cerebral circulation is to envision a parallel system of rigid pipes where Ohm's law would apply

$$F = \frac{P_i - P_o}{R} \qquad (1)$$

where

F = Flow
P_i = Input pressure
P_o = Outflow pressure
R = Resistance

The term $(P_i - P_o)$ is usually referred to as cerebral perfusion pressure (CPP) and is calculated as mean arterial pressure minus the outflow pressure. The cerebral venous system is compressible and may act as a "Starling resistor." Therefore P_o is whichever pressure is higher, intracranial or venous pressure. True cerebral perfusion pressure often is overestimated because a small gradient exists between systemic and cerebral vessels.[66] This may be particularly important in patients with cerebral AVMs.[69]

It is useful to conceptualize pressure and resistance as independent variables in the preceding equation and flow as the dependent variable (i.e., the pressure or resistance is affected by disease or treatment, and flow follows suit). For example, drugs exert effects on CBF by changing CPP and CVR (directly for vasodilators and indirectly by metabolic depressants).

Circulatory resistance can be modelled in terms of the Hagen-Poiseuille relationship (Equation 2). As is the case for Ohm's law, when applying this equation to an intact vascular system, a number of critical assumptions are clearly not met. The equation applies to Newtonian fluids during nonturbulent flow through rigid tubes; circulation, in contrast, is pulsatile with capacitance and the potential for turbulence.

$$R = \frac{8l\mu}{r^4} = \frac{P_i - P_o}{F} \qquad (2)$$

where

l = Length of conduit
μ = Blood viscosity
r = Radius of vessel
R = Resistance

Other symbol definitions are given previously.

From a purely practical standpoint, examination of the previous relationship leaves little question as to why vessel diameter evolved into the preeminent mode of vascular regulation. Although viscosity and vessel length influence resistance in a linear manner, the fact that flow is proportional to the fourth power of the conduit radius makes this the most efficient means of controlling resistance.

In normal individuals, CBF is constant between a CPP of approximately 50 to 150 mm Hg (Fig. 2-4). As the ability of the cerebral vasculature to respond to changes in pressure is exhausted, CBF passively follows changes in CPP. At the extremes, resistance probably does not stay fixed. Vessel collapse and passive vascular dilation may actually potentiate the predicted decline or increase caused by CPP changes: resistance does not remain linearly related to pressure.

As important as is the general concept put forth in Fig. 2-4, it is only a statistical description of how the general population responds, and a value of 50 mm Hg, even in a nonhypertensive individual, does not guarantee that a particular patient remains within the "autoregulatory plateau." Individual responses vary widely.[247]

Note that increases in CBF are qualitatively proportionate to increases in cerebral blood volume (CBV) (Fig. 2-4). In fact, CBV changes in a quantitatively different fashion than CBF.[87,221] For example, increasing systemic blood pressure decreases CBV in the process of maintaining CBF constant. This effect may be exploited in the setting of decreased intracranial compliance with or without an attendant increase in ICP.[218] However, the physiology of CBV is less well known than that of CBF.

There is a time constant associated with autoregulatory changes. Fig. 2-5, *A*, depicts the response of a simple tube (or a dysregulating vascular bed) to a step change in pressure. Because resistance does not change (assuming nonturbulent flow), flow passively follows the change in pressure. Fig. 2-5, *B*, depicts the response that is typical of a normal circulatory bed. With the step change in pressure, there is an instantaneous drop in flow, but as the bed actively autoregulates and resistance decreases, flow gradually increases and returns to baseline. When the pressure is returned to normal, there is a transient period of hyperemia while the resistance is reset.[70]

Venous Physiology. The influence of the cerebral venous system on overall autoregulation is unclear, primarily because of the difficulty of direct observation. The smooth muscle content and the innervation of the venous system are less extensive than those of the arterial system, and many believe that the venous system is a passive recipient of the "regulated" arterial inflow. Because the venous system contains most of the cerebral blood volume, however, slight changes in vessel diameter may have a profound effect on intracranial blood volume. Available evidence suggests the venous system may be regulated more by neurogenic than by myogenic or metabolic factors.[43]

Pulsatile Perfusion. Both a fast and slow component to the myogenic response to changes in perfusion pressure have been proposed.[251] This is of particular interest in the cardiac surgical patient.[111] During cardiopulmonary bypass the pulsatile variations in blood pressure transmitted to the cerebral vasculature appear to influence CBF, perhaps by

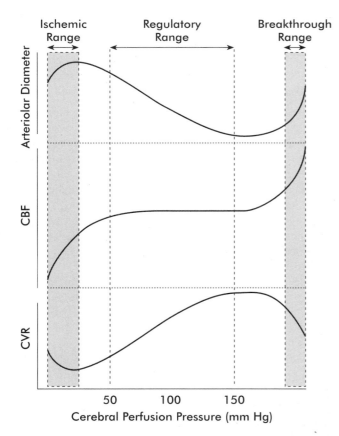

FIG. 2-4 Idealized depiction of pressure autoregulation in terms of CBF, cerebrovascular resistance, and arteriolar diameter. See text for further explanation. *(From Young W: Clinical neuroscience lectures, Munster, Ind, 1991, Cathenart Publishing.)*

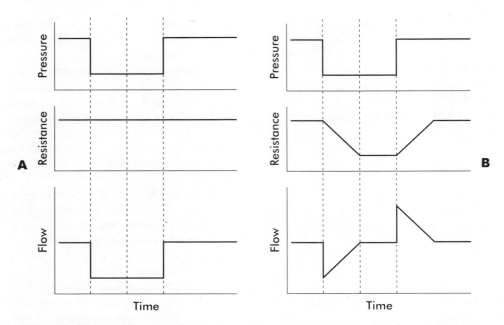

FIG. 2-5   Flow, resistance, and pressure as a function of time. The dotted vertical lines represent a time scale of "minutes." **A,** In a rigid pipe (or a totally vasoparalyzed circulation), a step decrease in pressure leads to an instantaneous fall in flow, as resistance stays fixed. **B,** In a conduit that autoregulates, a step decrease in pressure is first met with an instantaneous fall in flow. As resistance falls, however, flow increases toward baseline. With the step restoration of pressure to control level, there is an instantaneous hyperemic response, and subsequently flow decreases as resistance decreases toward control levels. *(From Young W:* Clinical neuroscience lectures, *Munster, Ind, 1991, Cathenart Publishing.)*

interaction with endothelium-derived mediators of vascular tone.[175] Although the importance of these effects has not been completely determined, the loss of pulsatility may worsen the outcome of a cerebral ischemic event.[258] Sudden restoration of pulsatile perfusion to a previously dampened circulatory bed may be a mechanism to explain certain instances of cerebral hyperemia.[282]

Cardiac Output.   It has been proposed that cardiac output may be responsible for improved CBF and outcome after subarachnoid hemorrhage (SAH). However, there is little evidence for this as an operative mechanism of improving cerebral perfusion.[31] Improved perfusion by volume loading is indirectly accomplished by improving blood rheology and directly accomplished by increasing systemic blood pressure and preventing occult decreases in systemic pressure in a patient population that is already subject to volume depletion (that is, decreased circulating blood volume).[237]

Studies examining the possible relationship between a change in cardiac output and a change in CBF have, for the most part, assessed the effect of drugs that increase cardiac output during either normotension or induced hypertension. There is some suggestion, however, during deliberate drug-induced hypotension, that a decrease in cardiac output might be reflected by a decrease in CBF, even when blood pressure is maintained above the lower autoregulatory threshold.[190]

Rheologic Factors

Clinically, hematocrit is the main influence on blood viscosity,[78] and, as shown in Equation 2, blood viscosity is a major determinant of vascular resistance. Muizelaar et al. have proposed that viscosity directly participates in hemodynamic autoregulation.[173,174] As will be discussed, viscosity may be the only determinant of cerebrovascular resistance subject to manipulation in certain settings. There is an inverse relationship between hematocrit and CBF. A continuing controversy is whether this is, in fact, purely rheologic or a function of changes in oxygen delivery to the tissue.[255]

The Hagen-Poiseuille model does not accurately describe the behavior of flow at the microcirculatory level.[46,291] When red blood cells flow near vessel walls, they create *shear* forces, which add resistance. (The shear rate is the change in velocity moving from the wall towards center of vessel.) Therefore in all vessels the red cell velocity is faster in the center of the vessel and slower at the periphery. In small vessels, cells move faster than the plasma (Fahraeus effect), and this reduces microvascular hematocrit. Because of this reduction in hematocrit, there is a reduction in viscosity (Fahraeus-Lindqvist effect). Another contribution of the smaller microvascular hematocrit is that, as the vessels become progressively smaller, the relative size of the annular periphery (with reduced flow velocity) becomes larger.

Cerebral hematocrit in humans is approximately 75% but is affected by $Paco_2$[221] and presumably other vasoactive influences. Relative hypercapnia reduces cerebral hematocrit and, presumably, so do other vasodilators.

Metabolic and Chemical Influences

Carbon Dioxide. CO_2 is a powerful modulator of cerebrovascular resistance. At one time CO_2 was thought to be the "coupler" between flow and metabolism[148] because an increase in metabolism generates CO_2 and therefore releases a cerebral vasodilator into the local environment. Rapid diffusion across the blood-brain barrier (BBB) allows CO_2 to modulate extracellular fluid pH and affect arteriolar resistance.[134] Metabolically induced changes in pH in the systemic circulation do not result in the same effect in the presence of an intact BBB, but metabolic production of H^+ released into the CSF or extracellular space from ischemic lactic acidosis does.

By active, though somewhat sluggish, exchange of HCO_3^-, the CSF eventually buffers itself against alterations in pH by CO_2 diffusion. Although CO_2-induced cerebral vasoconstriction wanes over a period of 6 to 10 hours;[212] this can be variable in an individual patient. Also important in this regard are chronic states of either hypocapnia or hypercapnia because sudden normalization of $Paco_2$ can result in relative hypoperfusion or hyperperfusion.

At normotension, there is a nearly linear response of CBF between a $Paco_2$ of 20 and 80 mm Hg (CBF changes about 2% to 4% for each mm Hg change in $Paco_2$). The linearity of the response breaks down as $Paco_2$ approaches the extremes. The values quoted for either percentage-change or absolute levels in CBF change per unit CO_2 are highly variable depending on the methodology employed and whether one is measuring hemispheric or cortical flow.[10,132] In general, doubling $Paco_2$ from 40 to 80 mm Hg doubles CBF, and halving $Paco_2$ from 40 to 20 mm Hg halves CBF. This highly reproducible cerebrovascular CO_2 response is frequently used as a method of validating and comparing different CBF methodologies.[10]

In a fashion analogous to blood pressure autoregulation, the CO_2 response is limited by either maximal vasodilation at extreme hypercapnia or maximal vasoconstriction at extreme hypocapnia. Hypocapnia, however, may adversely affect cellular metabolism and shift the oxyhemoglobin dissociation curve to the left.[232] Severe hypocapnia ($\approx$ 10 mm Hg) can result in anaerobic glucose metabolism and lactate production.[9,273] Although clinical experience clearly demonstrates impaired mentation with less severe degrees of hyperventilation, it is not clear whether this represents impairment of tissue oxygenation or some effect of tissue alkalosis and transcellular ionic shifts. Clinically, it is almost never necessary to induce such extreme levels of hypocapnia, and $Paco_2$ levels below 25 mm Hg are best avoided except under extraordinary circumstances. The use of induced hypocapnia in neurosurgical settings is bound to undergo careful scrutiny in the near future.[172]

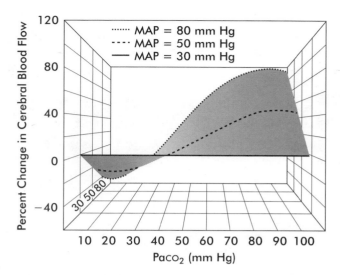

FIG. 2-6 The influence of blood pressure on the CBF response to $Paco_2$. The effects of alteration in $Paco_2$ on cortical blood flow in dogs with normotension (mean arterial pressure: 80 mm Hg, *upper trace*), moderate hypotension (50 mm Hg, *middle trace*), and severe hypotension (30 mm Hg, *lower trace*). *(From Harper AM: Acta Neurol Scand 41(suppl 14):94, 1965. Modified from McCulloch J. In Knezevic S, Maximilian VA, Mubrin Z et al, editors: Handbook of regional cerebral blood flow, Hillsdale, NJ, 1988, Lawrence Erlbaum Associates, p 1, using data from Harper AM: J Neurol Neurosurg Psychiatry 29:398, 1966.)*

Arteriolar tone, set by the systemic arterial blood pressure, modulates the effect of $Paco_2$ on CBF. Moderate hypotension blunts the ability of the cerebral circulation to respond to changes in $Paco_2$, and severe hypotension abolishes it altogether[104] (Fig. 2-6). Conversely, $Paco_2$ modifies pressure autoregulation, and from hypercapnia to hypocapnia there is a widening of the "autoregulatory plateau" (Fig. 2-7).[194]

$Paco_2$ responsiveness varies by region.[225] This may be due to the relative metabolic requirements present in each area, but this mechanism is not understood. Decreased CO_2 reactivity can be a function of local decreases in CPP distal to a spastic or stenotic vessel. In addition, it may reflect deranged metabolism or structural damage in a number of disease states, including head injury,[62] SAH,[124,229] and ischemic cerebrovascular disease.[41]

Oxygen. Within physiologic ranges, Pao_2 does not affect CBF. Hypoxemia, however, is a potent stimulus for arteriolar dilation.[39] This is a result of tissue hypoxia and concomitant lactic acidosis although the precise mechanism is unclear. CBF begins to increase at a Pao_2 of about 50 mm Hg and roughly doubles at a Pao_2 of 30 mm Hg. States that impair CO_2 reactivity are likely to interfere with O_2 reactivity as well. The response of CBF to both changes in Pao_2 and the oxygen content of blood is shown in Fig. 2-8. Hyperoxia decreases CBF, producing a modest 10% to 15% decrease at 1 atmosphere.[132] Hyperbaric oxygenation may further decrease CBF.

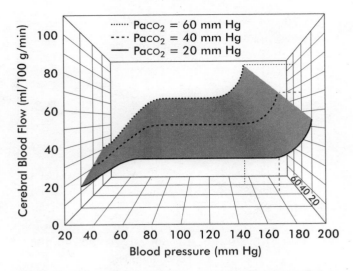

FIG. 2-7 The influence of Pa_{CO_2} on pressure autoregulation of CBF. *(Modified from Paulson OB, Strandgaard S, Edvinsson L: Cerebrovasc Brain Metab Rev 2:161, 1990.)*

Temperature. As is true for other organ systems, cerebral metabolism decreases with decreasing temperature. For each 1° C decrease in body temperature, CMR_{O_2} decreases by approximately 7%. Alternatively, this relationship may be characterized by the metabolic temperature coefficient, Q_{10}, which is defined as the ratio of CMR_{O_2} at temperature T, divided by the CMR_{O_2} at a temperature that is 10 degrees lower (T − 10). The value for cerebral Q_{10} in the physiologic range of 27° to 37° C is between 2.0 and 3.0.[243] Below 27° C, however, Q_{10} increases to near 4.5. This has been explained on the basis of the neuroelectrical effects, wherein the major suppression of neuronal function occurs between 17 and 27° C. Thus the lower Q_{10} between 27° and 37° C simply reflects the decrease in the rates of biochemical reaction, and the higher Q_{10} between 17 and 27° C is due to the additive effect of the decrease in neuronal function.[161]

Because the regulation of CBF is known to be closely coupled to cerebral metabolism, it is not surprising that this hypothermia-induced reduction in CMR_{O_2} is reflected by a parallel decrease in CBF. There is some heterogeneity in this response, however, so that CBF changes are most apparent in the cerebral and cerebellar cortex, less apparent in the thalamus, and not significant in the hypothalamus and brainstem.[119]

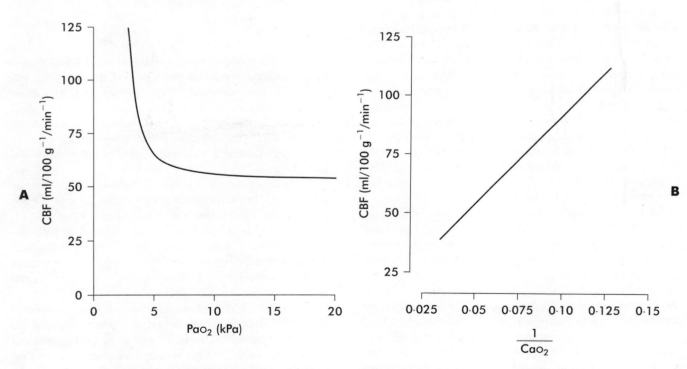

FIG. 2-8 Influence of oxygen content (Ca_{O_2}) and Pa_{O_2} on CBF. **A,** CBF is inversely proportional to Ca_{O_2}. **B,** Replotting the straight line in **A** by applying a sigmoid O_2 dissociation curve and taking the reciprocal produces the more familiar asymptotic curve of Pa_{O_2} vs. CBF, which disguises the dependence of CBF on Ca_{O_2}. 5 kPa is approximately 40 mm Hg. *(Redrawn by Lesser PJA, Jones JG. In Scurr C, Feldman S, Soni N, editors: Scientific foundations of anaesthesia: the basis of intensive care, ed 2, Chicago, 1990, Year Book Medical Publishers, p 205, from original data by Brown MM, Wade JPH, Marshall J: Brain 108[pt 1]:81, 1985.)*

Intraoperative hypothermia is most often encountered during cardiopulmonary bypass. CBF in this setting has been shown to correlate with nasopharyngeal temperature, with a maximum 55% reduction in CBF occurring, in one study, at the lowest measured temperature of 26° C. This corresponds to a 56% calculated reduction in $CMRo_2$.[86] $CMRo_2$ continues to decrease with further lowering of temperature up to the point of EEG silence. In dogs, this is reached at 18° C.[243]

The effects of hypothermia and anesthetic drugs may be additive to the point at which EEG activity ceases.[243] Thiopental administered during hypothermia in doses that enhance the hypothermia-induced suppression of EEG activity produces a further reduction in $CMRo_2$, which is paralleled by an additional decrease in CBF. Although similar effects on $CMRo_2$ can be effected by isoflurane, there appears to be no additional drop in CBF.[274]

Autoregulation, as well as CO_2 reactivity, is well preserved during cardiopulmonary bypass at moderate hypothermia.[86] There is some suggestion, however, that autoregulation may become impaired if the CO_2 content of blood is allowed to rise. This can occur when exogenous CO_2 is administered to provide a "normal" $Paco_2$ corrected to the patient's actual temperature during pH-stat management.[113] Recalculating the $Paco_2$ at 37° C for "alpha-stat" management reveals these patients to be markedly hypercarbic, which explains the grossly elevated levels of CBF reported in some cardiopulmonary bypass studies.[109,245]

Pharmacology. Dose-related anesthetic or drug effects (e.g., isoflurane[120]) can alter vasoactive responses just as BP and CO_2 do (Fig. 2-9).[156,157] The vasodilatory influence of isoflurane is apparent. Higher MAC levels can blunt the CO_2 response or render CBF pressure-passive. Vasoactive drugs may affect different aspects of autoregulatory behavior, as illustrated by recent evidence that nitroprusside impairs the ability of the circulation to maintain CBF when CPP is lowered but not when CPP is increased.[242]

Apparently independent of autoregulatory impairment,[8] anesthesia with volatile drugs appears to result in a trend for CBF to decrease over time in animal models, compared with control values.[37,259,270] It does not, however, involve an effect on CSF pH.[270] Not only do absolute flow levels decrease, but CO_2 changes responsiveness as well.[158] This time-dependent CBF decrease has been proposed to be operative during cardiopulmonary bypass in humans.[216]

The etiology of these flow decreases (or possibly return to "normal") has not been adequately explained. Evidence that flow does not decrease in other carefully controlled studies raises the question that this time effect may be a methodologic artifact.[30,215,227] In conditions of temperature flux, declines in CBF during the initial period of cardiopulmonary bypass with the skull closed probably reflect temperature equilibration in the brain. But, interestingly, with the skull open and direct monitoring of cortical temperature, there does not appear to be a lag during cooling and rewarming during cardiopulmonary bypass.[246]

Neurogenic Influences

One of the most striking differences between the systemic and cerebral circulations is the relative lack of humoral and autonomic influences on normal cerebrovascular tone. The

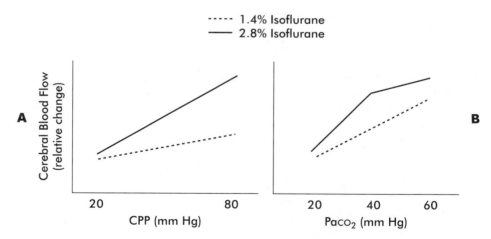

FIG. 2-9 Influence of vasodilators on blood pressure autoregulation and CO_2 reactivity in the isoflurane-anesthetized dog. Comparing 1 and 2 MAC isoflurane: With changing CPP **(A)**, autoregulation for blood pressure is not as efficient, and CBF flow appears to increase more between 20 and 40 mm Hg than between 40 and 60 mm Hg. However, CBF **(B)** increases at each of the three levels of $Paco_2$ (at 1 MAC isoflurane). With 2 MAC isoflurane, CBF increases only between 20 and 40 mm Hg. Presumably the circulation is maximally vasodilated at 2.0 MAC isoflurane and a $Paco_2$ of 40 mm Hg, so that increasing $Paco_2$ to 60 mm Hg has less of an effect on total cardiovascular resistance. *(Redrawn from data in McPherson RW, Brian JE, Traystman RJ: Anesthesiology 70843, 1989.)*

systemic circulation is regulated to a large extent by sympathetic nervous activity, but autonomic factors do not appear to control the cerebral circulation. Thus autonomic nerves are not *necessary* for regulatory responses, but they may *modify* these responses in several important ways.

The innervation of the cerebral vasculature is extensive[60,231] and involves serotonergic, adrenergic, and cholinergic systems of both intracranial and extracranial origin. The physiologic significance of this intricate and extensive system of innervation is not fully understood. One confounding factor in the interpretation of experimental studies is a marked interspecies difference in the CBF response to sympathetic stimulation.[108] Thus, in monkeys, acute sympathetic *denervation* has no effect on CBF but acute sympathetic *stimulation* reduces CBF during normotension and during hypertension. In cats and dogs, by contrast, sympathetic *stimulation* has no effect during normotension. However, when acute hypertension is induced in cats by aortic ligation, electrical stimulation of the cervical sympathetic chain attenuates the increase in CBF and decreases disruption of the blood-brain barrier.[25]

Under normal circumstances, the presence of baseline sympathetic tone exerted on the cerebral vasculature in humans is controversial. The lack of baseline tone is supported by studies demonstrating that phentolamine-induced alpha blockade does not affect CBF.[234] In contrast, Hernandez et al.[110] have demonstrated, in monkeys, that unilateral superior cervical ganglion excision leads to a 34% increase in CBF on the affected side, with no effect on autoregulation.

The effect of increased sympathetic tone on CBF in altered physiologic states, on the other hand, is well recognized. For example, using intense stimulation of the stellate ganglion in dogs, D'Alecy[51] could produce a decrease in CBF greater than 60%. Thus acute sympathetic stimulation can shift the autoregulatory curve to the right. Reflex increases in sympathetic tone have been shown to attenuate the transient increases in CBF that are observed during severe hypertensive episodes.[107] Sympathetic stimulation is also associated with a small decrease in the hyperemia seen during hypercapnia in normotensive rabbits.[24] The cerebrovascular effects are more pronounced during bilateral sympathetic nerve stimulation.[42]

These effects are seen in spite of acidosis, which inhibits the release of noradrenaline.[209,262] Sympathetic stimulation probably constricts the larger conductance and pial vessels, thereby interposing an additional "resistor" proximal to the arterioles. In those situations where an increase in CBF occurs as a result of an increase in cerebral metabolic rate (i.e., seizures), even bilateral activation of sympathetic nerves has no effect on CBF. In such situations, metabolic factors are the overwhelming determinants of CBF, with only a minimal contribution from the sympathetic nervous system.[64]

At the lower limits of autoregulation, sympathetic activity modifies the autoregulatory response of CBF to a decrease in arterial blood pressure (Fig. 2-10). At equivalent

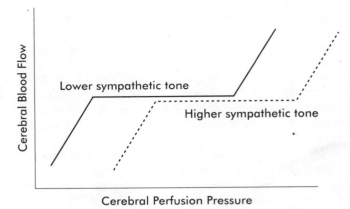

FIG. 2-10   Autonomic effects on autoregulation. Higher sympathetic tone, by adding a "proximal resistor" to the arteriolar bed, shifts the upper and lower ends of autoregulation to the right.

blood pressures, CBF is lower during hemorrhagic hypotension than during pharmacologically induced hypotension.[68] Thus when reflex sympathetic constriction of larger cerebral arteries in response to hypotension is prevented by acute surgical sympathectomy or alpha receptor blockade, CBF is better maintained because autoregulation is preserved to a mean arterial pressure that is 35% of control, in contrast to 65% of control pressure in untreated baboons. This explains why drug-induced hypotension during anesthesia is better tolerated than hypotension resulting from hemorrhagic shock. Although never studied, the sympathetic stimulation that occurs with severe pain may also shift the autoregulatory curve to the right.

Parasympathetic fibers surround the vessels of the Circle of Willis as well as the cortical pial vessels. These fibers contain a wide variety of vasodilatory mediators, which include substance P, neurokinin A, and calcitonin gene-related protein. Stimulation of these fibers promotes a vasodilatory reaction to ischemia. Thus, in rats rendered ischemic by branch occlusion of the MCA, sectioning of these nerves has recently been shown to lead to a greater cerebral infarction volume.[129] Any protective effect, however, may be overshadowed by an increase in postischemic hyperemia mediated by stimulation of these same fibers.[170] Because of species differences these results cannot reasonably be extrapolated to humans. In summary, despite extensive innervation of the intracerebral vessels, the purpose of these pathways currently remains baffling.

Other Clinical Considerations

The Hypertensive Patient.   Chronic hypertension is accompanied by a rightward shift of the autoregulation curve. Although this has some effect in protecting the brain against "breakthrough" by surpassing the upper limit of autoregulation, it occurs at the expense of the lower limit.

In contrast with normotensive individuals, in whom CBF is preserved as long as mean arterial pressure remains above

60 mm Hg, the lower limit of autoregulation in uncontrolled hypertensive patients may occur at a mean arterial pressure as high as 120 mm Hg or more. Thus, although symptoms of cerebral hypoxia do not generally occur with a mean arterial pressure above 35 to 40 mm Hg in the normotensive patient, these symptoms may occur at significantly higher blood pressures in the chronic hypertensive.[140] In one study, cerebral ischemia became apparent at an average mean arterial blood pressure of 68 mm Hg.[247] Both the lower limit of autoregulation and the blood pressure at which cerebral hypoxia occurs appear to correlate with the degree to which the resting blood pressure is elevated.

The significance of this rightward shift of the lower autoregulatory threshold is that, with decreases in blood pressure—whether caused by hemorrhage, shock, overly aggressive antihypertensive therapy, or deliberate hypotension—hypertensive patients may suffer cerebral ischemia at blood pressure levels well tolerated by normal patients. The mechanism responsible for the shift of the curve is not precisely known. Vascular hypertrophy, accompanied by an increase in media thickness and a resulting decrease in the size of the intravascular lumen (thicker wall-to-lumen ratio), increases proximal conductance vessel resistance.[180] Neurogenic factors may also contribute.[220] Thus, when cerebrovascular dilation in the resistance vessels is maximal, total vascular resistance is higher in the hypertensive subject, similar to the case with acute sympathetic stimulation. Despite the autoregulatory shift seen with chronic hypertension, CO_2 reactivity in this group is no different than in the normotensive population.[257] This underscores the probable difference in mechanisms between CO_2-induced and blood pressure–induced cerebral vasomotion.

The significance of this rightward shift of the upper autoregulatory threshold is that the hypertensive patient is provided with a protective mechanism whereby increases in blood pressure, which in normal patients would increase CBF, possibly compromising the competence of the blood-brain barrier or leading to hypertensive encephalopathy, have little effect. Cerebral vessel hypertrophy resists the tendency toward forced vasodilation, which is most apparent in the smaller arterioles. Anesthetics that diminish cerebrovascular tone (e.g., halothane) have been shown to attenuate this protective effect during extreme elevations of blood pressure.[72]

The vascular changes and autoregulatory shift induced by chronic hypertension are modified by long-term antihypertensive therapy.[121,263] The degree of reversal appears to be related to the length of treatment and correlates with the resultant fall in blood pressure.[77]

With regard to acute antihypertensive therapy, the questions of whether the method of blood pressure reduction in the chronically hypertensive subject has an effect on the resultant CBF has been studied by several investigators.[189] One may attribute the net effect of any antihypertensive drug to some combination of the predicted fall in CBF that is due to autoregulatory failure and the direct pharmaco-logic effect of the drug on the cerebral vasculature.[21,117,118,196] Barry and Strandgaard[21] have proposed a system for categorizing the effects of antihypertensive agents on autoregulatory phenomena, as follows:

1. Systemic direct vasodilators—without an action on cerebrovascular smooth muscle
2. Systemic direct vasodilators—with an action on cerebrovascular smooth muscle
3. Alpha-adrenergic and ganglionic blocking agents
4. Converting enzyme inhibitors

Their studies and others suggest that groups 1 and 3 should not have an effect on cerebrovascular autoregulation, in that they do not independently influence cerebrovascular tone. On the other hand, vasodilators that affect either the conductance or resistance vessels in the brain, such as hydralazine, sodium nitroprusside, nitroglycerin, and calcium channel blockers, may influence autoregulation. As discussed by Paulson et al.[194] and Michenfelder,[165] determining the exact interaction and extent of pharmacologic and autoregulatory vasomotion is currently an imprecise science.

Captopril appears to foreshorten the autoregulatory plateau, but it shifts the autoregulatory curve to the left. This probably accounts for patients with congestive heart failure tolerating lower perfusion pressure without evidence of cerebral ischemia.[19,20,192] This may be due to a direct involvement of the renin-angiotensin system in maintaining some influence on resting cerebrovascular tone.

The Elderly Patient. Normal resting hemispheric cerebral blood flow in humans is known to decrease with increasing age.[178,248,277] The significance of this decreased perfusion is unclear. In the absence of brain electrical activity (i.e., high-dose barbiturates), $CMRo_2$ has been demonstrated to be decreased in elderly rats. Thus one reason proposed for a decrease in CBF with age may be a decrease in metabolic demand for nonelectrical neuronal function.[23]

Accompanying this change in total CBF is a redistribution of rCBF: relative frontal hyperemia in the young contrasts with a more uniformly distributed gray matter flow in the elderly. (This CBF pattern is called "hyperfrontality" and is considered normal.) Thus the total CBF decrease with age is primarily a result of a rapid decrement of flow in the frontal regions, an intermediate decrement in the parietal regions, and a minor decrement in occipital rCBF.[248] This anterior circulation predominance of age-related changes correlates with previously demonstrated increases in regional cerebral vascular resistance and a decrease in gray matter weight in the middle cerebral artery territory.[178]

One may question whether the decreased resting CBF in the elderly represents a similar decrease in cerebrovascular reserve. In a recent study, CBF in newborn and juvenile pigs was 48 and 44 ml/100 g/min, respectively, compared with 27 ml/100 g/min in adults. CBF reserve was also shown to be lower in adult pigs, with EEG flattening occurring at significantly higher levels of CBF than in juveniles and newborns.[100]

Concerning cerebrovascular reactivity, the cerebral vasoconstrictive response to hypocarbia in humans becomes diminished with advancing age. Thus CO_2 reactivity at age 65 is roughly half that at age 20. This change in CO_2 reactivity is seen whether CO_2 reactivity is expressed as an absolute value or as a percentage change in CBF. It has been postulated that this change in reactivity may be due to minor atherosclerosis or the loss of cerebral vascular elasticity. Alternatively, this finding may simply be due to the fact that at normocapnia, CBF in the elderly is significantly lower than it is in the young. Thus, with hypocapnia, cerebrovascular constriction in the elderly is more likely to reduce CBF to the ischemic threshold. Below this level of CO_2, compensatory mechanisms may prevent the further reduction of CBF, yielding an artifactual impression of reduced CO_2 reactivity.[277]

The vasodilatory response to hypercarbia is also altered in the elderly. Yamamoto et al.[278] found that the decline in this response parallels the baseline decrease in CBF seen with advancing age. In normal subjects, however, when CO_2 reactivity is expressed as percentage change in CBF rather than absolute change, the age-related differences found in response to hypercarbia are minimal in healthy patients. Regional impairment of vasodilatory responsiveness to hypercarbia becomes increasingly more significant as one progresses across the spectrum from normal patients to patients with risk factors for cerebrovascular disease and, finally, to patients with symptomatic cerebral ischemia. Both resting CBF and the hyperemic response to hypercarbia may, however, be well preserved in patients with angiographically documented cerebrovascular occlusion.[248]

Although, as mentioned previously, most studies have shown a decrease in CBF as well as a deterioration in the regulation of CBF with advancing age, this premise is not universally accepted. This is because it is often difficult to isolate age as an independent factor. Thus one recent study demonstrated no change in CBF between the ages of 50 and 85 despite the presence of an age-related increase in brain atrophy. Of significance, in this combined stable xenon CT and positron emission tomography (PET) study, patients were carefully screened to exclude those with any brain lesions or mental deterioration as determined by psychologic examination. These older patients may thus be characterized as the fittest of the fit.[125] Earlier studies, however, have shown that, although risk factors for stroke enhance the age-related reduction in CBF, a reduction in CBF in the elderly is demonstrable even without the presence of these confounding factors.[178]

AUTOREGULATORY FAILURE

Cerebral autoregulation is disturbed in a number of disease states. Most diseases that affect the CNS will, in one way or another, affect the ability of the circulation to regulate itself. Examples include acute ischemia, mass lesions, trauma, inflammation, prematurity, neonatal asphyxia, and diabetes mellitus. In spite of a wide range of etiologies, the final common pathway of dysfunction, in its most extreme state, may be termed vasomotor paralysis.

What causes autoregulation to fail? The simplistic approach is to invoke tissue acidosis or local accumulation of "noxious metabolites," but this does not account for all cases. Localized damage that results in loss of autoregulation at sites distant from the injury is more difficult to explain.[230] Furthermore, Paulson et al.[128] coined the term "dissociated vasoparalysis" to describe retained CO_2 responsiveness with loss of autoregulatory capacity to changes in blood pressure. This can be observed in regions contralateral to tumor or infarction,[193] or during hyperperfusion after AVM resection.[286] Such a dissociation between two preeminent vasomotive stimuli emphasizes that pressure regulation is much more vulnerable than is loss of CO_2 reactivity or possibly other metabolic influences on regulatory mechanisms. Total loss of CO_2 responsiveness is probably a preterminal event. A related phenomenon is "diaschisis," which is the occurrence of hypoperfusion and hypometabolism remote from a damaged area.[11,159]

An additional phenomenon is "false autoregulation." This has been described in the setting of head injury.[49,62] In a paralyzed circulatory bed, pressure-passive increases in CBF may result in local pressure gradients in the most damaged areas. Local swelling may then maintain CBF constant despite increasing systemic pressures.

Autoregulatory failure (Fig. 2-11) can be divided into "right sided" (hyperperfusion) and "left sided" (hypoperfusion) autoregulatory failure. Although the following sections discuss the parenchymal consequences of dysregulation in a homogeneous light, there are differing regional susceptibilities to ischemia and circulatory breakthrough. Portions of the hippocampus, for example, are exquisitely sensitive to ischemia. Previously this was thought to be simply a function of the basal metabolic state of the tissue, that is, the higher the metabolic rate the more susceptible to ischemia, however, this sensitivity undoubtedly involves other mechanisms (see Choi[47]).

Hypoperfusion and Ischemia

Hypoperfusion leads to cerebral ischemia. However, there is no reason to suspect that the fundamental metabolic consequences of reduced CBF to the neurons are any different for any of the various modes of flow reduction. The distinction of complete vs. incomplete ischemia, however, may have metabolic consequences, and, most important, regional or focal ischemia carries with it the possibility of collateral supply of CBF.

Fig. 2-11 is an idealized expansion of the left side of the autoregulatory curve shown in Fig. 2-4. As CPP decreases toward the lower limit of autoregulation (approximately 50 mm Hg), arteriolar resistance vessels dilate and CBV increases. At the lower limit of autoregulation, however, the ability to vasodilate is exhausted, the circulation cannot decrease resistance further to maintain flow, and

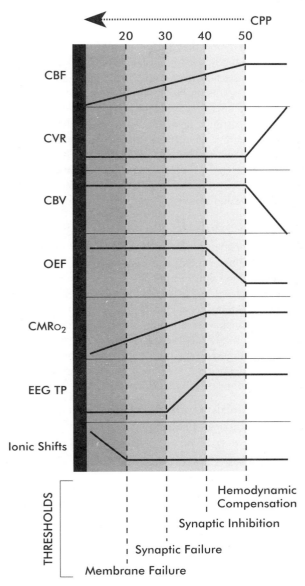

FIG. 2-11 Autoregulatory failure. The left side of Fig. 2-4 is expanded here to show idealized changes in various physiologic functions (some of the pathophysiologic events indicated overlap). The values for CPP are only approximate, and many of the changes in the various covariates may overlap. They are stylized here for the sake of clarity. *CBF* (cerebral blood flow), *CVR* (cerebrovascular resistance), *CBV* (cerebral blood volume), *OEF* (oxygen extraction fraction), *CMRo2* (cerebral metabolic rate for oxygen), *EEG TP* (total power of the cortical EEG signal), and *ionic shift* (e.g., water and Na^+ into the cells and K^+ out of the cells) are shown along the left of the figure. The various CBF thresholds are indicated by the broken lines and labeled at the bottom of the figure. The functional state between each threshold is shown along the abscissa. In this figure the loss of EEG power is still above the line for membrane failure. Clinically, any event that results in EEG signs of ischemia should be assumed to represent the potential for irreversible damage and should be treated accordingly. *(From Young W: Clinical neuroscience lectures, Munster, Ind, 1991, Cathenart Publishing.)*

CBF begins to decline passively as CPP decreases further. At first, an increase in oxygen extraction compensates for the passive decline in CBF. When oxygen extraction is maximum, $CMRo_2$ begins to decrease. Accordingly, synaptic transmission becomes impaired and eventually fails completely, as manifested by an isoelectric EEG. At this point, there is sufficient energy available to keep the neurons alive, but neuronal "work" is abolished. Proceeding to even lower flow levels results in "membrane failure" (Na^+, Ca^{2+}, and water enter, and K^+ exits the cell; i.e., cytotoxic edema). Such reductions in CBF are in the lethal range and result in infarction if not corrected.

The development of cerebral infarction depends on both the degree and duration at which flow is reduced to ischemic levels (Fig. 2-12).[128] Neuronal tissue can receive flow at a level that prevents normal function but does not result in permanent damage. If flow is returned to adequate levels, function returns. As shown in Fig. 2-12, two such states may exist, the *penlucida*, from which tissue recovers function irrespective of the ischemic time, and *penumbra*, from which tissue is salvageable only if flow is restored within a certain time. The term *penumbra*, which means "almost shadow," was introduced by Branston et al.[35] They originally used the term to denote all such tissue that was nonfunctional but that had the capacity to regain function. To make the distinction between tissue that survives without

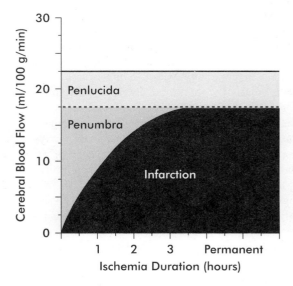

FIG. 2-12 Interaction of degree and duration of flow reductions on neurologic function. Tissue receiving flow between approximately 18 and 23 ml/100 g/min is functionally inactive, but function can be restored at any time with reinstitution of increased perfusion *(penlucida)*. For tissue perfused at lower blood flows, the development of infarction is a function of time. If tissue is restored to adequate perfusion before the time limit for infarction, it will recover function *(penumbra)*. *(Modified from data in Jones TH, Motawetz RB, Crowell RM et al.: J Neurosurg 54:773, 1981. From Young W: Clinical neuroscience lectures, Munster, Ind, 1991, Cathenart Publishing.)*

intervention and tissue that succumbs if left untended, Drummond et al. designated the former as ischemic penlucida ("almost light").[57]

Although any clinical event that results in EEG changes suggesting ischemia should be assumed to represent a threat for irreversible damage and be treated accordingly, many such events probably reflect flow reduction to the penumbral range (Fig. 2-11). An example of this phenomenon is the patient undergoing carotid endarterectomy in whom EEG changes suggesting ischemia develop after carotid clamping. With shunt placement, the EEG normalizes and the patient awakens without sequelae.

Hyperperfusion and Circulatory Breakthrough

If CPP exceeds the upper limit of autoregulation, flow initially increases with a fixed maximal arteriolar resistance. At some point, the arteriolar bed dilates under the increasing pressure, and the resistance falls as well. Clinically, one may observe brain swelling from this intravascular engorgement, vasogenic edema from opening of the blood-brain barrier, and intracerebral hemorrhage from vessel rupture.[194,226,286] The different types of brain swelling and their primary fluid compartment alterations are shown in Table 2-1.

To explain the occurrence of postoperative brain swelling and intracerebral hemorrhage after AVM resection, the concept "normal pressure perfusion breakthrough" (NPPB)[240] or "circulatory breakthrough"[181] has been proposed. This theory holds that the low-resistance AVM shunt system results in arterial hypotension and venous hypertension in the relatively normal circulatory beds irrigated by vessels in continuity with feeding arteries and draining veins adjacent to the lesion. Regional CBF in these neighboring areas is maintained in a normal range by appropriate autoregulatory vasodilation. This longstanding state of maximal dilation may result in vasomotor paralysis; the resistance vessels may no longer be able to autoregulate should perfusion pressure increase. When the AVM fistula is interrupted, the pressure "normalizes" in the neighboring circulation. However, the presence of a vasomotor paralysis in newly normotensive circulatory beds prevents the appropriate increase in cerebrovascular resistance necessary to maintain flow at a constant level, and cerebral hypere-

TABLE 2-1
Types of Brain Swelling

Type of Swelling	Primary Fluid Compartment Alteration
Cytotoxic	Shift of fluid from extracellular to intracellular space
Vasogenic	Shift of fluid from intravascular to extracellular space
Interstitial	Shift of CSF into extracellular space
Hyperemic	Increase in intravascular volume

mia occurs. This hyperperfusion and abrupt increase in perfusion pressure may result in swelling and hemorrhage although the precise mechanism is speculative. Postoperative swelling and hemorrhage after carotid endarterectomy[226] and after obliteration of a jugular-carotid fistula[94] are probably mechanistically related to NPPB. Many of the aspects concerning "perfusion breakthrough" are controversial and supported by anecdotal evidence only. Although the syndromes that result in postoperative catastrophes are clearly a clinical problem, the precise mechanisms and relative importance of the contributing circulatory physiology remain to be elucidated.[289] There is increasing interest in the contribution of neuroeffector mechanisms in the pathogenesis of hyperperfusion injury.[149]

Reperfusion Injury

Many of the pathophysiologic events leading to irreversible neuronal damage probably are due to injury sustained during reperfusion of the ischemic tissue, perhaps as a result of reoxygenation.[96] Specifically regarding CBF, there is the syndrome of delayed hypoperfusion.[210] The significance of the hypoperfusion in relation to neuronal damage is not clear. Most likely CBF is grossly and appropriately coupled to a decreased metabolic rate after ischemia[162]; however, certain areas of the brain may be left with a mismatched CBF-to-metabolism ratio.[210]

Hemodynamic Considerations During Autoregulatory Failure
Cerebrovascular Reserve

If cerebral vessels are stenotic, there may be region-specific areas with reduced inflow pressure. These regions frequently follow the distribution of a main arterial supply, such as the anterior, middle, or posterior cerebral arteries, or may be limited to a smaller distribution. Distal to an area of stenosis, there is a drop in perfusion pressure, and, thus, even at normal systemic blood pressure, the arterial bed distal to the stenosis is relatively hypotensive and may operate near or on the pressure-passive area of the autoregulatory curve (see Figs. 2-4 and 2-11). The resting flow to a tissue bed may be normal, but there is no further potential for vasodilation should there be a drop in perfusion pressure. Therefore these areas have an exhausted "cerebrovascular reserve," that is, the capacity to further vasodilate and maintain flow at appropriate levels. A way to assess cerebrovascular reserve is by challenging the circulation with a vasodilator. Clinically, both acetazolamide and carbon dioxide are used. In structurally normal regions (i.e., on routine MRI or CT scan) that have decreased vasodilatory response to such challenges, one may infer that the perfusion pressure is decreased.

Application of this sort of testing has been proposed, for example, to determine which patients might benefit from extracranial-to-intracranial revascularization procedures or to assess the effects of an acute arterial occlusion. Use of such methods, however, is still in its infancy in clinical practice. PET[203] and SPECT[205] methods may ultimately provide a more sensitive measure by simultaneously determining the ratio of CBF to CBV as an index of cerebrovascular reserve.

Patients with cerebrovascular disease have reductions in CBF, compared with control levels. In fact, patients with only risk factors for cerebrovascular disease have reductions in CBF and CO_2 reactivity.[278] These reductions do not necessarily depend on the presence of angiographically demonstrable vessel occlusions. The mechanism of these flow reductions and impaired vasomotion remains to be elucidated.

Newer theories on the pathogenesis of stroke in sickle cell disease combine elements of the concepts discussed in this and previous sections concerning hemodynamic regulation. Pavlakis et al.[195,208] have proposed that the pathogenesis of infarcts in patients with sickle cell disease is due to large proximal vessel occlusion with resultant drop in distal perfusion pressure; the distal irrigation of major vascular territories (e.g., MCA) is rendered hypotensive. These patients, however, have already exhausted their arteriolar vasodilatory capacity to compensate for decreased oxygen delivery from the anemia. Watershed infarcts are the clinical result.

Cerebral Steal

A related concept to "reserve" is cerebral "steal." *Steal* is a colorful but physiologically misleading term.[264] It refers to the decreased flow to ischemic areas caused by blood vessel dilation in nonischemic areas, such as can be induced by hypercapnia.[33] Blood is "stolen" from one area to another only if there is a pressure gradient between the two circulatory beds.

If an ischemic area is maximally vasodilated, addition of CO_2 vasodilates normal adjacent brain regions and may result in a net decrease in flow, presumably by lowering local input pressure, to the ischemic focus. Conversely, vasoconstriction in the normal brain may result in redistribution of blood to ischemic regions. This has been referred to as the "inverse steal" or "Robin Hood phenomenon." This mechanism may also be operative for other cerebral vasodilators, such as volatile anesthetics and systemic vasodilators such as nitroprusside, hydralazine, and nitroglycerin although data are lacking on the clinical importance of all such interactions.

Vessel Length and Viscosity

After exhaustion of vasodilatory capacity, flow is both pressure passive and highly dependent on vessel length and blood viscosity (primarily determined by hematocrit).[78] Thus, with maximal distal vasodilation, the areas with the lowest pressure are those farthest from the arterial input. These regions therefore have the highest resistance and the lowest flow. This concept is important clinically because brain regions that are farthest from their arterial input, watershed areas (such as the border between the arterial distribution of the middle and anterior cerebral arteries), are the regions most likely to become ischemic during systemic hypotension.

Viscosity reduction is also pertinent to the prevention or treatment of cerebral vasospasm in patients with aneurysmal subarachnoid hemorrhage (SAH).[236] Although the conductance vessels (as visualized angiographically) are seen to be in spasm (with a large pressure drop across constricted segments), the distal resistive bed may be maximally vasodilated.[91] Referring to Equation 2, the resistance term can no longer be influenced by changing vessel caliber. Because the vessel length term stays fixed, only blood viscosity can potentially affect cerebrovascular resistance, providing that oxygen-carrying capacity is not adversely affected.[78] In the clinical setting, however, the relative influence of hemodilution on the improved outcome from volume loading remains to be determined.

Excessive hemoglobin concentration may produce a hyperviscous state. Although polycythemia decreases CBF and is a risk factor for thromboembolic stroke, uniform guidelines for phlebotomy are lacking in clinical practice. Certainly patients with hematocrits above 60 should be anesthetized only in urgent circumstances.

Collateral Failure

After carotid occlusion in a patient with a normal cerebral circulation, the vessels in the ipsilateral hemisphere experience a fall in input pressure; accordingly, the resistance network of arteriolar vessels vasodilates. This allows collateral blood flow from a patent Circle of Willis or other channels to compensate and restore perfusion. However, if these channels do not exist, or the affected resistance vessels are already maximally vasodilated, no compensation occurs and a condition of cerebral ischemia ensues.

THERAPY FOR ENHANCING PERFUSION
Induced Hypertension
Rationale

Maintenance of a high perfusion pressure, in concert with optimal viscosity and oxygen delivery, may reduce cell death in a threatened vascular territory. As reviewed by Young and Cole,[282] there is ample experimental evidence for this strategy in the form of improvements in cerebral perfusion, electrophysiologic evoked responses, and histopathologic and neurologic outcomes. By augmenting systemic perfusion pressure, one can mitigate the pressure drop across a stenotic vessel or collateral pathway to an ischemic area (Fig. 2-13). Even small increases in CBF may shift a region from the penumbra (destined for infarction) to the penulucida and perhaps to a level of perfusion enabling normal function. However, the hazards of induced hypertension include worsening ischemic (vasogenic) edema and transforming a pale infarct into a hemorrhagic one. If blood pressure is used to increase CPP during brief periods of carotid or intracranial artery occlusion,[32,288] these concerns are less important. However, pharmacologically induced hypertension and any attendant tachycardia would increase the risk of cardiac ischemia.

Applications

Application of induced hypertension during acute thromboembolic stroke is controversial[282] but has relevance to anesthetic practice. Elevation of blood pressure during carotid endarterectomy has been discussed for some time;[32,61,73] many authors have recommended keeping blood pressure elevated during the period of temporary occlusion of the carotid artery. Both anastomotic cerebral perfusion pressure,[61,73] as measured in the distal stump of the carotid artery after clamping, and CBF[32] are increased by elevating systemic pressure. Fortunately, phenylephrine-induced hypertension does not seem to adversely affect CPP because venous sinus pressure is only minimally increased.[73] Despite claims that distal stump pressures do not correlate with

CBF changes during carotid endarterectomy,[155] the technique is a simple, low-risk, and cost-effective method to assess the adequacy of cerebral perfusion pressure.[14] False negatives may occur (i.e., normal stump pressure with inadequate CBF). However, if the angiogram demonstrates normal intracranial vessels, then a severe stump pressure reduction (i.e., <20 mm Hg) is potentially useful information.

A more recently evolving practice during neurovascular surgery is the use of temporary vascular occlusion to secure cerebral aneurysms.[22] Temporary occlusion techniques require some modification of the traditional anesthetic management of cerebral aneurysm clipping.[40,288] During temporary vascular occlusion of a major intracranial artery, not only must systemic hypotension be avoided, but blood pressure augmentation may be necessary.[56,271,282]

Induced hypertension has been used in the management

FIG. 2-13   Induced hypertension model. **A,** Normal. The arrow indicates the operating point on the autoregulatory curve; in this case, the circulatory bed is in the mid-position in the full range of autoregulation. The lower limit of autoregulation is the knee of the curve. The dotted vertical line represents the ischemic flow threshold. **B,** Inflow occlusion. If a major inflow channel to this vascular territory is interrupted, input pressure drops in the resistive bed. Autoregulatory function now adjusts for this decrease in input pressure by vasodilation of the bed. How much the input pressure falls after the major inflow occlusion is determined by the number and caliber of available collateral vascular pathways. In the example shown, there is sufficient collateral perfusion pressure to maintain the operating point above the threshold for ischemia although the operating point has entered the pressure-passive range (i.e., this bed is maximally vasodilated). **C,** Inflow occlusion with collateral failure. If one assumes atresia or stenosis of the collateral pathways (high collateral resistance), then, with occlusion of the major inflow channel, the input pressure drops to a much lower level distal to the occlusion. CBF is lower because the drop in pressure has exhausted the ability of the resistive bed to compensate by further vasodilation. Now the operating point is below the ischemic threshold. This situation demands treatment. **D,** Augmentation of collateral perfusion pressure. At this point systemic mean arterial pressure is increased. The pressure transmitted across the collateral pathways, although not sufficient to restore normal pressure in the ischemic bed, is sufficient to raise input pressure, allowing CBF to increase to just above the ischemic threshold (albeit still on the pressure-passive point on the curve). This small shift above the ischemic threshold may be crucial in determining the final extent of the infarct and the ultimate functional outcome after an ischemic event. *(From Young W: Clinical neuroscience lectures, Munster, Ind, 1991, Cathenart Publishing.)*

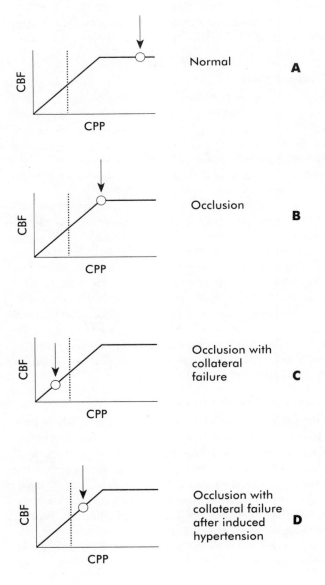

of aneurysmal SAH.[17,130,171] In this setting, hypertension is employed in conjunction with hypervolemic hemodilution; thus the relative contribution made by increasing perfusion pressure is not well defined.

Inverse Steal

There is no doubt that inverse steal can redistribute CBF to ischemic areas, with unequivocal studies documenting its clinical relevance.[269] Ideally, treatment should be tailored to individual patients' responses, which are probably variable. A practical problem is the lack of bedside methods to assess regional cerebral perfusion.

Hypocapnia

The concept that hypocapnia can favorably influence CBF during ischemia is not new,[238,239] but not all investigators have been able to demonstrate favorable flow redistribution.[58] Many of the early studies did not support a beneficial effect of hypocapnia (see Artru[15]). Early animal models used prolonged ischemia.[163] Furthermore, human studies showing trends of improved outcome with hypocapnia lacked sufficient statistical power.[18,48] As in the case of induced hypertension in the setting of carotid endarterectomy, there appears to be an improvement in collateral perfusion pressure in the presence of hypocapnia.[33,73,167,201,202] Therefore it is reasonable to consider a modest induced hypocapnia as an adjunct to induced hypertension.

Pharmacologic Manipulation

Vasoactive drugs that cause constriction of the normal vasculature may produce a favorable intracerebral redistribution of CBF to an ischemic focus, and vasodilators would be expected to work in a fashion analogous to hypercapnia. There is, however, no good evidence for improved outcome produced by such an effect.

One of the mechanisms proposed for the salutary effects of barbiturates on focal ischemia has been the redistribution of CBF from normal to ischemic areas.[34,185] In spite of this, the clinical role of barbiturates remains a controversial topic. Except for cardiopulmonary bypass, outcome studies are lacking, if not impractical.[254] Notwithstanding, most authors would agree that, in the intraoperative setting, barbiturates are to be recommended in the setting of acute temporary focal ischemia. Whether steal or inverse steal have any bearing on clinical anesthetic management is open to debate.[284] Other than agents such as propofol and etomidate (which have not been convincingly demonstrated to be cerebroprotective), there currently are no other pharmacologic agents that can accomplish inverse steal.

MEASUREMENT OF CEREBRAL BLOOD FLOW

The choice of CBF measurement method depends on many considerations: local availability of equipment and expertise, cost, subject (human vs. animal), desired anatomic resolution, and so on. The method used is important because it determines the range of normal and pathologic values, the anatomic specificity or resolution, and the set of assumptions necessary for interpreting the data. A particularly important consideration is the ability to perform repeated measures in a given patient or subject. For a general review of CBF methods, including historical aspects, see Bell.[26] A summary of CBF methods is presented in Table 2-2.

Kety-Schmidt (Arteriovenous Difference Method)

Although attempts had been made earlier, measurement of brain tissue perfusion was perfected by the pioneering work of Kety and Schmidt.[131] All CBF techniques in use today are either conceptually derived from their method or have been validated by some variation of it. Their work was based on the principle first described by Fick that the amount of tracer taken up by an organ per unit time *(Qb)* must equal the amount of tracer delivered to the organ via the arterial blood *(F · Ca)* less that recovered by the venous effluent *(F · Cv)* in the same amount of time, thus:

$$Qb = F \cdot (Ca - Cv) \qquad (3)$$

After the administration of a tracer, but before the attainment of steady state, for any small time epoch, Δt, the quantity of tracer within the organ increases by an amount that can be expressed as:

$$\Delta Qb = [C_a(t) - C_v(t)] \, (F) \, (\Delta t) \qquad (4)$$

Similarly, the total quantity of tracer present in the organ at steady state is determined by the integral:

$$Qb = \int F[C_a(t) - C_v(t)]dt \qquad (5)$$

This integration encompasses the time period beginning with the commencement of tracer input and ends with the attainment of steady state.

Manipulation of Equation 5 yields:

$$F(ml/min) = \frac{Qb(mg)}{\int [C_a(t) - C_v(t)]dt(mg/ml \; min)} \qquad (6)$$

Therefore CBF is equal to the equilibrium brain tracer content divided by the integral of the arteriovenous concentration differences.

The amount of tracer in the brain is equal to its concentration *(Cb)* times brain weight *(Wb)*:

Substituting in the previous equation:

$$Qb = Cb \cdot Wb \qquad (7)$$

$$F = \frac{Cb \cdot Wb}{\int [C_a(t) - C_v(t)] \, dt} \qquad (8)$$

However, this equation requires determination of absolute cerebral concentration and weight, which is not feasible in humans. At equilibrium, however, the venous and brain concentrations are no longer changing, and the brain

TABLE 2-2
A Comparison of CBF Methodologies

	Human or Animal	Relative Price*	Resolution	Time Scale	Repeated Measurement	Invasive	Tracers	Radiation	Relative Flow Values† (ml/100 g/min unless noted)
Hemispheric									
Kety-Schmidt	H	+	Hemispheric	15 min	Yes	Jugular puncture	N₂O, ¹³³Xe, ⁸³Kr	No, yes, yes	50
AVDo₂	H	+	Hemispheric	<1 min	Yes	Jugular puncture	N/A	No	Relative change
Two-Dimensional Clearance									
Intracarotid ¹³³Xe	H	+	3-4 cm cortical‡	<1 min (gray) 3-11 min (white)	Yes	Carotid puncture or transfemoral catheter	¹³³Xe	Yes	80 Gray (fg) 20 White 50 Initial Slope Index (ISI) (Mean Hemispheric Flow)
Intravenous ¹³³Xe	H	+	3-4 cm cortical	3-11 min	Yes	IV	¹³³Xe	Yes	As intracarotid ¹³³Xe
Inhaled ¹³³Xe	H	+	3-4 cm cortical	3-11 min	Yes	No	¹³³Xe	Yes	As intracarotid ¹³³Xe
Thermal clearance	H	+	<1-2 cm cortical	<1 min	Yes	Exposed cortex	Heat	No	Relative change
Hydrogen clearance	A	+	<5 mm cortical	<1 min	Yes	Exposed cortex, electrode placement	H₂	No	150-220
Tomographic (Three-Dimensional)									
Cold xenon	H	+++	<1 cm, three-dimensional	Several minutes per section level	Limited	No	sXe	Yes§	

Method		Cost*	Spatial resolution	Temporal resolution	Quantitation‡	Route	Tracer	Energy	Normal values†
PET	H	++++++	<1 cm, three-dimensional	Several minutes per section level	Limited	IV	Short $t_{1/2}$, lighter weight positron emitters; see text	Yes	50–70 Gray 20 White
SPECT	H	+++	<1 cm, three-dimensional	Several minutes per section level	Limited	IV	(1) longer $t_{1/2}$, heavier weight gamma emitters or (2) ^{127}Xe; ^{133}Xe; see text	Yes	Relative change for gamma; quantitative change for xenon
MRI	H‖	+++	<1 cm, three-dimensional	Several minutes per section level	Limited	IV	Paramagnetic agents	Magnetic	Relative change
Autoradiography	A	++	<5 mm, three-dimensional	<1 min	No¶	Sacrifice	^{3}H, ^{14}C, ^{18}F	Yes	90–150 Gray 20–30 White
Other Methods									
Microspheres	A	+++	<1 cm	<1 min	Yes	Sacrifice	^{153}Gd, ^{57}Co, ^{141}Ce, ^{51}Cr, ^{113}Sn, ^{103}Ru, ^{46}Sc, ^{85}Sr, ^{95}Nb	Yes	50–70 Gray 20 White
Doppler									
Laser Doppler	H	+	<5 mm	<1 min	Yes	Exposed cortex	N/A	Light	Relative changes
Transcranial Doppler ultrasound	H	+	Hemispheric	<1 min	Yes	No	N/A	Ultrasound	40–80 cm/sec
Mix									
Sagittal sinus outflow	A	+	Hemispheric	<1 min	Yes	Sagittal sinus cannulation	N/A	No	50

*Does not separate equipment investment from individual study cost.
†Values are approximate normal values for rough comparisons between methods.
‡Depends on detector size and collimator angle.
§No radiation from tracer, only from the CT scan itself.
‖No clinically approved tracers for tissue perfusion; current paramagnetic tracers are for transit time with rapid sampling MRI.
¶With single label techniques.
Various values and parameters listed are for the purpose of comparison only; for precise details, refer to citations in text.

and venous concentrations are thus related by the partition coefficient, λ, where

$$\lambda = \frac{Cb_{eq}}{Cv_{eq}} \qquad (9)$$

Substituting for lambda:

$$F = \frac{Cv_{eq} \cdot \lambda \cdot Wb}{\int [C_a(t) - C_v(t)]dt} \qquad (10)$$

where F is the flow to the entire organ.

If one divides each side of the equation by the weight of the brain, the blood flow per gram of brain tissue can be determined. Multiplying both sides of the equation by 100 introduces the well-known units for CBF of milliliters per 100 g per minute, and this "flow" is usually written with a lower-case f, to distinguish it from the upper case F denoting total brain blood flow in milliliters per minute.

$$f(ml/100\ g/min) = \frac{100\ \lambda \cdot Cv_{eq}}{\int [C_a(t) - C_v(t)]dt} \qquad (11)$$

Kety and Schmidt initially used nitrous oxide as the best available approximation of an inert, freely diffusible tracer. Subjects breathed a gas mixture containing 15% N_2O for 10 to 15 minutes. Blood samples were taken intermittently from a peripheral artery and the jugular bulb for determination of tracer concentration (Fig. 2-14). This method measures *hemispheric* CBF, and, because of the confluence of sinuses, it is really a global measure of CBF. There is "contamination" from the contralateral hemisphere, as each jugular bulb represents roughly one third of the contralat-

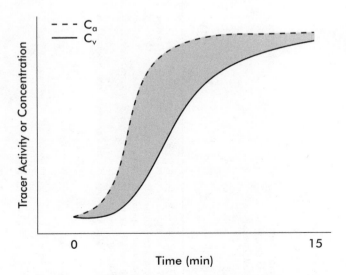

FIG. 2-14 Graphic depiction of the Kety-Schmidt CBF technique. A freely diffusible tracer is given until (theoretically) equilibrium exists between the arterial (Ca) and venous (Cv) concentrations. The area between the two curves is proportional to CBF.

eral hemispheric drainage. There is a small (<5%) extracerebral component as well.[144] Because nitrous oxide is not truly an inert tracer, later modifications of this CBF technique used radioactive tracers such as [85]krypton and [133]xenon, which are truly inert in the quantity used. One may measure arterial and venous *desaturation* rather than *saturation* curves; this may be easier to apply in certain clinical settings.

The Kety-Schmidt method has the disadvantage of being cumbersome and invasive; it requires puncture or retrograde catheterization of the jugular bulb and direct sampling of the arterial blood. CBF may be overestimated in the case of low perfusion states, where brain and venous blood may not equilibrate during the measurement interval.

After CBF is known, the arteriovenous difference of glucose and oxygen content across the brain can be calculated. The cerebral metabolic rate for a given substrate (oxygen or glucose) is calculated as CBF multiplied by the arteriovenous difference for substrate (milligrams per/100 ml):

$$CMR = CBF(Ca - Cv) \qquad (12)$$

Arteriovenous Difference in Oxygen Content (AVDo₂)

If cerebral metabolic activity remains constant, the relative changes in the AVDo₂ must reflect global CBF (Fig. 2-15), and a "CBF equivalent" can be calculated:

$$CBF = \alpha(Ca - Cv) \qquad (13)$$

where α is the proportionality constant.

This is a great leap of faith in most circumstances and should always be interpreted cautiously. It is, however, a practical way of assessing CBF changes where metabolism is expected to stay constant (e.g., examination of CO_2 reactivity) if a "calibration" has been done with another method (see Madsen et al.[150]). The AVDo₂ can be used to monitor changes in patients through placement of an oximetric catheter in the jugular bulb, but this is a case where the assumption of an unchanged underlying metabolic rate is tenuous. Nonetheless, AVDo₂ monitoring can be useful as an "early warning system" for disturbances in flow-metabolism coupling.[250] It has particular relevance to ICU care of the head-injured patient when adjusting minute ventilation to reduce brain volume,[50] because inducing hypocapnia after head injury without regard to CBF may adversely affect outcome.[172]

Radioactive Xenon
Intraarterial ¹³³Xe Methods

Based on Kety's work, the method of CBF determination described by Lassen and Ingvar allowed progression from "one-dimensional" (i.e., global measurements) to two-dimensional maps of cortical CBF patterns.[142,143] The technique involves injecting a radioactive tracer ([85]krypton or [133]xenon) as a bolus directly into the cerebral arterial sup-

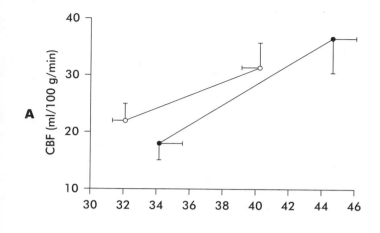

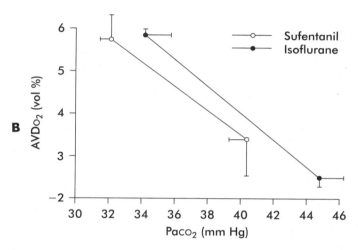

FIG. 2-15 Simultaneous CBF and AVDo₂ measurements. Comparison of cerebral blood flow (CBF) and arteriovenous difference in oxygen content (AVDo₂) values for sufentanil *(open circles)* and isoflurane *(closed circles)* anesthesia. The abscissa is Paco₂ for both **A** and **B**. There was a significant effect of Paco₂ concentration on the increase of CBF (p < 0.0001) and the decrease in AVDo₂ (p < 0.001); the product of CBF and AVDo₂, which reflects cerebral metabolic oxygen consumption, remained constant (p = 0.364). There was no significant effect between anesthetics. *(From Young WL, Prohovnik I, Correll JW et al: Anesthesiology 71:863 1989.)*

ply and following the cerebral washout with external scintillation counters placed over the skull, thus making it possible to perform regional determination of CBF. The higher energy of [133]xenon makes it preferable to [85]krypton, whose lower energy beta emissions do not effectively penetrate the skull.

Conceptually, the rate at which the tracer washes out of the brain is proportional to CBF. An important assumption here is that the bolus delivers all molecules of tracer to the tissue at the same time, before washout begins. In its simplest form (i.e., a single-compartment system), the radioactive count rate decays from a maximum value, C(0), as a single exponential whose rate constant is proportional to the flow rate:

$$C(t) = C(/0)e^{-kt} = C(0)e^{-ft/\lambda} \qquad (14)$$

where

k = f/λ or flow/position coefficient

Absolute tissue weight, absolute tracer amounts, and blood volume are not needed for calculation of CBF. Because under many circumstances the washout of tracer from the brain is bicompartmental, reflecting gray (fast-clearing) and white (slow-clearing) compartments, the previous equation may be expanded. Compartmental analysis is described elsewhere,[184] but conceptually it is illustrated in Fig. 2-16.

How to extract a usable number from these equations depends on the time scale of the measurement (rapid vs. slow) and the inclination of the user. Possible variations include the initial slope technique (suggested by Olesen et al.[188]), which uses the logarithm of the previous equation and differentiating:

$$f/\lambda = dlnC(t)/dt \qquad (15)$$

This method is useful for 1 to 2 minutes of tracer washout. Because of the mathematical instability of compartmental analysis, stochastic methods (i.e., height-over-area) have also been developed (see Appendix at the end of this chapter for a discussion of transit time and its relation to CBF).

Problems with intraarterial ^{133}Xe include the necessity for carotid artery injection, which currently in humans is feasible only during carotid surgery or cerebral angiography. The technique also requires the use of a volatile radionuclide.

Any method that uses isotope clearance techniques has an inherent weakness in that areas that are not perfused remain invisible—the "look-through phenomenon." "Look-through" results when a region in the field of view for a detector is not perfused, but adjacent or underlying regions are normally irrigated. This means that while the isotope is not delivered to the ischemic area, it does reach adjacent regions. The ischemic region is "invisible" to the detector because no (or little) washout is recorded from it, and the detector registers only normal washout from adjacent regions. Obrist and Wilkinson[184] have discussed some mathematical approaches to minimizing this problem of invisibility, but it remains of practical significance in the application of washout techniques to regional mapping of focal cerebral ischemia. How can one measure hemispheric CBF after the carotid occlusion? One method would be to inject the tracer bolus into the carotid artery, allow a few seconds for it to wash into the hemisphere, and then occlude.[249] The washout then is determined by the availability, if any, of collateral perfusion.

Scattered radiation is a problem for all CBF techniques using external counting of radioactive decay. Compton scattering describes the situation where relatively low-energy photons emitted from the isotope pass through the tissue

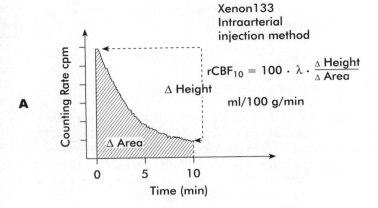

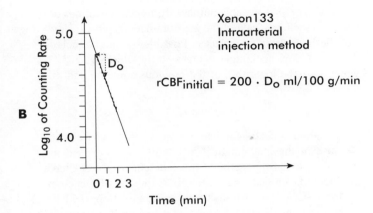

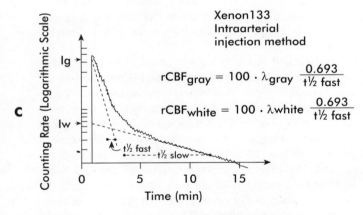

FIG. 2-16   Depiction of CBF calculations for the intracarotid ^{133}Xe method. Cerebral blood flow indices utilized by the intracarotid method. **A,** Height-over-area determination of mean flow, based on integration of the area under the curve to 10 minutes. **B,** Initial slope estimate of gray matter flow obtained from the first minute of clearance on a semilog plot. The constant, 200, represents 100 times the product of λ (assumed to be 0.87) and the factor for converting base 10 to natural logarithms. **C,** Compartmental analysis, where the curve is resolved into fast-clearing (gray matter) and slow-clearing (white matter) components, calculated from the half-times (t 1/2) on a semilog plot. *(From Obrist WD, Wilkinson WE: Cerebrovasc Brain Metab Rev 2:283, 1990.)*

and collide with molecules, producing a change in direction and some loss of energy. Because the detection device is set to measure photons at a specific energy (81 keV in the case of ^{133}Xe), true activity is underestimated.

Finally, the partition coefficient for xenon changes with both physiologic and pathologic conditions. The most important determinants are temperature and hematocrit.[45] The assumption, however, is made frequently that lambda does not change with pathologic states, and this must be considered as a potential source of error.

Intravenous and Inhaled Xenon Methods

Intravenous and inhaled ^{133}Xe methods are often lumped together under the rubric of "noninvasive" techniques because carotid artery puncture is not necessary. These methods use mathematical models developed primarily by Obrist[182] and later modified by Prohovnik.[206]

The inhalation method[183] employs a 1-minute period of ^{133}Xe inhalation followed by a 10-minute washout period. External scintillation detection is performed as for intracarotid injection techniques. The kinetics of tracer washout from the brain are similar to those obtained with intraarterial injection, with one important difference; instead of an instantaneous input of tracer to the brain, there is a "smeared" input, owing to mixing of the tracer in the heart and lungs. By using the tracer concentration in end-tidal expired gas as an estimate of arterial concentration, the "history" of the arterial input function is obtained and transformed into a series of weighted impulses. Because the total time-activity response of a linear system to such a series of weighted impulse inputs equals the sum of all responses to the component inputs, a mathematical technique known as *deconvolution* can be used to determine the input function. A "virtual" intracarotid washout curve is then obtained, and thereafter the slow and fast components of flow are determined in a manner conceptually similar to direct intracarotid injection.

Data analysis for intravenous injection of ^{133}Xe in saline is handled in exactly the same manner. The primary differences between systemic and intracarotid administration of ^{133}Xe are summarized in Fig. 2-17. Strictly speaking, the algorithms used for noninvasive methods render them compartmental, in that they are based on slope analysis. Because the slow compartment (corresponding to white matter flow for the intracarotid method) is contaminated by extracranial clearance (primarily muscle, skin, and connective tissue), the noninvasive methods are most suited for either gray matter flow or gray-weighted indices such as the Initial Slope Index.[214]

In the inhaled method, an artifact is introduced because of high radioactivity in the air passages. This is present to a much lesser extent with the intravenous method, where there is only exhaled activity. With endotracheal intubation, the contribution becomes even more negligible. The Obrist method for bicompartmental curve-fitting process involved

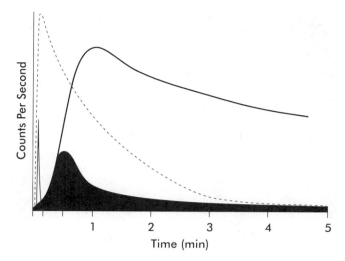

FIG. 2-17 Idealized input functions and washout curves recorded at the scalp after intracarotid and intravenous injection of ^{133}Xe. The intracarotid head curve *(dotted line)* is shown with its input function *(shaded spike)*, which is considered to be instantaneous and purely cerebral. The intravenous head curve *(dark solid line)* is accompanied by its input function (as recorded from continuous end-tidal sampling of expired ^{133}Xe), which is shared by extracerebral compartments. Note that the input function *(shaded curve underneath)* is delayed (and smeared). This results in a slower rise and decay of head curve activity after intravenous injection. Solutions for calculating CBF rely on deconvolution of the head curve by the delayed input function. *(From Young WL, Prohovnik I, Schroeder T et al: Anesthesiology 73:637, 1990.)*

a "Start-Fit Time,"[183] which was introduced to exclude data obtained during the first 60 to 90 seconds of data collection. This model delays curve-fitting until the peak activity of the end-tidal air curve has decreased to 20% of its maximal value. The model calculates the tissue transfer function by solving for four unknowns (two rate constants and two weight coefficients). To achieve solution of even the earliest parts of the clearance curve and eliminate the statistical variability associated with the Start-Fit Time, Prohovnik et al.[206] expanded the model to include two additional linear unknowns representing tracer concentrations in air and blood compartments. The curve-fitting procedure with this model, termed *M2,* is performed on the entire head curve.

With these common rate constants and weight coefficients, a value for CBF may be generated. Unfortunately, a bewildering number of different indices have been proposed for reporting CBF data.[184,204] Strictly compartmental indices such as the slope of the fast compartment *(fg),* are prone to inaccuracy because of a mathematical instability of compartmental analysis, sometimes referred to as *slippage,* in which too much relative weight is assigned to one or another compartment (see Prohovnik[204]). Although *fg* is the most sensitive flow index and conceptually the easiest to understand, it is the least stable of the indices.

The Initial Slope Index (ISI) (not the initial slope as described under intraarterial method) was originally proposed by Risberg et al.[214] and is the monoexponential slope of the deconvoluted clearance curve between minutes 2 and 3 of tracer washout. Prohovnik modified the ISI calculation to use the curve between 0.5 and 1.5 minutes[207] in order to reduce noise and increase sensitivity. The ISI reflects clearance from both fast and slow compartments but is dominated by the fast compartment. Because of its use of both compartments, it is inherently more stable, although less sensitive, than *fg.*[207,214] Strictly speaking, the ISI is a rate constant, but it can be expressed in milliliters per 100 g per minute, assuming a xenon λ of 1 for the perfused tissue, a mixture of gray (λ = 0.82) and white (λ = 1.5) matter.

Another useful model was proposed by Wyper.[275,276] It only uses the first 3 minutes of tracer washout. This method has application where physiologic conditions are not likely to remain in a steady state for 11 minutes.[285]

The noninvasive ^{133}Xe methods have many advantages. Like the intracarotid method, they provide reproducible information primarily about cortical perfusion. Repeated studies are easily done and are limited only by cumulative radiation exposure, which, in comparison with routine radiologic procedures, is minimal. CBF may be measured over both hemispheres and in the posterior fossa with a fair degree of spatial (two-dimensional) resolution because the isotope is delivered to all perfused areas of the brain. The inhalation and intravenous methods may be less reliable in the presence of pulmonary disease because end-tidal concentration of tracer may not reflect arterial concentration.[99] Although contamination of the head clearance by the extracranial tissue compartment may result in underestimation of CBF results, this is rarely a significant problem. Errors caused by isotope recirculation (which are small) are handled by quantitation of the arterial input function.

During most circumstances the noninvasive techniques yield information similar to that obtained by the intracarotid method.[287] An important caveat is that under extremely low flow states, especially at ischemic levels, they have not been validated and may not give equivalent quantitative information. This is important because many studies examining the flow thresholds for ischemia have used direct carotid injection.[35,164]

Hydrogen Clearance

This method is primarily confined to animal experimentation and is conceptually similar to the methods previously described in that it depends on washin and washout of a tracer, in this case molecular hydrogen.[280] It is a polarographic method. Typically, a platinum electrode is inserted into the brain. A current is used to polarize the electrode, positive with respect to a reference electrode. Molecular hydrogen (H_2) is administered and then is allowed to wash out. The H_2 in the vicinity of the reference electrode (the electron donor, or cathode) is oxidized into two protons and two electrons, the latter being accepted by the platinum electrode (the electron acceptor, or anode), thus generating current flow that is proportional to the relative concentration of H_2 in the vicinity of the electrode. As with the isotope techniques, measurement of absolute concentration is not required. The algorithms for CBF calculation are conceptually identical.

Advantages include the possibility of multiple repeated measures in a single subject, simple data analysis, low cost, and the ability to measure other physiologic events such as pH or K^+ in proximity. The tissue partition coefficient is relatively stable, compared to xenon. Disadvantages include the requirement for an exposed cortex, measurement of an unknown tissue volume, and tissue damage by the probe.[256]

Autoradiography

Autoradiographic determination of experimental animal CBF is based on Kety and Schmidt's original work and was developed in Kety's laboratory. Modern techniques use an inert, freely diffusible nonmetabolized tracer that is trapped in the tissue.[223] The most common tracer is ^{14}C-labelled iodoantipyrine, although others, such as ^3H-labelled nicotine[256] have been used. The tracer is infused intravenously (usually over 45 seconds) and the arterial "history" of the tracer is recorded by sampling arterial blood. Thin sections of brain are placed against photographic film along with standards of known radioactivity. The tracer trapped in tissue exposes the film (thus *autoradiography*). By calculating the optical density of brain against known standards, one can deduce tissue activity. Knowing the tissue activity and arterial input function, one can solve for CBF. Data are frequently presented by constructing a color lookup table (Fig. 2-18).

A variation of this method, "indicator fractionation," assumes the tracer enters the tissue and the brain is removed after all tracer has arrived but before any of it leaves.[191] The calculation of CBF is similar to that used for microspheres, which will be described in the next section. Indicator fractionation is best avoided during high-flow states.

The primary advantage of autoradiography is outstanding anatomic resolution, even in small laboratory animals. Disadvantages are expense, radiation concerns (although usually beta emitters as opposed to higher energy gamma emitters are used for many of these techniques), and the need to sacrifice the animal. The long turn-around time for cutting the brains, developing the film, and conducting computerized optical density analysis is a relative disadvantage. Repeat studies currently are not practical. Double labelling can provide for simultaneous measurement of CBF and another physiologic variable, such as cerebral glucose metabolism.

A hybrid of autoradiography and microspheres (see following discussion) might be termed the "chunk" method. The experiment is done exactly the same as one would for

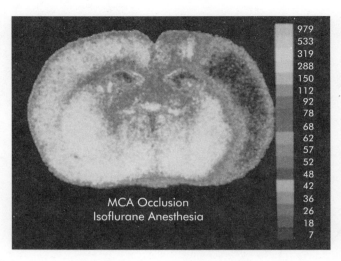

FIG. 2-18   Example of cerebral autoradiography. This coronal section of brain is from a rat that was subjected to middle cerebral artery occlusion during isoflurane anesthesia. The lookup table, shown on the right side of the figure, corresponds to flow units of ml/100 g/min. Note that the low-flow cortical infarct area is sharply delineated from the remainder of the section. *(Courtesy Dr. David S. Warner, University of Iowa.)*

autoradiography, except that instead of using optical density to infer tissue activity, one uses direct counting of cerebral tissue samples.[283] In this instance, one may use tracers that are cheaper but not suited for autoradiography because of volatility, such as ^{14}C butanol. Butanol is more freely diffusible at high flow rates than is iodoantipyrine.[261]

Microspheres

The radioactive microsphere technique is a widely used method for determining not only CBF but also flow in other organs. It is an embolic technique that relies on delivery of particles into capillary beds, where they are trapped. Typically, 15-μm latex spheres are used. The tissue being investigated is removed and counted in a gamma counter. Although there are a number of different approaches, the usual design and calculation involves setting up an "artificial organ," usually by withdrawing blood with a pump from a femoral artery at a known rate. Knowing the reference "artificial organ" flow and activity in the sample, C(reference), and the activity C(brain), in the region of interest, one then can solve for CBF, F(brain):

$$\frac{F(brain)}{F(reference)} = \frac{C(brain)}{C(reference)} \qquad (16)$$

Critical assumptions for the method include complete mixing of the microspheres in the circulation, complete trapping in the tissues, and an adequate number of particles in the counted tissue. Repeated measurements are limited by the number of isotope labels. The radionuclides currently used include ^{153}Gd, ^{57}Co, ^{141}Ce, ^{51}Cr, ^{113}Sn, ^{103}Ru, ^{46}Sc, ^{85}Sr, and ^{95}Nb. They can be discriminated from one another because each isotope has a unique emission "signature," that is, the emitted photons' energy peaks in different energy ranges. Depending on the size of the brain involved, regional measures of perfusion are possible. Disadvantages include high cost, the need to sacrifice the animal precluding outcome studies, and use of radioisotopes.

Xenon-Enhanced Computed Tomography (sXe-CT)

Nonradioactive or stable xenon (sXe) in sufficiently high concentrations is radiodense. Therefore it may also be used in conjunction with rapid sequential CT scanning to quantitate CBF.[92] In contrast to radionuclide studies, which use emission CBF tracers, sXe is used as a transmission tracer.

The advantages of this technique include relative availability because CT scanners are widely available and the fact that this technique is fully quantitative. Regions of interest for the quantitative determination of rCBF are easily selected visually from the anatomic delineation of known structures on the CT scans. Besides the ability to quantitate rCBF, the CT images enable one to qualitatively visualize changes in CBF. In addition, visualization of delayed images permits the qualitative evaluation of blood-brain barrier disruption. The disadvantages are an unfavorable signal/noise ratio (possibly degrading the inherently superior spatial resolution), difficulty in determining absolute flow values, possible anesthetic effects from the dose of xenon used, significant radiation exposure, the current limitation of analysis of only three CT slices at a time, and the requirement that the patient remain still for 7 to 9 minutes.

Mathematically, sXe-CT is based on the Kety algorithm and as such differs little from the previously mentioned radioisotope techniques. Instead of quantitating the washout of radioactivity, the estimated concentration of cold xenon is quantitated in terms of CT enhancement $[\Delta Ct(t)]$. Unlike radionuclide techniques that use standardized λ values, this method computes tissue-specific partition coefficients, which may help minimize errors and may have some diagnostic implications.[169] Major sources of error result from CT noise, tissue heterogeneity, and inaccuracies in the estimation of arterial xenon concentration. The degree of inaccuracy or error appears to be inversely related to the size of the area of interest.[84] Thus there is a tradeoff between resolution and accuracy.

The validity of sXe-CT would be questionable if it could be shown that sXe itself modifies CBF. In addition, any sXe-induced increase in intracranial pressure would severely limit the usefulness of this technique. Thus, for some time, sXe-CT was controversial. Several reports have implied that the concentration of xenon utilized (approximately 33%) might increase intracranial pressure by augmenting CBF.[93] This now appears, in fact, not to be a matter of concern. A recent study in monkeys with cortical freeze injury has shown that when the conditions under which CBF is measured are well controlled, ICP is not affected by 33% xenon, despite a small decrease in mean ar-

terial pressure attributed to the anesthetic effect of xenon.[52]

sXe-CT suffers from many of the shortcomings of previously mentioned CBF techniques. There is great variation in the relative contribution of gray and white matter to the flows obtained in different regions of interest. Even so, the technique has been shown to be useful in delineating rCBF changes within a given patient after pharmacologic intervention and has been validated for the determination of rCBF during low-flow states.[253] Until recently, because the technique was somewhat controversial, there was no standardized technique for the conduct of xenon-enhanced CT analysis, so that the delineation of normal reference values is just now beginning.[279]

PET (Positron Emission Tomography)

Current PET technology allows for precise imaging of glucose and oxygen utilization, cerebral blood volume, CBF, pH, numerous presynaptic and postsynaptic receptor and transmitter events, and protein synthesis.[76,203] Its great disadvantages, compared with all other techniques, are cost and complexity. Few anesthesiologists have used this technique.[12]

Certain unstable radioisotopes decay by producing positrons, which are equal in mass to an electron but have the opposite charge. After a few millimeters' travel through the tissue, the positron encounters an electron and mutual annihilation takes place. This collision results in the formation of two gamma energy photons, which are emitted in exactly opposite directions. By recording the simultaneous arrival of these photons on each side of the head with electronically linked coincidence detectors, it becomes possible to reconstruct tomographic, three-dimensional images of tracer activity. An advantage to this method is that it controls for tissue scattering because random deflections result in the loss of coincidence.

The resolution of PET is excellent ($\leq$ 1 cm), but limitations of current instruments include the fact that point sources of tracer activity cannot be perfectly separated. Reconstruction of the image results in partial volume averaging, that is, the radioactivity is smeared somewhat and any activity in a region of interest is partially contaminated by adjacent regions. The ability to discern point sources in brain imaging is referred to as Full Width, Half Maximum (FWHM), which denotes the separation between two point sources required for the instrument to discern them.

Isotopes currently used are those that can be incorporated into naturally occurring organic molecules (e.g., ^{11}C, ^{13}N, or ^{15}O) or isotopes that can be used to label biologically occurring molecules, such as ^{18}F. The positron-emitters are all short-lived and, except for ^{18}F, require on-site production with a cyclotron. The short half-life allows repeat studies and enables large doses to be used without excessive patient radiation exposure.

Measurement of CBF has been described using several tracers and techniques. The earliest method developed used inhaled ^{15}O-labeled CO_2. The ^{15}O ($T_{1/2}$ = 123 s) is rapidly transferred to $H_2{}^{15}O$ by carbonic anhydrase in the red blood cells. After 10 minutes, tracer entry to brain is in equilibrium with venous outflow and radioactivity decay. The arterial input function is assessed from peripheral blood. Using the model described previously for tissue autoradiography, CBF can be calculated. A variation of this approach is to use an intravenous infusion, thus avoiding air passage artifact. Several variations using bolus injections also have been proposed. Alternative tracers include ^{18}F-fluromethane and ^{15}O-butanol.[28] Albumin microspheres have also been used.[38] There are many methodologic issues beyond the scope of this chapter, but partition coefficient and the flow-limitations of $H_2{}^{15}O$ as a tracer are some of the drawbacks of current PET CBF studies.

SPECT (Single Photon Emission Computed Tomography)

SPECT is the image produced by gamma scintillation counting (like two-dimensional ^{133}Xe methods) that is reconstructed in three dimensions by some form of rotating or moving camera (Fig. 2-19).[260] It is a general term, and any camera that views an organ from more than one angle and uses a computer to achieve tomographic reconstruction may be considered SPECT. Most nuclear medicine depart-

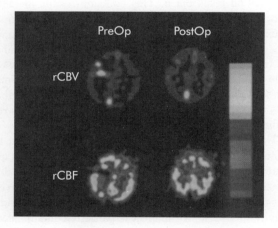

FIG. 2-19 Example of single photon emission computed tomography (SPECT). Double-label methodology used to simultaneously image both CBF (Spectamine, ^{131}I-iodoamphetamine) and cerebral blood volume (^{99}mTc-labeled RBC). The lookup table is relative, and the lighter shades reflect increasing flow or volume. Flow and volume imaging currently cannot be quantitated (as opposed to PET techniques). This patient had a temporal cerebral arteriovenous malformation, and these scans were done preoperatively. The CBF was normal except for a flow defect that corresponded to the AVM location demonstrated on MR imaging. The CBF tracer does not image the fistula because there are no capillaries. In the CBV image, one sees a hot spot on the posterior midline that represents the sagittal sinus. The larger temporal enhancement is the AVM nidus; the smaller one is a large draining vein. (*Courtesy Isak Prohovnik, Ph.D., and W.L. Young, M.D., Columbia University.*)

ments have rotating gamma cameras that fulfill this definition. Recently, however, dedicated brain scanners that are specifically optimized for the intracranial cavity have become increasingly available. SPECT technology offers slightly less resolution than PET yet has formidable anatomic specificity. Although it requires expensive hardware and software, it is significantly cheaper than PET. The FWHM with newer generation devices (7 to 9 mm) approaches that of PET scanners. Scattered radiation problems and partial volume effects produce inherent problems with data analysis.

For perfusion imaging, the only tracer that currently can reliably be quantitated is Xe. Although ^{133}Xe can be used, it provides poor resolution, and ^{127}Xe is preferable because of its higher energy. Unfortunately, however, ^{127}Xe has a significantly longer t 1/2. Administration and CBF calculations are roughly similar to the two-dimensional ^{133}Xe methods.

One may also use lipophilic tracers that are taken up by the tissue in proportion to flow and then trapped or bound. These include, at present, Spectamine (N-isopropyl-^{123}I-*p*-iodoamphetamine) and Ceretec (^{99}mTc-HM-PAO, a propylene amine oxime).[141] SPECT tracers are generally heavier metallic elements with longer half-lives (hours) that decay by single-photon gamma emission, as opposed to PET tracers, which are low-atomic-number organic elements with short half-lives (minutes) decaying by positron-emission short half-lives (minutes).

SPECT imaging will become increasingly commonplace in the management of cerebrovascular disease, allowing early assessment of the hemodynamic effects of cerebral thromboembolism and assessment of cerebrovascular reserve using CO_2 or acetazolamide.[290] It is being used with increasing frequency for assessing the adequacy of collateral circulation before surgical procedures where the internal carotid artery must be sacrificed, such as skull base tumor resection.

In addition to CBF, cerebral blood volume can be assessed by plasma or red blood cell labeling.[221] Some units can image ^{18}F, providing the possibility of studying receptor systems and CMRgl. Several single-photon-emitting receptor ligands are now becoming available for SPECT (for instance, dopaminergic [D_2], cholinergic, muscarinic, and some types of benzodiazepine and opiate receptors).[18]F has a longer half-life than most positron emitters, which makes it appealing for use in centers with no on-site cyclotron.

Magnetic Resonance (MR) Imaging

MR will become increasingly important to the study of vascular anatomy as MR angiography begins to supplant standard contrast x-ray techniques. By using paramagnetic tracers that can be excited in a magnetic field, one may directly examine cerebral perfusion. Capillary transit time can be assessed by currently available intravascular tracers, such as gadolinium-labeled agents, thus providing an indirect index of cerebral blood flow and cerebral blood volume.[27,59]

More important, with development of freely diffusible paramagnetic drugs, it will be possible to determine washin and washout in ways similar to current radioisotope methods.[63] MR resolution and the ability to correlate CBF information with structural information could make this the "gold standard" in years to come. MR also can image other cerebral physiologic functions, such as hemoglobin saturation, intracellular energy stores, sodium, and pH.[146,211]

Thermal Clearance

Thermal clearance is a well-known technique for quantitating cardiac output. Bolus thermal techniques applied to the brain, however, introduce artifact because of the effects of temperature on physiologic function (e.g., CO_2 reactivity).[116] However, thermal conductivity of cortical tissue varies proportionally with CBF, and measurement of thermal gradients (diffusion) at the cortical surface can be used for quantitative CBF determination.[44] The probe is placed directly on the cortical surface but away from large surface vessels or areas of direct brain retraction. There are several measurement variations. In one system, a large gold disk at the tip of the probe is equipped with an active temperature sensor and a heater, while a smaller disk is equipped with a neutral thermistor temperature sensor. When power is applied to the heater, the temperature of the gold disk increases while the temperature of the smaller disk remains at brain temperature. The difference in temperature between the two disks is inversely proportional to the thermal conductivity of the brain tissue.

The resulting thermal gradient would be maximal when there is no flow through the opposing cerebral cortex. As CBF increases, the temperature difference (recorded in millivolts) decreases in proportion to CBF, so that:

$$lCoCBF = \phi \left(\frac{1}{\Delta V} - \frac{1}{\Delta Vo} \right) \qquad (17)$$

where

    lCoCBF = Local cortical CBF

        ϕ = Constant value used as a scale factor

    ΔVo = Maximum temperature difference at zero blood flow

     ΔV = Actual temperature difference

The thermal diffusion CBF technique has been used to describe autoregulatory dysfunction in a number of operative settings, including cerebral aneurysm and arteriovenous malformation (AVM) surgery. The greatest strength of thermal diffusion is the ability to obtain continuous quantitative assessment of cortical perfusion. The time resolution is 1 to 2 seconds. There are currently no commercial units sufficiently reliable for routine use. If CBF changes take place in an entire vascular supply territory (e.g., middle cerebral artery [MCA]), the focal flow changes in the probe's area should reflect the regional changes.

Extraneous thermal influences, such as operating room lights, electrocautery interference, and irrigation of the surgical field, may result in erroneous CBF measurements. Another problem is frequent separation of the probe from the cortical surface. Therefore any detected CBF change must be carefully related to activity in the operative field.

Several assumptions are made in deriving the CBF values. First, the thermal conductivity of tissue from patient to patient is assumed constant. Thermal conductivity depends on the chemical composition of normal cortical tissue and appears to be constant within many different species, including humans. Proper calibration depends on knowledge of the ΔVo term in Equation 17, which represents no flow. Although this has been experimentally determined in animals, it cannot be done in the clinical setting. Therefore the nature of the CBF information is probably better viewed as a reflection of relative changes in perfusion rather than the frequently reported absolute values. Because the methodology does not require sophisticated equipment, does not use ionizing radiation, and is theoretically easy to use, it deserves further development for use during neurosurgery.[186]

Doppler Techniques
Transcranial Doppler Ultrasound

Transcranial Doppler (TCD) was introduced by Aaslid et al.[1,4] in 1982. Doppler-based devices are in wide use for clinical imaging, and the general methodology is similar for all applications. TCD uses a 2-MHz probe and is rangegated; therefore the ultrasonic beam can be focused on a target volume at a specific depth. No actual image of the vessel is obtained, as with "duplex" devices. The probe is placed over low-density bone regions of the skull, and the beam is focused on the desired vessel. The Doppler shift of the ultrasonic beam after its reflection on the moving blood column within the vessel is proportional to blood flow velocity.

This technique can provide continuous assessment of the systolic, diastolic, and mean flow velocities in the target vessel. There is evidence that the downstream vascular resistance is proportional to the difference between systolic and diastolic velocities. Several resistance indices have been proposed; a currently popular one is the "pulsatility index," defined as[85]:

$$PI = \frac{\text{Systolic velocity} - \text{Diastolic velocity}}{\text{Mean velocity}} \qquad (18)$$

Flow velocity in large vessels in the Circle of Willis and its major branches can be determined. The signals obtained document the direction and velocity of the vessel flow insonated by the beam. Additionally, spectrum analysis of the signal allows estimation of the degree of stenosis in a way similar to extracranial duplex Doppler. To insonate the distal internal carotid, anterior cerebral, middle cerebral, and posterior cerebral arteries, the probe is positioned above the zygomatic arch from 1 to 5 cm in front of the ear, the so-called temporal bone window. The basilar artery is insonated by directing the probe through the foramen magnum suboccipitally over the first cervical vertebra. For intraoperative application, a probe can be affixed to the temporal bone window with a strap. During craniotomy, adhesive can be used to directly mount a small probe against the skin.

TCD does *not* measure CBF; rather it determines velocity and direction of the moving column of blood in a major artery (Fig. 2-20). The bulk flow (*F* [ml/min], not *f* [ml/100 g/min]) is the product of the diameter of the vessel (*d*) and the velocity (*v*),

$$F = dv \qquad (19)$$

There are ample criticisms of the technique.[136] The question of what TCD measures is further muddled by choice of terminology, such as "cerebral blood flow velocity." Although correct in the strictest sense, it only serves to confuse by implying measurement of CBF. If flow in the MCA is being described, then "MCA velocity" is preferable. TCD measures large conductance vessel flow, not *tissue* perfusion rates.

Although tissue perfusion is relatively constant between similar patient populations, there is a much greater

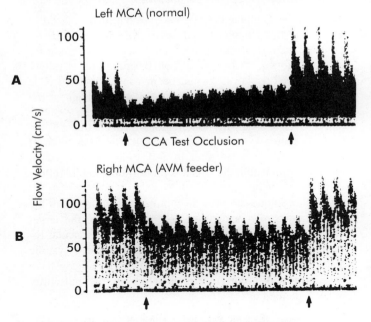

FIG. 2-20   TCD studies in a patient with an AVM. **A,** Carotid compression of the ipsilateral normal carotid artery yields a drop in MCA velocity. Gradually over the course of the compression, flow is recruited from collateral pathways. With release of compression there is a brief period of hyperemia. **B,** The MCA examined also feeds a large AVM. The low-resistance fistula of the AVM results in much higher flow velocities through the MCA stem. The ratio of systolic to diastolic velocities is different, with the diastolic velocity being much higher in relation to systolic velocity, indicating decreased pulsatility (see text). There is no apparent autoregulatory recruitment of collateral flow and no reperfusion increase in flow velocity in comparison with the ipsilateral, normal side. *(From Aaslid R: Transcranial Doppler sonography, New York, 1986, Springer-Verlag.)*

between-subject variation with TCD velocities because of varying proportions of hemispheric flow carried by the different vessels and the natural variability in arterial diameters. When used to monitor clinical changes with repeated measurement, the key assumption is that the diameter of the insonated vessel remains the same. Although this is probably true in the vast majority of cases[122] (B. Bissonnette, unpublished data), it requires further study. With currently available instruments, vessel diameter cannot be assessed.

Other problems with TCD relate to the inherent error in the natural variability of the exact angle of insonation. The error is proportional to the cosine of the angle of insonation, and, with less then 20-degree angles, this error is negligible in normal patients. Nonetheless, in certain neurosurgical patients with distorted intracranial anatomy, this error can become significant.[67] Another problem is difficulty in finding the vessel. With experience, this should occur less than 5% to 10% of the time, but it depends on the patient population.[95]

TCD's greatest advantages are that it is relatively inexpensive, noninvasive, and nonradioactive, and it furnishes beat-to-beat (i.e., continuous) information about the cerebral circulation. It has proved valuable to the neurologist in the diagnosis of intracranial stenoses and abnormal collateral blood flow patterns.[145,166] It might have potential as a powerful monitoring method during anesthesia and critical care. Also, it can be used to noninvasively study functional[2] and pressure[3] autoregulatory phenomena on a beat-to-beat basis. Finally, it may provide information about the venous circulation[5].

Some authors have proposed absolute values for TCD that correspond to EEG ischemic thresholds during carotid endarterectomy.[97] As with many other methods, however, TCD information is best considered in relative terms. Flow information is most reproducible when coupled with a physiologic challenge such as CO_2.[29] Relative CO_2 reactivity of TCD velocities is roughly similar to those reported for CBF.[152,200] Possible routes of development for TCD, in addition to monitoring hemispheric perfusion, include noninvasive ICP monitoring,[139] determining the adequacy of pulsatile perfusion during cardiopulmonary bypass,[176] and detection of intracranial arterial air emboli.[7]

Other Ultrasound Methods

With a 20 MHz probe, direct interrogation of surface vessels exposed during neurosurgical procedures is possible.[80,105] This has potential application during neurovascular surgery, including revascularization, aneurysm clipping, and AVM resection.

Experiments suggest use of albumin "microspheres" will allow increased sensitivity over existing techniques and will open up the possibility of quantitatively measuring intravascular transit time. Furthermore, it may be possible to simulate "autoradiography" of the exposed brain by interrogating a field of view during passage of the tracer.[213]

Laser Doppler

Laser Doppler is another CBF technique that can register CBF from the surface of exposed cortex at surgery. It detects the Doppler shift of laser light reflected off red blood cells moving in a small volume of cortical tissue. The cortical area interrogated by the probe is probably only several cubic millimeters in diameter. Similar to thermal diffusion, the technique is relatively inexpensive and nonradioactive, and furnishes continuous information. In addition, one can adjust the time resolution to examine events with a very short time constant, such as the effects of pulsatile pressure on local flow.[160] It is noninvasive in the sense that it may be used during an open skull operation with no additional preparation. It is well suited to animal studies[55] and, with improved probe design, may be adaptable for routine human use.[160,244] Although current instruments claim to be calibrated in terms of absolute flow (ml/100 g/min), relative changes are probably the most meaningful.

Other CBF Methods

Isolation of the sagittal sinus outflow and quantitation by either timed collection or flowmeters is a widely used experimental method.[16] Conceptually, the global outflow method is easy to understand (what exits must equal what enters), permits rapid repeated or continuous measures, and allows for simultaneous blood samples for metabolic calculations. However, it involves a fair degree of physiologic trespass because obliteration of accessory outflow tracts is required. Physiologic or pharmacologic manipulations may recruit additional accessory outflow pathways and thus confound interpretation of results.[265] A variation on this technique involves determining regional venous efflux, particularly for phenomena with a short time constant,[251] but this has been largely replaced by newer methods such as laser Doppler.

Umbelliferone, a hydroxycoumarin, is a pH-sensitive tracer that can be used to investigate highly focal areas of perfusion in the exposed cortex of the brain.[10] Various plethysmographic techniques have also been proposed for the indirect evaluation of cerebral perfusion (e.g., ocular plethysmography in adult patients and head plethysmography in neonates).[106] An emerging clinical methodology is transcranial measurement of cerebral hemoglobin saturation using the technique of near infrared spectrophotometry.[153,179]

Synthesis and Comment

An often-confusing aspect of the medical literature in general and CBF techniques in particular is that different methodologies often appear to be in competition. However, different methodologies examine different aspects of the same or related biologic phenomena, and different techniques may be required to completely elucidate a process. Examples of complementary methodologies are shown in Figs. 2-19 to 2-21.

SPINAL CORD BLOOD FLOW (SCBF)

Compared with the voluminous literature regarding regulation of cerebral blood flow, there has been limited experience in delineating the determinants of SCBF. Technology readily applicable to measurement of CBF has not yet had a major effect on the study of SCBF. Some of the difficulties encountered are (1) the lack of a suitable site for the venous sampling in light of the complexity and small size of the spinal cord venous drainage system, (2) difficulty in cannulating and tendency for vasospasm with radicular artery injection, and (3) difficulty in isolating spinal cord tissue and the resultant low count rates with external scintillation detectors.[235] An often-asked question is whether the spinal cord is a vascular microcosm of the brain.[112]

Measurement Techniques

The first measurements of SCBF historically were obtained with autoradiography. Because this methodology requires the sacrifice of the animal for the generation of flow values, repeated measurements in the same subject over a prolonged period of time are not possible. Thus this technique offers little in the ability to detect changes caused by drug administration or other provocative challenges. SCBF values obtained by this technique have varied from 10 to 20 ml/100 g/min for white matter and from 41 to 63 for gray matter.[224]

A variation of the ^{133}Xenon clearance technique was used by Smith to study SCBF in goats.[235] An isotope was injected directly into the spinal cord, with tissue washout measured using external scintillation detectors. Using this technique, the response to manipulation of Pa_{CO_2} could be demonstrated as an increase in SCBF with hypercarbia and a decrease with hypocarbia.

The same technique was used to systematically study the effect of changes in Pa_{O_2}, Pa_{CO_2}, and blood pressure on SCBF in dogs.[88-90] White matter flow values during anesthesia were relatively independent of the spinal cord segment at which the isotope was injected and varied from 10 to 30 ml/100 g/min. Under halothane anesthesia, an increase in Pa_{CO_2} from 43 to 80 mm Hg led to a 57% increase in SCBF. In a fashion analogous to CBF, SCBF does not change with decreased O_2 tension unless Pa_{O_2} decreases below 60 mm Hg, at which point there is a rise in SCBF. The response of SCBF during hemorrhagic hypotension was also investigated. In normocarbic, normoxic dogs, SCBF was well maintained to a mean arterial blood pressure of 60 mm Hg. Below this level, blood flow decreased with further reduction of pressure. With concurrent hypoxia, autoregulation was usually, but not invariably, impaired. In some cases, the lower limit of autoregulation was shifted to 110 mm Hg. With hypercarbia to a Pa_{CO_2} of 80 mm Hg, autoregulation was either markedly impaired or absent, with SCBF becoming blood-pressure passive. This series of studies, however, did not examine the response to increases in blood pressure, so the upper limit of SCBF autoregulation could not be determined.

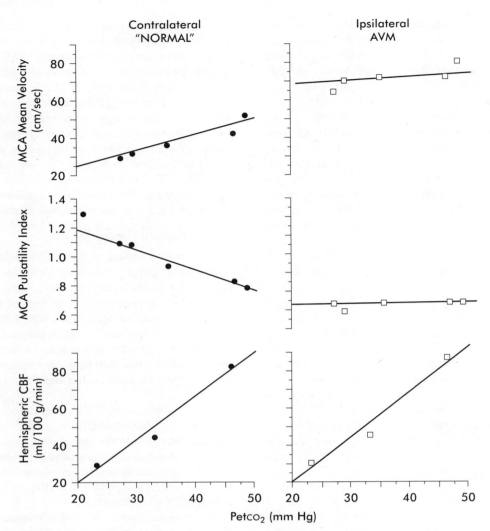

FIG. 2-21 Intraoperative ^{133}Xe CBF and TCD studies in a patient with an AVM fed by the middle cerebral artery. CBF was measured 5 to 6 cm away from the AVM nidus and in an equivalent homologous site over the contralateral hemisphere. TCD mean velocity was recorded from the proximal MCA via the temporal bone window. These data illustrate the different nature of the information obtained from these two complementary imaging techniques. As shown by the ^{133}Xe CBF study, Paco$_2$ reactivity was preserved in both hemispheres. ^{133}Xe washout measures tissue perfusion in the cortex underlying the detectors and was similar in both hemispheres. The TCD responses to increased Paco$_2$ are similar on the contralateral hemisphere, in that MV increases and the pulsatility index decreases, reflecting vasodilation of the resistance vessels with increasing Petco$_2$. TCD examination of the ipsilateral hemisphere reveals a different response. Because there is a large shunt in parallel with the normal resistance bed, its effect overshadows that of the normal adjacent circulation. The law of parallel resistances states that R_{normal} decreases with increasing Paco$_2$:

$$\frac{1}{R_{total}} = \frac{1}{R_{AVM}} + \frac{1}{R_{normal}}$$

The extremely low resistance of the AVM (R_{AVM}) shunt, however, completely masks resistance changes in the adjacent circulation. Although a high baseline mean velocity (MV) and low PI are present, these remain relatively constant with increased Paco$_2$ because (R_{total}) changes so little. *(From Young W: Clinical neuroscience lectures, Munster, Ind, 1991, Cathenart Publishing.)*

Intraspinal injection of xenon has been criticized for several reasons. It is often difficult to determine the anatomic location of the injection or to characterize the variable contributions of gray and white matter. Spinal cord damage may result from intramedullary injection, and this may affect the flow measurements. In addition, this method is limited to flow measurement in one small cord area at a time.

The application of the noninvasive radioisotope technology (intravenous or inhalational) for the measurement of SCBF is primarily limited by the necessity of a reasonable count rate, which can only be assured by the use of large doses of isotope. Were this practical, separation of the region of interest from surrounding tissue and background would still be difficult.

Attempts made to circumvent these problems in the early 1970s involved the placement of detectors close to the spinal cord. These include small vacuum mass spectrometer probes for the aspiration of cold argon tracer and miniature platinum electrodes for the detection of clearance of hydrogen gas that had been added to the inspired gas mixture. Neither of these techniques has had widespread acceptance.[224]

SCBF Compared To CBF

Sato et al.[225] obtained simultaneous recordings of blood flow from different parts of the cat central nervous system using hydrogen clearance during ketamine–nitrous oxide anesthesia. SCBF of 46 ml/100 g/min during normocapnia and normotension was significantly lower than the 86 ml/100 g/min recorded in the cerebrum. In the spinal cord, gray-matter blood flow is approximately five times greater than white-matter flow.

Regional differences in blood flow exist for the spinal cord in much the same way as they do in the brain. Thus mean blood flow in the cervical and lumbar segments is approximately 40% higher than in the thoracic segments. This is most likely related to the relative paucity of gray matter in the thoracic cord.[151] SCBF is metabolically linked to the local level of electrical activity. Thus unilateral stimulation of the sciatic and femoral nerves is reflected by a 50% increase in flow in the ipsilateral lumbosacral gray matter.[151]

Blood Pressure

Autoregulation of SCBF has been demonstrated in a number of species. Using hydrogen clearance in the monkey, Kobrine et al.[133] determined that, as a result of compensatory vasoconstriction, there was no change in SCBF with mean arterial blood pressures between 50 and 135 mm Hg. Below 50 mm Hg, the vasculature became maximally dilated, leading to a passive drop in SCBF with decreasing blood pressure. After the upper autoregulatory limit of 135 mm Hg was exceeded, vascular resistance actually decreased, presumably because of physical dilation resulting from high intraluminal pressure. This was accompanied by a marked increase in SCBF. Hickey et al.[112] demonstrated that, during thiopental anesthesia, autoregulation in several

regions of the rat spinal cord roughly mirrors regional autoregulation in the brain.

Comparing autoregulation in the spinal cord to that in the cerebrum, Sato[225] found that the upper and lower limits of the autoregulatory plateau were strikingly similar for the two regions in cats. Despite this finding, simultaneously obtained evoked potential data during blood pressure reduction below the autoregulatory minimum suggest that the spinal cord is less susceptible to ischemic damage as a result of reductions in regional blood flow than is the brain.

Carbon Dioxide and Oxygen Tension

As mentioned previously, SCBF increases with hypercarbia and decreases with hypocarbia.[89] Inasmuch as baseline blood flow levels are lower in the spinal cord than in the cerebrum, the absolute change in CBF per unit change in carbon dioxide tension (between 20 and 80 mm Hg) is greater than the corresponding change in SCBF. Blood flow changes expressed as percentage change are, however, the same for the two regions.[225] The manipulation of SCBF by regulation of arterial CO_2 tension seems to have no beneficial effect on the outcome of spinal cord injury. Therefore it has been proposed that the complex phenomena of steal and inverse-steal known to exist in the brain probably exist in the spinal cord as well.[71]

Temperature

Recent studies have confirmed that SCBF decreases with hypothermia.[222] Local spinal cord hypothermia within 4 hours of injury has been advocated for limiting the progression of spinal cord injury.[6]

Neurogenic Control

There is a paucity of data regarding autonomic control of SCBF. Neither chemoreceptor nor baroreceptor stimulation seems to affect SCBF in dogs, despite the fact that spinal cord blood vessels are richly innervated.[151]

Anesthetics

SCBF is affected by anesthetics in much the same way as CBF. Thus thiopental administered to dogs in a dose sufficient to induce EEG burst suppression reduced SCBF by 50%, prompting the investigators to suggest that barbiturate coma may provide spinal cord protection.[114] Pentobarbital–nitrous oxide anesthesia in sheep resulted in a decrease in SCBF, which became more apparent with longer exposure times (up to 3 hours).[115]

Although not as completely studied as CBF, SCBF measurement suggests that SCBF in many ways mimics CBF. The gray-matter-to-white-matter flow ratio of 5-to-1 is similar to that seen in the CNS. Autoregulation maintains both CBF and SCBF relatively constant, despite wide blood pressure fluctuations. Regional differences in both rCBF and rSCBF can be elicited in response to variations in local metabolic activity. Carbon dioxide tension is the single most significant physiologic variable affecting both CBF and SCBF.

SUMMARY

CBF measurements have been available for more than 40 years, and an enormous amount of research has been done using them. A Medline search in 1993 over the last 5 years resulted in 3329 articles on CBF and 140 articles on CBV. Furthermore CBF monitoring has elucidated mechanisms in a number of specific disease states and offered a means to instigate and monitor treatment effects for SAH, AVM, head injury, and thromboembolic stroke. CBF monitoring has also been used as an adjunct in the determination of brain death. In spite of this, the methodology must realistically be viewed as remaining in its infancy regarding the clinical care of patients.[281]

In the care of the anesthetized or critically ill patient, the clinician must either make an educated guess as to what is happening to the cerebral circulation or resort to logistically improbable imaging modalities (transport to the radiology department for angiography or SPECT). However, with the development of bedside methods, discussed previously, physicians will be able to more rationally care for the brain-injured or threatened patient. One particular bias in the anesthesia community that has held back the development of such methods is the somewhat unreasonable expectation that CNS monitoring must have absolute prognostic meaning rather than simple descriptive utility. The cost or risk benefit cannot be fully addressed here, but the following should be considered. No practicing physician demands that, for example, ECG or cardiac output monitoring have absolute prognostic algorithms associated with it. Monitoring the cerebral circulation should be held to the same standards. With the development of reasonably priced methodologies to assess cerebral perfusion at the bedside, physicians will no longer be faced with a plethora of questions regarding patient management, particularly those of blood pressure and ventilation. Empiricism will yield to rational titration of therapeutic measures.

Acknowledgements

The authors would like to thank Bennett M. Stein, M.D.; John Pile-Spellman, M.D.; Isak Prohovnik, Ph.D., Dale Pelligrino, Ph.D., and Daniel J. Cole, M.D. for helpful insights and Joyce Ouchi for expert assistance in preparation of the manuscript. Supported in part by NIH grant RO1-NS27713.

References

1. Aaslid R: *Transcranial Doppler sonography,* New York, 1986, Springer-Verlag, p 177.
2. Aaslid R: Visually evoked dynamic blood flow response of the human cerebral circulation, *Stroke* 18:771, 1987.
3. Aaslid R, Lindegaard K-F, Sorteberg W et al: Cerebral autoregulation dynamics in humans, *Stroke* 20:45, 1989.
4. Aaslid R, Markwalder T-M, Nornes H: Noninvasive transcranial Doppler ultrasound recording of flow velocity in basal cerebral arteries, *J Neurosurg* 57:769, 1982.
5. Aaslid R, Newell DW, Stooss R et al: Assessment of cerebral autoregulation dynamics from simultaneous arterial and venous transcranial Doppler recordings in humans, *Stroke* 22:1148, 1991.
6. Albin MS: Resuscitation of the spinal cord, *Crit Care Med* 62:70, 1978.
7. Albin MS, Hantler CB, Mitzel H et al: Aeric microemboli and the transcranial Doppler (TCD): episodic frequency and timing in 62 cases of open heart surgery, *Anesthesiology* 75:A53, 1991.
8. Albrecht RF, Miletich DJ, Madala LR: Normalization of cerebral blood flow during prolonged halothane anesthesia, *Anesthesiology* 58:26, 1983.
9. Alexander SC, Smith TC, Strobel G et al: Cerebral carbohydrate metabolism of a man during respiratory and metabolic alkalosis, *J Appl Physiol* 24:66, 1968.
10. Anderson RE, Sundt TM Jr, Yaksh TL: Regional cerebral blood flow and focal cortical perfusion: a comparative study of ^{133}Xe, ^{85}Kr, and umbelliferone as diffusible indicators, *J Cereb Blood Flow Metab,* 7:207, 1987.
11. Andrews RJ: Transhemispheric diaschisis: a review and comment, *Stroke* 22:943, 1991.
12. Archer DP, Labrecque P, Tyler JL et al: Measurement of cerebral blood flow and volume with positron emission tomography during isoflurane administration in the hypocapnic baboon, *Anesthesiology* 72:1031, 1990.
13. Archer DP, Shaw DA, Leblanc RL et al: Haemodynamic considerations in the management of patients with subarachnoid haemorrhage, *Can J Anaesth* 38:454, 1991.
14. Archie JR Jr: Technique and clinical results of carotid stump backpressure to determine selective shunting carotid endarterectomy, *J Vasc Surg* 13:319, 1991.
15. Artru AA, Merriman HG: Hypocapnia added to hypertension to reverse EEG changes during carotid endarterectomy, *Anesthesiology* 70:1016, 1989.
16. Artru AA, Michenfelder JD: Effects of hypercarbia on canine cerebral metabolism and blood flow with simultaneous direct and indirect measurement of blood flow, *Anesthesiology* 52:466, 1980.
17. Awad IA, Carter LP, Spetzler RF et al: Clinical vasospasm after subarachnoid hemorrhage: response to hypervolemic hemodilution and arterial hypertension, *Stroke* 18:365, 1987.
18. Baker WH, Rodman JA, Barnes RW et al: An evaluation of hypocarbia and hypercarbia during carotid endarterectomy, *Stroke* 7:451, 1976.
19. Barry DI, Jarden JO, Paulson OB et al: Cerebrovascular aspects of converting-enzyme inhibition. I. Effects of intravenous captopril in spontaneously hypertensive and normotensive rats, *J Hypertens* 2:589, 1984.
20. Barry DI, Paulson OB, Jarden JO et al: Effects of captopril on cerebral blood flow in normotensive and hypertensive rats, *Am J Med* 76:79, 1984.
21. Barry DI, Strandgaard S: Acute effects of antihypertensive drugs on autoregulation of cerebral blood flow in spontaneously hypertensive rats, *Prog Appl Microcirc* 8:206, 1985.
22. Batjer HH, Frankfurt AI, Purdy PD et al: Use of etomidate, temporary arterial occlusion, and intraoperative angiography in surgical treatment of large and giant cerebral aneurysms, *J Neurosurg* 6:8234, 1988.
23. Baughman VL, Hoffman WE, Miletich DJ et al: Effects of phenobarbital on cerebral blood flow and metabolism in young and aged rats, *Anesthesiology* 65:500, 1986.
24. Beausang-Linder M: Effects of sympathetic stimulation on cerebral and ocular blood flow, *Acta Physiol Scand* 114:217, 1982.
25. Beausang-Linder M, Bill A: Cerebral circulation in acute arterial hypertension—protective effects of sympathetic nervous activity, *Acta Physiol Scand* 111:193, 1981.
26. Bell BA: A history of the study of the cerebral circulation and the measurement of cerebral blood flow (review article), *Neurosurgery* 14:238-246, 1984.
27. Belliveau JW, Kennedy DN, McKinstry RC et al: Functional mapping of the human visual cortex by magnetic resonance imaging, *Science* 254:716, 1991.
28. Berridge MS, Adler LP, Nelson AD et al: Measurement of human cerebral blood flow with [^{15}O]butanol and positron emission tomography, *J Cereb Blood Flow Metab* 11:707, 1991.
29. Bishop CCR, Powell S, Rutt D et al: Transcranial Doppler measurement of middle cerebral artery blood flow velocity: a validation study, *Stroke* 17:913, 1986.
30. Bissonnette B, Leon JE: Cerebrovascular stability during isoflurane anaesthesia in children, *Can J Anaesth* 39:128, 1992.
31. Bouma GJ, Muizelaar JP: Relationship between cardiac output and cerebral blood flow in patients with intact and with impaired autoregulation, *J Neurosurg* 73:368, 1990.
32. Boysen G, Engell HC, Henriksen H: The effect of induced hypertension on internal carotid artery pressure and regional cerebral blood flow during temporary carotid clamping for endarterectomy, *Neurology* 22:1133, 1972.
33. Boysen G, Ladegaard-Pedersen HJ, Henriksen HL et al: The effects of $Paco_2$ on regional cerebral blood flow and internal carotid arterial pressure during carotid clamping, *Anesthesiology* 35:286, 1971.
34. Branston NM, Hope DT, Symon L: Barbiturates in focal ischemia of primate cortex: effects on blood flow distribution, evoked potential and extracellular potassium, *Stroke* 10:647, 1979.
35. Branston NM, Strong AJ, Symon L: Extracellular potassium activity, evoked potential and tissue blood flow: relationships during progressive ischaemia in baboon cerebral cortex, *J Neurol Sci* 32:305, 1977.

36. Bredt DS, Snyder SH: Nitric oxide, a novel neuronal messenger (review), *Neuron* 8:3, 1992.

37. Brian JE Jr, Traystman RJ, McPherson RW: Changes in cerebral blood flow over time during isoflurane anesthesia in dogs, *J Neurosurg Anesth* 2:122, 1990.

38. Brooks DJ, Frackowiak RSJ, Lammertsma AA: A comparison between regional cerebral blood flow measurements obtained in human subjects using ^{11}C-methylalbumin microspheres, the $C^{15}O_2$ steady-state method, and positron emission tomography, *Acta Neurol Scand* 73:415, 1986.

39. Brown MM, Wade JPH, Marshall J: Fundamental importance of arterial oxygen content in the regulation of cerebral blood flow in man, *Brain* 108:81, 1985.

40. Buckland MR, Batjer HH, Giesecke AH: Anesthesia for cerebral aneurysm surgery: use of induced hypertension in patients with symptomatic vasospasm, *Anesthesiology* 69:116, 1988.

41. Bullock R, Mendelow AD, Bone I et al: Cerebral blood flow and CO_2 responsiveness as an indicator of collateral reserve capacity in patients with carotid arterial disease, *Br J Surg* 72:348, 1985.

42. Busija DW, Heistad DD: Effects of activation of sympathetic nerves on cerebral blood flow during hypercapnia in cats and rabbits, *J Physiol* 347:195, 1974.

43. Capra NF, Kapp JP: Anatomic and physiologic aspects of the venous system. In Wood JH, editor: *Cerebral blood flow: physiologic and clinical aspects,* New York, 1987, McGraw-Hill, p 37.

44. Carter LP: Surface monitoring of cerebral cortical blood flow, *Cerebrovasc Brain Metab Rev* 3:246, 1991.

45. Chen RYZ, Fan F-C, Kim S et al. Tissue-blood partition coefficient for xenon: temperature and hematocrit dependence, *J Appl Physiol* 49:178, 1980.

46. Chien S, Usami S, Skalak R: Blood flow in small tubes. In Renkin EM, Michel CC, Geiger SR, editors: *Handbook of physiology: a critical comprehensive presentation, vol 4,* Bethesda, Md, 1984, American Physiological Society, p 217.

47. Choi DW: Cerebral hypoxia: some new approaches and unanswered questions, *J Neurosci* 10:2493, 1990.

48. Christensen MS, Paulson OB, Olesen J et al: Cerebral apoplexy (stroke) treated with or without prolonged artificial hyperventilation. 1. Cerebral circulation, clinical course, and cause of death, *Stroke* 4:568, 1973.

49. Cold G, Christensen M, Schmidt K: Effect of two levels of induced hypocapnia on cerebral autoregulation in the acute phase of head injury coma, *Acta Anaesth Scand* 25:397, 1981.

50. Cruz J, Miner ME, Allen SJ et al: Continuous monitoring of cerebral oxygenation in acute brain injury: injection of mannitol during hyperventilation, *J Neurosurg* 73:725, 1990.

51. D'Alecy LG: Relation between sympathetic cerebral vasoconstriction and CSF pressure, *Europ Neurol* 6:180, 1971/72.

52. Darby JM, Nemoto EM, Yonas H et al: Stable xenon does not increase intracranial pressure in primates with freeze-injury–induced intracranial hypertension, *J Cereb Blood Flow Metab* 11:522, 1991.

53. Day AL: Arterial distributions and variants. In Wood JH, editor: *Cerebral blood flow: physiologic and clinical aspects,* New York, 1987, McGraw-Hill, p 19.

54. DeWitt DS, Prough DS, Colonna DM et al: Nitric oxide synthase inhibitors decrease cerebral blood flow but do not affect pressure autoregulation in rats (abstract), *J Neurosurg Anesth* 4:303, 1992.

55. Dirnagl U, Pulsinelli W: Autoregulation of cerebral blood flow in experimental focal brain ischemia, *J Cereb Blood Flow Metab* 10:327, 1990.

56. Drummond JC: Deliberate hypotension for intracranial aneurysm surgery: changing practices, *Can J Anaesth* 38:935, 1991.

57. Drummond JC, Oh Y-S, Cole DJ et al: Phenylephrine-induced hypertension reduces ischemia following middle cerebral artery occlusion in rats, *Stroke* 20:1538, 1989.

58. Drummond JC, Ruta TS, Cole DJ et al: The effect of hypocapnia on cerebral blood flow distribution during middle cerebral artery occlusion in the rat, *J Neurosurg Anesth* 1:163, 1989.

59. Edelman RR, Mattle HP, Atkinson DJ et al: Cerebral blood flow: assessment with dynamic contrast-enhanced T_2-weighted MR imaging at 1.5 T, *Radiology* 176:211, 1990.

60. Edvinsson L, Owman C, Siesjö B: Physiological role of cerebrovascular sympathetic nerves in the autoregulation of cerebral blood flow, *Brain Res* 117:519, 1976.

61. Ehrenfeld WK, Hamilton FN, Larson CP Jr et al: Effect of CO_2 and systemic hypertension on downstream cerebral arterial pressure during carotid endarterectomy, *Surgery* 67:87, 1970.

62. Enevoldsen EM, Jensen FT: Autoregulation and CO_2 responses of cerebral blood flow in patients with acute severe head injury, *J Neurosurg* 48:689, 1978.

63. Ewing JR, Branch CA, Butt SM et al: Quantitative imaging of regional cerebral blood flow in cats using trifluoromethane and ^{19}F NMR detection, *J Cereb Blood Flow Metab* 11(suppl 2):S777, 1991.

64. Faraci FM, Mayhan WG, Werber AH et al: Cerebral circulation: Effects of sympathetic nerves and protective mechanisms during hypertension, *Circ Res* 61(suppl II):102, 1987.

65. Faraci FM: Role of endothelium-derived relaxing factor in cerebral circulation: large arteries vs. microcirculation, *Am J Physiol* 261:H1038, 1991.

66. Fein JM, Lipow K, Marmarou A: Cortical artery pressure in normotensive and hypertensive aneurysm patients, *J Neurosurg* 59:51, 1983.

67. Finn JP, Quinn MW, Hall-Craggs MA et al: Impact of vessel distortion on transcranial Doppler velocity measurements: Correlation with magnetic resonance imaging, *J Neurosurg* 73:572, 1990.

68. Fitch W, Ferguson GG, Sengupta D et al: Autoregulation of cerebral blood flow during controlled hypotension in baboons, *J Neurol Neurosurg Psychiatry* 39:1014, 1976.

69. Fleischer LH, Young WL, Rho T et al: Effect of arteriovenous fistulas on cerebral arterial pressures (abstract), *J Neurosurg Anesth* 4:307, 1992.

70. Florence G, Seylaz J: Rapid autoregulation of cerebral blood flow: a laser-Doppler flowmetry study, *J Cereb Blood Flow Metab* 12:674, 1992.

71. Ford RWJ, Malm DN: Therapeutic trial of hypercarbia and hypocarbia in acute experimental spinal cord injury, *J Neurosurg* 61:925, 1984.

72. Forster A, Van Horn K, Marshall LF et al: Anesthetic effects on blood-brain barrier function during acute arterial hypertension, *Anesthesiology* 49:26, 1978.

73. Fourcade HE, Larson CP Jr, Ehrenfield WK et al: The effects of CO_2 and systemic hypertension on cerebral perfusion pressure during carotid endarterectomy, *Anesthesiology* 33:383, 1970.

74. Francois-Dainville E, Buchweitz E, Weiss HR: Effect of hypoxia on percent of arteriolar and capillary beds perfused in the rat brain, *J Appl Physiol* 60:280, 1986.

75. Frankel H, Dribben J, Kissen I et al: Effect of carbon dioxide on the utilization of brain capillary reserve and flow, *Microcirc Endoth Lymphatics* 5:391, 1989.

76. Frost JJ, Wagner HN Jr: *Quantitative imaging: neuroreceptors, neurotransmitters, and enzymes,* New York, 1990, Raven Press.

77. Fujishima M, Ibayashi S, Fujii K et al: Effects of long-term antihypertensive treatment on cerebral, thalamic and cerebellar blood flow in spontaneously hypertensive rats (SHR), *Stroke* 17:985, 1986.

78. Gaehtgens P, Marx P: Hemorheological aspects of the pathophysiology of cerebral ischemia, *J Cereb Blood Flow Metab* 7:259, 1987.

79. Garcia-Roldan J-L, Bevan JA: Flow-induced constrictions and dilation of cerebral resistance arteries, *Circ Res* 66:1445, 1990.

80. Gilsbach J, Hassler W: Intraoperative Doppler and real time sonography in neurosurgery, *Neurosurg Rev* 7:199, 1984.

81. Gobel U, Theilen H, Kuschinsky W: Congruence of total and perfused capillary network in rat brains, *Circ Res* 56:271, 1990.

82. Gobel U, Theilen H, Schrock H et al: Dynamics of capillary perfusion in the brain, *Blood Vessels* 28:190, 1991.

83. Gonzalez C, Estrada C: Nitric oxide mediates the neurogenic vasodilation of bovine cerebral arteries, *J Cereb Blood Flow Metab* 11:366, 1991.

84. Good WF, Gur D, Yonas H et al: Errors in cerebral blood flow determinations by xenon-enhanced computed tomography due to estimation of arterial xenon concentrations, *Med Phys* 14:377, 1987.

85. Gosling RG, King DH: Arterial assessment by Doppler-shift ultrasound, *Proc Roy Soc Med* 67:447, 1974.

86. Govier AV, Reves JG, McKay RD et al: Factors and their influence on regional cerebral blood flow during nonpulsatile cardiopulmonary bypass, *Ann Thorac Surg* 38:592, 1984.

87. Greenberg JH, Alavi A, Reivich M et al: Local cerebral blood volume response to carbon dioxide in man, *Circ Res* 43:324, 1978.

88. Griffiths IR: Spinal cord blood flow in dogs. 1. The 'normal' flow, *J Neurol Neurosurg Psychiatry* 36:34, 1973.

89. Griffiths IR: Spinal cord blood flow in dogs. 2. The effects of the blood gases, *J Neurol Neurosurg Psychiatry* 36:42, 1973.

90. Griffiths IR: Spinal cord blood flow in dogs: the effect of blood pressure, *J Neurol Neurosurg Psychiatry* 36:914, 1973.

91. Grubb RL, Raichle ME, Eichling JO et al: Effects of subarachnoid hemorrhage on cerebral blood volume, blood flow, and oxygen utilization in humans, *J Neurosurg* 46:446, 1977.

92. Gur D, Yonas H, Good WF: Local cerebral blood flow by xenon-enhanced CT: current status, potential improvements, and future directions, *Cerebrovasc Brain Metab Rev* 1:68, 1989.

93. Gur D, Yonas H, Jackson DL et al: Measurements of cerebral blood flow during xenon inhalation as measured by the microsphere method, *Stroke* 16:871, 1985.

94. Halbach V, Higashida RT, Hieshima G et al: Normal perfusion pressure breakthrough occurring during treatment of carotid and vertebral fistulas, *Am J Neuroradiol* 87:51, 1987.

95. Halsey JH: Effect of emitted power on waveform intensity in trancranial Doppler, *Stroke* 211:573, 1990.

96. Halsey JH Jr, Conger KA, Garcia JH et al: The contribution of reoxygen-

ation to ischemic brain damage, *J Cereb Blood Flow Metab* 11:994, 1991.

97. Halsey JH, McDowell HA, Gelmon S et al: Blood velocity in the middle cerebral artery and regional cerebral blood flow during carotid endarterectomy, *Stroke* 20:53, 1989.

98. Halsey JH Jr, McFarland S: Oxygen cycles and metabolic autoregulation, *Stroke* 5:219, 1974.

99. Hansen M, Jakobsen M, Enevoldsen E et al: Problems in cerebral blood flow calculation using xenon-133 in patients with pulmonary diseases, *Stroke* 21:745, 1990.

100. Harada J, Takaku A, Endo S, et al: Differences in critical cerebral blood flow with age in swine, *J Neurosurg* 75:103, 1991.

101. Harder DR: Pressure-dependent membrane depolarization in cat middle cerebral artery, *Circ Res* 55:197, 1984.

102. Harder DR, Kauser K, Lombard JH et al: Pressure-induced activation of renal and cerebral arteries depends upon an intact endothelium. In Rubanyi GM, Vanhoutte PM, editors: *Endothelium-derived contracting factors,* Basel, Switzerland, 1980, Karger AG, p 8.

103. Harp JR, Wollman H: Cerebral metabolic effects of hyperventilation and deliberate hypotension, *Br J Anaesth* 45:256, 1973.

104. Harper AM: Autoregulation of cerebral blood flow: influence of the arterial blood pressure on the blood flow through the cerebral cortex, *J Neurol Neurosurg Psychiatry* 29:398, 1966.

105. Hassler W: Hemodynamic aspects of cerebral angiomas, *Acta Neurochir (Wien)* [Suppl 37] 1, 1986.

106. Hayes AC, Baker WH, Reichman OH: Non-invasive evaluation of patients with extracranial to intracranial bypass, *Stroke* 13:365, 1982.

107. Heistad DD: Summary of Symposium on Cerebral Blood Flow: Effect of nerves and neurotransmitters, Cardiovascular Center, University of Iowa, Iowa City, Iowa, June 16-18, 1981, *J Cereb Blood Flow Metab* 1:447, 1981.

108. Heistad DD, Marcus ML, Abboud FM: Role of large arteries in regulation of cerebral blood flow in dogs, *J Clin Invest* 62:761, 1978.

109. Henriksen L, Hjelms E, Lindeburgh T: Brain hyperperfusion during cardiac operations. Cerebral blood flow measured in man by intra-arterial injection of xenon 133: evidence suggestive of intraoperative microembolism, *J Thorac Cardiovasc Surg* 8:6202, 1983.

110. Hernandez MJ, Raichle ME, Stone HL: The role of the sympathetic nervous system in cerebral blood flow autoregulation, *Europ Neurol* 6:175, 1971/72.

111. Hickey PR, Buckley MJ, Philbin DM: Pulsatile and nonpulsatile cardiopulmonary bypass. Review of a counterproductive controversy, *Ann Thorac Surg* 36:720, 1983.

112. Hickey R, Albin MS, Bunegin L et al: Autoregulation of spinal cord blood flow: is the cord a microcosm of the brain? *Stroke* 17:1183, 1986.

113. Hindman BJ, Funatsu N, Harrington J et al: Differences in cerebral blood flow between alpha-stat and pH-stat management are eliminated during period of decreased systemic flow and pressure: a study during cardiopulmonary bypass in rabbits, *Anesthesiology* 74:1096, 1991.

114. Hitchon P, Kassell N, Hill T et al: The response of spinal cord blood flow to high-dose barbiturates, *Spine* 7:41, 1982.

115. Hitchon P, Lobosky J, Yamada T et al: Effect of laminectomy and anesthesia upon spinal cord blood flow, *J Neurosurg* 61:545, 1984.

116. Hoehner PJ, Dean JM, Rogers MC et al: Comparison of thermal clearance measurement of regional cerebral blood flow with radiolabelled microspheres, *Stroke* 18:606, 1987.

117. Hoffman WE, Albrecht RF, Miletich DJ: The influence of aging and hypertension on cerebral autoregulation, *Brain Res* 214:196, 1981.

118. Hoffman WE, Albrecht RF, Miletich DJ: Nitroglycerin induced hypotension will maintain CBF in hypertensive rats, *Stroke* 13:225, 1982.

119. Hoffman WE, Albrecht RF, Miletich DJ: Regional cerebral blood flow changes during hypothermia, *Cryobiology* 19:640, 1982.

120. Hoffman WE, Edelman G, Kochs E et al: Cerebral autoregulation in awake versus isoflurane-anesthetized rats, *Anesth Analg* 73:753, 1991.

121. Hoffman WE, Miletich DJ, Albrecht RF et al: Cerebrovascular response to hypotension in hypertensive rats: effect of antihypertensive therapy, *Anesthesiology* 58:326, 1983.

122. Huber P, Handa J: Effect of contrast material, hypercapnia, hyperventilation, hypertonic glucose and papaverine on the diameter of the cerebral arteries: angiographic determination in man, *Invest Radiol* 2:17, 1967.

123. Iadecola C: Does nitric oxide mediate the increases in cerebral blood flow elicited by hypercapnia? *Proc Natl Acad Sci USA* 89:3913, 1992.

124. Ishii R: Regional cerebral blood flow in patients with ruptured intracranial aneurysms, *J Neurosurg* 50:587, 1979.

125. Itoh M, Hatazawa J, Miyazawa H et al: Stability of cerebral blood flow and oxygen metabolism during normal aging, *Gerontology* 36:43, 1990.

126. Jones RA: EDRF/nitric oxide: the endogenous nitrovasodilator and a new cellular messenger (editorial), *Anesthesiology* 75:927, 1991.

127. Johns RA, Moscicki JC, DiFazio CA: Nitric oxide synthase inhibitor dose-dependently and reversibly reduces the threshold for halothane anesthesia, *Anesthesiology* 77:779, 1992.

128. Jones TH, Motawetz RB, Crowell RM et al: Thresholds of focal cerebral ischemia in awake monkeys, *J Neurosurg* 54:773, 1981.

129. Kano M, Moskowitz MA, Yokota M: Parasympathetic denervation of rat pial vessels significantly increases infarction volume following middle cerebral artery occlusion, *J Cereb Blood Flow Metab* 11:628, 1991.

130. Kassell NF, Peerless SJ, Durward QJ et al: Treatment of ischemic deficits from vasospasm with intravascular volume expansion and induced arterial hypertension, *Neurosurgery* 11:337, 1982.

131. Kety SS, Schmidt CF: The determination of cerebral blood flow in man by the use of nitrous oxide in low concentrations, *Am J Physiol* 14:353, 1945.

132. Kety SS, Schmidt CF: The effects of altered arterial tensions of carbon dioxide and oxygen on cerebral blood flow and cerebral oxygen consumption of normal young men, *J Clin Invest* 27:484, 1948.

133. Kobrine A, Doyle T, Rizzoli H: Spinal cord blood flow as affected by changes in systemic arterial blood pressure, *J Neurosurg* 44:12, 1976.

134. Koehler RC, Traystman RJ: Bicarbonate ion modulation of cerebral blood flow during hypoxia and hypercapnia, *Am J Physiol* 243:H33, 1982.

135. Koenig HM, Pelligrino DA, Albrecht RF: Halothane vasodilation and nitric oxide in rat pial vessels (abstract), *J Neurosurg Anesth* 4:301, 1992.

136. Kontos HA: Validity of cerebral arterial blood flow calculations from velocity measurements, *Stroke* 20:1, 1989.

137. Kontos HA, Wei EP, Navari RM et al: Responses of cerebral arteries and arterioles to acute hypotension and hypertension, *Am J Physiol* 234:H371, 1978.

138. Kozniewska E, Oseka M, Stys T: Effects of endothelium-derived nitric oxide on cerebral circulation during normoxia and hypoxia in the rat, *J Cereb Blood Flow Metab* 12:311, 1992.

139. Lam AM, Manninen PH, Ferguson GG et al: Monitoring electrophysiologic function during carotid endarterectomy: a comparison of somatosensory evoked potentials and conventional electroencephalogram, *Anesthesiology* 75:15, 1991.

140. Lassen NA: Cerebral blood flow and oxygen consumption in man, *Physiol Rev* 39:183, 1959.

141. Lassen NA, Blasberg RG: Technetium-99m-*d*,l-HM-PAO, the development of a new class of ^{99m}Tc-labeled tracers: an overview, *J Cereb Blood Flow Metab* 8:S1, 1988.

142. Lassen NA, Ingvar DH: The blood flow of the cerebral cortex determined by radioactive krypton[85], *Experientia* 17:42, 1961.

143. Lassen NA, Ingvar DH, Skinhoj E: Brain function and blood flow: changes in the amount of blood flowing in areas of the human cerebral cortex, reflecting changes in the activity of those areas, are graphically revealed with the aid of a radioactive isotope, *Sci Am* 239:62, 1978.

144. Lassen NA, Lane MH: Validity of internal jugular blood for study of cerebral blood flow and metabolism, *J Appl Physiol* 16:313, 1961.

145. Lindegaard K-F, Grolimund P, Aaslid R et al: Evaluation of cerebral

AVMs using transcranial Doppler ultrasound, *J Neurosurg* 65:335, 1986.

146. Litt L, Gonzalez-Mendez R, Severinghaus JW et al: Cerebral intracellular changes during supercarbia: an in vivo 31P nuclear magnetic resonance study in rats, *J Cereb Blood Flow Metab* 5:537, 1985.

147. Long CJ, Berkowitz BA: What is the relationship between the endothelium derived relaxant factor and nitric oxide? *Life Sci* 45:1, 1989.

148. Lou HC, Edvinsson L, MacKenzie ET: The concept of coupling blood flow to brain function: Revision required? *Ann Neurol* 22:289, 1987.

149. Macfarlane R, Moskowitz MA, Sakas DE et al: The role of neuroeffector mechanisms in cerebral hyperperfusion syndromes, *J Neurosurg* 75:845, 1991.

150. Madsen JB, Cold GE, Hansen ES et al: The effect of isoflurane on cerebral blood flow and metabolism in humans during craniotomy for small supratentorial cerebral tumors, *Anesthesiology* 66:332, 1987.

151. Marcus ML, Heistad DD, Ehrhardt JC et al: Regulation of total and regional spinal cord blood flow, *Circ Res* 41:128, 1977.

152. Markwalder T-M, Grolimund P, Seiler RW et al: Dependency of blood flow velocity in the middle cerebral artery on end-tidal carbon dioxide partial pressure—a transcranial ultrasound Doppler study, *J Cereb Blood Flow Metab* 4:368, 1984.

153. McCormick PW, Stewart M, Ray P et al: Measurement of regional cerebrovascular haemoglobin oxygen saturation in cats using optical spectroscopy, *Neurol Res* 13:65, 1991.

154. McDowall DG: Induced hypotension and brain ischaemia, *Br J Anaesth* 57:110, 1985.

155. McKay RD, Sundt TM, Michenfelder JD et al: Internal carotid artery stump pressure and cerebral blood flow during carotid endarterectomy: modification by halothane, enflurane, and innovar, *Anesthesiology* 45:390, 1976.

156. McPherson RW, Brian JE, Traystman RJ: Cerebrovascular responsiveness to carbon dioxide in dogs with 1.4% and 2.8% isoflurane, *Anesthesiology* 70:843, 1989.

157. McPherson RW, Traystman RJ: Effects of isoflurane on cerebral auto-

regulation in dogs, *Anesthesiology* 69:493, 1988.

158. McPherson RW, Traystman RJ: Effect of time on cerebrovascular responsivity to $Paco_2$ during isoflurane anesthesia, *Anesthesiology* 71:A105, 1989.

159. Meyer JS: Does diaschisis have clinical correlates? *Mayo Clin Proc* 66:430, 1991.

160. Meyerson BA, Gunasekera L, Linderoth B et al: Bedside monitoring of regional cortical blood flow in comatose patients using laser Doppler flowmetry, *Neurosurgery* 29:750, 1991.

161. Michenfelder JD, Milde JH: The relationship among canine brain temperature, metabolism, and function during hypothermia, *Anesthesiology* 75:130, 1991.

162. Michenfelder JD, Milde JH, Katusic ZS: Postischemic canine cerebral blood flow is coupled to cerebral metabolic rate, *J Cereb Blood Flow Metab* 11:611, 1991.

163. Michenfelder JD, Sundt TM Jr: The effect of $Paco_2$ on the metabolism of ischemic brain in squirrel monkeys, *Anesthesiology* 38:445, 1973.

164. Michenfelder JD, Sundt TM, Fode N et al: Isoflurane when compared to enflurane and halothane decreases the frequency of cerebral ischemia during carotid endarterectomy, *Anesthesiology* 67:336, 1987.

165. Michenfelder JD: *Anesthesia and the brain: clinical, functional, metabolic and vascular correlates,* New York, 1988, Churchill-Livingstone, pp 155-158.

166. Mohr JP, Petty GW, Sacco RL: Recent advances in cerebrovascular disease, *Curr Neurol* 9:77, 1989.

167. Mohr LL, Smith LL, Hinshaw DB: Blood gas and carotid pressure: factors in stroke risk, *Ann Surg* 184:723, 1976.

168. Moore L, Kirsch J, Helfaer M et al: Isoflurane induced cerebral hyperemia: role of prostanoids and nitric oxide in pigs (abstract), *J Neurosurg Anesth* 4:304, 1992.

169. Moossy J, Martinez J, Hanin I et al: Thalamic and subcortical gliosis with dementia. *Arch Neurol* 44:510, 1987.

170. Moskowitz MA, Sakas DE, Wei EP et al: Postocclusive cerebral hyperemia is markedly attenuated by chronic trigeminal ganglionectomy, *Am J Physiol* 257:H1736, 1989.

171. Muizelaar JP, Becker D: Induced hypertension for the treatment of cerebral ischemia after subarachnoid hemorrhage, *Surg Neurol* 25:317, 1986.

172. Muizelaar JP, Marmarou A, Ward JD et al: Adverse effects of prolonged hyperventilation in patients with severe head injury: a randomized clinical trial, *J Neurosurg* 75:731, 1991.

173. Muizelaar JP, Wei EP, Kontos HA et al: Mannitol causes compensatory cerebral vasoconstriction and vasodilation in response to blood viscosity changes, *J Neurosurg* 59:822, 1983.

174. Muizelaar JP, Wei EP, Kontos HA et al: Cerebral blood flow is regulated by changes in blood pressure and in blood viscosity alike, *Stroke* 17:44, 1986.

175. Murkin JM, Farrar JK: The influence of pulsatile vs nonpulsatile cardiopulmonary bypass on cerebral blood flow and cerebral metabolism, *Anesthesiology* 71:A41, 1989.

176. Murkin JM, Lee DH: Transcranial Doppler verification of pulsatile cerebral blood flow during cardiopulmonary bypass (abstract), *Anesth Analg* 72:S194, 1991.

177. Nakai K, Imai H, Kamei I et al: Microangioarchitecture of rat parietal cortex with special reference to vascular "sphincters": scanning electron microscopic and dark field microscopic study, *Stroke* 12:653, 1981.

178. Naritomi H, Meyer JS, Sakai F et al: Effects of advancing age on regional cerebral blood flow: studies in normal subjects and subjects with risk factors for atherothrombotic stroke, *Arch Neurol* 36:410, 1979.

179. Nioka S, Chance B, Smith DS et al: Cerebral energy metabolism and oxygen state during hypoxia in neonate and adult dogs, *Pediatr Res* 28:54, 1990.

180. Nordborg C, Johansson BB: Morphometric study on cerebral vessels in spontaneously hypertensive rats, *Stroke* 11:266, 1980.

181. Nornes H, Wikeby P: Cerebral arterial blood flow and aneurysm surgery. part 1. Local arterial flow dynamics, *J Neurosurg* 47:810, 1977.

182. Obrist WD, Thompson HK Jr, King CH et al: Determination of regional cerebral blood flow by inhalation of 133-xenon, *Circ Res* 20:124, 1967.

183. Obrist WD, Thompson HK Jr, Wang

HS et al: Regional cerebral blood flow estimated by ^{133}xenon inhalation, *Stroke* 6:245, 1975.

184. Obrist WD, Wilkinson WE: Regional cerebral blood flow measurement in humans by xenon-133 clearance, *Cerebrovasc Brain Metab Rev* 2:283, 1990.

185. Ochiai C, Asano T, Takakura K et al: Mechanisms of cerebral protection by pentobarbital and nizofenone correlated with the course of local cerebral blood flow changes, *Stroke* 13:788, 1982.

186. Ohmoto T, Nagao S, Mino S et al: Monitoring of cortical blood flow during temporary arterial occlusion in aneurysm surgery by the thermal diffusion method, *Neurosurgery* 28:49, 1991.

187. Olesen J: Contralateral focal increase of cerebal blood flow in man during arm work, *Brain* 94:635, 1971.

188. Olesen J, Paulson OB, Lassen NA: Regional cerebral blood flow in man determined by the initial slope of the clearance of intraarterially injected ^{133}Xe: theory of the method, normal values, error of measurement, correction for remaining radioactivity, relation to other flow parameters and response to Paco$_2$ changes, *Stroke* 2:519, 1971.

189. Ooboshi H, Sadoshima S, Fujii K et al: Acute effects of antihypertensive agents on cerebral blood flow in hypertensive rats, *Eur J Pharmacol* 179:253, 1990.

190. Ornstein E, Young WL, Prohovnik I et al: Effect of cardiac output on CBF during deliberate hypotension, *Anesthesiology* 73A:169, 1990.

191. Patlak CS, Blasberg RG, Fenstermacher JD: An evaluation of errors in the determination of blood flow by the indicator fractionation and tissue equilibration (Kety) methods, *J Cereb Blood Flow Metab* 4:47, 1984.

192. Paulson OB, Jarden JO, Vorstrup S et al: Effect of captopril on the cerebral circulation in chronic heart failure, *Eur J Clin Invest* 16:124, 1986.

193. Paulson OB, Olesen J, Christensen MS: Restoration of autoregulation of cerebral blood flow by hypocapnia, *Neurology* 22:286, 1972.

194. Paulson OB, Strandgaard S, Edvinsson L: Cerebral autoregulation, *Cerebrovasc Brain Metab Rev* 2:161, 1990.

195. Pavlakis S, Bello J, Prohovnik I et al: Brain infarction in sickle cell anemia: magnetic resonance imaging correlates, *Ann Neurol* 23:125, 1988.

196. Pearson RM, Griffith DNW, Woollard M et al: Comparison of effects on cerebral blood flow of rapid reduction in systemic arterial pressure by diazoxide and labetalol in hypertensive patients: preliminary findings, *Br J Clin Pharmacol* 8:195S, 1979.

197. Pelligrino DA, Koenig HM, Albrecht RF: The role of nitric oxide in regional cerebral blood flow responses to hypoxia and hypercapnia in rats (abstract), *J Neurosurg Anesth* 4:303, 1992a.

198. Pelligrino DA, Miletich DJ, Albrecht RF: Diminished muscarinic receptor−mediated cerebral blood flow response in streptozotocin-treated rats, *Am J Physiol* 262:E447, 1992b.

199. Petersen SE, Fox PT, Snyder AZ et al: Activation of extrastriate and frontal cortical areas by visual words and word-like stimuli, *Science* 249:1041, 1990.

200. Pilato MA, Bissonnette B, Lerman J: Transcranial Doppler: response of cerebral blood-flow velocity to carbon dioxide in anaesthetized children, *Can J Anaesth* 38:37, 1991.

201. Pistolese GR, Citone G, Faraglia V et al: Effects of hypercapnia on cerebral blood flow during the clamping of the carotid arteries in surgical management of cerebrovascular insufficiency, *Neurology* 21:95, 1971.

202. Pistolese GR, Faraglia V, Agnoli A et al: Cerebral hemispheric "countersteal" phenomenon during hyperventilation in cerebrovascular diseases, *Stroke* 3:456, 1972.

203. Powers WJ, Raichle ME: Positron emission tomography and its application to the study of cerebrovascular disease in man, *Stroke* 16:361, 1985.

204. Prohovnik I: Data quality, integrity and interpretation. In Knezevic S, Maximilian VA, Mubrin Z et al, editors: *Handbook of regional cerebral blood flow*, Hillsdale, New Jersey, 1988, Lawrence Erlbaum Associates, p 51.

205. Prohovnik I, Huang J, Young WL et al: Simultaneous SPECT CBF/CBV imaging with imperfect energy resolution, *J Cereb Blood Flow Metab* 13(Suppl 1):5321, 1993.

206. Prohovnik I, Knudsen E, Risberg J: Accuracy of models and algorithms for determination of fast-compartment flow by noninvasive ^{133}Xe clearance. In Magistretti PL, editors: *Functional radionuclide imaging of the brain,* New York, 1983, Raven Press, p 87.

207. Prohovnik I, Knudsen E, Risberg J: Theoretical evaluation and simulation test of the Initial Slope Index for noninvasive rCBF. In Hartmann A, Hoyer S, editors: *Cerebral blood flow and metabolism measurement,* Berlin, 1985, Springer Verlag, p 56.

208. Prohovnik I, Pavlakis SG, Piomelli S et al: Cerebral hyperemia, stroke, and transfusion in sickle cell disease, *Neurology* 39:344, 1989.

209. Puig M, Kirpekar SM: Inhibitory effect of low pH on norepinephrine release, *J Pharmacol Exp Ther* 176:134, 1967.

210. Pulsinelli WA, Levy DE, Duffy TE: Regional cerebral blood flow and glucose metabolism following transient forebrain ischemia, *Ann Neurol* 11:499, 1982.

211. Ra JB, Hilal SK, Oh CH et al: In vivo magnetic resonance imaging of sodium in the human body, *Magn Reson Med* 7:11, 1988.

212. Raichle ME, Posner JB, Plum F: Cerebral blood flow during and after hyperventilation, *Arch Neurol* 23:394, 1970.

213. Rampil IJ: Cerebral perfusion mapping with ultrasound contrast, *Anesthesiology* 75A:1006, 1991.

214. Risberg J, Ali Z, Wilson EM et al: Regional cerebral blood flow by ^{133}xenon inhalation, *Stroke* 6:142, 1975.

215. Roald OK, Forsman M, Steen PA: The effects of prolonged isoflurane anaesthesia on cerebral blood flow and metabolism in the dog, *Acta Anaesthesiol Scand* 33:210, 1989.

216. Rogers AT, Stump DA, Gravlee GP et al: Response of cerebral blood flow to phenylephrine infusion during hypothermic cardiopulmonary bypass: influence of Paco$_2$ management, *Anesthesiology* 69:547, 1988.

217. Rosenblum WI: Endothelium-derived relaxing factor in brain blood vessels is not nitric oxide, *Stroke* 23:1527, 1992.

218. Rosner MJ: Cerebral perfusion pressure link between intracranial pressure and systemic circulation. In Wood JH, editor: *Cerebral blood flow physiologic and clinical aspects,*

New York, 1987, McGraw-Hill, p 425.

219. Roy CS, Sherrington CS: On the regulation of the blood-supply of the brain, *J Physiol* 11:85, 1890.

220. Sadoshima S, Fujii K, Yao H et al: Regional cerebral blood flow autoregulation in normotensive and spontaneously hypertensive rats—effects of sympathetic denervation, *Stroke* 17:981, 1986.

221. Sakai F, Nakazawa K, Tazaki Y et al: Regional cerebral blood volume and hematocrit measured in normal human volunteers by single-photon emission computed tomography, *J Cereb Blood Flow Metab* 5:207, 1985.

222. Sakamoto T, Monafo WW: Regional blood flow in the brain and spinal cord of hypothermic rats, *Am J Physiol* 257:H785, 1989.

223. Sakurada O, Kennedy C, Jehle J et al: Measurement of local cerebral blood flow with iodo[^{14}C]antipyrine, *Am J Physiol* 234:H59, 1978.

224. Sandler AN, Tator CH: Review of the measurement of normal spinal cord blood flow, *Brain Res* 118:181, 1976.

225. Sato M, Pawlik G, Heiss W-D: Comparative studies of regional CNS blood flow autoregulation and responses to CO_2 in the cat: effects of altering arterial blood pressure and Paco$_2$ on rCBF of cerebrum, cerebellum, and spinal cord, *Stroke* 15:91, 1984.

226. Schroeder T: Hemodynamic significance of internal carotid artery disease, *Acta Neurol Scand* 77:353, 1987.

227. Schwartz AE, Michler RE, Young WL: Cerebral blood flow during low-flow hypothermic cardiopulmonary bypass in baboons, *Anesth Analg* 74:S267, 1992.

228. Shapiro HM, Stromberg DD, Lee DR et al: Dynamic pressures in the pial arterial microcirculation, *Am J Physiol* 221:279, 1971.

229. Shinoda J, Kimura T, Funakoshi T et al: Acetazolamide reactivity on cerebral blood flow in patients with subarachnoid haemorrhage, *Acta Neurochir (Wien)* 109:102, 1991.

230. Shiokawa O, Sadoshima S, Kusuda K et al: Cerebral and cerebellar blood flow autoregulations in acutely induced cerebral ischemia in spontaneously hypertensive rats—transtento-

rial remote effect, *Stroke* 17:1309, 1986.

231. Siesjö BK: Cerebral circulation and metabolism, *J Neurosurg* 60:883, 1984.

232. Siesjö BK: *Brain energy metabolism,* New York, 1978, John Wiley & Sons, p 297.

233. Siesjö BK: Pathophysiology and treatment of focal cerebral ischemia. Part II. Mechanisms of damage and treatment (review article), *J Neurosurg* 77:337, 1992.

234. Skinhoj E: The sympathetic nervous system and the regulation of cerebral blood flow, *Europ Neurol* 6:190, 1971/72.

235. Smith A, Pernder J, Alexander S: Effects of Pco$_2$ in spinal cord blood flow, *Am J Physiol* 216:1158, 1969.

236. Solomon RA, Fink ME, Lennihan L: Prophylactic volume expansion therapy for the prevention of delayed cerebral ischemia after early aneurysm surgery, *Arch Neurol* 45:325, 1988.

237. Solomon RA, Post KD, McMurtry JG: Depression of circulating blood volume in patients after subarachnoid hemorrhage. Implications for the management of symptomatic vasospasm, *Neurosurg* 15:354, 1984.

238. Soloway M, Moriarty G, Fraser JG et al: Effect of delayed hyperventilation on experimental cerebral infarction, *Neurology* 21:479, 1971.

239. Soloway M, Nadel W, Albin MS et al: The effect of hyperventilation on subsequent cerebral infarction, *Anesthesiology* 29:975, 1968.

240. Spetzler RF, Wilson CB, Weinstein P et al: Normal perfusion pressure breakthrough theory, *Clin Neurosurg* 25:651, 1978.

241. Squire L, Ojemann J, Miezin F et al: A functional anatomical study of human memory, *Soc Neurosci Abst* 17:4, 1991.

242. Stånge K, Lagerkranser M, Sollevi A: Nitroprusside-induced hypotension and cerebrovascular autoregulation in the anesthetized pig, *Anesth Analg* 73:745, 1991.

243. Steen PA, Newberg L, Milde JH et al: Hypothermia and barbiturates: individual and combined effects on canine cerebral oxygen consumption, *Anesthesiology* 58:527, 1983.

244. Steinmeier R, Fahlbusch R, Powers AD et al: Pituitary microcirculation: physiological aspects and clinical implications. A laser-Doppler flow

study during transsphenoidal adenomectomy, *Neurosurgery* 29:47, 1991.

245. Stephan H, Sonntag H, Lange H et al: Cerebral effects of anaesthesia and hypothermia, *Anaesthesia* 44:310, 1989.

246. Stone JG, Young WL, Smith CR et al: Do temperatures recorded at standard monitoring sites reflect actual brain temperature during deep hypothermia? *Anesthesiology* 75:A483, 1991.

247. Strandgaard S, Olesen J, Skinhoj E et al: Autoregulation of brain circulation in severe arterial hypertension, *Br Med J* 3:507, 1973.

248. Sullivan HG, Kingsbury TB IV, Morgan ME et al: The rCBF response to Diamox in normal subjects and cerebrovascular disease patients, *J Neurosurg* 67:525, 1987.

249. Sundt TM, Sharbrough FW, Piepgras DG et al: Correlation of cerebral flood flow and electroencephalographic changes during carotid endarterectomy, *Mayo Clin Proc* 56:533, 1981.

250. Sutton LN, McLaughlin AC, Dante S et al: Cerebral venous oxygen content as a measure of brain energy metabolism with increased intracranial pressure and hyperventilation, *J Neurosurg* 73:927, 1990.

251. Symon L, Held K, Dorsch NWC: A study of regional autoregulation in the cerebral circulation to increased perfusion pressure in normocapnia and hypercapnia, *Stroke* 4:139, 1973.

252. Tanaka K, Gotoh F, Gomi S et al: Inhibition of nitric oxide synthesis induces a significant reduction in local cerebral blood flow in the rat, *Neurosci Let* 127:129, 1991.

253. Tarr RW, Johnson DW, Rutigliano M et al: Use of acetazolamide-challenge xenon CT in the assessment of cerebral blood flow dynamics in patients with arteriovenous malformations, *Am J Neuroradiol* 11:441, 1990.

254. Todd MM, Hindman BJ, Warner DS: Barbiturate protection and cardiac surgery: a different result, *Anesthesiology* 74:402, 1991.

255. Todd MM, Weeks JB, Warner DS: The effects of hemodilution on the relationships between cerebral blood flow, blood volume, and cerebral tis-

sue hematocrit, *J Cereb Blood Flow Metab* 11(suppl 2):S85, 1991.

256. Tomida S, Wagner HG, Klatzo I et al: Effect of acute electrode placement on regional CBF in the gerbil: a comparison of blood flow measured by hydrogen clearance, [^{3}H]nicotine, and [^{14}C]iodoantipyrine techniques, *J Cereb Blood Flow Metab* 9:79, 1989.

257. Tominaga S, Strandgaard S, Uemura K et al: Cerebrovascular CO_2 reactivity in normotensive and hypertensive man, *Stroke* 7:507, 1976.

258. Tranmer BI, Gross CE, Kindt GW et al: Pulsatile versus nonpulsatile blood flow in the treatment of acute cerebral ischemia, *Neurosurgery* 19:724, 1986.

259. Turner DM, Kassell NF, Sasaki T et al: Time-dependent changes in cerebral and cardiovascular parameters in isoflurane-nitrous oxide–anesthetized dogs, *Neurosurgery* 14:135, 1984.

260. Van Heertum RL, Tikofsky RS: *Advances in cerebral SPECT imaging: an atlas and guideline for practitioners*, Philadelphia, 1989, Lea & Febriger, p 62.

261. Van Uitert RL, Sage JI, Levy DE et al: Comparison of radio-labeled butanol and iodoantipyrine as cerebral blood flow markers, *Brain Res* 222:365, 1981.

262. Verhaeghe RH, Lorenz RR, McGrath MA et al: Metabolic modulation of neurotransmitter release— adenosine, adenine nucleotides, potassium, hyperosmolarity, and hydrogen ion, *Fed Proc* 37:208, 1978.

263. Vorstrup S, Barry DI, Jarden JO et al: Chronic antihypertensive treatment in the rat reverses hypertension-induced changes in cerebral blood flow autoregulation, *Stroke* 15:312, 1984.

264. Wade JPH, Hachinski VC: Cerebral steal: robbery or maldistribution? In Wood JH, editor: *Cerebral blood flow: physiologic and clinical aspects*, New York, 1987, McGraw-Hill, p 467.

265. Wagner EM, Traystman RJ: Cerebral venous outflow and arterial microsphere flow with elevated venous pressure, *Am J Physiol* 244:H505, 1983.

266. Waldemar G, Paulson OB, Barry DI et al: Angiotensin converting enzyme inhibition and the upper limit of ce-

rebral blood flow autoregulation. Effect of sympathetic stimulation, *Circ Res* 64:1197, 1989.

267. Walker DAJ, Isley MR, Lucas WJ et al: Cerebral blood flow velocity is coupled to EEG activity during hypothermic cardiopulmonary bypass, *Anesthesiology* 75:A177, 1991.

268. Wang Q, Paulson OB, Lassen NA: Effect of nitric oxide blockage by N^G-nitro-L-arginine on cerebral blood flow response to changes in carbon dioxide tension, *J Cereb Blood Flow Metab* 12:947, 1992.

269. Warner DS, Hansen TD, Vust L et al: Distribution of cerebral blood flow during deep isoflurane vs. pentobarbital anesthesia in rats with middle cerebral artery occlusion, *J Neuro Anesth* 1:219, 1989.

270. Warner DS, Turner DM, Kassell NF: Time-dependent effects of prolonged hypercapnia on cerebrovascular parameters in dogs' acid-base chemistry, *Stroke* 18:142, 1987.

271. Wasnick JD, Conlay LA: Induced hypertension for cerebral aneurysm surgery in a patient with carotid occlusive disease, *Anesth Analg* 70:331, 1990.

272. Wei EP, Kontos HA: Increased venous pressure causes myogenic constriction of cerebral arterioles during local hyperoxia, *Circ Res* 55:249, 1984.

273. Wollman H, Smith TC, Stephen GW et al: Effects of extremes of respiratory and metabolic alkalosis on cerebral blood flow in man, *J Appl Physiol* 24:60, 1968.

274. Woodcock TE, Murkin JM, Farrar JK et al: Pharmacologic EEG suppression during cardiopulmonary bypass: cerebral hemodynamic and metabolic effects of thiopental or isoflurane during hypothermia and normothermia, *Anesthesiology* 67:218, 1987.

275. Wyper DJ, Lennox GA, Rowan JO: Two minute slope inhalation technique for cerebral blood flow measurement in man. 1. Method, *J Neurol Neurosurg Psychiatry* 39:141, 1976.

276. Wyper DJ, Lennox GA, Rowan JO: Two minute slope inhalation technique for cerebral blood flow measurement in man. 2. Clinical appraisal, *J Neurol Neurosurg Psychiatry* 39:147, 1976.

277. Yamaguchi F, Meyer JS, Sakai F et al: Normal human aging and cerebral vasoconstrictive responses to hypocapnia, *J Neurolog Sci* 44:87, 1979.

278. Yamamoto M, Meyer JS, Sakai F et al: Aging and cerebral vasodilator responses to hypercarbia: responses in normal aging and in persons with risk factors for stroke, *Arch Neurol* 37:489, 1980.

279. Yonas H, Darby JM, Marks EC et al: CBF measured by Xe-CT approach to analysis and normal values, *J Cereb Blood Flow Metab* 11:716, 1991.

280. Young W: H_2 clearance measurement of blood flow: a review of technique and polarographic principles, *Stroke* 11:552, 1980.

281. Young WL: Neuroanesthesia: a look into the future, *Anesth Clin North Am* 10:727, 1992.

282. Young WL, Cole DJ: Deliberate hypertension: rationale and application for augmenting cerebral blood flow. In *Problems in anesthesia,* Philadelphia, JB Lippincott, 7:140, 1993.

283. Young WL, Josovitz K, Morales O et al: The effect of nimodipine on post-ischemic cerebral glucose utilization and blood flow in the rat, *Anesthesiology* 67:54, 1987.

284. Young WL, Prohovnik I, Correll JW et al: Cerebral blood flow and metabolism in patients undergoing anesthesia for carotid endarterectomy: a comparison of isoflurane, halothane, and fentanyl, *Anesth Analg* 68:712, 1989.

285. Young WL, Prohovnik I, Ornstein E et al: Rapid monitoring of intraoperative cerebral blood flow using ^{133}Xe, *J Cereb Blood Flow Metab* 8:691, 1988.

286. Young WL, Prohovnik I, Ornstein E et al: The effect of arteriovenous malformation resection on cerebrovascular reactivity to carbon dioxide, *Neurosurgery* 27:257, 1990.

287. Young WL, Prohovnik I, Schroeder T et al: Intraoperative ^{133}Xe cerebral blood flow measurements by intravenous versus intracarotid methods, *Anesthesiology* 73:637, 1990.

288. Young WL, Solomon RA, Pedley TA et al: Direct cortical EEG monitoring during temporary vascular occlusion for cerebral aneurysm surgery, *Anesthesiology* 71:794, 1989.

289. Young WL, Kader A, Prohovnik I et al: Pressure autoregulation is intact after arteriovenous malformation resection, *Neurosurgery* 32:491, 1993.

290. Yudd AP, Van Heertum RL, Masdeu JC: Interventions and functional brain imaging, *Semin Nuclear Med* 21:153, 1991.

291. Zweifach BW, Lipowsky HH: Pressure-flow relations in blood and lymph microcirculation. In Renkin EM, Michel CC, Geiger SR, editors: *Handbook of physiology: a critical comprehensive presentation,* vol 4, Bethesda, Md, American Physiological Society, p 251.

APPENDIX 1

Transit Time

A more simplistic approach can be taken if one assumes that at any given time the concentration of isotope, *c(t)*, within the region of interest is homogeneous. In this case, the amount of blood that leaves (or enters) this region in a small increment of time, *dt*, is defined by the product of the flow rate and time, $F \times dt$. The amount of isotope carried away from the region by this departing blood is described as $c(t) \times F \times dt$. Again, by conservation of mass, the dose of isotope injected into the region of interest, *q*, must be the same as the amount leaving during all subsequent time periods:

$$q = \int c(t)F\,dt \qquad (20)$$

Rearranging this equation, one finds that flow can be described as the initially injected tracer dose within the region of interest divided by the area under the curve of the concentration vs. time relationship:

$$F = \frac{q}{\int c(t)\, dt} \qquad (21)$$

Taking the relationship derived in Equation 21 a step further, the rate at which tracer leaves the region of interest is the product of the flow rate and the concentration of isotope in the departing blood at that given time, $F \times c(t)$. At this point, it is useful to define the frequency function as:

$$h(t) = \frac{F\,c(t)}{q} \qquad (22)$$

The frequency function, simply stated, describes the fractional rate at which tracer leaves the region of interest. Because all tracer must ultimately leave:

$$\int h(t)\,dt = 1 \qquad (23)$$

For any small time interval between *t* and $t + dt$, the fraction of the original tracer leaving the system is thus $h(t) \cdot dt$. The quantity of tracer leaving is thus $q \times h(t) \cdot dt$. By virtue of the fact that the tracer is assumed to follow the same kinetics as the tracee, a similar analysis can

be made regarding the volume of blood (tracee) entering into the region of interest per unit time, *F*. The fraction of this blood leaving between *t* and $t + dt$ is again, $h(t) \cdot dt$. Thus, the blood that is present in the region of interest leaves at a rate of $F \cdot h(t) \cdot dt$ until the time when all such particles have left. Transforming from rates to volumes, the volume of blood that departs from the region of interest between *t* and $t + dt$, denoted as *dV*, is the product of the egress rate and the time required for this blood to leave, $t \cdot F \cdot h(t) \cdot dt$. Integrating over all time intervals, one obtains:

$$\int dV = \int tFh(t)\,dt = F\int t\,h(t)\,dt \qquad (24)$$

Because *h(t)* is the frequency function of the transit times of the tracer, the integral expression $\int th(t)\, dt$ is simply the mean transit time, $\bar{t}$, which statistically defines the average time that any particle of tracer, or for that matter tracee (blood), remains within the system. Substituting Equation 22 and then Equation 20 into the expression for $\bar{t}$:

$$\bar{t} = \int_{t=0}^{\infty} th(t)\,dt = \frac{\int_{t=0}^{\infty} t\,F\,c(t)\,dt}{q} = \frac{\int_{t=0}^{\infty} t\,c(t)\,dt}{\int_{t=0}^{\infty} c(t)\,dt} \qquad (25)$$

Mean transit time can thus easily be calculated from the concentration vs. time curve. Once again, invoking conservation of mass, it is clear that for any time interval, the volumes of blood entering and leaving a region of interest are equal. For the inert gas system being discussed, the mean transit time of the inert gas particles (the tracer), is equal to the mean transit time of the blood particles (the tracee). Thus the blood volume contained in the region of interest is equal to the product of the blood flow into (or out of) this region and the mean transit time through the region of interest:

$$rCBV = rCBF \times \bar{t} \text{ or (Flow)} \qquad (26)$$

3

Pathophysiology of Metabolic Brain Injury

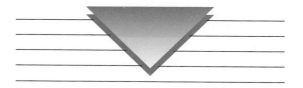

Leslie Newberg Milde
Margaret R. Weglinski

The purpose of this chapter is to present current knowledge regarding pathophysiology and the biochemical changes that occur during and after metabolic brain injury and which may contribute to ultimate neurologic outcome and to present current and future therapeutic measures designed to prevent or ameliorate cerebral damage resulting from such injury.

ISCHEMIA

Ischemia is the major cause of metabolic brain injury. It is hypothesized that specific biochemical disturbances that occur both during ischemia and after the restoration of circulation contribute to the ultimate neurologic damage.[239] Ischemia results when a decrease in tissue perfusion exceeds the tissue's ability to increase oxygen extraction from the blood[171] and consists of inadequate oxygen delivery, inadequate removal of carbon dioxide, increased intracellular lactic acid production, decreased stores of high-energy phosphates (phosphocreatine and adenosine triphosphate

[ATP]), decreased production of ATP, release of excitatory amino acid neurotransmitters, and disruption of the blood-brain barrier (BBB) (Box 3-1).[171,236]

Ischemia can be global, affecting the whole brain, or focal. Global ischemia may be complete or incomplete, but focal ischemia is incomplete (Table 3-1). Complete global ischemia occurs with cardiac arrest and results in the cessation of oxidative phosphorylation within 15 to 20 seconds.[3] Anaerobic metabolism with glycolysis supplying ATP continues until the intracellular stores of glucose have been exhausted. Anaerobic glycolysis produces lactic acid, causing a decrease in intracellular pH, which peaks a few minutes after the onset of ischemia. When intracellular ATP concentrations reach zero and glycolysis stops, all energy requiring reactions of the neurons cease and the cells soon die. Ischemia by itself will ultimately produce cell death if the duration and severity of the ischemia is sufficient to do so (Fig. 3-1).

Incomplete ischemia may be more damaging than short periods of complete ischemia because the oxygen supply is

▼

BOX 3-1
COMPONENTS OF ISCHEMIA

Decreased tissue perfusion
Increased oxygen extraction
Inadequate delivery of oxygen
Inadequate removal of carbon dioxide
Anaerobic metabolism
Increased intracellular lactic acid production
Decreased stores of high-energy phosphates
Decreased production of high-energy phosphates
Release of excitatory amino acid neurotransmitters
Disruption of the blood-brain barrier

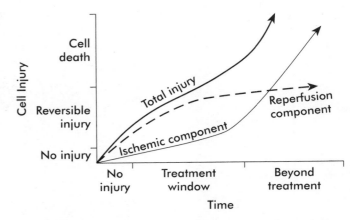

FIG. 3-1   The relationship between ischemic and reperfusion cellular changes leading to irreversible cell death.

TABLE 3-1
Types of Cerebral Ischemia

Focal	Global
Single-vessel stenosis or occlusion, vasospasm	Incomplete: Shock Hypotension Complete: Cardiac arrest

inadequate, resulting in anaerobic metabolism, and the continued but reduced supply of glucose is metabolized to lactic acid, producing a greater intracellular acidosis.[240]

In focal ischemia the decrease in cerebral blood flow depends on the existence of collateral vessels and local perfusion pressure.[9] It is hypothesized that a topographic gradient exists in which a center of dense ischemia is surrounded by areas of variable levels of perfusion.[11] These areas are potentially viable if blood flow to the area can be increased. Residual flow to the ischemic area depends on perfusion pressure because of loss of autoregulation in that area. Hemodynamic manipulation to support or increase the regional residual perfusion during ischemia can diminish the amount of neurologic damage that occurs as a result of focal ischemia.

FLOW THRESHOLDS

The functional state of the neuron depends on adequate cerebral blood flow (CBF) for the delivery of oxygen and glucose. When CBF decreases below a certain threshold, neuronal function becomes impaired.[125] Ischemic flow thresholds refer to the level of blood flow at which energy-requiring functions of the cell fail. Descriptions of such thresholds must include not only blood flow (supply) but also the functional and metabolic state of the cell (demand). The upper ischemic threshold is that flow at which neuronal function or electrical activity ceases. However, at this

blood flow there is enough blood supply to maintain the structural integrity of the cell. If CBF increases above this upper ischemic threshold, there can be full recovery of all neuronal function. The lower ischemic threshold is that CBF at which there is ATP depletion and membrane and mitochondrial failure. This flow threshold is associated with irreversible cell death. The differences in absolute blood flow between the upper and lower thresholds may be so small that any increase in regional CBF may improve neurologic function or any decrease in CBF may irreversibly destroy neurons.

SECONDARY CONSEQUENCES OF ISCHEMIA

Ischemic injury may occur as a result of the ischemia itself or during the period of reperfusion (Figs. 3-1 and 3-2). The *secondary* consequences of ischemia are those that occur after the cerebral circulation has been restored and may be termed *postischemic* or *reperfusion injury*. These include tissue edema, vasospasm, and red cell sludging, all of which can reduce blood flow, causing postischemic hypoperfusion; intracellular acidosis; release of excitatory amino acid neurotransmitters; increased catecholamine release; hypermetabolism; secondary depression of previously recovered metabolic activity; intracellular calcium overload, initiating calcium-mediated processes; changes in normal chelation and compartmentalization of free metals; and altered oxygen metabolism, leading to the production of free radicals, initiating free radical damage and lipid peroxidation (Box 3-2).[45,136]

If much of the tissue injury does not take place until the time of resuscitation, the therapeutic implications could be profound. Drugs presently under investigation for their ability to block reperfusion injury include calcium entry blockers, excitatory amino acid neurotransmitter antagonists, free radical scavengers, antagonists to the arachidonic acid cascade, and agents that block lipid peroxidation of cellular

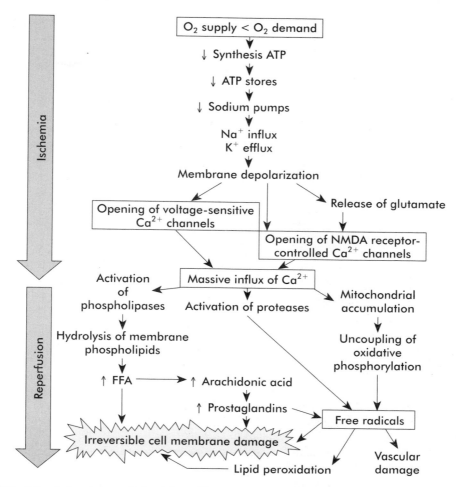

O_2 supply < O_2 demand

↓ Synthesis ATP

↓ ATP stores

↓ Sodium pumps

Na^+ influx
K^+ efflux

Membrane depolarization

Opening of voltage-sensitive Ca^{2+} channels

Release of glutamate

Opening of NMDA receptor-controlled Ca^{2+} channels

Activation of phospholipases

Massive influx of Ca^{2+}

Activation of proteases

Mitochondrial accumulation

Hydrolysis of membrane phospholipids

Uncoupling of oxidative phosphorylation

↑ FFA → ↑ Arachidonic acid

↑ Prostaglandins

Free radicals

Irreversible cell membrane damage

Lipid peroxidation

Vascular damage

Ischemia

Reperfusion

FIG. 3-2   Ischemic/reperfusion injury. Two components of tissue injury contribute to the ultimate neurologic damage. The ischemic component includes the processes of tissue damage occurring during ischemia. Cell death caused by the ischemic component alone depends on the severity and duration of ischemia. The secondary consequences of ischemia include the biochemical changes that take place at the time of reperfusion and reoxygenation after ischemia. The duration of these secondary processes and the extent to which they contribute to ultimate neurologic damage determine the therapeutic window during which treatment administered after ischemia may be effective. *(Modified from Bulkley GW:* Br J Cancer *[suppl] 55:66, 1987.)*

and mitochondrial membranes. In general, the utility of postischemic therapy for the treatment of tissue injury resulting from ischemia is proportionally related to the amount of injury that is due to reperfusion, vs. the amount caused by the ischemia itself.[40]

SELECTIVE VULNERABILITY

The concept of selective vulnerability applies to the *range* of responses in various regions of the brain, occurring in response to the same ischemic insult. Regions especially vulnerable to *ischemic* damage include the limbic system, primarily the pyramidal cells of the CA_1 region of the hippocampus, Purkinje cells of the cerebellum, and the small and medium-sized neurons of striatum and layers three,

five, and six of the cortex.[136] Damage to these selectively vulnerable neurons impairs cognition, motor function, coordination, recent memory, emotion, and drive. This accounts for the poor functional neurologic outcome of survivors of cardiac arrest.[60] It is hypothesized that the selective vulnerability of neurons may be due to a combination of specific neuroanatomic connections, synaptic organization, membrane properties, and patterns of neurotransmitters and receptors.[136]

OTHER CAUSES OF METABOLIC BRAIN INJURY

Ischemia, hypoglycemia, and epilepsy are very different disorders that affect the brain to produce superficially similar damage,[15] in that all three disorders seem to produce

BOX 3-2
SECONDARY CONSEQUENCES OF ISCHEMIA

Vascular Changes

Vasospasm
Red cell sludging
Hypoperfusion

Neuronal Changes

Intracellular acidosis
Release of excitatory amino acid neurotransmitters
Intracellular calcium overload
Calcium-mediated processes
Arachidonic acid cascade
Changes in chelation and compartmentalization of free
    metals
Altered oxygen metabolism
Production of free radicals (free radical damage)
Lipid peroxidation
Secondary depression of metabolism

similar neuronal necrosis. All three are disorders of cerebral energy metabolism in that they either stop or impede aerobic cellular energy production (ischemia and hypoglycemia) or enhance cellular energy consumption (epilepsy).

Ischemia produces a decrease in the cerebral circulation such that there is decreased delivery of oxygen and glucose and decreased removal of cellular waste products. Without the ability to produce ATP, the cellular concentrations of ATP decrease rapidly to near zero within 5 to 7 minutes after ischemia. Without ATP the transmembrane energy-dependent ion pumps fail, resulting in sodium (Na^+), chloride (Cl^-), and calcium (Ca^{2+}) influx, and potassium (K^+) efflux. As a result of ATP depletion and calcium influx, lipolytic and proteolytic reactions occur, and there is presynaptic release of excitatory neurotransmitters with an increase in glutamate and aspartate. During ischemia, increased amounts of intracellular lactic acid are formed. Permanent structural damage can occur with as little as 5 to 15 minutes of ischemia. However, the amount of time after ischemia before neuronal necrosis occurs is approximately 1 to 2 days, resulting in a long therapeutic window.

Like ischemia, hypoglycemia interferes with cerebral energy production, resulting in membrane depolarization, loss of ion homeostasis, lipolysis, and release of the excitatory amino acid neurotransmitters. In hypoglycemic coma (unlike ischemia), aspartate is released into the extracellular fluid much more than glutamate. Hypoglycemia can be tolerated for up to 60 minutes with full functional recovery although some neurons may die. Neuronal necrosis occurs within 2 to 6 hours of hypoglycemia,[14] much more rapidly than after ischemia. This allows a therapeutic window of only a few hours.

Epilepsy does not produce cerebral energy failure, even

during prolonged status epilepticus.[15] Tissue catabolism is less severe than in hypoglycemia. Although anaerobic glycolysis and tissue lactic acid production are stimulated during status epilepticus,[78] the accumulation of intracellular lactic acid is less than in ischemia.[265] The minimum duration of status epilepticus required to produce any neuronal necrosis is 45 to 60 minutes, a much longer duration than ischemia.[206] However, neuronal necrosis occurs very rapidly within 1 hour after the cessation of prolonged seizure activity.[139] This allows only a short therapeutic window after the cessation of prolonged seizures.

The excitotoxic theory of neuronal death (neuronal death is due to release within the brain of endogenous excitatory compounds that bind to excitatory surface receptors on neurons and ultimately cause necrosis) has been implicated in the selective death of neurons in all three disorders (ischemia,[23] hypoglycemia,[13,321] and epilepsy[109,216]). However, the brain damage produced by these insults is not equal and does not occur in the same areas. Ischemia produces necrosis in all middle laminae of the cortex, CA_4 and CA_1 neurons of the hippocampus, and the thalamic reticular nucleus in the thalamus. Hypoglycemia produces neuronal necrosis in the superficial layer of the cortex, the medial subiculum of the hippocampus, and the caudoputamen. Epilepsy produces necrosis in lamina three and four of the cortex but spares the caudate nucleus. Therefore the selectively vulnerable regions of brain are different with the three insults.

Given the preceding information, one can no longer conclude that these three insults produce similar damage (Table 3-2). However, basic mechanisms occurring in all three insults include selective neuronal necrosis, excess release of excitatory amino acids, and excess tissue acidosis.

PATHOPHYSIOLOGY OF ISCHEMIA
Vascular Changes

The principal vascular change after cerebral ischemia is delayed postischemic hypoperfusion.[8,136] When the circulation is restored after complete ischemia, there is a 15- to 20-minute period of reactive hyperemia. This occurs because the viscosity of the blood washing through the microcirculation is decreased relative to that of the stagnant blood pooled in the vascular beds[136] and because vascular tone is temporarily decreased by vasoactive substances released during ischemia. After this period of reactive hyperemia, postischemic hypoperfusion develops. The severity and duration of the postischemic hypoperfusion depends on the severity and duration of the ischemic insult. There is limited evidence that this postischemic hypoperfusion contributes to the ultimate neurologic damage occurring after ischemia[137,219] and that postischemic hypoperfusion in areas of increased functional (and metabolic) activity may contribute to the selective vulnerability of neurons in that area.

It is hypothesized that this postischemic hypoperfusion

TABLE 3-2
Differences Between Ischemia, Hypoglycemia, and Epilepsy

	Ischemia	Hypoglycemia	Epilepsy
Energy stores	Depleted	Reduced	Normal
Excitotoxin release	Glutamate	Aspartate	Unknown
Source of excitotoxins	Neurotransmitter pool	Metabolic pool	Neurotransmitter pool
Lactic acidosis	Mild to severe (dependent on blood glucose)	None	Mild
Duration of insult required to produce selective neuronal necrosis	2-10 min	10-20 min	45-120 min
Timing of neuronal death	Up to 2-4 days	1-8 hr	1-2 hr
Distribution of neuronal necrosis	Nuclear/laminar	Subnuclear, CSF	Transsynaptic
CBF during insult	Decreased	Increased	Increased
CBF after insult	Increased then decreased	Decreased	Unknown

CBF = cerebral blood flow; CSF = cerebrospinal fluid.
Modified from Auer RN, Siesjo BK: *Ann Neurol* 24:699, 1988.

is due in part to vasoconstriction caused by calcium ion (Ca^{2+}) activation of the contractile mechanisms in endothelial cells. An increase in intracellular Ca^{2+} in vascular smooth muscle cells occurring during ischemia activates myosin light-chain kinase, which in turn catalyzes the phosphorylation of myosin. This increases the actin-myosin interaction, resulting in contraction.[303] An increased production of thromboxane A_2, a potent vasoconstrictor, made from arachidonic acid during the recirculation and reoxygenation period after ischemia, may also contribute to the hypoperfusion. This hypoperfusion cannot be influenced by sympathomimetic vasoconstrictor substances or sympatholytic, direct-acting, or ganglionic blocking vasodilating substances but can be ameliorated by some calcium entry blockers and inhibitors of prostaglandin synthesis.

Membrane Changes

With complete cerebral ischemia, the high-energy phosphate stores of phosphocreatine are depleted within 1 minute, glucose and glycogen stores within 4 minutes, and ATP stores within 5 to 7 minutes.[263] This exhaustion of energy stores leads to failure of the membrane sodium pumps, allowing influx of Na^+ and Cl^-, efflux of K^+, and membrane depolarization.[236,263] The influx of Na^+ and Cl^- is accompanied by H_2O, which produces cell swelling.[263] When the extracellular K^+ concentration increases, changes in the plasma membrane potential open voltage-dependent Ca^{2+} channels, and increased concentrations of extracellular glutamate open receptor-controlled channels, resulting in a massive intracellular influx of Ca^{2+}.[27,236,263] It is hypothesized that failure of membranes to maintain normal ion gradients characterizes irreversible cell injury.

Mitochondria

Mitochondrial dysfunction also characterizes irreversible cell injury. The primary factors believed to cause cerebral mitochondrial damage during ischemia include intracellular lactic acidosis, Ca^{2+}-activated degradative enzymes, mitochondrial Ca^{2+} overload, and free-radical–induced membrane lipid peroxidation. Intracellular acidosis inhibits both mitochondrial respiration and Ca^{2+} sequestration by the mitochondria.[117,129] Calcium-activated degradative enzymes, including phospholipases and proteases, destroy phospholipids and proteins within cell and mitochondrial membranes. Mitochondrial sequestration of Ca^{2+} damages the mitochondrial electron transport chain and prevents the synthesis of ATP.

Glucose

It is a well-known clinical and laboratory phenomenon that hyperglycemia and increases in brain glucose worsen the cerebral injury after a period of complete or near-complete ischemia.* Perhaps less appreciated is the fact that the preischemic blood glucose level or the amount of glucose administered before ischemia need not be out of the clinically relevant range to augment postischemic cerebral injury.[153,233] In contrast to the situation of complete cerebral ischemia, the effect of hyperglycemia on postischemic outcome after focal cerebral ischemia is less well-defined. Studies in humans have shown either worse neurologic function[24,44,145,233,327] or no effect on function,[2,64] and animal studies have shown either worse† or improved infarct size.[101,149,333] Equally unsettled is the mechanism by which glucose affects cerebral injury after ischemia. With the exception of the effect of hyperglycemia on cerebral injury after a period of complete ischemia, relatively little is definitely known about the effect of glucose on the brain during ischemia.

The high energy demands of the brain are supplied by the utilization of ATP, which is produced by the oxidation of glucose through the Embden-Meyerhof pathway in the cytosol and the tricarboxylic acid cycle in the mitochondria (Fig. 3-3).[3] In the presence of oxygen, glucose is ini-

---

*References 153, 159, 160, 199, 228, 234, 235, 260.
†References 37, 69, 201, 202, 229, 330.

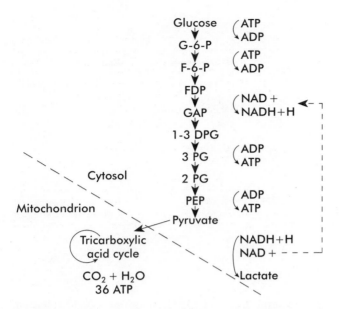

FIG. 3-3 Embden-Meyerhof pathway of glycolysis. During ischemia, pyruvate is metabolized to lactate to replenish the NAD+ supply for glycolysis. *(From Cucchiara RF, Michenfelder JD, editors: Clinical neuroanesthesia, New York, 1990, Churchill-Livingstone, p 175.)*

tially metabolized to pyruvate in the cytosol via the Embden-Meyerhof pathway, which produces 2 mol of ATP per mol of glucose. Pyruvate is then metabolized to carbon dioxide and water within the mitochondria via the tricarboxylic acid cycle. This produces 36 mol of ATP per mol of glucose.[3] During ischemia the cell must rely on both its reserves of high-energy phosphate bond energy and on glycolysis for the production of ATP. To continue glycolysis, pyruvate is converted to lactate to replenish the supply of nicotinamide adenine dinucelotide (NAD+). It is this production of lactate that underlies the most commonly proposed mechanism by which hyperglycemia aggravates cerebral ischemic injury. The mechanism is as follows: During periods of hyperglycemia, glucose diffuses across the blood-brain barrier, producing increases in brain glucose concentrations.[153,259,316] During ischemia, the brain anaerobically metabolizes glucose to lactic acid. If the ischemic insult occurs during a period of elevated brain glucose, lactic acid formation will be increased,[228,316] creating a pathologically acidic intracellular environment. It appears that ischemic brain lactate levels must increase to greater than 20 µmol/g to produce irreversible cell damage.[228,261] Below this lactate level, increased lactate accumulation is not associated with increased cerebral ischemic damage.[240] Hyperglycemia-enhanced injury could therefore be described as a threshold effect with no increase in ischemic damage occurring until ischemic brain lactate accumulation surpasses 20 µmol/g. Intracellular pH has been shown to remain stable until brain lactate reaches 17 µmol/g, at

which point it markedly decreases (from 6.9 to 6.2) as brain lactate rises beyond this level. These large decreases in brain intracellular pH may be responsible for the enhanced ischemic damage associated with high lactate levels.[52,61] This may also help to explain the finding that lactic acidosis may augment brain pathology more than other types of acidosis.[238] The molecular basis by which the increased cellular acid load produces irreversible cell damage is unknown. It has been hypothesized that the acidic reduction of ferric to ferrous iron and its subsequent release from organic stores may catalyze the formation of free oxygen radicals, with subsequent lipid peroxidation of cell membranes.[232]

Although the mechanism of hyperglycemia-enhanced cerebral ischemic injury commonly is proposed to be due to a rise in lactate production and concomitant tissue acidosis,[150,234] whether acidosis plays an important role in the pathogenesis of ischemic brain damage remains controversial.[218] In addition, there are data that challenge the association between increases in brain lactate and subsequent tissue damage or neurologic deficits.[133,134] Investigators recently proposed another significant contributing factor leading to the increased cerebral ischemic injury associated with hyperglycemia. It has been reported that hyperglycemia significantly attenuates the increase in brain tissue and cerebral spinal fluid (CSF) adenosine during ischemia[138,225] in animals. Adenosine, a purine nucleotide, is a cerebral vasodilator[25] that can inhibit the release of excitatory amino acids[63] and suppress neutrophil-endothelium interactions.[66] Theoretically, these cerebroprotective actions of adenosine would decrease the amount of ischemic damage and, conversely, attenuation of ischemic brain adenosine levels could potentiate the degree of damage.[138] It is proposed that this attenuation of cerebral adenosine production may be a factor in the pathogenesis of enhanced ischemic brain injury associated with hyperglycemia.[138]

Elevated blood glucose before ischemia has also been reported to be a direct cerebral vasoconstrictor that significantly reduces regional cerebral blood flow (rCBF) and increases heterogenicity in postischemic cerebral perfusion.[77,102,119,142] This postischemic regional heterogeneity of blood flow contrasts with the more regionally uniform alteration of flow caused by ischemia alone.[102] From these animal studies of hyperglycemia during global cerebral ischemia, one can conclude that preischemic blood glucose concentration, to the extent that it reflects intracellular glucose, lactate concentration, and pH and to the extent that it reduces rCBF, can significantly affect recovery from cerebral ischemia.

In five of five animal studies of glucose and complete cerebral ischemia,[67,153,199,200,234] elevated glucose in the blood or brain was associated with a worse postischemic outcome (Table 3-3). Of particular interest is the fact that the preischemic blood glucose levels in the glucose-administered animals in the majority of these studies were only moderately elevated,[67,153,200,234] and in one study

TABLE 3-3

Glucose and Neurologic Outcome After Global Cerebral
Ischemia

Authors	Species	Glucose Effect
Myers and Yamaguchi[199]	Monkeys	Worse function and histology*
Pulsinelli et al[234]	Rats	Worse histology
Longstreth et al[159]	Humans	Worse function
Longstreth and Inui[160]	Humans	Worse function
D'Alecy et al[67]	Dogs	Worse function
Lanier et al[153]	Monkeys	Worse function and histology
Nakakimura et al[200]	Cats	Worse function†

*This study contained the first report of glucose-induced enhancement of ischemic neurologic injury. The number of subjects was insufficient for statistical comparisons.

†There was a tendency toward more severe histologic injury in glucose-treated subjects (P = 0.07) in this study.

From Lanier WL: *Anesth Analg* 72:423, 1991.

TABLE 3-4

Glucose and Neurologic Outcome After Focal Cerebral
Ischemia

Authors	Species	Glucose Effect
Pulsinelli et al[233]	Humans	Worse function
Brint et al[37]	Rats	Worse infarct size
Candelise et al[44]	Humans	Worse function and lesion size*
Berger and Hakim[24]	Humans	Worse function and CT observations
Cox and Lorains[64]	Humans	No effect on function
Ginsberg et al[101]	Rats	Improved infarct size
Nedergaard and Diemer[202]	Rats	Worse histology; worse or no change in infarct size
Nedergaard[201]	Rats	Worse infarct size†
Woo et al[327]	Humans	Worse function
Adams et al[2]	Humans	No effect on function or CT lesion size‡
De Courten-Myers et al[69]	Cats	Worse infarct size
Prado et al[229]	Rats§	Worse cortical infarct size
Prado et al[229]	Rats§	No effect on cortical infarct size
Kiers et al[145]	Humans	Worse function and infarct size*
Zasslow et al[333]	Cats	Improved size of injury‖
Kraft et al[149]	Rabbits	Improved size of injury‖
Hoffman et al[134]	Rats¶	Worse function
Yip et al[330]	Rats	Worse infarct size

*Ischemic lesion size was determined using CT scans.

†Histology was described as more abnormal in glucose-treated rats, but data were not subjected to statistical analysis.

‡All patients received high-dose naloxone therapy.

§This study reported on two models of focal cerebral ischemia having differing severity of cortical ischemia.

‖Using a histologic assessment of size of injury.

¶This model is primarily of focal cerebral ischemia; however, it also includes an incomplete global ischemia component.

Modified from Lanier WL: *Anesth Analg* 72:423, 1991.

there was no significant difference in the preischemic blood glucose levels between groups treated with dextrose and with lactated Ringer's solution.[153] This suggests that even moderately increased blood glucose levels can augment postischemic neurologic injury. Death rates are also increased in animals receiving dextrose.[67] Moderate hyperglycemia has also worsened neurologic outcome in spinal cord ischemia.[75]

Of the two clinical studies that correlated blood glucose and neurologic outcome after complete cerebral ischemia, both are retrospective studies of patients surviving cardiac arrest. The first study was an attempt to develop a model that would forecast neurologic recovery after out-of-hospital cardiac arrest.[159] In this model, one of the four variables associated with a greater probability of awakening was an admission blood glucose level less than 300 mg/dl.[159] In the second study, all of the patients had received dextrose-containing solutions during resuscitation. The mean blood glucose level on hospital admission was found to be significantly higher in patients who never awakened (341 ± 13 mg/dl) than in patients who did awaken from coma (262 ± 7 mg/dl). Among those who awakened, the patients with persistent neurologic deficits had significantly higher mean glucose levels on admission (286 ± 15 mg/dl) than did those without deficits (251 ± 7 mg/dl).[160] Although acknowledging other explanations for the glucose–brain-injury association, such as the level of hyperglycemia being related to the stress of cardiac arrest and resuscitation or altered glucose metabolism in brain-damaged patients, the authors concluded that an elevated blood glucose level is a risk indicator for increased neurologic injury after cardiac arrest. They recommended that glucose infusions be avoided during and immediately after resuscitation in patients suffering cardiac arrest unless a low blood glucose level could be documented.[160] This recommendation has now been expanded to include all patients present-

ing to the emergency room with altered mental status. It is suggested that 50% dextrose be administered only to those patients in whom hypoglycemia is demonstrated.[39]

There is no consensus regarding the effect of increased blood glucose during focal cerebral ischemia although 12 of 18 cited studies of focal cerebral ischemia reveal an association between glucose and worse postischemic outcome* (Table 3-4). An excellent analysis of the six studies of focal cerebral ischemia that did not identify this association has been presented elsewhere.[152] The first human study of the effect of blood glucose on neurologic outcome in focal ischemia was a retrospective study of stroke patients.[233] Patients with diabetes, whose mean blood glucose level at hospital admission was 259 ± 125 mg/dl, had a significantly worse neurologic outcome and higher death rates than did nondiabetic patients (admission blood glucose 106 ± 19 mg/dl). A separate nondiabetic population with ischemic stroke was prospectively analyzed. Although the difference did not quite reach statistical significance be-

*References 24, 37, 44, 64, 69, 134, 145, 201, 202, 229, 233, 327.

cause of the small numbers involved (p = 0.061), patients with blood glucose levels >120 mg/dl had a worse neurologic outcome than patients with blood sugar levels <120 mg/dl.[233]

The question of whether aggressive therapy to normalize blood glucose levels before, during, or after a potentially ischemic event will improve neurologic outcome remains to be answered. A study of the effect of plasma glucose on infarct size in focal cerebral ischemia in rats showed that insulin treatment before ischemia in fed rats reduced hyperglycemic responses and infarct volume.[330] Timing of insulin treatment was critical: there was no significant difference in infarct volume between fed rats given insulin 30 minutes before ischemia and those receiving no treatment. However, rats given insulin 50 minutes before ischemia had significantly smaller infarct volumes than those treated 30 minutes before ischemia. Another study in rats found that treatment with insulin after transient forebrain ischemia significantly improved neurobehavioral performance and reduced ischemic neuronal necrosis.[305] Although these studies are promising, more work is needed to further define the effects and the timing of insulin treatment on blood glucose, intracellular lactate and pH, infarct size, and ultimate neurologic outcome in situations of focal or global ischemia.

There remains a large body of convincing data that high

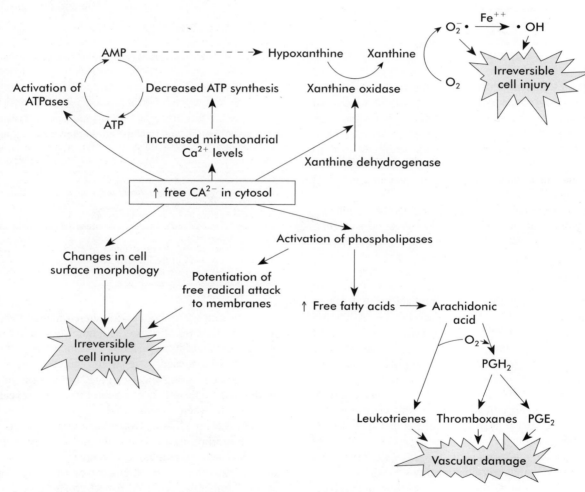

FIG. 3-4   Relationship among energy supply, cellular calcium regulation, the arachidonic acid cascade, the formation of prostaglandins, and the formation of free radicals. During ischemia, cellular stores of ATP are metabolized to AMP and ultimately to hypoxanthine. Increased cellular concentrations of Ca^{2+} activate proteases, converting xanthine dehydrogenase to xanthine oxidase, which catalyzes the metabolism of hypoxanthine to xanthine with superoxide radicals $(O_2^-\bullet)$ as a byproduct. Increased intracellular Ca^{2+} also activates phospholipases to release free fatty acids from cell membranes. During the reperfusion period, within the presence of oxygen, the primary free fatty acid, arachidonic acid, is metabolized to prostaglandins and leukotrienes. Free radicals and prostaglandins are responsible for cell injury after ischemia. (*Modified from Fuller BJ, Gower JD, Green CJ: Cryobiology 25:377, 1988.*)

blood glucose levels before and/or during an ischemic event in patients at risk for ischemia, either global or focal, may be deleterious and actually worsen neurologic outcome. Such patients include those resuscitated from cardiac arrest, those suffering from shock or severe dysrhythmias, those with vascular disease, those with evolving strokes, or those undergoing cardiac or cerebrovascular surgery. In these patients it is recommended that blood glucose levels be routinely monitored and that glucose-containing solutions not be used unless there is a risk of hypoglycemia.

Calcium

During ischemia, Ca^{2+} enters the cells through both voltage-dependent and agonist receptor–controlled channels and accumulates in the cytosol. This intracellular Ca^{2+} overload appears to be one of the common pathways leading to irreversible cell damage and death (Fig. 3-4). Calcium influx activates proteases that destroy cell membranes, resulting in receptor dysfunction and the failure of intracellular transport mechanisms. Increased intracellular Ca^{2+} also activates phospholipases A_1, A_2, and C, which hydrolyze phospholipids within mitochondrial and cell membranes to physically disrupt these membranes. These enzymes do not require oxygen or energy and so may function during or after ischemia. Hydrolysis of the membrane phospholipids releases free fatty acids (FFAs), which have detergent properties that can destroy the lipid portions of all membranes. The major FFA is arachidonic acid, which can be metabolized to free radicals, prostaglandins, and leukotrienes,[236,319] which can produce further changes in membrane permeability and ion distribution.[236] The normal

mechanisms for the control of intracellular Ca^{2+} concentration include the cell-membrane ATP-dependent Ca^{2+} translocase, the cell-membrane Ca^{2+}/Na^+ exchange pump, the ATP-dependent Ca^{2+} uptake of Ca^{2+} into the endoplasmic reticulum, and the sequestration of Ca^{2+} by the mitochondria at the expense of oxidative phosphorylation (Fig. 3-5).[263] All require energy and consume any ATP reserves or prevent further ATP synthesis. Only mitochondrial sequestration is available to the ischemic cell.

The calcium entry blockers form a heterogenous group of drugs, including derivatives of papaverine, dihydropyridine, and piperazine. These drugs block the influx of Ca^{2+} through the voltage-sensitive ion channels into the cells[302] and can block intracellular flux of calcium into mitochondria.[6,264] They are structurally and operationally distinct from the antagonists of excitatory neurotransmitters, which also block the entry of Ca^{2+} into the cell but through the excitatory amino-acid neurotransmitter receptor–controlled ion channels.

The calcium entry blockers vary in their effects on the myocardium and on the vasculature. The calcium entry blockers, which have been studied for brain protection, have been chosen because of their preferential effect on cerebral vessels. These include lidoflazine, nimodipine, and nicardipine. Protection by these drugs has been studied in focal ischemia and in complete global ischemia secondary to cardiac arrest.

Lidoflazine

Lidoflazine has been investigated only for its use in the prevention of neurologic damage from complete global isch-

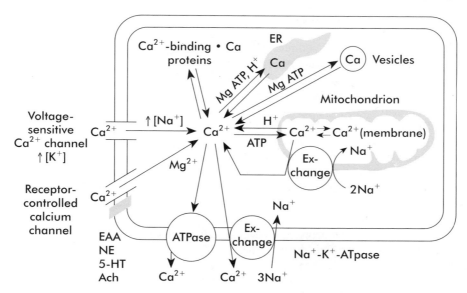

FIG. 3-5 Calcium transport processes. Calcium influx through cell membranes is passive down a concentration gradient through voltage-sensitive and NMDA receptor–controlled Ca^{2+} channels. Calcium efflux is via a Ca^{2+} translocase, and a Na^+-Ca^{2+} exchange mechanism, both of which require energy. Calcium uptake into cellular organelles (endoplasmic reticulum, vesicles, mitochondria) requires energy. (*Modified from Milde LN: Crit Care Clin 5:729, 1989.*)

emia after cardiac arrest. In animal models of cardiac arrest, the results with lidoflazine have been contradictory. One study reported improvement in postischemic hypoperfusion,[320] but subsequent studies have failed to demonstrate any effect of lidoflazine on postischemic cerebral blood flow.[84,325] Two animal studies have reported improvement in neurologic outcome with lidoflazine after complete cerebral ischemia,[325,297] but three studies have failed to demonstrate any improvement in neurologic outcome.[83,84] The only randomized *clinical* trial studied lidoflazine administered to patients remaining comatose after resuscitation from cardiac arrest. Lidoflazine produced no improvement in the proportion of patients who died, in the proportion who survived with good neurologic function, or in the proportion who survived with poor neurologic function.[35] From this one can conclude that lidoflazine, by itself, has no effect in ameliorating neurologic damage that occurs after prolonged cardiac arrest.

Nimodipine

Nimodipine, a dihydropyridine derivative, is the calcium entry blocker most extensively studied for its protective effects against cerebral ischemia. It has been studied in animal models of focal ischemia and in patients with acute strokes or after subarachnoid hemorrhage. It has also been studied in animal models of complete cerebral ischemia and in patients surviving cardiac arrest. Studies on the effect of nimodipine on rCBF when treatment is begun after the onset of focal ischemia are contradictory. Two studies reported improvement in regional cerebral blood flow to the ischemic areas, accompanied by a decrease in infarct size and an improvement in neurologic recovery.[100,172] However, one study reported that treatment with nimodipine failed to modify the pattern of rCBF distribution and had no effect on infarct size.[107]

In a study of patients with acute stroke, nimodipine produced a significant improvement in rCBF to the ischemic hemisphere, indicating that nimodipine produced an inverse (or Robin Hood) steal.[97] In two randomized, blinded, placebo-controlled trials of patients with acute strokes, treatment with nimodipine orally (120 mg daily) for 1 month after the stroke resulted in significantly less mortality and significantly faster and better improvement in neurologic function.[98,99] However, nimodipine had a differential effect on recovery. Neurologic recovery was greater in those patients whose initial deficits were mild to moderate. If the initial deficits were severe, nimodipine produced no improvement.[99] These studies on rCBF and neurologic outcome suggest that improvement in neurologic function is correlated with improvement in rCBF to the ischemic area and its penumbra. If the ischemia is mild, nimodipine may improve rCBF enough to restore normal neurologic function. If the ischemia is so severe that rCBF is below the threshold for cell survival, treatment with nimodipine will have no effect. These clinical trials are promising and suggest that nimodipine may be of benefit if started within 24 hours of the onset of stroke and administered in addition to standard treatment.

Nimodipine has been most extensively studied for its role in the treatment of vasospasm after subarachnoid hemorrhage (SAH). Several prospective, randomized, blinded, placebo-controlled studies on the use of nimodipine in patients after SAH* reported that patients treated with nimodipine had a significantly lower incidence of delayed ischemic deficits or death or had significantly better neurologic outcome than those patients given placebo. Although the number of patients in each of these studies was small, a metaanalysis of these studies clearly demonstrated that nimodipine treatment administered after SAH significantly decreased the incidence of delayed ischemic defects.[242] However, nimodipine has had no demonstrable effect on the extent and severity of vasospasm as determined by cerebral angiography. Similar to its effects in patients after stroke, nimodipine seemed to produce the most improvement in patients with moderate symptoms and produced little or no improvement in patients with severe symptoms.[223] The mechanism(s) of action of nimodipine in the amelioration of neurologic damage after SAH remains unclear. Nimodipine may be affecting the vasculature but does not seem to prevent vasospasm (at least as determined grossly by angiography) although it may lessen the severity of the vasospasm. It may be acting through its effects on neurons by preventing Ca^{2+} entry into the cells, Ca^{2+} sequestration by mitochondria, and subsequent alterations in metabolism of free fatty acid and the arachidonic acid cascade. Based on the previously mentioned studies, nimodipine, orally, (60 mg four times a day) is now recommended for patients with mild-to-moderate symptoms after subarachnoid hemorrhage caused by aneurysm rupture.

Nimodipine has also been studied for a possible protective effect in complete cerebral ischemia. Nimodipine has been reported to significantly ameliorate postischemic hypoperfusion.[144,194,283] This flow enhancement by nimodipine is regionally heterogeneous but tends to redistribute blood flow such that areas of low flow receive a greater increase in rCBF than areas of high flow, another example of a Robin Hood steal.[274] Nimodipine has also been shown to significantly improve neurologic recovery.[280] Because nimodipine improved both postischemic hypoperfusion and neurologic outcome, it has been concluded that postischemic hypoperfusion does contribute to the ultimate neurologic damage occurring after complete global ischemia. A prospective, randomized, blinded, placebo-controlled clinical trial of low-dose nimodipine in a small number of patients after cardiac arrest demonstrated that nimodipine significantly improved postischemic cerebral blood flow and shortened the time to awaken from coma but did not improve ultimate neurologic outcome.[87] A larger prospective, randomized, placebo-controlled study of patients re-

*References 7, 204, 215, 223, 224, 226.

▼

BOX 3-3
MECHANISMS OF ACTION OF CALCIUM ENTRY
BLOCKERS

Vasculature
  Vasodilation
  Prevention of vasospasm
Neuronal tissue
  Prevention of calcium entry into cells
  Prevention of calcium sequestration by mitochondria
    Alter free fatty acid metabolism
    Alter arachidonic acid cascade

---

suscitated from cardiac arrest reported that there was no improvement in survival rate or neurologic function in those patients receiving nimodipine. However, in a subset of patients in whom advanced life support measures were delayed 10 minutes or more from the onset of cardiac arrest, treatment with nimodipine significantly improved survival rate.[244,245]

Nicardipine, another dihydropyridine derivative, has been reported to decrease histopathologic damage after ischemia in cats[151] and rats.[111] Nicardipine does increase CBF after complete cerebral ischemia but does not improve neurologic outcome.[251]

These studies suggest that calcium entry blockers may be able to provide limited protection of, or improvement in, neurologic function when given to treat cerebral ischemia. Whether the major mechanism of action for this protection is an effect on the cerebral vasculature causing improvement in or redistribution of CBF or whether it is due to other subcellular neuronal effects has yet to be determined (Box 3-3).

Excitatory Amino Acid Neurotransmitters

The dicarboxylic amino acids, glutamate and aspartate, are excitatory neurotransmitters in many brain regions.[50,167] Glutamate normally is stored in vesicles in presynaptic terminals of neurons and released when the presynaptic axon is depolarized by calcium influx. Glutamate then acts at receptors on the postsynaptic neuron.[53,86] Normally the *extracellular* concentrations of glutamate increase only very briefly during synaptic transmission because of reuptake mechanisms in nerve terminals[288] and glia.[127] During cerebral ischemia, there is increased synaptic release[74] and impaired cellular reuptake of glutamate,[74] resulting in rapid increases in extracellular glutamate.[53,266] This increased extracellular concentration of glutamate then becomes neurotoxic.

Currently three postsynaptic receptors for the excitatory neurotransmitters are known: the N-methyl-D-aspartate (NMDA) receptor, the quisqualate [α-amino-3-hydroxy-5-methyl-4-isoxazole, AMPA] receptor, and the kainate re-

ceptor.[17] NMDA receptors occur in layers three, five, and six of the cerebral cortex, the thalamus, the striatum, the Purkinje and granule cell layers of the cerebellum, and the CA_1 region of the hippocampus. This indicates that there are high concentrations of this receptor in those brain regions that show selective vulnerability to ischemia. AMPA receptors occur in deep layers of cerebral cortex, thalamus, the striatum, the molecular layer of the cerebellum, and in the pyramidal cell layer and striatum lucidum of the hippocampus. Kainate receptors have been found only in the striatum lucidum of the hippocampus. Glutamate acts on all three receptors, but aspartate acts only on the NMDA receptor. All three receptors are linked to membrane cation channels. The kainate and AMPA receptors are linked to membrane channels that allow the influx of Na^+,[50] and the NMDA receptor is linked to membrane channels that allow the influx of Na^+ and Ca^{2+}.

Much research has focused on the NMDA receptor–controlled ion channel complex (Fig. 3-6).[5] The NMDA receptor is coupled to a membrane channel permeable to either Na^+ or Ca^{2+} influx, which can be blocked by magnesium (Mg^{2+}) attached within the channel. It is theorized that Mg^{2+} ions retain water and, in this bulky state, block the NMDA channel.[17] Zinc (Zn^+) can act as an antagonist of Mg^{2+} by attaching to the Mg^{2+} binding sites within the ion channel. Both chemical and electric signals affect the activity of the NMDA receptor–channel complex. Glutamate and aspartate excite the NMDA receptor. Glycine, usually an inhibitory transmitter, binds at a different site on the NMDA receptor to allow activation by glutamate. If glycine is not present, normal concentrations of glutamate do not open the NMDA receptor–controlled ion channels. The electrical action potential of the neuron also regulates the NMDA receptor and its ion channel activity. At a normal resting membrane potential, the NMDA ion channel is closed so that glutamate binding to the receptor induces little ion flux. Depolarization excites the NMDA receptor and dislodges the Mg^{2+} ions that block the NMDA channel when the cell is at rest. Activation of the NMDA receptor by glutamate then takes place to open the ion channel, allowing influx of Na^+ and/or Ca^{2+} into the neuron.

Under certain pathologic conditions, including ischemia, glutamate can become a neurotoxin to produce both immediate injury and delayed neuronal death. Immediate neuronal injury occurs after severe ischemia with energy depletion and is due to acute cell swelling. Increased concentrations of extracellular glutamate released during ischemia activate the NMDA receptor to open the membrane ion channels, allowing an influx of Na^+, membrane depolarization, a secondary passive influx of Cl^-, and with it, water, to produce cell swelling.[49,51,217,247] The cell swelling eventually causes lysis of the cell membrane and death.[247]

There is also a more slowly evolving neuronal degeneration in which neuronal injury after ischemia may not be apparent for up to 24 hours. Ca^{2+} can enter the cell through several routes: voltage-sensitive channels acti-

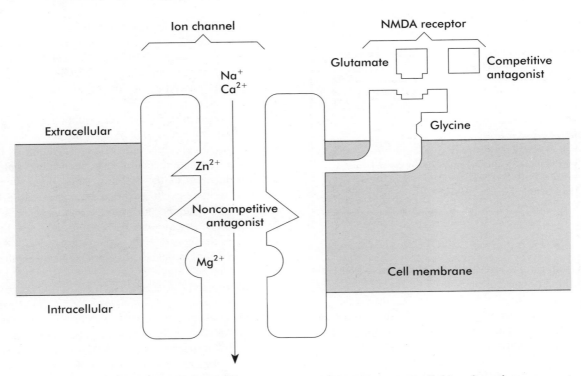

FIG. 3-6 Speculative schematic diagram of the NMDA receptor–controlled ion channel complex. Glutamate binding is facilitated by glycine and antagonized by competitive antagonists. Magnesium (Mg^{2+}), zinc (Zn^{2+}), and noncompetitive antagonists block the ion channel at specific binding sites. (*Modified from Albers GW: Clin Neuropharm 13:177, 1990.*)

vated by membrane depolarization, nonspecific leak conductance associated with cell swelling, or reverse operation of the Na^+-Ca^{2+} exchange mechanism, but the membrane channels controlled by NMDA receptors appear to be the most important for glutamate-related injury— that involving the selectively vulnerable regions of the brain.[198] The NMDA receptor–controlled channel may allow the highest percentage of calcium influx of any Ca^{2+} channel. It is theorized that the resultant increase in intracellular Ca^{2+} starts a cascade of reactions ultimately responsible for neuronal degeneration. Calcium entry into neuronal postsynaptic terminals can also increase the release of glutamate, thereby further propagating injury via a positive-feedback loop. This late propagation, in conjunction with the intrinsically delayed nature of the calcium-dependent glutamate injury, may account for the fact that ischemic neurologic injury can require nearly 24 to 72 hours to fully develop.[146,222,231]

Glutamate has been implicated as a mediator of neuronal damage during ischemia in the following way (Box 3-4)[59]:

1. The distribution of excitatory neurotransmitter receptors occurs primarily in those areas of the brain that are considered to be selectively vulnerable to ischemia.
2. Ischemia is associated with an increased concentration of glutamate in the extracellular space within a few minutes after cessation of blood flow.[23]
3. There is increased neuronal firing in the hippocampus produced by excitatory amino acids for up to 24 hours after ischemia.[289]
4. The interruption of glutaminergic nerve tracts to areas of high concentration of glutamate receptors has been reported to protect against ischemic injury.[322]
5. High concentrations of Mg^{2+}, which block synaptic transmission in general and NMDA receptor–controlled ion channels specifically, decrease ischemic neuronal injury.[143,246]
6. Pharmacologic blockade of postsynaptic NMDA receptors attenuates ischemic neurologic injury.[51]
7. In the first few minutes of reperfusion Ca^{2+} accumulates in neurons in a nonselective pattern presumably caused by entry through the voltage-dependent channels and impaired outward pumping of calcium. When energy metabolism is restored, the less vulnerable neurons rapidly return to normal appearance, whereas the neurons in the regions vulnerable to ischemia continue accumulation of Ca^{2+}, leading to neuronal damage.[269] This is hypothesized to be a consequence of burst firing brought about through the activation of NMDA receptors and Ca^{2+} influx through the NMDA receptor–controlled channels.[168]

▼

BOX 3-4
EVIDENCE FOR THE MEDIATION OF NEURONAL INJURY BY GLUTAMATE

High concentration of glutamate receptors occurs in areas of brain selectively vulnerable to ischemia

Increased concentrations of glutamate occur during ischemia

Increased neuronal firing occurs after ischemia

Interruption of glutaminergic nerve tracts to areas of high concentration of glutamate receptors decreases ischemic injury

High concentrations of Mg^{2+}, which block NMDA receptor–controlled ion channels, decreases ischemic injury

Pharmacologic blockade of NMDA receptor–controlled ion channels, decreases ischemic injury

Toxic intracellular calcium accumulation occurs in areas of brain selectively vulnerable to ischemia

▼

BOX 3-5
SITES OF ANTAGONISM ON THE NMDA RECEPTOR–CONTROLLED ION CHANNEL

Glutamate binding site (competitive)
Glycine binding site (noncompetitive)
Ion channel binding sites (noncompetitive)
    Magnesium binding site
    Zinc binding site
    Phencyclidine binding site
    Other sites (dextorphan, dextromethorphan)
Interference with secondary effects of glutamic excitatory neurotransmission

There are several types of antagonists to the NMDA receptor–ion channel complex (Box 3-5). The action of glutamate can be antagonized *competitively* by compounds that compete for the glutamate receptor binding site. Normally occurring competitive antagonists are highly polar molecules with poor BBB penetration. Competitive antagonists have been synthesized that do cross the BBB and therefore can act after systemic administration. However, because of the difficulty in making a nontoxic competitive antagonist with adequate BBB penetration that is effective in low concentrations, most biochemical research has concentrated on the noncompetitive antagonists.

The action of glutamate can also be antagonized *noncompetitively* by compounds that bind within the ion channel, thereby impeding ion flux through the channel. These include Mg^{2+}, Zn^+, and other compounds that bind to a separate phencyclidine binding site within the channel, including dizocilipine maleate and the dissociative anesthetics, ketamine and phencyclidine, which block the NMDA-receptor–associated ion channel in the open state. Dextorphan and dextromethorphan are also noncompetitive antagonists that block the ion channel in the closed state.[50] Noncompetitive antagonists are lipid soluble, easily cross the BBB, tend to concentrate in the brain, and have short half-lives. The effect of the noncompetitive antagonists cannot be overcome by increasing concentrations of glutamate, which would displace competitive antagonists. Noncompetitive NMDA antagonists have significant side effects, including non-NMDA-mediated excitatory synaptic transmission, impairment of learning,[58] morphologic neuronal changes, and psychomimetic and adverse behavioral properties.[4,248]

NMDA receptor antagonists have been studied to determine their effect on neurologic outcome after ischemia.

However, the results have been conflicting.[179,270] Improved outcome has been reported when NMDA antagonists were given after the onset of ischemia.[51,88,164,268,285] Many of these reported improvements were based only on histologic changes, emphasizing areas of known NMDA receptor concentration, the selectively vulnerable areas. Studies on the effects of NMDA antagonists in global ischemia have produced mixed results.[4,30,31,323] In those studies reporting improvement after complete ischemia, the noncompetitive receptor antagonist, dizocilipine maleate, was given.[30,31,323] This drug is known to decrease body temperature if not aggressively maintained, so decreases in brain temperature could have provided the observed neurologic protection rather than the dizocilipine maleate itself.

Antagonists to the glycine binding site have also been synthesized.[4] These too have been shown to prevent some neuronal injury after ischemia.[120,220] Drugs that interfere with the secondary effects of excessive NMDA activation or inhibit glutamate release during ischemia are also being investigated. In the future, these compounds might prove advantageous because they do not interfere with normal NMDA-mediated neuronal transmission.

Recent investigation has centered on the quisqualate or AMPA receptor–controlled ion channel complex. AMPA receptor activation causes depolarization of the plasma membrane, allowing Na^+ influx. AMPA receptor stimulation may activate voltage-dependent ion channels and may reverse the Na^+/Ca^{2+} exchange mechanism. It has been demonstrated that an antagonist to the AMPA receptor, NBQX [2,3-dihydroxy-6-nitro-7-sulfamoyl-benzo (F) quinoxaline], readily crosses the BBB and can decrease ischemic neuronal injury even when administered after ischemia. The exact intracellular mechanisms whereby AMPA receptor activation contributes to cell injury are unknown. However, blockade of this receptor may become an important therapeutic intervention against brain damage from cerebral ischemia in the future.

Present evidence suggests that selective neuronal death after transient cerebral ischemia involves excitatory neurotransmitters. NMDA or AMPA antagonists may offer a new strategy for the treatment of ischemic brain injury. This new approach is supported scientifically by some promising results with therapy in a variety of animal models of ischemia. The identification of several different classes of drugs that can block excitation at postsynaptic receptors opens the possibility for prevention and treatment of cerebral ischemia. Further studies should identify active compounds and their possible use in preventing or ameliorating the neurologic damage produced by ischemia.

Prostaglandins

Prostaglandins are products of the interaction between molecular oxygen and FFAs (Fig. 3-7). Accessible phospholipids from cell membranes are converted by hydrolysis to FFAs by phospholipase A_2. FFAs are normally converted to acyl-CoA by an ATP-dependent ligase and then enter into the tricarboxylic acid cycle. However, during ischemia this metabolism of FFAs cannot take place because of the depletion of ATP. Therefore the concentration of FFAs increases. High concentrations of FFAs can be deleterious to mitochondrial function because they uncouple oxidative phosphorylation, cause efflux into the cytosol of K^+ and Ca^{2+} ions stored within the mitochondria, and increase prostaglandin synthesis.

The most common FFA is arachidonic acid, the precursor of the prostaglandins. The concentration of arachidonic acid in normal tissues is near zero. An increase in arachidonic acid concentration can be stimulated by a variety of conditions, including trauma, hypoxia, severe hypoglycemia, pyrogen fever, convulsions, tissue dissection, or ischemia.[326] With reperfusion and reoxygenation after ischemia, arachidonic acid is converted by cyclo-oxygenase to the endoperoxides PGG_2 and PGH_2, which are short-lived intermediates (Fig. 3-7). PGG_2 is the precursor of prostacyclin (PGI_2) made in vascular endothelial cells, and PGH_2

is the precursor of thromboxane A_2 (TxA_2) synthesized in platelets. Arachidonic acid is also converted by lipoxygenase in leukocytes to leukotrienes, which are the slow reactive substances of anaphylaxis (SRS-A), and by lipoxygenase in platelets to hydroperoxy acids (HPETE) and peroxy acids (HETE).[324] It is hypothesized that during and immediately after ischemia the endoperoxide intermediates inactivate prostacyclin synthetase that is in the wall of the ischemic cerebral vessels so that relatively less prostacyclin (a potent vasodilator) is made.[80] The reduced synthesis of prostacyclin then results in increased synthesis of thromboxane A_2,[299] a potent vasoconstrictor, which may contribute to postischemic hypoperfusion.

Arachidonic acid itself, the short-lived endoperoxides, and thromboxane A_2 are potent platelet aggregators that can contribute to hypoperfusion. The endoperoxides are also potential free radicals, and an increase in their production may elicit a cascade of harmful reactions, including cross-linking reactions of membrane phospholipids and proteins and peroxidation of the polyunsaturated fatty acids in cell membranes. These reactions have the potential to irreversibly change cell structure such that cell and mitochondrial membrane function are altered.

It has been hypothesized that inhibitors of the arachidonic acid cascade might attenuate postischemic hypoperfusion and thereby ameliorate neuronal damage after ischemia. The production of prostaglandins can be blocked by the cyclo-oxygenase inhibitor, indomethacin, if it is given before the ischemic event such that postischemic hypoperfusion is prevented.[71] Another inhibitor of prostaglandin synthesis, ibuprofen, has been reported to improve CBF after complete global ischemia.[108] However, inhibition of prostaglandin synthesis by indomethacin given after ischemia has no effect on postischemic hyperperfusion or on neurologic outcome.[34,115] Although ischemia increases the

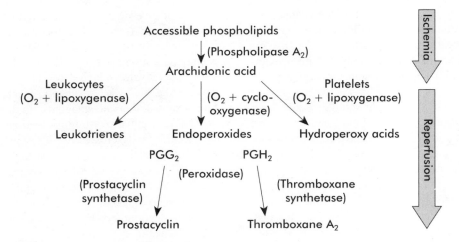

FIG. 3-7   Role of arachidonic acid in the production of leukotrienes, endoperoxides, hydroperoxy acids, and prostaglandins with reperfusion and reoxygenation after ischemia. *(From Milde LN: Crit Care Clin 5:729, 1989.)*

concentration of thromboxane,[72,148] research on specific inhibitors of thromboxane has failed to improve cerebral perfusion or neurologic outcome following ischemia.[230]

Free Radicals

Most molecules have chemical bonds consisting of a pair of electrons. The two electrons spin in opposite directions, thereby canceling each other's magnetic field, resulting in a low-energy state. Free radicals are molecules with an odd number of electrons formed by a break in a covalent bond. The bond splits symmetrically, and both fragments of the molecule retain a single electron. This unpaired electron has a magnetic field that produces a high-energy state, making the molecule highly reactive and unstable with a very short half-life.[281] Because of this, free radicals exist only in very low concentration and do not travel far from their site of formation. Such molecules react with adjacent nonradical molecules to produce a stable molecule and a new free radical. This starts a chain reaction of free radical generation until it is terminated by the random collision of two free radicals to form a molecule with a stable bond or until quenched by a free radical scavenger molecule, a molecule with a structure that imparts chemical stability to the free radical.

Free radicals are produced in small amounts in normal cellular processes.[253] Free radicals can be generated during oxidative phosphorylation in the mitochondrial electron transport system in which production of ATP is linked to the reduction of molecular oxygen to water.[54] Under normal conditions the mitochondrial electron transport system adds four electrons at once to O_2, reducing it to H_2O. However, leaks in the mitochondrial electron transport allow the acceptance of single electrons. If the four electrons are acquired singly, a series of free radical intermediates are formed (superoxide, $O_2^-\bullet$; hydrogen peroxide, H_2O_2; and the hydroxyl radical, $\bullet OH$).[54] These free radicals usually remain tightly bound within the mitochondrial membrane so that they can donate electrons further down the mitochondrial electron transport system. Normally they present no threat to the cell. Some leak of the free radicals does occur, but this is usually controlled by scavenging mechanisms. Free radicals can also be produced during the synthesis of prostaglandins, by autooxidation of small molecules, including the catecholamines, and by the microsomal cytochrome P-450 reductase system.[93]

Superoxide is the first free radical formed by univalent reduction (adding one electron) to molecular oxygen. Under normal conditions, superoxide radicals dismutate spon-

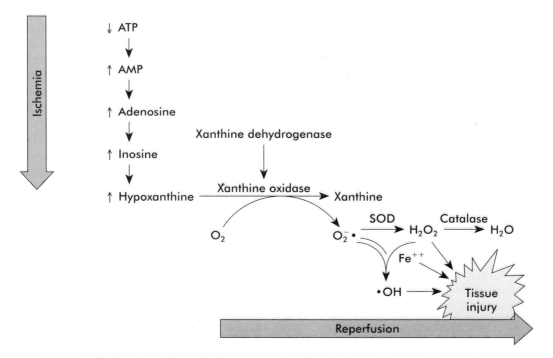

FIG 3-8 Mechanism of free radical generation in ischemic tissues after reperfusion and reoxygenation. With the onset of ischemia, ATP is metabolized to the adenine nucleotides and ultimately to the purine bases, causing accumulation of hypoxanthine. During ischemia, xanthine dehydrogenase is converted to xanthine oxidase. During reperfusion and reoxygenation, hypoxanthine is converted to xanthine by xanthine oxidase, which produces superoxide radicals ($O_2^-\bullet$) as a byproduct. Using ferrous iron (Fe^{++}) released during ischemia, superoxide radicals are converted to the more highly reactive hydroxyl radicals ($\bullet OH$) in the Fenton reaction. Free radicals can destroy cellular membranes, causing irreversible tissue damage.

taneously to hydrogen peroxide.[94] Hydrogen peroxide is a weak oxidizing agent and can react catalytically with transitional metals (iron and copper) to form the hydroxyl radical in a reaction known as the Fenton reaction.[85] Hydroxyl radicals are the most reactive of the free radicals and react with almost any intracellular molecule: carbohydrates, lipids, proteins, or nucleic acid bases. Polyunsaturated fatty acids are particularly susceptible to hydroxyl radical attack, forming lipid radicals. This is the initial step in the chain reaction of lipid peroxidation.[312] Lipid radicals react with oxygen to form lipid hydroperoxides and other products (alkanes, alkenes, hydroxy and epoxy derivatives, ketones, and polyhydroperoxides). Most of these radical products are toxic to cells even in small quantities.

During ischemia, several events take place that predispose to the formation of free radicals (Fig. 3-8). Ischemia stops the production of ATP, and the existing stores of ATP are rapidly metabolized for energy. With depletion of the cell's energy stores, transmembrane ion gradients cannot be maintained. This allows a massive influx of calcium. The metabolism of ATP also increases the cellular concentrations of AMP (adenosine monophosphate). AMP is metabolized to adenosine and inosine intermediates, and then to hypoxanthine. The elevated cytosolic calcium concentration activates the protease, calpain, which converts xanthine dehydrogenase to xanthine oxidase. In addition, sulfhydryl oxidation in ischemic tissues can convert xanthine dehydrogenase to xanthine oxidase. Xanthine oxidase converts the hypoxanthine that has accumulated in the cells during ischemia to xanthine, reducing O_2 to the superoxide radical as a byproduct. This appears to be the major source of superoxide radicals in postischemic tissues.

The formation of superoxide radicals is increased during the reperfusion period after ischemia because of the abundance of reducing equivalents, such as nicotinamide adenine dinucleotide phosphate (NADPH), which are produced in excess during ischemia, the action of xanthine oxidase, and the availability of molecular oxygen.[70] Intracellular levels of free iron may increase during ischemia because of Ca^{2+}-mediated mitochondrial injury releasing stores of mitochondrial iron and because of the release of free iron from ferritin.[318] This increased free iron concentration catalyzes the conversion of the superoxide radicals to the more highly reactive and toxic hydroxyl radicals.[48,253] With reperfusion free radicals can also be generated as byproducts of the oxidation of arachidonic acid (released from membrane phospholipids during ischemia) to produce prostaglandins and leukotrienes.

It is *hypothesized* that cellular damage that occurs after ischemia may be due in part to biochemical alterations produced by superoxide and hydroxyl radicals.[318] Neuronal membranes, rich in polyunsaturated fatty acids, are especially susceptible to attack by free radicals at carbon-carbon double bonds. Peroxidation of the polyunsaturated fatty acids in the membranes severely damages them. Potential consequences of damage to membranes include changes in fluidity and permeability and in the orientation of proteins embedded within the membranes, altering their function.[38,116] The end products of lipid peroxidation are aldehydes, hydrocarbon gases, and other residue that can cause cytotoxic and vasogenic cell edema, alter vascular endothelial and BBB permeability, and produce inflammation and chemotaxis.[276,277] Superoxide radicals themselves can elicit an inflammatory response with a resultant influx of neutrophils that will respond by secreting oxygen radicals of their own and by forming vascular plugs, thereby increasing cellular edema.[312]

The normal defense systems against free radical damage include spatial separation of radical-generating reactions and target molecules, enzymatic systems that quench free radicals, and antioxidative enzymes that scavenge free radicals.[262] Free radical scavengers include the superoxide dismutases directed against superoxide, catalase and glutathione peroxidase directed against H_2O_2, and vitamin E and ceruloplasmin directed against those radicals in lipid and aqueous phases. Vitamin E neutralizes free radicals by donating hydrogen atoms, leaving an unpaired electron on the vitamin E molecule, but this free radical is harmless. Vitamin C exists as a relatively unreactive free radical, which, by combining with the superoxide or hydroxyl radicals, prevents further propagation of chain reactions. Uric acid can scavenge hydroxyl radicals and can bind transitional metals to prevent hydroxyl radical formation. Transferrin can bind free iron, and plasma ceruloplasmin can convert free iron to ferric iron. It is the free iron that catalyzes the Fenton reaction to form hydroxyl radicals. Superoxide dismutase catalyzes the conversion of two superoxide radicals to hydrogen peroxide and water. Catalase converts hydrogen peroxide into O_2 and H_2O, and glutathione peroxidase uses hydrogen peroxide to oxidize glutathione. The brain contains only small concentrations of the free radical scavengers: superoxide dismutase, catalase, glutathione peroxidase, and vitamin E. Therefore, during reperfusion after ischemia, superoxide dismutase and catalase, capable of destroying the superoxide radicals formed during normal aerobic metabolism, are overwhelmed. This results in an increased concentration of superoxide radicals, some of which are converted to hydroxyl radicals by iron-catalyzed reactions.[16]

Therapy designed to prevent ischemic damage by free radicals includes anoxic reperfusion to deliver free radical scavengers before reoxygenation; administration of specific free radical scavengers, such as superoxide dismutase or catalase, or the nonspecific scavenger, vitamin E, to scavenge free radicals and block the chain reaction formation of more free radicals; the binding of free iron by iron chelators, such as deferoxamine, to prevent the formation of hydroxyl radicals and the subsequent cell damage initiated by them; and inhibition of xanthine oxidase by allopurinol to block the formation of xanthine and the subsequent formation of superoxide radicals.

Currently, free radical damage as a cause of neuronal

cell injury or death is only a hypothesis. Although in vitro studies have reported that free radicals are capable of damaging central nervous system tissue, it is still unclear whether and where free radicals contribute to cerebral ischemic damage in vivo. It is difficult to directly observe superoxide and hydroxyl radicals in biologic systems because they are extremely short-lived and are produced only in minute quantity. Free radical damage must be demonstrated in vivo before it can be determined that early application of effective anti-free-radical or antiperoxidative agents can promote survival and neurologic recovery after central nervous system injury. The efficacy of the administration of protective enzymes or free radical scavengers in ameliorating neurologic injury after cerebral ischemia is the subject of much investigation. The beneficial effect, if any, of such use of scavenging agents depends on the possibility of mediation of the pathology produced by free radicals, the biologic compatibility of the scavenging agents, the dosage used, and the ability to deliver the scavenger to act at the cellular site where the free radicals are causing injury.[277]

Steroids

Certain glucocorticoid steroids in high concentrations have been shown to inhibit lipid peroxidation of cell membranes and to protect susceptible fatty acids within the membranes from peroxidative attack by oxygen free radicals.[112] A new class of steroids, the 21-aminosteroids, lack glucocorticoid activity.[163] The 21-aminosteroids readily cross the BBB and are extremely potent inhibitors of iron-catalyzed lipid peroxidation. If free radical destruction of membranes via lipid peroxidation contributes significantly to irreversible cell damage after ischemia, 21-aminosteroids may provide protection from these secondary consequences of ischemia. It remains to be shown whether the 21-aminosteroids actually reduce free radical generation or lipid peroxidation in vivo. A few animal studies have investigated the efficacy of 21-aminosteroids in preventing neurologic injury after focal and complete global cerebral ischemia. U74006F and U74500A, when given after ischemia, have been shown to protect some selectively vulnerable CA_1 hippocampal neurons and certain neocortical areas against ischemia and to improve survival,[113] reduce ischemic brain edema,[331] and attenuate postischemic hypoperfusion.[114] U74500A can also bind iron, which may explain its greater efficacy against lipid peroxidation.

Hypothermia

The capacity of hypothermia to protect the brain and other vital organs during periods of decreased or absent oxygen delivery is well known and used daily during cardiac surgery. Total circulatory arrest is commonly induced in patients for up to 60 minutes at 15 to 18° C without any subsequent neurologic injury.[291] The classic mechanism proposed for protection by hypothermia is an inhibition of oxygen and glucose consumption sufficient to permit tolerance of prolonged periods of oxygen interruption. Hypothermia decreases the energy requirements of the brain by decreasing both the activation metabolism required for neuronal function, as indicated by electroencephalogram (EEG) activity, and the residual metabolism necessary for the maintenance of cellular integrity. However, the relationship of temperature to the cerebral metabolic rate for oxygen consumption must be known in order to predict the cerebral protection that can be anticipated at any given temperature if total cerebral protection is due to alterations in metabolic rate alone. The relationship between temperature and cerebral metabolism is expressed by the temperature coefficient Q_{10}, which is the ratio of the rates of oxygen consumption separated by 10° C.[184] However, the relationship between temperature and cerebral oxygen consumption is not a single exponential because hypothermia affects both components of neuronal oxygen metabolism: neuronal function and the reactions necessary for cellular integrity. A Q_{10} of approximately 2.2 to 2.4 between the temperatures of 37° C and 27° C is consistent with the Q_{10} for most biologic reactions, with little effect on neuronal function.[182,184,284] However, between 27° C and 14° C, the Q_{10} is approximately 4.5.[184,284] The large increase in Q_{10} that occurs in this temperature range is accompanied by cessation of neuronal function (the EEG is progressively suppressed and eventually becomes isoelectric). Below 14° C with the total cessation of neuronal function, the Q_{10} is approximately 2.2 to 2.4 again.[184] Thus, if a decrease in cerebral metabolism were the only mechanism by which hypothermia protected the brain, knowledge of the Q_{10} would permit calculation of the duration of tolerable ischemia.

However, recent studies have indicated that a decrease in cerebral metabolism may not be the only mechanism by which hypothermia provides protection from ischemia. Animal studies have demonstrated that small differences in brain temperature can critically determine the extent of neuronal injury. It has been reported[41] that decreases of 2 to 6° C in brain temperature markedly attenuated or abolished histopathologic damage in selectively vulnerable areas of the brain after incomplete global ischemia. These dramatic changes in histopathology occurred despite the fact that these differences in brain temperature had no significant influence on cerebral metabolism as indicated by concentrations of cerebral metabolites. This study was confirmed by another[196] in which spontaneous cooling of the brain to approximately 32° C or deliberate cooling of the brain to 35 or 33° C significantly attenuated the ischemic damage in the brain regions vulnerable to ischemia. A third study[252] also reported that a decrease in brain temperature of 3° C during incomplete global ischemia significantly reduced the histologic damage in the brain regions selectively vulnerable to ischemia. In a model of fluid percussion brain injury, a decrease in brain temperature of 6° C significantly reduced mortality and neurologic deficit.[55] These studies indicate that mechanisms other than a reduction in cerebral metabolism are operative in protection from ischemic damage by hypothermia. However, an earlier study reported[26]

▼

BOX 3-6
PROPOSED MECHANISMS OF PROTECTION BY HYPOTHERMIA

Decrease in cerebral metabolism
Maintenance of the integrity of membrane ion channels
Preservation of ion homeostasis
Decrease in excitatory neurotransmission
Decrease in calcium flux
Prevention of lipid peroxidation
Maintenance of the blood-brain barrier

▼

BOX 3-7
COMPLICATIONS OF DEEP HYPOTHERMIA

Cardiovascular Complications
Myocardial depression
Dysrhythmias including ventricular fibrillation
Hypotension
Inadequate tissue perfusion
Ischemia

Coagulation
Thrombocytopenia
Fibrinolysis
Platelet dysfunction
Increased bleeding

Metabolism
Slowed metabolism of anesthetic agents
Prolonged neuromuscular blockade
Increased protein catabolism

Shivering
Increased oxygen consumption
Increased carbon dioxide production
Increased cardiac output
Arterial oxygen desaturation
Hemodynamic instability

that small, 1 to 3° C differences in body (rectal) temperature (brain temperature was not measured and may have varied more than rectal temperature) during incomplete global ischemia significantly reduced the amount of anaerobic metabolism that occurred as measured by concentrations of cerebral metabolites. Because this is the only evidence that small changes in brain temperature significantly alter cerebral metabolism, other mechanisms for the observed protective effect have been proposed. These include effects on ion homeostasis, excitatory neurotransmission,[43] calcium flux, membrane lipid peroxidation, and permeability of the blood-brain barrier (Box 3-6). If these protective effects of small decreases in brain temperature can be substantiated with other animal studies of neurologic function or outcome after focal and complete global cerebral ischemia, mild hypothermia may become a very useful clinical technique. The significant side effects occurring with deep hypothermia are attenuated or avoided with mild hypothermia.

Deep hypothermia of less than 27° C requires cardiopulmonary bypass with surgery, general anesthesia, and support of the circulation because the heart commonly fibrillates at temperatures below 26 to 28° C. Complications of deep hypothermia include myocardial depression, dysrhythmias, hypotension, and tissue injury caused by inadequate tissue perfusion. Metabolic acidosis may result from decreased perfusion caused by inadequate blood flow and temperature gradients between core and periphery. Hypothermia may also produce bleeding disorders such as thrombocytopenia,[292] fibrinolysis,[106] and platelet dysfunction[298] with increased blood loss. Even mild hypothermia slows drug metabolism and prolongs neuromuscular blockade.[123,124] Deep hypothermia increases protein catabolism[46] and produces hypokalemia[32] after surgery. Postoperative complications include shivering with increased oxygen consumption and carbon dioxide production, hemodynamic instability, arterial oxygen desaturation because of changes in the oxy-hemoglobin desaturation curve, increased oxygen solubility at low temperatures, and inhibition of hypoxic pulmonary vasoconstriction (Box 3-7).

Anesthetics
Barbiturates

Anesthetic drugs that have been used to protect the brain from ischemia can exert their protective effects in three ways[3,27,171]: (1) reduction in oxygen demand, (2) increase in oxygen delivery, and (3) inhibition of deleterious pathologic intracellular processes. These categories are not mutually exclusive, as any one agent may provide protection via more than one mechanism.

Barbiturates have served as the prototype for anesthetic protection against cerebral ischemia. Their primary mechanism of protection is attributed to their ability to decrease the cerebral metabolic rate for oxygen (CMR_{O_2}), thereby increasing the ratio of oxygen supply to oxygen demand. Specifically, it has been proposed that the barbiturates selectively decrease the energy expenditure required for synaptic transmission and neuronal function, while maintaining the energy required for basic neuronal integrity.[175,185,281] The reduction in cerebral oxygen consumption that parallels the reduction in neuronal function reaches a plateau when neuronal function is abolished as seen by an isoelectric EEG.[173] This decrease in CMR_{O_2} is accompanied by a parallel decrease in CBF and cerebral blood volume, which is the mechanism by which the barbiturates

▼

BOX 3-8
Proposed Mechanisms of Barbiturate Protection

Decrease in cerebral metabolic requirements
Improvement in distribution of rCBF
Suppression of seizures
Suppression of catecholamine-induced hyperactivity
Anesthesia, deafferentation, immobilization
Loss of thermoregulation
Decrease in ICP
Decrease in cerebral edema
Decrease in CSF secretion
Scavenging of free radicals
Stabilization of membranes
Blockade of calcium channels
Alteration in fatty acid metabolism

From Cucchiara RF, Michenfelder JD, editors: *Clinical neuroanesthesia*, New York, 1990, Churchill-Livingstone, p 193.

▼

BOX 3-9
Experimental Models of Cerebral Ischemia

I. Focal ischemia
  A. Selective arterial occlusion
    1. Permanent (stroke)
    2. Temporary (intraoperative ischemia)
  B. Arterial embolization
  C. Subarachnoid hemorrhage with vasospasm
II. Incomplete global ischemia
  A. Arterial occlusion with hypoxia
  B. Arterial occlusion with systemic hypotension
  C. Severe drug-induced hypotension
  D. Exsanguination
  E. Intracranial hypertension
III. Complete global ischemia
  A. Cardiac arrest
    1. Ventricular fibrillation
    2. Administration of KCl
    3. Cardiopulmonary bypass — stop pump
  B. Aortic occlusion
  C. Neck tourniquet inflation with hypotension
  D. Exsanguination
  E. Intracranial hypertension

From Cucchiara RF, Michenfelder JD, editors: *Clinical neuroanesthesia*, New York, 1990, Churchill-Livingstone, p 191.

decrease intracranial pressure (ICP). It is also the mechanism by which barbiturates may redistribute rCBF and possibly shunt blood from normal areas of brain to ischemic areas.[36,82] Both of these mechanisms may contribute secondarily to the protective effect of barbiturates. Other proposed mechanisms of barbiturate protection during cerebral ischemia are listed in Box 3-8.

Before discussing the potential for cerebral protection with barbiturates (and other anesthetics), it is important to differentiate between reports concerning focal or incomplete ischemia or hypoxia as opposed to those concerning complete ischemia or asphyxia (anoxia). A more detailed list of the animal experimental models for each condition can be found in Box 3-9. With the onset of complete global ischemia, brain function, as reflected by EEG activity, is abolished within 15 to 30 seconds and basal metabolism is almost immediately induced, precluding any further metabolic suppression by anesthetics. Complete global ischemia also obviously precludes any vascular effects in the form of redistribution of cerebral blood flow, which are possible with regional or incomplete ischemia. By contrast, during focal ischemia or hypoxemia wherein neuronal function is not completely abolished and the ischemic area continues to consume energy at greater than basal levels, anesthetics such as barbiturates can decrease metabolism down to basal levels and perhaps either prolong the brain's tolerance for the injury or prevent infarction altogether.[173] Because barbiturates are also capable of constricting normal vessels, they might shunt blood flow toward the ischemic area (inverse steal) and thereby provide protection.[62] This latter mechanism could not be operative in models of global ischemia or hypoxia. If barbiturate-induced brain

protection is determined solely by its ability to decrease cerebral metabolic demand associated with neuronal function and/or favorably redistribute cerebral blood flow, then it is not surprising that cerebral protection is not demonstrable in the event of complete ischemia, but a beneficial effect is demonstrable in models of focal ischemia.[177]

There are no confirmed studies demonstrating that barbiturates provide any cerebral protection after complete global ischemia in either experimental animal models of cardiac arrest (Table 3-5) or in humans resuscitated from cardiac arrest. Three initial reports from animal models of complete cerebral ischemia that high-dose barbiturate treatment administered before (pentobarbital),[104] during (methohexital),[329] or after (thiopental)[29] cardiac arrest improved neurologic outcome were refuted by subsequent studies in the same[103,282] or other[275] animal models of complete global ischemia. Although postischemic treatment with thiopental failed to improve neurologic outcome in survivors of a ventricular fibrillation model of cardiac arrest, it did demonstrate improved survival rate with thiopental therapy.[293]

In humans, the only well-conducted, multiinstitutional, randomized clinical trial showed that treatment with thiopental in patients who remained comatose after resuscitation from cardiac arrest showed no beneficial effect on neu-

TABLE 3-5
Barbiturate Protection/Amelioration in Global Brain Anoxia

Author	Species	Barbiturate	Protection/Amelioration
Goldstein et al,[104] 1966	Dog	Pentobarbital (before)	Yes
Yatsu et al,[329] 1972	Rabbit	Methohexital (during)	Yes
Bleyaert et al,[29] 1978	Rhesus	Thiopental (after)	Yes
Steen et al, [282] 1979	Dog	Pentobarbital (before)	No
Snyder et al,[275] 1979	Dog	Thiopental (after)	No
Todd et al,[293] 1982	Cat	Thiopental (after)	No
Gisvold et al,[103] 1984	Pigtail	Thiopental (after)	No

From Michenfelder JD: *Anesthesia and the brain*, New York, 1988, Churchill-Livingstone, p 102.

rologic outcome as compared with those receiving standard therapy.[1] This report combined with the recent consistently negative animal studies led to the conclusion that the use of barbiturates is not justified in an attempt to prevent irreversible anoxic and ischemic brain injury after cardiac arrest.[328]

In contrast is the positive experimental evidence in laboratory animals that barbiturates provide protection from neurologic injury after focal cerebral ischemia.* Some of these reports, however, are contradictory and confusing, probably because of the many variables besides the barbiturates influencing outcome in these studies. The effectiveness of barbiturate protection in focal ischemia can be affected by the experimental model; species differences; the type of barbiturate; the dose, timing, and duration of administration[157]; the temporary or permanent nature of cerebral vascular occlusion; cardiovascular and respiratory responses to barbiturates; glucose levels; and incidence of seizures.

One of the first reports to draw attention to the beneficial effects of thiopental in regional ischemia used a *canine* model of permanent middle cerebral artery (MCA) occlusion. Pretreatment with pentobarbital (56 mg/kg) or thiopental (40 mg/kg), or thiopental given after MCA occlusion resulted in significantly less neurologic injury and less cerebral infarction than in animals receiving 1 to 2 minimum alveolar concentration (MAC) halothane anesthesia.[271] In a similar study of permanent MCA occlusion in *primates*,[131] large doses of pentobarbital (60 to 120 mg/kg) administered before ischemia significantly decreased infarct size when compared with halothane-anesthetized animals, but there were no differences in neurologic outcome between the groups. This lack of improvement in outcome despite a reduction in infarct size produced by the barbiturates may have been due to the small number of animals in each group or to the cardiovascular and respiratory complications occurring in the barbiturate group that were not aggressively treated. Cerebral protection has also been provided by smaller initial doses of barbiturate followed by intermittent doses. Pentobarbital treatment (14 mg/kg followed by 7 mg/kg every 2 hours for 48 hours) after permanent MCA occlusion in Java monkeys produced significantly better neurologic outcome, less cerebral infarction, and better survival than in control animals.[183] In another study of permanent MCA occlusion in cats, pentobarbital (25 mg/kg) given for the first 3 days after vessel occlusion resulted in significantly less cerebral infarction than in controls.[214] Although neurologic outcome was not studied, it was demonstrated that rCBF to the ischemic regions was significantly improved in those animals given pentobarbital. One study reported a dose-related decrease in infarct size with pentobarbital in doses of 10 to 40 mg/kg given 1 hour after permanent MCA occlusion in dogs, but that higher doses failed to provide a beneficial effect.[62] None of the dogs was given any cardiovascular or respiratory support, and at higher doses (50 and 80 mg/kg) the respiratory depressant effects of the barbiturates resulted in death.

All of the previous reports produced *permanent* focal ischemia and lead to the conclusion that either a massive bolus dose or a smaller bolus dose followed by a continuous infusion of pentobarbital to suppress neuronal function and reduce cerebral energy demand,[181,211,212] redistribute or increase CBF,[36,214] and inhibit the formation of cerebral edema[154,267,272] provides some level of protection by decreasing neurologic injury, by increasing neuronal survival time, or by reducing infarct size. Applying the results of these animal studies to clinical trials of intraoperative focal ischemia or stroke to evaluate the effects of barbiturates may be difficult because of the large doses needed for protection in the animal studies and their associated cardiovascular and respiratory complications.[180]

Reports of barbiturate protection for *temporary* focal ischemia are also contradictory. In a primate study of 6 hours of MCA occlusion followed by reperfusion, *postischemic* treatment with pentobarbital (30 mg/kg plus infusion) to maintain an isoelectric EEG (continued for 96 hours) throughout the period of cerebral edema formation was reported to protect from ischemic injury.[255] Reperfusion in the control group was associated with elevated ICP that was thought to result from cerebral edema. This was attenuated by the barbiturate coma. It was shown that bar-

* References 28, 118, 131, 183, 255, 271.

biturate coma during MCA occlusion significantly reduced CBF in the contralateral hemisphere but had less effect in the occluded hemisphere, resulting in a redistribution of rCBF to the ischemic region. In another study pentobarbital (70 mg/kg) given after temporary focal ischemia led to less histologic cell changes of ischemia, but there was no difference in neurologic injury between the two groups.[157] In a study of cats given a single bolus of thiopental in a dose sufficient to produce burst suppression on the EEG before temporary MCA occlusion, histologic neuronal injury resulting from the ischemia was not reduced in the animals receiving thiopental.[96]

Clinical studies describing the protective effects of thiopental are mostly anecdotal, and there is little clinical evidence for the efficacy of barbiturates in preventing or treating focal ischemia. In humans only one prospective randomized clinical study[213] has demonstrated improved neurologic function after focal ischemia. In a series of patients undergoing open-heart cardiac procedures using normothermic perfusion, thiopental administered in doses sufficient to produce burst suppression on the EEG during the peribypass period (40 mg/kg) significantly improved postoperative neuropsychiatric outcome but was associated with a longer time for awakening postoperatively, a longer time required for postoperative tracheal intubation and ventilation, and an increased requirement for inotropic support to terminate bypass. The cerebral protective effects of thiopental are specific to this patient population. Thiopental reportedly does not reduce the number of strokes in patients undergoing coronary artery bypass grafting.[290]

Despite the relatively few studies demonstrating the efficacy of barbiturates in protecting against temporary focal ischemia, prophylactic barbiturate therapy continues to be recommended for cerebral protection when a possible transient ischemic episode is anticipated, such as during carotid endarterectomy,[110,128,166,279] aneurysm procedures requiring transient occlusion of the parent artery,[22,73,132] extracranial-to-intracranial bypass procedures,[155,278] profound induced hypotension,[174] and cardiopulmonary bypass procedures requiring an open ventricle.[213] Concern that large doses of barbiturates produce cardiovascular depression and drug-induced coma, delaying evaluation of neurologic function postoperatively, has resulted in the recommendation of small single doses of barbiturate.* The appropriate dose of barbiturate is thought to be one that produces burst suppression on the EEG. Normal anesthetizing doses of thiopental (3 to 7 mg/kg) produce burst suppression on the EEG for less than 5 to 10 minutes,[96] and larger doses of thiopental (10 to 25 mg/kg) produce burst suppression on the EEG that lasts only 10 minutes.[110] However, in the event that significant ischemia results from vessel occlusion, it has been speculated that the delivered thiopental does not wash out and the metabolic suppression and protection is maintained for a longer time.[174] This speculation

*References 73, 132, 155, 166, 173, 197, 278.

has been challenged by the results of a feline study in which a single bolus dose of thiopental failed to provide protection during temporary MCA occlusion.[96]

If a sufficient dose of thiopental (3 to 5 mg/kg) is given to produce burst suppression on the EEG, the vessel can be clamped within 10 to 15 seconds.[174] Ideally the occluded vessel should be briefly opened every 5 to 10 minutes (if possible and despite hemorrhage) for subsequent small doses of thiopental (1 to 2 mg/kg) to reach the region of ischemia.[174] If this is not possible, a continuous infusion of thiopental (3 to 5 mg/kg/hr) should be given to maintain burst suppression throughout the ischemic period.[18] Ideally the EEG should be monitored to ascertain the proper dose of thiopental needed to produce burst suppression in each patient. If necessary, blood pressure should be maintained within normal limits with a phenylephrine infusion.

Etomidate

Although barbiturates have been proposed for brain protection during cardiac surgery involving an open ventricle, the high doses required to achieve and maintain an isoelectric EEG result in a prolonged duration of tracheal intubation (19 or more hours)[213] and profound hypotension requiring vasopressor support.[213,294] Partly for these reasons, etomidate has gained some favor as an induction drug and possible neuroprotective drug. Etomidate is a nonbarbiturate imidazole derivative that has minimal cardiovascular side effects[65,89,105,290] and a shorter half-life, allowing a shorter time to awakening than high-dose thiopental.

Etomidate is similar to thiopental[173] in that it produces a dose-related decrease in neuronal function with an accompanying decrease in $CMRo_2$ and CBF.[56,57,193,241] Etomidate is also a direct cerebral vasoconstrictor with the ability to significantly decrease CBF. This effect on CBF is independent of its effect on cerebral metabolism.[193] Although CBF is markedly decreased by etomidate, CO_2 reactivity remains intact.[56,57,241,296]

Proposed mechanisms by which etomidate may provide protection against ischemia include the previously mentioned decrease in $CMRo_2$; reduction in intracranial blood volume; decrease in ICP;[68,193] decrease or redistribution of CBF;[313] membrane stabilization; and inhibition of free-fatty-acid liberation.[205] Several studies in animal models have shown that etomidate provides protection during incomplete global ischemia[190,296,314] and severe hypoxemia.[273] However, one study in rats that examined neurologic outcome after a period of regional ischemia found that the animals receiving etomidate showed a tendency toward greater neurologic deficit and mortality than those treated with methohexital or midazolam, but less than those animals receiving only N_2O.[21] Postischemic application of etomidate also has been reported to have no beneficial effect on recovery after complete cerebral ischemia in the rat.[33]

Despite the advantages of producing greater cardiovascular stability and having a shorter half-life than thiopental, enthusiasm for use of etomidate has been dampened by its producing a high incidence of myoclonic movements and suppression of adrenal cortical function. Etomidate's ability to cause adrenal cortical suppression is of concern because it might attenuate a patient's ability to withstand intraoperative and postoperative stress.[158] In normal patients undergoing elective surgery, a single dose of etomidate can produce adrenal cortical suppression lasting 24 hours or more.[90,334] This effect is dose-related and also more pronounced if infusions are used.[306,307] There have been no reports of increased morbidity or mortality after an induction dose of etomidate, and the initial reports of etomidate-induced adrenal cortical suppression were in critically ill patients receiving continuous infusions of etomidate for long-term sedation.[156] Etomidate appears to affect the synthesis of cortisol, corticosterone, aldosterone, and 17 alpha-hydroxyprogesterone,[91,307] but not the response of the receptors, so that supplemental administration of exogenous steroids should prevent the adverse effects of adrenal cortical suppression. This becomes even less of an issue in most neurosurgical patients who routinely receive intravenous glucocorticoids to minimize cerebral edema and ICP.

Although more randomized controlled studies are needed to further define the ability of etomidate to act as a protective drug for intraoperative ischemia, etomidate may prove to be an option to the barbiturates.

Propofol

Propofol, 2,6 diisopropylphenol is a new intravenous hypnotic anesthetic drug[141] used both for the induction of anesthesia[243] and as a total intravenous anesthetic for the maintenance of anesthesia,[95] and has been widely used as an anesthetic for neurosurgical patients.[92,169] In animals[237,300] and in humans propofol has been reported to decrease neuronal activity on the EEG with an accompanying decrease in $CMRo_2$ and CBF and an increase in cerebrovascular resistance (CVR).[161,227,286,301] Because its effects on neuronal activity, $CMRo_2$, and CBF appear to be similar to those of thiopental, it has been hypothesized that propofol could provide some degree of cerebral protection against ischemia.

The following studies sought to measure a possible protective effect of propofol. Models of hypoxia are crude screening tests for possible protection. The most common of these exposes groups of mice to a hypoxic atmosphere, usually 5% oxygen, and measures their survival rate. One study[304] reported that pretreatment with intraperitoneal propofol significantly prolonged survival of mice exposed to hypoxia. This prolongation of survival was similar to that found for pentobarbital by other investigators.[254] Three studies have been done on the effect of propofol during incomplete global ischemia produced by hypotension. When propofol was given to cats[315] in doses sufficient to produce an isoelectric EEG, it significantly lowered CBF, which was further lowered by hypotension induced by trimethaphan and hemorrhage. The magnitude of these

changes was similar to that obtained with thiopental. During the recovery period from hypotension, the CBF in the animals receiving propofol was significantly higher than that of the untreated animals and that of the animals receiving thiopental. When extracellular electrolytes and pH were measured in this model, there was less evidence of ischemia with propofol or thiopental than in the untreated group. This indicates that propofol may protect against anaerobic metabolism during hypotension, thereby protecting against incomplete global ischemia, and may provide better CBF in the postischemic period, a time when CBF is usually depressed and may produce an additional period of ischemia that could also contribute to the ultimate neurologic outcome. In a second study, the protective effects of propofol administered in a dose sufficient to suppress EEG activity in rats were compared with those of a control group receiving fentanyl/N_2O anesthesia.[147] Neurologic status was evaluated for 3 days. Neurologic outcome was significantly improved in the group receiving propofol compared with the group receiving fentanyl/N_2O. However, there were significant differences in the blood glucose levels between the two groups. The hormonal stress response to hemorrhagic hypotension was not blunted in the animals receiving fentanyl/N_2O, but it was blunted in the animals receiving propofol. Increased blood glucose levels in the fentanyl/N_2O group may have contributed to the ultimate neurologic damage. In a third study, the effect of propofol during incomplete ischemia was compared with thiopental or fentanyl in dogs.[195] Propofol and thiopental were given to produce burst suppression on the EEG. This resulted in a significant decrease in CBF and $CMRo_2$. Severe hypotension was then induced by hemorrhage, which further decreased CBF in all groups. The decreases in CBF in the thiopental and fentanyl groups could not sustain normal aerobic metabolism, resulting in a significant increase in cerebral lactate concentration. In the group receiving propofol, CBF was adequate to maintain aerobic metabolism. From these studies one can conclude that propofol does convey some amount of cerebral protection. This protection may be due to a decrease in $CMRo_2$, a maintenance or redistribution of CBF, or the prevention of large increases in blood glucose, which may be associated with a worse neurologic outcome when it occurs during cerebral ischemia.[187] These results are promising, but studies in other animal models and clinical studies should be done to confirm these findings before one can recommend that propofol be used for brain protection.

Isoflurane

Any anesthetic drug that decreases neuronal function with an accompanying decrease in cerebral metabolism presumably may provide cerebral protection during focal or incomplete global ischemia insofar as it provides metabolic suppression without causing hemodynamic compromise. Isoflurane is unique among the volatile anesthetics in that 2 MAC isoflurane (2.4%) can induce a level of anesthesia in humans that is characterized by an isoelectric EEG and is well tolerated hemodynamically.[287] Like many other general anesthetics, isoflurane produces a dose-related decrease in cortical electrical activity and thus reduces that portion of the $CMRo_2$ that is associated with neuronal function.[207] Maximal cerebral metabolic suppression correlates with the onset of an isoelectric EEG and is approximately 40% to 50% of normal awake values in animals[208] and humans.[210] This effect is identical to that of thiopental[173] and is proposed to be the primary mechanism by which isoflurane imparts its protective effect.

If the primary mechanism by which isoflurane provides cerebral protection during ischemia is a reduction in neuronal function and cerebral metabolism, one would expect it would be protective during focal and incomplete ischemia but not during complete global ischemia, during which neuronal function is abolished by the ischemia itself. In two animal models of incomplete global ischemia, isoflurane was shown to provide protection;[207,209] in a model of near-complete global ischemia, however, it did not provide protection.[308] The level of protection provided in these models is similar to that provided by the barbiturates.[186] In *animal* studies of regional ischemia, there are conflicting results on the effect of isoflurane as a protective drug.

The protection provided by thiopental in regional cerebral ischemia may be produced not only by metabolic suppression, but also possibly by an advantageous redistribution of cerebral blood flow secondary to the vasoconstriction produced in the nonischemic brain areas.[176] Because of its vasodilatory properties, this latter effect is not possible with isoflurane, and theoretically an opposite effect may occur.[176] A study of temporary focal ischemia in primates reported a significantly lower incidence of cerebral infarction and less neurologic damage in animals anesthetized with high-dose thiopental (with burst suppression on the EEG as the end point) than with comparable doses of isoflurane.[203] However, a major flaw of the study was that the mean arterial pressure was significantly different between the two treatment groups such that the higher pressure in the thiopental-treated animals might have redistributed rCBF to the ischemic regions, thereby favorably influencing the outcome.[122,135] When a similar primate study was performed with arterial pressure equally maintained, there were no differences in either neurologic outcome or infarct size between the thiopental-treated animals and the isoflurane-treated animals.[189] In another animal study comparing the protective effects of barbiturates and isoflurane during temporary focal ischemia, the possibility of cerebral vascular steal during isoflurane anesthesia was examined.[311] Rats underwent 2 hours of reversible MCA occlusion while receiving deep methohexital, isoflurane, or halothane anesthesia. While isoflurane did not cause cerebrovascular steal, there was no difference in neurologic outcome between the groups, and mean infarct volume was significantly less in the methohexital group.

There is, however, evidence in humans that isoflurane provides some protection in incomplete regional ischemia, but only when compared with the effects of halothane and enflurane. No comparison with the barbiturates or benzodiazipines has been made. In studies of patients undergoing carotid endarterectomy, the critical CBF (that blood flow below which the majority of patients developed ipsilateral EEG changes of ischemia within 3 minutes of carotid occlusion) was significantly lower during isoflurane anesthesia[170] than during anesthesia with halothane,[165,256,295] enflurane,[165] or Innovar.[166] This suggests that, through its ability to reduce cerebral metabolism significantly more than the other volatile anesthetics at the clinical concentrations (0.5 to 1 MAC) used and thereby preserve the ratio of oxygen supply to oxygen demand, isoflurane increased the tolerance of the brain to low blood flows. Another study demonstrated a significantly lower incidence of EEG ischemic changes during carotid endarterectomy with isoflurane anesthesia (18%) than with either halothane (25%) or enflurane (26%).[178] The decreased incidence of intraoperative ischemia in those patients receiving isoflurane occurred despite the fact that their preoperative risk status was greater than those patients receiving halothane or enflurane. From these studies one can conclude that isoflurane provides better protection than other volatile anesthetics from incomplete regional ischemia in humans.

Nitrous Oxide

Nitrous oxide (N_2O) has been reported to have an effect in cerebral protection. The literature is confusing concerning the effects of N_2O on CBF and $CMRo_2$ because of species variations in potency and response. The MAC of N_2O varies from 82% to 275%. This potency variation cannot be corrected by adjustment of dose, so most studies have used 70% N_2O despite this potency variation among species. N_2O has little effect on $CMRo_2$ and CBF in the rat.[47] In dogs,[192,249] pigs,[162] goats,[221] and rabbits,[76] N_2O significantly increases CBF and $CMRo_2$. In humans N_2O is a potent cerebral vasodilator in the absence of other anesthetics.[126] This effect of N_2O on CBF and $CMRo_2$ appears to be due to stimulation of sympathetic activity by N_2O.[79] Because of these species-specific effects on CBF and $CMRo_2$, the literature on the effect of N_2O on brain protection is also confusing. It has been reported that exposure to N_2O abolished the protective effect of thiopental in mice exposed to hypoxia,[121] but a subsequent study reported that N_2O, either alone or in combination with thiopental, had no positive or detrimental effect on survival of hypoxia; it reported that the findings of the previous study had been influenced by uncontrolled body temperature.[188] In rats it has been reported that N_2O alone, through its effect on sympathetic activity, can significantly worsen neurologic outcome in a model of severe incomplete global ischemia.[317] In the same animal model it was reported that either halothane or isoflurane provided significantly better neurologic and histologic outcomes than did the N_2O control and that this effect may have been due to the ability of halothane or isoflurane to both decrease CMR_{O_2} and to blunt the sympathetic hyperactivity associated with N_2O.[19] This conclusion was further supported by a similar study of the interactions of isoflurane and N_2O in the same rat model of incomplete cerebral ischemia.[20] A subsequent study in rats failed to demonstrate any detrimental effect by N_2O, although all animals were deeply anesthetized with methohexital, which could have blunted any effect the N_2O might have had on either CMR_{O_2} or sympathetic activity.[310] From these studies one can conclude that N_2O may have a detrimental effect if used alone when there is a risk of cerebral ischemia. Clinically this seldom occurs because other potent anesthetics are used in addition to N_2O. Many of these may modify the effect of N_2O. Its varying potency and subsequent metabolic effect in different animal species and its effect on sympathetic activity should be considered before using N_2O as the control in animal models of cerebral ischemia and studies of brain protection.

Local Anesthetics

Lidocaine is the local anesthetic most frequently used in studies examining the cerebral effects of local anesthetics. It significantly reduces CMR_{O_2} when administered in both subepileptogenic doses[140,250] and massive doses above the seizure threshold.[12] As a local anesthetic producing blockade of nerve conduction, its action involves blocking the sodium channels in the cell membrane, which inhibits both Na^+ influx and K^+ efflux. By restricting these ion fluxes, lidocaine may decrease the work of the cell membrane ATP-dependent ion pumps and the associated energy requirements necessary to maintain ion homeostasis.[10] This would appear as a decrease in cerebral metabolism in the normal brain, whereas this decrease in energy requirement might theoretically provide some protection in the ischemic brain.

Evidence of a possible cerebral protective effect for lidocaine was reported by Evans et al.[81] using an experimental model of cerebral ischemia in cats produced by arterial air embolism. Ischemic depression of cortical somatosensory evoked responses was shown to be markedly attenuated by prophylactic administration of lidocaine 5 mg/kg. A beneficial effect for lidocaine in focal cerebral ischemia was also shown by Shokunbi et al.[258] Using a continuous infusion of lidocaine during temporary MCA occlusion in cats, they found that the lidocaine-treated cats had an enhanced preservation of somatosensory evoked potentials, significant reduction in the size of the infarct, and relative preservation of blood flow in the ischemic zones. However, a study from this same group 4 years earlier using the same model of focal cerebral ischemia found no cerebral protective effect for lidocaine when administered at a dose 15 times greater and large enough to maintain an isoelectric EEG.[257] They attributed this lack of effect to the hypotension produced by such large doses of lidocaine. If circulation is supported by cardiopulmonary bypass, massive doses of lidocaine (160 mg/kg) have been shown to reduce

CMR_{O_2}.[12] Part of this decrease in CMR_{O_2}, however, may be due to a direct toxic effect on oxidative phosphorylation because it is accompanied by a disturbance in cerebral high-energy metabolites.[191] Therefore any decrease in cerebral metabolism produced by large doses of lidocaine may be due to a variety of factors both protective and toxic, including membrane stabilization, inhibition of neuronal function, and uncoupling of oxidative phosphorylation. A study of transient near-complete global ischemia in rats using clinically relevant doses of lidocaine before ischemia failed to show any protective effect.[309] Until more studies are done that show lidocaine to be a cerebral protective drug, it should not be used in this capacity.

Clinical Recommendations

When a temporary episode of incomplete or focal ischemia is anticipated intraoperatively, such as during carotid endarterectomy, aneurysm procedures requiring transient occlusion of the parent artery, extracranial-to-intracranial bypass procedures, profound induced hypotension, and cardiopulmonary bypass procedures requiring an open ventricle, several factors can be optimized in the perioperative period to maximize cerebral protection. These include anesthetic drug, mean arterial pressure, blood glucose level, and temperature.

During focal or incomplete cerebral ischemia, electrical activity persists, and drugs that reduce cerebral metabolism by decreasing neuronal activity should provide some protective effects. Thiopental is the only anesthetic drug in humans that has been shown in a prospective, randomized clinical study to improve neurologic function after focal ischemia.[213] Its prophylactic use has been recommended for brain protection in situations of possible temporary focal or incomplete ischemia.[110,132,155,174,213] Administering thiopental for cerebral protection is associated with several undesirable side effects: The large doses required can result in hemodynamic compromise, a longer time for awakening postoperatively, and a prolonged period of postoperative tracheal intubation and ventilation.[213] Many of these side effects can be avoided with the use of the volatile anesthetic isoflurane because of the ability to rapidly terminate its action and vary its concentration.[203] Isoflurane has been reported to be associated with a significantly decreased incidence of EEG ischemic changes in patients undergoing carotid endarterectomy when compared with the other volatile anesthetics.[178] Isoflurane has not been compared with thiopental in clinical studies. Isoflurane is recommended for use during carotid endarterectomy. Thiopental remains the drug of choice for brain protection during aneurysm clipping, extracranial-to-intracranial bypass procedures, and open ventricle cardiac surgery.

Induced hypertension has been demonstrated to provide some degree of protection during focal ischemia. During ischemia autoregulation may be lost and CBF becomes passively dependent on cerebral perfusion pressure. It is recommended that the mean arterial blood pressure be increased by 10% to 20% with phenylephrine in an attempt to increase regional cerebral blood flow.

Another important consideration during the perioperative period is the blood (and thus the brain) glucose level. Grossly elevated glucose levels appear to aggravate the effects of cerebral ischemia.[233,235] Although it was commonly believed that blood glucose levels must exceed 250 mg/dl to cause damage, a recent study demonstrated that even preischemic blood glucose levels below 200 mg/dl, if preceded by a glucose infusion, can result in a significantly worse neurologic outcome.[153] Therefore it is recommended that patients at risk for temporary focal or incomplete ischemia not receive glucose-containing solutions in the perioperative period and that blood glucose levels be routinely monitored. Whether administration of insulin to normalize blood glucose levels before, during, or after a potentially ischemic event improves neurologic outcome is uncertain.

Cerebral protection provided by hypothermia has recently come under further scrutiny. Profound hypothermia has traditionally been used to prolong ischemic tolerance during complete circulatory arrest and cardiopulmonary bypass. Deep hypothermia is not without its own complications, however, and has very limited usefulness in neurosurgical patients. Although discovered about 30 years ago,[130] not until recently was it definitively shown that even small (1 to 3° C) reductions in brain temperature could provide a protective effect during cerebral ischemia in animals.[41] There is even evidence that postischemic induction of moderate brain hypothermia also may offer protection.[42] If these protective effects can be substantiated with additional animal studies of not only histopathology but also neurologic outcome after focal and complete global brain ischemia, hypothermia may become a very useful therapeutic intervention in the perioperative period.

Intraoperative complete global ischemia is fortunately uncommon. Currently little can be done to improve neurologic outcome after complete ischemia other than prompt and aggressive resuscitation. During episodes of either complete or focal ischemia one must not overlook the basics of adequate oxygenation and ventilation and cardiovascular stability.

▼

SUMMARY

Following ischemic injury, the brain is limited in its regenerative ability. Medical research has searched for methods to prevent or ameliorate such injury. This research has centered on the prevention or amelioration of brain injury as evidenced by abnormalities in metabolism, neurotransmission, histopathology, or neurologic function occurring after an hypoxic or ischemic event. This chapter presents current information on pathophysiology and biochemical changes occurring during and following cerebral ischemia (changes that may contribute to the ultimate neurologic outcome) and discusses current and *future* therapeutic measures hypothesized to prevent or ameliorate both the primary and secondary injury resulting from ischemia. It includes both clinical and experimental strategies, acknowledging that information gained in the future may significantly alter understanding of the mechanism of cerebral injury and efficacious therapy.

References

1. Abramson NS, Safar P, Detre DM et al: Randomized clinical study of thiopental loading in comatose survivors of cardiac arrest. Brain resuscitation clinical trial I study group, *N Engl J Med* 314:397, 1986.
2. Adams HP Jr, Olinger CP, Marler JR et al: Comparison of admission serum glucose concentration with neurologic outcome in acute cerebral infarction: a study in patients given naloxone, *Stroke* 19:455, 1988.
3. Aitkenhead A: Cerebral protection, *Br J Hosp Med* 35:290, 1986.
4. Albers GW: Potential therapeutic uses of N-methyl-D aspartate antagonists in cerebral ischemia, *Clin Neuropharmacol* 13:177, 1990.
5. Albers GW, Goldberg MP, Choi DW: N-methyl-D-aspartate antago-

nists: ready for clinical trial in brain ischemia? *Ann Neurol* 25:398, 1989.
6. Allen GS: Role of calcium antagonists in cerebral arterial spasm, *Am J Cardiol* 55:149B, 1985.
7. Allen GS, Ahn HS, Preziosi TJ et al: Cerebral arterial spasm—a controlled trial of nimodipine in patients with subarachnoid hemorrhage, *N Engl J Med* 308:619, 1983.
8. Ames A, Wright RL, Kowada M et al: Cerebral ischemia. II. The no-reflow phenomenon, *Am J Pathol* 52:437, 1968.
9. Astrup J: Energy requiring cell functions in the ischemic brain. Their critical supply and possible inhibition in protective therapy, *J Neurosurg* 56:482, 1982.
10. Astrup J, Skovsted P, Gjerris F et al:

Increase in extracellular potassium in the brain during circulatory arrest. Effects of hypothermia, lidocaine, and thiopental, *Anesthesiology* 55:256, 1981.
11. Astrup J, Siesjo BK, Symon L: Thresholds in cerebral ischemia—the ischemic penumbra, *Stroke* 12:723, 1981.
12. Astrup J, Sorensen P, Sorensen HR: Inhibition of cerebral oxygen and glucose consumption in the dog by hypothermia, pentobarbital, and lidocaine, *Anesthesiology* 55:263, 1981.
13. Auer RN, Kalimo H, Olsson Y et al: The dentate gyrus in hypoglycemia: pathology implicating excitotoxic-mediated neuronal necrosis, *Acta Neuropathol* 67:279, 1985.
14. Auer RN, Kalimo H, Olsson Y et al:

The temporal evolution of hypoglycemic brain damage: I. Light and electron microscopic findings in the rat cerebral cortex, *Acta Neuropathol* 67:13, 1985.

15. Auer RN, Siesjo BK: Biological differences between ischemia, hypoglycemia, and epilepsy, *Ann Neurol* 24:699, 1988.

16. Babbs CF: Role of iron ions in the genesis of reperfusion injury following successful cardiopulmonary resuscitation: preliminary data and a biochemical hypothesis, *Ann Emerg Med* 14:777, 1985.

17. Barnes DM: NMDA receptors trigger excitement, *Science* 239:254, 1988.

18. Barson WG: Pharmacologic therapeutic modalities: barbiturates, *Crit Care Q* 5:63, 1983.

19. Baughman VL, Hoffman WE, Miletich DJ et al: Neurologic outcome in rats following incomplete cerebral ischemia during halothane, isoflurane, or N_2O, *Anesthesiology* 69:192, 1988.

20. Baughman VL, Hoffman WE, Thomas C et al: The interaction of nitrous oxide and isoflurane with incomplete cerebral ischemia in the rat, *Anesthesiology* 70:767, 1989.

21. Baughman VL, Hoffman WE, Miletich DJ et al: Neurologic outcome following regional cerebral ischemia with methohexital, midazolam, and etomidate (abstract), *Anesthesiology* 67:A582, 1987.

22. Belopavlovic M, Buchthal A, Beks JWF: Barbiturates for cerebral aneurysm surgery, *Acta Neurochir* 76:73, 1985.

23. Beneviste H, Drejer J, Schousboe A et al: Elevation of the extracellular concentrations of glutamate and aspartate in rat hippocampus during transient cerebral ischemia monitored by intracellular microdialysis, *J Neurochem* 43:1369, 1984.

24. Berger L, Hakim A: The association of hyperglycemia with cerebral edema in stroke, *Stroke* 17:865, 1986.

25. Berne RM, Rubio R, Curnish RR: Release of adenosine from ischemic brain, *Circ Res* 35:262, 1974.

26. Berntman L, Welsh FA, Harp JR: Cerebral protective effect of low-grade hypothermia, *Anesthesiology* 55:495, 1981.

27. Bircher NG: Ischemic brain protection, *Ann Emerg Med* 14:784, 1985.

28. Black KL, Weidler DJ, Jallad NS et al: Delayed pentobarbital therapy of acute focal cerebral ischemia, *Stroke* 9:245, 1978.

29. Bleyaert AL, Nemoto EM, Safar P et al: Thiopental amelioration of brain damage after global ischemia in monkeys, *Anesthesiology* 49:390, 1978.

30. Boast CA, Gerhardt SC, Pastor G et al: The N-methyl-D-aspartate antagonists CGS 19755 and CPP reduce ischemic brain damage in gerbils, *Brain Res* 442:345, 1988.

31. Boast CA, Gerhardt SC, Janak P: Systemic AP7 reduces ischemic brain damage in gerbils. In Hicks TP, Lodge D, McLennan H, editors: Excitatory amino acid transmission, New York, 1987, Alan R Liss, p 249.

32. Boelhouwer R, Bruining H, Ong G: Correlations of serum potassium fluctuations with body temperature after major surgery, *Crit Care Med* 15:310, 1987.

33. Bohrer H, Hoyer S, Krier C: The influence of etomidate upon cerebral metabolites after complete brain ischemia in the rat, *Eur J Anaesth* 8:233, 1991.

34. Boulu RG, Plotkine M, Gueniau C et al: Effect of indomethacin in experimental cerebral ischemia, *J Pathol Biol* 30:278, 1982.

35. Brain resuscitation clinical trial group: A randomized clinical study of a calcium entry blocker (lidoflazine) in the treatment of comatose survivors of cardiac arrest, *N Engl J Med* 324:1225, 1991.

36. Branston NM, Hope DT, Symon L: Barbiturates in focal ischemia of primate cortex: effects on blood flow distribution, evoked potential, and extracellular potassium, *Stroke* 10:647, 1979.

37. Brint S, Kraig R, Kiessling M et al: Hyperglycemia augments infarct size in focal experimental brain ischemia (abstract), *Ann Neurol* 18:127, 1985.

38. Brown K, Fridovich I: Superoxide radical and superoxide dismutase: threat and defense, *Acta Physiol Scand*, Suppl 492:9, 1980.

39. Browning RG, Olson DW, Stueven HA et al: 50% Dextrose: antidote or toxin? *Ann Emerg Med* 19:683, 1990.

40. Bulkey GB: Free radical-mediated reperfusion injury: a selective review, *Br J Cancer* 55(suppl VIII):66, 1987.

41. Busto R, Dietrich WD, Globus MY et al: Small differences in intra-ischemic brain temperature critically determine the extent of ischemic neuronal injury, *J Cereb Blood Flow Metab* 7:729, 1987.

42. Busto R, Dietrich WD, Globus MY et al: Postischemic moderate hypothermia inhibits CA1 hippocampal ischemic neuronal injury, *Neurosci Lett* 101:299, 1989.

43. Busto R, Globus MY, Dietrich WD et al: Effect of mild hypothermia on ischemia-induced release of neurotransmitters and free fatty acids in rat brain, *Stroke* 20:904, 1989.

44. Candelise L, Landi G, Orazio EN et al: Prognostic significance of hyperglycemia in acute stroke, *Arch Neurol* 42:661, 1985.

45. Cao W, Carney JM, Duchon A et al: Oxygen free radical involvement in ischemia and reperfusion injury to the brain, *Neurosci Lett* 88:233, 1988.

46. Carli F, Emery P, Freemantle C: Effect of perioperative normothermia on postoperative metabolism in elderly patients undergoing hip arthroplasty, *Br J Anaesth* 63:276, 1989.

47. Carlsson C, Hagerdal M, Siesjo BK: The effect of nitrous oxide on oxygen consumption and blood flow in the cerebral cortex of the rat, *Acta Anaesthesiol Scand* 20:91, 1976.

48. Cerchiari EL, Hoel TM, Safar P et al: Protective effects of combined superoxide dismutase and deferoxamine on recovery of cerebral blood flow and function after cardiac arrest in dogs, *Stroke* 18:869, 1987.

49. Choi DW: Ionic dependence of glutamate neurotoxicity in cortical cell culture, *J Neurosci* 7:369, 1987.

50. Choi DW: Glutamate neurotoxicity and diseases of the nervous system, *Neuron* 1:623, 1988.

51. Choi DW, Koh J, Peters S: Pharmacology of glutamate neurotoxicity in cortical cell culture attenuation by NMDA antagonists; *J Neurosci* 8:185, 1988.

52. Chopp M, Frinak S, Walton DR et al: Intracellular acidosis during and after cerebral ischemia: in vivo nuclear magnetic resonance study of hyperglycemia in cats, *Stroke* 18:919, 1987.

53. Clark GD: Role of excitatory amino acids in brain injury caused by hypoxia-ischemia, status epilepticus,

and hypoglycemia, *Clin Perinatol* 16:459, 1989.

54. Clark IA, Cowden WB, Hunt NH: Free radical-induced pathology, *Med Res Rev* 5:297, 1985.

55. Clifton GL, Jiang JL, Lyeth BG et al: Marked protection by moderate hypothermia after experimental traumatic brain injury, *J Cereb Blood Flow Metab* 11:114, 1991.

56. Cold GE, Eskesen V, Eriksen H et al: CBF and CMRo$_2$ during continuous etomidate infusion supplemented with N$_2$O and fentanyl in patients with supratentorial cerebral tumor. A dose response study, *Acta Anaesthesiol Scand* 29:490, 1985.

57. Cold GE, Eskesen V, Eriksen H et al: Changes in CMRo$_2$, EEG, and concentration of etomidate in serum and brain tissue during craniotomy with continuous etomidate supplemented with N$_2$O and fentanyl, *Acta Anaesthesiol Scand* 30:159, 1986.

58. Collingridge GL, Bliss TV: NMDA receptors—their role in long term potentiation, *Trends Neurosci* 10:288, 1988.

59. Collins RC: Selective vulnerability of brain: new insights from the excitatory synapse, *Metab Br Dis* 1:231, 1986.

60. Collins RC, Dobkin BH, Choi DW: Selective vulnerability of the brain: new insights into the pathophysiology of stroke, *Ann Intern Med* 110:992, 1989.

61. Combs DJ, Dempsey RJ, Maley M et al: Relationship between plasma glucose, brain lactate, and intracellular pH during cerebral ischemia in gerbils, *Stroke* 21:936, 1990.

62. Corkill G, Sivalingam S, Reitan JA et al: Dose dependency of the post-insult protective effect of pentobarbital in the canine experimental stroke model, *Stroke* 9:10, 1978.

63. Corradetti R, Lo Conte G, Moroni F et al: Adenosine decreases aspartate and glutamate release from rat hippocampal slices, *Eur J Pharmacol* 104:19, 1984.

64. Cox NH, Lorains JW: The prognostic value of blood glucose and glycosylated haemoglobin estimation in patients with stroke, *Postgrad Med J* 62:7, 1986.

65. Criado A, Maseda J, Navarro E et al: Induction of anaesthesia with etomidate: haemodynamic study of 36 patients, *Br J Anaesth* 52:803, 1980.

66. Cronstein BN, Rosenstein ED, Kramer SB et al: Adenosine: a physiologic modulator of superoxide anion generation by human neutrophils. Adenosine acts via an A2 receptor on human neutrophils, *J Immunol* 135:1366, 1985.

67. D'Alecy LG, Lundy EF, Barton KJ et al: Dextrose containing intravenous fluid impairs outcome and increases death after eight minutes of cardiac arrest and resuscitation in dogs, *Surgery* 100:505, 1986.

68. Dearden NM, McDowall DG: Comparison of etomidate and althesin in the reduction of increased intracranial pressure after head injury, *Br J Anaesth* 57:361, 1985.

69. DeCourten-Myers G, Myers RE, Schoolfield L: Hyperglycemia enlarges infarct size in cerebrovascular occlusion in cats, *Stroke* 19:623, 1988.

70. DelMaestro RF: An approach to free radicals in medicine and biology, *Acta Physiol Scand* 492:153, 1980.

71. Dempsey RJ, Roy MW, Meyer KL et al: Indomethacin-mediated improvement following middle cerebral artery occlusion in cats. Effects of anesthesia, *J Neurosurg* 62:874, 1985.

72. DeWitt DS, Kong DL, Lyeth BG et al: Experimental traumatic brain injury elevates brain prostaglandin E$_2$ and thromboxane B$_2$ levels in rats, *J Neurotrauma* 5:303, 1988.

73. Ditmore QM, Samson DS, Beyer CW: Traumatic middle cerebral artery aneurysm: case report, *Neurosurgery* 6:293, 1980.

74. Drejer J, Benveniste H, Diemer NH et al: Cellular origin of ischemia-induced glutamate release from brain tissue in vivo and in vitro, *J Neurochem* 45:145, 1985.

75. Drummond JC, Moore SS: The influence of dextrose administration on neurologic outcome after temporary spinal cord ischemia in the rabbit, *Anesthesiology* 70:64, 1989.

76. Drummond JC, Scheller MS, Todd MM: The effect of nitrous oxide on cortical cerebral blood flow during anesthesia with halothane and isoflurane with and without morphine in the rabbit, *Anesth Analg* 66:1083, 1987.

77. Duckrow RB, Beard DC, Brennan RW: Regional cerebral blood flow decreased during chronic and acute hyperglycemia, *Stroke* 18:52, 1987.

78. Duffy TE, Howse DC, Plum F: Cerebral energy metabolism during experimental status epilepticus, *J Neurochem* 24:925, 1975.

79. Ebert TJ, Kampine JP: Nitrous oxide augments sympathetic outflow: direct evidence from human peroneal nerve endings, *Anesth Analg* 69:444, 1989.

80. Egan RW, Paxton J, Kuehl FA: Mechanism for irreversible self deactivation of prostaglandin synthetase, *J Biol Chem* 257:7329, 1976.

81. Evans DE, Catron PW, McDermott JJ et al: Effect of lidocaine after experimental cerebral ischemia induced by air embolism, *J Neurosurg* 70:97, 1989.

82. Feustal PJ, Ingvar MC, Severinghaus JW: Cerebral oxygen availability and blood flow during middle cerebral artery occlusion: effects of pentobarbital, *Stroke* 12:858, 1981.

83. Fleischer JE, Lanier WL, Milde JH et al: Lidoflazine does not improve neurologic outcome when administered after complete cerebral ischemia in primates, *J Cereb Blood Flow Metab* 7:366, 1987.

84. Fleischer JE, Lanier WL, Milde JH et al: Effect of lidoflazine on cerebral blood flow and neurologic outcome when administered after complete cerebral ischemia in dogs, *Anesthesiology* 66:304, 1987.

85. Floyd RA: Role of oxygen free radicals in carcinogenesis and brain ischemia, *FASEB J* 4:2587, 1990.

86. Fonnum F: Glutamate: a neurotransmitter in mammalian brain, *J Neurochem* 42:1, 1984.

87. Forsman M, Aarseth HP, Nordby HK et al: Cerebral blood flow, intracranial pressure and neurologic outcome after cardiac arrest. Effects of nimodipine, *Anesth Analg* 68:436, 1989.

88. Foster AC, Gill R, Iverson LL et al: Systemic administration of MK-801 protects against ischaemia-induced hippocampal neurodegeneration in the gerbil, *Br J Pharmacol* 90:9P, 1987.

89. Fragen RJ, Caldwell N, Brunner EA: Clinical use of etomidate for anesthesia induction: a preliminary report, *Anesth Analg* 55:730, 1976.

90. Fragen RJ, Shanks CA, Molteni A et al: Effects of etomidate on hormonal responses to surgical stress, *Anesthesiology* 61:652, 1984.

91. Fraser R, Watt I, Gray CE et al: The effect of etomidate on adrenocortical function in dogs before and during hemorrhagic shock, *Endocrinology* 6:2266, 1984.

92. Freedman M, Levy ER: Propofol intravenous anaesthesia for neurosurgery, *S Afr Med J* 74:10, 1988.

93. Freeman BA, Crapo JD: Biology of disease: Free radicals and tissue injury, *Lab Invest* 47:412, 1982.

94. Fuller BJ, Gower JD, Green CJ: Free radical damage and organ preservation: fact or fiction? *Cryobiology* 25:377, 1988.

95. Galletly DC, Short TG: Total intravenous anaesthesia using propofol infusion—50 consecutive cases, *Anaesth Intens Care* 16:150, 1988.

96. Gelb AW, Floyd P, Lok P et al: A prophylactic bolus of thiopentone does not protect against prolonged focal cerebral ischaemia, *Can Anaesth Soc J* 33:173, 1986.

97. Gelmers HJ: Effect of nimodipine on post-ischaemic cerebrovascular reactivity as revealed by measuring regional cerebral blood flow, *Acta Neurochir* 63:283, 1982.

98. Gelmers HJ: The effects of nimodipine on the clinical course of patients with acute ischaemic stroke, *Acta Neurol Scand* 69:232, 1984.

99. Gelmers HJ, Gorter K, de Weerdt CJ et al: A controlled trial of nimodipine in acute ischemic stroke, *N Engl J Med* 318:203, 1988.

100. Germano IM, Bartkowski HM, Cassel ME et al: The therapeutic value of nimodipine in experimental focal cerebral ischemia. Neurological outcome and histopathological findings, *J Neurosurg* 67:81, 1987.

101. Ginsberg MD, Prado R, Dietrich WD et al: Hyperglycemia reduces the extent of cerebral infarction in rats, *Stroke* 18:570, 1987.

102. Ginsberg MD, Welsh FA, Budd WW: Deleterious effects of glucose pretreatment on recovery from diffuse cerebral ischemia in the cat, *Stroke* 11:347, 1980.

103. Gisvold SE, Safar P, Hendrickx HHL et al: Thiopental treatment after global brain ischemia in pigtailed monkeys, *Anesthesiology* 60:88, 1984.

104. Goldstein A Jr, Wells BA, Keats AS: Increased tolerance to cerebral anoxia by pentobarbital, *Arch Int Pharmacodyn* 161:138, 1966.

105. Gooding JM, Weng J-T, Smith RA et al: Cardiovascular and pulmonary responses following etomidate induction of anesthesia in patients with demonstrated cardiac disease, *Anesth Analg* 58:40, 1979.

106. Goto H, Nonami R, Hamasaki Y et al: Effect of hypothermia on coagulation, *Anesthesiology* 63:A107, 1985.

107. Gotoh O, Mohamed AA, McCulloch J et al: Nimodipine and the haemodynamic and histopathological consequences of middle cerebral artery occlusion in the rat, *J Cereb Blood Flow Metab* 6:321, 1986.

108. Grice SC, Chappell ET, Prough DS et al: Ibuprofen improves cerebral blood flow after global cerebral ischemia in dogs, *Stroke* 18:787, 1987.

109. Griffiths T, Evans MC, Meldrum BS: Intracellular calcium accumulation in rat hippocampus during seizures induced by biculline or L-allyglycine, *Neuroscience* 10:385, 1983.

110. Gross CE, Adams HP Jr, Sokoll MD et al: Use of anticoagulants, electroencephalographic monitoring, and barbiturate cerebral protection in carotid endarterectomy, *Neurosurgery* 9:1, 1981.

111. Hadani M, Young W, Flamm ES: Nicardipine reduces calcium accumulation and electrolyte derangements in regional cerebral ischemia in rats, *Stroke* 19:1125, 1988.

112. Hall ED, Braughler JM: Central nervous system trauma and stroke: II. Physiological and pharmacological evidence for involvement of oxygen radicals and lipid peroxidation, *Free Rad Biol Med* 6:303, 1989.

113. Hall ED, Pazara E, Braugler JM: 21-Aminosteroid lipid peroxidation inhibitor U74006F protects against cerebral ischemia in gerbils, *Stroke* 19:997, 1987.

114. Hall ED, Yonkers PA: Attenuation of postischemic cerebral hypoperfusion by the 21-aminosteroid U47006F, *Stroke* 19:340, 1988.

115. Hallenbeck JM, Furlow TW: Prostaglandin I_2 and indomethacin prevent impairment of post-ischemic brain reperfusion in the dog, *Stroke* 10:629, 1979.

116. Halliwell B, Gutteridge JMC: Oxygen free radicals and the nervous system, *Trends Neurosci* 8:22, 1985.

117. Hamud F, Fiskum G: Loss of maximal respiratory and Ca^{++} uptake capacities by rat brain mitochondria during cerebral ischemia, *Biophys J* 47:414a, 1985.

118. Hankinson HL, Smith AL, Nielsen SL et al: Effect of thiopental on focal cerebral ischemia in dogs, *Surg Forum* 25:445, 1974.

119. Harik SI, LaManna JC: Vascular perfusion and blood-brain glucose transport in acute and chronic hyperglycemia, *J Neurochem* 51:1924, 1988.

120. Hartley DM, Monyer H, Colamarino SA et al: 7-Chloro-kynurenate blocks NMDA receptor-mediated neurotoxicity in cortical cell cultures, *Soc Neurosci Abstr* 15:762, 1989.

121. Hartung J, Cottrell JE: Nitrous oxide reduces thiopental-induced prolongation of survival in hypoxic and anoxic mice, *Anesth Analg* 66:47, 1987.

122. Hayashi S, Nehls DG, Kieck CF et al: Beneficial effects of induced hypertension on experimental stroke in awake monkeys, *J Neurosurg* 60:151, 1984.

123. Heier T, Caldwell JE, Sessler DI et al: The relationship between adductor pollicis twitch tension and central, skin, and muscle temperature during nitrous oxide/isoflurane anesthesia in humans, *Anesthesiology* 71:381, 1989.

124. Heier T, Caldwell JE, Sessler DI et al: Mild intraoperative hypothermia increases duration of action and recovery time of vecuronium, *Anesth Analg* 70:S153, 1990.

125. Heiss W-D: Flow thresholds of functional and morphologic damage of brain tissue, *Stroke* 14:329, 1983.

126. Henricksen HG, Jorgensen PB: The effect of nitrous oxide and intracranial pressure in patients with intracranial disorders, *Brit J Anaesth* 45:486, 1973.

127. Hertz L: Functional interactions between neurons and astrocytes. I. Turnover and metabolism of putative amino acid transmitters, *Prog Neurobiol* 13:277, 1979.

128. Hicks RG, Kerr DR, Horton DA: Thiopentone cerebral protection under EEG control during carotid endarterectomy, *Anaesth Intens Care* 14:22, 1986.

129. Hillered L, Ernster L, Siesjo BK: Influence of in vitro lactic acidosis and hypercapnia on respiratory activity of isolated rat brain mitochondria, *J*

Cereb Blood Flow Metab 4:430, 1984.

130. Hirsch H, Muller HA: Funktionelle und histologische Veranderungen des Kaninchengehirns nach kompletter Gehirnischamie, *Pflugers Arch* 275:277, 1962.

131. Hoff JT, Smith AL, Hankinson HL et al: Barbiturate protection from cerebral infarction in primates, *Stroke* 6:28, 1975.

132. Hoff JT, Pitts LH, Spetzler R et al: Barbiturates for protection from cerebral ischemia in aneurysm surgery, *Acta Neurol Scand Suppl* 56:158, 1977.

133. Hoffman WE, Harrington SL, Braucher E et al: Brain lactate and neurologic outcome following incomplete ischemia in hypo- and hyperglycemic rats, *Anesth Rev* 15:92, 1988.

134. Hoffman WE, Braucher E, Pelligrino DA et al: Brain lactate and neurologic outcome following incomplete ischemia in fasted, nonfasted, and glucose-loaded rats, *Anesthesiology* 72:1045, 1990.

135. Hope DT, Branston NM, Symon L: Restoration of neurological function with induced hypertension in acute experimental cerebral ischemia, *Acta Neurol Scan Suppl* 64:506, 1977.

136. Hossmann KA: Post-ischemic resuscitation of the brain: selective vulnerability versus global resistance, *Prog Brain Res* 63:3, 1985.

137. Hossmann KA, Zimmermann V: Resuscitation of the monkey brain after 1 hour complete ischemia. I. Physiological and morphological observations, *Brain Res* 81:49, 1974.

138. Hsu SS, Meno JR, Zhou JG et al: Influence of hyperglycemia on cerebral adenosine production during ischemia and reperfusion, *Am J Physiol* 261:H398, 1991.

139. Ingvar M, Morgan PF, Auer RN: The nature and timing of excitotoxic neuronal necrosis in the cerebral cortex, hippocampus, and thalamus due to flurothyl-induced status epilepticus, *Acta Neuropathol* 75:362, 1988.

140. Ingvar M, Shapiro HM: Selective metabolic activation of the hippocampus during lidocaine-induced pre-seizure activity, *Anesthesiology* 54:33, 1981.

141. James R, Glen JB: Synthesis, biological evaluation and preliminary structure-activity considerations of a series of alkyphenols as intravenous anaesthetic agents, *J Med Chem* 23:1350, 1980.

142. Kagstrom E, Smith M-L, Siesjo BK: Recirculation in the rat brain following incomplete ischemia, *J Cereb Blood Flow Metab* 3:183, 1983.

143. Kass IS, Lipton P: Mechanisms involved in irreversible anoxic damage to the in vitro hippocampal slice, *J Physiol* 332:459, 1982.

144. Kazda S, Hoffmeister F, Garthoff B et al: Prevention of the post-ischemic impaired reperfusion of the brain by nimodipine, *Acta Neurol Scand Suppl* 60:302, 1979.

145. Kiers L, Davis SM, Larkins RG et al: Pathogenesis and outcome of stroke in diabetes and hyperglycemia (abstract), *Stroke* 20:138, 1989.

146. Kironi T: Delayed neuronal death in the gerbil hippocampus following ischemia, *Brain Res* 239:57, 1982.

147. Kochs E, Hoffman WE, Werner C et al: The effects of propofol on neurologic outcome from incomplete cerebral ischemia in the rat, *Anesthesiology* 73:A718, 1990.

148. Kong DL, Prough DS, Whitley JM et al: Hemorrhage and intracranial hypertension in combination increase cerebral production of thromboxane A$_2$, *Crit Care Med* 19:532, 1991.

149. Kraft SA, Larson CP Jr, Shuer LM et al: Effect of hyperglycemia on neuronal changes in a rabbit model of focal cerebral ischemia, *Stroke* 21:447, 1990.

150. Kraig RP, Chesler M: Astrocytic acidosis in hyperglycemia and complete ischemia, *J Cereb Blood Flow Metab* 10:104, 1990.

151. Kucharczyk J, Chew W, Derugin N et al: Nicardipine reduces ischemic brain injury. Magnetic resonance imaging/spectroscopy study in cats, *Stroke* 20:268, 1989.

152. Lanier WL: Glucose management during cardiopulmonary bypass: cardiovascular and neurologic implications, *Anesth Analg* 72:423, 1991.

153. Lanier WL, Stangland KJ, Scheithauer BW et al: The effects of dextrose infusion and head position on neurologic outcome after complete cerebral ischemia in primates: examination of a model, *Anesthesiology* 66:39, 1987.

154. Lawner P, Laurent J, Simeone F et al: Attenuation of ischemic brain edema by pentobarbital after carotid ligation in the gerbil, *Stroke* 10:644, 1979.

155. Lawner PM, Simeone FA: Treatment of intraoperative middle cerebral artery occlusion with pentobarbital and extracranial-intracranial bypass, *J Neurosurg* 51:710, 1975.

156. Ledingham IM, Watt I: Influence of sedation on mortality in multiple trauma patients, *Lancet* 2:1270, 1983.

157. Levy DE, Brierley JB: Delayed pentobarbital administration limits ischemic brain damage in gerbils, *Ann Neurol* 5:59, 1979.

158. Longnecker DE: Stress free: to be or not to be, *Anesthesiology* 61:643, 1984.

159. Longstreth WT Jr, Diehr P, Inui TS: Prediction of awakening after out-of-hospital cardiac arrest, *N Engl J Med* 308:1378, 1983.

160. Longstreth WT Jr, Inui TS: High blood glucose level on hospital admission and poor neurologic recovery after cardiac arrest, *Ann Neurol* 15:59, 1984.

161. Madsen JB, Guldager M, Jensen PM: CBF and CMRo$_2$ during neuroanesthesia with continuous infusion of propofol, *Acta Anaesth Scand* 33(suppl 91):143, 1989.

162. Manohar M: Impact of 70 percent nitrous oxide administration on regional distribution of brain blood flow in unmedicated healthy swine, *J Cardiovasc Pharmacol* 7:463, 1985.

163. McCall JM, Braughler JM, Hall ED: A new class of compounds for stroke and trauma: effects of 21-aminosteroids on lipid peroxidation, *Acta Anaesth Belg* 38:417, 1987.

164. McDonald JW, Silverstein FS, Johnston MV: MK-801 protects the neonatal brain from hypoxic-ischemic damage, *Eur J Pharmacol* 140:359, 1987.

165. McKay RD, Sundt TM, Michenfelder JD et al: Internal carotid artery stump pressure and cerebral blood flow during carotid endarterectomy: modification by halothane, enflurane, and Innovar, *Anesthesiology* 45:390, 1976.

166. McMeniman WJ, Fletcher JP, Little JM: Experience with barbiturate therapy for cerebral protection during carotid endarterectomy, *Ann R Coll Surg Engl* 66:361, 1984.

167. Meldrum B: Possible therapeutic ap-

plications of antagonists of excitatory amino acid neurotransmitters, *Clin Sci* 68:113 1985.

168. Meldrum BS, Evans MC, Swan JH et al: Protection against hypoxic/ischaemic brain damage with excitatory amino acid antagonists, *Med Biol* 65:153, 1987.

169. Merckx L, Van Hemelrijck J, Van Aken H et al: Total intravenous anaesthesia using propofol and alfentanil infusion in neurosurgical patients, *Anesthesiology* 69:A576, 1988.

170. Messick JM Jr, Casement B, Sharbrough FW et al: Correlation of regional cerebral blood flow (rCBF) with EEG changes during isoflurane anesthesia for carotid endarterectomy: critical rCBF, *Anesthesiology* 66:344, 1987.

171. Messick JM Jr, Milde LN: Brain protection. In Stoelting RK, editor: *Advances in anesthesia*, Chicago, 1987, Year Book Medical Publishers.

172. Meyer FB, Anderson RE, Yaksh TL et al: Effect of nimodipine on intracellular brain pH, cortical blood flow, and EEG in experimental focal cerebral ischemia, *J Neurosurg* 64:617, 1986.

173. Michenfelder JD: The interdependency of cerebral functional and metabolic effects following massive doses of thiopental in the dog, *Anesthesiology* 41:231, 1974.

174. Michenfelder JD: Cerebral preservation for intraoperative focal ischemia, *Clin Neurosurg* 32:105, 1985.

175. Michenfelder JD: A valid demonstration of barbiturate-induced brain protection in man—at last, *Anesthesiology* 64:140, 1986.

176. Michenfelder JD: *Anesthesia and the brain*, New York, 1988, Churchill-Livingstone, p. 79.

177. Michenfelder JD: *Anesthesia and the brain*, New York, 1988, Churchill-Livingstone, p 95.

178. Michenfelder JD, Sundt TM, Fode F et al: Isoflurane when compared to enflurane and halothane decreases the frequency of cerebral ischemia during carotid endarterectomy, *Anesthesiology* 67:336, 1987.

179. Michenfelder JD, Lanier WL, Scheithauer BW et al: Evaluation of the glutamate antagonist dizocilipine maleate (MK-801) on neurologic outcome in a canine model of complete cerebral ischemia: correlation with hippocampal histopathology, *Brain Res* 481:228, 1989.

180. Michenfelder JD, Milde JH: Cerebral protection by anesthetics during ischemia (review), *Resuscitation* 4:219, 1975.

181. Michenfelder JD, Milde JH: Influence of anesthetics on metabolic, functional, and pathologic responses to regional cerebral ischemia, *Stroke* 6:405, 1975.

182. Michenfelder JD, Milde JH: The relationship among canine brain temperature, metabolism, and function during hypothermia, *Anesthesiology* 75:130, 1991.

183. Michenfelder JD, Milde JH, Sundt TM Jr: Cerebral protection by barbiturate anesthesia use after middle cerebral artery occlusion in Java monkeys, *Arch Neurol* 33:345, 1976.

184. Michenfelder JD, Theye RA: Hypothermia: effect on canine brain and whole body metabolism, *Anesthesiology* 29:1107, 1968.

185. Michenfelder JD, Theye RA: The effects of anesthesia and hypothermia on canine cerebral ATP and lactate during anoxia produced by decapitation, *Anesthesiology* 33:430, 1970.

186. Michenfelder JD, Theye RA: Cerebral protection by thiopental during hypoxia, *Anesthesiology* 39:510, 1973.

187. Milde LN: Brain protection. In Cucchiara RF, Michenfelder JD editors: *Clinical neuroanesthesia*, New York, 1990, Churchill-Livingstone, p 188.

188. Milde LN: The hypoxic mouse model for screening cerebral protective agents: a re-examination, *Anesth Analg* 67:917, 1988.

189. Milde LN, Milde JH, Lanier WL et al: Comparison of the effects of isoflurane and thiopental on neurologic outcome and neuropathology after temporary focal cerebral ischemia in primates, *Anesthesiology* 69:905, 1988.

190. Milde LN, Milde JH: Preservation of cerebral metabolites by etomidate during incomplete cerebral ischemia in dogs, *Anesthesiology* 65:272, 1986.

191. Milde LN, Milde JH: The detrimental effect of lidocaine on cerebral metabolism measured in dogs anesthetized with isoflurane, *Anesthesiology* 67:180, 1987.

192. Milde LN, Milde JH, Gallagher WJ: Effects of sufentanil on cerebral circulation and metabolism in dogs, *Anesth Analg* 70:138, 1990.

193. Milde LN, Milde JH, Michenfelder JD: Cerebral functional, metabolic, and hemodynamic effects of etomidate in dogs, *Anesthesiology* 63:371, 1985.

194. Milde LN, Milde JH, Michenfelder JD: Delayed treatment with nimodipine improves cerebral blood flow after complete cerebral ischemia in the dog, *J Cereb Blood Flow Metab* 6:332, 1986.

195. Milde LN, Milde JH, Michenfelder JD: The comparative cerebral protective effects of propofol, thiopental and fentanyl in a canine model of incomplete global cerebral ischemia, *Anesthesiology* (in press).

196. Minamisawa H, Nordstrom CH, Smith ML et al: The influence of mild body and brain hypothermia on ischemic brain damage, *J Cereb Blood Flow Metab* 10:365, 1990.

197. Moffat JA, McDougall MJ, Brunet D et al: Thiopental bolus during carotid endarterectomy-rational drug therapy? *Can Anaesth Soc J* 30:615, 1983.

198. Murphy SN, Thayer SA, Miller RJ: The effects of excitatory amino acids on intracellular calcium in single mouse striatal neurons in vitro, *J Neurosci* 7:4145, 1987.

199. Myers RE, Yamaguchi S: Nervous system effects of cardiac arrest in monkeys, *Arch Neurol* 34:65, 1977.

200. Nakakimura K, Fleischer JE, Drummond JC et al: Glucose administration before cardiac arrest worsens neurologic outcome in cats, *Anesthesiology* 72:1005, 1990.

201. Nedergaard M: Transient focal ischemia in hyperglycemic rats is associated with increased cerebral infarction, *Brain Res* 408:79, 1987.

202. Nedergaard M, Diemer NH: Focal ischemia of the rat brain, with special reference to the influence of plasma glucose concentration, *Acta Neuropathol* 73:131, 1987.

203. Nehls DG, Todd MM, Spetzler RF et al: A comparison of the cerebral protective effects of isoflurane and barbiturates during temporary focal ischemia in primates, *Anesthesiology* 66:453, 1987.

204. Neil-Dwyer G, Mee E, Dorrance D et al: Early intervention with nimo-

dipine in subarachnoid haemorrhage, *Eur Heart J* 8:41, 1987.

205. Nemoto EM, Shiu GK, Bleyaert AL: Efficacy of therapies and attenuation of brain free fatty acid liberation during global ischemia, *Crit Care Med* 9:397, 1981.

206. Nevandeer G, Ingvar M, Auer R et al: Status epilepticus in well oxygenated rats causes neuronal necrosis, *Ann Neurol* 18:281, 1985.

207. Newberg LA, Michenfelder JD: Cerebral protection by isoflurane during hypoxemia or ischemia, *Anesthesiology* 59:29, 1983.

208. Newberg LA, Milde JH, Michenfelder JD: The cerebral metabolic effects of isoflurane at and above concentrations that suppress cortical electrical activity, *Anesthesiology* 59:23, 1983.

209. Newberg LA, Milde JH, Michenfelder JD: Systemic and cerebral effects of isoflurane-induced hypotension in dogs, *Anesthesiology* 60:541, 1984.

210. Newman B, Gelb AW, Lam AM: The effect of isoflurane-induced hypotension on cerebral blood flow and cerebral metabolic rate for oxygen in humans, *Anesthesiology* 64:307, 1986.

211. Nilsson L, Siesjo BK: The effect of phenobarbital anesthesia on blood flow and oxygen consumption in the rat brain, *Acta Anesthesiol Scand Suppl* 57:18, 1975.

212. Nordstrom C-H, Rehncrona S, Siesjo BK: Effects of phenobarbital in cerebral ischemia. Part II. Restitution of cerebral energy state, as well as glycolytic metabolites, citric acid cycle intermediates and associated amino acids, *Stroke* 9:335, 1978.

213. Nussmeier NA, Arlund C, Slogoff S: Neuropsychiatric complications after cardiopulmonary bypass: cerebral protection by a barbiturate, *Anesthesiology* 64:165, 1986.

214. Ochai C, Asano T, Takakura K et al: Mechanisms of cerebral protection by pentobarbital and nizofenone correlated with the course of local cerebral blood flow changes, *Stroke* 13:788, 1982.

215. Ohman J, Heiskanen O: Effect of nimodipine on the outcome of patients after aneurysmal subarachnoid haemorrhage and surgery, *J Neurosurg* 69:683, 1988.

216. Olney JW, de Gubareff T, Sloviter RS: "Epileptic" brain damage in rats induced by sustained electrical stimulation of the perforant path: II. ultrastructural analysis of acute hippocampal pathology, *Brain Res Bull* 10:699, 1983.

217. Olney JW, Price MT, Samson L et al: The role of specific ions in glutamate neurotoxicity, *Neurosci Lett* 65:65, 1986.

218. Paljarvi L, Soderfeldt B, Kalimo H et al: The brain in extreme respiratory acidosis. A light- and electron-microscopic study in the rat, *Acta Neuropathol* 58:87, 1982.

219. Paschen W, Djuricic BM, Bosma HJ et al: Biochemical changes during graded ischemia in gerbils. Part 2. Regional evaluation of cerebral blood flow and brain metabolites, *J Neurol Sci* 58:37, 1983.

220. Patel JB, Ross LE, Duncan B et al: Administration of glycine antagonists, HA-966 and 7-chlorokynurenic acid reduce ischemic brain damage in gerbils, *Soc Neurosci Abstr* 15:43, 1989.

221. Pelligrino DA, Miletich DJ, Hoffman WE et al: Nitrous oxide markedly increases cerebral cortical metabolic rate and blood flow in the goat, *Anesthesiology* 60:405, 1984.

222. Petito CK, Feldmann E, Pulsinelli WA et al: Delayed hippocampal damage in humans following cardiac arrest, *Neurology* 37:1281, 1987.

223. Petruk KC, West M, Mohr G et al: Nimodipine treatment in poor-grade aneurysm patients: Results of a multicenter double-blind placebo-controlled trial, *J Neurosurg* 68:505, 1988.

224. Philippon J, Grob R, Dagreou F et al: Prevention of vasospasm in subarachnoid hemorrhage. A controlled study with nimodipine, *Acta Neurochir* 82:110, 1986.

225. Phillis JW, Simpson RE, Walter GA: The effect of hyperglycemia on extracellular levels of adenosine in the hypoxic rat cerebral cortex, *Brain Res* 524:336, 1990.

226. Pickard JD, Murray GD, Illingworth R et al: Effect of oral nimodipine on cerebral infarction and outcome after subarachnoid haemorrhage: British aneurysm nimodipine trial, *Br Med J* 298:636, 1989.

227. Pinaud M, Lelausque JN, Fauchoux N et al: Effects of propofol on cerebral hemodynamics and metabolism in patients with head trauma, *Anesthesiology* 69:1569, 1988.

228. Plum F: What causes infarction in ischemic brain?: The Robert Wartenberg lecture, *Neurology* 33:222, 1983.

229. Prado R, Ginsberg MC, Dietrich WD et al: Hyperglycemia increases infarct size in collaterally perfused but not end-arterial vascular territories. *J Cereb Blood Flow Metab* 8:186, 1988.

230. Prough DS, Kong D, Watkins WD et al: Inhibition of thromboxane A_2 production does not improve postischemic brain hypoperfusion in the dog, *Stroke* 17:1272, 1986.

231. Pulsinelli WA, Brierly JB, Plum F: Temporal profile of neuronal damage in a model of transient forebrain ischemia, *Ann Neurol* 11:491, 1982.

232. Pulsinelli WA, Kraig RP, Plum F: Hyperglycemia, cerebral acidosis, and ischemic brain damage. In Plum F, Pulsinelli WA, editors: *Cerebrovascular diseases. 14th Research Princeton-Williamsburg Conference,* New York, 1985, Raven Press, p 201.

233. Pulsinelli WA, Levy DE, Sigsbee B et al: Increased damage after ischemic stroke in patients with hyperglycemia with or without established diabetes mellitus, *Am J Med* 74:540, 1983.

234. Pulsinelli WA, Waldman S, Rawlinson D et al: Moderate hyperglycemia augments ischemic brain damage: a neuropathologic study in the rat, *Neurology* 32:1239, 1982.

235. Pulsinelli W, Waldman S, Sigsbee B et al: Experimental hyperglycemia and diabetes mellitus worsen stroke outcome, *Trans Am Neurol Assoc* 105:21, 1980.

236. Raichle ME: The pathophysiology of brain ischemia, *Ann Neurol* 13:2, 1983.

237. Ramani R, Todd MM, Warner DS: Dose-related changes in CBF and $CMRo_2$ during propofol infusions in rabbits, *Anesthesiology* 73:A702, 1990.

238. Rehncrona S, Hauge HN, Siesjo BK: Enhancement of iron-catalyzed free radical formation by acidosis in brain homogenates: difference in effect by lactic acid and CO_2, *J Cereb Blood Flow Metab* 9:65, 1989.

239. Rehncrona S, Kagstrom E: Tissue lactic acidosis and ischemic brain damage, *Am J Emerg Med* 1:168, 1983.

240. Rehncrona S, Rosen I, Siesjo BK: Excessive cellular acidosis: an important mechanism of neuronal damage in the brain? *Acta Physiol Scand* 110:435, 1980.

241. Renou AM, Vernheit J, Macrez P et al: Cerebral blood flow and metabolism during etomidate anaesthesia in man, *Br J Anaesth* 50:1047, 1978.

242. Robinson MJ, Teasdale GM: Calcium antagonists in the management of subarachnoid haemorrhage, *Cerebrovasc Brain Metab Rev* 2:205, 1990.

243. Rogers KM, Adam HK, Dewar KMS et al: ICI 35868, a new i.v. anaesthetic: preliminary findings in 20 patients, *Br J Anaesth* 52:230, 1980.

244. Roine RO, Kaste M, Kinnunen A et al: Safety and efficacy of nimodipine in resuscitation of patients outside hospital, *Br Med J* 294:20, 1987.

245. Roine RO, Kaste M, Kinnunen A et al: Nimodipine after resuscitation from out-of-hospital ventricular fibrillation. A placebo-controlled, double-blind, randomized trial, *JAMA* 264:3171, 1990.

246. Rothman SM: Synaptic activity mediates death of hypoxic neurons, *Science* 220:536, 1983.

247. Rothman SM: The neurotoxicity of excitatory amino acids is produced by passive chloride influx, *J Neurosci* 5:1483, 1985.

248. Rothman SM, Olney JW: Glutamate and the pathophysiology of hypoxic-ischemic brain damage, *Ann Neurol* 19:105, 1986.

249. Sakabe T, Kuramoto T, Inoue S et al: Cerebral effects of nitrous oxide in the dog, *Anesthesiology* 48:195, 1978.

250. Sakabe T, Maekawa T, Ishikawa T et al: The effects of lidocaine on canine cerebral metabolism and circulation related to the electroencephalogram, *Anesthesiology* 40:433, 1974.

251. Sakabe T, Nagai T, Ishikawa T et al: Nicardipine increases cerebral blood flow but does not improve neurologic recovery in a canine model of complete cerebral ischemia, *J Cereb Blood Flow Metab* 6:684, 1986.

252. Sano T, Patel PM, Drummond JC et al: A comparison of the cerebral protection effects of isoflurane and mild hypothermia in a model of incomplete forebrain ischemia, *Anesthesiology* 75:A602, 1991.

253. Schmidley JW: Free radicals in central nervous system ischemia, *Stroke* 21:1086, 1990.

254. Secher O, Wilhjelm B: The protective action of anesthetics against hypoxia, *Can Anaesth Soc J* 15:423, 1968.

255. Selman WR, Spetzler RF, Roessmann UR et al: Barbiturate-induced coma therapy for focal cerebral ischemia, effect after temporary and permanent MCA occlusion, *J Neurosurg* 55:220, 1981.

256. Sharbrough FW, Messick JM Jr, Sundt TM Jr: Correlation of continuous electroencephalograms with cerebral blood flow measurements during carotid endarterectomy, *Stroke* 4:674, 1973.

257. Shokunbi MT, Gelb AW, Peerless SJ et al: An evaluation of the effect of lidocaine in experimental focal cerebral ischemia, *Stroke* 17:962, 1986.

258. Shokunbi MT, Gelb AW, Wu XM et al: Continuous lidocaine infusion and focal feline cerebral ischemia, *Stroke* 21:107, 1990.

259. Siemkewicz E, Gjedde A: Postischemic coma in rat: effect of different pre-ischemic blood glucose levels on cerebral metabolic recovery after ischemia, *Acta Physiol Scand* 110:225, 1980.

260. Siemkewicz E, Hansen AJ: Clinical restitution following cerebral ischemia in hypo-, normo-, and hyperglycemic rats, *Acta Neurol Scand* 58:1, 1978.

261. Siesjo BK: Cell damage in the brain: a speculative synthesis, *J Cereb Blood Flow Metab* 1:155, 1981.

262. Siesjo BK: Brain cell death in aging and ischemia: are free radicals involved? *Monogr Neurol Sci* 11:1, 1984.

263. Siesjo BK: Cerebral circulation and metabolism, *J Neurosurg* 60:883, 1984.

264. Siesjo BK: Historical overview: calcium, ischemia, and death of brain cells, *Ann NY Acad Sci* 522:638, 1988.

265. Siesjo BK, Bendek G, Koide T et al: Influence of acidosis on lipid peroxidation in brain tissues in vitro, *J Cereb Blood Flow Metab* 5:253, 1985.

266. Silverstein FS, Buchanan K, Johnston MV: Perinatal hypoxia-ischaemia disrupts striatal high-affinity [3H] glutamate uptake into synaptosomes, *J Neurochem* 47:1614, 1982.

267. Simeone F, Frazer G, Lawner P: Ischemic brain edema: comparative effects of barbiturates and hypothermia, *Stroke* 10:8, 1979.

268. Simon RP, Bartkowski H, Roman R: Attenuation of infarct size by pharmacologic inhibition of excitatory amino acid neurotransmission by specific NMDA antagonist administered 15 minutes after stroke, *Neurology* 38:147, 1988.

269. Simon RP, Griffiths T, Evans MC et al: Calcium overload in selectively vulnerable neurons of the hippocampus during and after ischaemia: an electron microscopy study in the rat, *J Cereb Blood Flow Metab* 4:350, 1984.

270. Simon RP, Swan JH, Griffiths T et al: Blockage of N-methyl-D-aspartate receptors may protect against ischemic damage in the brain, *Science* 226:850, 1984.

271. Smith AL, Hoff JT, Nielsen SL et al: Barbiturate protection in acute focal ischemia, *Stroke* 5:1, 1974.

272. Smith AL, Marque J: Anesthetics and cerebral edema, *Anesthesiology* 45:64, 1976.

273. Smith DS, Keykhah MM, O'Niell JJ et al: The effect of etomidate pretreatment on cerebral high energy metabolites, lactate, and glucose during severe hypoxia in the rat, *Anesthesiology* 71:438, 1989.

274. Smith M-L, Kagstrom E, Rosenn I et al: Effect of the calcium antagonist nimodipine on the delayed hypoperfusion following incomplete ischemia in the rat, *J Cereb Blood Flow Metab* 3:543, 1983.

275. Snyder BD, Ramirez-Lassepas M, Sukhum P et al: Failure of thiopental to modify global anoxic injury, *Stroke* 10:135, 1979.

276. Southorn PA, Powis G: Free radicals in medicine. I. Chemical nature and biologic reactions, *Mayo Clin Proc* 63:381, 1988.

277. Southorn PA, Powis G: Free radicals in medicine. II. Involvement in human disease, *Mayo Clin Proc* 63:390, 1988.

278. Spetzler RF, Selman WR, Roski RA et al: Cerebral revascularization dur-

ing barbiturate coma in primates and humans, *Surg Neurol* 17:111, 1982.

279. Spetzler RF, Martin N, Hadley MN et al: Microsurgical endarterectomy under barbiturate protection: a prospective study, *J Neurosurg* 65:63, 1986.

280. Steen PA, Gisvold SE, Milde JH et al: Nimodipine improves outcome when given after complete cerebral ischemia in primates, *Anesthesiology* 62:406, 1985.

281. Steen PA, Michenfelder JD: Mechanisms of barbiturate protection, *Anesthesiology* 53:183, 1980.

282. Steen PA, Milde JH, Michenfelder JD: No barbiturate protection in a dog model of complete cerebral ischemia, *Ann Neurol* 5:343, 1979.

283. Steen PA, Newberg LA, Milde JH et al: Cerebral blood flow and neurologic outcome when nimodipine is given after complete cerebral ischemia in the dog, *J Cereb Blood Flow Metab* 4:82, 1984.

284. Steen PA, Newberg LA, Milde JH et al: Hypothermia and barbiturates: individual and combined effects on canine cerebral oxygen consumption, *Anesthesiology* 58:527, 1983.

285. Steinberg GK, Saleh J, Kunis D: Delayed treatment with dextromethorphan and dextorphan reduces cerebral damage after transient focal ischemia, *Neurosci Lett* 89:193, 1988.

286. Stephan H, Sonntag H, Schenk HD et al: Einflus von Disoprivan (propofol) auf die Durchblutung und den Sauerstoffverbrauch des Gehirns und die CO_2-Reaktivität der Hirngefase beim Menschen, *Anaesthetist* 36:60, 1987.

287. Stockard J, Bickford R: The neurophysiology of anesthesia, *Monogr Anaesthesiol* 2:3, 1975.

288. Storm-Mathisen J, Iversen L: Uptake of [3H] glutamic acid in excitatory nerve endings: light and electron microscopic observations in the hippocampal formation of the rat, *Neuroscience* 4:1237, 1987.

289. Suzuki R, Yamaguchi T, Li CL et al: The effects of 5-minute ischemia in mongolian gerbils. II. Changes of spontaneous neuronal activity in cerebral cortex and CA1 sector of hippocampus, *Acta Neuropathol* 60:217, 1983.

290. Tarnow J, Hess W, Klein W: Etomidate, alfathesin and thiopentone as induction agents for coronary artery surgery, *Can Anaesth Soc* J 27:338, 1986.

291. Tharion J, Johnson DC, Celermajor JM et al: Profound hypothermia with circulatory arrest: Nine years clinical experience, *J Thorac Cardiovasc Surg* 84:66, 1982.

292. Thomas R, Hessel EA 2d, Harker LA et al: Platelet function during and after deep surface hypothermia, *J Surg Res* 31:314, 1981.

293. Todd MM, Chadwick HS, Shapiro HM et al: The neurologic effects of thiopental therapy following experimental cardiac arrest in cats, *Anesthesiology* 57:76, 1982.

294. Todd MM, Drummond JC, Hoi Sang U: The hemodynamic consequences of high-dose thiopental anesthesia, *Anesth Analg* 64:681, 1985.

295. Trojaborg W, Boysen G: Relation between EEG, regional cerebral blood flow and internal carotid artery pressure during carotid endarterectomy, *Electroencephalogr Clin Neurophysiol* 34:61, 1973.

296. Tulleken CAF, van Dieren A, Jonkman J et al: Clinical and experimental experience with etomidate as a brain protective agent, *J Cereb Blood Flow Metab*, (suppl) 2:592, 1982.

297. Vaagenes P, Cantadore R, Safar P et al: Amelioration of brain damage by lidoflazine after prolonged ventricular fibrillation cardiac arrest in dogs, *Crit Care Med* 12:846, 1984.

298. Valeri CR, Feingold H, Cassidy G et al: Hypothermia-induced reversible platelet dysfunction, *Ann Surg* 205:175, 1987.

299. Van den Kerckhoff W, Hossmann KA, Hossmann V: No effect of prostacyclin on blood flow, regulation of blood flow and blood coagulation following global cerebral ischemia, *Stroke* 14:724, 1983.

300. Van Hemelrijck J, Fitch W, Mattheussen M et al: Effect of propofol on cerebral circulation and autoregulation in the baboon, *Anesth Analg* 71:49, 1990.

301. Vandensteene A, Trempont V, Engelman E et al: Effect of propofol on cerebral blood flow and metabolism in man, *Anaesthesia* 43(suppl):42, 1988.

302. Vanhoutte PM: Calcium entry blockers and vascular smooth muscle, *Circulation* (suppl) 65:11, 1982.

303. Vanhoutte PM: Calcium entry blockers, vascular smooth muscle, and systemic hypertension, *Am J Cardiol* 55(suppl B): 17-23, 1985.

304. Varner PD, Vinik HR, Funderburg C: Survival during severe hypoxia and propofol or ketamine anesthesia in mice, *Anesthesiology* 69:A571, 1988.

305. Voll CL, Whishaw IQ, Auer RN: Postischemic insulin reduces spatial learning deficit following transient forebrain ischemia in rats, *Stroke* 20:646, 1989.

306. Wagner RL, White PF, Kan PB et al: Inhibition of adrenal steroidogenesis by the anesthetic etomidate, *N Engl J Med* 310:1415, 1984.

307. Wagner RL, White PF: Etomidate inhibits adrenocortical function in surgical patients, *Anesthesiology* 61:647, 1984.

308. Warner DS, Deshpande JK, Wieloch T: The effect of isoflurane on neuronal necrosis following near-complete forebrain ischemia in the rat, *Anesthesiology* 64:19, 1986.

309. Warner DS, Godersky JC, Smith M: Failure of pre-ischemic lidocaine administration to ameliorate global ischemic brain damage in the rat, *Anesthesiology* 68:73, 1988.

310. Warner DS, Zhou J, Ramani R et al: Nitrous oxide does not alter infarct volume in rats undergoing reversible middle cerebral artery occlusion, *Anesthesiology* 73:686, 1990.

311. Warner DS, Zhou JG, Ramani R et al: Reversible focal ischemia in the rat: effects of halothane, isoflurane, and methohexital anesthesia, *J Cereb Blood Flow Metab* 11:794, 1991.

312. Watson BD, Ginsberg MD: Ischemic injury in the brain: role of oxygen radical-mediated processes, *Ann NY Acad Sci* 559:269, 1989.

313. Wauquier A: Brain protective properties of etomidate and flunarizine, *J Cereb Blood Flow Metab* (suppl) 2:553, 1982.

314. Wauquier A, Ashton D, Clincke G et al: Antihypoxic effects of etomidate, thiopental, and methohexital, *Arch Int Pharmacodyn Ther* 249:330, 1981.

315. Weir DL, Goodchild CS, Graham DZ: Propofol: effects on indices of cerebral ischemia, *J Neurosurg Anesth* 1:284, 1989.

316. Welsh FA, Ginsberg MD, Rieder W

et al: Deleterious effect of glucose pretreatment on recovery from diffuse cerebral ischemia in the cat. II. Regional metabolite levels, *Stroke* 11:355, 1980.

317. Werner C, Hoffman WE, Thomas C et al: Ganglionic blockade improves neurologic outcome from incomplete ischemia in rats: partial reversal with exogenous catecholamines, *Anesthesiology* 73:923, 1990.

318. White BC, Aust SD, Arfors KE et al: Brain injury by ischemic anoxia: Hypothesis extension—a tale of two ions? *Ann Emerg Med* 13:862, 1984.

319. White BC, Wiegenstein JG, Winegar CD: Brain ischemic anoxia. Mechanisms of injury, *JAMA* 251:1586, 1984.

320. White BC, Winegar CD, Wilson RF et al: Calcium blockers in cerebral resuscitation, *J Trauma* 23:788, 1983.

321. Wieloch T: Hypoglycemia-induced neuronal damage prevented by N-methyl-D-aspartate antagonist, *Science* 230:681, 1985.

322. Wieloch T, Gusafsson I, Westerberg E: MK-801 does not protect against brain damage in a rat model of cerebral ischemia, *Neurochem Int* 12:24, 1988.

323. Wieloch T, Lindvall O, Blomquist P et al: Evidence for amelioration of ischemic neuronal damage in hippocampal formation by lesions of the perforant path, *Neurol Research* 7:24, 1985.

324. Wieloch T, Siesjo BK: Ischemic brain injury: the importance of calcium, lipolytic activities, and free fatty acids, *J Pathol Biol* 5:269, 1982.

325. Winegar CP, Henderson O, White BC et al: Early amelioration of neurologic deficit by lidoflazine after fifteen minutes of cardiopulmonary arrest in dogs, *Ann Emerg Med* 12:471, 1983.

326. Wolfe LS: Eicosanoids: prostaglandins, thromboxanes, leukotrienes, and other derivatives of carbon-20 unsaturated fatty acids, *J Neurochem* 38:1, 1982.

327. Woo E, Chan YW, Yu YL et al: Admission glucose level in relation to mortality and morbidity outcome in 252 stroke patients, *Stroke* 19:185, 1988.

328. Yatsu FM: Cardiopulmonary-cerebral resuscitation, *N Engl J Med* 314:440, 1986.

329. Yatsu FM, Diamond I, Graziano C et al: Experimental brain ischemia: pro-

tection from irreversible damage with a rapid acting barbiturate (methohexital), *Stroke* 3:726, 1972.

330. Yip PK, He YY, Hsu CY et al: Effect of plasma glucose on infarct size in focal cerebral ischemia-reperfusion, *Neurology* 41:899, 1991.

331. Young W, Wojak JC, DeCrescito V: 21-Aminosteroid reduces ion shifts and edema in rat middle cerebral artery occlusion model of regional ischemia, *Stroke* 19:1013, 1988.

332. Zarden JR, Klochany A, Martin WM et al: Effect of thiopental on neurologic outcome following coronary artery bypass grafting, *Anesthesiology* 74:406, 1991.

333. Zasslow MA, Pearl RG, Shuer LM et al: Hyperglycemia decreases acute neuronal ischemic changes after middle cerebral artery occlusion in cats, *Stroke* 20:519, 1989.

334. Zurick AM, Sigurdsson H, Koehler LS et al: Magnitude and time course of perioperative adrenal suppression with single dose etomidate in male adult cardiac surgical patients. *Anesthesiology* 65:A248, 1986.

4

Cerebrospinal Fluid

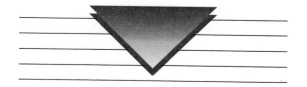

ALAN A. ARTRU

Brain and spinal cord well-being during anesthesia, surgery, and critical care is supported by cerebrospinal fluid (CSF). CSF provides mechanical protection, subserves nutriative and transport functions, and clears unwanted and harmful substances from neural tissue. These CSF functions are influenced by the dynamic aspects of CSF—that is, the rate of CSF formation ($\dot{V}_f$), resistance to reabsorption of CSF (R_a), and the manner in which they affect and are affected by CSF pressure. Research on CSF physiology and dynamics is ongoing, with the aim of better understanding this system and how it can best be managed in patients at risk for brain or spinal cord injury.

The first section of this chapter reviews CSF with respect to its anatomy, physiology, and effects of anesthetics and other influences. The second section of this chapter reviews the relationship between CSF dynamics and intracranial pressure (ICP), anesthetics and drug-induced changes in CSF dynamics that increase or decrease ICP, and clinical situations wherein therapy to alter CSF dynamics may affect neurologic outcome. This chapter provides comprehensive information about the regulation of fluid and chemicals in the brain and spinal cord and also provides a background for understanding the relation of those systems to the later chapters on clinical care.

ANATOMY OF THE CSF SPACES AND PROPERTIES OF CSF

CSF is formed in the brain and circulates through macroscopic and extracellular fluid (ECF) spaces that are in con-

TABLE 4-1
CSF Pressure and Volume in Humans

	Range of CSF Values*
CSF Pressure (mm Hg)	
Children	3.0-7.5
Adults	4.5-13.5
Volume (ml)	
Infants	40-60
Young children	60-100
Older children	80-120
Adult	100-160

*Values based on references 45, 55, 82, 132, 203.

tinuity. The macroscopic CSF spaces include two lateral ventricles, the third (cerebral) ventricle, the aqueduct of Sylvius, the fourth (cerebellar) ventricle, the central canal of the spinal cord, and the subarachnoid space. The total volume of these spaces ranges from 50 ml in infants to 140 to 150 ml in adults (Table 4-1). Ventricular volume composes about 16% to 17% of macroscopic CSF volume in adults.[55] The ECF space is that which surrounds the neuronal and glial elements of the central nervous system (CNS). Brain ECF volume is about 300 to 350 ml in adults.

Macroscopic Spaces

The choroid plexuses (CPs) of the lateral ventricles extend from the inferior horn to the central part of the ventricle. The CPs of the two lateral ventricles and the third ventricle become continuous with each other at the interventricular foramina. Each CP is supported on vascular invaginations of the pia mater called the tela choroidea. The CPs in the body of the lateral and third ventricles receive their blood supply from the posterior and anterior choroidal arteries, respectively. The CPs in the temporal horns and the fourth ventricle are supplied by the superior and posterior inferior cerebellar arteries, respectively.[127] The nervous supply to the CPs includes branches of the vagus, glossopharyngeal, and sympathetic nerves.

Most of the macroscopic CSF spaces are lined by a single layer of epithelial cells. In contrast, the ventricles and central canal of the spinal cord are lined by ependyma, a ciliated, low-columnar epithelium. There are tight junctions between ependymal cells where they cover the CP but not elsewhere. An "open" mesothelium, formed inwardly by the pia and outwardly by a loose investment of arachnoid cells, covers the cisterns and sulci of the subarachnoid space.

ECF Spaces

The ECF spaces of the brain and spinal cord, unlike those of other organs in the body, are small in diameter (180 Å). These narrow, interconnecting channels are anatomically continuous with the adjoining macroscopic CSF spaces. Exchange between cerebral capillaries and the ECF is limited, because the capillary membrane is highly impermeable. This "blood-brain barrier" (BBB) consists of two elements. First, the cells of the cerebral capillary endothelium are joined by tight junctions (zonulae occludentae) that restrict the intercellular movement of molecules having a diameter of 20 Å or more.[29,66,158] Second, astrocyte foot processes surround the capillaries. This architecture is unique to cerebral blood vessels and is found in all areas of the brain except at the CP (and several other small regions).

There is evidence that the ECF spaces communicate with lymphatic channels. Up to 30% of labeled CSF or tracers injected into the brain can be recovered in the deep cervical lymph system.[31,49,50] CSF may reach these lymphatics via the cribriform plate. The arachnoid of the plate joins with olfactory perineurium composed of fibroblasts and large intercellular spaces.[119] CSF and its contents may thus enter the nasal submucosa and from there pass into the deep cervical lymph nodes via afferent ducts.

COMPOSITION OF CSF

CSF is a clear aqueous solution that, compared with plasma, contains higher concentrations of sodium, chloride, and magnesium and lower concentrations of glucose, proteins, amino acids, uric acid, potassium, bicarbonate, calcium, and phosphate (Table 4-2). The concentration of these and other substances in the macroscopic spaces varies according to the sampling site, because diffusion between CSF and ECF occurs as CSF passes through the ventricles and subarachnoid spaces.[55] Differences between the composition of CSF and an ultrafiltrate of plasma indicate that active secretion occurs during CSF formation. Regional variations in potassium, urea, albumin, globulin, and amino acids indicates that transport of solutes into and out of the CSF occurs at sites other than the CP.[73] For example, the concentrations of calcium, bicarbonate, and potassium are lower, and the concentration of chloride is greater in mixed CSF than in freshly formed CSF. In the case of calcium, its movement out of CSF is reported to occur by a transport mechanism and to be concentration independent.[62] The higher concentration of protein in lumbar CSF relative to cisternal CSF probably reflects net addition of CNS metabolites to CSF as it drains toward sites of absorption.[129]

CSF FORMATION

The rate of CSF formation is about 0.35 to 0.40 ml/min or 500 to 600 ml/day in humans. Approximately 0.25% of total adult CSF volume is replaced by freshly formed CSF each minute. The turnover time for total CSF volume is 5 to 7 hours, yielding a turnover rate of about four times per day.[132] About 40% to 70% of CSF enters the macroscopic spaces via the CP, whereas 30% to 60% of CSF enters across the ependyma and pia.[170]

TABLE 4-2
Composition of CSF and Plasma in Humans

	Mean CSF Concentration*	Mean Plasma Concentration*
Specific gravity	1.007	1.025
Osmolality (mOsm/kg H_2O)	289	289
pH	7.31	7.41
P_{CO_2} (mm Hg)	50.5	41.1
Sodium (mEq/L)	141	140
Potassium (mEq/L)	2.9	4.6
Calcium (mEq/L)	2.5	5.0
Magnesium (mEq/L)	2.4	1.7
Chloride (mEq/L)	124	101
Bicarbonate (mEq/L)	21	23
Glucose (mg/100 ml)	61	92
Protein (mg/100 ml)	28	7000
Albumin	23	4430
Globulin	5	2270
Fibrinogen	0	300

*Average values based on references 45, 55, 82, 132, 203.

CSF Formation at the Choroid Plexus

Unlike the capillary endothelium of other cerebral vessels, the capillary endothelium of the CP does not possess tight junctions between its cells. Instead, the capillary endothelium of the CP is fenestrated. Blood entering CP capillaries is filtered across this endothelium and forms a protein-rich fluid within the CP stroma that is similar in composition to interstitial fluid in other tissues of the body. The CP stroma is separated from the macroscopic CSF spaces by the CP epithelial cells. These contain apical tight junctions that restrict passive solute exchange and constitute a "blood-CSF barrier" at the CP.[35] Epithelial-cell enzymes that are involved with the active, bidirectional transport of substances between plasma and CSF[27,129,130,206] and pinocytotic vesicles and lysosomes also contribute to this "barrier."[54,131]

Selected constituents of the stromal fluid are transported across the relatively impermeable CP epithelium by the combined processes of ultrafiltration and secretion.[129,130] Stroma fluid enters clefts between the CP epithelial cells due to hydrostatic pressure and bulk flow (Fig. 4-1). Adenosine triphosphate (ATP)–dependent membrane pumps on the abluminal surface move sodium ions into the cell and potassium and hydrogen ions into the stroma as counter ions.[90,91,177,205] Water moves into the cell along the resultant osmolar gradient, and chloride ions—coupled with sodium ions—move into the cell. Bicarbonate and hydrogen ions are formed within the epithelial cell by the action of carbonic anhydrase on carbon dioxide created within the cell as a result of cellular metabolism or diffusing into the cell from capillary blood. ATP-dependent membrane pumps on the secretory surface of the cell move sodium ions into the CSF and potassium ions in the direction of the stroma. Water entering the epithelial cell along the osmotic gradient established by active sodium secretion continues along that gradient and passes into the ventricle. Water may also move from the stroma into the CSF via "leaky" tight junctions. Chloride and bicarbonate anions in the epithelial cell move passively into the CSF along an electrochemical gradient. Some chloride anions and the ions found in low concentrations in the CSF (such as calcium and magnesium) also pass through "leaky" tight junctions.

Extrachoroidal CSF Formation

Sixty percent of extrachoroidal CSF formation results from oxidation of glucose by the brain, and 40% results from ultrafiltration from cerebral capillaries.[155] In most of the cerebral vasculature, passage of large and polar molecules across the "blood-ECF" interface is restricted by capillary tight junctions and specialized heterolytic vesicles within endothelial cells. Water, electrolytes, glucose, amino acids, urea, lipid-soluble materials, and a number of small nonelectrolytes pass more freely across this interface.[97,145] Some of these substances may be actively transported by the astrocyte layer that envelopes the capillary endothelium, while others may diffuse into the brain ECF.[143] This glucose-rich and protein-poor "lymph" diffuses through the ECF space toward the macroscopic CSF spaces (Fig. 4-2). In addition, beyond the capillary-glial complex and downstream from the "blood-ECF" interface are transport systems that further modify the chemical composition of substances entering the macroscopic CSF spaces. These systems include not only sodium and potassium pumps associated with neurons,[77] but also specialized transport mechanisms possessed by the ventricular ependyma.[97,128]

Movement of Glucose

The concentration of glucose in CSF at the CP or in mixed samples is approximately 60% of that in blood.[168] This ratio remains constant unless blood glucose increases to above 15 to 20 mM (270 to 360 mg/dl). Glucose in blood enters CSF by facilitated transport, so that glucose crosses the "blood-CSF barrier" more quickly than would be predicted on the basis of its lipid solubility.[83] Transport follows saturable kinetics, with the rate being directly related to serum glucose concentration and independent of the serum-to-CSF glucose concentration gradient.[84] At normoglycemia, diffusion of glucose from blood is insignificant.[23] Glucose moves into CSF, independent of $\dot{V}_f$, along the downhill blood-CSF glucose concentration gradient needed for facilitated diffusion.

Movement of glucose in the opposite direction, from the cerebral ventricles into the surrounding brain and blood, occurs via oubain-sensitive and -insensitive fluxes and diffusion.[36] One transport site may be located at the CP.[37,47] Periventricular tissue clears and metabolizes 50% of the glucose in CSF.[84] As glucose is cleared from the CSF, it is replaced by glucose from serum in an amount that is about 25% of the serum glucose concentration.

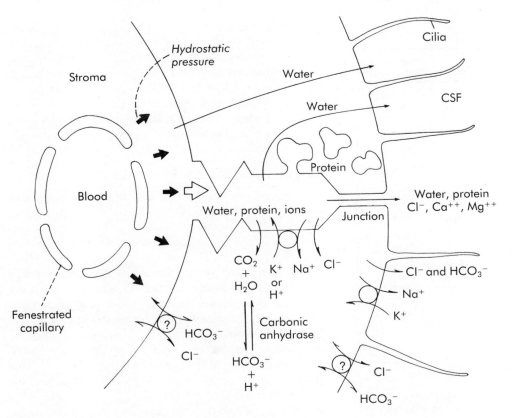

FIG. 4-1 Some of the processes involved in CSF formation at the choroid plexus are shown in schematic form. ATP-dependent membrane "pumps" transport Na^+ across the abluminal surface to within the choroid plexus cell and across the secretory surface, into the macroscopic CSF space, in exchange for K^+ and H^+. Water moves from the stroma into CSF as it follows the concentration gradient produced by the ionic "pumps." *(From Cucchiara RF, Michenfelder JD, editors:* Clinical neuroanesthesia, *New York, 1990, Churchill-Livingstone.)*

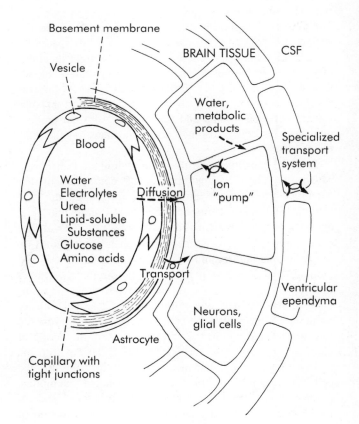

FIG. 4-2 Water and other constituents of plasma cross the BBB (capillary endothelial cells, basement membrane, and astrocyte foot processes) into the brain ECF space by diffusion or transport. This fluid diffuses toward the macroscopic CSF space and subarachnoid space. Water and other cellular metabolites are added to the ECF from neurons and glial cells.

Movement of Protein

Protein entry into CSF from blood at the CP and extrachoroidal sites is limited, so that CSF protein concentrations are normally 0.5% or less of the respective plasma or serum concentrations. Entry rates at CP and extrachoroidal sites for many proteins remain to be determined.[34,35,55,156] If a structural barrier between the brain ECF and the macroscopic CSF space is absent, proteins entering the brain ECF drain into the macroscopic CSF space by bulk flow. Once in CSF, proteins are transported along with CSF through the macroscopic pathways and are cleared from the CSF space into dural venous sinuses. This "sink effect" of flowing CSF keeps the CSF and brain protein concentration low and far from equilibrium with blood.[55,67,70,155] In normal infants and adults, CSF protein concentrations are lowest in the ventricles (about 26 mg/100 ml), intermediate in the cisterna magna (about 32 mg/100 ml), and highest in the lumbar sac (42 mg/100 ml).[195] The lumbar:ventricular CSF concentration ratio for albumin is 2.2:1, for immunoglobulin (Ig)G, it is 2.6:1; and for prealbumin, it is 0.7:1. Albumin and IgG in CSF derive from blood, whereas prealbumin is produced in part by nervous tissue or is transported actively into CSF. It has been speculated that the increased concentration of protein in the lumbar subarachnoid compartment (56% of total CSF compartment volume), as compared with the ventricular and cisternal compartments (26% and 18% of total volume respectively), is related to decreased CSF flow and washout rate in the lumbar space.[108]

Under normal conditions, 60% of protein entry into CSF occurs at the CP and 40% occurs at extrachoroidal sites.[85] At the CP, stromal protein may enter into CSF between epithelial cells because the apical tight junctions of these cells are less restrictive than most cerebrovascular tight junctions.[30,43] Proteins within the CP stroma may also enter the CSF by vesicular transport across the CP epithelium.[26,33] Further, stromal proteins may diffuse into CSF at the edge of the CP, where a functional leak exists at the border between CP epithelium and ventricular ependyma.[33] Models have been proposed to explain the reported negative relationship between the steady state CSF:blood concentration ratio and the hydrodynamic ratio of blood derived proteins. A heterogenous model of aqueous pores with a 117-Å radius, as well as transfer by pinocytotic vesicles with an assumed radius of 25 Å, has been proposed as the most likely model.[157]

Effects of Increased ICP on CSF Formation

The negative correlation between $\dot{V}_f$ and increased ICP is weak; the relationship between $\dot{V}_f$ and cerebral perfusion pressure (CPP) is somewhat stronger.[147] Increase of ICP to 20 mm Hg produces no change in $\dot{V}_f$, so long as CPP remains above ~70 mm Hg.[42,197] When CPP is reduced below ~70 mm Hg, whether by arterial hypotension or by combining arterial hypotension with increased ICP, $\dot{V}_f$ decreases.

These $\dot{V}_f$ results are consistent with reported effects of changes in CPP on cerebral blood flow (CBF), lateral ventricle CP blood flow (CPBF), and fourth ventricle CPBF.[147] A decrease of CPP to 70 mm Hg by arterial hypotension, combined with increased ICP, reduces CBF and CPBF. A decrease of CPP to 50 mm Hg causes a further decline in CPBF when CPP is reduced by an even greater increase of ICP, but not when CPP is reduced solely by arterial hypotension. These results indicate that $\dot{V}_f$ and CPBF are directly related to CPP. That CPBF is lower when CPP is decreased by combining arterial hypotension with increased ICP than when CPP is decreased solely by arterial hypotension may be due to an increase in CP vascular resistance (due to CP compression), as well as to changes in hydrostatic forces within the CP vascular bed.[147] Both factors reduce filtration from CP capillaries.

CIRCULATION OF CSF

CSF moves through the macroscopic spaces from sites of formation to sites of reabsorption. Several factors contribute to that movement. The hydrostatic pressure of CSF formation, 15 cm H_2O, produces CSF flow where it is freshly formed.[55] Cilia on ependymal cells generate currents that propel CSF toward the fourth ventricle and its foramina into the subarachnoid spaces.[44] Respiratory variations and vascular pulsations of the cerebral arteries and CP cause ventricular excursions, supplying additional momentum for CSF movement. The pressure difference between mean CSF pressure, 15 cm H_2O, and superior sagittal sinus pressure, 9 cm H_2O, provides a 6 cm H_2O pressure gradient for passage of CSF across the arachnoid villi.[32,126,129] The high velocity of blood flow through the fixed diameter of the sinuses and the low intraluminal pressure that develops at the circumference of the sinus wall where the arachnoid villi enter causes a "suction-pump" action that may explain how the circulation of the CSF continues through a wide range of postural pressures.[126]

After its formation in the two lateral ventricles, CSF passes through the paired interventricular foramina of Monro into the midline third ventricle. CSF then flows caudally through the aqueduct of Sylvius and fourth ventricle and into the subarachnoid space by one of three exits. Two are the paired lateral foramina of Luschka, from which CSF flows around the brain stem into the cerebellopontine angle and prepontine cisterns. The third exit is the midline foramen of Magendie, from which CSF flows through the vallecula into the cisterna magna. A small portion of CSF may also leave the fourth ventricle through the central canal of the spinal cord.[58]

CSF follows three paths out of the cisterna magna. CSF may pass superiorly into the subarachnoid space surrounding the cerebellar hemisphere. CSF may pass inferiorly into the spinal subarachnoid space. Here CSF flows in a caudal direction dorsal to the cord (posterior to the dentate ligaments) to the lumbar theca and then in a cephalad direction

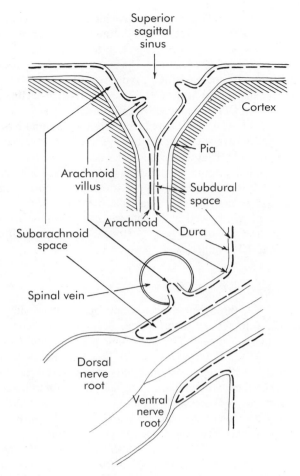

Superior
sagittal
sinus

Cortex

Pia

Arachnoid
villus

Subdural
space

Arachnoid   Dura

Subarachnoid
space

Spinal vein

Dorsal
nerve
root

Ventral
nerve
root

FIG. 4-3   CSF is reabsorbed via arachnoid villi at the sagittal sinus and at spinal veins on dorsal nerve roots. *(From Cucchiara RF, Michenfelder JD, editors:* Clinical neuroanesthesia, *New York, 1990, Churchill-Livingstone.)*

ventral to the cord to the basilar cisterns.[58,126] A third path is for cisternal CSF to move cephalad, into the premedullary, pontine, and interpeduncular cisterns. CSF flows in two directions out of these basilar cisterns. One course is inferiorly, through the interpeduncular cistern, Sylvian fissure, and prechiasmatic cisterns, to the subarachnoid space of the lateral and frontal cerebral cortex. A second course is dorsomedially, through the ambient cisterns and cisterna venae magnae cerebri, to the subarachnoid space of the medial and posterior aspects of the cerebral cortex. CSF circulation concludes with reabsorption across arachnoid villi into the superior sagittal sinus and spinal dural sinusoids located on dorsal nerve roots (Fig. 4-3).

Radioisotope studies indicate that labelled CSF flows from the ventricles to the basal cisterns within a few minutes and collects along the superior sagittal sinus area at 12 to 24 hours.[57] CSF enters the low cervical–high thoracic region at 10 to 20 minutes, the thoracolumbar area at 30 to 40 minutes, the lumbosacral *cul de sac* at 60 to 90 minutes, and the basal cisterns at 2 to 2.5 hours.[59] About 20%

to 33% of the labelled CSF reaches the intracranial cavity within 12 hours. Circulation of CSF is not substantially altered by posture or ambulation, although physical activity disturbs CSF concentration gradients by promoting CSF mixing,[153] and coughing causes spinal CSF to flow toward the cisterna magna.[199]

REABSORPTION OF CSF

CSF passes from the subarachnoid space into venous blood through microscopic arachnoid villi and macroscopic arachnoid granulations. Intracranial arachnoid villi are located within the dural wall bordering the superior sagittal sinus and venous lacunae, and spinal arachnoid villi are located within the dural wall bordering dural sinusoids on dorsal nerve roots.[198] Under usual conditions, 85% to 90% of CSF is reabsorbed at intracranial sites and 10% to 15% of CSF is reabsorbed at spinal sites.

The arachnoid villus or granulation is composed of arachnoid cells protruding from the subarachnoid space into and through the wall of an adjacent venous sinus[187] (Fig 4-4). Elsewhere, the arachnoid membrane that covers the subarachnoid space is made up of several layers of arachnoid cells. Tight junctions between these cell layers form a barrier that prevents the transfer of CSF from the subarachnoid space into the dura.[139] In contrast, at the arachnoid villus, large spaces are present between the inner layers of arachnoid cells; this loose arrangement does not constitute an effective barrier. CSF in the subarachnoid space passes readily into the villus, the center of which contains a maze of loosely arranged arachnoid cells and intercellular spaces. Other than lacking tight junctions, the arachnoid cells within the villus are structurally similar to those of the rest of the subarachnoid space.[139] Collagen fibers—either singly or, more frequently, in bundles—are located in the open spaces within the villus. In addition, occasional myelinated and unmyelinated nerves are present within those spaces. Under normal conditions, an endothelium composed of arachnoid cells joined by tight junctions covers the villus. In adults, this endothelial covering may be multilayered.

Normal ICP

The endothelium covering the villus acts as a CSF-blood "barrier" that limits the rate of passage of CSF and solute into venous blood. The rate at which CSF passes through the subarachnoid space and arachnoid villi and across the endothelium is determined by (1) the transvillus hydrostatic pressure gradient (CSF pressure minus venous sinus pressure) and (2) a pressure-sensitive resistance to CSF outflow at the arachnoid villus. Because the endothelium is highly permeable, transvillus osmotic differences probably do not play a major role in determining CSF movement through arachnoid villi.

CSF may exit the villus by passing between or through endothelial cells. Although endothelial cells are usually connected by tight junctions, there are some cell junctions

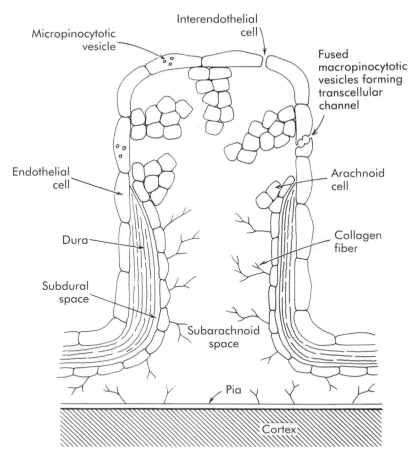

FIG. 4-4 Schematic drawing of the microscopic anatomy of an arachnoid villus. *(From Cucchiara RF, Michenfelder JD, editors:* Clinical neuroanesthesia, *New York, 1990, Churchill-Livingstone.)*

with no areas of membrane fusion or significant focal narrowing of the intercellular space. These intercellular spaces form open channels extending from the abluminal to the luminal surface of the cell, allowing CSF to diffuse from the subarachnoid space into blood. CSF may pass through endothelial cells via pinocytotic vesicles and transcellular openings formed by chains of fused vesicles extending from one surface of the epithelium to the other.[179,180] These vesicles transport macromolecular tracers, as well as fluid, from CSF to blood. Although at resting CSF pressure, micropinocytotic vesicles appear to be the primary route of CSF transport, both pathways contribute to the total resistance to CSF outflow.

Increased ICP

The rate of reabsorption of CSF ($\dot{V}_a$) increases as the pressure gradient across the villus (CSF pressure minus venous sinus pressure) increases. R_a remains close to "normal" as CSF pressure increases to above 30 cm H_2O. Thereafter, with further increases in CSF pressure, R_a declines.[92,93,113,114] An increase in the size and number of endothelial vesicles was reported when CSF pressure was increased from 9 to 30 cm H_2O.[40] At CSF pressures of greater than 30 cm H_2O, increasing numbers of transcellular channels were present concurrent with progressive increases in steady-state pressures and decreases in R_a. Comparison of the outflow-resistance curve (as a function of increasing CSF pressure) with these structural changes suggests that the decrease in R_a at the arachnoid villus is primarily related to the formation of open transcellular channels. Presumably, this transition from micropinocytotic vesicles to larger pinocytotic vesicles and transendothelial channels permits transfer of a proportionately greater volume of fluid across the endothelium with progressively increased steady state CSF pressure.[201,202] In addition, increased CSF pressure may increase CSF outflow from the villus by facilitating passage through existing intercellular clefts and by opening closed intercellular spaces that, at resting CSF pressure, appear occluded by tight junctions.

Clearance of Brain Interstitial Fluid
Normal ICP

Under normal conditions, there is relatively little bulk flow across cerebral capillaries and through the parenchyma of the brain.[69] Molecules in the brain ECF move through that space primarily by diffusion. The rate at which molecules exit the brain ECF relates to their molecular size, tissue concentration gradients, and the ability of the molecules to cross the BBB and reenter the vascular system.

Cerebral Edema

Vasogenic brain edema results from damage to cerebral vessels. This type of edema is frequently associated with tumors, trauma, and infection. Increased cerebrovascular permeability allows serum constituents to pass into the brain ECF under the hydrostatic pressure of the systemic circulation. The formation and spread of vasogenic brain edema in white matter is not by diffusion but by bulk flow, with molecules of significantly different sizes all moving at the same rate for the same distance.[160]

Vasogenic edema resolves in part by passage of edema fluid into ventricular CSF. One factor favoring fluid movement out of brain ECF is the pressure gradient between edematous brain tissue and CSF. A second factor favoring fluid movement out of brain ECF is the "sink" action of CSF.[124,160,161] Clearance of edema fluid was reported to increase when ICP was decreased, presumably due to an increase in the pressure gradient between edematous brain tissue and CSF.[162] Clearance of brain ECF proteins occurs by intraglial uptake, and this step is believed to play an important role in the resolution of vasogenic brain edema.[98]

FUNCTION OF CSF

The varied and complex functions of CSF include protection, support, and chemical regulation of the brain. The low specific gravity of CSF (1.007) relative to that of the brain (1.040) reduces the effective mass of a 1400-g brain to only 47 g.[48] In continuity with the brain ECF, CSF provides a stable supply of substrates, primarily glucose, even though concentrations of substrates in plasma are continuously changing. CSF maintains a chemically precise environment required for neurotransmission and removes metabolic products, unwanted drugs, and harmful substances resulting from CNS injury.

Protection of Brain and Spinal Cord

CSF cushions neural tissue from external forces applied to the rigid skull and spinal column. The buoyancy provided by CSF prevents the brain's full weight from producing traction on emerging nerve roots, blood vessels, and delicate membranes.[48] When CSF is replaced by air, the reduction of brain effective mass provided by CSF is lost and most patients experience pain.

Nutrition

Certain nutritive and other substrates for the brain are actively transported by systems in the capillary-glial complex. Simple sugars, certain vitamins, eicosanoids, monosaccharides, neutral and basic amino acids (brain tissue does not appear to contain an acidic amino acid transport system), and monocarboxylic acids are transported by specialized

pump mechanisms (equilibrating carriers) between blood and brain ECF.[1,28,69,154,164] Also, CSF may mediate uptake of certain vitamins such as ascorbic acid.[183]

Control of the Chemical Environment

Exchange between CSF and neural tissue ECF occurs readily because the maximum distance for diffusion between CSF and any brain area in humans is 15 mm and the interstitial space of the brain and spinal cord is continuous with the macroscopic CSF spaces.[48] The acid-base characteristics of CSF influence respiration, CBF, autoregulation of CBF, and cerebral metabolism.[101] CSF calcium, potassium, and magnesium influence heart rate, blood pressure, vasomotor and other autonomic reflexes, respiration, muscle tone, and emotional states. Calcium, potassium, magnesium, and bicarbonate ions are actively transported by "primary pumps," whereas hydrogen and chloride ions are passively transferred by "secondary pumps."[69] Within limits, CSF composition of larger molecules is regulated by the BBB with the almost total exclusion of toxic or potentially toxic large, polar, and lipid-insoluble drugs, humoral agents, and metabolites.

Excretion

Accumulation of metabolites and substances in brain ECF is prevented by their passage into CSF, cerebral veins, or cervical lymphatics. While passage into CSF may occur by two mechanisms, net diffusion and bulk flow of ECF, bulk flow accounts for the majority of passage of many substrates of different molecular weights.[48,49] Bulk flow is reported to account for clearance of substances entering the brain, as well as substances synthesized by the brain. It is particularly important for clearing lipid-insoluble substances such as inulin,[52] mannitol,[52] sulfanilic acid,[52] urea,[51] albumin,[85] globulin,[86] dopamine,[76,150,151] homovanillic acid,[150] serotonin,[76] and norepinephrine.[174] For other substances, less than 20% of solute clearance from the ECF is accounted for by drainage into CSF.[49] Many of these substances—such as penicillin, methotrexate, and neurotransmitter acid metabolites—are absorbed into the veins of the CP using a probenecid-sensitive transport mechanism.[24] Prolactin is taken up and bound by the CP. This may reflect a role for prolactin in regulating CSF composition, or it might serve to transport prolactin from blood to CSF, permitting prolonged delivery of prolactin to hypothalamic receptor neurons.[71]

Intracerebral Transport

Because CSF circulates to regions of the brain known to participate in neuroendocrine activity, it serves as a convenient vehicle for intracerebral transport of neurotransmitters. Neurohormone-releasing factors are synthesized in the hypothalamus and released into the brain ECF and CSF by neurons having axonal contact with specialized cells of the ependyma.[5,190,191] These factors are carried by the CSF to the median eminence, where they stimulate the dendrites of receptor neurons.[190] Median eminence factors may also be taken up by certain ependymal cells, tanycytes; pass to the abluminal surface; and be released into the pituitary-hypothalmic portal system to stimulate hormone release from the pituitary gland.[148,155] Injection of dopamine into the third ventricle also stimulates release of pituitary hormones.[149] Opioid effects—such as analgesia and respiratory depression—may be mediated by third-ventricle cellular elements in contact with CSF because electrical stimulation of the medial thalamus or periaqueductal gray increases the level of beta-endorphins in ventricular CSF.[2,88,89] Adenohypophyseal hormones are present in CSF in quantities suggesting that they reach CSF by a saturable active transport system rather than by simple diffusion.[163] Conditions that release vasopressin from the neurohypohysis increase antidiuretic activity in CSF.[193] Release of antidiuretic hormone during perfusion of the cerebral ventricles with hypertonic saline suggests that CSF alterations may affect CNS osmoreceptors.[163] CSF vasopressin may also influence memory and learning or regulate the formation of CSF.[100] CSF melanin concentration exhibits a diurnal rhythm. It also increases in response to stimuli that increase blood melanin and may mediate reproductive function via hypothalamic receptors bathed in CSF.[159] Patients with pituitary tumors may have symptoms of hormone imbalance when hormone concentrations in CSF are elevated but concentrations in plasma are normal.[152]

Effects of Anesthetics and Other Influences on Formation and Reabsorption of CSF

Methods of Determining $\dot{V}_f$ and R_a

Experimental Animals

Three currently used methods for determining $\dot{V}_f$, R_a, and other CSF dynamics in animals are ventriculocisternal perfusion, manometric infusion, and volume injection/withdrawal. Ventriculocisternal perfusion was first described by Pappenheimer, Heisey, and colleagues in the early 1960's.[80,144] The method requires placement of cannulae in one or both lateral ventricles and in the cisterna magna. Labelled, mock CSF is infused into the ventricles, and a mixed sample composed of labelled, mock CSF and native CSF is collected from the cisterna magna. A portion of the continuous outflow of mock-native CSF from the cisternal cannula is collected and the volume of the sample determined. The concentration of the label in the outflow sample is measured, and the time over which the sample was obtained is noted. $\dot{V}_f$ is calculated according to the formula:

$$\dot{V}_f = \dot{V}_i \left(\frac{C_i - C_o}{C_o} \right)$$

where

$\dot{V}_i$ = Mock CSF inflow rate
C_i = Concentration of the label in mock CSF

C_o = Concentration of the label in the mixed outflow solution

$\dot{V}_a$ is calculated either by the following formula:

$$\dot{V}_a = \frac{\dot{V}_i C_i - \dot{V}_o C_o}{C_o}$$

where

$\dot{V}_o$ = Outflow rate of CSF from the cisternal cannula

Or it is calculated by the formula:

$$\dot{V}_a = \dot{V}_i + \dot{V}_f - \dot{V}_o$$

R_a is a reciprocal measure of the slope relating $\dot{V}_a$ to CSF pressure. To calculate R_a, $\dot{V}_a$ must be determined at several CSF pressures. If the slope relating $\dot{V}_a$ to CSF pressure is linear, a single R_a value adequately describes the data. If the $\dot{V}_a$/CSF pressure slope is not linear, multiple R_a values must be calculated. For any CSF pressure, the corresponding R_a value is the inverse of tangent to the $\dot{V}_a$/CSF pressure slope.

Manometric infusion, as it is currently used, was described by Maffeo and by Mann et al. in the late 1970s.[110,113] For this technique, a manometric infusion device is inserted into the spinal or supracortical subarachnoid space. Mock CSF is infused into the subarachnoid space, and CSF pressure is measured at the same site as the infusion. Each steady state CSF pressure (P_s) is paired with its associated $\dot{V}_i$. Next, each pair of $\dot{V}_i : P_s$ values is plotted on a semilog plot of $\dot{V}_i$ versus P_s. A linear slope is then fit through the three to six data points. To determine $\dot{V}_f$, the linear slope is extrapolated toward the origin (to the left). The $\dot{V}_i$ value at resting CSF pressure (P_o)—that is, the $\dot{V}_i$ value corresponding to the intersection of a perpendicular from P_o and the extrapolated semilog plot—is considered to be $\dot{V}_f$. R_a is determined using observed values and two calculated, species-dependent parameters: M (transport capacity) and P_R (pressure at maximum resistance). These species-dependent parameters are calculated based on the following formula:

$$\dot{V}_i = \frac{1}{M} e \, P_s / P_R$$

Simultaneously solving this equation for the three to six pairs of $\dot{V}_i : P_s$ values used to calculate $\dot{V}_f$ yields one unique pair of M and P_R values. R_a is then calculated according to the following formula:

$$R_a = M P_e - P_s / P_R$$

In addition, the compliance (C) of the CSF compartment can be calculated according to this formula:

$$C = \frac{\dot{V}_i}{\Delta P / \Delta t}$$

where

P = CSF pressure

t = Time

$\Delta P/\Delta t$ = Slope of the linear rise in CSF pressure during infusion of mock CSF

Volume injection/withdrawal was described by Marmarou, Shulman, and colleagues and Miller and colleagues in the mid-1970s.[120-122,133-137,178] A ventricular or spinal subarachnoid catheter is inserted to permit injection or withdrawal of CSF and measurement of the CSF pressure change that accompanies injection/withdrawal. P_o is determined, and then a known volume of CSF (ΔV) is injected into (or withdrawn from) the catheter while a timed recording of CSF pressure is made. $\dot{V}_f$ and R_a are determined by first calculating the pressure volume index (PVI) as follows:

$$PVI = \Delta V/[\log P_P/P_O]$$

where

P_p = Peak CSF pressure (increase after volume injection and decrease after volume withdrawal)

R_a is then calculated based on the following formula:

$$R_a = \frac{t \cdot P_o}{PVI \cdot \log_{10}\left(\frac{P_2(P_p - P_o)}{P_p(P_2 - P_o)}\right)}$$

where

P_2 = CSF pressure measured sometime between P_p and the return of CSF pressure to P_o

t = Time from volume injection/withdrawal to P_2

$\dot{V}_f$ is calculated based on the formula:

$$P_o = P_v - (R_a \cdot \dot{V}_f)$$

which can be rewritten as follows:

$$\dot{V}_f = \frac{P_v - P_o}{R_a}$$

where

P_v = Venous blood pressure of the sagittal sinus

C is calculated based on the formula:

$$C = \frac{0.4343 \cdot PVI}{P_o}$$

Humans

Ventriculocisternal perfusion, manometric infusion, and volume injection/withdrawal have also been used to calculate $\dot{V}_f$, R_a, and C in patients.[113] For ventriculocisternal perfusion, the outflow catheter may be placed in the lumbar subarachnoid space, and ventricular and spinal CSF pressures are closely monitored to be sure that CSF pressure does not increase to potentially hazardous levels due to obstructed perfusion. For manometric infusion, the number of infusions is reduced and infusion rates are limited to 1.5 to 15 times the $\dot{V}_f$—that is, 0.01 to 0.1 ml/sec. Infusions are restricted to 20 to 60 sec, being discontinued at CSF pressures of 60 to 70 cm H_2O and/or if a rapid rise in CSF pressure with no apparent tendency toward stabilization is ob-

served. The procedures and formulas for calculation of $\dot{V}_f$, R_a, and C are the same as those for experimental animals.

Because of the hazards associated with prolonged infusion of mock CSF, ventriculocisternal perfusion and manometric infusion are less commonly used in patients than is volume injection/withdrawal. An obvious advantage of this latter method is that when ICP is of concern, CSF withdrawal is therapeutic—as well as useful for calculating $\dot{V}_f$, R_a, and C. The risk of infection is minimized, because the system can remain completely closed. For repeated testing, CSF can be alternately withdrawn and then injected, with the net change of CSF volume being made according to the patient's ICP responses. Calculation of CSF dynamics requires only a single change of CSF volume and pressure lasting for several minutes. In constrast, with ventriculocisternal perfusion, >1 h infusion of mock CSF may be needed for tracer equilibration, and the manometric technique requires multiple infusions.

Anesthetic and Drug-Induced Changes in $\dot{V}_f$ and R_a and Transport of Various Molecules into CSF and CNS

Anesthetics

Anesthetics influence many aspects of CSF dynamics (Table 4-3). Early studies with enflurane reported that 1 minimum alevolar concentration (MAC) increased $\dot{V}_f$ by 50% to 80% on initial exposure in rats and dogs.[21,116] $\dot{V}_f$ gradually returned to normal over a period of several hours. Enflurane also increased R_a, but R_a did not return to normal when administration of enflurane was continued for several hours.[12,116] Enflurane produced these alterations of CSF dynamics when administered with either nitrogen (60% to 70%) or nitrous oxide (60% to 70%) in oxygen. More recent studies with enflurane reported that its effects on $\dot{V}_f$ and R_a are dose related. High concentrations of enflurane (2.6% and 3.5% end-expired) increased $\dot{V}_f$ (by about 40% when corrected for the effects of time), whereas low con-

TABLE 4-3
Effects of Inhaled Anesthetics on CSF Dynamics

Inhaled Anesthetics	$\dot{V}_f$	R_a	Predicted Effect on ICP
Desflurane	0, + #	0	0, + #
Enflurane			
Low concentration	0	+	+
High concentration	+	0	+
Halothane	−	+	+
Isoflurane			
Low concentration	0	0, + *	0, + *
High concentration	0	−	−
Nitrous oxide	0	0	0
Sevoflurane	−	+	?

V_f, rate of CSF formation; R_a, resistance to reabsorption of CSF; +, increase; *0*, no change; −, decrease; #, effect occurs only during hypocapnia combined with increased CSF pressure; *, effect dependent on dose; *?*, uncertain.

centrations (0.9% and 1.8%) did not.[7] Conversely, low concentrations increased R_a, but high concentrations did not. Halothane (1 MAC) generally is reported to decrease $\dot{V}_f$[6,112,188] and increase R_a.[13,112] In addition, halothane enhances transport of glucose into brain[140] and movement of albumin and IgG[78,146] and sodium, chloride, and water[18,175] into CSF. Nitrous oxide (66%) is reported to produce no change in R_a or $\dot{V}_f$[6,8] and to decrease brain glucose influx and efflux.[3] Early studies with isoflurane reported that 1 MAC of that anesthetic decreased R_a and caused no change in $\dot{V}_f$.[12,14] More recent studies with isoflurane reported that its effects on R_a are dose related. R_a was normal at 0.6% (end-expired) isoflurane, increased at 1.1%, and decreased at 1.7% and 2.2%.[7] At 2% (inspired) isoflurane, the BBB transfer coefficient for small hydrophilic molecules was decreased.[46] Sevoflurane (1 MAC) is reported to decrease $\dot{V}_f$ by about 40% and to increase R_a, as compared with a comparison group of cats anesthetized with 50% nitrous oxide in oxygen.[184] Studies with desflurane reported that its effects on $\dot{V}_f$ are related to CSF pressure and P_aCO_2. At normocapnia and normal CSF pressure, normocapnia and increased CSF pressure, and hypocapnia and normal CSF pressure, both 0.5 and 1 MAC desflurane caused no change in $\dot{V}_f$ or R_a.[17] However, at hypocapnia and increased CSF pressure, both concentrations of desflurane increased R_a.

Ketamine (40 mg · kg^{-1} · h^{-1}) increases R_a but does not alter $\dot{V}_f$ (Table 4-4).[116] In addition, ketamine (150 mg/kg) decreases the transport of small hydrophilic molecules across the BBB.[172] Low doses of etomidate (0.86 mg/kg, followed by 0.86 or 1.72 mg · kg^{-1} · h^{-1}) do not alter R_a or $\dot{V}_f$, whereas high doses (2.58 or 3.44 mg · kg^{-1} · h^{-1})

decrease both R_a and $\dot{V}_f$.[11] Low doses of thiopental (6 mg/kg, followed by 6 or 12 mg · kg^{-1} · h^{-1}) increase or do not alter R_a and do not alter $\dot{V}_f$, whereas high doses (18 or 24 mg · kg^{-1} · h^{-1}) decrease both R_a and $\dot{V}_f$.[11] Propofol (6 mg/kg, followed by 12, 24, and 48 mg · kg^{-1} · h^{-1}) and pentobarbital (40 mg/kg) produce no change in R_a or $\dot{V}_f$.[16,116] In addition, pentobarbital decreases transport of glucose,[75] amino acids,[169] and small hydrophilic molecules[172] into brain. Among the sedative-hypnotic drugs, the effects of midazolam appear to be the most variable. Low doses of midazolam (1.6 mg/kg, followed by 0.5 mg · kg^{-1} · h^{-1}) increase R_a and do not alter $\dot{V}_f$, intermediate doses (1.0 to 1.5 mg · kg^{-1} · h^{-1}) cause no change, and high doses (2.0 mg · kg^{-1} · h^{-1}) increase R_a and decrease $\dot{V}_f$.[11] The benzodiazepine antagonist flumazenil caused no change in $\dot{V}_f$ when given to dogs receiving midazolam (1.6 mg/kg, followed by 1.25 mg · kg^{-1} · h^{-1}) or dogs not receiving midazolam.[9] Low-dose flumazenil (0.0025 mg/kg) caused no change in R_a, and high-dose flumazenil (0.16 mg/kg) decreased R_a. In dogs receiving midazolam, low-dose flumazenil increased R_a (perhaps due to partial reversal of midazolam so that CSF dynamics approximated those of low-dose midazolam), whereas after high-dose flumazenil, R_a returned to normal (that is, to values characteristic of dogs not receiving midazolam).

Early studies with fentanyl reported that 60.0 μg/kg, followed by 0.2 μg · kg^{-1} · min^{-1} decreased R_a[13] and did not alter $\dot{V}_f$.[6] More recent studies reported that its effects on $\dot{V}_f$ and R_a are dose related (Table 4-5). High doses of fentanyl decreased $\dot{V}_f$, whereas low doses did not.[8] R_a was decreased at the two low doses, normal at one high dose, and increased at the highest dose. All doses of sufentanil studied caused no change in $\dot{V}_f$.[8] R_a was decreased at the two low doses, increased at one high dose, and normal at

TABLE 4-4
Effects of Intravenous Drugs on CSF Dynamics

Sedative-Hypnotics and other Intravenous Drugs	$\dot{V}_f$	R_a	Predicted Effect on ICP
Etomidate			
Low dose	0	0	0
High dose	−	0, −*	−
Flumazenil			
Low dose	0	0	0
High dose	0	−	−
Ketamine	0	+	+
Midazolam#			
Low dose	0	+, 0*	+, 0*
High dose	−	0, +*	−, ?*
Pentobarbital	0	0	0
Propofol	0	0	0
Thiopental			
Low dose	0	+, 0*	+, 0*
High dose	−	0, −*	−

$\dot{V}_f$, rate of CSF formation; R_a, resistance to reabsorption of CSF; +, increase; 0, no change; −, decrease; *, effect dependent on dose; #, partial reversal with flumazenil causes CSF dynamics similar to lowest dose of midazolam; complete reversal with flumazenil causes CSF dynamics similar to pre-midazolam (control) values; ?, uncertain.

TABLE 4-5
Effects of Opioid Anesthetics on CSF Dynamics

Opioids	$\dot{V}_f$	R_a	Predicted Effect on ICP
Alfentanil			
72 μg/kg	0	−	−
144 μg/kg	0	−	−
432 μg/kg	0	0	0
1292 μg/kg	0	0	0
Fentanyl			
8 μg/kg	0	−	−
16 μg/kg	0	−	−
48 μg/kg	−	0	−
144 μg/kg	−	+	?
Sufentanil			
1.5 μg/kg	0	−	−
3.5 μg/kg	0	−	−
9.0 μg/kg	0	+	+
29.0 μg/kg	0	0	0

$\dot{V}_f$, rate of CSF formation; R_a, resistance to reabsorption of CSF; +, increase; 0, no change; −, decrease; ?, uncertain.

the highest dose. In addition, sufentanil (0.5 μg/kg, followed by 0.1 μg · kg^{-1} · h^{-1}) combined with thiopental (2 to 5 mg/kg, followed by 1 to 4 mg · kg^{-1} · h^{-1}) caused no increased movement of albumin or IgG into CSF.[146] None of the doses of alfentanil studied caused a change in $\dot{V}_f$.[8] R_a was decreased at the two low doses and normal at the two high doses.

The mechanism(s) by which inhalational and intravenous anesthetics alter CSF dynamics is uncertain. Increase of $\dot{V}_f$ with enflurane may result from an enflurane-induced increase of CP metabolism.[125] Decrease of $\dot{V}_f$ with halothane may result from halothane-induced stimulation of vasopressin receptors.[111]

Diuretics

While diuretics differ in their mechanism of action, most are reported to decrease $\dot{V}_f$. Acetazolamide reduces $\dot{V}_f$ by up to 50%.[118] Acetazolamide inhibits carbonic anhydrase, the enzyme that catalyzes the hydration of intracellular carbon dioxide, which decreases the amount of hydrogen ions available for exchange with sodium on the abluminal border of the epithelial cell.[186] Acetazolamide may also decrease $\dot{V}_f$ by an indirect action on ion transport mediated by an effect on bicarbonate.[192] Another view is that acetazolamide constricts CP arterioles, reducing CPBF.[109] Methazolamide, another carbonic anhydrase inhibitor, also is reported to reduce $\dot{V}_f$ by up to 50%.[141] The effects of carbonic anhydrase inhibitors are additive with those produced by drugs that work by other mechanisms. For example, the combination of acetazolamide and ouabain decreases $\dot{V}_f$ by 95%.[181]

Ethacrynic acid decreases $\dot{V}_f$, presumably by inhibiting the exchange of sodium ions for potassium or hydrogen at the abluminal border of the cell.[138,181] Spironolactone and amiloride decrease $\dot{V}_f$, probably by minimizing the entry of sodium into cells at the abluminal transport site.[56] Furosemide decreases $\dot{V}_f$, either by reducing sodium or chloride transport, which is linked to sodium transport on the abluminal surface but follows an electrochemical gradient on the luminal surface.[39] Mannitol decreases $\dot{V}_f$ because of reduced CP output and reduced ECF flow from cerebral tissue to the macroscopic CSF compartment.[166,167,171]

Steroids

Numerous steroids are reported to alter R_a and $\dot{V}_f$. With increased R_a secondary to pneumococcal meningitis, methylprednisolone reduced R_a to a value that was intermediate between control and untreated animals.[53] It was speculated that methylprednisolone improved CSF flow in the supracortical subarachnoid space and/or arachnoid villi. When R_a was increased due to pseudotumor cerebri, prednisone decreased R_a to a value that was intermediate between pretreatment and normal values for patients.[115] CSF reabsorption may have increased, because impaired transport across arachnoid epithelial cells was improved or metabolically in-

duced changes in the structure of the villi were reversed. Cortisone was reported to decrease $\dot{V}_f$.[74] Rapid uptake of radioactive-labelled hydrocortisone into the CP suggests that cortisone exerts its action at the CP rather than at extrachoroidal sites.[176] Dexamethosone decreases $\dot{V}_f$ by up to 50%,[173,196] probably because it inhibits sodium-potassium-ATPase, thereby reducing the activity of the sodium-potassium pump at the CP epithelial membrane.

Other Drugs

A number of other drugs are reported to alter $\dot{V}_f$ and R_a. Theophylline increases $\dot{V}_f$, presumably because inhibition of phosphodiesterase elevates CP cyclic adenosine monophosphate levels, stimulating the CP epithelial sodium-potassium pump.[207] Cholera toxin is also reported to increase $\dot{V}_f$.[165] Vasopressin decreases $\dot{V}_f$, perhaps by constricting CP blood vessels.[56] Others contend that physiologic doses of vasopressin provide insufficient CP vascular effect to explain the observed decrease of $\dot{V}_f$.[204,207] Vasopressin also decreases R_a.[165] Hypertonic saline (3%) decreases $\dot{V}_f$, presumably by reducing the osmolality gradient for movement of fluid out of plasma and into the CP stroma or across brain tissue and into CSF.[72] Hypertonic saline increases R_a at some doses but not others. Dinitrophenol decreases $\dot{V}_f$, probably as a result of its action to uncouple oxidative phosphorylation, thereby reducing the energy available for active secretory and transport processes, such as the membrane pumps. Atrial natriuretic peptides decrease $\dot{V}_f$ by stimulating production of cyclic guanine monophosphate.[165] Digoxin[181] and oubain[189] decrease $\dot{V}_f$ by inhibition of the sodium-potassium-ATPase of the CP epithelial sodium-potassium pump.

In contrast to the aforementioned drugs, both succinylcholine (continuous infusion) and vecuronium (continuous infusion) produce no change in $\dot{V}_f$ or R_a.[15]

Neurogenic Regulation of $\dot{V}_f$ and R_a
Structural Aspects

Adrenergic nerves form networks around the small arteries and veins of the CP, and their nerve terminals are located between the CP endothelium and the underlying fenestrated capillaries.[61,102] Adrenergic nerve density is greatest in the third ventricle, least in the fourth ventricle, and intermediate in the lateral ventricles. For the most part these adrenergic nerves originate in the superior cervical ganglia, though some fibers in the CP of the fourth ventricle derive from lower ganglia.[61-63,103] Innervation of the lateral ventricles is unilateral, whereas innervation of the midline ventricles is bilateral.[61]

Cholinergic nerves also form networks around the small arteries and veins of the CP, with terminals located between the endothelium and adjacent capillaries.[64,104] The CP of the third ventricle is richly supplied by cholinergic nerves, whereas the fourth ventricle is almost devoid of cholinergic innervation. The origin of the cholinergic nerve supply to the CP is uncertain. Adrenergic and cholinergic terminals have been identified at the base of choroid epithelial cells, in the clefts between cells, and near the smooth muscle cells of the choroid arterioles.

Peptidergic nerves are also found in the CP, but the density of these nerves is less than that of adrenergic and cholinergic nerves.[99] Similar to the former networks, peptidergic nerves are located between the small blood vessels of the CP and the overlying CP epithelium.[105] Peptidergic nerves contain vasoactive intestinal peptide or substance P, both potent dilators of cerebral vessels.

Functional Aspects

Studies of the effects of adrenergic stimulation on isolated anterior CP arteries suggest that the adrenergic system plays a role in regulating CPBF.[60] Constriction with norepinephrine, phenylephrine, and isoproterenol—in that order of potency—was blocked by phentolamine and so presumably occurs via alpha-adrenergic receptors. In vessels in which active tone was first induced by prostaglandin F_{2a}, relaxation with isoproterenol, norepinephrine, epinephrine, and terbutaline—in that order of potency—was blocked with propranolol and so presumably occurs via beta-adrenergic receptors. The adrenergic system also appears to exert a functional influence on CP epithelial cells. Carbonic anhydrase activity increased by 125% to 150% in CP homogenate after sympathectomy achieved by surgical removal of the superior cervical ganglion or injection of reserpine.[62] In another study, sympathetic denervation altered epithelial cell transport of organic acids and bases in isolated CP.[200]

In addition, the adrenergic system is reported to alter $\dot{V}_f$. Cervical sympathetic stimulation decreased $\dot{V}_f$ by 32%,[79,103,106] and bilateral excision of the superior cervical ganglia increased $\dot{V}_f$ by 33%.[61,63] Intraventricular perfusion with norepinephrine caused a dose-related decrease of $\dot{V}_f$ that was reversed by intraventricular perfusion of phentolamine or propranolol or intravenous infusion of phentolamine.[106] In contrast, intravenous infusion of propranolol potentiated the reduction of $\dot{V}_f$. It was suggested that low norepinephrine concentrations decreased $\dot{V}_f$ by a beta-adrenoreceptor–mediated effect on the secretory epithelium, while the reduction at high concentrations represents alpha-adrenoreceptor–mediated CP vasoconstriction. In additional studies, intraventricular perfusion with a $beta_1$-adrenoreceptor stimulator decreased $\dot{V}_f$, whereas intraventricular perfusion with a $beta_2$ stimulator or intravenous infusion with either a $beta_1$ or $beta_2$ stimulator had little or no effect. Thus the beta-induced decrease of $\dot{V}_f$ appears to derive from a direct, inhibitory action on the CP epithelium via $beta_1$-adrenoreceptors.

The cholinergic system is also reported to alter $\dot{V}_f$. Intraventricular perfusion with carbacholine or with acetylcholine in the presence of the cholinesterase inhibitor neostigmine reduced $\dot{V}_f$ by 25% to 55%.[107] Cholinergic receptors presumably are muscarinic, because the effect of carbachol is blocked by atropine but is not altered by hexamethonium. The site of action of cholinergic agonists or

antagonists is uncertain. It is believed that they act on the CP epithelium, rather than on the CP vasculature, because carbacholine has no vasomotor effect on isolated anterior choroidal arteries.[65]

Metabolic Regulation of $\dot{V}_f$ and R_a

Alterations in metabolism or physiologic status affect $\dot{V}_f$ and $\dot{V}_a$. Hypothermia decreases $\dot{V}_f$, probably by reducing the activity of active secretory and transport processes and by reducing CBF.[55] Each 1° C reduction in temperature between 41° C and 31° C decreases $\dot{V}_f$ by 11%.[182] Hypercapnia increases $\dot{V}_f$ to normal values if $\dot{V}_f$ was decreased at normocapnia but does not change $\dot{V}_f$ if it was normal at normocapnia.[81] Normalization of $\dot{V}_f$ by hypercapnia may have occurred because CPBF improved. In contrast, hypocapnia acutely decreases $\dot{V}_f$, either due to reduced CPBF or reduced hydrogen ion availability for exchange with sodium at the abluminal surface of the CP epithelial cells.[4] After several hours of hypocapnia, $\dot{V}_f$ returns to normal values.[21,123] Prolonged hypercapnia or hypocapnia does not significantly change $\dot{V}_f$.[21,81] Metabolic acidosis does not change $\dot{V}_f$, but metabolic alkalosis decreases $\dot{V}_f$, presumably due to a pH effect unrelated to ion or substrate availability.[142]

Reduced osmolarity of ventricular CSF or increased osmolarity of serum decreases $\dot{V}_f$.[87] Similarly, increased osmolarity of ventricular CSF or reduced osmolarity of serum increases $\dot{V}_f$.[87,194] The increase or decrease of $\dot{V}_f$ caused by change in serum osmolarity was four times greater than that caused by a comparable change in ventricular fluid osmolarity. It was suggested that the changes in $\dot{V}_f$ resulting from altered ventricular fluid osmolarity occurred at the CP, whereas the changes resulting from altered serum osmolarity occurred at extrachoroid sites.

CSF DYNAMICS AND ICP
Equilibrium Between CSF Formation and Reabsorption

Within limits, $\dot{V}_f$ is not affected by increase or decrease of ICP. Thus $\dot{V}_f$ remains "normal" whether ICP is 2 cm H_2O or 22 cm H_2O (Fig. 4-5). Only when ICP increases sufficiently to reduce CPP below ~70 mm Hg will $\dot{V}_f$ decrease. In contrast, $\dot{V}_a$ is quite sensitive to change of ICP. At ICPs below ~7 cm H_2O, minimal reabsorption occurs.[38] At ICPs of greater than ~7 cm H_2O, $\dot{V}_a$ increases directly as ICP increases. The relationship between $\dot{V}_a$ and ICP is linear for ICPs up to ~30 cm H_2O. The equilibrium pressure is that at which the plots of $\dot{V}_f$/ICP and $\dot{V}_a$/ICP intersect. At that ICP, $\dot{V}_f$ equals $\dot{V}_a$ and no net change in CSF volume occurs.

Anesthetic- and Drug-induced Changes in ICP

Treatments that alter $\dot{V}_f$ and/or $\dot{V}_a$ will alter ICP. For example, theophylline is reported to increase $\dot{V}_f$.[207] Assum-

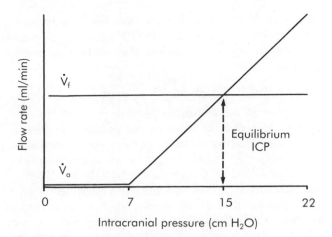

FIG. 4-5 $\dot{V}_f$ and $\dot{V}_a$ are plotted as a function of ICP. So long as CPP remains above ~70 mm Hg, $\dot{V}_f$ is unaffected by ICP. At ICP <7 cm H_2O, $\dot{V}_a$ is minimal. At 7 cm H_2O <ICP <25 to 30 cm H_2O, R_a is relatively constant and $\dot{V}_a$ is linearly related to ICP. ICP stabilizes at a value where $\dot{V}_f$ equals $\dot{V}_a$. *(From Cucchiara RF, Michenfelder JD, editors:* Clinical neuroanesthesia, *New York, 1990, Churchill-Livingstone.)*

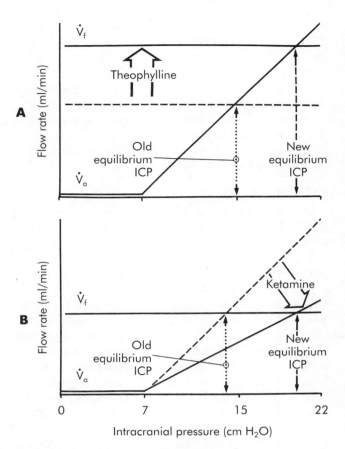

FIG. 4-6 Theophylline **(A)** increases $\dot{V}_f$ ("elevating" the $\dot{V}_f$/ICP slope) and ketamine **(B)** increases R_a ("flattening" the $\dot{V}_f$/ICP slope). With both treatments $\dot{V}_f$ equals $\dot{V}_a$ at increased ICP. *(From Cucchiara RF, Michenfelder JD, editors:* Clinical neuroanesthesia, *New York, 1990, Churchill-Livingstone.)*

ing no change in $\dot{V}_a$, the plots of $\dot{V}_f$/ICP and $\dot{V}_a$/ICP after administration of theophylline will intersect at an ICP value that is higher than "normal" (Fig. 4-6, *A*). Stated another way, theophylline increases $\dot{V}_f$ so that the volume of CSF formed each minute exceeds the volume reabsorbed each minute. As a result, CSF volume expands, causing ICP to increase. ICP continues to increase as CSF volume expands, and as ICP increases it provides an increasingly greater "driving force" for reabsorption of CSF. $\dot{V}_a$ increases as ICP increases until $\dot{V}_a$ equals $\dot{V}_f$. A new equilibrium state is achieved when formation and reabsorption are equal and no net change in CSF volume or further change of ICP occurs. The net effect of these changes is that by increasing $\dot{V}_f$, theophylline should cause an increase of ICP, provided that other CSF dynamics are not altered.

Ketamine is reported to increase R_a.[116] By definition R_a is the inverse of the slope of the relationship between $\dot{V}_a$ and ICP. Increased R_a produces a "flattening" of the $\dot{V}_a$/ICP regression line. Assuming no change in $\dot{V}_f$, the plots of $\dot{V}_f$/ICP and $\dot{V}_a$/ICP after administration of ketamine will intersect at an ICP that is higher than normal (Fig. 4-6, *B*). Stated another way, ketamine reduces $\dot{V}_a$ because "normal" ICP does not provide sufficient "driving force" to cause usual amounts of CSF to be reabsorbed now that R_a has increased. As a result the volume of CSF formed each minute exceeds the volume reabsorbed each minute. CSF volume expands, causing ICP to increase. ICP continues to increase as CSF volume expands, and as ICP increases it provides a progressively greater "driving force" for reabsorption of CSF. $\dot{V}_a$ increases as ICP increases, until $\dot{V}_a$ equals $\dot{V}_f$. A new equilibrium is achieved, where forma-

tion and reabsorption are equal and no net change in CSF volume or further change of ICP occurs. The net effect of these changes is that by increasing R_a, ketamine should cause an increase of ICP, provided that other CSF dynamics are not altered.

Enflurane alters ICP because it increases both $\dot{V}_f$ and R_a.[7,12,22] An increase of $\dot{V}_f$ "elevates" the $\dot{V}_f$/ICP regression line, and an increase of R_a "flattens" the $\dot{V}_a$/ICP regression line. Thus the plots of $\dot{V}_f$/ICP and $\dot{V}_a$/ICP after administration of enflurane intersect at an ICP that is higher than "normal" (Fig. 4-7, *A*). As a result of these changes in $\dot{V}_f$ and R_a, moderate concentrations of enflurane should cause a substantial increase in ICP, provided that other CSF dynamics are not altered.

Halothane also has combined effects on $\dot{V}_f$ and R_a.[6,13] However, unlike enflurane, its effects are opposing rather than additive. A decrease of $\dot{V}_f$ "lowers" the $\dot{V}_f$/ICP regression line, whereas an increase of R_a "flattens" the $\dot{V}_f$/ICP regression line. In a "closed" cranium model, it was concluded that the expansion of CSF volume caused by halothane-induced increase of R_a was greater than the con-

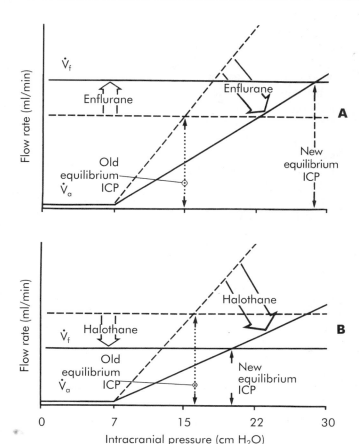

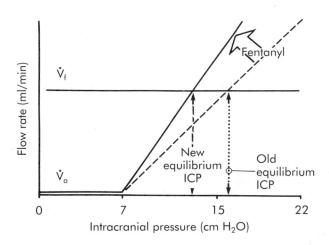

FIG. 4-7 Enflurane **(A)** at intermediate concentrations increases both $\dot{V}_f$ ("elevating" the $\dot{V}_f$/ICP slope) and R_a ("flattening" the $\dot{V}_a$/slope). Halothane **(B)** decreases $\dot{V}_f$ ("lowering" the $\dot{V}_f$/ICP slope) and increases R_a. With both anesthetics $\dot{V}_f$ equals $\dot{V}_a$ at increased ICP. *(From Cucchiara RF, Michenfelder JD, editors:* Clinical neuroanesthesia, *New York, 1990, Churchill-Livingstone.)*

traction of CSF volume caused by halothane-induced decrease of $\dot{V}_f$ (Fig. 4-7, *B*).[20] As a result, halothane should cause an increase in ICP, provided that other CSF dynamics are not altered.

Fentanyl is an example of a drug that decreases ICP. Fentanyl decreases R_a, so that the $\dot{V}_a$/ICP regression line becomes "steeper" (Fig. 4-8).[8] Consequently, "normal" ICP, the "driving force" for reabsorption of CSF, is in excess of what is needed for "normal" $\dot{V}_a$. $\dot{V}_a$ is greater than $\dot{V}_f$, causing a contraction of CSF volume and reduction of ICP. ICP gradually decreases, resulting in a lesser "driving force" for reabsorption of CSF. $\dot{V}_a$, initially greater than $\dot{V}_f$, gradually decreases until at some reduced ICP $\dot{V}_a$ is lowered to a value that matches $\dot{V}_f$. A new equilibrium between formation and reabsorption is achieved, and ICP decreases no further.

Furosemide is another example of a drug that decreases ICP. Furosemide decreases $\dot{V}_f$, "lowering" the $\dot{V}_f$/ICP regression line (Fig. 4-9, *A*). As a result, at "normal" ICP $\dot{V}_a$ exceeds $\dot{V}_f$, causing a contraction of CSF volume and reduction of ICP. ICP continues to decrease, providing a lesser "driving force" for reabsorption of CSF. At some re-

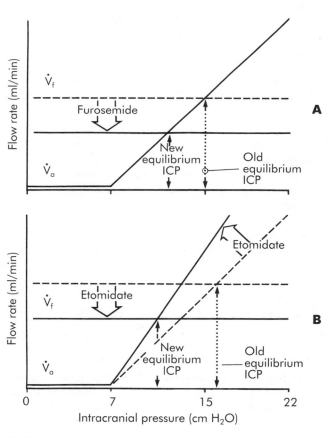

FIG. 4-9 Furosemide **(A)** decreases $\dot{V}_f$ ("lowering" the $\dot{V}_f$/ICP slope), and etomidate **(B)** in high doses decreases $\dot{V}_f$ and R_a ("steepening" the $\dot{V}_a$/ICP slope). With both treatments $\dot{V}_f$ equals $\dot{V}_a$ at decreased ICP. *(From Cucchiara RF, Michenfelder JD, editors:* Clinical neuroanesthesia, *New York, 1990, Churchill-Livingstone.)*

FIG. 4-8 Fentanyl in low doses decreases R_a ("steepening" the $\dot{V}_a$/ICP slope). As a result $\dot{V}_f$ equals $\dot{V}_a$ at decreased ICP.

duced ICP, $\dot{V}_a$ is decreased enough to match the reduced $\dot{V}_f$. Formation and reabsorption are in equilibrium at that reduced ICP, and no further decrease of ICP occurs.

High doses of etomidate reduce ICP by combined effects on $\dot{V}_f$ and R_a.[11] Etomidate decreases $\dot{V}_f$, so that the $\dot{V}_f$/ICP regression line is "lowered" and decreases R_a, so that the $\dot{V}_a$/ICP regression line becomes "steeper" (Fig. 4-9, B). At initial ICP, $\dot{V}_a$ exceeds the reduced $\dot{V}_f$, and CSF volume contracts. Reduction of CSF volume decreases ICP. ICP equilibrates at a low value, because when R_a is reduced only a small ICP is needed to provide a "driving force" for reabsorption of CSF.

CSF Volume Change to Compensate for Intracranial Volume Change

When the volume of intracranial blood, brain tissue, gas, and so on increases, CSF volume contracts by translocation of intracranial CSF to the spinal subarachnoid space and by reabsorption of CSF. Conversely, when the volume of intracranial blood, brain tissue, gas, and so on decreases, CSF volume expands by cephalad translocation and a temporary decrease in $\dot{V}_a$. CSF volume and ICP responses to increases or decreases of intracranial volume are easily illustrated using the $\dot{V}_f$/ICP and $\dot{V}_a$/ICP relationships discussed previously. For example, subdural hematoma adds volume to the intracranial contents thereby increasing ICP (Fig. 4-10, A). Increased ICP (A) provides a "driving force" for reabsorption of CSF, so that $\dot{V}_a$ increases (B) to a value greater than $\dot{V}_f$ (which does not change). Consequently, the volume of CSF reabsorbed each minute exceeds the volume of CSF formed each minute. Gradually CSF volume contracts and, as it does, total intracranial volume decreases, causing ICP to fall (C) from its increased level. As ICP approaches "normal," $\dot{V}_a$ falls toward "normal" and the mismatch between $\dot{V}_a$ and $\dot{V}_f$ becomes progressively reduced. When ICP returns to prehematoma values, $\dot{V}_f$ and $\dot{V}_a$ once again are in equilibrium and no further change of CSF volume or ICP occurs. At the new equilibrium state, ICP and total intracranial volume are much the same as before the subdural hematoma, but cerebral blood volume (CBV) (part of it in the form of the hematoma) is increased and CSF volume is decreased.

Conversely, surgical removal of brain tissue reduces intracranial volume, thereby decreasing ICP (Fig. 4-10, B). Reduced ICP (D) provides only a weak "driving force" for reabsorption of CSF, so that $\dot{V}_a$ (E) is less than $\dot{V}_f$ (which does not change). Thus over the ensuing minutes the volume of CSF reabsorbed is less than the volume formed. Gradually CSF volume expands and, as it does, total intracranial volume increases, causing ICP to rise (F) from its reduced level. Increasing ICP stimulates $\dot{V}_a$. When ICP reaches presurgical values, $\dot{V}_f$ and $\dot{V}_a$ once again are in equilibrium and no further change of CSF volume or ICP occurs. At the new equilibrium state, ICP and total intracranial volume are much the same as before surgical removal of brain tissue, but brain tissue volume is decreased and CSF volume is increased.

Drugs and treatments that alter $\dot{V}_f$ and/or $\dot{V}_a$ affect the expansion or contraction of CSF volume in response to a change of intracranial volume. Hypercapnia (and other drugs/treatments that may increase $\dot{V}_f$) or low doses of thiopental (and other drugs and treatments that may increase R_a) oppose the contraction of CSF volume that occurs in response to increased intracranial volume (such as subdural hematoma). Mannitol (and other drugs and treatments that decrease $\dot{V}_f$) or low doses of fentanyl (and other drugs and treatments that decrease R_a) enhance the contraction of CSF volume that occurs in response to increased intracranial volume. Conversely, acetazolamide (and other drugs and treatments that decrease $\dot{V}_f$) will oppose the expansion of CSF volume that occurs in response to decreased intracranial volume (such as after surgical removal of brain tissue).

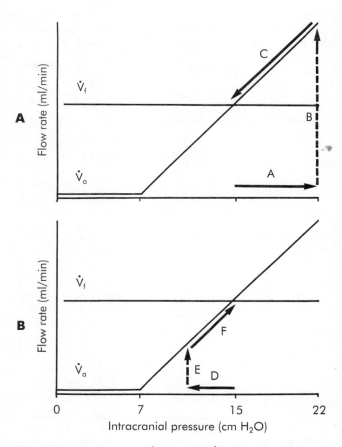

FIG. 4-10   The plots of $\dot{V}_f$/ICP and $\dot{V}_a$/ICP show how CSF volume changes to offset changes in intracranial volume, thereby minimizing ICP changes. **A,** An increase of intracranial volume increases ICP (A). At increased ICP, $\dot{V}_a$ (B) exceeds $\dot{V}_f$, so CSF volume decreases. As CSF volume decreases, ICP decreases (C) until $\dot{V}_f$ equals $\dot{V}_a$. If $\dot{V}_f$ and R_a are not altered, ICP returns to "normal." **B,** A decrease of intracranial volume decreases ICP (D). At decreased ICP, $\dot{V}_a$ (E) is less than $\dot{V}_f$, so CSF volume increases. As CSF volume increases, ICP increases (F) until $\dot{V}_f$ equals $\dot{V}_a$. If $\dot{V}_f$ and R_a are not altered, ICP returns to "normal." *(From Cucchiara RF, Michenfelder JD, editors:* Clinical neuroanesthesia, *New York, 1990, Churchill-Livingstone.)*

Limits to Linear Modeling of CSF Dynamics

The linear models of CSF dynamics discussed previously serve to illustrate the equilibrium between $\dot{V}_f$ and $\dot{V}_a$, contraction and expansion of CSF volume, and the manner in which drugs and treatments affect these aspects of CSF physiology. However, these linear models do not accurately predict ICP in all circumstances. There are several reasons for this. One reason is that concurrent treatments or conditions may also alter CSF dynamics. For example, in dogs it was reported that inflation of an intracranial, epidural balloon increased R_a.[21] Thus, in the example of the epidural hematoma given previously, the hematoma may increase R_a and so prevent adequate CSF volume contraction. As a result, ICP may not return to prehematoma levels. Another reason that these linear models may not accurately predict ICP is that treatments or conditions may have a certain effect on $\dot{V}_f$ and/or $\dot{V}_a$ when pretreatment $\dot{V}_f/\dot{V}_a$ are "normal," but have a quite different effect when pretreatment $\dot{V}_f/\dot{V}_a$ are not "normal." For example, it was reported that hypercapnia had no effect on $\dot{V}_f$ when $\dot{V}_f$ was "normal" before hypercapnia but increased $\dot{V}_f$ when $\dot{V}_f$ was low before hypercapnia.[81]

A third reason that these linear models of CSF dynamics may not accurately predict ICP is that when ICP is substantially increased, the $\dot{V}_f/ICP$ and $\dot{V}_a/ICP$ relationships change. $\dot{V}_f$ is independent of ICP and mean arterial blood pressure (MAP) when ICP is low or MAP is high. $\dot{V}_f$ becomes inversely related to ICP and/or directly related to MAP when ICP increases and/or MAP decreases sufficiently to reduce CPP below ~70 mm Hg. R_a, which is independent of MAP and ICP when ICP is low, decreases as ICP increases to above 25 to 30 cm H_2O (Fig. 4-11).[92]

This decrease in R_a corresponds with formation of macropinocytotic vesicles and transcellular channels across the arachnoid villus endothelium, as well as pressure-facilitated diffusion of CSF through (1) open intercellular spaces and (2) transient opening of closed intercellular spaces that, at resting ICP, are functionally occluded by tight junctions. Decreased R_a is expressed as a several-fold increase in the slope of the $\dot{V}_a/ICP$ regression line at ICPs between 25 and 50 cm H_2O.

CONDITIONS WHERE ALTERED CSF DYNAMICS CHANGE ICP
Responses to Increased ICP

Recent work in animal models and in clinical studies demonstrates how $\dot{V}_f$ and R_a affect CSF volume and contribute to ICP change in clinically relevant ways.[10]

Intracranial Mass

Rapid expansion of an intracranial mass causes an increase of ICP followed by compensatory decreases of CBV, CSF volume, and/or brain tissue volume. To delineate these changes and the contribution of $\dot{V}_f$ and R_a, three groups of dogs were studied.[19] It was reported that hypocapnia initially decreased CBV and that, during 4 h hypocapnia, CBV reexpanded and CSF volume changed reciprocally (group 1). In group 2, increase of ICP with an intracranial balloon caused a decrease of CBV and increase of R_a that was stable for 4 h. In group 3, balloon inflation decreased CBV, hypocapnia caused a further decrease of CBV, and, during 4 h hypocapnia, CBV reexpanded and CSF volume changed reciprocally. Brain tissue composition was not different between groups.

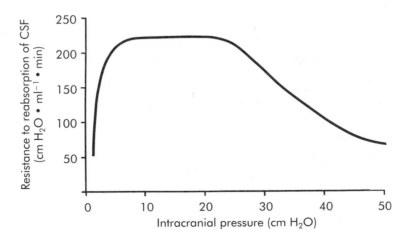

FIG. 4-11   Resistance to reabsorption of CSF (R_a) is plotted as a function of ICP. R_a is relatively constant at "normal" ICP, but decreases as ICP increases above 25 to 30 cm H_2O. As a result, the $\dot{V}_a/ICP$ slope is no longer linear but assumes more of the characteristics of an exponential curve. *(From Cucchiara RF, Michenfelder JD, editors:* Clinical neuroanesthesia, *New York, 1990, Churchill-Livingstone.)*

Effects of Anesthetics

Anesthetics may affect the initial increase of ICP and subsequent compensatory decrease of CBV, CSF volume, and/or brain tissue volume caused by rapid expansion of an intracranial mass. To examine these changes and the contribution of $\dot{V}_f$ and R_a, five groups of dogs were anesthetized with inhalational or intravenous agents while an intracranial mass was present, and hypocapnia was used to decrease ICP.[18] With enflurane- and halothane-induced anesthesia, $\dot{V}_f$ and/or R_a were high and ICP progressively increased because CSF volume did not contract to the same extent that CBV reexpanded. With isoflurane-, fentanyl-, or thiopental-induced anesthesia, $\dot{V}_f$ and R_a were normal and ICP did not progressively increase because reexpansion of CBV was minimal (fentanyl) or because CSF volume contracted to the same extent that CBV reexpanded (isoflurane and thiopental).

Causes for Increased ICP

A number of clinical conditions are accompanied by an increase in ICP. Recent laboratory and clinical studies demonstrate the role of altered $\dot{V}_f$ and/or R_a in clinical conditions where ICP is increased.

Acute Subarachnoid Hemorrhage

Acute subarachnoid hemorrhage frequently results in increased ICP. To examine the effect of blood components on $\dot{V}_f$ and $\dot{V}_a$ and to determine the effects of $\dot{V}_f$ and $\dot{V}_a$ on ICP, animals were intrathecally given (1) heparinized whole blood, (2) plasma, (3) dialysate of plasma, (4) serum (fibrinogen free), and (5) saline.[41,93,94,113] $\dot{V}_f$ and $\dot{V}_a$ were determined by manometric infusion. Whole blood and plasma increased ICP and produced a 3- to 10-fold increase in R_a. Electron microscopic examination of the arachnoid villi revealed decreased numbers of transendothelial channels and fibrin deposits within the villi.

Chronic Changes after Subarachnoid Hemorrhage

Hydrocephalus often follows subarachnoid hemorrhage. In both animals and patients examined at various time intervals after subarachnoid hemorrhage, scanning electron microscopic studies of the CSF pathways and arachnoid villi revealed extensive fibrosis resulting from blood within these spaces.[185] It was concluded that after subarachnoid hemorrhage, as well as after other clinical conditions in which leptomeningeal scarring exists, chronic obstruction to CSF outflow results from functional narrowing or block of CSF outflow pathways. By this mechanism, R_a is increased within both the subarachnoid space and the arachnoid villi.

Bacterial Meningitis

Bacterial meningitis is frequently accompanied by increased ICP. To examine the effect of meningitis on $\dot{V}_f$ and $\dot{V}_a$ and to determine the effects of $\dot{V}_f$ and $\dot{V}_a$ on ICP, animals were intrathecally given (1) Streptococcus pneumoniae or (2) Escherichia coli.[53] $\dot{V}_f$ and $\dot{V}_a$ were determined before inoculation, 16 to 24 h after inoculation, and after therapy. ICP increased in both groups. R_a was increased 25-fold with Str. pneumoniae and 36-fold with E. coli and, although antibiotic therapy sterilized the CSF and prevented mortality, R_a remained elevated at 2 weeks posttreatment. Methylprednisolone reduced R_a to a value that was intermediate between control and infected animals.

Pseudotumor Cerebri

It has been speculated that the increased ICP seen in pseudotumor cerebri results from either (1) increased R_a, (2) increased $\dot{V}_f$, (3) increased water movement into brain across cerebral capillaries, (4) increased CBF and CBV, or (5) glial and/or neuronal cellular edema.[115] Currently, most evidence favors altered CSF dynamics as the principal cause for increased ICP.[95] To determine the role of CSF dynamics, $\dot{V}_f$ and R_a were determined in both control patients and patients with pseudotumor cerebri.[117] Resting ICP was 33 cm H_2O in patients with pseudotumor cerebri and 14 cm H_2O in controls. Maximal R_a was 10 times greater, and R_a at resting ICP was 6 times greater in the pseudotumor patients than in controls. $\dot{V}_f$ was decreased 39% in the pseudotumor patients, as compared with controls. These results are comparable with results previously reported by others and support the view that in pseudotumor patients impaired CSF reabsorption is a principal mechanism leading to increased ICP.[96] Prednisone decreased R_a to a value that was intermediate between controls and untreated pseudotumor patients.

Head Injury

Head injury frequently results in increased ICP. In a recent study the PVI was used to determine $\dot{V}_f$, R_a, and the contribution of altered $\dot{V}_f$ and R_a to increased ICP in head-injured patients.[25] It was found that R_a was increased but $\dot{V}_f$ was within normal limits for 75% of the patients studied. It was calculated that about 20% of the ICP increase in this population derived from $\dot{V}_f$ and R_a.

Summary

CSF plays a key role in brain well-being. It cushions the brain, provides pathways for nutrients and other substrates, regulates the concentrations of ions and other chemicals, provides routes of clearance for unwanted substances, and transports neurohormones and neurotransmitters. Alteration of $\dot{V}_f$ causes a change in ICP, with increase (or decrease) of $\dot{V}_f$ causing an increase (or decrease) of CSF volume. Alteration of R_a not only causes a change in ICP, but also determines the pressure-buffering capacity of the CSF "compartment," with increase of R_a causing a decreased ability of CSF volume to contract in response to increased intracranial volume and vice versa. Studies in animal models of increased ICP report that anesthetic-induced changes in $\dot{V}_f$ and R_a significantly alter the effectiveness of treatments employed to lower ICP. Studies in patients with increased ICP report that $\dot{V}_f$ and R_a may be significant (though not the major) factors altering the effectiveness of treatments to lower ICP.

References

1. Agnew WF, Crone C: Permeability of brain capillaries to hexoses and pentoses in the rabbit, *Acta Physiol Scand* 70:168-175, 1967.

2. Akil H, Richardson DE, Borchas JD et al: Appearance of β-endorphin-like immunoreactivity in human ventricular cerebrospinal fluid upon analgesic electrical stimulation, *Proc Natl Acad Sci USA* 75:5170-5172, 1978.

3. Alexander SC et al: Effects of general anesthesia on canine blood-brain barrier glucose transport. In Harper M, Jennett B, Miller O et al, editors: *Blood flow and metabolism in the brain,* Edinburgh, 1975, Churchill-Livingstone, p 9.37.

4. Ames A III, Higashi K, Nesbett FB: Effects of P_{CO_2}, acetazolamide and oubain on volume and composition of choroid-plexus fluid, *J Physiol (London)* 181:516-524, 1965.

5. Anton-Tay R, Wurtman RJ: Regional uptake of ^{3}H-melatonin from blood or cerebrospial fluid by rat brain, *Nature (London)* 222:474-475, 1969.

6. Artru AA: Effects of halothane and fentanyl on the rate of CSF production in dogs, *Anesth Analg* 62:581-585, 1983.

7. Artru AA: Concentration-related changes in the rate of CSF formation and resistance to reabsorption of CSF during enflurane and isoflurane anesthesia in dogs receiving nitrous oxide, *J Neurosurg Anesth* 1:256-262, 1989.

8. Artru AA: Dose-related changes in the rate of CSF formation and resistance to reabsorption of CSF during administration of fentanyl, sufentanil, or alfentanil in dogs, *J Neurosurg Anesth* 3:283-290, 1991.

9. Artru AA: The rate of CSF formation, resistance to reabsorption of CSF, and aperiodic analysis of the EEG following administration of flumazenil to dogs, *Anesthesiology* 72:111-117, 1990.

10. Artru AA: Cerebrospinal fluid dynamics. In Cucchiara RF, Michenfelder JD, editors: *Clinical neuroanesthesia,* New York, 1990, Churchill-Livingstone, pp 41-76.

11. Artru AA: Dose-related changes in rate of cerebrospinal fluid formation and resistance to reabsorption of cerebrospinal fluid following administration of thiopental, midazolam, and etomidate in dogs, *Anesthesiology* 69:541-546, 1988.

12. Artru AA: Effects of enflurane and isoflurane on resistance to reabsorption of cerebrospinal fluid in dogs, *Anesthesiology* 61:529-533, 1984.

13. Artru AA: Effects of halothane and fentanyl anesthesia on resistance to reabsorption of CSF, *J Neurosurg* 60:252-256, 1984.

14. Artru AA: Isoflurane does not increase the rate of CSF production in the dog, *Anesthesiology* 60:193-197, 1984.

15. Artru AA: Muscle relaxation with succinylcholine or vecuronium does not alter the rate of CSF production or resistance to reabsorption of CSF in dogs, *Anesthesiology* 68:392-396, 1988.

16. Artru AA: Propofol combined with halothane or with fentanyl/halothane does not alter the rate of CSF formation or resistance to reabsorption of CSF in rabbits, *J Neurosurg Anesth* 5:250-257, 1993.

17. Artru AA: Rate of cerebrospinal fluid formation, resistance to reabsorption of cerebrospinal fluid, brain tissue water content, and electroencephalogram during desflurane anesthesia in dogs, *J Neurosurg Anesth* 5:178-186, 1993.

18. Artru AA: Reduction of cerebrospinal fluid pressure by hypocapnia: changes in cerebral blood volume, cerebrospinal fluid volume and brain tissue water and electrolytes. II. Effects of anesthetics, *J Cereb Blood Flow Metabol* 8:750-756, 1988.

19. Artru AA: Reduction of cerebrospinal fluid pressure by hypocapnia: changes in cerebral blood volume, cerebrospinal fluid volume and brain tissue water and electrolytes, *J Cereb Blood Flow Metabol* 7:471-479, 1987.

20. Artru AA: Relationship between cerebral blood volume and CSF pressure during anesthesia with halothane or enflurane in dogs, *Anesthesiology* 58:533-539, 1983.

21. Artru AA, Hornbein TF: Prolonged hypocapnia does not alter the rate of CSF production in dogs during halothane anesthesia or sedation with nitrous oxide, *Anesthesiology* 67:66-71, 1987.

22. Artru AA, Nugent M, Michenfelder JD: Enflurane causes a prolonged and reversible increase in the rate of CSF production in the dog, *Anesthesiology* 57:255-260, 1982.

23. Atkinson AJ, Weiss MF: Kinetics of blood-cerebrospinal fluid glucose transfer in the normal dog, *Am J Physiol* 216:1120-1126, 1969.

24. Baramy EH: Inhibition by hippurate and probenicid of in vitro uptake of iodipamide and O-iodohippurate: a composite uptake system for iodipamide in choroid plexus, kidney cortex and anterior uvea of several species, *Acta Physiol Scand* 86:12-27, 1972.

25. Becker DP: *Isolation of factors leading to raised ICP in head-injured patients: a preliminary report* (abstract), annual meeting of the American Association of Neurological Surgeons, 1985.

26. Becker NH, Almazon R: Evidence for the functional polarization of micropinocytotic vesicles in the rat choroid plexus, *J Histochem Cytochem* 16:278-280, 1968.

27. Becker NH, Sutton CH: Histochemistry of the choroid plexus. In Netsky MB, Shuangshoti S, editors: *The choroid plexus in health and disease,* Charlottesville, Va, 1975, University of Virginia Press, p 67.

28. Bito LZ: Absorptive transport of prostaglandins and other eicosanoids across the blood-brain barrier system and its physiological significance. In Suckling AJ, Rumsby MG, Bradbury MWB, editors: *The blood brain barrier in health and disease,* Chichester, England, 1986, Ellis Horwood Ltd, pp 109-121.

29. Bodenheimer TS, Brightman MW: A blood-brain barrier to peroxidase in capillaries surrounded by perivascular spaces, *Am J Anat* 122:249-267, 1968.

30. Bouldin TW, Krigman MR: Differential permeability of cerebral capillary and choroid plexus to lanthanum ion, *Brain Res* 99:444-448, 1975.

31. Bradbury MWB: Lymphatic and the central nervous system, *Trends Neurosci* 4:100-101, 1981.

32. Bradley KC: Cerebrospinal fluid pressure, *J Neurol Neurosurg Psychiatry* 33:387-397, 1970.

33. Brightman MW: Ultrastructural characteristics of adult choroid plexus: relation to the blood-cerebrospinal fluid barrier to proteins. In Netsky MG, Shuangshoti S, editors: *The choroid plexus in health and disease,* Charlottesville, Va, 1975, University Press of Virginia, p 86.

34. Brightman MW, Reese TS: Junctions between intimately apposed cell membranes in the vertebrate brain, *J Cell Biol* 40:648-677, 1969.

35. Brightman MW, Reese TS, Feder N: Assessment with the electron microscope of the permeability to peroxidase of cerebral endothelium and epithelium in mice and sharks. In Crone C, Lassen NA, editors: *Capillary permeability,* New York, 1970, Academic Press, p 468-476.

36. Bronsted HE: Ouabain-sensitive carrier-mediated transport of glucose from the cerebral ventricles to surrounding tissue in the cat, *J Physiol (London)* 209:187-208, 1970.

37. Bronsted HE: Transport of glucose, sodium, chloride and potassium between the cerebral ventricles and surrounding tissues in cats, *Acta Physiol Scand* 79:523-532, 1970.

38. Brumback RA: Anatomic and physiologic aspects of the cerebrospinal fluid space. In Herndon RM, Brumback RA, editors: *The cerebrospinal fluid,* Boston, 1989, Kluwer Academic Publishers, pp 15-43.

39. Buhrley LE, Reed DJ: The effect of furosemide on sodium-22 uptake into cerebrospinal fluid and brain, *Exp Brain Res* 14:503-510, 1972.

40. Butler AB et al: Mechanisms of cerebrospinal fluid absorption in normal and pathologically altered arachnoid villi. In Wood JH, editor: *Neurobiology of cerebrospinal fluid 2,* New York, 1983, Plenum Press, p 707-726.

41. Butler AB et al: Impaired absorption of CSF during experimental subarachnoid hemorrhage: effects of blood components on vesicular transport in arachnoid villi. In Shulman K, Marmarou A, Miller JD et al, editors: *Intracranial pressure IV,* New York, 1980, Springer-Verlag, p 45.

42. Carey ME, Vela AR: Effect of systemic arterial hypotension on the rate of CSF formation in dogs, *J Neurosurg* 41:350-355, 1974.

43. Castel M, Sahar A, Erlij D: The movement of lanthanum across diffusion barriers in the choroid plexus of the cat, *Brain Res* 67:178-184, 1974.

44. Cathcart RS, Worthington WC: Ciliary movement in the rat cerebral ventricles, clearing action and directions of currents, *J Neuropathol Exp Neurol* 23:609-618, 1964.

45. Cerebrospinal fluid. In Lentner C, editor: *Geigy Scientific Tables,* Basel, 1981, Ciba-Geigy, p 165.

46. Chi OZ et al: Effects of isoflurane anesthesia on the blood-brain barrier transport, *Anesthesiology* 73:A682, 1990.

47. Csaky TZ, Rigor BM: The choroid plexus as a glucose barrier, *Prog Brain Res* 29:147-158, 1967.

48. Cserr HF: Physiology of the choroid plexus, *Physiol Rev* 51:273-311, 1971.

49. Cserr HF, Cooper DM, Milhort TJ: Flow of cerebral interstitial fluid as indicated by the removal of extracellular markers from rat caudate nucleus, *Exp Eye Res Suppl* 25:461-473, 1977.

50. Cserr HF, Cooper DM, Suri PK et al: Efflux of radiolabeled polyethylene glycols and albumin from rat brain, *Am J Physiol* 240:F319-F328, 1981.

51. Cserr HF, Fenstermacher JD, Rall DP: Permeabilities of the choroid plexus and blood-brain barrier to urea. In Schmidt-Neilsen B et al, editors: *International Colloquy on Urea and the Kidney, Int. Congr. Ser.,* No. 195, Amsterdam, 1970, Excerpta Medica, pp 127-134.

52. Cserr HF, Rall DP, Fenstermacher JD: Studies relating to the function of cerebrospinal fluid in *Squalus acanthus, Bull Mt Desert Isl Biol Lab* 7:16-18, 1967.

53. Dacey RG Jr, Scheld WM, Winn HR: Bacterial meningitis: selected aspects of cerebrospinal fluid pathophysiology. In Wood JH, editor: *Neurobiology of cerebrospinal fluid 2,* New York, 1983, Plenum Press, pp 727-738.

54. Davis DA, Milhorat TH: The blood-brain barrier of the rat choroid plexus, *Anat Rec* 181:779-788, 1975.

55. Davson H: *Physiology of cerebrospinal fluid,* London, 1967, Churchill-Livingstone.

56. Davson H, Segal MB: The effects of some inhibitors and accelerators of sodium transport on the turnover of ^{22}Na in the cerebrospinal fluid and the brain, *J Physiol (London)* 209:131-153, 1970.

57. DiChiro G: Movement of the cerebrospinal fluid in human beings, *Nature (London)* 204:290-291, 1964.

58. DiChiro G: Observations on the circulation of the cerebrospinal fluid, *Acta Radiol Diagn* 5:988-1002, 1966.

59. DiChiro G, Hammock MK, Bleyer WA: Spinal descent of cerebrospinal fluid in man, *Neurology* 26:1-8, 1976.

60. Edvinsson L, Lindvall M: Autonomic vascular innervation and vasomotor reactivity in the choroid plexus, *Exp Neurol* 62:394-404, 1978.

61. Edvinsson L et al: Adrenergic innervation of the mammalian choroid plexus, *Am J Anat* 139:299-302, 1974.

62. Edvinsson L et al: Ultrastructural and biochemical evidence for a sympathetic neural influence on the choroid plexus, *Exp Neurol* 48:241-251, 1975.

63. Edvinsson L et al: Concentration of noradrenaline in pial vessels, choroid plexus, and iris during two weeks after sympathetic ganglionectomy or decentralization, *Acta Physiol Scand* 85:201-206, 1972.

64. Edvinsson L, Nielsen KC, Owman C: Cholinergic innervation of choroid plexus in rabbits and cats, *Brain Res* 63:500-503, 1973.

65. Edvinsson L, Owman C, West KA: Changes in continuously recorded intracranial pressure of conscious rabbits at different time-periods after superior cervical sympathectomy, *Acta Physiol Scand* 83:42-50, 1971.

66. Feder N, Reese TS, Brightman MW: Microperoxidase, a new tracer of low molecular weight: a study of the interstitial compartments of the mouse brain, *J Cell Biol* 43:35A-36A, 1969.

67. Felgenhauer K: Protein size and cerebrospinal fluid composition, *Klin Wochenschr* 52:1158-1164, 1974.

68. Fenstermacher JD, Patlak CS: The movement of water and solutes in the brain of mammals. In Pappius HM, Feindel W, editors: *Dynamics of brain edema*, New York, 1976, Springer-Verlag, p 87.

69. Fenstermacher JD, Rall DP: Physiology and pharmacology of cerebrospinal fluid. In Capri A, editor: *Pharmacology of the cerebral circulation*, New York, 1972, Pergamon Press, pp 41-72.

70. Ferguson RK, Woodbury DM: Penetration of ^{14}C-inulin and ^{14}C-sucrose into brain, cerebrospinal fluid and skeletal muscle of developing rats, *Exp Brain Res* 7:181-194, 1969.

71. Firemark HM: Choroid-plexus transport of enkephalins and other neuropeptides. In Wood JH, editor: *Neurobiology of cerebrospinal fluid 2*, New York, 1983, Plenum Press, pp 77-81.

72. Foxworthy JC IV, Artru AA: Cerebrospinal fluid dynamics and brain tissue composition following intravenous infusion of hypertonic saline in anesthetized rabbits, *J Neurosurg Anesth* 2:256-265, 1990.

73. Franklin GM, Dudzinski DS, Cutler RWP: Amino acid transport into the cerebrospinal fluid of the rat, *J Neurochem* 24:367-372, 1975.

74. Garcia-Bengochea F: Cortisone and the cerebrospinal fluid of noncastrated cats, *Am Surg* 31:123-127, 1965.

75. Gjedde A, Rasmussen M: Pentobarbital anesthesia reduces blood-brain glucose transfer in the rat, *J Neurochem* 35:1382-1387, 1980.

76. Guldberg HC, Yates CM: Some studies of the effects of chlorpromazine, reserpine and dihydroxyphenylalanine on the concentrations of homovanillic acid, 3,4-dihydroxyphenyl acetic acid and 5-hydroxyindo-3-ylacetic acid in ventricular cerebrospinal fluid of the dog using the technique of serial sampling of the cerebrospinal fluid, *Br J Pharmacol* 33:457-471, 1968.

77. Hamberger A, Blomstrand C, Lehninger AL: Comparative studies on mitochondria isolated from neuron-enriched and glia-enriched fractions of rabbit and beef brain, *J Cell Biol* 45:221-234, 1970.

78. Hannan CJ Jr et al: Blood-brain barrier permeability during hypocapnia in halothane-anesthetized monkeys, *Ann NY Acad Sci* 529:172-174, 1988.

79. Haywood JR, Vogh BP: Some measurements of autonomic nervous system influence on production of cerebrospinal fluid in the cat, *J Pharmacol Exp Ther* 208:341-346, 1979.

80. Heisey SR, Held D, Pappenheimer JR: Bulk flow and diffusion in the cerebrospinal fluid system of the goat, *Am J Physiol* 203:775-781, 1962.

81. Heisey SR, Adams T, Fisher MJ, et al: Effect of hypercapnia and cerebral perfusion pressure on cerebrospinal fluid production in cat, *Am J Physiol* 244:R224-F227, 1983.

82. Hochwald GM: Cerebrospinal fluid mechanisms. In Cottrell JRE, Turndorf H, editors: *Anesthesia and neurosurgery,* St Louis, 1986, Mosby–Year Book, pp 33-53.

83. Hochwald GM, Gandhi M, Goldman S: Transport of glucose from blood to cerebrospinal fluid in the cat, *Neuroscience* 10:1035-1040, 1983.

84. Hochwald GM, Magee J, Ferguson V: Cerebrospinal fluid glucose: turnover and metabolism, *J Neurochem* 44:1832-1837, 1985.

85. Hochwald GM, Wallenstein MC: Exchange of albumin between blood, cerebrospinal fliud, and brain in the cat, *Am J Physiol* 212:1199-1204, 1967.

86. Hochwald GM, Wallenstein MC: Exchange of alpha-globulin between blood, cerebrospinal fluid and brain in the cat, *Exp Neurol* 19:115-126, 1967.

87. Hochwald GM et al: The effects of serum osmolarity on cerebrospinal fluid volume flow, *Life Sci* 15:1309 1316, 1974.

88. Hosobuchi Y, Rossier J, Bloom FE et al: Stimulation of human periaqueductal gray for pain relief increases immunoreactive β-endorphin in ventricular fluid, *Science* 203:279-281, 1979.

89. Jeffcoate WJ et al: β-endorphin in human cerebrospinal fluid, *Lancet* 2:119-121, 1978.

90. Johanson CE: The choroid plexus-arachnoid membrane-cerebrospinal fluid system. In Boulton AA, Baker GB, Walz W, editors: *Neuromethods: the neuronal microenvironment,* Clifton, NJ, 1988, The Humana Press, p 33.

91. Johanson CE, Parandoosh Z, Smith QR: Chloride-bicarbonate exchange in the choroid plexus: analysis by the DMO method for cell pH, *Am J Physiol* 249:F470-F477, 1985.

92. Johnson RN et al: Intracranial hypertension in experimental animals and man: quantitative approach to system dynamics of circulatory cerebrospinal fluid. In Wood JH, editor: *Neurobiology of cerebrospinal fluid 2,* New York, 1983, Plenum Press, pp 697-706.

93. Johnson RN et al: A comparative model of cerebrospinal fluid systems, *Life Sci* 8:79, 1978.

94. Johnson RN et al: Mechanism for intracranial hypertension during experimental subarachnoid hemorrhage: acute malfunction of arachnoid villi by components of plasma, *Trans Am Neurol Assoc* 103:138-142, 1978.

95. Johnston I: The definition of a reduced CSF absorption syndrome: a reappraisal of benign intracranial hypertension and related syndromes, *Med Hypoth* 1:10-14, 1975.

96. Johnston I, Paterson A: Benign intracranial hypertension. II. CSF pressure and circulation, *Brain* 97:301-312, 1974.

97. Katzman R, Pappius HM: *Brain electrolytes and fluid metabolism,* Baltimore, 1973, Williams & Wilkins.

98. Klatzo I et al: Resolution of vasogenic brain edema (VBE), *Adv Neurol* 28:359-373, 1980.

99. Larsson LI, Edvinsson L, Fohrenkrug J et al: Immunohistochemical localization of a vasodilatory peptide (VIP) in cerebrovascular nerves, *Brain Res* 113:400-404, 1976.

100. Leurssen TG, Robertson GL: Cerebrospinal fluid vasopressin and vasotocin in health and disease. In Wood JH, editor: *Neurobiology of cerebrospinal fluid 1,* New York, 1980, Plenum Press, pp 613-623.

101. Leusen IR, Weyne JJ, Demeester GM: Regulation of acid-base equilibrium of cerebrospinal fluid. In Wood JH, editor: *Neurobiology of cerebrospinal fluid 2,* New York, 1983, Plenum Press, pp 25-42.

102. Lindvall M: Fluorescence histochemical study on regional differences in the sympathetic nerve supply of the choroid plexus from various laboratory animals, *Cell Tissue Res* 198:261-267, 1979.

103. Lindvall M, Edvinsson L, Owman C: Sympathetic nervous control of cerebrospinal fluid production from the choroid plexus, *Science* 201:176-207, 1978.

104. Lindvall M, Edvinsson L, Owman C: Histochemical study on regional differences in the cholinergic nerve supply of the choroid plexus from various laboratory animals, *Exp Neurol* 55:152-159, 1977.

105. Lindvall M et al: Peptidergic (VIP) nerves in the mammalian choroid plexus, *Neurosci Lett* 9:77-82, 1978.

106. Lindvall M, Edvinsson L, Owman C: Effect of sympathomimetic drugs and corresponding receptor antagonists on the rate of cerebrospinal fluid production, *Exp Neurol* 64:132-148, 1979.

107. Lindvall M, Edvinsson L, Owman C: Reduced cerebrospinal fluid formation through cholinergic mechanisms, *Neurosci Lett* 10:311-316, 1978.

108. Lups S, Haan AMFH: *The cerebrospinal fluid,* Amsterdam, 1954, Elsevier.

109. Macri FJ et al: Preferential vasoconstrictor properties of acetazolamide on the arteries of the choroid plexus, *Int J Neuropharmacol* 5:109-115, 1966.

110. Maffeo CJ et al: Constant flow perfusion of the cerebrospinal fluid system of rat, dog, and man: a mathematical model. In Saha S, editor: *Proceedings of the Fourth New England Bioengineering Conference,* New York, 1976, Pergamon Press, p 447.

111. Maktabi MA, El Bokl FF, Todd MM: Effect of halothane anesthesia on production of cerebrospinal fluid: possible role of vasopressin V_1 receptors, *J Cereb Blood Flow Metabol* 11:S268, 1991 (abstract).

112. Mann ES, Cookson SL, Mann JD: Effects of enflurane and halothane on CSF dynamics in the rat, *Anesthesiology Suppl 3* 51:54-57, 1979.

113. Mann JD et al: Regulation of intracranial pressure in rat, dog, and man, *Ann Neurol* 3:156-165, 1978.

114. Mann JD, Butler AB, Johnson RN, et al.: Clearance of macromolecular and particulate substances from the cerebrospinal fluid system of the rat, *J Neurosurg* 50:343-348, 1979.

115. Mann JD et al: Cerebrospinal fluid circulatory dynamics in pseudotumor cerebri and response to steroid therapy. In Wood JH, editor: *Neurobiology of cerebrospinal fluid 2,* New York, 1983, Plenum Press, pp 739-751.

116. Mann JD, Mann ES, Cookson SL: Differential effect of pentobarbital, ketamine hydrochloride, and enflurane anesthesia on CSF formation rate and outflow resistance in the rat. In Miller JD, Becker DP, Hochwald G et al, editors: *Intracranial pressure IV,* New York, 1980, Springer-Verlag, p 466.

117. Mann JD et al: Impairment of cerebrospinal fluid circulatory dynamics in pseudotumor cerebri and response to steroid treatment, *Neurology* 29:550-554, 1979.

118. Maren TH: Carbonic anhydrase: chemistry, physiology and inhibition, *Physiol Rev* 47:595-781, 1967.

119. Maren TH: Ion secretion into cerebrospinal fluid, *Exp Eye Res Suppl* 25:157-159, 1977.

120. Marmarou A, Shulman K, LaMorgese J: Compartmental analysis of compliance and outflow resistance of the cerebrospinal fluid system, *J Neurosurg* 43:523-534, 1975.

121. Marmarou A, Shapiro K, Shulman K: Isolating factors leading to sustained elevations of the ICP. In Beks JWF, Bosch DA, Brock M, editors: *Intracranial pressure III,* New York, 1976, Springer-Verlag, pp 33-35.

122. Marmarou A, Shulman K, LaMorgese J: A compartmental analysis of compliance and outflow resistance and the effects of elevated blood pressure. In Lundberg N, Ponten U, Brock M, editors: *Intracranial pressure II,* New York, 1975, Springer-Verlag, pp 86-88.

123. Martins AN, Doyle TF, Newby N: P_{CO_2} and rate of formation of cerebrospinal fluid in the monkey, *Am J Physiol* 231:127-131, 1976.

124. Matsen FA III, West CR: Supracortical fluid: a monitor of albumin exchange in normal and injured brain, *Am J Physiol* 222:532-539, 1972.

125. Meyer RR, Shapiro HM: Paradoxical effect of enflurane on choroid plexus metabolism: clinical implications (abstract), *American Society of Anesthesiologists,* 1978, pp 489-490.

126. Milhorat TH: *Hydrocephalus and the cerebrospinal fluid,* Baltimore, 1972, Williams & Wilkins.

127. Milhorat TH: Pediatric neurosurgery. In Plum F, McDowell FH, editors: *Contemporary neurology series,* vol 16, Philadelphia, 1978, FA Davis, pp 91-135.

128. Milhorat TH: Structure and function of the choroid plexus and other sites of cerebrospinal fluid formation, *Int Rev Cytol* 47:225-288, 1976.

129. Milhorat TH: The third circulation revisited, *J Neurosurg* 42:628-645, 1975.

130. Milhorat TH, Davis DA, Hammock MK: Localization of ouabain-sensitive NaD-K-ATPase in frog, rabbit, and rat choroid plexus, *Brain Res* 99:170-174, 1975.

131. Milhorat TH, Davis DA, Lloyd BJ: Two morphologically distinct blood-brain barriers preventing the entry of cytochrome c into the cerebrospinal fluid, *Science* 180:76-78, 1973.

132. Milhorat TH, Hammock MK: Cerebrospinal fluid as reflection of internal milieu of brain. In Wood JH, editor: *Neurobiology of cerebrospinal fluid 2,* New York, 1983, Plenum Press, pp 1-23.

133. Miller JD: Intracranial pressure-volume relationships in pathological conditions, *J Neurosurg Sci* 20:203-209, 1976.

134. Miller JD: Volume and pressure in the craniospinal axis. In Wilkins RH, editor: *Clinical neurosurgery,* vol 22, Baltimore, 1975, Williams & Wilkins, pp 76-105.

135. Miller JD, Garibi J: Intracranial volume-pressure relationships during continuous monitoring of ventricular fluid pressure. In Brock M, Deitz H, editors: *Intracranial pressure,* New York, 1972, Springer-Verlag, pp 270-274.

136. Miller JD, Garibi J, Pickard JD: The effects of induced changes of cerebrospinal fluid volume during continuous monitoring of ventricular pressure, *Arch Neurol* 28:265-269, 1973.

137. Miller JD, Leech PJ, Pickard JD: Volume-pressure response in various experiments and clinical conditions. In Lundberg N, Ponten U, Brock M, editors: *Intracranial pressure II,* New York, 1975, Springer-Verlag, pp 97-100.

138. Miner LC, Reed DJ: The effect of ethacrynic acid on Na^+ uptake into the cerebrospinal fluid of the rat, *Arch Intern Pharmacodynam Ther* 190:316-321, 1971.

139. Nabeshima S et al: Junctions in the meninges and marginal glia, *J Comp Neurol* 164:127-134, 1975.

140. Nemoto EM, Stezoski SW, Mac-Murdo D: Glucose transport across the rat blood-brain barrier during anesthesia, *Anesthesiology* 49:170-176, 1978.

141. Oppelt WW, Patlak CS, Rall DP: Effect of certain drugs on cerebrospinal fluid production in the dog, *Am J Physiol* 206:247-250, 1964.

142. Oppelt WW et al: Effects of acid-base alterations on cerebrospinal fluid production, *Proc Soc Exp Biol Med* 114:86-96, 1963.

143. Pappenheimer JR: On the location of the blood-barrier. In *Proceedings of the Wales Symposium on the Blood-Brain Barrier,* London, 1970, Oxford, p 66.

144. Pappenheimer JR et al: Perfusion of the cerebral ventricular system in unanesthetized goats, *Am J Physiol* 203:763-774, 1962.

145. Pappius HM, Oh JB, Dossetor JB: The effects of rapid hemodialysis on brain tissues and cerebrospinal fluid in dogs, *Can J Physiol Pharmacol* 45:129-147, 1967.

146. Pashayan AG et al: Blood-CSF barrier function during general anesthesia in children undergoing ventriculoperitoneal shunt placement, *Anesth Rev* 15:30-31, 1988 (abstract).

147. Pollay M, Stevens FA, Roberts PA: Alteration in choroid-plexus blood flow and cerebrospinal fluid formation by increased ventricular pressure. In Wood JH, editor: *Neurobiology of cerebrospinal fluid 2,* New York, 1983, Plenum Press, pp 687-695.

148. Porter JC: Neuroendocrine systems: the need for precise identification and rigorous description of their operation, *Prog Brain Res* 39:1-6, 1973.

149. Porter JC, Kamberi IA, Ondo JG: Role of biogenic amines and cerebrospinal fluid in the neurovascular transmittal and hypophysiotrophic substances. In Knigge KM, Scott DE, Weindl A, editors: *Brain-Endocrine interaction, median eminence: structure and function (Proceedings of the International Symposium on Brain-Endocrine Interaction, Munich, 1971),* Basel, 1972, S. Karger, pp 245-253.

150. Portig PJ, Sharman DF, Vogt M: Release by tubocurarine of dopamine and homovanillic acid from the superfused caudate nucleus, *J Physiol (London)* 194:565-572, 1968.

151. Portig PJ, Vogt M: Activation of a dopaminergic nigro-striatal pathway, *J Physiol (London)* 197:20P-21P, 1968.

152. Post KD, Biller BJ, Jackson IMD: Cerebrospinal fluid pituitary hormone concentrations in patients with pituitary tumors. In Wood JH, editor: *Neurobiology of cerebrospinal fluid 1,* New York, 1980, Plenum Press, pp 591-604.

153. Post RM, Allen FH, Ommaya AK: Cerebrospinal fluid flow and iodide[131] transport in the spinal subarachnoid space, *Life Sci* 14:1885-1894, 1974.

154. Pratt OE, Greenwood J: Movement of vitamins across the blood-brain barrier. In Suckling AJ, Rumsby MG, Bradbury MWB, editors: *The blood brain barrier in health and disease,* Chichester, England, 1986, Ellis Horwood Ltd, pp 87-97.

155. Rapoport SI: *The blood-brain barrier in physiology and medicine,* New York, 1976, Raven Press, pp 43-86.

156. Rapoport SI: A mathematical model for vasogenic brain edema, *J Theor Biol* 74:439, 1978.

157. Rapoport SI: Passage of proteins from blood to cerebrospinal fluid: model for transfer by pores and vesicles. In Wood JH, editor: *Neurobiology of cerebrospinal fluid 2,* New York, 1983, Plenum Press, pp 233-245.

158. Reese TS, Karnovsky MJ: Fine structural localization of a blood-brain barrier to exogenous peroxidase, *J Cell Biol* 34:207-217, 1967.

159. Reppert SM, Perlow MJ, Klein DC: Cerebrospinal fluid melanin. In Wood JH, editor: *Neurobiology of cerebrospinal fluid 1,* New York, 1980, Plenum Press, pp 579-589.

160. Reulen HJ, Graham R, Spatz M et al: Role of pressure gradients and bulk flow in dynamics of vasogenic brain edema, *J Neurosurg* 46:24-35, 1977.

161. Reulen HJ, Kreysch KG: Measurement of brain tissue in cold induced cerebral edema, *Acta Neurochir* 29:29-40, 1973.

162. Reulen HJ et al: Clearance of edema fluid into cerebrospinal fluid: mechanisms for resolution of vasogenic brain edema. In Wood JH, editor: *Neurobiology of cerebrospinal fluid 2,* New York, 1983, Plenum Press, pp 777-787.

163. Rodriguez EM et al: Evidence for the periventricular localization of the hypothalamic osmoreceptors. In Knowles F, Vollrath L, editors: *Neurosecretion—the final neuroendocrine pathway,* New York, 1973, Springer-Verlag, pp 319-320.

164. Rosenberg GA: Glucose, amino acids, and lipids. In Rosenberg GA, editor: *Brain fluids and metabolism,* New York, 1990, Oxford University Press, pp 119-144.

165. Rosenberg GA: Physiology of cerebrospinal and interstitial fluids. In Rosenberg GA, editor: *Brain fluids and metabolism,* New York, 1990, Oxford University Press, pp 36-57.

166. Rosenberg GA, Kyner WT: Effect of mannitol-induced hyperosmolarity on transport between brain interstitial fluid and cerebrospinal fluid. In Wood JH, editor: *Neurobiology of cerebrospinal fluid 2,* New York, 1983, Plenum Press, pp 765-775.

167. Rosenberg GA, Kyner WT, Estrada E: Bulk flow of brain interstitial fluid under normal and hyperosmolar conditions, *Am J Physiol* 238:F42-F49, 1980.

168. Sadler K, Welch K: Concentration of glucose in new choroidal cerebrospinal fluid of the rabbit, *Nature* 215:884-885, 1967.

169. Sage JI, Duffy TE: Pentobarbital anesthesia: influence on amino acid transport across the blood-brain barrier, *J Neurochem* 33:963-965, 1979.

170. Sahar A: Choroidal origin of cerebrospinal fluid, *Isr J Med Sci* 8:594, 1972.

171. Sahar A, Tsipstein E: Effects of mannitol and furosemide on the rate of formation of cerebrospinal fluid, *Exp Neurol* 60:584-591, 1978.

172. Saija A, Princi P, Pasquale R et al: Modifications of the permeability of the blood-brain barrier and local cerebral metabolism in pentobarbital- and ketamine-anaesthetized rats, *Neuropharmacol* 28:997-1002, 1989.

173. Sato O, Hara M, Asai T et al: The effect of dexamethasone phosphate on the production rate of cerebrospinal fluid in the subarachnoid space of dogs, *J Neurosurg* 39:480-484, 1973.

174. Schanberg SM, Breese GR, Schildkraut JJ: 3-Methoxy-4-hydroxyphenylglycol sulfate in brain and cerebrospinal fluid, *Biochem Pharmacol* 17:2006-2008, 1968.

175. Schettini A, Furniss WW: Brain water and electrolyte distribution during the inhalation of halothane, *Br J Anaesth* 51:1117-1124, 1979.

176. Schwartz ML, Tator CH, Hoffman HJ: The uptake of hydrocortisone in mouse brain and ependymoblastoma, *J Neurosurg* 36:178-183, 1972.

177. Segal MB, Pollay M: The secretion of cerebrospinal fluid, *Exp Eye Res Suppl* 25:127-148, 1977.

178. Shulman K, Marmarou A: Pressure-volume considerations in infantile hydrocephalus, *Dev Child Neurol (Suppl 25)* 13:90-95, 1971.

179. Simionescu N, Simionescu M, Palade GE: Permeability of muscle capillaries to small hemepeptides: evidence for the existence of patent transendothelial channels, *J Cell Biol* 64:586-607, 1975.

180. Simionescu N, Simionescu M, Palade GE: Structural basis of permeability in sequential segments of the microvasculature of the diaphragm. II. Pathways followed by microperoxidase across the endothelium, *Microvasc Res* 15:17-36, 1978.

181. Smith RV, Roberts PA, Fisher RG: Alteration of cerebrospinal fluid production in the dog, *Surg Neurol* 2:267-270, 1974.

182. Snodgrass SR, Lorenzo AV: Temperature and cerebrospinal fluid production rate, *Am J Physiol* 222:1524-1527, 1972.

183. Spector R, Lorenzo AV: Specificity of ascorbic acid transport system of the central nervous system, *Am J Physiol* 226:1468-1473, 1974.

184. Sugioka S: Effects of sevoflurane on intracranial pressure and formation and absorption of cerebrospinal fluid in cats, *Masui (Jap J Anesth)* 41:1434-1442, 1992.

185. Suzuki S, Ishii M, Iwabuchi T: Post-haemorrhagic subarachnoid fibrosis in dogs: scanning electron microscopic observation and dye perfusion study, *Acta Neurochir* 46:105-117, 1979.

186. Tschirgi RC, Frost RW, Taylor JL: Inhibition of cerebrospinal fluid formation by a carbonic anhydrase inhibitor, 2-Acetylamino-1,3,4-Thiadiazole-5-sulfonamide (Diamox), *Proc Soc Exp Biol Med* 87:373-376, 1954.

187. Upton ML, Weller RO: The morphology of cerebrospinal fluid drainage pathways in human arachnoid granulations, *J Neurosurg* 63:867-875, 1985.

188. Van Landingham KE et al: Cerebrospinal fluid dynamics in the cat under halothane and pentobarbital anesthesia, *Soc Neurosci* 7:89, 1981 (abstract).

189. Vates TS, Bonting SJ, Oppelt WW: Na-K-activated adenosine triphosphatase formation of cerebrospinal fluid in the cat, *Am J Physiol* 206:1165-1172, 1964.

190. Vigh B, Vigh-Teichman I: Comparative ultrastructure of the cerebrospinal fluid contacting neurons. In Bourne GH, Danielli JF, editors. *International review of cytology*, vol 35, New York, 1973, Academic Press, pp 189-251.

191. Vigh-Teichman I, Vigh B: Structure and function of the liquor contacting neurosecretory system. In Bargmann W, Scharrer B, editors: *Aspects of neuroendocrinology*, New York, 1970, Springer-Verlag, pp 329-337.

192. Vogh BP, Maren TH: Sodium, chloride and bicarbonate movement from plasma to cerebrospinal fluid in cats, *Am J Physiol* 228:673-685, 1975.

193. Vorherr H, Bradbury MW, Hoghoughi M et al: Antidiuretic hormone in cerebrospinal fluid during endogenous and exogenous changes in its blood levels, *Endocrinology* 83:246-250, 1968.

194. Wald A, Hochwald GM, Gandhi M: Evidence for the movement of fluid, macromolecules and ions from the brain extracellular space to the CSF, *Brain Res* 151:283-290, 1978.

195. Weisner B, Bernhardt W: Protein fractions of lumbar, cisternal and ventricular cerebrospinal fluid, *J Neurol Sci* 37:205-214, 1978

196. Weiss MH, Nulsen FE: The effect of glucocorticoids on CSF flow in dogs, *J Neurosurg* 32:452-458, 1970.

197. Weiss MH, Wertman N: Modulation of CSF production by alterations in cerebral perfusion pressure, *Arch Neurol* 35:527-529, 1978.

198. Welch MH, Pollay M: The spinal arachnoid villi of the monkeys cercopithecus aethiops sabaeus and macacairus, *Anat Rec* 145:43-48, 1963.

199. Williams B: Cerebrospinal fluid pressure changes in response to coughing, *Brain* 99:331-340, 1976.

200. Winbladh B, Edvinsson L, Lindvall M: Effect of sympathectomy on active transport mechanisms in choroid plexus in vitro, *Acta Physiol Scand* 102:85A, 1978.

201. Wolff J: On the meaning of vesiculation in capillary endothelium, *Angiologica* 4:64-68, 1967.

202. Wolff JR: Ultrastructure of the terminal vascular bed as related to function. In Kaley G, Altura BM, editors: *Microvascular circulation*, vol I, Baltimore, 1977, University Park Press, p 95.

203. Wood JH: Physiology, pharmacology, and dynamics of cerebrospinal fluid. In Wood JH, editor: *Neurobiology of cerebrospinal fluid 1*, New York, 1980, Plenum Press, p 1-16.

204. Wood JH et al: Normal-pressure hydrocephalus: diagnosis and patient selection for shunt surgery, *Neurology* 24:517-526, 1974.

205. Woodbury JW: An epilogue, an hypothetical model for CSF formation and blood-brain barrier function. In Siesjo BK, Sorensen SC, editors: *Ion homeostasis of the brain*, Copenhagen, 1971, Munksgaard, pp 465-471.

206. Wright EM: Mechanisms of ion transport across the choroid plexus, *J Physiol (London)* 226:545-571, 1972.

207. Wright EM: Transport processes in the formation of cerebrospinal fluid, *Rev Physiol Biochem Pharmacol* 83:1-34, 1978.

5

Intracranial Pressure Monitoring

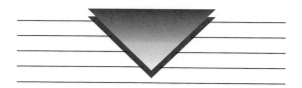

JEFFREY S. SCHWEITZER
MARVIN BERGSNEIDER
DONALD P. BECKER

The increasingly demanding procedures that neurosurgeons and neuroanesthesiologists are required to implement and the complex problems of patients whom they are called on to manage require sophisticated monitoring strategies. While the monitoring of intracranial pressure (ICP) is not a new concept (first having been proposed some 40 years ago[29]), the situations in which such monitoring may be beneficial, the techniques used to perform the monitoring, and the analysis and interpretation of the data acquired are all subject to continuing investigation and refinement.

In the care of the critically ill neurosurgical patient, the head-injured patient, and the patient undergoing craniotomy, the neurosurgeon and neuroanesthesiologist, equipped with an understanding of ICP and the techniques available to assess it and to intervene based on this assessment, are able to make the greatest contribution toward preserving life

and neurologic function. Significant clinical changes in ICP do not occur in isolation, and we wish here to place special emphasis on the interactions between ICP, cerebral perfusion, and pathologic anatomy. It is our purpose to give an overview of the current understanding of how ICP is modulated, both normally and pathophysiologically; how its measurement is best accomplished and interpreted; and the way in which neurosurgical and neuroanesthesia teams may best work together to apply this knowledge in clinical practice.

HISTORICAL ASPECTS

While a rudimentary understanding of the phenomena underlying changes in ICP dates back at least 200 years,[38,50,76] the realization that abnormalities of ICP play a critical role in neurologic dysfunction was first formalized in the pioneering studies of Harvey Cushing, who—at the turn of the century—studied the effects of saline infused into the cerebrospinal fluid (CSF) space on respiratory and cardiovascular function of animals. This work demonstrated hypertension, bradycardia, and respiratory changes as CSF pressure approached systemic arterial pressure.[19] The significance of these changes—which we commonly refer to as the "Cushing response" or "Cushing reflex"—long remained controversial because their clinical application and significance were not clear. Cushing himself believed the changes to be due to medullary ischemia.[19] Early attempts to measure ICP in human patients were done by lumbar puncture—i.e., by measurement of lumbar subarachnoid CSF pressure; pressure measured this way was seldom observed to reach the levels Cushing described.* Today, with an improved understanding of intracranial pathology and CSF hydrodynamics, the clinician is seldom faced with the "classic" Cushing triad, and such changes are of more academic than practical value.

Key to the development of our modern understanding of intracranial pressure dynamics was the work of Meyer,[65] Kernohan and Woltman,[40] and Moore and Stern[77] in the 1920s and 1930s. These investigators described the pathologic changes associated with intracranial brain shift and herniation in autopsy specimens. With such findings came the realization that the intracranial and intraspinal spaces

_____
*References 12, 27, 32, 33, 62, 63.

were not uniform and equivalent in terms of pressure and, that, not only did pressure gradients exist, but they were of critical clinical significance. It was realized that many of the early workers who failed to find elevated pressures with lumbar puncture in the presence of known supratentorial mass lesions had, in fact, been measuring pressure in the presence of foramen magnum herniation with resultant block and that the lumbar puncture itself could be a contributing factor to the development of such herniation.[23,34,91]

A better understanding of the relationships between CSF pressure and the effects of varying intracranial blood volume, CSF volume, respiratory function, systemic blood pressure, and serum osmolality emerged through a series of clinical investigations conducted on human patients by Henry Ryder and his group in the 1950s.[99-105] While these studies did not immediately lead to an appreciation of the usefulness of ICP measurement in the presence of mass lesions, they complemented the development of methods for continuous monitoring of ventricular CSF pressure pioneered by Guillaume and Janny in 1951 and continued by Lundberg in 1960.[29,49] The investigations and clinical observations of Lundberg and his colleagues began the modern era of ICP monitoring.

Lundberg first described rhythmic and other variations in ventricular fluid pressure and attempted to correlate these with their physiologic or pathologic mechanisms. His work described the presence of different classes of pressure

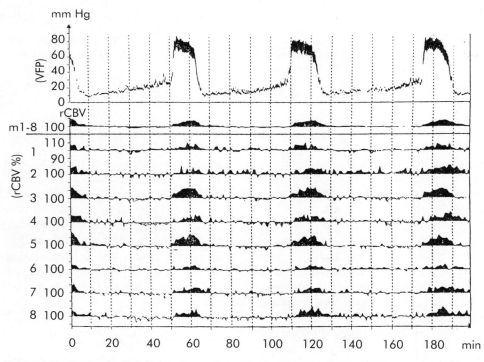

FIG. 5-1 Plateau waves. Recordings of ventricular fluid pressure (VFP), together with regional cerebral blood volume (rCBV) at the indicated locations. This illustrates the concept that the rCBV changes are etiologically related to the plateau waves. *(From Risberg J, Lundberg N, Ingrav DH: J Neurosurg 31:303-310, 1969.)*

"waves," which he labeled "A," "B," and "C." While B and C waves were associated with respiratory and blood pressure phenomena and were of limited clinical usefulness, A waves—now more commonly known as "plateau waves" (Fig. 5-1)—were often associated with significant neurologic manifestations.[41,49,51] Although the basis of these plateau waves was and still remains somewhat obscure, the demonstration that they could be prevented by CSF drainage or diuretic administration led Lundberg to suggest that ICP monitoring could be a valuable tool in the management of patients with intracranial pathology involving raised ICP.[49,51,52]

The laboratory studies of Langfitt,[46] Pappenheimer,[20,31] and others introduced the mechanisms of cerebral hemodynamics and CSF hydrodynamics into the emerging understanding of ICP regulation. In addition, Langfitt formalized the concept of the intracranial pressure-volume relationship[45,46] (Fig. 5-2). With these advances came renewed interest in and understanding of the relationship between (1) intracranial hypertension and intracranial mass lesions and (2) cerebral metabolism and blood flow, as well as the role of therapeutic maneuvers in these interrelationships.

INTRACRANIAL PRESSURE AND ITS REGULATION
Pathophysiology of Intracranial Hypertension

In the absence of disease, ICP may undergo quite marked rises without ill effect. Sneezing, coughing, and straining result in elevations of ICP by 60 mm Hg or more but seldom result in neurologic impairment. Patients with benign intracranial hypertension can endure significantly elevated pressures over long periods. The work of Ryder et al.[105] involving artificial elevation of CSF pressure in human patients by saline infusion showed that pressures as high as 110 mm Hg might be tolerated. It is therefore not the ambient pressure per se within the calvarium, but its interaction with other pathology, that produces the symptomatology of raised ICP.

Mechanical shifts and deformations may have direct disruptive effects on neuronal function, particularly when lateral movement is involved.[94,95] However, most of the damage produced by slower mechanical shifts—e.g., that produced by large masses or resulting from generalized paren-

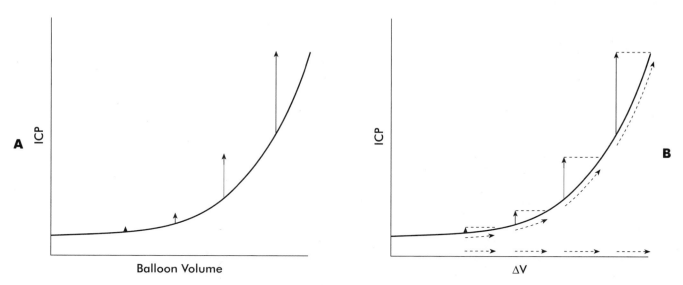

FIG. 5-2 The intracranial pressure-volume relationship. The plots illustrate concepts derived from the experiments of Langfitt and colleagues.[46] **A,** Plot of ICP vs. the volume of an expanding epidural balloon. The arrows indicate the ICP changes noted with hypercarbia, induced hypertension, or rapid saline addition to the supratentorial CSF space. With larger balloon volumes, these perturbations result in much larger ICP increases, an indication of reduced intracranial compliance. **B,** Extrapolation of the experimental findings to a general concept of an intracranial pressure-volume curve. Here the perturbations in blood pressure — P_{CO_2} or CSF volume — are treated as volume additions themselves, as though each represented equivalent expansion of the experimental epidural balloon from the plot in **A.** The dotted lines and arrows indicate the point to which these volume additions shift the system along the single pressure-volume curve. This proposal assumes that a single curve prevails for all intracranial components and that volume additions to any component are equivalent and additive with additions to any other. Though conceptually useful, these assumptions are an oversimplification, as discussed in the text.

chymal swelling—is ischemic damage due to reduction of local or global cerebral perfusion pressure (CPP). The CPP is the pressure gradient across the capillary bed and is the difference between mean systemic arterial pressure and ICP (except in circumstances where venous outflow pathology raises venous pressure above ICP). Blood flow is determined by both the CPP and vascular tone (resistance). When elevated ICP or other causes result in a fall in cerebral blood flow—globally or regionally—below metabolic demands, a progression of pathologic events takes place at the cellular level, which may lead to eventual cell death.[17,123] These events may be reversible if blood flow is restored and cell metabolic requirements met before a point of irreversible metabolic destabilization. Within this window of reversibility, medical or surgical interventions—including correction of elevated ICP—may rescue or preserve neurologic function. Recent data on the role of ischemia in head injury has underscored the clinical importance of the ICP-CPP relationship.[10,54,81] Some have argued that the role of diminished perfusion as a mechanism of neuronal damage due to elevated ICP is so critical that clinical treatment of intracranial hypertension should be directed at increasing CPP, rather than at reducing ICP per se.[98,109,112]

Normal and Pathologic Determinants of Intracranial Pressure

The term *intracranial pressure* is usually construed as defining a uniform pressure within the cranial vault. This as-

sumption of uniformity is in many cases not valid as is apparent both from a consideration of static and dynamic mechanical principles, as well as from actual clinical observations of pressures measured simultaneously in multiple locations.[37,96,120] In situations in which ICP gradients exist, monitoring of pressure at a single site will provide only limited information, and an understanding of the mechanical and anatomic factors contributing to the measured ICP is therefore essential to the correct interpretation of the measured data.

In the adult the rigid skull establishes the cranial vault as an essentially fixed volume. Classically the contents of this fixed volume have been considered as consisting of three components: brain parenchyma, CSF, and intravascular or blood volume (Fig. 5-3). Pathologic circumstances may introduce a fourth component, the mass lesion, which may constitute tumor, abscess, hematoma, contusion, or other material and which may behave differently from the three normal components. Within the cranial vault, changes in the volume of one component will necessitate compensatory changes in volume of one or more of the other components if the ICP is to remain constant. This principle has been termed the Monro-Kellie hypothesis.[38,50,76]

The *brain parenchyma* component may be divided into cellular and extracellular compartments. Within the cellular compartment, the contribution of cell membranes and myelin may be considered fixed, whereas the intracellular fluid volume is maintained in equilibrium with the extracellular fluid volume by passive movement of water along

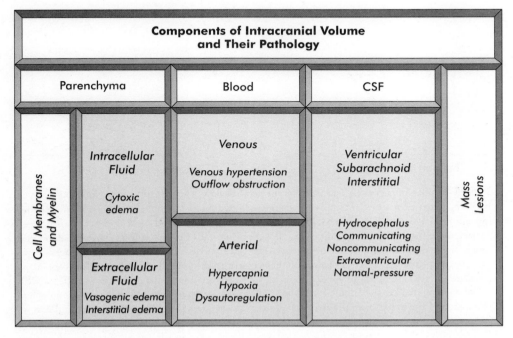

FIG. 5-3   Components of the intracranial volume. Shaded portions indicate those elements that undergo volume changes in pathologic states: examples of such conditions are given for each component.

osmotic gradients established across semipermeable cell membranes. Changes in either intracellular or extracellular fluid volume are common in pathologic states.[26] Where the blood-brain barrier is disrupted, as in the vicinity of abscesses or tumors, an increase in extracellular (interstitial fluid) volume is frequently seen and is known as *vasogenic edema*. Where the normal homeostatic mechanisms maintaining intracellular volume are disrupted, increased intracellular volume may result and is termed *cytotoxic edema*. This may be seen after trauma or infarction. Combinations of these circumstances may occur. The term *interstitial edema* is used to refer to extracellular fluid volume increases associated with changes in the CSF spaces, such as occurs in hydrocephalus. While therapy may be quite different depending on the cause of the edema, the overall contribution of brain parenchyma to changes in intracranial volume is determined by the sum of the intracellular and extracellular fluid volume changes.

The cerebrospinal fluid spaces are filled with fluid that is derived approximately 60% from the choroid plexus and 40% from transependymal movement of fluid from the extracellular space. The choroid plexus is located in the lateral third and fourth ventricles and produces CSF at a rate that is nearly constant, except in the setting of ventriculitis or possibly with extremely high intraventricular pressures. CSF resorption rate, on the other hand, is subject to control by numerous processes, including cerebral venous pressure and the rate of flow through the intraventricular and subarachnoid spaces. A decrease in resorption rate will thus lead to an increased CSF volume (hydrocephalus). In chronic situations this may be well tolerated for long periods, but severe acute hydrocephalus may be rapidly fatal.

Intracranial blood volume is determined largely through regulation of cerebral arterial and arteriolar caliber although

pressure and volume in the venous sinuses may also contribute to overall ICP. Cerebral arterial blood flow is subject to an incompletely understood homeostatic process known as autoregulation. Under normal circumstances, autoregulation serves to maintain a constant cerebral blood flow over a wide range of systemic arterial blood pressures through compensatory changes in cerebral vascular resistance (Fig. 5-4). This is accomplished efficiently by changes in vessel tone or caliber because resistance to flow is inversely proportional to the fourth power of vessel radius (Poiseuille's law). These changes in vessel lumen size will also modulate cerebral blood volume, which is directly proportional to the square of vessel radius. Autoregulation—the mechanism of which may be related to changing adenosine levels in response to the adequacy of tissue oxygenation[28,66]—is quite sensitive to arterial P_{O_2} and P_{CO_2}, and alterations in these parameters may therefore have major effects on cerebral blood volume. Failure of normal autoregulation may lead to significant alterations in cerebral blood volume and perfusion; such changes may include the "breakthrough" phenomenon after resection of certain arteriovenous malformations[111] and the hyperemia often seen after head injury, especially in children.[15,39,80,82] Because it affects not only intracranial blood volume and therefore ICP, but also CPP directly, autoregulation may play a critical role in intracranial pathophysiology.[39,80,82]

Intracranial mass lesions may occur either within the brain itself or extraaxially. It is valuable to consider them as a separate component of intracranial volume because they are usually not subject to the compensatory or regulatory mechanisms that govern the volume of the three "normal" components. The effect of such a lesion on ICP is determined not only by its volume but also by position; for example, a small lesion causing CSF obstruction may be more dangerous than a much larger lesion in a less inopportune position.

Pressure-Volume Relationships, Compliance, and Capacitance

The total contribution of brain parenchyma, CSF, and blood volume to the intracranial contents—together with mass lesions when present—will determine ICP. The relationship between volume and pressure in the intracranial space may be expressed as a *pressure-volume curve*.[45,46] In a series of studies, Langfitt[45,46] used an inflatable epidural balloon in rhesus monkeys and monitored pressure in the lateral ventricle. He plotted a curve of pressure vs. balloon volume, which was flat at low balloon volumes but became very steep at high balloon volumes (see Fig. 5-2), where small increases in balloon volume resulted in large increases in the monitored pressure.

The slope at any given point on this pressure-volume curve represents the degree of cerebral compliance. Standard physiologic nomenclature defines compliance as the change in volume for a given change in pressure ($\triangle V/\triangle P$). Some authors use the term *cerebral elastance* ($\triangle P/\triangle V$) in-

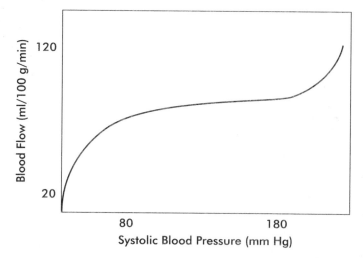

FIG. 5-4 Autoregulation. The nonlinear relationship between systemic blood pressure and cerebral blood flow allows the latter to be maintained in a narrow range *(flat portion of the curve)* over a wide range of input pressures.

stead. However, with respect to the brain, most authors have historically used the term *compliance* in association with the pressure-volume relationship. This quantity reflects both the viscoelastic properties, or stiffness, of the intracranial contents and the functioning of compensatory mechanisms available to reduce ICP at any given point on the curve. Another clinically significant property may be referred to as *cerebral capacitance*. This quantity describes the rate at which the brain can accommodate changes in intracranial volume and is determined by time-dependent derivatives of the same variables determining cerebral compliance. Thus traumatic intracranial hematomas that grow rapidly may result in rapid pressure increases and fatal cerebral herniation, while a meningioma may slowly grow to a much larger size in a similar location with few symptoms (Fig. 5-5). We are not aware of any experimental or clinical trials to date that attempt to quantify cerebral capacitance.

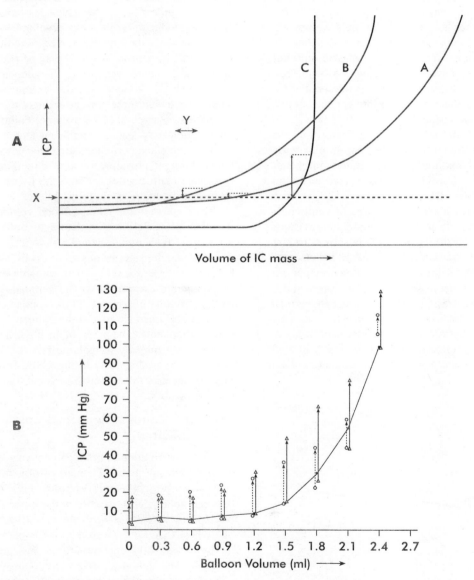

FIG. 5-5   Multiple pressure-volume curves. **A,** Different pressure-volume curves give different values of volume-pressure response (VPR) at a single ICP or CSF pressure. In practice, the shape of the pressure-volume curve varies with cerebral compliance and capacitance. Arrows indicate pressure change caused by the addition of fixed volume. **B,** Volume additions to different intracranial components do not produce equivalent pressure changes. The heavy curve is a plot of ICP vs. epidural balloon volume, as in Fig. 5-2. Solid arrows and triangles indicate the result of volume addition to the balloon, whereas dotted arrows and circles represent equivalent volume addition to the CSF space (at a rate fast enough to preclude significant CSF absorption). *(A, from Wilkins RA, editor:* Clin Neurosurg *22:75-105, 1975;* **B,** *from Sullivan HG, Miller JD, Griffin RL et al:* Am J Phys *234:12167-171, 1978.)*

Many factors involving all components of the intracranial contents may affect changes in cerebral compliance. Quantity and location of CSF and its rate of resorption, the extent of cerebral tissue edema, and the presence of pathologic lesions will all affect this parameter. The relationship between cerebral blood volume and compliance is more complex. This was investigated by Lundberg,[92] who measured CBF and regional cerebral blood volume (rCBV) during plateau waves, which he interpreted as being an indicator of low cerebral compliance. He found that during these periods there occurred an increase in rCBV and a decrease in CBF (see Fig. 5-1). This suggested that the pathologic plateau waves might be triggered by regional increases in cerebral blood volume during the low compliance state. Lundberg proposed that vasodilation causes a rapid rise in ICP with concomitant obstruction of cerebral venous drainage, thus resulting in the increased rCBV and decreased CBF. Other changes in rCBV and CBF are also closely linked to the preservation or failure of cerebral vascular autoregulation, which may thus affect compliance. Muizelaar[79] has shown that in patients with severe head injuries who have intact autoregulation, administration of mannitol decreased ICP by 27%, while CBF remained unchanged. The improved blood rheology provided by the mannitol permitted autoregulatory vasoconstriction while maintaining blood flow and tissue oxygenation at this reduced cerebral blood volume. In patients with defective autoregulation, the decrease in ICP with mannitol administration was limited to 5%, while CBF actually increased 18% because no reflexive vasoconstriction was possible.

Compensatory mechanisms available in the presence of rising ICP or an expanding intracranial mass may involve any of the intracranial components. Pappenheimer's and Cutler's work[20,31] produced early evidence that changes in CSF distribution and bulk flow were the initial compensatory responses. CSF may be displaced into the spinal subarachnoid space, or its resorption rate may increase. Reductions in cerebral tissue and blood volume may follow but are obviously more limited. In the presence of autoregulatory dysfunction, changes in systemic blood pressure or other factors affecting cerebral blood volume may have significant effects on cerebral compliance and ICP.[54,79,80] The size and rate of expansion of intracranial masses and degree of cerebral edema influence cerebral compliance and capacitance and therefore the effectiveness of other compensatory mechanisms.

Measurement of Intracranial Compliance

An ability to quantify cerebral compliance would provide a means of determining the current position of a patient's intracranial contents on the cerebral pressure-volume curve. A fall in compliance to a critical level could provide warning of imminent decompensation. Miller[67,68,71-73] first attempted to quantify cerebral compliance by injecting a small volume of fluid into a patient's intraventricular catheter and then measuring the resultant change in intraventricular pressure. The *volume-pressure response* (VPR) was defined as the change in ICP measured after injection or withdrawal of 1 ml of CSF over 1 second. A normal VPR was found to be less than 2 mm Hg/ml, whereas a VPR of greater than 5 mm Hg/ml indicated a critical reduction in the volume-buffering capacity of the brain.[74] It was found that VPR could change independently of the baseline intraventricular pressure. In clinical terms, the combination of a normal intraventricular pressure and an elevated VPR almost always indicated the presence of a previously unexpected intracranial mass lesion.[69] Thus the VPR served as a sensitive indicator of impaired cerebral compliance. However, the usefulness of VPR was limited; 17% of 160 patients studied by Miller[69] went on to die of malignant intracranial hypertension, despite a low VPR.

Marmarou[53,56-58] subsequently defined a *pressure-volume index* (PVI), which corresponded to the calculated volume and—when added to the intracranial contents—produced a tenfold increase in ICP. Over the pressure range of 0 to 50 mm Hg and the volume range of 3% of intracranial volume, the CSF pressure–CSF volume relationship was exponential.[114] A PVI of 22 to 30 ml was considered normal, below 18 ml was pathologic, and of 13 ml or less indicated a critically low cerebral compliance.[107] However, this index was no more sensitive than ICP itself in indicating the presence of experimental mass lesions (epidural balloons in cats), and, above the limited exponential range noted previously, PVI actually increased with increasing balloon volumes, further casting doubt on its use.[113,114]

Both VPR and PVI calculations require manipulation of the ICP monitoring device, with attendant risks of infection or malfunction. Both require a substantial period of time to acquire and calculate and thus are not suitable for moment-to-moment monitoring. More recently, attempts to derive a useful predictive indicator of cerebral compliance changes have focused on the waveform analysis of intrinsic, rhythmic ICP perturbations, such as those produced by pulse and respiration. ICP is not a constant quantity. Rather, it is a complex cyclic waveform, and what is commonly referred to as ICP is, in effect, the mean value of this waveform. From a systems analysis viewpoint, the intracranial cavity may be considered a "black box," with the cerebral arterial pressure signal as input and the ICP signal as output (because respiratory effects on cerebral venous pressure and arterial P_{CO_2} affect ICP with a frequency nearly an order of magnitude slower than arterial pulse pressure, their effects on this input-output relationship may, in most circumstances, be ignored.)[47] The relationship between the arterial pressure input signal and the ICP output signal may be termed the *intracranial transfer function,* which—in effect—defines the frequency response for the intracranial cavity (Fig. 5-6). This, in turn, reflects the hydrodynamic and physiologic properties of the intracranial contents. All physical materials have an intrinsic fundamental frequency that will be elicited if the material is perturbed; properties of the material that determine this fre-

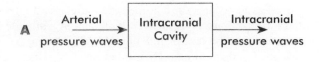

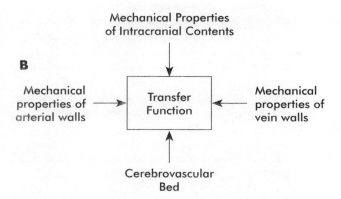

FIG. 5-6   ICP determination as viewed by systems analysis. A, The intracranial cavity as a "black box" with arterial pressure waves as input and ICP waves as output. B, Factors determining the transfer function operating inside the black box. *(From Lin ES, Poon W, Hutchinson RC et al: Br J Anaesth 66:476-482, 1991.)*

quency include density, geometric shape, and external forces. Changes within the intracranial vault—such as the presence of mass lesions, elevation of ICP, and diminution of cerebral compliance—will thus alter the fundamental frequency, along with associated harmonic frequencies. This changes the intracranial transfer function, and thus the ICP waveform response, to a given arterial pressure waveform input.

Changes in the ICP waveform seen in pathologic conditions include an increased ICP pulse pressure, with elevated mean ICP and a marked change in the waveform pattern of individual ICP peaks. These changes are distinct from the Lundberg type A, B, and C patterns, which describe trends in mean ICP occurring over minutes.[49,51] Shifts in the fundamental and harmonic frequencies of the intracranial contents will cause corresponding, predictable shifts in the frequency components of the ICP waveform. These shifts in frequency response (the transfer function) may thus be used to estimate changes in intracranial physical properties, chiefly compliance. Bray and Robertson[13,93] used a bedside computer to periodically estimate the frequency components of the ICP waveform via a fast Fourier transform. A power-weighted average frequency (termed the *high-frequency centroid*, or HFC) was determined, indicating the predominant frequency component. It was hoped that this

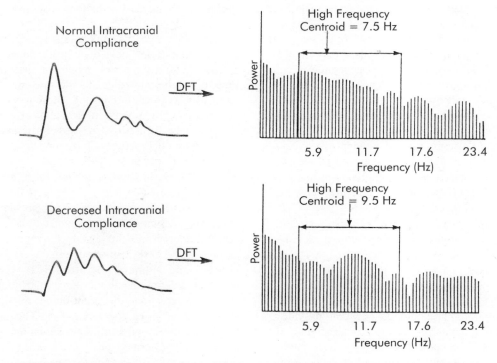

FIG. 5-7   Power-spectrum analysis of the intracranial pressure waveform. Changes in intracranial compliance were found to cause shifts in the power-density spectrum generated by discrete Fourier transform. These shifts occurred in the 4- to 15-Hz range, and a "high-frequency centroid" could be calculated to quantify the change. *DFT*, digital Fourier transformation. *(From Robertson C, Narayan RK, Contant CF, et al: J Neurosurg 71:673-680, 1989.)*

value would provide a clinically useful estimate of cerebral compliance. In experimental studies, HFC showed the expected inverse relationship to PVI, with a normal HFC of 6.5 to 7 Hz and an HFC of 9 Hz corresponding to a reduction in PVI to 13 ml, indicative of critically low compliance (Fig. 5-7). Unfortunately, as with PVI itself, HFC proved less useful in clinical application than had been hoped. Although in some patients the presence of a mass lesion was heralded by a shift in the HFC to 9 Hz before a rise in ICP, the method showed poor sensitivity, specificity, and positive or negative predictive values. HFC and ICP were not statistically related overall. Thus, while ICP waveform analysis holds the promise of providing a continuous, low-risk method for early detection of impending intracranial decompensation, further work will be required before this promise is fulfilled.[30]

ICP Measurement and Intracranial Compartmentalization

We have noted that while ICP is usually conceived as a measure of global intracranial conditions, in many—or perhaps most—clinical situations, this is untrue. The intracranial space is normally nonuniform; it contains irregularly shaped CSF spaces with distinct flow patterns and is subdivided by bony, dural, and arachnoidal barriers. Asymmetry is further introduced by the presence of mass lesions.

The supratentorial and infratentorial spaces are divided by a semirigid tentorium, which allows only limited craniocaudal displacement. Below it, the infratentorial space may be considered a single compartment, with limited connection to the supratentorial space via the tentorial notch and to the spinal subarachnoid space via the foramen magnum. The supratentorial space is, in turn, partially divided by another semirigid barrier, the falx cerebri. In addition, the anterior temporal lobes are effectively surrounded by the sphenoid wing superiorly and anteriorly, the temporal bone laterally and inferiorly, and the tentorium medially, so that they may be considered as belonging to yet another partially isolated compartment. Within each of these anatomic compartments exists not only brain tissue, but an internal CSF space, consisting of the various horns of the lateral ventricles, the third and fourth ventricles, and the narrow foramina and aqueducts that connect them to each other and to the subarachnoid space. Finally, the different compartments contain varying amounts of gray and white matter, the compliance of which may differ. The viscoelasticity of the brain substance exerts tangential forces that also diminish radial transmission of pressure inequalities.

Under normal conditions, the various compartments communicate via the CSF channels, both within and outside the brain substance. In the presence of a pathologic condition, this situation may be quite different. Focal pathologic lesions may cause obstruction of CSF flow and blockage of CSF egress from one portion of the ventricular system but not from another; this may result in supratentorial "noncommunicating" hydrocephalus when the aqueduct of

Sylvius is affected, or in the phenomenon of the "trapped ventricle" or "trapped temporal horn" frequently seen with hemispheric lesions in different locations. Under these circumstances, a catheter placed in one ventricular space may not accurately reflect pressure in another.[37,96] Focal brain pathologic conditions may not only raise pressure within the affected compartment by direct volume effect but may alter the viscoelastic properties of the injured brain as well. Finally, the different intracranial components differ in capacitance and may therefore react to pressure changes at different rates.[89]

When pressure gradients become large enough to overcome the resistance of brain tissue to distortion, shift of intracranial contents from one compartment to another occurs. This is known as herniation (Fig. 5-8). The hemispheres may herniate under the falx (subfalcine herniation), the supratentorial contents may herniate through the tentorial notch (transtentorial herniation), or the cerebellar tonsils may herniate through the foramen magnum. Movement will continue until the pressure gradient is eliminated or until the physical properties of the herniating tissue prevent further movement, even though a pressure gradient remains (Fig. 5-9). Thus, after cerebellar tonsillar herniation, intracranial and spinal subarachnoid pressures will no longer be equal, and after subfalcine herniation in the presence of a cerebral hemispheric lesion (sometimes accompanied by ventricular trapping), pressures on the two sides of the falx

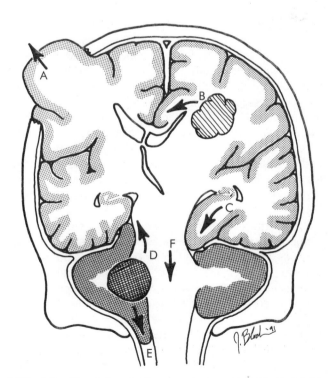

FIG. 5-8 Herniation syndromes. *A,* transcalvarial, *B,* subfalcine, *C,* transtentorial (uncal), *D,* transtentorial ("upward"), *E,* tonsillar, and *F,* transtentorial (central, or "coning").

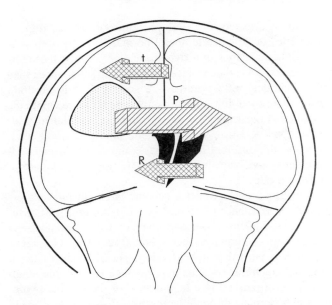

FIG. 5-9 Schematic diagram of intracranial forces in the presence of a mass lesion. *P,* pressure gradient resulting from the presence of a hemispheric mass lesion; *t,* tentorial resistance force normal to this pressure gradient; *R,* composite force representing the sum of elastic, tangential, and other forces acting in various directions with components normal to the pressure gradient and opposite in sign. The system will be in equilibrium when P = t + R. This illustrates why a pressure gradient may be measured between the two hemispheres, even when equilibrium is reached.

may remain unequal. A small posterior fossa hematoma may block the aqueduct of Sylvius while expanding the posterior fossa volume, resulting in unequal pressures above and below the tentorium. In all these instances, it can be that the brain shift and movement itself, through tissue distortion or vascular compression, is more deleterious than the elevated ICP.[1,25,94,95] Moreover, the pressures measured by an ICP monitor in a single compartment may not accurately reflect conditions in other compartments.[37,89,96] This is illustrated by the situation in which an expanding temporal lobe mass lesion may result in disastrous uncal herniation, despite a "normal" ICP measured in the frontal horn of the lateral ventricle.

Compartmentalization also introduces a theoretic reservation into analytic measures, such as VPR and PVI. Both methods derive data from a ventricular catheter in the frontal horn of the lateral ventricle. Thus what is actually measured is the compliance of this ventricular compartment. It is readily apparent that blockage of CSF outflow anywhere along the intraventricular course decreases the effective volume being measured, which results in a decreased compliance calculation whether or not a mass lesion is present. A distant mass lesion in an isolated compartment, conversely, might produce no significant change in the VPR at the location at which it is measured.

In this era of neuroimaging with magnetic resonance (MR) and computed tomography (CT), situations in which the possibility of intercompartmental pressure differences exists are usually apparent. The selection of a suitable site for ICP monitor placement and the correct interpretation of the monitored data must be influenced by an appreciation of these nonuniformities.

INDICATIONS FOR ICP MONITORING

As monitoring techniques have grown safer and more sophisticated and as our understanding of intracranial pathophysiology has improved, the range of situations in which knowledge of ICP serves a useful therapeutic role has expanded. The decision to monitor ICP is usually made on a dual basis; the clinical situation must provide indications, and radiologic imaging studies must corroborate the indications and confirm the safety of the proposed monitor placement. With the availability of high-resolution, noninvasive imaging techniques, particularly CT and MR, these studies themselves may be the chief determining factor in deciding to initiate ICP monitoring and in following the response to ICP treatment. They also provide warning of situations, such as mass lesions of the temporal lobes, in which ICP measurement may fail to reflect the progression of pathologic events.

Tumor

Expanding intracranial tumors that do not announce their presence through the production of neurologic deficits or seizures often present with symptoms and signs of raised ICP, such as headache, nausea, sixth nerve palsies, and papilledema. This may be due either to direct effects of a large intracranial mass or to obstruction of the CSF pathways, producing hydrocephalus. When relatively slow-growing hemispheric lesions cause signs of intracranial hypertension, they often do so at surprisingly large volumes, as slow compression of the intracranial content shifts the volume-pressure curve to the right or "flattens" it, an expression of capacitance (see Fig. 5-5). In these circumstances, the onset of symptoms indicate that all available compensatory mechanisms have been exhausted and that any additional intracranial volume increase is likely to be tolerated poorly. In contrast, when obstructive hydrocephalus occurs as a relatively acute event, it may result in large rises in ICP with relatively small CSF volume increases.

The primary goal in treating tumors that are producing decompensation is elimination of the mass, be it through surgery, radiation, or chemotherapy. Where obstructive hydrocephalus has occurred, its prompt relief is usually indicated, either by means of a permanent CSF diversion or via ventriculostomy. Obstructive hydrocephalus is especially common with posterior fossa tumors that compress the aqueduct of Sylvius. In addition to relief of intracranial hypertension by CSF drainage, the ventricular catheter may be used for monitoring ICP during nonoperative therapy, so as to judge when and if permanent diversion is needed, or for monitoring and control of CSF pressure during induction of anesthesia or conduct of surgery. With easy access to CT and MR, the role of ICP monitoring in the presence of large intraparenchymal tumors without hydrocephalus is quite limited. In special situations, ventricular or intraparenchymal catheter monitoring of ICP may be useful during induction of anesthesia or for monitoring postoperative changes in patients who remain comatose after surgery because of either their underlying pathologic condition or the use of barbiturates for cerebral protection.

Hydrocephalus and Benign Intracranial Hypertension

Because CSF production is relatively constant, obstruction to CSF flow at any point in the intraventricular or subarachoid space—or inadequate resorption at the arachnoid villi—may result in the development of increased CSF pressure and expansion of the CSF space at the expense of parenchymal and vascular volume. These conditions, of varying causes, are grouped together under the diagnosis of hydrocephalus. In addition, the phenomenon of increased CSF volume with apparently normal CSF pressure, or normal pressure hydrocephalus, is diagnosed with considerable frequency and must often be distinguished from "true" hydrocephalus. Benign intracranial hypertension, or pseudotumor cerebri, is a condition commonly associated with obesity, certain hormonal abnormalities, vitaminoses, and hypercoagulable states. In many cases it probably is a result of thrombosis of major cerebral draining veins.[2] It consists of elevated ICP without a significant pathologic condition seen on imaging studies (except for vascular abnormalities as noted), and typically the presenting symptom is severe headache.

Treatment of classic hydrocephalus consists of CSF diversion, and ICP monitoring is usually not necessary. However, CSF diversion techniques are subject to many difficulties, among which is excessive shunting. The symptoms of this problem may be difficult to distinguish from that of shunt failure, and when radiologic studies are inconclusive, ICP monitoring may help differentiate the two conditions. In our hands this is usually done via the insertion of an intraparenchymal ICP monitor. Such monitoring may also be useful in evaluating the proper functioning of the shunt in patients with benign intracranial hypertension who continue to complain of headache after shunt placement. Finally, the use of invasive monitoring of the ICP—and trial CSF drainage to test for clinical improvement—may be accomplished in patients being considered for CSF diversion procedures for normal pressure hydrocephalus. At our institution, this is usually accomplished by placement of a lumbar subarachnoid catheter, which is less invasive than is intraventricular monitoring.

Trauma

It was in the care of trauma patients that the earliest attempts to measure ICP were undertaken. The studies of Jackson,[33]

McCreery and Berry,[63] and Browder and Myers[14] examined lumbar CSF pressure in large numbers of patients with traumatic brain injury and attempted to correlate the measurements with other findings. Most of the measurements were low, even in severely injured patients, a finding that most likely relates to occlusion of the foramen magnum by the herniating brain. It was not until well after this phenomenon was recognized that ICP monitoring was definitively introduced as a useful tool in the care of the patient with a brain injury.[52] In the quarter century which has passed since this report, an understanding of the pathology of brain trauma has progressed. It is clear that the cycle of trauma, brain swelling, intracranial hypertension, cerebral hypoperfusion, and further tissue damage is—in large part—responsible for poor outcome in these patients.* With the use of ICP monitoring, medical and surgical efforts at control of intracranial hypertension can be continuously evaluated and adjusted. Through ventricular catheters, CSF may be therapeutically drained or VPR estimated. ICP monitoring—even in the age of CT and MRI—remains the most effective means of early detection of untoward intracranial events, and efforts to improve the predictive value of the data obtained are continuing.

We feel that ICP monitoring should generally be instituted in all patients with head injuries whose presenting signs include Glasgow coma scores of 8 or less,[55] unless circumstances clearly indicate an imminent and irreversible fatal outcome. Patients with these low Glasgow coma scores are potentially salvageable, but a change in the neurologic examination cannot be relied on to warn of worsening intracranial conditions. The ICP data is used in close concert with the initial CT scan and follow-up scans at appropriate intervals to aid in assessing the effectiveness of medical management and the indications for surgical intervention. There is clear evidence that in trauma patients, a sustained ICP of greater than 20 mm Hg is associated with a significantly worse clinical outcome.[54,59,60,84]

Vascular Anomalies

Intracranial arterial aneurysms and arteriovenous malformations present numerous surgical and medical management problems. Although many of these difficulties are directly connected with such cerebrovascular processes as vasospasm, ICP monitoring may play a role in the perioperative management of these patients. Hydrocephalus after the hemorrhage may result from decreased CSF resorption at the arachnoid villi or from obstruction of CSF flow by an intraventricular clot or an intraparenchymal clot, causing shift. This is often treated with a preoperative ventriculostomy, which may serve during anesthesia induction as a monitor of ICP and during surgery as a CSF drainage device to enhance brain relaxation. During the interval leading up to surgical control of the aneurysm, careful control of ICP is essential because an elevated pressure may result

*References 8, 10, 44, 54, 60, 69, 74, 123.

in neurologic impairment, whereas an unduly lowered pressure could presumably promote rerupture of the aneurysm due to increase in the structure's transmural pressure.[5] In the patient who has recovered, subarachnoid hemorrhage may lead to communicating hydrocephalous and placement of a temporary or permanent CSF diversion.

ICP management is frequently used with other forms of invasive and noninvasive monitoring in the care of patients with postoperative arteriovenous malformation (AVM). Changes in cerebral blood flow patterns and pressures—as well as postoperative anatomic changes in CSF spaces—may contribute to increases in ICP, the detection of which is critical.

ICP Monitoring and CSF Drainage

As alluded to previously, ventricular drains are frequently placed therapeutically, both for primary care of conditions requiring CSF drainage for lowering ICP or as an adjunct to surgery. Certain situations call for placement of lumbar subarachnoid drains for similar indications. In these situations, proper functioning of the CSF drainage system requires frequent determination of the pressure in the system. When the CSF spaces are thus externalized, CSF flow rate and pressure are closely linked, and overdrainage resulting in excessively low or even negative pressure may be nearly as dangerous as increased pressure.

Other Pathology

The circumstances mentioned previously do not constitute a comprehensive list of all situations in which ICP monitoring should be considered. Other clinical situations in which increased ICP may develop, where its treatment may improve outcome, and in which noninvasive monitoring techniques (such as the neurologic examination) are unable to provide information on ongoing intracranial pathology may also call for these measures. Examples include cases of metabolic coma with cerebral edema, certain cases of viral hepatitis or fulminant hepatic encephalopathy, or patients in controlled barbiturate coma for *status epilepticus* or other indications. It seems likely that with continuing advances in therapy and changes in diagnostic techniques, the indications for ICP monitoring will continue to change as it proves useful in new situations or unneeded in others.

ICP MONITORING TECHNIQUES

A large variety of techniques have been developed for chronic ICP measurement in the more than 30 years since Lundberg's original work.[3,35] These techniques vary somewhat in their accuracy, the ease of device insertion and pressure measurement, and relative risks. Choice of technique depends largely on the clinical indications and on the experience and preferences of the surgeon. Techniques may be classified as supratentorial, infratentorial, or lumbar; and, in the supratentorial compartment, they may be epidural, subdural-subarachnoid, intraventricular, or intraparenchymal.

Supratentorial Monitors

Supratentorial ICP monitors are by far the most commonly indicated and employed. Until a few years ago, these were basically all hollow fluid-filled devices opening into the compartment being monitored and connected to an external pressure transducer.[35] The devices vary as to which intracranial spaces or potential spaces are monitored, and a tacit assumption is made—which may not be correct in all conditions—that intracranial pressures are equal in all these spaces. Epidural monitors were more widely used in the past[3,22,84] but are now rarely indicated. Placement in this potential space is technically more difficult, the risk of hemorrhage or creation of a mass effect is probably somewhat higher than with other techniques, and accuracy is questionable.[3,85,90] Subdural-subarachnoid monitoring devices usually constitute some type of hollow screw or "bolt" fixed to the calvarium, with the tip placed in direct communication with the intradural space (for the purposes of this type of monitoring, this placement would be considered subarachnoid, although in certain pathophysiologic circumstances, the subarachnoid space and subdural potential space may behave differently).[75,118] Advantages of these devices include ease of placement and insertion and low risk of injury to underlying structures. As with all fluid-filled devices, there is a risk of infection, and occlusion of the bolt lumen by brain tissue has been a significant problem. Nevertheless, subdural-subarachnoid monitors were the standard device for ICP monitoring during much of the 1970s and 1980s, and, among nonneurosurgeons, the term "bolt" seems to remain synonymous with ICP monitoring.* Ventricular catheters or ventriculostomies are the "gold standard" by which other techniques of CSF pressure and ICP monitoring are judged.[3,29,49,64,85] These are flexible plastic catheters placed percutaneously into the frontal horn of the lateral ventricles near the foramen of Monro (Fig. 5-10). Although the technique is not new,[29,49] it has perhaps been slower to gain widespread use because of its relatively more invasive nature. Potential placement sites are more restricted than for the devices mentioned previously because of the necessity of avoiding injury to underlying vessels and eloquent areas of the brain. More skill and experience is necessary for placement, compared with other techniques. With proper insertion, these catheters are safe and reliable and provide a potential therapeutic advantage, CSF drainage, that other techniques do not permit. Intrathecal antibiotics can be administered in situations that call for their use, and ventricular air contrast radiographic studies or cisternograms can be performed when indicated. Studies have shown the infection rate to be quite low for the first 4 days after placement,[4,61,97] and at our institution catheters are "rotated" to a new site every fifth day. Hemorrhage or neurologic impairment from ventriculostomy placement are rare,[4,97] probably because the blunt tip of the device separates—rather than divides—white matter tracts.

---

*References 3, 6, 64, 70, 75, 118.

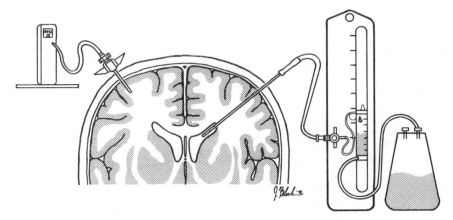

FIG. 5-10 Ventricular and intraparenchymal pressure monitoring systems. The stopcock on the ventricular monitoring system *(right)* is fixed and must be positioned at the same height as the tip of the intraventricular catheter to properly "zero" the system. The graduated cylinder may be adjusted vertically. The height at which the CSF fluid column just spills over into the cylinder, with respect to the zero value of the stopcock, is the ventricular fluid pressure. The intraparenchymal monitor *(left)* is "zeroed" before insertion, and the monitoring box position will not affect readings.

To ensure accurate measurement, the device must be calibrated by "zeroing" the transducer (analogous to an arterial line set-up), which should be positioned at the level of the external auditory canal (the level of the patient's ventricular system). Maintenance of this calibration can be problematic in the uncooperative or agitated patient. Furthermore, when the ventricular catheter system is opened for therapeutic drainage, concurrent ICP measurement cannot be accurately made.[121]

Optimally, a triphasic waveform should be obtained. A dampened waveform (monophasic, small "pulse pressure") signifies a partially occluded ventricular catheter due to debris, poor placement, or air in the fluid column between the ventricle and the transducer. Purging the air from the system simply consists of flushing the tubing from one access port to another with sterile saline (no preservatives). Meticulous sterile technique must be used since ventriculostomy-related ventriculitis carries serious morbidity.

Intraparenchymal ICP monitoring techniques are a relatively recent addition to the neurosurgical armamentarium.[16,18,87,89,115] Such devices as the Camino monitor consist of a fine fiberoptic cable with a miniature transducer at the tip[18,87] (see Fig. 5-10). The devices work by assessing the degree of phase shift of an externally generated laser beam reflected off a tiny deformable membrane in the transducer tip. These monitors are easier to insert than are ventriculostomies, are of smaller diameter and thus less disruptive of brain tissue, and do not require access to the ventricular system, which may be extremely difficult to enter in the presence of edema and ventricular compression. There is no fluid column, so the risk of infection is probably smaller. However, the device must be calibrated before insertion and cannot be recalibrated subsequently, so it is not possible to check for the occurrence of "drift" in the

mechanism. The fiberoptic cable is relatively fragile although technical improvements have alleviated this problem somewhat. Extraordinarily high measurements (e.g., 400 mm Hg) are always due to a system malfunction. Negative ICPs (down to −30 mm Hg) can occur and are real, especially in patients with shunts for hydrocephalus. Therapeutic drainage or CSF studies are not possible. Recently, devices that incorporate a fiberoptic monitor in a ventricular catheter have been developed.[16]

Infratentorial Subarachnoid Monitors

Pressure monitoring in the posterior fossa has not been widely adopted because of the inherent difficulties in percutaneous access to the area and the sensitive and fragile nature of the neural and vascular structures there. Placement of catheters at surgery has also been limited, probably because of anticipated complications, such as pseudomeningocele formation. Nevertheless, a report by Rosenwasser and colleagues[96] on their use of postsurgical infratentorial pressure monitoring revealed some significant differences between pressures recorded simultaneously above and below the tentorium and remarked on the safety of the technique in their limited series. It seems possible that this type of monitoring may become more widely adopted in the future.

Lumbar Subarachnoid Monitors

Early attempts at ICP monitoring were directed at measurement of the lumbar CSF pressure, with disappointing results. Only when the pathology of brain herniation was understood did the reasons for this become clear, and the risks apparent. Today, indwelling lumbar subarachnoid catheters are placed mainly for use as CSF drainage devices after surgery, to aid in the prevention of CSF leaks in difficult dural repairs, or as a method of achieving brain relaxation.

Measurement of pressure is used in these contexts chiefly to confirm that the device is functioning in the desired fashion. However, in circumstances where herniation is not a risk (meningitis, communicating hydrocephalus, benign intracranial hypertension), lumbar CSF pressure measurements via percutaneous lumbar puncture continue to be the most common method of ICP estimation. Long-term monitoring at this site is seldom used.

ANESTHETICS AND INTRACRANIAL PRESSURE

Nowhere is the role of the anesthesiologist in the total care of a perioperative patient more critical, and nowhere is an understanding action of anesthetic drugs more important, than in dealing with intracranial pathology. The anesthesiologist must take into account a variety of special neurosurgical considerations in addition to the more commonly monitored parameters involved in any surgical anesthetic. Chief among these is maintenance of CPP. This is determined by systemic arterial blood pressure, cerebral venous pressure, and ICP, all of which may be influenced in complex ways by the actions of anesthetic drugs. The effects of the proposed agents on cerebral blood flow and metabolic requirements must be weighed.* Their influence on ICP must be predicted, based on the known effects of the drugs on vasomotor tone, CSF production, and other factors, as well as on the nature of the patient's pathologic and neurologic conditions and responsiveness.

It is especially desirable that the anesthesia team play an early role in the care of emergency neurosurgery patients, particularly those with head trauma. Early assessment of the patient's condition and anesthetic requirements—as well as prompt, controlled, and smooth tracheal intubation and anesthesia induction—are particularly important in these patients, in whom time is precious and tolerance for secondary injury resulting from hypoxia, ischemia, seizures, or exacerbated intracranial hypertension is minimal. Communication between neurosurgical and anesthesia teams regarding patient condition, treatment plans, and moment-to-moment changes in clinical condition is vital to successful intervention. This type of preparation and continuing communication is also important during long and complex elective operations. Potential systemic problems apparent to the anesthesia team should be communicated to the surgeon, and the requirements for brain relaxation, fast or slow emergence from anesthesia at the end of the operation, or other special needs—such as induced hypotension or barbiturate coma—should be discussed in advance. Use of such drugs as mannitol, steroids, and barbiturates should be anticipated and prepared at the outset where possible.

TREATMENT OF INTRACRANIAL HYPERTENSION

Once the causes of raised ICP and the nature of the pressure-volume relationship are understood, the principles of treatment become reasonably straightforward. Reduction of ICP in the closed skull is equivalent to enhancement of "brain relaxation" with the open dura at surgery, where raised ICP may be manifested as brain stiffness or herniation out of the operative site. The measures taken to control the two phenomena are the same and can be classified according to which compartment they are designed to affect.

Blood volume can be reduced by ensuring adequate venous outflow and by promoting vasoconstriction (to the extent compatible with adequate cerebral perfusion). To achieve this, the head is positioned above the heart and oriented to prevent kinking or compression of the jugular veins, keeping in mind any cervical spine precautions that may be necessary. This reduces intracranial venous blood volume and also ensures that venous outflow pressure does not reduce the prolonged cerebral perfusion (> 48 hours) pressure gradient.

In the past, prolonged hyperventilation (>48 hours) to reduce arterial P_{CO_2}—and thereby produce cerebral vasoconstriction (with reduced cerebral blood volume)—was used extensively in the care of patients with head trauma and those with raised ICP.[7] In the presence of intact autoregulation, cerebral blood flow is reduced 3% to 4% per 1 mm Hg reduction in arterial P_{CO_2}.[86] As the significance of cerebral ischemia and its interactions with head injury and elevated ICP have become clearer,[10] the role of hyperventilation has been questioned. Muizelaar and colleagues[81] showed that there was a significantly worsened outcome among "good" head-injury patients (those with initial Glasgow motor scores of 4 to 5) who received hyperventilation, compared with control patients who did not. These authors therefore recommended against the prophylactic use of hyperventilation in those with a head injury. They further suggested that prolonged hyperventilation results in loss of CSF buffering capacity and cerebrovascular hypersensitivity to changes in P_{CO_2} and that, for those patients requiring hyperventilation for ICP control, this results in a more variable ICP, with increased periods of ICP above 20 mm Hg. In their study, administration of the buffering agent trimethamine (THAM) to increase CSF buffering reserve counteracted this ICP instability and improved outcome.[81] How these findings relate to the use of hyperventilation for ICP elevation resulting from nontraumatic conditions is as yet unclear. However, hyperventilation can no longer be regarded uncritically as a management tool for elevated ICP, and measurement of ICP should be considered more important than ever as a guide to the need for this therapy. Hyperventilation still plays a major role in the initial treatment of increased ICP and in reducing brain bulk in the operating room.

Finally, hypoxia—in addition to its directly harmful effects at the cellular level—is a potent vasodilator, and an adequate arterial P_{O_2} (usually greater than 60 mm Hg) is essential to the care of the patient with a head injury or with elevated ICP.

CSF volume may be reduced by catheter drainage,

---

*References 36, 42, 48, 78, 83, 117, 119.

generally via the lateral ventricles. A ventriculostomy provides both a means of measurement of ICP and a therapeutic intervention because it allows CSF drainage. An additional theoretic benefit of ventriculostomy is that drainage may alter the normal dynamics of CSF bulk flow. It could reduce or reverse CSF transudation across the ependyma and thus decrease tissue volume. There are few, if any, ill effects associated with removal of CSF, and this therapy is usually limited only by collapse of the ventricular system with occlusion of the catheter. Special considerations must be made when a large hemispheric mass or infratentorial mass might result in subfalcine herniation or "upward" transtentorial herniation in the presence of ventricular drainage.

Tissue volume, either brain parenchyma or mass lesions, may be reduced by mechanical means—e.g., surgical resection of tumor, abscess, hematoma, contusion, or infarct. A variation of this approach is subtemporal decompression, a time-honored technique to enlarge the intracranial volume by removal of temporal bone and dura to prevent uncal herniation. Tissue volume may also be reduced by measures that decrease brain swelling. Traditionally, hyperosmolar agents—such as urea or, more commonly, mannitol— have been used to increase intravascular osmotic pressure and thus promote resorption of interstitial fluid.[104] More recent work suggests that mannitol may work largely via a rheologic effect in that it decreases blood viscosity, allowing cerebral autoregulation to maintain the same flow rates at lower intravascular volumes.[9,79,116] With prolonged use (> 48 hours), mannitol itself enters the interstitial space, which can reduce or even reverse the osmotic gradient. Therefore, the patient should be weaned from mannitol gradually, with attention paid to ICP monitoring because sudden reduction in vascular osmolality while interstitial mannitol remains present could lead to intravascular fluid movement into the interstitial space with increased edema. Mannitol has a potent diuretic effect, and excessive administration may result in systemic hypotension and cerebral hypoperfusion. The goal of therapy should be to achieve a normovolemic, hyperosmolar state.

Corticosteroids, such as dexamethasone, are frequently used for intracranial hypertension because of vasogenic edema in the presence of tumor or abscess and are remarkably effective in this context. However, steroids have not been shown to be of any benefit in dealing with head trauma.[21] Although this may well change with future studies, at the present time steroids cannot be recommended in the management of increased ICP in patients with trauma. Obviously, steroids have numerous side effects, among which are hyperglycemia, which itself may contribute to worsened outcome after head trauma.[43]

Barbiturates continue to play a somewhat controversial role in the management of increased ICP resulting from head trauma. Although they may bring under control intracranial hypertension that is refractory to management by other measures,[24,88] a convincing demonstration that this results in improved clinical outcome is still lacking.

Pending the resolution of this issue, we feel justified in recommending the use of barbiturates to produce burst-suppression coma only when all other measures have failed to control ICP.[88,106,108,110,122] Such patients must have continuous central venous and systemic arterial pressure monitoring to allow detection and correction of the depressant effects of barbiturates on the cardiovascular system. Continuous EEG monitoring is an essential guide to this therapy.

Care of the trauma or perioperative patient with elevated ICP follows simple guidelines. Oxygenation and systemic hemodynamic stability are established and maintained. The cause of the raised ICP is determined; for tumor or abscess, steroids may be administered. During surgery or critical care, the head is elevated and mannitol is given at a dose of 0.5 to 1.5 gm/kg initially, with maintenance doses given to keep serum osmolality near 305 to 310 mOsm/kg. For elective craniotomy, mannitol is usually given just before skin incision. In anesthetized or comatose patients with elevated ICP, judicious use of hyperventilation may be instituted to maintain a PCO_2 of 30 mm Hg, with administration of THAM to be considered if prolonged use of hyperventilation seems likely.[81] ICP monitoring may be considered postoperatively after elective surgery, or an ICP monitoring device may be placed in the emergency ward, intensive care unit, or operating room to guide further therapy. Sedation and pharmacologic paralysis in more responsive patients are sometimes useful adjuncts to ICP control. Muscle relaxants should not be used without adequate sedation.

▼ SUMMARY

The cause and pathophysiology of intracranial hypertension are increasingly well understood, and the complex interactions between ICP, cerebral perfusion, and the anatomy and physical structure of the intracranial contents are gradually becoming more clear. Monitoring and control of raised ICP have become recognized as essential for the effective care of the neurosurgical patient. With this principle established, efforts currently continue (1) to improve monitoring techniques in terms of reliability, accuracy, and safety, (2) to develop better analytic tools to identify and predict the appearance of preventable intracranial pathology, based on ICP data, and (3) to establish new or improved therapeutic regimens to lower raised ICP and to preserve neuronal function in the face of decreased cerebral perfusion pressure. Success in these efforts will continue to broaden the range of neurosurgical problems amenable to effective treatment.

References

1. Adams H, Graham DI: The relationship between ventricular fluid pressure and the neuropathology of raised intracranial pressure. In Brock M, Deitz H, editors: *Intracranial pressure,* Berlin, 1972, Springer-Verlag, pp 250-253.
2. Adams RD, Victor M: Disturbances of cerebrospinal fluid circulation, including hydrocephalus and meningeal reactions. In *Principles of neurology,* ed 3, New York, 1985, McGraw-Hill, pp 468-469.
3. Allen R: Intracranial pressure: a review of clinical problems, measurement techniques and monitoring methods, *J Med Eng Technol* 10:299-320, 1986.
4. Aucoin PJ, Kotilainen HR, Gantz NM et al: Intracranial pressure monitors. Epidemiologic study of risk factors and infections, *Am J Med* 80:369-376, 1986.
5. Bailes JE, Spetzler RF, Hadley MN et al: Management morbidity and mortality of poor-grade aneurysm patients, *J Neurosurg* 72:559-566, 1990.
6. Barlow P, Mendelow AD, Lawrence AE et al: Clinical evaluation of two methods of subdural pressure monitoring, *J Neurosurg* 63:578-582, 1985.
7. Becker DP, Gardner S: Intensive management of head injury. In Wilkins RH, Rengachary SS, editors: *Neurosurgery,* vol 2, New York, 1985, McGraw-Hill, pp 1593-1599.
8. Becker DP, Miller JD, Ward JD et al: The outcome from severe head injury with early diagnosis and intensive treatment, *J Neurosurg* 47:491-502, 1977.
9. Bouma GJ, Muizelaar JP: Relationship between cardiac output and cerebral blood flow in patients with intact and with impaired autoregulation, *J Neurosurg* 73:368-374, 1990.
10. Bouma GJ, Muizelaar JP, Choi SC et al: Cerebral circulation and metabolism after severe traumatic brain injury: the elusive role of ischemia, *J Neurosurg* 75:685-693, 1991.
11. Bracken MB, Shepard MJ, Collins WE et al: A randomized, controlled trial of methylprednisolone or naloxone in the treatment of acute spinal cord injury. Results of the Second National Acute Spinal Cord Injury Study, *N Engl J Med* 322:1405-1411, 1990.
12. Brain WR: A clinical study of increased intracranial pressure in sixty cases of cerebral tumor, *Brain* 48:105, 1925.
13. Bray RS, Sherwood AM, Halter JA et al: Development of a clinical monitoring system by means of ICP waveform analysis. In Miller JD, Teasdale GM, Rowan JO et al, editors: *Intracranial pressure VI,* Berlin, 1986, Springer-Verlag, pp 260-264.
14. Browder J, Meyers R: Observations on behavior of the systemic blood pressure, pulse and spinal fluid pressure following craniocerebral injury, *Am J Surg* 31:403-427, 1936.
15. Bruce DA, Alavi A, Bilianuk L et al: Diffuse cerebral swelling following head injuries in children: the syndrome of "malignant brain edema," *J Neurosurg* 54:170-178, 1981.
16. Chambers IR, Mendelow AD, Sinar EJ et al: A clinical evaluation of the Camino subdural screw and ventricular monitoring kits, *Neurosurgery* 26:421-423, 1990.
17. Choi DW, Rothman SH: The role of glutamate neurotoxicity in hypoxic-ischemic neuronal death, *Ann Rev Neurosci* 13:171-182, 1990.
18. Crutchfield JS, Narayan RK, Robertson CS et al: Evaluation of a fiberoptic intracranial pressure monitor, *J Neurosurg* 72:482-487, 1990.
19. Cushing H: Some experimental and clinical observations concerning states of increased intracranial tension, *Ann J Med Sci* 124:375-400, 1902.
20. Cutler RWP, Page L, Galecich J et al: Formation and absorption of cerebrospinal fluid in man, *Brain* 91:707-720, 1968.
21. Dearden NM, Bibson JS, McDowall JG et al: Effect of high-dose dexamethasone on outcome from severe head injury, *J Neurosurg* 64:81-88, 1986.
22. Dorsch NWC, Symon L: A practical technique for monitoring extradural pressure, *J Neurosurg* 42:249-257, 1975.
23. Duffy GP: Lumbar puncture in the presence of raised intracranial pressure, *Br Med J* 1:407-409, 1969.
24. Eisenberg HM, Frankowski RF, Contant CF et al: High-dose barbiturate control of elevated intracranial pressure in patients with severe head injury, *J Neurosurg* 69:15-23, 1988.
25. Finney LA, Walker EA: *Transtentorial herniation,* Springfield, Ill, 1992, Charles C Thomas.
26. Fishman RA: Brain edema, *N Engl J Med* 293:706-711, 1975.
27. Fremont-Smith F, Hodgson JS: Combined ventricular and lumbar puncture in the diagnosis of brain tumor, *Assoc Res Nerv Dis Proc* 4:172-184, 1924.
28. Gray WJ, Rosner MJ: Pressure-volume index as a function of cerebral perfusion pressure. II. The effects of low cerebral perfusion pressure and autoregulation, *J Neurosurg* 67:377-380, 1987.
29. Guillaume J, Janny P: Manométrie intracranienne: continue interêt de la méthode et premiers résultats, *Rev Neurol* 84:131-142, 1951.
30. Hara K, Nakatani S, Ozaki K et al: Detection of B waves in the oscillation of intracranial pressure by fast Fourier transform, *Med Inform* 15:125-131, 1990.
31. Heisey SR, Held D, Pappenheimer JR: Bulk flow and diffusion in the cerebrospinal fluid system of the goat, *Am J Physiol* 203:775-781, 1962.
32. Hodgson JS: The relationship between increased intracranial pressure and increased intraspinal pressure: changes in cerebrospinal fluid in increased intracranial pressure, *Assoc Res Nerv Dis Proc* 8:182-188, 1927.
33. Jackson H: The management of acute cranial injuries by the early exact determination of intracranial pressure and its relief by lumbar drainage, *Surg Gynecol Obstet* 34:494-508, 1922.
34. Jefferson G: The tentorial pressure cone, *Arch Neurol Psychiatr* 40:857-875, 1938.
35. Jennett B, Teasdale G: *Epidural, subdural and ventricular monitors for management of head injuries,* Philadelphia, 1989, FA Davis.
36. Kaieda R, Todd MM, Weeks JB et al: A comparison of the effects of halothane, isoflurane, and pentobarbital anesthesia on intracranial pressure and cerebral edema formation following brain injury in rabbits, *Anesthesiology* 71:571-579, 1989.

37. Kaufmann GE, Clark K: Continuous simultaneous monitoring of the intraventricular and cervical subarachnoid cerebrospinal fluid pressures to indicate development of cerebral or tonsillar hernation, *J Neurosurg* 33:145-150, 1970.

38. Kellie G: An account of the appearances observed in the dissection of two or three individuals presumed to have perished in the storm of the 3rd, and whose bodies were discovered in the vicinity of Leith on the morning of the 4th November, 1821, with some reflections on the pathology of the brain, *Trans Med Chir Soc Edinb* 1:84-169, 1824.

39. Kelly JP, Nichols JS, Filley CM et al: Concussion in sports. Guidelines for the prevention of catastrophic outcome, *JAMA* 266:2867-2869, 1991.

40. Kernohan JW, Woltman HW: Incisure of the crus due to contralateral brain tumor, *Arch Neurol Psychiatr* 21:274-287, 1921.

41. Kjallgvist A, Lundberg N, Ponten U: Respiratory and cardiovascular changes during spontaneous variations of ventricular fluid pressure in patients with intracranial hypertension, *Acta Neurol Scand* 40:291-317, 1964.

42. Lagerkranser EG, Rudehill A, von Holst H: The effect of isoflurane on cerebrospinal fluid pressure in patients undergoing neurosurgery, *Acta Anaesth Scand* 32:108-112, 1988.

43. Lam AM, Winn HR, Cullen BF et al: Hyperglycemia and neurological outcome in patients with head injury, *J Neurosurg* 75:545-551, 1991.

44. Langfitt TW, Gennarelli TA: Can the outcome from head injury be improved? *J Neurosurg* 56:19-25, 1982.

45. Langfitt TW, Weinstein JD, Kassell NF: Cerebral vasomotor paralysis produced by intracranial hypertension, *Neurology* 15:622-641, 1965.

46. Langfitt TW, Weinstein JD, Kassel NF et al: Transmission of increased intracranial pressure. I. Within the craniospinal axis, *J Neurosurg* 21:989-997, 1964.

47. Lin ES, Poon W, Hutchinson RC et al: Systems analysis applied to intracranial pressure waveforms and correlation with clinical status in head injured patients, *Br J Anaesth* 66:476-482, 1991.

48. Lundar T, Lindegaard K-F, Refsum L et al: Cerebrovascular effects of isoflurane in man. Intracranial pressure and middle cerebral artery flow velocity, *Br J Anaesth* 59:1208-1213, 1987.

49. Lundberg N: Continuous recording and monitoring of ventricular fluid pressure in neurosurgical practice, *Acta Psychiatr Neurol Scand (Suppl 149)* vol 36, 1960.

50. Lundberg N: The sage of the Monro-Kellie doctrine. In Ishii S, Nagai H, Brock M, editors: *Intracranial pressure V,* Berlin, 1983, Springer-Verlag.

51. Lundberg N, Crongvist K, Jallquist A: Clinical investigations on interrelations between intracranial pressure and intracranial hemodyanmics. In Luyendijk W, editor: *Progress in brain research,* vol 30, Amsterdam, 1968, Elsevier, pp 69-75.

52. Lundberg N, Troupp H, Lorin H: Continuous recording of ventricular fluid pressure in patients with severe acute traumatic brain injury: a preliminary report, *J Neurosurg* 22:581-590, 1965.

53. Marmarou A: *A theoretical and experimental evaluation of the cerebrospinal fluid system,* PhD thesis, University of Pennsylvania, Philadelphia, 1973.

54. Maramarou A, Anderson RL, Ward JD et al: Impact of ICP instability and hypotension on outcome in patients with severe head trauma, *J Neurosurg* 75(suppl):S59-S66, 1991.

55. Marmarou A, Anderson RL, Ward JD et al: NINDS traumatic coma data bank: intracranial pressure monitoring methodology, *J Neurosurg* 75 (suppl):S21-S27, 1991.

56. Marmarou A, Shapiro K, Shulman K: Isolating factors leading to sustained elevations of ICP. In Beks JWF, Bosch DA, Brock M, editors: *Intracranial pressure III* Berlin, 1976, Springer-Verlag, pp 33-35.

57. Marmarou A, Shulman K, LaMorgese J: A compartmental analysis of compliance and outflow resistance and the effects of elevated blood pressure. In Lundberg N, Ponten U, Brock M, editors: *Intracranial pressure II,* Berlin, 1975, Springer-Verlag, pp 86-88.

58. Marmarou A, Shulman K, LaMorgese J: Compartmental analysis of compliance and outflow resistance of the cerebrospinal fluid system, *J Neurosurg* 43:523-534, 1976.

59. Marshall LF, Marshall SB, Klauber MR et al: A new classification of head injury based on computerized tomography, *J Neurosurg* 75(suppl): S14-S20, 1991.

60. Marshall LF, Smith RW, Shapiro HM: The outcome with aggressive treatment in severe head injuries. I. The significance of intracranial pressure monitoring, *J Neurosurg* 50:20-25, 1979.

61. Mayhall CG, Archer NH, Lamb VA et al: Ventriculostomy-related infections. A prospective epidemiologic study, *N Engl J Med* 310:553-559, 1984.

62. McClure RD, Crawford AS: The management of craniocerebral injuries, *Arch Surg* 16:451-468, 1928.

63. McCreery JA, Berry FB: A study of 520 cases of fracture of the skull, *Ann Surg* 88:890-901, 1928.

64. Mendelow AD, Rowan JO, Murray L et al: A clinical comparison of subdural screw pressure measurements with ventricular pressure, *J Neurosurg* 58:45-50, 1983.

65. Meyer A: Herniation of the brain, *Arch Neurol Psychiatr* 4:387-400, 1920.

66. Michenfelder JD, Miller JH, Katusic ZS: Postischemic canine cerebral blood flow is coupled to cerebral metabolic rate, *J Cereb Blood Flow Metab* 11:611-616, 1991.

67. Miller JD: Intracranial volume-pressure relationships in pathological conditions, *J Neurosurg Sci* 20:203-209, 1976.

68. Miller JD: Volume and pressure in the craniospinal axis. In Wilkins RH, editor: *Clinical neurosurgery,* vol 22, Baltimore, 1975, Williams & Wilkins, pp 76-105.

69. Miller JD, Becker DP, Ward JD et al: Significance of intracranial hypertension in severe head injury, *J Neurosurg* 47:503-516, 1977.

70. Miller JD, Bobo H, Kapp JP: Inaccurate pressure readings for subarachnoid bolts, *Neurosurgery* 19:253-255, 1986.

71. Miller JD, Garibi J: Intracranial volume-pressure relationships during continuous monitoring of ventricular fluid pressure. In Brock M, Deitz H, editors: *Intracranial pressure,* Berlin, 1972, Springer-Verlag, pp 270-274.

72. Miller JD, Garibi J, Pickard JD: The effects of induced changes of cerebrospinal fluid volume during continuous monitoring of ventricular pressure, *Arch Neurol* 28:265-269, 1973.

73. Miller JD, Leech PJ, Pickard JD: Volume-pressure response in various experiments and clinical conditions. In Lundberg N, Ponten U, Brock M, editors: *Intracranial pressure II,* Berlin, 1975, Springer-Verlag, pp 97-100.

74. Miller JD, Pickard JD: Intracranial volume-pressure studies in patients with head injury, *Injury* 5:265-269, 1974.

75. Mollman HD, Gaylan LR, Ford SE: A clinical comparison of subarachnoid catheters to ventriculostomy and subarachnoid bolts: a prospective study, *J Neurosurg* 68:737-741, 1988.

76. Monro A: *Observations on the structure and function of the nervous system,* Edinburgh, 1783, Creech & Johnson.

77. Moore MT, Stern K: Vascular lesions in brain stem and occipital lobe occurring in association with brain tumors, *Brain* 61:70-98, 1938.

78. Moss E: Volatile anaesthetic agents in neurosurgery, *Br J Anaesth* 63:4-6, 1989.

79. Muizelaar JP, Lutz HA, Becker DP: Effect of mannitol on ICP and CBF and correlation with pressure autoregulation in severely head-injured patients, *J Neurosurg* 61:700-706, 1984.

80. Muizelaar JP, Marmarou A, De-Salles AAF et al: Cerebral blood flow and metabolism in severely head injured children. I. Relationship with GCS score, outcome, ICP, and PVI, *J Neurosurg* 71:63-71, 1989.

81. Muizelaar JP, Marmarou A, Ward JD et al: Adverse effects of prolonged hyperventilation in patients with severe head injury: a randomized clinical trial, *J Neurosurg* 75:731-739, 1991.

82. Muizelaar JP, Ward JD, Marmarou A et al: Cerebral blood flow and metabolism in severely head injured children. II. Autoregulation, *J Neurosurg* 71:72-76, 1989.

83. Nilsson L: The influence of barbiturate anesthesia upon the energy state and upon acid-base parameters of the brain in arterial hypotension and asphyxia, *Acta Neurol Scand* 47:233-253, 1971.

84. Nordby HK, Gunnerod N: Epidural monitoring of the intracranial pressure in severe head injury characterized by non-localizing motor responses, *Acta Neurochir* 74:21-26, 1985.

85. North B, Reilly P: Comparison among three methods of intracranial pressure recording, *Neurosurgery* 18:730-732, 1986.

86. Obrist WD, Langfitt TW, Jaggi JL et al: Cerebral blood flow and metabolism in comatose patients with acute head injury: relationship to intracranial hypertension, *J Neurosurg* 61:241-253, 1984.

87. Ostrup RC, Luerssen TG, Marshall LE et al: Continuous monitoring of intracranial pressure with a miniaturized fiberoptic device, *J Neurosurg* 67:206-209, 1987.

88. Piatt JH, Goodkin R, Eisenberg HM et al: Barbiturates in severe head injury, *J Neurosurg* 70:501-503, 1989 (letter).

89. Piek J, Bock WJ: Continuous monitoring of cerebral tissue pressure in neurosurgical practice—experience with 100 patients, *Int Care Med* 16:184-188, 1990.

90. Powell MP, Crockard HA: Behavior of an extradural pressure monitor in clinical use. Comparison of extradural with intraventricular pressure in patients with acute and chronically elevated intracranial pressure, *J Neurosurg* 63:745-749, 1985.

91. Richards PG, Towu-Aghanste E: Dangers of lumbar puncture, *Br Med J* 292:605-606, 1986.

92. Risberg J, Lundberg N, Ingrav DH: Regional cerebral blood volume during acute rises of the intracranial pressure (plateau waves), *J Neurosurg* 31:303-310, 1969.

93. Robertson C, Narayan RK, Contant CF et al: Clinical experience with a continuous monitor of intracranial pressure, *J Neurosurg* 71:673-680, 1989.

94. Ropper AH: A preliminary study of the geometry of brain displacement and level of consciousness in patients with acute intracranial masses, *Neurology* 39:622-627, 1989.

95. Ropper AH: Lateral displacement of the brain and level of consciousness in patients with an acute hemispheral mass, *N Engl J Med* 314:953-958, 1986.

96. Rosenwasser RH, Kleiner LI, Krze-monski JP et al: Intracranial pressure monitoring in the posterior fossa. A preliminary report, *J Neurosurg* 71:503-505, 1989.

97. Rosner MJ, Becker DP: ICP monitoring: complications and associated factors, *Clin Neurosurg* 23:494-519, 1976.

98. Rosner MJ, Daughton S: Cerebral perfusion pressure management in head injury, *J Trauma* 30:933-941, 1990.

99. Ryder HW, Espey FF, Kimbell FD et al: Influence of changes in cerebral blood flow on the cerebrospinal fluid pressure, *Arch Neurol Psychiatr* 68:165-169, 1952.

100. Ryder HW, Espey FF, Kimbell FD et al: Modification of the effect of cerebral blood flow on cerebral spinal fluid pressure by variations in craniospinal blood volume, *Arch Neurol Psychiatr* 68:170-174, 1952.

101. Ryder HW, Espey FF, Kimbell FD et al: Effect of changes in systemic venous pressure on cerebrospinal fluid pressure, *Arch Neurol Psychiatr* 68:175-179, 1952.

102. Ryder HW, Espey FE, Kimbell FD et al: The mechanism of the change in cerebrospinal fluid pressure following an induced change in the volume of the fluid space, *J Lab Clin Med* 41:428-435, 1953.

103. Ryder HW, Espey FF, Kimbell FD et al: The elasticity of the craniospinal venous bed, *J Lab Clin Med* 42:944, 1953.

104. Ryder HW, Espey FF, Kimbell FD et al: The mechanism of the effect of changes in blood osmotic pressure on the cerebrospinal fluid pressure, *J Lab Clin Med* 41:543-549, 1953.

105. Ryder HW, Rosenauer A, Penka EJ et al: Failure of abnormal cerebrospinal fluid pressure to influence cerebral function, *Arch Neurol Psychiatr* 70:563-586, 1953.

106. Shapiro HM: Barbiturates in brain ischemia, *Br J Anaesth* 57:82-95, 1985.

107. Shapiro K, Maramarou A, Shulman K: Characterization of clinical CSF dynamics and neural axis compliance using the pressure-volume index. I. The normal pressure-volume index, *Ann Neurol* 7:508-514, 1980.

108. Smith DS, Rehncrona S, Siesjo BK: Barbiturates as protective agents in brain ischemia and as free radical scavengers *in vitro, Acta Physiol Scand* 492(suppl):129-134, 1980.

109. Smith HP, Kelly DL Jr, McWhorter JM et al: Comparison of mannitol regimens on patients with severe head injury undergoing intracranial pressure monitoring, *J Neurosurg* 65:820-824, 1986.

110. Spetzler RF, Martin N, Hadley MN et al: Microsurgical endarterectomy under barbiturate protection: a prospective study, *J Neurosurg* 65:63-73, 1986.

111. Spetzler RF, Wilson CB, Weinstein B et al: Normal perfusion pressure breakthrough theory, *Clin Neurosurg* 25:651-672, 1978.

112. Stuart GG, Merry GS, Smith JA et al: Severe head injury managed without intracranial pressure monitoring, *J Neurosurg* 59:601-605, 1983.

113. Sullivan HG, Miller JD, Becker DP et al: The physiological basis of ICP change with progressive epidural brain compression: an experimental evaluation in cats, *J Neurosurg* 47:532-550, 1977.

114. Sullivan HG, Miller JD, Griffith RL et al: CSF pressure transients in response to epidural and ventricular volume loading, *Am J Physiol* 234: R167-171, 1978.

115. Sundbarg G, Nordstrom CH, Messeter K et al: A comparison of intraparenchymatous and intraventricular pressure recording in clinical practice, *J Neurosurg* 67:841-845, 1987.

116. Suzuki M, Iwasaki Y, Yamamoto T et al: Sequelae of the osmotic blood-brain barrier opening in rats, *J Neurosurg* 69:421-428, 1988.

117. Van Hemelrijck J, van Aken H, Plets C et al: The effects of propofol on intracranial pressure and cerebral perfusion pressure in patients with brain tumors, *Acta Anaesth Belg* 40:95-100, 1989.

118. Vries JK, Becker DP, Young HF: A subarachnoid screw for monitoring intracranial pressure: technical note, *J Neurosurg* 39:416-419, 1973.

119. Walters FJM: Neuroanesthesia—a review of the basic principles and current practices, *Centr Afr J Med* 36:44-51, 1990.

120. Weaver DD, Winn HR, Jane JA: Differential intracranial pressure in patients with unilateral mass lesions, *J Neurosurg* 56:660-665, 1982.

121. Wilkinson HA, Yarzebski J, Wilkinson EC et al: Erroneous measurement of intracranial pressure caused by simultaneous ventricular drainage: a hydrodynamic model study, *Neurosurgery* 24:348-354, 1989.

122. Yatsu FM: Pharmacologic protection against ischemic brain damage, *Neurol Clin* 1:37-53, 1983.

123. Young WL, McCormick PC: Perioperative management of intracranial catastrophes, *Crit Care Clin* 5:821-844, 1989.

6

The Blood-Brain Barrier and Cerebral Edema

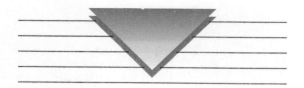

Thomas H. Milhorat

The central nervous system (CNS), which generates and conducts electrical impulses, is provided with a specialized environment that is watery in composition, chemically precise, and sheltered from the blood by the blood-brain barrier (BBB). The extracellular (EC) compartment of the CNS has two fluids: (1) the interstitial fluid (ISF) and (2) the cerebrospinal fluid (CSF). These fluids extend from the BBB through a series of 150- to 200-Å wide intercellular spaces to the cerebral ventricles, subarachnoid space, and absorptive channels (arachnoid villi and perineural lymphatics), which allow egress to the blood.

THE BLOOD-BRAIN BARRIER

The concept of a "Blüthirnschränke" (blood-brain barrier) derives from vital staining experiments that established the curious finding that when basic dyes are injected into blood, they tend to stain almost all the tissues of the body except the brain. Because dyes are bound immediately to plasma proteins,[93] their distribution in tissues reflects the movement of dye-protein complexes, rather than water-soluble markers. In a classic set of studies, Goldmann[33,34] demonstrated that whereas intravascularly injected trypan blue does not stain the brain except for the choroid plexuses and leptomeninges, when the dye is injected into the CSF there is heavy staining of the entire parenchyma, including the cellular elements. These observations proved conclusively that a barrier of some sort exists between the blood and brain although a detailed understanding of the BBB was not possible until the advent of electron microscopy. It is now established that there are two morphologically distinct barriers that guard the passage of plasma constituents into the EC compartment of the brain: (1) the capillary endothelium, and (2) the specialized ependyma of the circumventricular organs.[8,61,79]

Capillary Endothelium

The primary surface across which blood-tissue exchanges take place is the capillary endothelium. In most areas of the brain, the cells of the capillary endothelium differ from those found in other tissues of the body by the following distinctive features: (1) the absence of fenestrae, (2) the presence of tight junctions (zonulae occludentes) between adjacent cells, (3) the low cellular profile of plasmalemmal pits and vesicles, (4) the high cellular profile of mitochondria, and (5) a perivascular investment of closely applied astrocytic foot processes.

The intercellular tight junctions of the cerebral endothelium are pentalaminar (five-layered) adhesions that form a continuous belt of "spot welds" around the entire circumference of the capillary.[10,79] The integrity of the junctions can be shown graphically by examining the distribution of ultrastructural tracers. For example, following the intravascular injection of colloidal proteins, such as ferritin (mol. wt. 400,000) or horseradish peroxidase (mol. wt. 40,000), the tracers are confined within the capillary lumen and are halted in their movement into brain by the first tight junction on the luminal side of the endothelium. Limited uptake sometimes occurs in small pinocytotic pits along the luminal plasmalemma, but the tracers do not pass through cells or through their intercellular clefts to reach the pericapillary space.[10,61,79] When the tracers are injected into the ventricles or subarachnoid space, their distribution forms a "mirror image" of their distribution after intravascular injection, that is, the tracers pass with relative ease across the ependymal and pial surfaces to distribute widely throughout the extracellular compartment (EC) and pericapillary spaces but are halted in their outward movement by the first tight junction on the abluminal side of the endothelium. Taken together, these findings make it clear that the tight junctions of the cerebral endothelium impose an obligatory restraint on the movement of substances between blood and brain based on molecular size.

The "tightness" of the brain's capillaries has been the subject of considerable interest. Although the cerebral endothelium is unquestionably impermeable to large or polar molecules, it is highly permeable to most lipid soluble substances and exhibits variable permeability to ions, small nonelectrolytes, and urea.[44,68] When hyperosmotic agents—such as urea or mannitol—are injected intraarterially, there is a shrinkage of cerebral endothelial cells and a "reversible opening" of the tight junctions.[9,78] Other conditions that probably produce junctional uncoupling are hyperthermia, prolonged hypercarbia, and vasodilation associated with the loss of autoregulation.[75,78] On the basis of currently available data, it is estimated that the tight junctions of the cerebral endothelium are perforated by aqueous channels having a diameter of 6 to 8 Å.[26] If one accepts the lower limit of the estimate, this would permit the passage of only three molecules found in the body: H_2O, Na^+, and Cl^-.

The cells of the cerebral endothelium contain compara-

tively few pinocytotic pits and vesicles. These structures have been linked to transcellular vesicular transport in cardiac and skeletal endothelia, and their reduced profile in normal cerebral endothelium has been cited as an important feature of the BBB.[26] In vasogenic edema, greatly stimulated pinocytotic activity appears to be an important mechanism in the transport of serum proteins into the interstitial spaces.[46] Increased vesicular transport of proteins has also been observed in association with cerebral hypoxia, stroke, head injuries, infections, inflammatory and autoimmune reactions, intoxications, brain tumors, cold injury lesions, hyperthermia, prolonged hypercapnia, vasodilatation associated with the loss of cerebral autoregulation, and acute arterial hypertension.[41,46,75,78]

It is estimated that in regions of the brain possessing closed capillaries, mitochondria account for 8% to 11% of the endothelial cell volume, as compared with 2% to 5% in all other organs of the body.[69] Mitochondria are known to be involved with a variety of complex metabolic activities and appear to serve the brain-capillary barrier, both as a means for trapping certain substrates and for facilitating the transcapillary transport of others.[20] Thus dopa decarboxylase—a mitochondrial enzyme that converts L-DOPA into the highly impermeable solute dopamine—probably contributes to the exclusion of this biologically active neurotransmitter,[5] just as gamma aminobutyric acid (GABA) transaminase—also present in large amounts in the mitochondria of cerebral capillaries—is thought to exclude the passage from blood to brain of systemically administered GABA.[94] Other endothelial enzymes that probably contribute to the permeability characteristics of the brain-capillary barrier, either by restricting or by facilitating transcellular transport, include gamma glutamyl transpeptidase, adenosine triphosphatase, monoamine oxidase, acid phosphatase, alkaline phosphatase, nicotinamide adenine dinucleotide, and various glucose, glutamate, lactate, and succinate dehydrogenases.[6,75]

Immediately beyond the capillary tubule, and closely applied to its basement membrane, is a perivascular investment of astrocytic foot processes. This second layer of cells forms a complete cuff around the circumference of the vessel. It is mainly for this reason that early electron microscopists referred to a "capillary-glial membrane," which was thought to create a virtually impenetrable protoplasmic barrier. However, modern ultrastructural studies have shown that the pericapillary space and the intercellular clefts between astrocytic foot processes are open and communicating channels measuring approximately 150 to 200 Å in diameter.[10,79] Astrocytes contain high concentrations of certain important enzymes, including carbonic anhydrase (which is involved with water and sodium transport) and nucleoside phosphatase (which is crucial to adenosine triphosphate [ATP] energy systems). The latter enzyme is not found in endothelial cells; it is richly localized in foot processes of astrocytes and the pericapillary basement membrane.[92] Further evidence of glial-endothelial cell interaction comes from tissue culture experiments, which have established that gamma glutamyl transpeptidase—an enzyme involved with amino acid and peptide exchanges—is not found in pure cultures of endothelial cells but is produced in significant concentrations when the two cell types are grown together.[36] Astrocytic foot processes appear to have a capacity for making rapid and sensitive adjustments in the microchemical environment of EC fluid and thus contribute indirectly to the permeability characteristics of the BBB.[26,71]

Specialized Ependyma of Circumventricular Organs

In a few circumscribed areas of the brain, the cells of the capillary endothelium are not joined by tight junctions and the vessels are fenestrated or "open" like those in other organs of the body. Each of these areas border the cerebral ventricles, and all are involved with specific secretory activities that presumably require a direct contact with the plasma. On the basis of morphologic and functional similarities, structures possessing open capillaries have been described collectively as "the circumventricular organs." They include the following: the four choroid plexuses, the median eminence, the neural lobe of the hypophysis, the organum vasculosum lamina terminalis, the subfornical organ, the subcommissural organ, the pineal gland, and the area postrema.

Overlying each of the circumventricular organs and enclosing the zone of "functional capillary leakage" is a specialized epithelium, unlike ependyma found elsewhere, whose cells are joined by intercellular tight junctions. These junctions arise at the apical borders of contiguous cell membranes and form a continuous zonule or belt that is capable of restricting the passage of certain plasma constituents, including proteins, into CSF. After intravascular injection, colloidal proteins pass rapidly out of fenestrated capillaries and fill the perivascular spaces, the EC spaces, and the intercellular clefts between adjacent ependymal cells up to the apical tight junction.[8,61] The tracers do not pass beyond the apical tight junction and do not enter the CSF. Conversely, when colloidal proteins are injected into the cerebral ventricles, they easily pass between the cells of ordinary ependyma but are prevented from entering the intercellular clefts of the specialized ependyma by the apical tight junctions. Thus it is evident that these junctions, like the cerebral endothelium form an effective barrier to proteins and impose an obligatory restraint on the passage of substances based on molecular size.

A second morphologic feature that appears to contribute to the barrier characteristics of specialized ependyma is the abundance of intracellular organelles and lysosomes. In choroid plexus epithelium, ultrastructural studies have revealed an unusually high profile of mitochondria, pinocytotic pits and vesicles, Golgi, Golgi-derived vesicles (terminal vesicles), and multivesicular bodies.[21] When colloidal proteins are injected intravascularly, these large markers pass freely out of choroidal capillaries and are incorporated almost immediately into membrane-bound vesicles along the basal and lateral plasmalemmas of ependymal cells. Thereafter, the tracers are removed to multivesicular and dense bodies and are subsequently degraded by lysosomal enzymes. This heterolytic mechanism is probably an important feature of the brain's epithelial barrier and may limit diffusional leakage of substances into the CSF.[57]

Internal Milieu

An essential function of the BBB is to provide a specialized environment for nervous tissue. Within limits, the chemical composition of the brain EC fluid is carefully regulated, and a variety of substances—especially those which are large, polar, or lipid-insoluble—are almost totally excluded from the brain. In this manner, the CNS is protected from toxic or potentially toxic substances, and the CSF is maintained as a protein-poor product of the plasma.

The cells of the CNS are metabolically active. The milieu that surrounds them is responsible for a number of functions: (1) providing a large and continuous supply of substrates, primarily glucose, despite transient and often wide variations in the plasma concentrations of these substances, (2) maintaining a chemically precise environment that is suitable for the electrophysiologic needs of nervous tissue, and (3) removing products of metabolism and disease.

Little is known about the chemical regulation of nutrients entering the brain. For simple sugars (e.g., glucose), transport probably occurs by means of a specialized pump mechanism (equilibrating carrier) between the blood and brain.[63] A similar mechanism is probably responsible for transporting hexoses and pentoses, organic acids, serotonin, biogenic amines, penicillin, and a wide variety of drugs.[27,63,77]

The normal electrophysiologic activities of nervous tissue require that the concentration of inorganic ions be kept relatively constant. The concentrations of most ions in CSF exhibit sufficient variations with those in the blood to require that active transport mechanisms be present. The concentration of calcium ion (Ca^{2+}), for example, is considerably below that in the plasma, and the equilibration of intravenously injected ^{45}Ca between blood and CSF is a lengthy process that takes 5 to 6 hours or even longer to complete.[70] It is estimated that approximately two thirds of the Ca^{2+} concentration in CSF comes from the blood, and approximately one third comes from the brain.[37] A calcium influx "pump" is probably involved in the transport of this ion from the blood to the brain and subsequently to the CSF.

Potassium ion (K^+), which is also found in lower concentration in CSF than in plasma, exchanges extremely slowly (40 hr) between the blood and brain. Katzman[43] has shown that cardiac glycosides are capable of altering the concentration of K^+ in the brain, and, by perfusing the ventricles of dogs and cats with artificial CSF containing 10^{-4} and 10^{-5} M ouabain, a consistent decrease in the K^+ efflux and an increase in the K^+ concentration can be demonstrated.[27] Magnesium (Mg^{2+}) and chloride (Cl^{-1}) are found in slightly higher concentrations in CSF than in plasma, and both are known to play an important role in neuronal conduction. The failure of alterations in the Mg^{2+} and Cl ion concentrations to effect similar changes in CSF concentrations implies that the transport of these ions does not occur exclusively by passive means. Maren[51] has reported that the intravenous administration of acetazolamide in cats causes a proportional reduction in the rate of CSF formation and the entry of ^{36}Cl into the CSF. This finding suggests that the movement of chloride ion from blood to CSF is closely linked to CSF production although the exact mechanism has not been established.

Bicarbonate ion (HCO_3^-), which is concerned with the regulation of pH, plays an important role in the maintenance of electrical activity within the CNS. Under normal conditions, the CSF/plasma ratio of HCO_3 is about 0.8, and, in states of both alkalosis and acidosis, the CSF concentration of this ion is considerably below that predicted for electrochemical equilibration. Pappenheimer[72] has demonstrated that HCO_3 can be transported actively by means of either a primary HCO_3^- pump or a secondary ion pump (i.e., H^+ or Cl^-) between the brain interstitial fluid (ISF) and blood.

Davson[22] has summarized the specific details of sodium (Na^+) transport within the brain. There is no current evidence that ion is actively pumped. On the basis of experimental data, it is possible to conclude that (1) the concentration of Na^+ in newly formed CSF is similar to that in plasma, (2) the exchange of Na^+ between CSF and brain follows standard diffusion kinetics, (3) the uptake of Na^+ by the brain is restricted by the BBB, and (4) the exchange of water between the blood, brain, and CSF is exceedingly rapid. Bering[4] has reported a D_2O half-time of 12 to 25 sec between blood and brain and 3 to 8 min between blood and CSF. These exchanges appear to be limited only by the rate of blood flow to the brain.

If CSF is withdrawn from the cerebral ventricles, cisterna magna, and subarachnoid space, significant variations in chemical composition are encountered. The concentration of K^+—for example—decreases steadily as CSF passes from the cerebral ventricles to the subarachnoid space, and the opposite holds true for the concentrations of urea, albumin, and globulin. Franklin[28] has reported regional variations in the concentrations of a number of amino acids, including arginine, serine, glycine, lysine, alanine, taurine, and glutamine. On the basis of these findings, it is evident that sites other than the choroid plexuses must be involved with the transport of solutes into and out of the CSF.[63] The higher protein content of lumbar CSF, as compared with ventricular CSF, is probably the result of steady net additions of cerebral metabolites to the bulk circulation as it drains toward sites of absorption.[55]

Brain Extracellular Compartment

The EC spaces of the brain form a series of narrow, interconnecting channels that are anatomically continuous with the cerebral ventricles and subarachnoid space. Although closely spaced, the cellular elements of the brain are separated by distinct clefts that extend between the membranes of cell bodies and their processes (i.e., dendrites, axons, astrocytic foot processes). The intercellular clefts have a minimum width of 150 to 200 Å, which is also the standard measurement in densely packed areas, such as the cortex, gray matter nuclei, brainstem, and spinal cord. In the cerebral hemispheres, characteristic 150- to 200-Å wide gaps are found around the basement membrane of cerebral capillaries and between astrocytic foot processes, neurons and their subcellular extensions, and the cells of lining epithelia (ependyma and pia). In less dense areas of the white matter, the intercellular clefts tend to be larger and vary from characteristic 150-to-200-Å wide gaps to those with a diameter of 1000 to 2000 Å.[63]

The macroscopic CSF cavities consist of two main compartments: (1) an internal compartment, formed by the three cerebral ventricles, the aqueduct of Sylvius, the fourth (cerebellar) ventricle, and the central canal of the spinal cord, and (2) an external compartment formed by the cisterns, fissures, and sulci of the subarachnoid space. Each cavity is continuous with the next through one or more well-defined openings, and the pathway terminates at the level of the dural sinuses where expansions of the subarachnoid space—the arachnoid villi—protrude into the venous circulation.

In humans, the total volume of the CSF cavities is approximately 140 ml. The subarachnoid space, which is by far the larger of the two main compartments, contains approximately 118 to 120 ml of fluid, of which 30 ml belongs to the spinal subarachnoid space. The volume of the cerebral ventricles is given as 20 to 23 ml, with each lateral ventricle accounting for approximately 7.5 ml. It is estimated that the total brain EC (interstitial and CSF spaces) represents 10% to 15% of total brain volume, with a mean value of approximately 12%.[59]

Lymphatic-Like Function of Brain EC Fluid

The lymphatic-like function of brain EC fluid is fundamental to the study of EC edema and can be summarized as follows:

- The CSF formation rate in humans is approximately 0.37 ± 0.1 SD ml/min,[87] or 500 ml/day. Stated differently, because the total volume of the EC compartment is approximately 140 to 175 ml, the CSF volume is renewed every 8 hours.[55] Age does not affect the rate of CSF formation, which is also unaffected by intracranial pressures from -10 to 240 mm H_2O.
- CSF is formed by two mechanisms: (1) secretion of the choroid plexuses,* and (2) lymphatic-like drainage of brain ISF.[18,19,54,56,64] Although the exact contributions from these two sources remain to be determined, the percentage of ISF formed to the total rate of CSF formation has been variously given as 6% to

*References 22, 44, 51, 54, 56, 64, 78, 87.

$11\%^{18}$ to 30% to 40%.[55,84] The production of brain ISF fluid appears to involve the following steps:[63] (1) ultrafiltration and active transport by the cerebral endothelium, (2) formation of water from metabolism by the cellular elements of the brain, and (3) addition of metabolic wastes.

- The movement of brain ISF occurs by bulk flow through the narrow intercellular clefts of the neuropil and appears to be influenced by the hydrostatic pressure gradient between ISF and CSF.[59] The CSF flows in bulk from the cerebral ventricles into the subarachnoid space, from which it is absorbed across the arachnoid villi and perineural lymphatics. The following factors contribute to the circulatory movement of CSF: (1) the continuous outpouring of newly formed ventricular fluid, (2) the ventricular pulsations, representing the combined effects of respiratory variations and pulsations emanating from cerebral arteries and choroid plexuses, and (3) the pressure gradient across the arachnoid villi. In humans, the mean CSF pressure in the lateral recumbent position (150 mm saline) is considerably higher than the mean pressure of venous blood in the sagittal sinus (90 mm saline), jugular vein (40 mm saline), and right atrium of the heart (−4 mm saline). This differential is required to promote drainage and absorption across the arachnoid villi and doubtless contributes to the cephalic movement of the CSF.[55]

- The most clinically important lymphatic-like role of the CSF is to remove products of cerebral metabolism. To date, direct proof of net transport from brain ISF to CSF has been established for the following lipid-insoluble substances: inulin, mannitol, sulfanilic acid, urea, albumin, globulin, dopamine, homovanillic acid, serotonin, and norepinephrine.[56] The CSF concentrations of many substances exhibit circadian rhythms.[63] From a diagnostic standpoint, the chemical analysis of CSF has been shown to be helpful in assessing a wide range of neurologic conditions, including degenerative diseases, convulsive disorders, manic and depressive states, essential hypertension, organic pain syndromes, psychogenic pain, and schizophrenia.[99]

BRAIN SWELLING AND EDEMA

Cerebral edema may be defined as an increase in brain water content of sufficient magnitude to produce clinical symptoms. The disorder is associated with a wide variety of pathologic conditions, including neoplasms, infections, trauma, and ischemia. It is current practice to classify the cerebral edemas into two main types: (1) vasogenic edema, caused by increased permeability of the BBB, and (2) cytotoxic edema, characterized by an abnormal uptake of water by the cellular elements of the brain.[45] While useful, this classification equates cellular swelling with "edema" and fails to include a number of important types, such as

BOX 6-1
CLASSIFICATION OF BRAIN BULK ENLARGEMENT

Increased Vascular Volume
Arterial dilation
Venous obstruction

Cellular Swelling
Cytotoxic injuries
Metabolic storage

Extracellular Edema
Vasogenic edema
Osmotic edema
Compressive edema
Hydrocephalic edema

periventricular edema occurring with hydrocephalus and parenchymal edema occurring with water intoxication, plasma hypoosmolarity, and inappropriate secretion of antidiuretic hormone.

The difficulties encountered in distinguishing brain swelling and cerebral edema require an understanding of the primary types of brain bulk enlargement. Like other organs in the body, the brain has three anatomic compartments that can accumulate fluid in excessive amounts: (1) the vascular compartment, composed of arteries, capillaries, and veins, (2) the cellular compartment, composed of cells and their subcellular extensions, and (3) the EC compartment, composed of the ISF and the CSF spaces. Volumetric expansion of one or more of these compartments will lead to bulk enlargement of the brain. Box 6-1 summarizes the three primary types of brain bulk enlargement. Many diseases produce mixed types.[59]

BRAIN BULK ENLARGEMENT
Increased Vascular Volume

Volumetric expansion of the cerebrovascular bed can occur as a consequence of two mechanisms: (1) arterial dilation, which increases capillary blood flow and volume and ultimately venous volume, and (2) obstruction of venous outflow. With transient expansion of the cerebrovascular bed, the increase in the bulk of the brain is solely a function of increased blood volume. This results in some shift of fluid out of the EC compartment, as evidenced by the small size of the cerebral ventricles, which can dissipate the rise in intracranial pressure (ICP). However, with severe or prolonged expansions, compliance is lost, the ICP rises, and there is usually an alteration of brain capillary permeability that can lead to the formation of edema and hemorrhages.

Arterial Dilation

Under normal conditions, the cerebral circulation responds rapidly and precisely to the metabolic needs of the brain.

This control is vested in the cerebral arteries and arterioles whose smooth muscle cells respond in a sensitive manner to a variety of stimuli, including arterial P_{CO_2}, tissue P_{O_2}, extracellular pH, hydrostatic pressure, sympathetic innervation, and specific chemical and hormonal substances.[50,97] With a change in arterial diameter, there is a simultaneous change in blood flow and volume within the capillary bed. These adjustments are regulated on a regional basis to meet physiologic requirements but can be affected by pathologic processes that alter metabolic needs or directly disturb arterial tone and caliber. Pronounced arterial dilation leading to hyperemia and congestion may occur in association with any of the following conditions: malignant hypertension, global ischemia, prolonged hypercapnia, febrile infections, seizures, severe anemia, uremia, and the loss of cerebral autoregulation.[60]

Venous Obstruction

Obstruction of the cerebral veins or dural sinuses can occur with a wide variety of disorders, including bacterial meningitis, subdural abscess, severe dehydration, pregnancy, parasagittal tumors, head trauma, polycythemia, radical neck dissection, head and neck tumors, strangulation, superior vena cava syndrome, failure of the right side of the heart, and cor pulmonale. With acute occlusions, the brain is congested and the ventricles are small. There is an effort to restore normal venous volume and pressure by rerouting blood through collateral vessels, but this is far less successful than with slowly evolving thromboses (e.g., sagittal sinus invasion by meningiomas) or with extracranial obstructions that can take advantage of alternative routes to the heart (e.g., Batson's plexus). In morbid cases, the brain is congested and there is evidence of widespread venous stasis, interstitial edema, and hemorrhagic infarction.[42]

Cellular Swelling

The excessive uptake by cells of fluid or other abnormal substances can lead to varying degrees of brain swelling. This does not constitute edema in the strict sense of the term, and on cut sections the brain is dry and sticky.[101] There are two general types of cellular swelling (Box 6-1).

Cytotoxic Edema

The term *cytotoxic edema* was introduced by Klatzo[45] to describe a disturbance of cellular osmoregulation that results in the abnormal uptake of fluid within the cytoplasm of cells. The primary mechanism appears to be a disturbance of the energy-dependent Na^+/K^+ pump of the cell membrane, which serves to exclude Na^+—and hence water—from the intracellular compartment.[46] With the uptake of fluid from the EC compartment, the affected cells swell, reducing the EC space, whose solutes become concentrated.[32] Because a mere shift of fluid into the intracellular compartment will not produce an increase in brain mass, some EC fluid is replenished. This may occur by passive diffusion across the cerebral endothelium and possibly by

a reversal of ISF bulk flow according to the principle of brain volume regulation proposed by Bradbury.[7]

The most common clinical disorder to cause cytotoxic brain swelling is cerebral ischemia. As its name implies, cytotoxic injuries may be caused by a long list of intoxications. A selective swelling of astrocytes is typically seen after exposure to methionine sulfoximine, cuprizone, and isoniazid, and similar findings have been reported in Reye's syndrome and after infections with transmissable viruses. In triethyltin and hexachlorophene intoxications, the accumulation of water appears to be mainly in the intramyelinic clefts, and axonal swelling is particularly prominent after exposure to hydrogen cyanide. Other agents known to produce cytotoxic insults include 2,4 dinitrophenol, 6-aminonicatinamide, and lead.[59]

Metabolic Storage

The intracellular uptake of abnormal metabolites is common to a rare group of inherited disorders known collectively as the *storage diseases*. In these cases, the increase in parenchymal mass is due primarily to the "stuffing" of neurons and is most pronounced in the early stages of the disease before cell death and atrophy supervene. Some of the better known examples include the intracellular storage of glycogen (Pompe's disease), mucopolysaccharides (Hurler's disease), GM2 ganglioside (Tay-Sachs disease), glycosyl ceramide (Gaucher's disease), and sphingomyelin (Niemann-Pick disease).

EXTRACELLULAR EDEMA

Extracellular or "wet" brain edema includes four general types: (1) vasogenic, (2) osmotic, (3) compressive, and (4) hydrocephalic.

Vasogenic Edema

This is the most common type of EC edema. It occurs as a consequence of increased permeability of brain capillaries and hence is a frequent complication of clinically important disorders, such as head injuries, tumors, infections, inflammations, and certain types of cerebrovascular accidents. The mechanisms of increased brain capillary permeability include (1) structural injury of the cerebral endothelium leading to opening of tight junctions, increased pinocytosis, or disruption of cells; (2) metabolic impairment of endothelial transport systems; and (3) neovascularization by vessels lacking BBB characteristics.[59]

Regardless of the cause of brain capillary dysfunction, a significant increase in cerebrovascular permeability will lead to the formation of EC edema. The chemical composition of the extravasated fluid will vary with the magnitude of BBB breakdown, so that with major disturbances a protein-rich fluid is likely to be formed, representing a mixture of plasma, normal ISF, and the products of tissue damage. With experimental cold injury lesions, the chemical composition of edema fluid exhibits a sodium concentration (143 mEq/L) and a colloid osmotic pressure (14 mm

Hg) that are closer to those of plasma (146 mEq/L and 20 mm Hg, respectively). than to those of CSF (158 mEq/L and 0.6 mm Hg, respectively). These findings reflect the direct contribution of the plasma extravasate, whereas the higher potassium concentration of edema fluid (4.75 mEq/L)—as compared with plasma (3.94 mEq/L) or CSF (3.40 mEq/L)—can only be accounted for by the leakage of the ion from injured tissue.[32]

Edema Spread

The spread of vasogenic edema follows the normal pathways of ISF bulk flow. From the lesion site, the extravasated fluid extends ("like water seeping into soil from a broken pipe") through the pericapillary spaces, the intercellular clefts between astrocytic foot processes, and the 150- to 200-Å EC spaces that are anatomically continuous with the CSF spaces. The flooding of the parenchyma distends the EC compartment and results in a volumetric increase that can approach 45% in the immediate circumference of the injured area.[44] Because of the greater density of gray matter, edema fluid tends to spread preferentially through the white matter, whose meager cellularity and straighter EC clefts produce a lower resistance to flow.[82]

The driving force of vasogenic edema is the mean arterial pressure, which promotes the filtration of plasma into the EC compartment and governs its subsequent spread. The relationship is immediate and direct and can be stated as follows: with an increase in arterial pressure, there is a proportional increase in the volume of edema and its rate of spread; with a decrease in arterial pressure, there is a proportional decrease in both parameters.[47] The magnitude of edema formation depends on a number of other variables, including the severity of BBB dysfunction, the size of the lesion, and the duration of barrier opening.[83]

Pathophysiology of Edema

The filtration of plasma constituents into the brain results in a consistent reduction of local cerebral blood flow. This occurs as a consequence of volumetric flooding of the EC compartment, which increases local tissue pressure and leads to a compromise of the regional microcirculation. The formation of a congruent field of edema/ischemia can be shown to occur as a direct function of the systemic arterial pressure.[65]

In areas of brain invaded by edema, the spread of plasma constituents produces a number of secondary effects. For example, the extravasation of free radicals, lysosomal enzymes, and fatty acids is a likely cause of glial cell swelling.[3,75] Toxic substances may also contribute to the formation and spread of vasogenic edema by enhancing the permeability of regional cerebral capillaries.[3] With focal edematous lesions, there is a profound depression of local glucose utilization in the ipsilateral cerebral cortex, accompanied by a smaller depression in the cerebral cortex of the contralateral hemisphere, the bilateral subcortical structures, and the white matter of both cerebral hemi-

spheres.[73,74] This pattern of global metabolic depression has been attributed to the release of biologically active substances, including prostaglandins and catecholamines, from injured capillaries.[74,75]

From a clinical standpoint, the most important consequences of spreading edema are related to local mass effects. With expansion of the edematous field there is a rise in intracranial pressure and a compartmental shift of cerebral structures, which can lead to brainstem compression and signs of rostral-caudal deterioration, characterized by arterial hypertension, bradycardia, and cardiorespiratory collapse. Cerebral displacement is an inevitable consequence of large and rapidly expanding intracranial mass lesions.

Osmotic Edema

This type of edema has been emphasized by Go[31] and depends on the establishment of an unfavorable osmotic gradient between the plasma and the brain EC fluid. For osmotic edema to develop, the BBB must be intact; otherwise, an effective osmotic gradient could not be maintained. The action of mannitol and other dehydrating agents depends on this principle.

Decreased Plasma Osmolarity

Osmotic edema may occur in association with a number of hypoosmolar conditions, including the improper administration of intravenous fluids, compulsive drinking by psychiatric patients, inappropriate secretion of the antidiuretic hormone, pseudotumor cerebri, and excessive hemodialysis of uremic patients.[25,59] With a significant dilution of the plasma, water enters the brain and distributes evenly within the EC spaces of gray and white matter.[75] The electrolyte composition of the fluid tends to reflect the consequences of dilution, as modified by solvent drag. When the osmotic stress is prolonged, there is a real loss of brain K^+, presumably as a consequence of cellular adaptation.[31]

The spread of osmotically induced edema occurs by bulk flow along normal ISF pathways. After a 10% or greater reduction of plasma osmolarity, there is a pronounced increase in ISF volume flow, and extracellular markers are cleared into the CSF at an increased rate.[90] The formation of osmotic edema can lead to a significant increase in the rate of CSF formation,[24] without any contribution of the choroid plexuses. Because osmotic edema is vented rapidly, brain bulk enlargement tends to be modest.[96]

Increased Tissue Osmolarity

Osmotic edema can occur when the plasma osmolarity is normal if there is a significant increase in tissue osmolarity. In patients with intracerebral hemorrhage, the release of proteins from the "melting hematoma" can draw fluid to the circumference of the lesion across the intact BBB.[59] A similar mechanism may also play a role in the formation of peritumoral edema although this type of edema is usually associated with a dominant vasogenic or compressive component.

Compressive Edema

Any mass lesion that obstructs the bulk flow of brain ISF can cause compressive edema.[59] This type of edema is a common complication of benign tumors that do not alter BBB permeability (e.g., meningioma) and probably occurs to some extent with all large intracranial masses. Compressive edema can also occur with cerebral hernias or displacements in which the incarcerated tissue becomes swollen as a consequence of an obstructed flow of brain ISF, impaired venous drainage, or both.

Hydrocephalic Edema

The edema of hydrocephalus, more than any other type of cerebral edema, resembles lymphedema in the general body tissues. With few exceptions, both result from obstruction of the drainage channels, leading to distention of the cavities proximal to the block with retrograde flooding of the extracellular compartment. In acute hydrocephalus, the earliest finding involving the brain parenchyma is periventricular edema.[13] The invaded tissues are spongy in appearance, and there is evidence of widespread separation of glial cells and axons characteristic of EC edema. Astrocytes are particularly susceptible to EC edema and undergo selective swelling, followed by gradual atrophy and cell loss. In chronic hydrocephalus, the pathologic findings are destruction of axon collaterals, a gradual unraveling of the myelin sheath, and phagocytosis of lipid by the microglia.[55]

The formation of hydrocephalic edema probably involves two mechanisms: (1) stasis of brain ISF, occurring as a consequence of the reduced gradient for bulk flow into the cerebral ventricles, and (2) reflux of CSF into the periventricular tissues, occurring as a consequence of increased intraventricular pressure.[59] In patients with communicating hydrocephalus, isotope ventriculography typically demonstrates retrograde filling of the ventricular system and the presence of a "double-density" halo around the cerebral ventricles, representing migration of the radiopharmaceutical into the periventricular tissues.[62] With progressive or persistent periventricular edema, there is a significant reduction in local cerebral blood flow,[84] which probably contributes to the functional disturbances of hydrocephalus.[95]

TREATMENT OF CEREBRAL EDEMA

Table 6-1 summarizes the treatment modality options currently employed in the management of cerebral edema.

Surgical Excision

Surgical excision of mass lesions (e.g., tumors, abscesses, subdural hematoma) is effective in the treatment of compressive edema and the vasogenic component that attends neovascularization or increased capillary permeability. In addition to removing leaky capillaries, surgical excision reduces the release of potentially toxic substances—such as free radicals and prostaglandins—and usually improves local cerebral perfusion by reducing mass effect.

TABLE 6-1
Treatment of Cerebral Edema

Modality	Site of Action	Primary Mechanism of Action	Complications/Disadvantages
Surgical excision	Local	Removal of inciting lesion and area of leaky capillaries	Attendant to specific procedure
Head elevation	General	Reduction of ICP by lowering cerebrovenous pressure	Reduction of cerebral perfusion pressure
Hyperventilation	General	Reduction of ICP by vasoconstriction of normal brain vessels	Cerebral hypoxia and the accumulation of tissue lactic acid
Osmotherapy	General	Reduction of ICP by osmotic withdrawal of water from normal brain tissue	Electrolyte disturbances and renal failure
Steroids	Local/general	Reduction of local capillary leakage and reduction of global metabolic depression (? effect on catecholamine metabolism)	Gastrointestinal bleeding, electrolyte disturbances, reduced immunocompetence, hyperglycemia, mental disturbances
Antinflammatory drugs	Local	Reduction of local capillary leakage (? inhibition of arachidonic acid–prostaglandin cascade)	Awaiting clinical trials
Antihypertensive drugs	Local	Reduction of capillary leakage by lowering filtration pressure	Reduction of cerebral perfusion pressure
CSF drainage	Local/general	Reduction of ICP; transventricular clearance of edema fluid	Infection, obstruction
Barbiturate coma	Local/general	Reduction of capillary leakage by lowering blood pressure; reduction of cerebral metabolic needs	Loss of neurologic responses and requirement for complex clinical monitoring
Operative decompression	Local/general	Reduction of local mass effect; reduction of ICP	Treatment of last resort

Head Elevation

It is standard clinical practice to elevate the head of patients with cerebral edema to facilitate cerebrovenous drainage and reduce ICP. However, there is evidence that the cerebral perfusion pressure is maximal in the horizontal position and that elevation of the head above the heart reduces the hydrostatic force of the systemic arterial circulation.[86] While elevation of the head may be desirable as a means for reducing "filtration edema," a decrease in cerebral blood flow in the upright position has been linked to a "vasodilatory cascade," characterized by a paradoxical rise of ICP and abrupt deterioration of clinical status despite unchanged or reduced levels of ICP.[85] It is evident, therefore, that the benefits and risks of head elevation need to be carefully considered and that this is best done by continuously monitoring ICP and titrating its level to achieve an optimal clinical response.

Hyperventilation

Since cerebral vessels are exquisitely sensitive to changes in CO_2 tension, hyperventilation is an effective means for reducing ICP. This occurs by "blowing off" the P_{CO_2}, which vasoconstricts cerebral arteries and arterioles and leads to a commensurate reduction of cerebral blood flow and vascular volume. The consequences of hyperventilation are global in nature and do not affect the local lesion site, except to the extent that a reduction in cerebral perfusion potentially decreases edema formation by reducing filtration forces. Prolonged or excessive hyperventilation can lead to diffuse cerebral hypoxia and the accumulation of lactic acid within the parenchymal tissues.[44,76]

Osmotherapy

The use of hypertonic drugs (osmotherapy) is an effective means for producing a rapid reduction of brain water content. In the treatment of patients with increased ICP, mannitol (20% solution) has the widest clinical applicability and is usually given as an intravenous infusion in doses of 0.25 to 1.0 g/kg body weight over an interval of 60 to 90 min.[75,98] The clinical benefits of hypertonic drugs derive from their ability to withdraw water from tissues osmotically and not from their diuretic effect although the duration of action of osmotherapy can be prolonged by the use of loop diuretics (e.g., furosemide, ethacrynic acid), which preferentially excrete water as compared with solute.[75]

Contrary to popular belief, hypertonic drugs have little direct effect on edematous tissues and do not remove edema fluid per se. This is understandable when it is recalled that the efflux of fluid from tissues depends on the osmotic gradient that is established between the vascular and EC compartments at the distal end of capillaries (Starling's hypothesis) and that this process requires an intact capillary membrane across which osmotic gradients can be operative. In areas invaded by edema, but in which cerebral capillaries are intact, it is likely that some efflux of fluid occurs. Osmotic dehydration can also reduce the total volume of CSF,[91] which occurs by retrograde drainage into the EC compartment and subsequent efflux across cerebral capillaries according to the brain volume regulation model of Bradbury.[7]

Although hypertonic drugs have only a limited direct effect on edema fluid, they have been shown to reduce blood viscosity and tend to increase local cerebral blood flow.[39,53,66] If autoregulation is intact, such changes can potentially lead to some vasoconstriction with a reduction of "filtration edema" or to an increased efflux of fluid as a consequence of enhanced drug action.[66,67] The administration of hypertonic agents must be carefully monitored because severe or prolonged hyperosmolarity can produce a number of systemic complications, such as metabolic acidosis, hypokalemia, oliguria, and permanent renal damage.[49]

In patients with pseudotumor cerebri occurring in association with menarche, pregnancy, the use of oral contraceptives, menstrual disturbances, or the inappropriate secretion of antidiuretic hormone, it is desirable to restrict salt intake. Severe or refractory elevations of ICP can sometimes be treated effectively by Diamox or oral isosorbide.[59] In patients with osmotic edema resulting from iatrogenically induced plasma hypoosmolarity, fluid restriction and correction of the electrolyte imbalance usually results in prompt resolution of symptoms.

Steroids

To date, the most clearly established benefits of glucocorticoids center around their ability to influence the perifocal edema occurring with mass lesions.[29,49,75] In the management of patients with malignant brain tumors, it is not uncommon for subjects who are somnolent or stuporous on admission to respond within hours to a loading dose of dexamethasone (8 to 32 mg) and to appear alert and without neurologic deficits by the following day. A similar, but less consistent, response to steroids is observed in the treatment of perifocal edema associated with cerebral abscesses, bacterial meningitis, tuberculous infections, subdural hematoma, and postoperative cerebral swelling. A dramatic response to steroids is sometimes seen in patients with pseudotumor cerebri, but this is most apt to occur in those with vasogenically induced causes, such as Addison's disease, intoxications, and allergic reactions.[59]

Despite these generally favorable results, the administration of glucocorticoids appears to be relatively ineffective when cerebral autoregulation is impaired. Thus steroid therapy is rarely of benefit in the treatment of acute hemorrhagic conditions (e.g., intracerebral hematoma) and tends to produce equivocal results in the management of patients with severe closed head injuries.[1,16,88] Indeed, evidence has been presented that the use of steroids may actually be harmful to patients with hypoxic brain damage[48] or with traumatic brain injuries producing ischemia[23] because of the augmentation of metabolic needs and the tendency of glucocorticoids to induce hyperglycemia and to increase brain lactate levels. Steroid therapy is also of little benefit in the management of vascular swelling, cytotoxic swelling, or any of the EC edemas, except for vasogenic edema.

The mechanisms by which steroids influence vasogenic edema are thought to include one or more of the following: (1) stabilization of the cerebral endothelium, leading to a decrease of plasma filtration, (2) increase in lysosomal activity of cerebral capillaries, (3) inhibition of the release of potentially toxic substances, such as free radicals, fatty acids, and prostaglandins, (4) electrolyte shifts favoring transcapillary efflux of fluid, and (5) increase in local and global cerebral glucose use, leading to improved neuronal function.[12,59,74,100] In experimental cold injury edema, it has been shown that glucocorticoids do not inhibit the arachidonic acid–prostaglandin cascade and that the beneficial effects may be related to a modification of catecholamine metabolism.[74]

Antiinflammatory Agents

Because of the many recognized complications of steroid therapy, increasing attention has been focused on the potential use of nonsteroidal antiinflammatory drugs (e.g., indomethacin, probenecid, ibuprofen) in the treatment of vasogenic edema. These agents have long been used in the management of systemic inflammations and are comparatively safe and well tolerated by most patients. Indomethacin and ibuprofen significantly reduce the vascular permeability associated with experimental gliomas,[80] and a similar response has been reported in carrageenan-induced brain inflammations treated with probenecid.[30] The mechanism of action of nonsteroidal antiinflammatory drugs has not been fully elucidated but appears to be related to a direct inhibition of the arachidonic acid–prostaglandin cascade.[30,74] In experimental gliomas, the reduction of capillary leakage by antiinflammatory agents has been found to compare favorably with that occurring after dexamethasone administration.[80]

Antihypertensive Drugs

Because the formation and spread of vasogenic edema are directly related to the systemic arterial pressure, it is desirable to reduce any untoward elevations of blood pressure by the use of controlled hypotension.[44,75] In patients with severe spreading edema, it is usually appropriate to maintain the mean arterial pressure in a physiologic range by the intravenous infusion of nitroprusside (0.1 μg/kg/min). Even lower pressures may be tolerated by otherwise normal subjects, but caution must be exercised in patients who are elderly or who have hypertension because of the risk of impairing cerebral perfusion.

CSF Drainage

CSF shunting is effective in resolving periventricular edema associated with hydrocephalus and is sometimes required in the treatment of patients with refractory pseudotumor cerebri. There is convincing evidence that CSF drainage increases the clearance of EC edema by increasing the gradient for ISF bulk flow into the cerebral ventricles.[11,81,83] To date, there are conflicting reports about the therapeutic effectiveness of CSF drainage in the management of patients with severe head injuries.[2,11,40]

Barbiturates

The therapeutic benefits of high doses of barbiturates for metabolic suppression are difficult to assess because the treatment is often a choice of last resort and is used in conjunction with many other modalities. However, barbiturates have been shown to reduce the metabolic needs of the brain,[35,38,89] and their apparent usefulness in management of vasogenic edema[15,52,75] may be related to the ability to control systemic arterial pressure and hence to reduce the filtration of fluid across leaky capillaries. When used to achieve these goals, barbiturates are administered as a loading dose of pentobarbital (3 to 5 mg/kg) or thiopental (20 mg/kg), and the drugs are then titrated by constant intravenous infusion to achieve the desired effect. Objections to barbiturate coma include the following: (1) the reduction or elimination of neurologic responses, which are often crucial in following the patient's progress, and (2) the need for continuous physiologic monitoring (e.g., ICP, blood gas levels, central venous pressure, arterial pressure), assisted ventilation, and intravenous feedings in a critical care unit.

Operative Decompression

The creation of a cranial opening (external decompression), with or without the resection of brain tissue (internal decompression), is a time-honored way for combating massive brain swelling. While often a desperate gesture, operative decompression is particularly useful in the management of unilateral hemispheric swelling when there is evidence of progressive transtentorial herniation. It is desirable to perform a generous subtemporal decompression and open the dura. If the brain is devitalized, necrotic tissue should be removed, and resection of the temporal lobe tip may relieve compression of the brainstem. Experience has shown that operative decompression is far less effective in the treatment of diffuse swelling, as compared with focal swelling, even when such radical measures as bilateral hemicalvarectomy or circumferential craniotomy are performed.[14,17,58]

SUMMARY

Cerebral edema is a common clinical disorder that results from an abnormal increase in water content within the extracellular (EC) compartment of the brain. It is distinguished from two other types of brain bulk enlargement: (1) vascular swelling, caused by arterial dilatation or venous obstruction, and (2) cellular swelling, caused by cytotoxic injuries or metabolic storage. Under normal conditions, the EC compartment has two fluids, interstitial fluid (ISF) and cerebrospinal fluid (CSF), and extends from the blood brain barrier (BBB) through a series of 100 to 150-Å-wide intercellular spaces that are anatomically continous with the CSF spaces. There are four primary types of EC edema: (1) vasogenic edema, which results from an increase in brain capillary permeability and is governed by the interaction of systemic arterial pressure and tissue resistance; (2) osmotic edema, which results from an unfavorable osmotic gradient between the plasma and ISF across an intact BBB; (3) compressive edema, which results from obstruction of ISF bulk flow pathways; and (4) hydrocephalic edema, which results from obstruction of CSF bulk flow pathways. Many clinical disorders are associated with mixed types of brain swelling and edema. The available modalities for managing brain bulk enlargement are summarized.

References

1. Alexander E: Medical management of closed head injuries, *Clin Neurosurg* 19:240, 1972.
2. Auer L: Long term monitoring of ventricular fluid pressure in patients with head injury: problems and indications, *Neurosurg Rev* 2:73, 1979.
3. Baethmann A, Oettinger W, Rothenfusser W et al: Brain edema factors: current state with particular reference to plasma constituents and glutamate, *Adv Neurol* 28:171, 1980.
4. Bering EA: Water exchange of central nervous system and cerebrospinal fluid, *J Neurosurg* 9:279, 1952.
5. Bertler A, Falck B, Owman CH et al: The localization of monoaminergic blood-brain barrier mechanisms, *Pharmacol Rev* 18:369, 1966.
6. Betz AL, Goldstein GW: The basis for active transport at the blood-brain barrier. In Eisenberg HM, Suddith RL, editors: *The cerebral microvasculature: investigation of the blood-brain barrier,* New York, 1980, Plenum Press.
7. Bradbury MWB: *The concept of a blood-brain barrier,* Chichester, England, 1979, Wiley.
8. Brightman MW: The distribution within the brain of ferritin injected into cerebrospinal fluid compartments. I. Ependymal distribution, *J Cell Biol* 26:99, 1965.
9. Brightman MW, Hori M, Rapoport SI et al: Osmotic opening of tight junctions in cerebral endothelium, *J Comp Neurol* 152:317, 1973.
10. Brightman MW, Reese TS: Junctions between intimately opposed cell membranes in the vertebrate brain, *J Cell Biol* 40:648, 1969.
11. Cao M, Lisheng H, Shouzheng S: Resolution of brain edema in severe brain injury at controlled high and low intra-cranial pressures, *J Neurosurg* 61:707, 1984.
12. Chan PH, Fishman RA, Caronna J et al: Induction of brain edema following intracerebral injection of arachidonic acid, *Ann Neurol* 13:625, 1983.
13. Clark RG, Milhorat TH: Experimental hydrocephalus. III. Light microscopic findings in acute and subacute obstructive hydrocephalus in the monkey, *J Neurosurg* 32:400, 1970.
14. Clark K, Nash TM, Hutchison GC et al: The failure of circumferential craniotomy in acute traumatic cerebral swelling, *J Neurosurg* 29:367, 1968.
15. Clasen RA, Pandolfi S, Casey D: Furosemide and pentobarbital in cryogenic cerebral injury and edema, *Neurology* 24:642, 1974.
16. Cooper PR, Moody S, Clark WK et al: Dexamethasone and severe head injury. A prospective double-blind study, *J Neurosurg* 51:307, 1979.
17. Cooper PR, Rovit RL, Ransohoff J: Hemicraniectomy in the treatment of acute subdural hematoma: A reappraisal, *Surg Neurol* 5:25, 1976.
18. Cserr HF: Convection of brain interstitial fluid. In Shapiro K, Marmarou A, Portnoy H, editors: *Hydrocephalus,* New York, 1984, Raven Press.
19. Cserr HF, Cooper DN, Milhorat TH: Flow of cerebral interstitial fluid as indicated by the removal of extracellular markers from rat caudate nucleus, *Exp Eye Res* 25:461, 1977.
20. Cutler RWP: Neurochemical aspects of blood-brain-cerebrospinal fluid barriers. In Wood JH, editor: *Neurobiology of cerebrospinal fluid,* vol 1, New York, 1980, Plenum Press.
21. Davis DA, Milhorat TH: The blood-brain barrier of the rat choroid plexus, *Anat Rec* 181:779, 1975.
22. Davson H: The blood-cerebrospinal fluid and blood-brain barriers, *Ergeb Physiol* 52:20, 1963.
23. Deutschman CS, Konstantinides FN, Raup S et al: Physiological and metabolic response to isolated closed head injury. II. Effects of steroids on metabolism, *J Neurosurg* 66:388, 1987.
24. DiMattio J, Hochwald GM, Malhan C et al: Effects of changes in serum osmolarity on bulk flow of fluid into cerebral ventricles and on brain water content, *Pflugers Arch* 359:253, 1975.
25. Doczi T, Szerdahelyi P, Gulya K et al: Brain water accumulation after the central administration of vasopressin, *Neurosurgery* 11:402, 1982.
26. Fenstermacher JD, Gross P, Sposito N et al: Structural and functional variations in capillary systems within the brain. In Strand FL, editor: Fourth Colloquium in Biological Sciences: blood-brain transfer, *Ann NY Acad Sci* 529:21, 1988.
27. Fenstermacher JD, Rall DP: Physiology and pharmacology of cerebrospinal fluid. In Capri A, editor: *Pharmacology of the cerebral circulation,* New York, 1972, Pergamon Press.
28. Franklin GM, Dudzinski DS, Cutler RWP: Amino acid transport into the cerebrospinal fluid of the rat, *J Neurochem* 24:367, 1975.

6 *The Blood-Brain Barrier and Cerebral Edema* **147**

29. Galicich JH, French LA: Use of dexamethasone in the treatment of cerebral edema resulting from brain tumors and brain surgery, *Am Practit* 12:169, 1961.

30. Gamache DA, Ellis EF: Effect of dexamethasone, indomethacin, ibuprofen, and probenecid on carrageenan-induced brain inflammation, *J Neurosurg* 65:686, 1986.

31. Go KG: The classification of brain edema. In de Vlieger M, de Lange SA, Beks JWF, editors: *Brain edema,* New York, 1981, Wiley.

32. Go KG, Gazendam J, Van Zanten AK: The influence of hypoxia on the composition of isolated edema fluid in cold-induced brain edema, *J Neurosurg* 51:78, 1979.

33. Goldmann EE: Die aüssere und innere Sekretion des gesunden und kranken Organismus in Lichte der "vitalen Farbung," *Beitr Klin Chirurg* 64:192, 1909.

34. Goldmann EE: Vitalfärbung am Zentralnervensystem, *Abh Preuss Akad Wiss Phys-Math* 1:1, 1913.

35. Goldstein A, Wells BA, Keats AS: Increased tolerance to cerebral anoxia by pentobarbital, *Arch Int Pharm Ther* 161:138, 1966.

36. Goldstein GW: In vitro studies of glial-endothelial cell interactions. In Strand FL, editor: Fourth Colloquim in Biological Sciences: Blood-Brain Transfer, *Ann NY Acad Sci* 529:98, 1988.

37. Graziani LJ, Kaplan RK, Escriva A: Calcium flux into CSF during ventricular and ventriculocisternal perfusion, *Am J Physiol* 213:629, 1967.

38. Hoff JT, Smith AL, Hankinson HL et al: Barbiturate protection from cerebral infarction in primates, *Stroke* 6:28, 1975.

39. Jafar JJ, Johns LM, Mullan SF: The effect of mannitol on cerebral blood flow, *J Neurosurg* 64:754, 1986.

40. Jennett B, Teasdale G: *Management of head injuries,* Philadelphia, 1981, FA Davis.

41. Johansson BB, Linder LE: The blood brain barrier in renal hypertensive rats, *Clin Exp Hypertens* 2:983, 1980.

42. Kalbag RM, Woolf AL: *Cerebral venous thrombosis,* London, 1967, Oxford University Press.

43. Katzman R, Graziani LJ, Kaplan RK et al: Exchange of cerebrospinal fluid potassium with blood and brain, *Arch Neurol* 13:513, 1965.

44. Katzman R, Pappius HM: *Brain electrolytes and fluid metabolism,* Baltimore, 1973, Williams & Wilkins.

45. Klatzo I: Neuropathological aspects of brain edema, *J Neuropath Exp Neurol* 26:1, 1967.

46. Klatzo I, Chui E, Fujiwara K: Aspects of the blood-brain barrier in brain edema. In de Vlieger M, de Lange SA, Beks JWF, editors: *Brain edema,* New York, 1981, Wiley.

47. Klatzo I, Piraux A, Laskowski EJ: The relationship between edema, blood-brain barrier and tissue elements in a local brain injury, *J Neuropath Exp Neurol* 17:548, 1958.

48. Koide T, Wieloch TW, Siesjo BK: Chronic dexamethasone pretreatment aggravates ischemic neuronal necrosis, *J Cerebr Blood Flow Metab* 6:395, 1986.

49. Langfitt TW: Increased intracranial pressure and the cerebral circulation. In Youmans JR, editor: *Neurological surgery,* vol 2, Philadelphia, 1982, WB Saunders.

50. Langfitt TW, Kassell NF: Cerebral vasodilatation produced by brain stem stimulation: neurogenic control vs. autoregulation, *Am J Physiol* 215:90, 1968.

51. Maren TH, Broder LE: The role of carbonic anhydrase in anion secretion into cerebrospinal fluid, *J Pharmacol Exp Ther* 172:197, 1970.

52. Marshall LF, Bruce DA, Bruno LA et al: Role of intracranial pressure monitoring and barbiturate therapy in malignant intracranial hypertension, *J Neurosurg* 47:481, 1977.

53. Meyer FB, Anderson RE, Sundt TM et al: Treatment of experimental focal cerebral ischemia with mannitol. Assessment by intracellular brain pH, cortical blood flow, and electroencephalography, *J Neurosurg* 66:109, 1987.

54. Milhorat TH: Choroid plexus and cerebrospinal fluid production, *Science* 166:1514, 1969.

55. Milhorat TH: *Hydrocephalus and the cerebrospinal fluid,* Baltimore, 1972, Williams & Wilkins.

56. Milhorat TH: The third circulation revisited, *J Neurosurg* 42:628, 1975.

57. Milhorat TH: Structure and function of the choroid plexus and other sites of cerebrospinal fluid formation, *Int Rev Cytol* 47:225, 1976.

58. Milhorat TH: *Pediatric neurosurgery,* Philadelphia, 1978, FA Davis.

59. Milhorat TH: *Cerebrospinal fluid and the brain edemas,* New York, 1987, Neuroscience Society of New York.

60. Milhorat TH: Classification of cerebral edema with reference to hydrocephalus, *Child's Nerv Sys* 8:301, 1992.

61. Milhorat TH, Davis DA, Lloyd BJ: Two morphologically distinct blood-brain barriers preventing entry of cytochrome c into cerebrospinal fluid, *Science* 180:76, 1973.

62. Milhorat TH, Hammock MK: Isotope ventriculography. Interpretation of ventricular size and configuration in hydrocephalus, *Arch Neurol* 25:1, 1971.

63. Milhorat TH, Hammock MK: Cerebrospinal fluid as reflection of internal milieu of brain. In Wood JH, editor: *Neurobiology of cerebrospinal fluid,* vol 2, New York, 1983, Plenum Press.

64. Milhorat TH, Hammock MK, Fenstermacher JD et al: Cerebrospinal fluid production by the choroid plexus and brain, *Science* 173:330, 1971.

65. Milhorat TH, Johnson WD, Dow-Edwards DL: Relationship between oedema, blood pressure, and blood flow following local brain injury, *Neurol Res* 11:29, 1989.

66. Muizelaar JP, Lutz HA, Becker DP: Effect of mannitol on ICP and CBF and correlation with pressure autoregulation in severely head-injured patients, *J Neurosurg* 61:700, 1984.

67. Nath F, Galbraith S: The effect of mannitol on cerebral white matter content, *J Neurosurg* 65:41, 1986.

68. Oldendorf WH: Blood-brain barrier. In Himwich HE, editor: *Brain metabolism and cerebral disorders,* ed 2, New York, 1976, Spectrum Publications.

69. Oldendorf WH, Cornford ME, Brown WJ: The large apparent work capability of the blood-brain barrier: a study of the mitochondrial content of capillary endothelial cells in brain and other tissues of the rat, *Ann Neurol* 1:409, 1977.

70. Oppelt WW, Owens ES, Rall DP: Calcium exchange between blood and cerebrospinal fluid, *Life Sci* 2:599, 1963.

71. Pappenheimer JR: On the location of the blood-brain barrier. In Pappenheimer JR, editor: *Proceedings of the Wales Symposium on the Blood-*

Brain Barrier, London, 1970, Oxford University Press.

72. Pappenheimer JR, Fencl V, Heissy SR et al: Role of cerebral fluids in control of respiration in unanesthetized goats, *Am J Physiol* 208:436, 1965.

73. Pappius HM: Local cerebral glucose utilization in thermally traumatized rat brain, *Ann Neurol* 9:484, 1981.

74. Pappius HM, Wolfe LS: Functional disturbances in brain following injury: search for underlying mechanisms, *Neurochem Res* 8:63, 1983.

75. Pollay M: Blood-brain barrier; cerebral edema. In Wilkins RH, Rengachary SS, editors: *Neurosurgery,* vol 1, New York, 1985, McGraw-Hill.

76. Posner JB, Plum F: Independence of blood and cerebrospinal fluid lactate, *Arch Neurol* 16:492, 1967.

77. Rall DP, Stabenau JR, Zubrod CG: Distribution of drugs between blood and cerebrospinal fluid: general methodology and effect of pH gradients, *J Pharmacol Exp Ther* 125:185, 1959.

78. Rapoport SI: *Blood-brain barrier in physiology and medicine,* New York, 1976, Raven Press.

79. Reése TS, Karnovsky MJ: Fine structural localization of a blood-brain barrier to exogenous peroxidase, *J Cell Biol* 34:207, 1967.

80. Reichman HR, Farrell CL, Del Maestro RF: Effects of steroids and non-steroid anti-inflammatory agents on vascular permeability in a rat glioma model, *J Neurosurg* 65:233, 1986.

81. Reulen HJ, Graham R, Spatz M et al: Role of pressure gradients and bulk flow in dynamics of vasogenic brain edema, *J Neurosurg* 46:24, 1977.

82. Reulen HJ, Prioleau GR, Tsuyumu M et al: Clearance of edema fluid into cerebrospinal fluid, In Wood JH, editor: *Neurobiology of cerebrospinal fluid,* vol 2, New York, 1983, Plenum Press.

83. Reulen HJ, Tsuyumu M: Pathophysiology of formation and natural resolution of vasogenic brain edema. In de Vlieger M, de Lange SA, Beks JWF, editors: *Brain edema,* 1981, New York, Wiley.

84. Rosenberg GA, Kyner WT: Effect of mannitol-induced hyperosmolarity on transport between brain interstitial fluid and cerebrospinal fluid. In Wood JH, editor: *Neurobiology of cerebrospinal fluid,* vol 2, New York, 1983, Plenum Press.

85. Rosner MJ: Vasodilatory cascade and intracranial pressure waves: theory, physiology, and therapy. In Miller JD, Teasdale JO, editors: *Intracranial pressure,* New York, 1987, Springer-Verlag.

86. Rosner MJ, Coley IB: Cerebral perfusion pressure, intracranial pressure, and head elevation, *J Neurosurg* 65:636, 1986.

87. Rubin RC, Henderson ES, Ommaya AK et al: The production of cerebrospinal fluid in man and its modification by acetazolamide, *J Neurosurg* 25:430, 1966.

88. Saul TG, Ducker TB, Sakman M et al: Steroids in severe head injury. A prospective randomized clinical trial, *J Neurosurg* 54:596, 1981.

89. Shapiro HM, Wyte SR, Loeser J: Barbiturate-augmented hypothermia for reduction of persistent intracranial hypertension, *J Neurosurg* 40:90, 1974.

90. Stern J, Hochwald GM, Wald A et al: Visualization of brain interstitial fluid movement during osmotic disequilibrium, *Exp Eye Res* 25:475, 1977.

91. Takagi H, Saitoh T, Kitahara T et al: The mechanism of ICP reducing effect of mannitol. In Ishii S, Nagai H, Brock M, editors: *Intracranial pressure V,* New York, 1983, Springer-Verlag.

92. Torack RM, Barrnett RJ: The fine structural localization of nucleoside phosphatase activity in the blood-brain barrier, *J Neuropath Exp Neurol* 23:46, 1964.

93. Tschirgi RD: Protein complexes and the impermeability of the blood-brain barrier to dyes, *Am J Physiol* 163:756, 1950.

94. Van Gelder NM: A possible enzyme barrier for gamma-aminobutyric acid in central nervous system, *Prog Brain Res* 28:259, 1968.

95. Vorstrup S, Christensen J, Gjerris F et al: Cerebral blood flow in patients with normal pressure hydrocephalus before and after shunting, *J Neurosurg* 66:379, 1987.

96. Wasterlain CG, Torack RM: Cerebral edema in water intoxication, *Arch Neurol* 19:79, 1968.

97. Winn HR, Rubio GR, Berne RM: The role of adenosine in the regulation of cerebral blood flow, *J Cereb Blood Flow Metab* 1:239, 1981.

98. Wise BL, Chater N: The value of hypertonic mannitol solution in decreasing brain mass and lowering cerebrospinal fluid pressure, *J Neurosurg* 19:1038, 1962.

99. Wood JH: Neuroendocrinology of cerebrospinal fluid: peptides, steroids and other hormones, *Neurosurgery* 11:293, 1982.

100. Yamada K, Ushio Y, Hayakawa T et al: Effects of methylprednisolone on peritumoral brain edema. A quantitative autoradiographic study, *J Neurosurg* 59:612, 1983.

101. Zulch KJ: Neuropathological aspects and histological criteria of brain edema and brain swelling. In Klatzo I, Seitelberger F, editors: *Brain edema,* New York, 1967, Springer-Verlag.

7

Effects of Anesthetic Agents and Other Drugs on Cerebral Blood Flow, Metabolism, and Intracranial Pressure

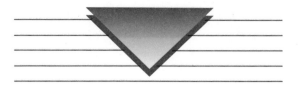

TAKEFUMI SAKABE
KAZUHIKO NAKAKIMURA

Major goals in neurosurgical anesthesia are to provide adequate tissue perfusion to the brain (and spinal cord) so that the regional metabolic demand is met and to provide adequate surgical conditions (a "relaxed brain"). The role of anesthetic drugs in achieving these goals will be discussed.

If anesthetic drugs or anesthetic techniques are improperly used, they can worsen the existing intracranial pathology and may produce new damage. Some anesthetics or anesthetic techniques may help protect the brain subjected to metabolic stress or even ameliorate damage from such an insult. Thus it is important to know the effects of anesthetics and anesthetic techniques on cerebral circulation, metabolism, and intracranial pressure (ICP) in both normal and pathologic conditions.

In this chapter, the basic aspects concerning regulation of cerebral blood flow (CBF) and ICP will be summarized. This will be followed by a review of the effects of anesthetics and other drugs on CBF, cerebral metabolism, and ICP. The clinical relevance of these issues to the practice of neurosurgical anesthesia will be discussed and applied not only to patients undergoing neurosurgery but also to patients who have neurologic disorders and are undergoing other types of surgery. Abbreviations frequently used in this chapter are summarized in Box 7-1.

149

▼

```
┌─────────────────────────────────────────────────┐
│                   BOX 7-1                         │
│                ABBREVIATIONS                      │
├─────────────────────────────────────────────────┤
│  CBF       Cerebral blood flow                    │
│  lCBF      Local cerebral blood flow              │
│  rCBF      Regional cerebral blood flow           │
│  CBV       Cerebral blood volume                  │
│  CMRO₂     Cerebral metabolic rate for oxygen     │
│  CMRgl     Cerebral metabolic rate for glucose    │
│  lCMRgl    Local cerebral metabolic rate for glucose │
│  MABP      Mean arterial blood pressure           │
│  CPP       Cerebral perfusion pressure            │
│  CVR       Cerebral vascular resistance           │
│  ICP       Intracranial pressure                  │
│  CSF       Cerebrospinal fluid                    │
│  CSFP      Cerebrospinal fluid pressure           │
│  Sch       Succinylcholine                        │
│  D-Tc      D-tubocurarine                         │
│  SNP       Sodium nitroprusside (nitroprusside)   │
│  TNG       Trinitroglyceride (nitroglycerine)     │
│  TMP       Trimethaphan                           │
└─────────────────────────────────────────────────┘
```

BASIC ASPECTS OF REGULATION OF CBF AND ICP

Regulation of CBF

Brain tissue perfusion is regulated through various mechanisms, including metabolic, chemical, and neurogenic regulation, and autoregulation. Rheologic changes are also relevant. These regulatory mechanisms may be attenuated or impaired by various pathologic conditions as well as by some anesthetic drugs.

Metabolic Regulation

Cerebral functional changes induced by voluntary movement of the extremities, psychologic tasks, sensory stimulation, anxiety, or stress are accompanied by increases in metabolism that are coupled to increases in CBF. This phenomenon is called metabolic regulation of CBF. Local tissue metabolites such as CO_2, lactate, H^+, K^+, Ca^{2+}, adenosine, and cyclic adenosine monophosphate are postulated as mediators that maintain tight coupling of neuronal activity (function), metabolism, and blood flow. However, the exact mechanisms that link flow and metabolism are unclear. In pathologic conditions, this regulatory mechanism is impaired either globally or regionally. Certain anesthetic drugs also alter this coupling.

Chemical Regulation

In general, CO_2 and O_2 are considered to be the chemical regulatory factors. CO_2 can produce marked changes in cerebrovascular resistance (CVR) and CBF. Over a range of $Paco_2$ of 20 to 80 mm Hg, for each 1 mm Hg increase or decrease in $Paco_2$ a 2% to 4% increase or decrease in CBF occurs. Compared with adults, children have less cerebral reactivity to CO_2 changes. Changes in the extracellular H^+ concentration have been considered a major regulatory factor for cerebrovascular reactivity to CO_2. At a $Paco_2$ level above 80 mm Hg, the CBF reactivity is diminished because the vasculature has reached maximal dilation. Below a $Paco_2$ of 20 mm Hg, the hypoxia from vasoconstriction prevents further vascular changes.

CO_2 reactivity is modified by time. For example, over a period of 5 hours, despite continued hyperventilation, CBF returns to previous levels because CSF pH gradually normalizes as a result of the renal extrusion of bicarbonate.[194] It has been reported that CSF pH adaptation has an estimated half-time of about 6 hours, and is complete within 30 hours. During chronic hypocapnia with spontaneous ventilation, CSF pH gradually declines to normal over 3 to 5 days, with concomitant return of CBF to normal. With chronic hypercapnia, bicarbonate is retained, maintaining CSF pH constant. These changes in reactivity to CO_2 should be considered while managing patients in the intensive care unit or during prolonged operations.

During acute hypoxia, CBF increases when Pao_2 falls below 50 mm Hg, provided that blood pressure is maintained. The mechanism for this increase in CBF may be due, in part, to an increase in lactate or adenosine in brain tissue. Hyperoxia, often seen in clinical practice, appears to have minimal effect on CBF.

Autoregulation and Cerebral Perfusion Pressure

CBF is maintained relatively constant despite changes in arterial blood pressure. This is called autoregulation. The upper and lower limits of autoregulation in adult humans are cerebral perfusion pressures (CPP) of approximately 150 and 50 mm Hg, respectively. In children, both the upper and lower limits of autoregulation are assumed to be lower than those of adult. Autoregulation does not work instantaneously; CBF changes for a few minutes after altering arterial pressure and then returns to the previous level.

When CPP (or mean arterial blood pressure, MABP) increases above the upper limit of autoregulation, an increase in CBF may be accompanied by a disruption of the blood-brain barrier, and plasma protein may leak into the tissue and cause brain edema. This "breakthrough" occurs more easily when cerebral vessels are dilated by hypercapnia or cerebral vasodilators.

In pathologic conditions, autoregulation may be diminished or completely abolished, either globally or regionally, and in this situation CBF becomes dependent on blood pressure. Chronic hypertensive subjects have higher upper and lower limits of autoregulation than do normotensive subjects. Thus hypertensive patients may not tolerate levels of hypotension tolerated by normotensive subjects. Similar shifts in the upper and lower limits of autoregulation are encountered when sympathetic nerves are stimulated. Therefore hemorrhagic hypotension, which is usually accompanied by sympathetic stimulation, causes a more pronounced reduction in CBF compared with that seen during drug-induced hypotension.

Neurogenic Control

The cerebral vessels receive substantial innervation from cholinergic, adrenergic, and serotonergic fibers, the density of nerve fibers being higher in the larger vessels than in the smaller ones. It has been suggested that the primary regulation of extraparenchymal vessels is neurogenic and that of intraparenchymal vessels is metabolic-chemical. Under normal conditions, the neurogenic influence is less obvious than that of the metabolic-chemical influence. However, it becomes more apparent during stressful situations.

Rheology

The Hagen-Poiseuille equation relates blood flow *(Q)* through vessels as a function of the pressure difference *(ΔP)*, vessel radius *(r)*, length *(L)*, and blood viscosity *(η)*.

$$Q = \frac{\Delta P \pi r^4}{8 L \eta}$$

However, because blood is a non-Newtonian fluid, the exact blood flow differs from that calculated by this equation. Nevertheless, it is true that changes in blood viscosity influence CBF, and hematocrit is the most important determinant of blood viscosity. Thus CBF increases with severe anemia, but it decreases with polycythemia. Optimal oxygen delivery is thought to be obtained with a hematocrit value of 30% to 34%. When cerebral vessel dilation is prevented by vessel spasm or stenosis, rCBF may be increased by decreasing blood viscosity. Thus hemodilution is often employed to improve regional CBF in patients with cerebrovascular occlusive diseases.

Regulation of ICP

During physiologic conditions, ICP is maintained in a fairly limited range (5 to 13 mm Hg). ICP is determined by brain tissue volume, cerebral blood volume (CBV), and cerebrospinal fluid (CSF) volume. These compartments normally account for approximately 85%, 5%, and 10% of the total intracranial volume, respectively. A decrease in the volume of any one of these compartments compensates for increases in intracranial volume. Decreasing the CSF volume by shifting CSF into the spinal subarachnoid space is the primary mechanism for compensation under most circumstances. Other compensatory mechanisms include reduction in CBV from compression of cerebral veins. Anesthetic drugs and techniques or changes in physiological variables (such as $Paco_2$, Pao_2, blood pressure, venous pressure, or intrathoracic pressure) influence CBV and ICP.

Changes in CBF and ICP Regulation with Pathologic Conditions

Brain tissue hypoxia, acidosis, and edema are the main pathological consequences of most brain disorders. In acute brain disorders, cerebral vasoparalysis occurs and coupling between blood flow and metabolism is impaired. As the injury becomes chronic, coupling tends to recover. During the period of vasoparalysis, CBF is usually greater than $CMRo_2$ if perfusion pressure is adequate ("luxury perfusion"). Under these circumstances, autoregulation and CO_2 reactivity are also disturbed, although disturbances in the former are more common than disturbances in the latter. Strict blood pressure control is important in the management of these patients because the failure in autoregulation makes cerebral perfusion tightly dependent on mean arterial blood pressure (MABP) in contrast with the normal situation.

CO_2 reactivity may be attenuated or abolished either globally or regionally. In the event of focal cerebral ischemia, a complex response to $Paco_2$ changes may result. During hypercapnia, the normal vessels dilate but the vessels in the damaged area do not respond to the change in $Paco_2$. Consequently blood flow is shunted from the ischemic to the normal area (intracerebral steal). Conversely, during hypocapnia, the normal vessels constrict and blood is diverted to the ischemic area (inverse intracerebral steal, or Robin Hood phenomenon). This is why hypocapnia has been recommended in acute stroke because it may increase CBF to functionally depressed but not irreversibly damaged areas (penumbra). However, the inverse steal does not predictably occur in every patient with focal ischemia, so normocapnia is recommended except on the occasion of severe life threatening intracranial hypertension where hypocapnia is required to decrease ICP. Hypercapnia should be avoided.

Although not confirmed for every anesthetic, experimental data in animals suggest that intracerebral steal or inverse steal may possibly be induced pharmacologically. Anesthetics that dilate vessels may produce the steal phenomenon by dilating the vessels in the normal brain tissue without changing the vessel diameter in the damaged area. Anesthetics that constrict the vessels have the opposite effect, resulting in inverse steal, and may protect the brain or ameliorate the damage.[28,62]

CO_2 and acetazolamide have been used to evaluate cerebral collateral capacity in patients with cerebrovascular occlusive disease.[182,264] In the patient at risk, CBF may decrease further in the poorly perfused areas if CO_2 is inhaled or acetazolamide is administered. Positive findings suggest that these patients would tolerate poorly a reduction of blood pressure.

When intracranial compensatory mechanisms are impaired, ICP tends to increase exponentially with small changes in CBV, and this may cause a decrease in CPP. Thus any drug or technique that produces an increase in CBF (CBV) has potential hazard. If an increase in CBF is unavoidable, preventive measures such as hyperventilation, concomitant use of vasoconstrictive anesthetics, and osmotic diuretics should be employed.

EFFECTS OF ANESTHETIC DRUGS AND OTHER DRUGS

General Considerations

Blood Flow and Metabolism Changes in Relation to Functional Changes

Anesthetics cause functional alterations in the central nervous system and produce metabolic changes. Anesthesia long has been believed to produce a state of functional depression that is accompanied by a reduction in $CMRo_2$. Although this is true for many anesthetics, the anesthetic state is not necessarily accompanied by a reduction in $CMRo_2$. Differences between drugs have become discernable with advances in techniques for measuring regional blood flow and metabolism. Some anesthetics increase metabolic rate in specific structures of the brain, reflecting an induced increase in functional activity. These metabolic increases are usually accompanied by a decrease in vascular resistance and an increase in CBF. Metabolic depression, in contrast, is accompanied by an increase in vascular resistance and a decrease in CBF. This coupling is maintained with most intravenous anesthetics. In contrast, with most inhalational anesthetics, CBF increases while $CMRo_2$ decreases. The increase in the ratio of CBF to $CMRo_2$ suggests a disturbance in coupling. The uncoupling is greater as anesthetic depth is increased. There is a positive correlation between MAC multiples and the $CBF/CMRo_2$ ratio for all volatile anesthetics. However, it is notable that there is a strong correlation between cerebral metabolic rate for glucose (CMRgl) and CBF within individual brain structures during either halothane or isoflurane anesthesia.[81] It has also been reported that seizure activity[142] or noxious stimuli[109] during anesthesia produces parallel increases in CBF and $CMRo_2$. These data suggest that the coupling is not lost but only altered during inhalation anesthesia.

Anesthesia alters ICP because of changes in CBV, and, in general, this appears to be proportional to the changes in CBF.[8,9] Thus an increase in CBF causes an increase of CBV and thus ICP. The magnitude of the increase in CBV is determined mainly by the cerebral vasodilatory potency of anesthetics as well as the changes in $Paco_2$ (and Pao_2). Blood pressure increases, especially when autoregulation is impaired, also produce an increase in CBV. Mechanical effects, such as patient's posture and respiratory pattern (by influencing intrathoracic pressure) also may influence ICP. Increases in central venous pressure are directly transmitted to the intracranial veins and result in an increase in cerebrospinal fluid pressure (CSFP). Thus inappropriate head-neck rotation, head-down position, excessive positive end expiratory pressure (PEEP), bucking, and straining should be avoided in patients with decreased intracranial compliance.

Anesthetic agents also affect ICP by changing the rate of production and absorption of CSF.[10-12] These effects, however, appear to be small compared with the effects of anesthetics on CBF (and CBV). Furthermore, when the dura is opened, CSF is drained and the increase in CSF production rate or decreased absorption is less important.

Normally the body compensates for an increase in ICP by displacement of CSF from the cranium. When compensatory mechanisms are exhausted, a small additional increase in intracranial volume produces dramatic increases in ICP. The increase in ICP may cause cerebral ischemia as well as localized compression or herniation that may be life-threatening. Even if the elevation in ICP has not reached this critical magnitude, it may lead to poor operating conditions because of a bulging brain.

Spinal Cord Blood Flow and Metabolism

Limited data are available concerning spinal cord blood flow and metabolism. However, there is no reason to suspect that they would differ from those of the brain.[119] Pharmacologic and physiologic principles discussed for the brain can also be applied in the case of spinal cord pathology.

EFFECTS OF SPECIFIC ANESTHETIC DRUGS AND OTHER DRUGS

Inhalational Anesthetics

In general, all the inhalational anesthetics can be considered to be more or less potent cerebral vasodilators and thus possess the capability of increasing ICP. Inhalational anesthetics, with the possible exception of nitrous oxide (N_2O), usually depress metabolism. Despite the dissociation of CBF and $CMRo_2$, changes in the magnitude of cerebral vasodilation still appear to be related to the level of tissue metabolism.

Nitrous Oxide (N_2O)

There are great variations in the reported effects of N_2O. One possible cause for these variations is that N_2O is often used in combination with other drugs that may modify its original effect. Another reason may be a species variation in MAC values. Theye and Michenfelder[248] observed increases in both CBF and $CMRo_2$ with 70% N_2O in dogs that had received vagotomy and total spinal anesthesia. Several subsequent studies in dogs confirmed that 60% N_2O increased both CBF and $CMRo_2$ by about 100% and 20%, respectively.[211] Reserpine pretreatment did not alter the effect of N_2O on CBF and $CMRo_2$, suggesting that the increases were not related to the sympathetic hyperactivity.[211] In the goat, N_2O was reported to increase CBF and $CMRo_2$ without producing any increase in plasma catecholamine.[191]

In mice and rats, most studies demonstrated no change in CBF and $CMRo_2$.[34,46] However, Baughman et al.[21] demonstrated that, in unanesthetized unrestrained rats, 70% N_2O produced a significant increase in CBF without affecting $CMRo_2$ or plasma catecholamine concentrations. Thus the inability to demonstrate the effect of N_2O in the previous studies of rats might have been due to the control situation in which the rats were restrained and the effect of N_2O might have been masked.

The interaction of N_2O with volatile anesthetics is complex. With addition of N_2O to 0.8% halothane in dogs, CBF and $CMRo_2$ increased by 60% and 10%, respectively, indicating that the increases were slightly attenuated compared with the 100% and 20% increases observed in dogs maintained with 0.2% halothane.[211] In swine an increase in CBF (and $CMRo_2$) has been reported for N_2O, whether given alone or in combination with various volatile anesthetics.[134] Seyde et al.[225] reported that in rats the addition of N_2O to a background halothane anesthetic was associated with dilation of cerebral vasculature (and an increase in ICP). In rabbits, the increase in CBF was greater when N_2O was added to a higher concentration of either halothane or isoflurane (0.5 MAC vs. 1.0 MAC).[56] Baughman et al.[20] have shown that in rats, the addition of N_2O to an isoflurane background anesthetic increased CBF, the increase being numerically greater at 0.5 MAC than at 1 MAC isoflurane. Roald et al.[202] recently demonstrated in dogs that N_2O, when added to 1 MAC isoflurane, produced an increase in CBF, but it did not do so when added to 2.2 MAC isoflurane. There were no significant changes in $CMRo_2$ when N_2O was added to both concentrations of isoflurane. It is not clear whether the differences in modification of N_2O-induced increases in CBF by volatile anesthetics are due to the differences in species, methodology, or the concentration ranges of the volatile anesthetics examined.

The interaction of N_2O with intravenous anesthetics also is complex. In dogs, cerebral circulatory and metabolic changes induced by N_2O were completely blocked by the pretreatment with thiamylal.[211] In rabbits, morphine, when added to 0.5 MAC of halothane or isoflurane, did not alter the cerebral vasodilating effect of N_2O.[56] Kaieda et al.[101] reported less increase in CBF from N_2O when it was given under a fentanyl and pentobarbital background anesthesic compared with a background of 1 MAC of halothane or isoflurane. In rats, when N_2O was combined with diazepam, a marked decrease in CBF and $CMRo_2$ has been reported, suggesting a synergistic effect.[35] Different results have been reported when N_2O was added to other benzodiazepines; one study showed that N_2O added to midazolam increased $CMRo_2$ with no change in CBF in rats,[91] and another study showed an increase in CBF with no change in $CMRo_2$ in dogs.[63] Again, it is not clear whether this discrepancy in the effects of N_2O combined with benzodiazepines is due to the differences in species, methodology, or the doses examined.

Regional metabolic studies in rats demonstrated that N_2O increased lCMRgl by 15% to 25% in subcortical structures.[95] N_2O increases lCMRgl in the brain and spinal cord.[45] An increased cerebral metabolism was observed in rats lightly anesthetized with pentobarbital after the addition of N_2O but not in rats anesthetized with doses of pentobarbital that produced a flat EEG,[213] indicating that during pentobarbital anesthesia N_2O acts as a cerebral metabolic stimulant in the presence of cortical function (EEG). Cole et al.[42] reported that increasing the N_2O concentration (while concurrently decreasing enflurane concentration to maintain a total anesthetic dose of 1.2 MAC) produced a biphasic metabolic response; 30% N_2O with enflurane produced a heterogenous increase in lCMRgl in the brain and a homogenous increase in the spinal cord, but with 60% N_2O, the increase in lCMRgl tended to be less. As CO_2 reactivity is preserved, the CBF increase produced by N_2O was usually reversed during hypocapnia. However, in rabbits, the increase in CBF and ICP observed when N_2O was added to 1 MAC halothane or isoflurane persisted despite hypocapnia.[101]

In humans, classic studies demonstrated that N_2O did not significantly affect CBF, although it decreased $CMRo_2$ by 2% to 23%.[229] However, these results might have been affected by premedication, anesthetic induction drugs, or body temperature. In patients anesthetized with 0.84% halothane, the addition of 60% N_2O significantly increased the CBF equivalent (reciprocal of $C(a-v)o_2$, which is equal to $CBF/CMRo_2$), suggesting that N_2O is a cerebral vasodilator.[210] The combined use of N_2O and morphine has been reported to have no significant effect on CBF and $CMRo_2$.[100] However, there is a possibility that the effect of N_2O can be antagonized by the effect of morphine.

An increase in ICP caused by N_2O has been repeatedly demonstrated in humans[167] and in animals.[3,211] The increase can be attenuated by prior administration of thiopental, diazepam, or morphine, or induction of hypocapnia.[192,211] Although, in some animal studies, this increase in CBF and ICP is not prevented by hypocapnia,[251] it is advisable to use hypocapnia and/or cerebral vasoconstricting drugs when N_2O is used, especially for induction of anesthesia in patients with decreased intracranial compliance. N_2O may also increase ICP when an intracranial air space exists because N_2O diffuses into air space more rapidly than N_2 diffuses out. N_2O should be avoided or immediately withdrawn during such occasions.

Some have proposed that N_2O has neurotoxic properties. In mice subjected to hypoxia, survival time has been reported to be either reduced[83] or unchanged.[154] The reason for the discrepancy between these two studies is not known. During incomplete ischemia, N_2O has been reported to attenuate the cerebral protective effects of isoflurane.[20] In that study, addition of N_2O to 0.5 MAC isoflurane attenuated the improvement in neurologic outcome and produced more histologic damage compared with isoflurane alone. It is difficult, based on current data, to determine whether N_2O should be avoided during operations on the central nervous system. Michenfelder[149] stated that "at the least it would seem clinically prudent in the event of a tight brain. . . that efforts to reduce brain mass should include discontinuation of N_2O whenever possible."

Halothane

In the majority of animal experiments,[4,230,240,250] halothane produces an increase in CBF in association with a decrease in CVR. The varying magnitude of the increase in CBF reported may be due not only to species differences but also to the level of CPP. If the blood pressure decrease that occurs with halothane is not corrected, the increase in CBF is less.

At low concentrations, the results with halothane are conflicting. Earlier studies described a decrease in CBF at concentrations of 0.5% or lower. A recent study by Brüssel et al.[30] demonstrated in primates that low concentrations of halothane (0.125% to 0.375%) produced a 10% to 20% reduction of CBF compared with the baseline value (phencyclidine and N_2O background anesthesia), suggesting that the decrease in CBF may result from the reduction in $CMRo_2$. An increase in CBF with concentrations of halothane above 0.375% was demonstrated, provided that the systemic blood pressure was maintained with a vasopressor. There is a possibility that an interaction between halothane and drugs used as the background anesthesia might have affected the results. Direct comparison may be difficult in these studies because of the differences in species, experimental design, or drugs used concomitantly. However, it is possible that at low concentration, the cerebral vasodilatory effect of halothane is weak and flow may be determined by the metabolic depressive effect. At higher concentration, the vasodilating effect overcomes this metabolism-dependent vasoconstrictive action and results in a net increase in CBF. Similar dose-related biphasic flow response has been reported for isoflurane.[259] Regional flow measurement in the rat demonstrated that vasodilation with halothane is more prominent in the cerebral cortex when compared with subcortical structures, but isoflurane dilates vessels in the subcortical structures.[81]

In humans, most studies demonstrated that halothane induces cerebral vasodilation and increases CBF, provided that the systemic blood pressure is maintained. Using the ^{133}Xe-clearance method, Eintrei et al.[58] demonstrated that the increase in rCBF in cerebral cortex close to cerebral tumors was greater with halothane than with enflurane or isoflurane at equiMAC concentrations.

Although the mechanism of the cerebral vasodilation produced by halothane (and other volatile anesthetics) is still obscure, it was proposed that the CBF alterations were produced as secondary responses to tissue Po_2.[230] However, this hypothesis may not be correct because the increase in CBF was observed a few minutes after anesthesia induction, before any change in $CMRo_2$. This may indicate that the direct effect of halothane on vascular smooth muscle occurs more rapidly than its effects on metabolic depression.[4] Several studies have demonstrated that the effect of halothane on CBF is time dependent[5,26,267] and CBF eventually returns to normal without a further decrease in $CMRo_2$. Thus a mechanism unrelated to cerebral metabolic rate could be responsible for changes in CBF. It has been suggested that a dose-related increase in brain cAMP has a causal relationship to the cerebrovasodilator effect of halothane.[123]

A dose-related cerebral metabolic depressive effect of halothane has been demonstrated repeatedly in both humans[229] and animals.[230,240,250] At clinical levels of anesthesia the decrease in $CMRo_2$ ranges from 10% to 30%,[229] but in some experimental animals clinical doses of halothane decreased $CMRo_2$ by 50%.[163] Regional differences in metabolic change during halothane have been reported. For example, lCMRgl decreased relatively more in the occipital lobe, brainstem, cerebellar cortex, and anterior commissure[226] compared with other parts of the brain. Michenfelder and Theye[144] administered halothane, up to 9% in dogs, while CBF was maintained by extracorporeal circulation. At about 4.5% inspired halothane, the EEG became flat and $CMRo_2$ decreased by 50%. Further increases in halothane concentration produced a progressive decrease in $CMRo_2$. There were measurable increases in brain lactate and decreases in brain phosphocreatine and ATP levels with halothane concentrations above 2.3%, these changes being exaggerated at concentrations above 4%. These results were interpreted as reflecting a toxic effect on oxidative phosphorylation produced by high concentrations of halothane. This toxic effect has not been observed for isoflurane[176] or barbiturates.[143]

Both in animals and humans, halothane increases ICP in a dose-related fashion, and the increase in ICP is parallel to the increase in CBF.[1,250] However, at 0.5 MAC or less, the effect on ICP is minimal. The increased ICP that, with halothane, often occurs in association with systemic hypotension, results in reduced CPP. This may augment the risk of cerebral ischemia.

Among the commonly used volatile anesthetics, halothane appears to be the most potent in producing an increase in ICP. Brain surface protrusion during craniotomy is most pronounced during anesthesia with halothane when compared with anesthesia using enflurane or isoflurane.[53] The protrusion is more prominent when blood pressure is supported with vasoactive drugs. The increased resistance to CSF outflow with halothane may in part contribute to the elevation in ICP.[9] This increase in ICP may be attenuated either by hyperventilation (induced before the introduction of the inhalational anesthetic) or by barbiturates.[1] However, the beneficial effects of hypocapnia may not be obtained when the initial ICP is very high or reactivity to CO_2 is globally lost.

An increase in CBF with halothane results in an increase in $CBF/CMRo_2$, the increase in this ratio being greater with halothane than with isoflurane.[53] This does not necessarily mean that halothane may have a protective effect against cerebral ischemia. In fact, after experimental focal ischemia (middle cerebral artery occlusion), neurologic outcome was worse and the infarcted area greater in animals anesthetized with halothane when compared with awake dogs, but pentobarbital significantly attenuated the deleterious effects of MCA occlusion.[89] Similar results have been reported by Michenfelder et al.[145]

In summary, there has been considerable discussion concerning the use of halothane during surgery for intracranial space-occupying lesions, and some recommend against the use of halothane. However, as discussed, halothane in low concentration (less than 1%) can be safely used in clinical neuroanesthesia practice, especially if $Paco_2$ is reduced and barbituates are also given.

Enflurane

In animal experiments, both increased and unchanged CBF has been reported with enflurane. These differences may be explained by different levels of CPP used in the various studies. CBF increased when blood pressure was supported[142] but remained unchanged when it was not supported.[209]

A dose-dependent decrease in $CMRo_2$ has been observed during enflurane anesthesia.[209,240] However, during seizures induced by hypocapnia or by auditory stimulation (hand clapping), precipitous increases in CBF and $CMRo_2$ were demonstrated in dogs.[142] In rats, enflurane produced a decrease in lCMRgl in many brain structures, but it produced an increase in lCMRgl in the hippocampus and other subcortical structures.[173] Nakakimura et al.[173] reported that 4% enflurane in rats produced a marked increase (31% to 70%) in lCMRgl in the hippocampal CA3 layer, ventrobasal (VB) area of the thalamus, and corpus callosum, when compared with lCMRgl during 0.5% or 2% enflurane. The increases in lCMRgl in the VB area and corpus callosum were obliterated after unilateral excision of the cerebral cortex. The results indicate that intercortical and corticothalamic pathways are metabolically activated during deep enflurane anesthesia, suggesting that the epileptogenic property of enflurane may be related to activation of these pathways. Although EEG seizure activity was not accompanied by perturbation of global cerebral energy metabolism,[223] regional oxygen supply-demand balance could be disturbed in some circumstances.

In humans, several reports have shown no change or even a decrease in CBF with enflurane.[197,203] However, in these studies, patients were premedicated, N_2O was also used, and the blood pressure fall was left untreated. If arterial blood pressure support was provided, CBF increased during enflurane anesthesia. The magnitude of CBF increase was less when compared with halothane but greater when compared with isoflurane. Sakabe et al.[212] demonstrated that enflurane, 3.5% inspired, produced frequent spiking and suppression of the EEG, an increase in CBF, and a decrease in $CMRo_2$. In contrast, 2% enflurane produced an insignificant increase in CBF (15%). In this study, MABP was maintained above 70 mm Hg. These CBF effects have been confirmed by Eintrei et al.[58] Madsen et al.[124] reported a dose-related decrease in $CMRo_2$ in craniotomy patients who were anesthetized with enflurane supplemented by N_2O and fentanyl. CBF was also decreased in this study.

ICP increases with enflurane appeared to be small in animals with normal ICP but significant in those with increased ICP.[27] In cats, brain surface protrusion through a craniotomy was less prominent with enflurane (or isoflurane) than with halothane.[53] However, the protrusion was greater with both enflurane and isoflurane when blood pressure falls were prevented. The increase in ICP with enflurane was not solely related to CBV and may be due in part to an increased production of CSF and an increased resistance to CSF absorption.[11]

As with the animal findings, in humans, enflurane increases ICP and decreases CPP.[168,239] The increase in ICP is small in the subjects with normal ICP but marked in patients with space-occupying lesions, especially when high enflurane concentrations are used.

In summary, enflurane, like halothane, is a cerebral metabolic depressant. Its cerebral vasodilatory properties are weak compared with those of halothane but are modified by systemic blood pressure and concomitant drug therapy. However, because of its potential effects on ICP and possible epileptogenic properties, high concentrations of enflurane should be avoided in patients at risk. Low doses of enflurane, in association with moderate hypocapnia and supplemental doses of barbiturates or narcotics, can be safely used during neurosurgery.

Isoflurane

In most animal experiments, isoflurane has been shown to produce an increase in CBF that is accompanied by a decrease in CVR and $CMRo_2$.[70,176,240,250] However, at low concentration (0.5%) isoflurane has been reported to decrease CBF, and at high concentration (0.95%) to increase CBF.[259] In this study, baboons were tranquilized with a phencyclidine and supplemented with N_2O, which might have affected the results. In general, the increase in global CBF is smaller with isoflurane than with halothane.[54,218,250] The cerebral vasodilating potency of isoflurane (and halothane) appear to depend on the $CMRo_2$ present before anesthetic administration. If the initial $CMRo_2$ is depressed by a high dose of pentobarbital, halothane and isoflurane have similar vasodilating potencies.[55] These reported smaller increases in CBF with isoflurane when compared with halothane may be due to a more potent cerebral metabolic depressive effect of isoflurane.

In regional CBF studies there are substantial differences in the response of CBF in the different regions. Flow increases in deep structures are greater than in the cortex.[132,134] Hansen et al.[80] reported that, in rats, cortical CBF was greater during halothane anesthesia, but subcortical CBF was greater during isoflurane anesthesia. In this study, hemispheric CBF was identical during both halothane and isoflurane anesthesia. The different flow responses may be related to different metabolic effects in various brain regions. A subsequent study demonstrated that isoflurane has disproportionate metabolic depressive effects on the neocortex.[81] At a given level of glucose use, isoflurane possesses greater cerebral vasodilating capabilities than halothane.[81]

In dogs, isoflurane decreased $CMRo_2$ in a dose-related

manner until the EEG became flat (2 MAC); thereafter, no further decrease in $CMRo_2$ was observed despite an increase in isoflurane to 4 MAC.[176] A brain-tissue biopsy revealed normal brain high-energy metabolites and a normal energy charge, indicating no toxic effect such as was reported with high-dose halothane. In rats, isoflurane produces a decrease in lCMRgl in the majority of brain structures,[132,187] but in limbic structures, lCMRgl was either increased[187] or unchanged.[132]

In humans, isoflurane produces no change in CBF and produces a decrease in $CMRo_2$.[6,126] In a report by Eintrei et al.,[58] isoflurane, when administered in combination with N_2O (total dose of 1.5 MAC), produced a small but insignificant decrease in CBF. Madsen et al.[126] reported no significant change in CBF in patients supplemented with N_2O when isoflurane concentration was increased from 0.75% to 1.5% inspired, but $CMRo_2$ was significantly decreased. No significant change in CBF was observed when isoflurane (0.85% inspired) was added to 65% N_2O.[6] During hypotension induced with isoflurane, CBF was unchanged but $CMRo_2$ was significantly decreased in association with EEG burst suppression.[127,180] Thus it seems that the increase in CBF, if present at all, is smaller while the decrease in $CMRo_2$ is greater than the changes observed with halothane or enflurane.

In animal experiments, isoflurane increases ICP minimally in normal subjects as well as those with intracranial hypertension.[3,250] However, a substantial increase in ICP has been reported when isoflurane and N_2O are used in combination.[3] ICP elevation with 1% isoflurane was partially blocked by hypocapnia.[218] CBV, which is an indirect measure of ICP, has been reported to be increased with isoflurane, even during hypocapnia.[8] Artru[10] reported that the increase in ICP from isoflurane only lasted for 30 minutes, but with halothane or enflurane the elevation lasted more than 3 hours. ICP elevation with isoflurane (and halothane) in rabbits subjected to cryogenic brain lesion was not prevented by prior induction of hypocapnia.[219] Edema formation after cryoinjury was greater in animals anesthetized with isoflurane than with halothane.[102] However, brain surface protrusion through a craniotomy in cats anesthetized with isoflurane was less than that with halothane.[53] Thus the different results are at least partly explained by species differences and differences in experimental models, that is, intact vs. injured brain.

In humans, several reports have shown an increase in ICP during isoflurane anesthesia. The increase, however, is prevented or partially blocked by hypocapnia (even if it is induced after introduction of isoflurane) or barbiturate administration.[2,32,75] In some reports of patients with space-occupying lesions, isoflurane increased ICP even during mild hypocapnia,[78] but in others ICP was not increased unless isoflurane inspired concentration was increased to 1.5%.[32] In these latter studies the increase was insignificant and even decreased with hypocapnia. In spite of the minimal increase in ICP observed, Grosslight et al.[78] con-

cluded that isoflurane may not be a benign anesthetic in patients known to be at risk for increases in ICP. However, from the data mentioned previously, one could conclude that isoflurane's ICP-elevating properties are weak when compared with halothane.

Because of the potent cerebral metabolic depressive effect, isoflurane was predicted to have cerebral protective effects similar to thiopental. In mice subjected to hypoxia, survival time was longer when the mice were anesthetized with isoflurane instead of N_2O.[177] Protective effects have been reported in a canine model of incomplete ischemia using severe hypotension,[178] but not in a forebrain ischemia model in rats, where the ischemia was nearly complete.[215,268] Seyde and Longnecker[224] reported significantly higher brain tissue Po_2 with isoflurane-induced hypotension when compared with hypotension induced by 2-chloroadenosine. The results of studies of regional ischemia are complex but not conclusive.[153,175] Baughman et al.[18,20] reported better outcome, after ischemia, in animals anesthetized with isoflurane compared to those anesthetized with N_2O.

In humans during carotid endarterectomy, the critical CBF below which ischemic EEG changes occur is greater in patients anesthetized with halothane than in patients anesthetized with isoflurane.[140] At a comparable level of regional CBF, the incidence of EEG ischemic changes with isoflurane has been reported to be significantly lower than that seen with either halothane or enflurane.[147] The data clearly favor the use of isoflurane over either halothane or enflurane if a volatile anesthetic is used in a patient who has or may develop regional cerebral ischemia.

In summary, isoflurane appears to produce a moderate increase in CBF and a pronounced decrease in cerebral metabolism. In neurosurgical patients, the increase in ICP caused by isoflurane, if it occurs, may be mild and can be prevented by hypocapnia even when it is induced after isoflurane introduction. Because of its potent cerebral metabolic depressive effects, isoflurane may have a cerebral protective effect and is a desirable anesthetic for many neurosurgical procedures, including carotid endarterectomy or when induced hypotension may be needed.

Sevoflurane, Desflurane

Sevoflurane has similar effects to those of isoflurane. It produces minimal to moderate increases in CBF and ICP and a decrease of $CMRo_2$ in association with EEG slowing.[220,221] The disadvantages of sevoflurane are that this drug is biodegradable and that the metabolites may be toxic in high concentrations. Although such toxicity has not yet been reported, prolonged anesthesia, which is often necessary for neurosurgical anesthesia, may increase the possibility of significant elevation of these metabolites.

Desflurane is reported in dogs to produce a dose-dependent cerebrovasodilation and a decrease in $CMRo_2$ with no significant effect on ICP.[121] Cerebrovascular reactivity to $Paco_2$ changes appears to be preserved.[122] During desflurane-induced hypotension, CBF decreased significantly. $CMRO_2$ also decreased, but cerebral metabolite concentrations of high-energy phosphates were within the normal range.[156] During hypocapnia ($Paco_2$ of 25 mm Hg) patients receiving desflurane (1 or 1.5 MAC) had CBF measured using [133]Xe (iv). Although the CBF at 1 MAC was lower, the CBF at 1.5 MAC was not significantly different from CBF measured during an equiMAC isoflurane anesthetic. Reactivity to changes in $Paco_2$ tended to be lower with desflurane than with isoflurane.[190] In patients with supratentorial mass lesions, 1 MAC desflurane (7%) has been reported to produce an increase in CSFP despite prior establishment of hypocapnia, but 1 MAC isoflurane did not produce an increase in CSFP.[172] However, another study in neurosurgical patients with supratentorial mass lesions showed that the administration of 0.5 MAC desflurane (3.5%) with 50% N_2O after establishment of hypocapnia had no effect on lumbar CSFP.[170]

In summary, limited information is available concerning the effects of sevoflurane and desflurane. However, it is probably appropriate to say that the cerebrovascular effects of sevoflurane and desflurane appear to be qualitatively similar to those of other volatile anesthetics.

Intravenous Anesthetics

Intravenous anesthetics in general cause a decrease in CBF and $CMRO_2$. However, these anesthetics might not be vasoconstrictors in a strict sense, because, in vitro barbiturates, for example, dilate isolated cerebral vessels. The decrease in CBF induced by most intravenous anesthetics appears to be the result of decreased cerebral metabolism secondary to cerebral functional depression. Among the intravenous anesthetics, ketamine may be unique, because it produces an increase in both CBF and $CMRO_2$.

Barbiturates

In animal experiments, thiopental produces a dose-dependent reduction in CBF and $CMRO_2$.[143,162,240] A similar reduction in CBF and $CMRO_2$ (or CMRgl) has also been reported with phenobarbital and pentobarbital.[88,181] In dogs, a dose-dependent reduction in CBF and $CMRO_2$ occurs until the EEG becomes flat. At the point of EEG isoelectricity, no further $CMRO_2$ reduction occurs despite further increases in barbiturate dose.[143,235] The maximal thiopental-induced $CMRO_2$ decrease is 55% to 60%. Thus, with barbiturates, functional depression appears to be coupled with the reduction in CBF and $CMRO_2$. This observation also suggests that barbiturates reduce the metabolic components linked to brain function and produce only minimal effects on metabolic function related to the maintenance of the cellular integrity. A similar reduction in spinal cord blood flow with plateau phenomenon has been reported with high-dose thiopental in dogs.[87] When thiopental is combined with hypothermia, which can reduce the metabolic component for maintaining cellular integrity, $CMRO_2$ is further reduced to 30% of control.[110] With mas-

sive doses of thiopental or pentobarbital, ATP, PCr, and lactate concentrations in the brain tissue remain normal.[77,143] This is in contrast to the changes with deep halothane anesthesia, suggesting that high doses of thiopental have no direct, deleterious effect on the brain.

Studies of lCMRgl reveal that the metabolic depression with barbiturates is homogeneous in the various brain structures, except in the habenulo-interpeduncular system, where lCMRgl was preserved or even increased.[85,88] The decrease in local glucose utilization with pentobarbital was smaller in the spinal cord than in the brain, possibly because of the lower cellular density in the former than the latter.[45]

In dogs, acute CNS tolerance to thiopental has been confirmed in terms of the response of CBF and $CMRO_2$. $CMRO_2$ was higher during thiopental infusion in dogs pretreated with a single induction dose of thiopental compared with nonpretreated dogs. In another study, during prolonged administration of pentobarbital, $CMRO_2$ increased with time despite a steady deep level of anesthesia with an unchanged EEG pattern (deep burst-suppression pattern) and constant blood levels of pentobarbital.[77] The clinical relevance of tolerance awaits further study. However, tolerance, if it occurs, may limit the degree of expected brain protection provided by barbiturates.

In humans, as in the animal experiments, a dose-dependent reduction in CBF and $CMRO_2$ occurs. Thiopental, in doses insufficient to produce unconsciousness, does not affect CBF and $CMRO_2$ but, in doses high enough to produce high-voltage, slow waves in the EEG, thiopental decreases CBF and $CMRO_2$ to about 50% of the awake value. The decrease in CBF is accompanied by an increase in CVR. When thiopental sufficient to produce a burst-suppression pattern on EEG is given, both CBF and $CMRO_2$ decrease to about 40% (near maximal reduction). Hypocapnia decreases CBF even more, to 30% of awake control values, but $CMRO_2$ remains unaffected.

ICP is reduced by barbiturates, possibly because of the reduction in CBF and CBV. This effect is used during the treatment of raised ICP in head-injured patients (although this use is controversial[266]), as well as in the induction of anesthesia in patients with decreased intracranial compliance. Barbiturates attenuate cerebral vasodilation produced by N_2O and ketamine and thus are useful as supplemental anesthetics.[49, 211]

Etomidate

A metabolic effect of etomidate, similar to barbiturates, has been reported in canine experiments.[150] During the infusion of etomidate, $CMRO_2$ decreased progressively until an isoelectric EEG appeared. As with thiopental, increasing doses of etomidate after EEG flattening did not produce further reduction in $CMRO_2$, and brain energy metabolism remained normal. Unlike the $CMRO_2$, CBF decreased precipitously with the start of the etomidate infusion. CBF achieved a maximal decrease before the $CMRO_2$ maximal decrease. This may suggest that etomidate causes vasoconstriction through a different mechanism (possibly by direct action) than do the barbiturates. A parallel decrease in ICP and CBF was observed.

The metabolic suppression caused by etomidate has regional variability. The decrease in lCMRgl is predominantly observed in forebrain structures, and the metabolic depression in the hindbrain is less.[47] The specific regional variation in the effect of etomidate suggests a mechanism of action involving a receptor-ligand interaction. Furthermore, there is no demonstrable dose dependency; all tested doses caused the same pattern and degree of metabolic suppression, suggesting that the receptors may have been occupied with the smallest doses examined.

In humans etomidate has been reported to induce almost parallel reductions in CBF and $CMRo_2$. With clinical doses, CBF and $CMRo_2$ were decreased by approximately 30% to 50%.[40,198] Reactivity to CO_2 is preserved during etomidate anesthesia.[40,198]

Etomidate effectively decreases ICP[193] without decreasing CPP.[50] In severely head-injured patients, etomidate decreased ICP while electrocortical activity was present but was not effective when cortical electrical activity was already maximally suppressed.[25] This indicates that the decrease in ICP may be caused by the reduction of CBF that is induced by functional (metabolic) depressant effects of etomidate.

During hypoxia and ischemia studies in animals etomidate has been reported to have substantial brain protective effects as judged from better survival or maintenance of high-energy metabolites in the brain tissue.[151,231,261,269] Furthermore, a recent report suggests the possibility that high-dose etomidate may preserve the cerebral metabolic state during induced hypotension.[67] However, poor outcome after incomplete cerebral ischemia treated with high doses of etomidate has also been reported.[19] The differing results in these studies may be due to differences in the degree of ischemia. Etomidate may have protective effect when ischemia is mild or moderate.

Adverse effects of this drug include adrenocortical suppression and frequent occurrence of involuntary muscle activity and seizure activity. Etomidate should be used with caution in patients with seizure histories.

Propofol

Propofol has been shown to decrease both CBF and $CMRo_2$ in humans in a parallel and dose-related manner.[236,260] CO_2 reactivity is preserved.[236] In vitro, propofol inhibits extracellular Ca^{2+} influx through voltage-gated Ca^{2+} channels.[38] Thus, like barbiturates, the decrease of CBF with propofol is opposite in direction from that expected from in vitro results, suggesting that the CBF decrease is attributable to its metabolic depressant effect.

Most studies have shown that propofol either decreases or does not change ICP.[82,195] At the same time, MABP is decreased by almost the same magnitude or more; thus CPP decreases in most circumstances.[82] However, Ravussine et al.[195] found that although lumbar CSF pressure during induction of anesthesia with propofol decreased by 32% and MABP also decreased, CPP remained above 70 mm Hg.

In summary, propofol seems to have similar cerebral hemodynamic and metabolic effects to those of the barbiturates. This drug may be useful in patients with intracranial pathology provided that hypotension is prevented. Further study may be needed before this drug can be widely applied to neuroanesthesia practice.

Ketamine

Ketamine is a phencyclidine derivative and is a unique anesthetic because it induces a catatonic state. Increases in CBF and $CMRo_2$ have been reported in animals.[37,48,49] Pretreatment with thiopental completely blocks these CBF and $CMRo_2$ effects.[49] Vasodilation by ketamine has been attributed, in part, to its metabolic stimulating effect. In addition, this drug has a direct dilating effect on cerebral arteries caused, in part, by interference with the transmembrane influx of Ca^{2+}.[69] Ketamine-induced increases in CBF are blocked with scopolamine and augmented with CO_2 or physostigmine.[196] Thus ketamine may increase CBF by a cholinergic mechanism. In goats, ketamine has been reported to have no significant effect on CBF.[222] Whether these discrepancies are caused by differences in background anesthesia (N_2O) or by a species difference is not clear. Cerebral metabolic effects of ketamine appear to vary among the various brain structures; lCMRgl is increased in the hippocampus and extrapyramidal structures, but it is decreased in the somatosensory and auditory systems.[37] Diazepam pretreatment attenuates the increase in lCMRgl in the hippocampus.[184]

In humans, intravenous ketamine (3 mg/kg) increases CBF by about 60% and reduces CVR. However, $CMRo_2$ does not change significantly.[241] The rCBF increases in frontal and parietooccipital areas are remarkable and might be related to the dreams or hallucinations peculiar to ketamine. It is suggested that the metabolic regulatory mechanisms are involved in the cerebrovascular response to ketamine.[92]

Ketamine markedly increases ICP.[13,217,271] Ketamine-induced increases in ICP can be blocked or attenuated by induced hypocapnia[217] or by administration of thiopental or a benzodiazepine.[13,271] However, some reports demonstrate failure to block ketamine-induced ICP elevation by secobarbital, droperidol, diazepam or midazolam.[24] Thus ketamine is not recommended during neuroanesthesia, especially in patients with elevated ICP or decreased intracranial compliance.

Benzodiazepines

The effects of diazepam on CBF and $CMRo_2$ are variable and species-dependent. Moderate decreases in CBF and $CMRo_2$ have been reported in dogs. Intravenous diazepam (0.25 mg/kg) decreased CBF and $CMRo_2$ by about 15%, and was accompanied by EEG slowing.[128] In rats, diazepam has been reported to decrease CBF by 30% with minimal change in CMR_{O_2}. However, the combination of diazepam and N_2O (70%) decreased CMR_{O_2} (and CBF) by about 40%, suggesting a synergistic interaction between diazepam and N_2O.[35] In dogs, the CMR_{O_2} decrease after diazepam was not attenuated by the addition of N_2O.[200]

In normal humans, diazepam in combination with fentanyl and N_2O produces parallel decreases in CBF and CMR_{O_2}. CO_2 reactivity is preserved.[262] In the head-injured patient, diazepam produces a proportional 25% decrease in CBF and CMR_{O_2}.[43] Contrary to the assumption that ICP would be decreased because of a lower CBF, diazepam (0.25 mg/kg) does not change ICP.[245] The effects of midazolam are similar. It produces a parallel reduction in CBF and CMR_{O_2}.[63,91] Metabolic suppression is less with midazolam than with barbiturates. In dogs, midazolam infusion produces parallel decreases in CBF and CMR_{O_2} by a maximum of 25%. Despite increasing dose, no further decreases in CBF and CMR_{O_2} occur. This plateau may reflect saturation of the benzodiazepam receptors.

In humans, midazolam (0.15 mg/kg) decreases CBF by approximately 30%[65,117] with a concomitant reduction in CMR_{O_2}.[65] This effect is completely blocked by the specific benzodiazepine antagonist Flumazenil.[66]

Midazolam has been reported to produce either a decrease[117] or no change[72] in ICP. In patients with brain tumors the induction of anesthesia with midazolam (0.25 mg/kg) was reported to have no effect on ICP, and this was comparable with that seen with thiopental.[72] Negative results may be due to the normal ICP before the administration of the drugs in this study. In patients with elevated ICP anesthetized with fentanyl and N_2O, midazolam administration (0.2 mg/kg) decreased ICP, but it had no significant effect in patients with normal ICP.[117] Midazolam has been shown to maintain better hemodynamic stability compared with thiopental when administered to patients with brain tumors. There is less fall in MABP, and CPP tends not to decrease. Midazolam may have protective effects against hypoxia or cerebral ischemia; the effects appear to be comparable with or slightly less than those of the barbiturates.[19,183]

Lorazepam, triazolam, and flurazepam seem to have effects similar to those of diazepam and midazolam.

Because a specific receptor antagonist is now available, benzodiazepine derivatives are useful as induction or supplemental drugs during neuroanesthesia. However, one must recognize that the competitive benzodiazepine receptor antagonist, flumazenil, also antagonizes the effects of midazolam on CBF, CMR_{O_2}, and ICP.[14,66] Thus one must use this drug cautiously when reversing benzodiazepine-induced sedation in patients with impaired intracranial compliance.

Droperidol

In dogs, droperidol alone produces a decrease in CBF while the CMR_{O_2} is unchanged.[141] When droperidol is used in combination with fentanyl, further decreases in CBF and CMR_{O_2} occur.[141]

In humans, droperidol with fentanyl produces no significant change in CBF and CMR_{O_2}.[216] When droperidol was used during hypocapnia in patients with supratentorial tumors anesthetized with N_2O and fentanyl, a parallel reduction in CBF and CMR_{O_2} (about 35%) occurred, and CO_2 reactivity was preserved.[41] Droperidol used either alone or in combination with fentanyl does not increase ICP if ventilation is controlled to avoid an elevation in Pa_{CO_2}.[158,161]

Narcotic Analgesics

The reported effects of narcotics on CBF, CMR_{O_2}, and ICP are variable. The variability appears to be due to the background anesthetic and not species differences. When vasodilating drugs are used as the background anesthetic, the narcotic effect is consistently that of a cerebral vasoconstrictor. Conversely, when vasoconstrictors are used as the background anesthetic or when no anesthetic is given, narcotics have either no effect or may even increase CBF. When N_2O is used, most narcotics decrease CMR_{O_2}.

Morphine

An early report found that morphine increased CBF, but this may have been due to an increase in Pa_{CO_2} secondary to respiratory depression. In more recent studies, incremental doses of morphine caused a progressive and parallel decrease in CBF and CMR_{O_2} in normocapnic dogs anesthetized with N_2O. A metabolic depressive effect that accompanied the decreased CBF was antagonized with N-allylnormorphine.[242] Several reports demonstrate that morphine does not significantly affect CBF and CMR_{O_2} (lCMRgl).

In nonanesthetized humans given 60 mg of morphine, Moyer et al.[169] reported a significant reduction in CMR_{O_2} with no change in CBF. In normocapnic human volunteers, morphine-N_2O anesthesia does not significantly affect CBF, CMR_{O_2}, or cerebral autoregulation.[99,100] It may be possible that the vasoconstrictive effect of morphine is counteracted by the vasodilating effect of N_2O.

Meperidine

This drug has effects similar to morphine. There was a modest decrease in CMR_{O_2} when N_2O was used as a background anesthetic.

Fentanyl

In dogs and rats, fentanyl, when given with an N_2O background anesthetic, causes a decrease in CBF and CMR_{O_2}.[36,138,141,207] In unanesthetized newborn lambs, fentanyl in doses as high as 4.4 mg/kg do not alter CBF or CMR_{O_2}.[273] Increases in CBF and CMR_{O_2} have been reported in rats when seizures were induced with high fentanyl doses.[36,207] However, the CBF increases were not comparable with the increases in CMR_{O_2}.[36] Whether the disproportionate increase in metabolism causes ischemic brain damage is not yet determined.

An autoradiographic study in rats revealed that when EEG spikes were induced by a dose of fentanyl of about 200 µg/kg, lCBF significantly increased in the superior colliculus, sensory motor cortex, and pineal body. With progression to seizures, lCBF increased in most of the brain structures.[131] A comparable study demonstrated that hypermetabolism occurs in the limbic structures during fentanyl-induced seizure activity.[252] Keykhah et al.[106] reported that high-dose fentanyl decreased global $CMRo_2$ in rats but failed to prevent the reduction in ATP and PCr or increase in lactate during hypoxemia.

In humans, the combined use of clinical doses of fentanyl (5 µg/kg) and droperidol (0.25 mg/kg) had no significant effect on CBF and $CMRo_2$.[216] In patients anesthetized with N_2O and diazepam, fentanyl decreased CBF by 25%, a reduction that may be attributed to the effect of diazepam. In another human study, fentanyl (10 µg/kg) in combination with diazepam and N_2O was found to decrease rCBF and $CMRo_2$.[262]

ICP is either not elevated or may be slightly decreased during neuroleptoanesthesia in normal patients. In patients with raised ICP, fentanyl alone[166] or in combination with droperidol[161] was found to produce no significant change in ICP. Reported ICP increases in patients with space-occupying lesions have been attributed to hypercapnia.[158] Herrick et al.[86] reported that fentanyl (sufentanil and alfentanil) did not affect brain retractor pressure in neurosurgical patients anesthetized with isoflurane and hyperventilated, suggesting these narcotics appeared safe for intraoperative administration after the cranium was open. However, a recent report has revealed that fentanyl and sufentanil increased ICP in head trauma patients despite hyperventilation.[233] The mechanism for the increase in ICP was unclear.

Sufentanil

In rats with an N_2O background anesthetic, sufentanil decreases CBF and $CMRo_2$.[105] High doses of sufentanil provoke epileptic seizure activity[105,274] and produce significant increases in lCMRgl in the limbic nuclei, particularly the amygdala.[274] In dogs, with no background anesthesia, sufentanil was reported to produce an increase in CBF in the absence of seizure activity, although it decreased $CMRo_2$.[155] Although ICP did not change in that study, a sudden increase in CBF may be detrimental, if it occurs, in subjects at risk. However, a recent report has demonstrated that in dogs anesthetized with isoflurane and N_2O, sufentanil decreased CBF in response to decreased metabolic demand without significantly affecting ICP.[270] The differences could be due to the differences in background conditions (unanesthetized vs. anesthetized).

Clinical studies are also contradictory. In patients undergoing elective excision of supratentorial tumors, sufentanil produced a significant increase in CSFP and a decrease in CPP.[137] In contrast, better cerebral relaxation with the combined use of sufentanil, N_2O, and isoflurane during craniotomy has been reported, suggesting that sufentanil probably has cerebrovasoconstrictive activity.[29] No significant change in brain retractor pressure in patients during craniotomy also has been reported.[86] However, in severe head trauma patients, an ICP increase with sufentanil has recently been reported, the mechanism for the increase being unclear.[233]

Alfentanil

In patients with supratentorial tumors, alfentanil increased lumbar CSFP and decreased MABP and CPP.[137] However, alfentanil has been used in neurosurgical anesthesia with satisfactory results.[68] Recently, the effects of alfentanil on ICP in children undergoing ventriculoperitoneal shunt revision have been reported. In contrast to adult patients, alfentanil did not increase ICP in pediatric patients with hydrocephalus who were anesthetized with isoflurane and N_2O.[135] Alfentanil has been shown to have no significant effect on brain retractor pressure during craniotomy.[86]

In summary, clinically used doses of most narcotics have minimal to modest depressive effects on CBF and $CMRo_2$. During narcotic-induced seizures there is a substantial increase in CBF and $CMRo_2$ (CMRgl). If adequate alveolar ventilation is instituted to maintain $Paco_2$ (and Pao_2) within the normal range and rigidity is prevented, narcotics have minimal or negligible effects on ICP. However, the possibility of an increase in ICP with fentanyl, sufentanil, and alfentanil cannot be completely excluded.

Muscle Relaxants
Succinylcholine (Sch)

In animals, many studies have demonstrated that succinylcholine elevates ICP.[44,113,249] Lanier et al.[113] found, in dogs anesthetized with 1 MAC halothane, that the increase in ICP with Sch was accompanied by muscle fasciculation, EEG arousal, and an increase in CBF. The increase in CBF was disproportionately greater than expected from the concomitant increase in $Paco_2$. In their subsequent study, they demonstrated that an increase in muscle spindle afferent activity paralleled the increase in CBF.[114] Fasciculation in the muscles of the neck, causing stasis in the jugular veins, might also be a factor contributing to increased ICP with Sch.[44] Pretreatment with nonparalyzing doses of pancuronium did not block the afferent muscle activity or the CBF response.[116] The increase in ICP was also not blocked by pretreatment with thiopental.[249]

Regardless of the presence or absence of space-occupying intracranial lesions, Sch in humans produces significant increases in ICP.[160,237] The increase in ICP was prevented or diminished by pretreatment with a nondepolarizing muscle relaxant.[160,237] This result is in contrast to the animal study cited previously in which pretreatment with pancuronium did not attenuate the Sch-induced increase in afferent muscle activity and CBF.[116]

It has also been reported that Sch induced ventricular fibrillation in patients with subarachnoid hemorrhage, an effect possibly caused by elevation of serum K^{+98}, although, some have demonstrated that the elevation of K^+ is not significant if patients received Sch at a relatively early stage (within 4 days).[133] Nevertheless, the use of Sch has been decreasing in clinical neuroanesthesia practice, with the exception of emergency situations, such as the patient with a full stomach in whom a rapid-sequence induction is recommended. In this situation, small doses of nondepolarizing muscle relaxants should be administered before the administration of Sch. Lidocaine administration may also be helpful.

D-tubocurarine (D-Tc)

In animal experiments, D-Tc produces an increase in CBF, but the increase in CBF was observed only when the blood-brain barrier had been opened with urea. Histamine release might be the cause for the increase in CBF. The increase in CBF is antagonized with cimetidine.[263] Pretreatment with diphenhydramine attenuated the CBF and P_{CO_2} responses to D-Tc, but CSF production remained increased.

In an early study in humans, D-Tc did not produce any significant change in CBF. However, a later study demonstrated that D-Tc produced a significant elevation in ICP and a decrease in thalamic baseline impedance, suggesting cerebral vasodilation, possibly caused by the release of histamine.[244] Because of its ganglionic blocking effect, D-Tc decreases blood pressure. If an ICP increase occurs concomitantly with a decrease in MABP, a substantial decrease in CPP may occur. Because other nondepolarizing muscle relaxants have no such adverse effects on ICP, it is reasonable to avoid the use of D-Tc in the patients at risk for ICP elevation.

Pancuronium

Pancuronium does not produce an increase in CBF, CMR_{O_2}, or ICP in dogs anesthetized with 1 MAC of halothane.[112] However, pancuronium frequently induces an increase in blood pressure and heart rate. This could be disadvantageous for certain patients, such as those with hypertension, especially if they have disturbed autoregulation. In these patients a substantial elevation of ICP could occur.

Atracurium

In animals, atracurium seems to have no significant effect on CBF, CMR_{O_2},[112] or ICP.[73,112] Its metabolite, laudanosine, has been reported to cross the blood-brain barrier readily and cause seizures. However, the blood level of laudanosine after clinical doses of atracurium should not cause undesirable consequences.[39,247] Lanier et al.[115] reported that there were no significant differences in seizure threshold for lidocaine in cats paralyzed with atracurium, pancuronium, or vecuronium. High doses of atracurium have the potential to release histamine, but the potential is consider-

ably less than that of D-Tc.[17] In humans, as in animals, atracurium has been shown to have no effect on ICP.[159,204]

Vecuronium

Vecuronium does not induce histamine release, nor does it change blood pressure or heart rate. In cats with elevated ICP, vecuronium did not induce a further ICP elevation.[74] In patients with brain tumors, vecuronium was found to have no or minimum effect on ICP.[205,238]

Pipecuronium

Pipecuronium, a new long-acting nondepolarizing neuromuscular blocking agent, has been reported to have no significant effect on ICP or CPP in patients with intracranial tumors when their ICP is not elevated at the time of administration.[206]

In summary, should succinylcholine be used, prior administration of small doses of a nondepolarizing muscle relaxant is recommended, as well as maintenance of adequate depth of anesthesia. With respect to the use of nondepolarizing muscle relaxants, in most clinical situations the changes in CBF and ICP are minimal if respiration is well controlled and an increase in Pa_{CO_2} is avoided.

Lidocaine

Lidocaine has been widely used as a local anesthetic, antidysrhythmic agent, and suppressant of the cough reflex. It produces unique CNS effects that depend on the blood concentration; at low concentration sedation occurs, but at higher concentration seizures may occur. Non–seizure-inducing doses of lidocaine produce a dose-related reduction of CMR_{O_2} and CBF. Large doses of lidocaine reduce CMR_{O_2} by a maximum of 30% in dogs. If seizures are induced by lidocaine, CMR_{O_2} increases, along with a concomitant increase in CBF.[208] Brain oxygenation seems to be adequate because there is a normal oxygen-glucose index. This index is the ratio of oxygen consumption to glucose consumption on a molar basis, and its reduction reflects anaerobic metabolism. No evidence of anaerobic metabolism has been observed in rats during the preseizure period or during the seizure itself.[130] In regional metabolism and blood flow studies, lidocaine infusion increased lCMRgl in the limbic structures, especially in the hippocampus, during the preconvulsive state, but it reduced lCMRgl in the majority of the other regions.[94,253] Because the lCBF in the hippocampus was unchanged, there is a possibility that some brain regions are not sufficiently perfused to meet regional metabolic demand.[253]

Intravenous lidocaine 1.5 mg/kg has been reported effective in preventing an elevation of ICP during tracheal intubation[23] or after application of a pin-type skull clamp or skin incision in craniotomy patients.[22] Lidocaine also prevents intracranial hypertension during endotracheal suctioning.[272]

Whether lidocaine possesses a cerebral protective effect is controversial. Astrup et al.[15] reported that lidocaine significantly reduced K^+ efflux during complete ischemia in dogs. When pentobarbital was given first to induce an iso-electrical EEG, CMR_{O_2} decreased further (by 15% to 20%) with lidocaine administration. When the two drugs were given in reverse sequence, pentobarbital had no effect on CMR_{O_2}.[16] The authors concluded that lidocaine, in addition to suppressing synaptic transmission, had a specific membrane-stabilizing effect, and they speculated that lidocaine may have more potent cerebral protective effects than do barbiturates. Lidocaine also has been reported to ameliorate the cerebral damage induced by air embolism.[61] In contrast, a recent canine study demonstrated that the addition of lidocaine during a period of EEG isoelectricity induced with isoflurane caused no further reduction in CMR_{O_2} but caused a significant reduction in ATP and energy charge along with an increase in the AMP concentration, possibly reflecting a toxic effect on oxidative phosphorylation rather than a protective effect.[152] The protective effects of lidocaine on the central nervous system are still controversial, and further studies are warranted.

Vasoactive Drugs
Sodium Nitroprusside (SNP)

SNP is a potent, direct-acting cerebral vasodilator that can produce an increase in CBV and ICP. Most of the reported literature has demonstrated an increase in ICP in both animals[33,96,164] and humans.[76,136] The reported CBF effects are variable, the CBF being either decreased[146] or unchanged.[33] This variability might be due to species differences, MABP, or the timing of the CBF measurements. In a study where both CBF and ICP were measured during SNP administration, ICP increased without a significant change in CBF.[33] The ICP elevation was attributed to the dilation of capacitance vessels, leading to an increase in CBV.[148]

Besides the ICP elevation, side effects of SNP include cyanide toxicity, tachyphylaxis, metabolic acidosis, and rebound hypertension. Blood-brain-barrier dysfunction has been associated with SNP in some circumstances.[97] However, brain-surface oxygen tensions during SNP-induced hypotension remain normal, but during trimethaphan (TMP)-induced hypotension they decrease.[129] In clinical practice, when blood pressure needs to be immediately controlled, SNP is the drug of choice because of its reliability, rapid action, and short duration. In patients at risk of an increase in ICP, hyperventilation, diuretics, or barbiturate therapy may be helpful to prevent unacceptable increases in ICP. With cessation of SNP, rebound hypertension occurs and is attributed to increased activity of renin and catecholamines.[108] This rebound hypertension can be prevented by captopril or beta adrenergic blocking drugs.[107]

Nitroglycerin (TNG)

TNG acts predominantly on capacitance vessels. In both animals and humans, TNG has been shown to increase ICP (or CSFP).[51,90,164] The increase in ICP is probably due to an increase in CBV from dilation of capacitance vessels. In rats and dogs, TNG in a dose that decreased MABP to 45 to 40 mm Hg did not induce significant change in CBF.[90] Brain-surface oxygen tension in cats has been reported to be better maintained with SNP than with TNG.[129] Because the ICP elevation induced with TNG seems greater than that induced by SNP, and the effects on blood pressure are somewhat unreliable, there is little role for TNG as a drug to induce hypotension in neurosurgical patients.

Trimethaphan (TMP)

TMP is a short-acting ganglionic blocking drug. Its hypotensive effect is primarily mediated by vasodilation caused by ganglion blockade, although it has some direct action. Theoretic problems associated with TMP include histamine release, which can dilate cerebral blood vessels and increase ICP. TMP-induced hypotension has been reported to disturb CBF, cortical P_{O_2}, EEG, cortical extracellular fluid pH, and potassium more than other drugs used to produce hypotension.[129,146,165] The ICP elevation with TMP has been shown to be smaller than that induced with SNP.[255] The somewhat unreliable effects on blood pressure and the fact that it produces pupillary dilation tend to make this drug less useful than SNP during neurosurgical anesthesia.

Adenosine Triphosphate (ATP) and Adenosine

Both ATP and adenosine are potent vasodilators, and their hypotensive effects have a rapid onset and a short duration. ATP is rapidly degraded to adenosine, and its hypotensive effects appear to be mediated by adenosine. Because ATP has some dysrhythmogenic properties, adenosine may be more useful than ATP in clinical practice. Advantages of adenosine include lack of toxicity, tachyphylaxis, or rebound hypertension.

During adenosine- or ATP-induced hypotension, CBF was either increased[59,232,257] or unchanged.[111,234] CBF was decreased when the blood pressure fall was extreme[104,179,257] or when extreme hypocapnia was induced.[265] Despite many reports showing lack of rebound hypertension after adenosine- or ATP-induced hypotension, there may be a risk of cerebral hyperperfusion for a period of time commencing soon after adenosine-induced hypotension is discontinued.[234] CMR_{O_2} has been reported to be unchanged or slightly decreased during adenosine- and ATP-induced hypotension.[104,111,179,234,257] Regional CMRgl was decreased significantly when hypocapnia was combined with adenosine-induced hypotension.[265] Effects of adenosine on ICP were inconsistent. ICP was increased in association with decreased intracranial compliance in one study[258] but was unchanged in another.[179] No clinical data concerning the effect of adenosine on ICP is available. However, adenosine, like other vasodilators, should be used cautiously in patients with elevated ICP or decreased intracranial compliance.

Sympatholytic Agents

Alpha-adrenergic receptor blocking agents *phentolamine* and *phenoxybenzamine* have been shown to be without effect on resting CBF, but they reduce the blood flow response to phenylephrine, adrenaline, and noradrenaline.[57]

Beta-adrenergic receptor blocking agents such as *propranolol* have been shown to cause a slight decrease in CBF and $CMRo_2$ in rats.[84] CO_2 response of the cerebral circulation was decreased by propranolol.[7]

Labetalol, a combined alpha- and beta-adrenergic receptor blocking drug, has been used for the treatment of hypertension and induced hypotension. This drug has advantages such as lack of toxicity, tachyphylaxis, or rebound hypertension. In dogs anesthetized with pentobarbital and fentanyl, labetalol, given in a dose sufficient to produce a reduction in MABP of about 45%, produced no significant change in CBF.[79] During neuroleptanesthesia, labetalol given to dogs with or without intracranial hypertension caused no significant changes in ICP despite a MABP reduction of 27% to 38%.[256] In this study ventricular volume pressure response curves were identical both before and after labetalol, irrespective of whether baseline ICP was elevated, suggesting that labetalol produces no change in compliance or elastance. Because of the wide variation in drug response and the difficulty of producing deeper hypotension, this drug may not be the drug of choice when used alone to induce hypotension.[256]

In patients with AVM or aneurysm, labetalol, given after surgery, permitted either weaning off SNP or substantial reduction in SNP requirement, improved CPP, and decreased ICP.[188] Satisfactory control of hypertension with labetalol after intracranial surgery also has been reported.[171]

Esmolol, an ultrashort-acting beta-adrenergic receptor blocking drug, has been shown to be useful during neurosurgical anesthesia.[171,189] Esmolol has no significant effects on CBF or ICP.[31] In a recent study labetalol and esmolol were compared for the control of hypertension during emergence from anesthesia after intracranial surgery. Both drugs proved effective in the control of blood pressure and were discontinued 10 minutes after extubation. Labetalol produced a higher incidence of bradycardia in the postanesthesia care unit than did esmolol. These findings suggest that the effects of labetalol may persist into the postoperative period and create unwanted cardiovascular effects. Thus esmolol may be the better drug for control of blood pressure in this situation.[171]

Calcium Entry Blockers

A cerebral protective effect of some calcium entry blockers has been reported in various models of experimental ischemia.[214,227] Thus a calcium entry blocker may be a drug of choice for induced hypotension. However, only limited data are available. Data from studies in which these drugs were used to control hypertension show that nifedipine and nicardipine elevate ICP.[71,246] Whether the elevation of ICP can be prevented by hyperventilation or other clinically applicable interventions awaits further study.

Angiotensin

Angiotensin is used to test autoregulation because it is believed to have no direct effects on CBF and $CMRo_2$. This

is probably true in humans. However, in animals, it is uncertain whether angiotensin has a direct effect. In rabbits, when angiotensin is given into one carotid artery, regional CBF decreases.[199] In isolated canine brain preparations with fixed CBF, angiotensin increases the perfusion pressure secondary to an increase in CVR.[120] A significant decrease in $CMRo_2$ also has been reported with angiotensin infusion during 1.4% isoflurane anesthesia.[202] These results are in contrast to a report in cats demonstrating no angiotensin affect on $CMRo_2$ during isoflurane anesthesia.[250]

Phenylephrine

Phenylephrine has been reported to have no effect on CBF or $CMRo_2$.[229] However, Newberg et al.[176] reported that phenylephrine in a dose producing a 15 mm Hg rise in MABP during 1.4% (end-tidal) isoflurane anesthesia produces a significant decrease in CBF, an increase in CVR, but no change in $CMRo_2$.

Epinephrine, Norepinephrine

It is generally accepted that systemic administration of epinephrine or norepinephrine does not produce significant changes in CBF or $CMRo_2$ unless it gains access to the brain through a disrupted blood-brain barrier or unless the blood pressure exceeds the upper limit of autoregulation. However, epinephrine appears to have an indirect effect, which may increase CBF, because it produces anxiety and arousal. Norepinephrine decreases CBF, and there is no change in $CMRo_2$.[57]

In summary, among the drugs used to control hypertension or to induce hypotension, sodium nitroprusside is the drug of choice. Calcium entry blockers, because of their potential protective effects against brain ischemia, may be alternatives. Combinations of other drugs with low concentrations of inhalational anesthetics also can be used with careful observation. Because it is difficult to predict the blood pressure at which ischemic events occur, one should maintain the cerebral perfusion pressure above 60 mm Hg in normotensive patients and keep the duration of induced hypotension as short as possible. Blood pressure should be returned slowly to normal after induced hypotension.

ANESTHETIC INTERACTIONS

Modification of autoregulation and CO_2 responses with anesthetics is important because these changes lead to unsatisfactory operative conditions and a potentially poor clinical outcome. Other important aspects are the interaction of anesthetics with surgical stimulation and time (duration of anesthesia).

Autoregulation during Anesthesia

Evaluation of autoregulation of blood pressure during anesthesia necessitates induced changes in CPP (MABP) while a constant anesthetic depth is maintained. In most studies, angiotensin, phenylephrine, and norepinephrine have been used to elevate blood pressure, while trimethaphan, nitroprusside, and withdrawal of blood have been used to decrease blood pressure. Some of these methods are without direct effect on the cerebral vasculatures.

Autoregulation appears to be impaired with volatile anesthetics, especially at high concentrations.* In baboons rendered severely hypotensive by deep halothane for more than 2 hours (MABP of 33 mm Hg), autoregulation was lost even after the depth of anesthesia was decreased.[185] Such findings suggest that normalization of blood pressure after induced hypotension should not be rapid. There are reports showing that autoregulation is partly preserved with isoflurane at 1 to 2 MAC.[250]

Autoregulation is influenced not only by the anesthetic itself but also by the level of Pa_{CO_2}.[157,186] It was found in dogs that with 2 mg/kg morphine, autoregulation was maintained irrespective of the level of Pa_{CO_2}. However, with 1.5% halothane, autoregulation was impaired during hypercapnia, but it was maintained during normocapnia and hypocapnia.[186] During halothane or enflurane anesthesia, Miletich et al.[157] reported disturbed autoregulation during normocapnia and hypercapnia; they reported that it was restored with the introduction of hypocapnia. This finding suggests that when cerebral vessels have been already dilated by hypercapnia or vasodilating drugs, compensatory vasodilation may not occur when arterial pressure decreases. N_2O alone or in combination with morphine does not appear to disturb autoregulation.[99,228,229] Barbiturates and fentanyl, either alone or in combination, also preserve autoregulation.[52,138]

Autoregulation is usually impaired in patients with intracranial space-occupying lesions.[60] When autoregulation is lost or disturbed, sudden blood pressure changes can produce ischemia or brain edema. Therefore deep inhalational anesthesia and/or hypercapnia should definitely be avoided. A study by Engberg et al.[60] showed that during surgical incision and after extubation, there was a decrease in the arterial-cerebral venous blood oxygen content difference ($AVDO_2$) during either neuroleptoanesthesia or 0.45% to 0.9% halothane anesthesia supplemented with N_2O, suggesting that an increase in MABP may increase the CBF in such situations. Thus careful management of blood pressure is critical in patients with intracranial pathology.

Cerebrovascular Reactivity to CO_2

At clinical levels of anesthesia, cerebrovascular responses to alterations in Pa_{CO_2} are preserved, although the magnitude of response may vary depending on the anesthetic and anesthetic depth. In general, the increase in CBF seen in response to each 1 mm Hg change in Pa_{CO_2} appears to be greater when vasodilatory anesthetics are used, compared with when vasoconstrictor drugs are used. The percentage change of CBF for each 1 mm Hg change in Pa_{CO_2} ranges

from 1.5% to 3.4% during halothane, enflurane, or N_2O in dogs.[243] Scheller et al.[218] demonstrated that in the rabbit halothane increased CBF at all Pa_{CO_2} levels examined (20, 40, and 50 mm Hg). In contrast, with isoflurane, CBF decreased during hypocapnia, it was unchanged during normocapnia, and it increased during hypercapnia. Drummond and Todd[54] demonstrated that CO_2 reactivity is greater with isoflurane than with halothane. At a Pa_{CO_2} of 18 to 20 mm Hg, CBF was significantly less with isoflurane than with halothane. This could be due to greater cerebral metabolic depression compared with the ability to dilate cerebral vessels. In humans, CO_2 reactivity was maintained at 1 MAC of isoflurane and enflurane.[118] CO_2 reactivity is impaired or lost when blood pressure decreases during high concentrations of inhalational anesthetics.[139,259]

Intravenous anesthetics in general preserve CO_2 reactivity. Thiopental in large doses attenuates but does not abolish CO_2 reactivity in dogs.[103] In humans, CO_2 reactivity is maintained to barbiturate concentrations that produce burst suppression. During narcotic anesthesia, CO_2 reactivity was reported to be intact.[100,105,138,242,262] Diazepam,[262] etomidate,[40] propofol,[236] and ketamine[217] preserve CO_2 reactivity. CO_2 reactivity is preserved also during neuroleptanesthesia.[41]

The level of arterial blood pressure is a factor that may affect the reactivity to CO_2. In baboons whose MABP was decreased below 60 mm Hg with deep halothane, reactivity to CO_2 was lost, but it was restored with return of MABP produced by decreasing the depth of anesthesia.[185] Similar modulation of CO_2 reactivity by a reduction in blood pressure has been reported for isoflurane.[259] It is not clear, however, whether the loss of reactivity to CO_2 is due to the anesthetic itself or to the hypotension.

Reactivity to CO_2 has been shown to be present in anesthetized patients with intracranial space-occupying lesions.[58,125] This is contrary to the concept that cerebral autoregulation is generally impaired in patients with a space-occupying lesion. This is why hyperventilation is recommended in patients with increased ICP or decreased intracranial compliance. CO_2 reactivity also varies by region, as already discussed.

Surgical Stimulation

It is important to know the changes in CBF, CMR_{O_2}, and ICP that occur during surgical stimulation. Nevertheless, not much information is available. Kuramoto et al.[109] examined the effects of sciatic nerve stimulation on CBF and CMR_{O_2} in dogs. During 0.5% and 1.0% halothane, stimulation produced a coupled increase in CBF and CMR_{O_2}, accompanied by EEG desynchronization. During 1.4% halothane, stimulation produced an increase in CBF without a change in CMR_{O_2} or EEG, or an increase in arterial blood pressure. During morphine anesthesia (0.5 mg/kg and 1.5 mg/kg with or without N_2O), nerve stimulation produced almost parallel increases in CBF and CMR_{O_2} and was accompanied by EEG desynchronization. During light thio-

---

*References 30, 64, 157, 163, 185, 259.

pental anesthesia, sciatic nerve stimulation produced increases in CBF and CMR_{O_2} in association with EEG desynchronization, but during deep thiopental anesthesia did not change CBF, CMR_{O_2}, or EEG by stimulation.[162] Therefore, irrespective of anesthetic depth, there is tight coupling among changes in CBF, CMR_{O_2}, and EEG with stimulation during thiopental anesthesia.

These results suggest that anesthetics that possess cerebral vasodilator effects disturb the coupling between flow and metabolism with stimulation, whereas cerebral vasoconstrictor drugs tend to maintain it. In humans anesthetized with 3.5% enflurane, no apparent increases in CBF or CMR_{O_2} were observed with surgical stimulation despite changes in EEG.[212] However, in that study, CBF and CMR_{O_2} were measured by the Kety-Schmidt method, and the regional changes in CBF and CMR_{O_2} with stimulation may not have been detected.

Through autoradiographic techniques, cerebral vasodilation elicited by focal stimulation within the medullary reticular formation in rats anesthetized with alpha-chloralose has been reported, and this effect appears to be mediated by intrinsic pathways of the central nervous system.[93] Nakakimura et al.[174] examined the changes in local glucose utilization in the brain and lumbar spinal cord produced by unilateral sciatic nerve stimulation in rats anesthetized with 0.5%, 2%, and 4% enflurane. Sciatic nerve stimulation produced a 70% to 110% increase in glucose utilization in the ipsilateral dorsal horn of the lumbar spinal cord at all anesthetic concentrations examined. Stimulation also produced a 30% to 50% increase in glucose use in the hindlimb projection area of the contralateral somatosensory cortex at the two lowest concentrations (0.5% and 2%). At 4% enflurane no stimulation-induced increase in glucose utilization was observed. The results show that there is a threshold at which enflurane suppresses the metabolic responses to peripheral stimulation in the somatosensory cortex but not in the spinal cord. If electrical stimulation is regarded as analogous to surgical stimulation, a considerable increase in spinal cord metabolism may occur during surgery, even in a deeply anesthetized subject, although the cerebral cortical responses are blocked with high anesthetic concentrations. One must consider the possibility that, during light anesthesia, surgical stimulation provokes a CBF increase in association with metabolic activation and may cause an increase in ICP.

Interactions With Time

CBF responses change during prolonged anesthesia with volatile anesthetics. The increase in CBF (54%) in goats caused by 1% halothane returned to the preanesthetic level over a 150-minute period of anesthesia in association with a moderate increase in CVR (and CMR_{O_2}).[4] Similar time-dependent decreases in CBF were observed in dogs anesthetized with 1% halothane. CBF decreased by half during the 2- to 7-hour period of exposure.[267] In a different study in dogs, a steady-state CBF was achieved 3 hours after introduction of 1.3 MAC isoflurane and 5 hours after introduction of 1.7 MAC halothane.[26] Use of 1.7 MAC isoflurane produced a larger initial increase in CBF and a more prolonged period (5 hours) to reach a final steady-state CBF. In dogs anesthetized with 70% N_2O and paralyzed, a 35% decrease in CBF at 3 hours has been reported.[242] The mechanism for this gradual return of CBF to preanesthetic level is not clear. However, this phenomenon could not be modified by prior administration of alpha- and beta-receptor blocking drugs. In addition, it is not related to time-dependent changes in autoregulation or CSF pH.[267] Because time-dependent decreases in CBF have been observed (5%/hr) in both anesthetized and unanesthetized dogs, Raichle et al.[194] concluded that these phenomena were related to the possible effects of immobilization and/or mechanical ventilation. However, it is insufficient to attribute these time-dependent decreases in CBF to immobilization because the results concerning the effects of prolonged anesthesia with isoflurane are not consistent. Turner et al.[254] reported gradual declines in CBF over a period of hours during isoflurane anesthesia. In contrast, Roald et al.,[201] using a modified sagittal sinus outflow measurement technique, reported that CBF and CMR_{O_2} during isoflurane anesthesia of 3 to 4 hours' duration remained unchanged. With this model, CBF was stable over time and the results obtained were different from the original studies demonstrating CBF decreases as a function of time.[240,242] Time-dependent changes in CBF so far have not been directly examined in humans.

SUMMARY

Anesthetic drugs and techniques influence cerebral circulation, metabolism, and ICP. The data discussed in the present chapter are important for the anesthetic management of both neurosurgical patients and non-neurosurgical patients with cerebrovascular disease. The severely damaged brain cannot be restored. Anesthetic management thus should focus on preventing the propagation of damage, preventing new damage, and providing appropriate surgical conditions. If a potent cerebral vasodilatory anesthetic is used in patients with intracranial space-occupying lesions or decreased intracranial compliance, marked increase in ICP may occur. Induction of cerebral hyperemia in a patient with a space-occupying intracranial lesion therefore should always be avoided. Induction of vasoconstriction, by hyperventilation and/or concomitant use of vasoconstricting anesthetics such as barbiturates, decreases and stabilizes the ICP. During carotid endarterectomy and bypass surgery, normocapnia may be recommended because the regional CBF response of an ischemic area to altered Pa_{CO_2} cannot

Continued.

be accurately predicted in individual patients. Autoregulation may be impaired by pathologic conditions as well as deep inhalational anesthesia. Furthermore, the CPP necessary to maintain adequate cerebral perfusion cannot be easily determined in an individual patient. Thus, during surgery for ischemic cerebrovascular deceases, arterial blood pressure should be maintained no lower than the lowest preoperative pressure. Isoflurane may be a good choice if an inhalational anesthetic is deemed desirable. The metabolic depressive effect of barbiturates and other intravenous anesthetics may also be beneficial in such situations. Noxious stimuli under inadequate anesthesia or seizure activity can also produce undesirable events, such as increased metabolism, CBV, and ICP. Narcotics and supplemental local anesthetics are recommended.

References

1. Adams RW, Gronert GA, Sundt TM et al: Halothane, hypocapnia, and cerebrospinal fluid pressure in neurosurgery, *Anesthesiology* 37:510-517, 1972.

2. Adams RW, Cucchiara RF, Gronert GA et al: Isoflurane and cerebrospinal fluid pressure in neurosurgical patients, *Anesthesiology* 54:97-99, 1981.

3. Albin MS, Bunegin L, Gelineau J: ICP and CBF reactivity to isoflurane and nitrous oxide during normocapnia, hypocapnia and intracranial hypertension. In Miller JD, Teasdale GM, Rowan JO et al, editors: *Intracranial pressure VI*, Berlin, 1986, Springer, pp 719-724.

4. Albrecht RF, Miletich DJ, Rosenberg R et al: Cerebral blood flow and metabolic changes from induction to onset of anesthesia wth halothane or pentobarbital, *Anesthesiology* 47:252-256, 1977.

5. Albrecht RF, Miletich DJ, Madala LR: Normalization of cerebral blood flow during prolonged halothane anesthesia, *Anesthesiology* 58:26-31, 1983.

6. Algotsson L, Messeter K, Nordström CH et al: Cerebral blood flow and oxygen consumption during isoflurane and halothane anesthesia in man, *Acta Anaesthesiol Scand* 32:15-20, 1988.

7. Aoyagi M, Deshmukh VD, Meyer JS et al: Effects of beta-adrenergic blockade with propranolol on cerebral blood flow, autoregulation and CO_2 responsiveness, *Stroke* 7:291-295, 1976.

8. Archer DP, Labrecque P, Tylor JL et al: Cerebral blood volume is increased in dogs during administration of nitrous oxide or isoflurane, *Anesthesiology* 67:642-648, 1987.

9. Artru AA: Relationship between cerebral blood volume and CSF pressure during anesthesia with halothane or enflurane in dogs, *Anesthesiology* 58:533-539, 1983.

10. Artru AA: Isoflurane does not increase the rate of CSF production in the dog, *Anesthesiology* 60:193-197, 1984.

11. Artru AA: Effects of enflurane and isoflurane on resistance to reabsorption of cerebrospinal fluid in dogs, *Anesthesiology* 61:529-533, 1984.

12. Artru AA: Effects of halothane and fentanyl anesthesia on resitance to reabsorption of CSF, *J Neurosurg* 60:252-256, 1984.

13. Artru AA, Katz RA: Cerebral blood volume and CSF pressure following administration of ketamine in dogs; modification by pre- or posttreatment with hypocapnia or diazepam, *J Neurosurg Anesthesiol* 1:8-15, 1989.

14. Artru AA: Flumazenil reversal of midazolam in dogs: dose-related changes in cerebral blood flow, metabolism, EEG, and CSF pressure, *J Neurosurg Anesthesiol* 1:46-55, 1989.

15. Astrup J, Skovsted P, Gjerris F et al: Increase in extracellular potassium in the brain during circulatory arrest: effects of hypothermia, lidocaine, and thiopental, *Anesthesiology* 55:256-262, 1981.

16. Astrup J, Sørensen PM, Sørensen HR: Inhibition of cerebral oxygen and glucose consumption in the dog by hypothermia, pentobarbital, and lidocaine, *Anesthesiology* 55:263-268, 1981.

17. Basta SJ, Savarese JJ, Ali HH et al: Histamine-releasing potencies of atracurium, dimethyl tubocurarine and tubocurarine, *Br J Anaesth* 55:105S-106S, 1983.

18. Baughman VL, Hoffman WE, Miletich DJ et al: Neurologic outcome in rats following incomplete cerebral ischemia during halothane, isoflurane, or N_2O, *Anesthesiology* 69:192-198, 1988.

19. Baughman VL, Hoffman WE, Miletich DJ et al: Cerebral metabolic depression and brain protection produced by midazolam and etomidate in the rat, *J Neurosurg Anesthesiol* 1:22-28, 1989.

20. Baughman VL, Hoffman WE, Thomas C et al: The interaction of nitrous oxide and isoflurane with incomplete cerebral ischemia in the rat, *Anesthesiology* 70:767-774, 1989.

21. Baughman VL, Hoffman WE, Miletich DJ et al: Cerebrovascular and cerebral metabolic effects of N_2O in unrestrained rats, *Anesthesiology* 73:269-272, 1990.

22. Bedford RF, Persing JA, Pobereskin L et al: Lidocaine or thiopental for rapid control of intracranial hypertension? *Anesth Analg* 59:435-437, 1980.

23. Bedford RF, Winn HR, Tyson G et al: Lidocaine prevents increased ICP after endotracheal intubation. In Shulman K, Marmarou A, Miller JD, et al, editors: *Intracranial pressure IV*, Berlin, 1980, Springer, pp 595-598.

24. Belapavovic M, Buchthal A: Modification of ketamine-induced intracranial hypertension in neurosurgical patients by pretreatment with midazolam, *Acta Anaesth Scand* 26:458-462, 1982.

25. Bingham RM, Procaccio F, Prior PF et al: Cerebral electrical activity influences the effects of etomidate on cerebral perfusion pressure in traumatic coma, *Br J Anaesth* 57:843-848, 1985.

26. Boarini DJ, Kassel NF, Coester HC et al: Comparison of systemic and cerebrovascular effects of isoflurane and halothane, *Neurosurgery* 15:400-409, 1984.
27. Boop WC, Knight R: Enflurane anesthesia and changes of intracranial pressure, *J Neurosurg* 48:228-231, 1978.
28. Branston NH, Hone DT, Symon L: Barbiturates in focal ischemia of primate cortex: effects on blood flow distributron, evoked potential, and extracellular potassium, *Stroke* 10:647-653, 1979.
29. Bristow A, Shalev D, Rice B et al: Low-dose synthetic narcotic infusions for cerebral relaxation during craniotomies, *Anesth Analg* 66:413-416, 1987.
30. Brüssel T, Fitch W, Brodner G et al: Effects of halothane in low concentrations on cerebral blood flow, cerebral metabolism, and cerebrovascular autoregulation in the baboon, *Anesth Analg* 73:758-764, 1991.
31. Bunegin L, Albin MS, Gelineau EF: Effect of esmolol on cerebral blood flow during intracranial hypotension and hemorrhagic hypovolemia, *Anesthesiology* 67:A424, 1987.
32. Campkin TV: Isoflurane and cranial extradural pressure, a study in neurosurgical patients, *Br J Anaesth* 56:1083-1087, 1984.
33. Candia GJ, Heros RC, Lavyne MH et al: Effect of intravenous sodium nitroprusside on cerebral blood flow and intracranial pressure, *Neurosurgery* 3:50-53, 1978.
34. Carlsson C, Hagerdal M, Siesjö BK: The effect of nitrous oxide on oxygen consumption and blood flow in the cerebral cortex of the rat, *Acta Anaesthesiol Scand* 20:91-95, 1976.
35. Carlsson C, Hagerdal M, Kaasik AE et al: The effects of diazepam on cerebral blood flow and oxygen consumption in rats and its synergistic interaction with nitrous oxide, *Anesthesiology* 45:319-325, 1976.
36. Carlsson C, Smith DS, Keykhah MN et al: The effects of high dose fentanyl on cerebral circulation and metabolism in rats, *Anesthesiology* 57:375-380, 1982.
37. Cavazzuti M, Porro CA, Biral GP et al: Ketamine effects on local cerebral blood flow and metabolism in the rat, *J Cereb Blood Flow Metab* 7:806-811, 1987.
38. Chang KSK, Laey MO, Davis RF: Propofol produces vasodilation by a calcium channel antagonist action, *Anesthesiology* 75:A553, 1991.
39. Chapple DJ, Miller AA, Ward JB et al: Cardiovascular and neurological effects of laudanosine, *Br J Anaesth* 59:218-225, 1987.
40. Cold GE, Eskesen V, Eriksen H et al: CBF and CMR_{O_2} during continuous etomidate infusion supplemented with N_2O and fentanyl in patients with supratentorial cerebral tumours. A dose response study, *Acta Anaesthesiol Scand* 29:490-494, 1985.
41. Cold GE, Christensen KJS, Nordentoft J et al: Cerebral blood flow, cerebral metabolic rate of oxygen and relative CO_2 reactivity during neurolept anesthesia in patients subjected to craniotomy for supratentorial cerebral tumors, *Acta Anaesthesiol Scand* 32:310-315, 1988.
42. Cole DJ, Shapiro HM: Different 1.2 MAC combinations of nitrous oxide-enflurane cause unique cerebral and spinal cord metabolic responses in the rat, *Anesthesiology* 70:787-792, 1989.
43. Cotev S, Shalit MN: Effects of diazepam on cerebral blood flow and oxygen uptake after head injury, *Anesthesiology* 43:117-122, 1975.
44. Cottrell JE, Hartung J, Giffin JP et al: Intracranial and hemodynamic changes after succinylcholine administration in cats, *Anesth Analg* 62:1006-1009, 1983.
45. Crosby G, Crane AM, Sokoloff L: A comparison of local rates of glucose utilization in spinal cord and brain in conscious and nitrous oxide- or pentobarbital-treated rats, *Anesthesiology* 61:434-438, 1984.
46. Dahlgren N, Ingvar M, Yokoyama H et al: Influence of nitrous oxide on local cerebral blood flow in awake, minimally restrained rats, *J Cereb Blood Flow Metab* 1:211-218, 1981.
47. Davis DW, Mans AM, Biebuyck JF et al: Regional brain glucose utilization in rats during etomidate anesthesia, *Anesthesiology* 64:751-757, 1986.
48. Davis DW, Mans AM, Biebuyck JF et al: The influence of ketamine on regional brain glucose use, *Anesthesiology* 69:199-205, 1988.
49. Dawson B, Michenfelder JD, Theye RA: Effect of ketamine on canine cerebral blood flow and metabolism: modification by prior administration of thiopental, *Anesth Analg* 50:443-447, 1971.
50. Dearden NM, McDowall DG: Comparison of etomidate and althesin in the reduction of increased intracranial pressure after head injury, *Br J Anaesth* 57:361-368, 1985.
51. Dohi S, Matsumoto M, Takahashi K: The effects of nitroglycerin on cerebrospinal fluid pressure in awake and anesthetized humans, *Anesthesiology* 54:511-514, 1981.
52. Donegan JH, Traystman RJ, Koehler RC et al: Cerebrovascular, hypoxic, and autoregulatory responses during reduced brain metabolism, *Am J Physiol* 249:H421-H429, 1985.
53. Drummond JC, Todd MM, Toutant SM et al: Brain surface protrusion during enflurane, halothane and isoflurane anesthesia in cats, *Anesthesiology* 59:288-293, 1983.
54. Drummond JC, Todd MM: The response of the feline cerebral circulation to Pa_{CO_2} during anesthesia with isoflurane and halothane and during sedation with nitrous oxide, *Anesthesiology* 62:268-273, 1985.
55. Drummond JC, Todd MM, Scheller MS et al: A comparison of the direct cerebral vasodilating potencies of halothane and isoflurane in the New Zealand white rabbit, *Anesthesiology* 65:462-467, 1986.
56. Drummond JC, Scheller MS, Todd MM: The effect of nitrous oxide on cortical blood flow during anesthesia with halothane and isoflurane, with and without morphine, in the rabbit, *Anesth Analg* 66:1083-1089, 1987.
57. Edvinsson L, Mac Kenzie ET: Amine mechanisms in the cerebral circulation, *Pharmacol Rev* 28:275-348, 1977.
58. Eintrei C, Leszniewski W, Carlsson C: Local application of ^{133}Xenon for measurement of regional cerebral blood flow (rCBF) during halothane, enflurane, and isoflurane anesthesia in humans, *Anesthesiology* 63:391-394, 1985.
59. Eintrei C, Carlsson C: Effects of hypotension induced by adenosine on brain surface oxygen pressure and cortical cerebral blood flow in the pig, *Acta Physiol Scand* 126:463-469, 1986.
60. Engberg M, Øberg B, Christensen KS et al: The cerebral arterio-venous oxygen content differences($AV_{D_{O_2}}$)

during halothane and neurolept anesthesia in patients subjected to craniotomy, *Acta Anaesthesiol Scand* 33:642-646, 1989.

61. Evans DE, Kobrine AI, LeGrys DC et al: Protective effect of lidocaine in acute cerebral ischemia induced by air embolism, *J Neurosurg* 60:257-263, 1984.

62. Feustel PJ, Ingvar MC, Severinghaus JW: Cerebral oxygen availability and blood flow during middle cerebral artery occlusion; effects of pentobarbital, *Stroke* 12:858-863, 1981.

63. Fleischer JE, Milde JH, Moyer TP et al: Cerebral effects of high-dose midazolam and subsequent reversal with RO 15-1788 in dogs, *Anesthesiology* 68:234-242, 1988.

64. Forster A, Van Horn K, Marshall LF et al: Anesthetic effects on blood-brain barrier function during acute arterial hypertension, *Anesthesiology* 49:26-30, 1978.

65. Forster A, Juge O, Morel D: Effects of midazolam on cerebral blood flow in human volunteers, *Anesthesiology* 56:453-455, 1982.

66. Forster A, Juge O, Louis M et al: Effects of a specific benzodiazepine antagonist (RO15-1788) on cerebral blood flow, *Anesth Analg* 66:309-313, 1987.

67. Frizell RT, Meyer YJ, Borchers DJ et al: The effects of etomidate on cerebral metabolism and blood flow in a canine model for hypoperfusion, *J Neurosurg* 74:263-269, 1991.

68. From RP, Warner DS, Todd MM et al: Anesthesia for craniotomy: a double-blind comparison of alfentanil, fentanyl, and sufentanil, *Anesthesiology* 73:896-904, 1990.

69. Fukuda S, Murakawa T, Takeshita H et al: Direct effects of ketamine on isolated canine cerebral and mesenteric arteries, *Anesth Analg* 62:553-558, 1983.

70. Gelman S, Fowler KC, Smith LR: Regional blood flow during isoflurane and halothane anesthesia, *Anesth Analg* 63:557-565, 1984.

71. Giffin JP, Cottrell JE, Hartung J et al: Intracranial pressure during nifedipine-induced hypotension, *Anesth Analg* 62:1078-1080, 1983.

72. Giffin JP, Cottrell JE, Shwiry B et al: Intracranial pressure, mean arterial pressure, and heart rate following midazolam or thiopental in humans with

brain tumors, *Anesthesiology* 60:491-494, 1984.

73. Giffin JP, Litwak B, Cottrell JE et al: Intracranial pressure, mean arterial pressure and heart rate after rapid paralysis with atracurium in cats, *Can Anaesth Soc J* 32:618-621, 1985.

74. Giffin JP, Hartung J, Cottrell JE et al: Effect of vecuronium on intracranial pressure, mean arterial pressure and heart rate in cats, *Br J Anaesth* 58:441-443, 1986.

75. Gordon E, Lagerkranser M, Rudehill A et al: The effect of isoflurane on cerebrospinal fluid pressure in patients undergoing neurosurgery, *Acta Anaesthesiol Scand* 32:108-112, 1988.

76. Griswold WR, Roznik V, Mendoza SA: Nitroprusside induced intracranial hypertension, *JAMA* 246:2679-2680, 1981.

77. Gronert GA, Michenfelder JD, Sharbrough FW et al: Canine cerebral metabolic tolerance during 24 hours deep pentobarbital anesthesia, *Anesthesiology* 55:110-113, 1981.

78. Grosslight K, Foster R, Colohan AR et al: Isoflurane for neuroanesthesia: risk factors for increases in intracranial pressure, *Anesthesiology* 63:533-536, 1985.

79. Gustafson C, Ahlgren I, Aronsen K-F et al: Haemodynamic effects of labetalol-induced hypotension in the anaesthetized dog, *Br J Anaesth* 53:585-590, 1981.

80. Hansen TD, Warner DS, Todd MM et al: Distribution of cerebral blood flow during halothane versus isoflurane anesthesia in rats, *Anesthesiology* 69:332-337, 1988.

81. Hansen TD, Warner DS, Todd MM et al: The role of cerebral metabolism in determining the local cerebral blood flow effects of volatile anesthetics: evidence for persistent flow-metabolism coupling, *J Cereb Blood Flow Metab* 9:323-328, 1989.

82. Hartung HJ: Intracranial pressure after propofol and thiopental administration in patients with severe head trauma, *Anaesthetist* 36:285-287, 1987.

83. Hartung J, Cottrell JE: Nitrous oxide reduces thiopental-induced prolongation of survival in hypoxic and anoxic mice, *Anesth Analg* 66:47-52, 1987.

84. Hemmingsen R, Hertz MM, Barry DI: The effect of propranolol on ce-

rebral oxygen consumption and blood flow in the rat: measurement during normocapnia and hypercapnia, *Acta Physiol Scand* 105:274-281, 1979.

85. Herkenham M: Anesthetics and the habenulo-interpeduncular system: selective sparing of metabolic activity, *Brain Res* 210:461-466, 1981.

86. Herrick IA, Gelb AW, Manninen PH et al: Effects of fentanyl, sufentanil, and alfentanil on brain retractor pressure, *Anesth Analg* 72:359-363, 1991.

87. Hitchon PW, Kassell NF, Hill TR et al: The response of spinal cord blood flow to high-dose barbiturates, *Spine* 7:41-45, 1982.

88. Hodes JE, Soncrant TT, Larson DM et al: Selective changes in local cerebral glucose utilization induced by phenobarbital in the rat, *Anesthesiology* 63:633-639, 1985.

89. Hoff J, Schmith A, Nielsen S et al: Effects of barbiturate and halothane anaesthesia on focal cerebral infarction in the dog, *Surg Forum* 24:449-452, 1973.

90. Hoffman WE, Albrecht RF, Miletich DJ: Nitroglycerin induced hypotension will maintain CBF in hypertensive rats, *Stroke* 13:225-228, 1982.

91. Hoffman WE, Miletich DJ, Albrecht RF: The effects of midazolam on cerebral blood flow and oxygen consumption and its interaction with nitrous oxide, *Anesth Analg* 65:729-733, 1986.

92. Hougaard K, Hansen A, Brodersen P: The effect of ketamine on regional cerebral blood flow in man, *Anesthesiology* 41:562-567, 1974.

93. Iadecola C, Nakai M, Arbit E et al: Global cerebral vasodilatation elicited by focal electrical stimulation within the dorsal medullary reticular formation in anesthetized rat, *J Cereb Blood Flow Metab* 3:270-279, 1983.

94. Ingvar M, Shapiro HM: Selective metabolic activation of the hippocampus during lidocaine-induced pre-seizure activity, *Anesthesiology* 54:33-37, 1981.

95. Ingvar M, Siesjö BK: Effect of nitrous oxide on local cerebral glucose utilization in rats, *J Cereb Blood Flow Metab* 2:481-486, 1982.

96. Ishikawa T, Funatsu N, Okamoto K et al: Cerebral systemic effects of hypotension induced by trimethaphan

and nitroprusside in dogs, *Acta Anaesthesiol Scand* 26:643-648, 1982.

97. Ishikawa T, Funatsu N, Okamoto K et al: Blood-brain barrier function following drug-induced hypotension in the dog, *Anesthesiology* 59:526-531, 1983.

98. Iwatsuki N, Kuroda N, Amaha K et al: Succinylcholine-induced hyperkalemia in patients with ruptured cerebral aneurysms, *Anesthesiology* 53:64-67, 1980.

99. Jobes DR, Kennell E, Bitner R et al: Effects of morphine-nitrous oxide anesthesia on cerebral autoregulation, *Anesthesiology* 42:30-34, 1975.

100. Jobes DR, Kennell E, Bush GL et al: Cerebral blood flow and metabolism during morphine-nitrous oxide anesthesia in man, *Anesthesiology* 47:16-18, 1977.

101. Kaieda R, Todd MM, Warner DS: The effects of anesthetics and Pa_{CO_2} on the cerebrovascular, metabolic, and electroencephalographic responses to nitrous oxide in the rabbit, *Anesth Analg* 68:135-143, 1989.

102. Kaieda R, Todd MM, Weeks JB et al: A comparison of the effects of halothane, isoflurane, and pentobarbital anesthesia on intracranial pressure and cerebral edema formation following brain injury in rabbits, *Anesthesiology* 71:571-579, 1989.

103. Kassell NF, Hitchon PW, Gerk MK et al: Influence of changes in arterial Pco_2 on cerebral blood flow and metabolism during high dose barbiturate therapy in dogs, *J Neurosurg* 54:615-619, 1981.

104. Kassell NF, Boarini DJ, Olin JJ et al: Cerebral and systemic circulatory effects of arterial hypotension induced by adenosine, *J Neurosurg* 58:69-76, 1983.

105. Keykhah MM, Smith DS, Carlsson C et al: Influence of sufentanil on cerebral metabolism and circulation in the rat, *Anesthesiology* 63:274-277, 1985.

106. Keykhah MM, Smith DS, O'Neill JJ et al: The influence of fentanyl upon cerebral high-energy metabolites, lactate, and glucose during severe hypoxia in the rat, *Anesthesiology* 69:566-570, 1988.

107. Khambutta HJ, Stone JG, Matteo RS et al: Propranolol premedication blunts stress response to nitroprusside hypotension, *Anesth Analg* 63:125-128, 1984.

108. Knight PR, Lane GA, Hensinger RN et al: Catecholamine and renin-angiotensin response during hypotensive anesthesia induced by sodium nitroprusside or trimethaphan camsylate, *Anesthesiology* 59:248-253, 1983.

109. Kuramoto T, Oshita S, Takeshita H et al: Modification of the relationship between cerebral metabolism, blood flow, and electroencephalogram by stimulation during anesthesia in the dog, *Anesthesiology* 51:211-217, 1979.

110. Lafferty JJ, Keykhah MM, Shapiro HM et al: Cerebral hypometabolism obtained with deep pentobarbital anesthesia and hypothermia (30° C), *Anesthesiology* 49:159-164, 1978.

111. Lagerkranser M, Bergstrand G, Gordon E et al: Cerebral blood flow and metabolism during adenosine-induced hypotension in patients undergoing cerebral aneurysm surgery, *Acta Anaesthesiol Scand* 33:15-20, 1989.

112. Lanier WL, Milde JH, Michenfelder JD: The cerebral effects of pancuronium and atracurium in halothane-anesthetized dogs, *Anesthesiology* 63:589-597, 1985.

113. Lanier WL, Milde JH, Michenfelder JD: Cerebral stimulation following succinylcholine in dogs, *Anesthesiology* 64:551-559, 1986.

114. Lanier WL, Iaizzo PA, Milde JH: Cerebral blood flow and afferent muscle activity following IV succinylcholine in dogs, *Anesthesiol Rev* 14:60-6, 1987.

115. Lanier WL, Sharbrough FW, Michenfelder JD: Effects of atracurium, vecuronium or pancuronium pretreatment on lignocaine seizure thresholds in cats, *Br J Anaesth* 60:74-80, 1988.

116. Lanier WL, Iaizzo PA, Milde JH: Cerebral function and muscle afferent activity following intravenous sccinylcholine in dogs anesthetized with halothane: the effects of pretreatment with a defasciculating dose of pancuronium, *Anesthesiology* 71:87-95, 1989.

117. Larsen R, Hilfiker O, Radle J et al: The effects of midazolam on the general circulation, the cerebral blood flow and cerebral oxygen consumption in man, *Anaesthetist* 30:18-21, 1981.

118. Larsen R, Maurer I, Khambatta H: Cerebral blood flow and oxygen consumption during isoflurane and enflurane anesthesia in humans, *Anesthesist* 37:173-181, 1988.

119. Lassen NA: Cerebral and spinal cord blood flow. In Cottrell JE, Turndorf H, editors: *Anesthesia and neurosurgery,* ed 2, St Louis, 1986, CV Mosby.

120. Lowe RF, Gilboe DD: Canine cerebrovascular response to nitroglycerin, acetycholine, 5-hydroxytryptamine, and angiotensin, *Am J Physiol* 225:1333-1338, 1973.

121. Lutz LJ, Milde JH, Milde LN: The cerebral functional, metabolic, and hemodynamic effects of desflurane in dogs, *Anesthesiology* 73:125-131, 1990.

122. Lutz LJ, Milde JH, Milde LN: The response of the canine cerebral circulation to hyperventilation during anesthesia with desflurane, *Anesthesiology* 74:504-507, 1991.

123. MacMurdo SD, Nemoto EM, Nikki P et al: Brain cyclic-AMP and possible mechanisms of cerebrovascular dilation by anesthetics in rat, *Anesthesiology* 55:435-438, 1981.

124. Madsen JB, Cold GE, Eriksen HO et al: CBF and CMR_{O_2} during craniotomy for small supratentorial cerebral tumours in enflurane anaesthesia. A dose-response study, *Acta Anaesthesiol Scand* 30:633-636, 1986.

125. Madsen JB, Cold GE, Hansen ES et al: Cerebral blood flow, cerebral metabolic rate of oxygen and relative CO_2-reactivity during craniotomy for supratentorial cerebral tumours in halothane anaesthesia. A dose-response study, *Acta Anaesthesiol Scand* 31:454-457, 1987.

126. Madsen JB, Cold GE, Hansen ES et al: The effect of isoflurane on cerebral blood flow and metabolism in humans during craniotomy for small supratentorial cerebral tumors, *Anesthesiology* 66:332-336, 1987.

127. Madsen JB, Cold GE, Hansen ES et al: Cerebral blood flow and metabolism during isoflurane-induced hypotension in patients subjected to surgery for cerebral aneurysms, *Br J Anaesth* 59:1204-1207, 1987.

128. Maekawa T, Sakabe T, Takeshita H: Diazepam blocks cerebral metabolic and circulatory responses to local anesthetic-induced seizures, *Anesthesiology* 41:389-391, 1974.

129. Maekawa T, McDowall DG, Okuda

Y: Brain-surface oxygen tension and cerebral cortical blood flow during hemorrhagic and drug-induced hypotension in the cat, *Anesthesiology* 51:313-320, 1979.

130. Maekawa T, Oshibuchi T, Takeshita H et al: Cerebral energy state and glycolytic metabolism during lidocaine infusion in the cat, *Anesthesiology* 54:278-283, 1981.

131. Maekawa T, Tommasino C, Shapiro HM: Local cerebral blood flow with fentanyl induced seizures, *J Cereb Blood Flow Metab* 4:88-95, 1984.

132. Maekawa T, Tommasino C, Shapiro HM et al: Local cerebral blood flow and glucose utilization during isoflurane anesthesia in the rat, *Anesthesiology* 65:144-151, 1986.

133. Manninen PH, Mahendran B, Gelb AW et al: The effect of succinylcholine on serum potassium in patients with acutely ruptured cerebral aneurysms, *Anesth Analg* 68:S180, 1989.

134. Manohar M, Parks C: Regional distribution of brain and myocardial perfusion in swine while awake and during 1.0 and 1.5 MAC isoflurane anesthesia produced without and with 50% nitrous oxide, *Cardiovasc Res* 18:344-353, 1984.

135. Markovitz BP, Duhaime A-C, Sutton L et al: Effects of alfentanil on intracranial pressure in children undergoing ventriculoperitoneal shunt revision, *Anesthesiology* 76:71-76, 1992.

136. Marsh ML, Shapiro HM, Smith RW et al: Changes in neurologic status and intracranial pressure associated with sodium nitroprusside administration, *Anesthesiology* 51:336-338, 1979.

137. Marx W, Shah N, Long C et al: Sufentanil, alfentanil, and fentanyl: impact on cerebrospinal fluid pressure in patients with brain tumors, *J Neurosurg Anesthesiol* 1:3-7, 1989.

138. McPherson RW, Traystman RJ: Fentanyl and cerebral vascular responsivity in dogs, *Anesthesiology* 60:180-186, 1984.

139. McPherson RW, Brian JE, Traystman RJ: Cerebrovascular responsiveness to carbon dioxide in dogs with 1.4% and 2.8% isoflurane, *Anesthesiology* 70:843-850, 1989.

140. Messick JM, Casement B, Sharborough FW et al: Correlation of regional cerebral blood flow (rCBF) with EEG changes during isoflurane anesthesia for carotid endarterec-

tomy: critical rCBF, *Anesthesiology* 66:344-349, 1987.

141. Michenfelder JD, Theye RA: Effects of fentanyl, droperidol, and innovar on canine cerebral metabolism and blood flow, *Br J Anaesth* 43:630-636, 1971.

142. Michenfelder JD, Cucchiara RF: Canine cerebral oxygen consumption during enflurane anesthesia and its modification during induced seizures, *Anesthesiology* 40:575-580, 1974.

143. Michenfelder JD: The interdependency of cerebral functional and metabolic effects following massive doses of thiopental in the dog, *Anesthesiology* 41:231-236, 1974.

144. Michenfelder JD, Theye RA: In vivo toxic effects of halothane on canine cerebral metabolic pathways, *Am J Physiol* 229:1050-1055, 1975.

145. Michenfelder JD, Milde JH, Sundt JM Jr: Cerebral protection by barbiturate anesthesia. Use after middle cerebral artery occlusion in Java monkeys, *Arch Neurol* 33:345-350, 1976.

146. Michenfelder JD, Theye RA: Canine systemic and cerebral effects of hypotension induced by hemorrhage, trimethaphan, halothane, or nitroprusside, *Anesthesiology* 46:188-195, 1977.

147. Michenfelder JD, Sundt TM, Fode N et al: Isoflurane when compared to enflurane and halothane decreases the frequency of cerebral ischemia during carotid endarterectomy, *Anesthesiology* 67:336-340, 1987.

148. Michenfelder JD, Milde JH: The interaction of sodium nitroprusside, hypotension, and isoflurane in determining cerebral vasculature effects, *Anesthesiology* 69:870-875, 1988.

149. Michenfelder JD: *Anesthesia and the brain,* New York, 1988, Churchill-Livingstone, p 59.

150. Milde LN, Milde JH, Michenfelder JD: Cerebral functional, metabolic, and hemodynamic effects of etomidate in dogs, *Anesthesiology* 63:371-377, 1985.

151. Milde LN, Milde JH: Preservation of cerebral metabolites by etomidate during incomplete cerebral ischemia in dogs, *Anesthesiology* 65:272-277, 1986.

152. Milde LN, Milde JH: The detrimental effect of lidocaine on cerebral me-

tabolism measured in dogs anesthetized with isoflurane, *Anesthesiology* 67:180-184, 1987.

153. Milde LN, Milde JH, Lanier WL et al: Comparison of the effects of isoflurane and thiopental on neurologic outcome and neuropathology after temporary focal cerebral ischemia in primates, *Anesthesiology* 69:905-913, 1988.

154. Milde LN: The hypoxic mouse model for screening cerebral protective agents: a re-examination, *Anesth Analg* 67:917-922, 1988.

155. Milde LN, Milde JH, Gallagher WJ: Effects of sufentanil on cerebral circulation and metabolism in dogs, *Anesth Analg* 70:138-146, 1990.

156. Milde LN, Milde JH: The cerebral and systemic hemodynamic and metabolic effects of desflurane-induced hypotension in dogs, *Anesthesiology* 74:513-518, 1991.

157. Miletich DJ, Ivankovich AD, Albrecht RF et al: Absence of autoregulation of cerebral blood flow during halothane and enflurane anesthesia, *Anesth Analg* 55:100-109, 1976.

158. Miller R, Tausk HC, Starc DCC: Effect of innovar, fentanyl and droperidol on the cerebrospinal fluid pressure in neurosurgical patients, *Can Anaesth Soc J* 22:502-508, 1975.

159. Minton MD, Stirt JA, Bedford RF et al: Intracranial pressure after atracurium in neurosurgical patients, *Anesth Analg* 64:1113-1116, 1985.

160. Minton MD, Grosslight K, Stirt JA et al: Increases in intracranial pressure from succinylcholine: prevention by prior nondepolarizing blockade, *Anesthesiology* 65:165-169, 1986.

161. Misfeldt BB, Jörgensen PB, Spotoft H et al: The effects of droperidol and fentanyl on intracranial pressure and cerebral perfusion pressure in neurosurgical patients, *Br J Anaesth* 48:963-968, 1976.

162. Miyauchi Y, Sakabe T, Maekawa T et al: Responses of EEG, cerebral oxygen consumption and blood flow to peripheral nerve stimulation during thiopentone anaesthesia in the dog, *Can Anaesth Soc J* 32:491-498, 1985.

163. Morita H, Nemoto EM, Bleyaert AL et al: Brain blood flow autoregulation and metabolism during halothane anesthesia in monkeys, *Am J Physiol* 233:H670-676, 1977.

164. Morris PJ, Todd M, Philbin D: Changes in canine intracranial pressure in response to infusions of sodium nitroprusside and trinitroglycerin, *Br J Anaesth* 54:991-995, 1982.

165. Morris PJ, Heuser D, McDowall DG et al: Cerebral cortical extracellular fluid H$^+$ and K$^+$ activities during hypotension in cats, *Anesthesiology* 59:10-18, 1983.

166. Moss E, Powell D, Gibson RM et al: Effects of fentanyl on intracranial pressure and cerebral perfusion pressure during hypocapnia, *Br J Anaesth* 50:779-784, 1978.

167. Moss E, McDowall DG: ICP increases with 50% nitrous oxide in oxygen in severe head injuries during controlled ventilation, *Br J Anaesth* 51:757-761, 1979.

168. Moss E, Dearden NM, McDowall DG: Effects of 2% enflurane on intracranial pressure and cerebral perfusion pressure, *Br J Anaesth* 55:1083-1088, 1983.

169. Moyer JH, Pontius R, Morris G et al: Effect of morphine and n-allylnormorphine on cerebral hemodynamics and oxygen metabolism, *Circulation* 15:379-384, 1957.

170. Muzzi D, Daltner C, Losaso T et al: The effect of desflurane and isoflurane with N$_2$O on cerebrospinal fluid pressure in patients with supratentorial mass lesions, *Anesthesiology* 75:A167, 1991.

171. Muzzi DA, Black S, Losasso TJ et al: Labetalol and esmolol in the control of hypertension after intracranial surgery, *Anesth Analg* 70:68-71, 1990.

172. Muzzi DA, Losasso TJ, Dietz NM et al: The effect of desflurane and isoflurane on cerebrospinal fluid pressure in human with supratentorial mass lesions, *Anesthesiology* 76:720-724, 1992.

173. Nakakimura K, Sakabe T, Funatsu N et al: Metabolic activation of intercortical and corticothalamic pathways during enflurane anesthesia in rats, *Anesthesiology* 68:777-782, 1988.

174. Nakakimura K, Sakabe T, Takeshita H: Modulation of cerebrospinal metabolic responses to peripheral stimulation by enflurane anesthesia in rats, *J Neurosurg Anesthesiol* 1:333-338, 1989.

175. Nehls DG, Todd MM, Spetzler RF et al: A comparison of the cerebral protective effects of isoflurane and barbiturates during temporary focal ischemia in primates, *Anesthesiology* 66:453-464, 1987.

176. Newberg LA, Milde JH, Michenfelder JD: The cerebral metabolic effects of isoflurane at and above concentrations that suppress cortical electrical activity, *Anesthesiology* 59:23-28, 1983.

177. Newberg LA, Michenfelder JD: Cerebral protection by isoflurane during hypoxemia or ischemia, *Anesthesiology* 59:29-35, 1983.

178. Newberg LA, Milde JH, Michenfelder JD: Systemic and cerebral effects of isoflurane-induced hypotension in dogs, *Anesthesiology* 60:541-546, 1984.

179. Newberg LA, Milde JH, Michenfelder JD: Cerebral and systemic effects of hypotension induced by adenosine or ATP in dogs, *Anesthesiology* 62:429-436, 1985.

180. Newman B, Gelb AW, Lam AM: The effect of isoflurane-induced hypotension on cerebral blood flow and cerebral metabolic rate for oxygen in humans, *Anesthesiology* 64:307-310, 1986.

181. Nilsson L, Siesjö BK: The effect of phenobarbitone anaesthesia on blood flow and oxygen consumption in the rat brain, *Acta Anaesthesiol Scand Suppl* 57:18-24, 1975.

182. Norrving B, Nilsson B, Risberg J: RCBF in patients with carotid occlusion: resting and hypercapnic flow related to collateral pattern, *Stroke* 13:155-162, 1982.

183. Nugent M, Artru AA, Michenfelder JD: Cerebral metabolic, vascular and protective effects of midazolam maleate, *Anesthesiology* 56:172-176, 1982.

184. Oguchi K, Arakawa K, Nelson SR et al: The influence of droperidol, diazepam, and physostigmine on ketamine-induced behavior and brain regional glucose utilization in rat, *Anesthesiology* 57:353-358, 1982.

185. Okuda Y, McDowall DG, Ali MM et al: Changes in CO$_2$ responsiveness and in autoregulation of the cerebral circulation during and after halothane-induced hypotension, *J Neurosurg Psychiatry* 39:221-230, 1976.

186. Ono H: Autoregulation of cerebral blood flow during halothane and morphine anesthesia in dogs, *Bull Yamaguchi Med Sch* 28:99-104, 1981.

187. Ori C, Dam M, Pizzolato G et al: Effects of isoflurane anesthesia on local cerebral glucose utilization in the rat, *Anesthesiology* 65:152-156, 1986.

188. Orlowski JP, Shiesley D, Vidt DG et al: Labetalol to control blood pressure after cerebrovascular surgery, *Crit Care Med* 16:765-768, 1988.

189. Ornstein E, Young WL, Ostapkovich N et al: Deliberate hypotension in patients with intracranial arteriovenous malformations: esmolol compared with isoflurane and sodium nitroprusside, *Anesth Analg* 72:639-644, 1991.

190. Ornstein E, Young WL, Ostapkovich N et al: Comparative effects of desflurane and isoflurane on cerebral blood flow, *Anesthesiology* 75:A209, 1991.

191. Pelligrino DA, Miletich DJ, Hoffman WE et al: Nitrous oxide markedly increases cerebral cortical metabolic rate and blood flow in the goat, *Anesthesiology* 60:405-412, 1984.

192. Phirman JR, Shapiro HM: Modification of nitrous oxide-induced intracranial hypertension by prior induction of anesthesia, *Anesthesiology* 46:150-151, 1977.

193. Prior JGL, Hinds CJ, Williams J et al: The use of etomidate in the management of severe head injury, *Intensive Care Med* 9:313-320, 1983.

194. Raichle ME, Posner JB, Plum F: Cerebral blood flow during and after hyperventilation, *Arch Neurol* 23:394-403, 1970.

195. Ravussin P, Guinard JP, Ralley F et al: Effect of propofol on cerebrospinal fluid pressure and cerebral perfusion pressure in patients undergoing craniotomy, *Anesthesia* 43(suppl): 37-41, 1988.

196. Reicher D, Bohalla P, Rubinstein EH: Cholinergic cerebral vasodilation effect of ketamine in rabbits, *Stroke* 18:445-449, 1987.

197. Reinhold H, DeRood M: Cerebral blood flow under enflurane anesthesia, *Acta Anaesthesiol Belg* 27 (suppl): 250-258, 1976.

198. Renou AM, Vernhiet J, Macrez P et al: Cerebral blood flow and metabo-

lism during etomidate anaesthesia in man, *Br J Anaesth* 50:1047-1051, 1978.

199. Reynier-Rebuffel AM, Pinard E, Aubineau PF et al: Generalized cerebral vasoconstriction induced by intracarotid infusion of angiotensin II in the rabbit, *Brain Res* 269:91-101, 1983.

200. Roald OK, Steen PA, Milde JH et al: Reversal of the cerebral effects of diazepam in the dog by the benzodiazepine antagonist RO15-1788, *Acta Anaesthesiol Scand* 30:341-345, 1986.

201. Roald OK, Forsman M, Steen PA: The effects of prolonged isoflurane anaesthesia on cerebral blood flow and metabolism in the dog, *Acta Anaesthesiol Scand* 33:210-213, 1989.

202. Roald OK, Forsman M, Heier MS et al: Cerebral effects of nitrous oxide when added to low and high concentrations of isoflurane in the dog, *Anesth Analg* 72:75-79, 1991.

203. Rolly G, Van Aken J: Influence of enflurane on cerebral blood flow in man, *Acta Anaesthesiol Scand* 71(suppl):59-63, 1979.

204. Rosa G, Orfei P, Sanfilippo M et al: The effects of atracurium besylate (Tracrium) on intracranial pressure and cerebral perfusion pressure, *Anesth Analg* 65:381-384, 1986.

205. Rosa G, Sanfilippo M, Viardi V et al: Effects of vecuronium bromide on intracranial pressure and cerebral perfusion pressure, *Br J Anaesth* 58:437-440, 1986.

206. Rosa G, Sanfilippo M, Orfei P et al: The effects of pipecurium bromide on intracranial pressure and cerebral perfusion pressure, *J Neurosurg Anesthesiol* 3:253-257, 1991.

207. Safo Y, Young ML, Smith DS et al: Effects of fentanyl on local cerebral blood flow in the rat, *Acta Anaesthesiol Scand* 29:594-598, 1985.

208. Sakabe T, Maekawa T, Ishikawa T et al: The effects of lidocaine on canine metabolism and circulation related to the electroencephalogram, *Anesthesiology* 40:433-441, 1974.

209. Sakabe T: Effect of enflurane (Ethrane) on canine cerebral metabolism and circulation, *Masui* 24:323-331, 1975.

210. Sakabe T, Kuramoto T, Kumagae S et al: Cerebral responses to the addition of nitrous oxide to halothane in man, *Br J Anaesth* 48:957-961, 1976.

211. Sakabe T, Kuramoto T, Inoue S et al: Cerebral effects of nitrous oxide in the dog, *Anesthesiology* 48:195-200, 1978.

212. Sakabe T, Maekawa T, Fujii S et al: Cerebral circulation and metabolism during enflurane anesthesia in humans, *Anesthesiology* 59:532-536, 1983.

213. Sakabe T, Tsutsui T, Maekawa T et al: Local cerebral glucose utilization during nitrous oxide and pentobarbital anesthesia in rats, *Anesthesiology* 63:262-266, 1985.

214. Sakabe T: Calcium entry blockers in cerebral resuscitation, *Magnesium* 8:238-252, 1989.

215. Sano T, Drummond JC, Patel PM et al: A comparison of the cerebral protective effects of isoflurane and mild hypothermia in a model of incomplete forebrain ischemia in the rat, *Anesthesiology* 76:221-228, 1992.

216. Sari A, Okuda Y, Takeshita H: The effects of thalamonal on cerebral circulation and oxygen consumption in man, *Br J Anaesth* 44:330-334, 1972.

217. Sari A, Okuda Y, Takeshita H: The effect of ketamine on cerebrospinal fluid pressure, *Anesth Analg* 51:560-565, 1972.

218. Scheller MS, Todd MM, Drummond JC: Isoflurane, halothane, and regional cerebral blood flow at various levels of Paco$_2$ in rabbits, *Anesthesiology* 64:598-604, 1986.

219. Scheller MS, Todd MM, Drummond JC et al: The intracranial pressure effects of isoflurane and halothane administered following cryogenic brain injury in rabbits, *Anesthesiology* 67:507-512, 1987.

220. Scheller MS, Tateishi A, Drummond JC et al: The effects of sevoflurane on cerebral blood flow, cerebral metabolic rate for oxygen, intracranial pressure and electroencephalogram are similar to those of isoflurane in the rabbit, *Anesthesiology* 68:548-551, 1988.

221. Scheller MS, Nakakimura K, Fleischer JE et al: Cerebral effects of sevoflurane in the dog: comparison with isoflurane and enflurane, *Br J Anaesth* 65:388-392, 1990.

222. Schwedler M, Miletich DJ, Albrecht RF: Cerebral blood flow and metab-

olism following ketamine administration, *Can Anaesth Soc J* 29:222-226, 1982.

223. Seo K, Maekawa T, Takeshita H et al: Cerebral energy state and glycolytic metabolism during enflurane anesthesia in the rat, *Acta Anaesthesiol Scand* 28:215-219, 1984.

224. Seyde WC, Longnecker DE: Cerebral oxygen tension in rats during deliberate hypotension with sodium nitroprusside, 2-chloroadenosine, or deep isoflurane anesthesia, *Anesthesiology* 64:480-485, 1986.

225. Seyde WC, Ellis JE, Longnecker DE: The addition of nitrous oxide to halothane decreases renal and splanchnic flow and increases cerebral blood flow in rats, *Br J Anaesth* 58:63-68, 1986.

226. Shapiro HM, Greenberg JH, Reivich M et al: Local cerebral glucose uptake in awake and halothane-anesthetized primates, *Anesthesiology* 48:97-103, 1978.

227. Siesjö BK, Bengtsson F: Calcium fluxes, calcium antagonists, and calcium-related pathology in brain ischemia, hypoglycemia, and spreading depression: a unifying hypothesis, *J Cereb Blood Flow Metab* 9:127-140, 1989.

228. Smith AL, Neigh JL, Hoffman JC et al: Effects of general anesthesia on autoregulation of cerebral blood flow in man, *J Appl Physiol* 29:665-669, 1970.

229. Smith AL, Wollman H: Cerebral blood flow and metabolism: effects of anesthetic drugs and techniques, *Anesthesiology* 36:378-400, 1972.

230. Smith AL: The mechanism of cerebral vasodilation by halothane, *Anesthesiology* 39:581-587, 1973.

231. Smith DS, Keykhah MM, O'Neill JJ et al: The effect of etomidate pretreatment on cerebral high energy metabolites, lactate, and glucose during severe hypoxia in the rat, *Anesthesiology* 71:438-443, 1989.

232. Sollevi A, Ericson K, Eriksson L et al: Effect of adenosine on human cerebral blood flow as determined by positron emission tomography, *J Cereb Blood Flow Metab* 7:673-678, 1987.

233. Sperry RJ, Bailey PL, Reichman MV et al: Fentanyl and sufentanil increase intracranial pressure in head trauma patients, *Anesthesiology* 77:416-420, 1992.

234. Stånge K, Lagerkranser M, Rudehill A et al: Effects of adenosine-induced hypotension on cerebral blood flow and metabolism in the pig, *Acta Anaesthesiol Scand* 33:199-203, 1989.

235. Steen PA, Newberg L, Milde JH et al: Hypothermia and barbiturates: individual and combined effects on canine cerebral oxygen consumption, *Anesthesiology* 58:527-532, 1983.

236. Stephan H, Sonntag H, Schenk HD et al: Effects of disoprivan on cerebral blood flow, cerebral oxygen consumption, and cerebral vascular reactivity, *Anaesthesist* 36:60-65, 1987.

237. Stirt JA, Grosslight KR, Bedford RF et al: "Defasciculation" with metocurine prevents succinylcholine-induced increases in intracranial pressure, *Anesthesiology* 67:50-53, 1987.

238. Stirt JA, Maggio W, Haworth C et al: Vecuronium: effect on intracranial pressure and hemodynamics in neurosurgical patients, *Anesthesiology* 67:570-573, 1987.

239. Stullken EH, Sokoll MD: Anesthesia and subarachnoid intracranial pressure, *Anesth Analg* 54:494-500, 1975.

240. Stullken EH, Milde JH, Michenfelder JD et al: The nonlinear responses of cerebral metabolism to low concentrations of halothane, enflurane, isoflurane, and thiopental, *Anesthesiology* 46:28-34, 1977.

241. Takeshita H, Okuda Y, Sari A: The effects of ketamine on cerebral circulation and metabolism in man, *Anesthesiology* 36:69-75, 1972.

242. Takeshita H, Michenfelder JD, Theye RA: The effects of morphine and N-allylnormorphine on canine cerebral metabolism and circulation, *Anesthesiology* 37:605-612, 1972.

243. Takeshita H, Okuda Y, Ishikawa T: Cerebrovascular response to anesthetic agents and adjuvant drugs. In Hülsz E, Sánchez-Hernández JA, Vasconcelos G, editors: *Excerpta Medica International Congress Series No. 399: Anaesthesiology*, Amsterdam, 1976, Excerpta Medica, pp 223-230.

244. Tarkkanen L, Laitinen L, Johansson G: Effects of D-tubocuranine on intracranial pressure and thalamic electrical impedance, *Anesthesiology* 40:247-251, 1974.

245. Tateishi A, Maekawa T, Takeshita H et al: Diazepam and intracranial pressure, *Anesthesiology* 54:335-337, 1981.

246. Tateishi A, Sano T, Takeshita H et al: Effects of nifedipine on intracranial pressure in neurosurgical patients with arterial hypertension, *J Neurosurg* 69:213-215, 1988.

247. Tateishi A, Zornow MH, Scheller MS et al: Electroencephalographic effects of laudanosine in an animal model of epilepsy, *Br J Anaesth* 62:548-552, 1989.

248. Theye RA, Michenfelder JD: The effect of nitrous oxide on canine cerebral metabolism, *Anesthesiology* 29:1119-1124, 1968.

249. Thiagarajah S, Sophie S, Lear E et al: Effect of suxamethonium on the ICP of cats with and without thiopentone pretreatment, *Br J Anaesth* 60:157-160, 1988.

250. Todd MM, Drummond JC: A comparison of the cerebrovascular and metabolic effects of halothane and isoflurane in the cat, *Anesthesiology* 60:276-282, 1984.

251. Todd MM: The effects of Pa_{CO_2} on the cerebrovascular response to nitrous oxide in the halothane-anesthetized rabbit, *Anesth Analg* 66:1090-1095, 1987.

252. Tommasino C, Maekawa T, Shapiro HM: Fentanyl-induced seizures activate subcortical brain metabolism, *Anesthesiology* 60:283-290, 1984.

253. Tommasino C, Maekawa T, Shapiro HM: Local cerebral blood flow during lidocaine-induced seizures in rats, *Anesthesiology* 64:771-777, 1986.

254. Turner DM, Kassell NF, Sasaki T et al: Time-dependent changes in cerebral and cardiovascular parameters in isoflurane–nitrous oxide–anesthetized dogs, *Neurosurgery* 14:135-141, 1984.

255. Turner JM, Powell D, Gibson RM et al: Intracranial pressure changes in neurosurgical patients during hypotension induced with sodium nitroprusside or trimetaphan, *Br J Anaesth* 49:419-425, 1977.

256. Van Aken H, Puchstein C, Schweppe M-L et al: Effect of labetalol on intracranial pressure in dogs with and without intracranial hypertension, *Acta Anaesthesiol Scand* 26:615-619, 1982.

257. Van Aken H, Puchstein C, Fitch W et al: Haemodynamic and cerebral effects of ATP-induced hypotension, *Br J Anaesth* 56:1409-1416, 1984.

258. Van Aken H, Puchstein C, Anger C et al: Changes in intracranial pressure and compliance during adenosine triphosphate–induced hypotension in dogs, *Anesth Analg* 63:381-385, 1984.

259. Van Aken H, Fitch W, Graham DI et al: Cardiovascular and cerebrovascular effects of isoflurane-induced hypotension in the baboon, *Anesth Analg* 65:565-574, 1986.

260. Vandesteene A, Trempont V, Engelman E et al: Effect of propofol on cerebral blood flow and metabolism in man, *Anaesthesia*. 43[suppl]:42-43, 1988.

261. Van Reempts J, Borgers M, Van Eyndhoven J et al: Protective effects of etomidate in hypoxic-ischemic brain damage in the rat. A morphologic assessment, *Exper Neurol* 76:181-195, 1982.

262. Vernhiet J, Renou AM, Orgogozo JM et al: Effects of a diazepam-fentanyl mixture on cerebral blood flow and oxygen consumption in man, *Br J Anaesth* 50:165-169, 1978.

263. Vesely R, Hoffman WE, Gil KSL: Cerebrovascular effects of curare and histamine in the rat, *Anesthesiology* 65:A336, 1986.

264. Vorstrup S, Boysen G, Brun B et al: Evaluation of the regional cerebral vasodilatory capacity before carotid endarterectomy by the acetazolamide test, *Neurol Res* 9:10-18, 1987.

265. Waaben J, Hunsum B, Hansen AJ et al: Regional cerebral blood flow and glucose utilization during hypocapnia and adenosine-induced hypotension in the rat, *Anesthesiology* 70:299-304, 1989.

266. Ward JD, Becker DP, Miller JD et al: Failure of prophylactic barbiturate coma in the treatment of severe head injury, *J Neurosurg* 62:383-388, 1985.

267. Warner DS, Boarini DJ, Kassell NF: Cerebrovascular adaptation to prolonged halothane anesthesia is not related to cerebrospinal fluid pH, *Anesthesiology* 63:243-248, 1985.

268. Warner DS, Deshpande JK, Wieloch T: The effect of isoflurane on neuronal necrosis following near-complete forebrain ischemia in the rat, *Anesthesiology* 64:19-23, 1986.

269. Wauquier A, Achton D, Clincke G et al: Anti-hypoxic effects of etomidate, thiopental and methohexital, *Arch Int Pharmacodyn Ther* 249:330-334, 1981.

270. Werner C, Hoffman WE, Baughman VL et al: Effects of sufentanil on cerebral blood flow, cerebral blood flow velocity, and metabolism in dogs, *Anesth Analg* 72:177-181, 1991.

271. Wyte SR, Shapiro HM, Turner P et al: Ketamine-induced intracranial hypertension, *Anesthesiology* 36:174-176, 1972.

272. Yano M, Nishiyama H, Yokota H et al: Effect of lidocaine on ICP response to endotracheal suctioning, *Anesthesiology* 64:651-653, 1986.

273. Yaster M, Koehler RC, Traystman RJ: Effects of fentanyl on peripheral and cerebral hemodynamics in neonatal lambs, *Anesthesiology* 66:524-530, 1987.

274. Young ML, Smith DS, Greenberg J et al: Effects of sufentanil on regional cerebral glucose utilization in rats, *Anesthesiology* 61:564-568, 1984.

8

Neuroradiology

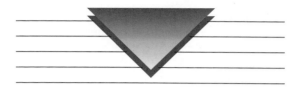

FRED J. LAINE
WENDY R.K. SMOKER

The radiologic armamentarium currently available for the investigation of pathology in patients with neurologic dysfunction is extensive. This chapter introduces the reader to the more commonly used procedures: plain radiographs, computed tomography (CT), magnetic resonance imaging (MR), cerebral angiography, and myelography. First, an introduction to technical factors is presented to give the reader a theoretical basis of image production. This is followed by a discussion of representative areas of normal anatomy, pathology, and basics of interpretation.

IMAGING MODALITIES
Plain Radiographs

X-rays are rays of short wavelength electromagnetic energy that travel in straight lines at the speed of light. When an x-ray beam passes through matter, its intensity is reduced by absorption. The denser the substance, the greater the absorption. Photographic film is affected by x-rays in the same way as it is by visible light. When film is placed behind an object through which an x-ray beam is passed, an image is produced in the film's emulsion that can be developed to produce an accurate representation of the various tissue densities. Therefore bones, because they absorb more radiation, appear as light areas surrounded by darker soft-tissue structures.

Plain radiographs, typically the first studies obtained when evaluating traumatic injuries (particularly cervical spine injuries), are a rapid, inexpensive, and accurate modality for evaluating osseous integrity and alignment. A major disadvantage of plain radiographs is that, although they provide an accurate image of osseous structures, they are inadequate for evaluating soft tissues. Radiographs of the skull and spine, helpful in identifying fractures, fail to provide significant information concerning intracranial or intraspinal parenchymal injury.

Computed Tomography

With the advent of high-resolution computed tomography (CT) scanners, axial cross-sectional images have enabled one to identify and evaluate intracranial parenchymal structures and spinal structures. CT images are generated by a variable number of radiation detectors, permanently fixed 360 degrees around the CT gantry.[55] The x-ray tube rotates in a circle, inside the detector ring, and emits a fan-shaped, collimated beam of ionizing radiation that passes through the body part positioned within the gantry opening. The detectors directly opposite the x-ray tube measure the amount of radiation that has passed through the intervening body part. For each image produced, the x-ray tube travels 360 degrees around the gantry. Thus one CT image is composed of many projections, each at a slightly different angle. The difference between the amount of radiation emitted and the amount detected is known as the *attenuation coefficient* and represents a measure of radio-absorbency. Attenuation therefore depends on the amount (voxel size) and type of tissue through which the x-ray beam has passed.

In CT, a cross-sectional layer of the body is divided into many tiny blocks or volume elements (voxels), and each block is assigned a number proportional to the degree to which it attenuates the x-ray beam. The CT scanner calculates, from the collected data, the attenuation coefficient and converts the value to a picture element (pixel).[22] Attenuation values (Hounsfield numbers) are recorded on a gray scale of *density* readings with values ranging from +1000 for cortical bone to −1000 for air, with 0 representing water. The projected image therefore is composed of various shades of gray, with the lightest (white) areas produced by high attenuation and darkest (black) areas produced by low attenuation.

With its widespread availability, noninvasiveness, and safety, CT is the primary imaging modality for almost all pathologic processes. A significant advantage of CT lies in a postprocessing procedure that permits evaluation of both osseous and soft tissue structures by varying the "window levels" at which the images are photographed. "Wide (bone) windows" optimally display osseous structures, and "narrow (soft tissue) windows" are best suited for evaluation of soft tissue structures. An additional feature of CT is its ability to reconstruct axial images into coronal and sagittal planes. Evaluation of fractures suspected on plain radiographs can, on occasion, only be demonstrated on the reconstructed views.

Normal and Abnormal CT Scans

The CSF spaces (ventricular system and subarachnoid cisterns), being composed predominantly of water, are the darkest areas identified on head CT studies (Fig. 8-1, *A*). Extracranially, air within the paranasal sinuses and fat within the subcutaneous tissues are the areas of lowest den-

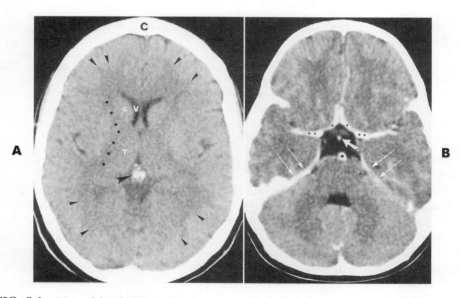

FIG. 8-1   Normal head CT. **A,** Non-contrast-enhanced study. CSF in frontal horns of the lateral ventricles *(V)* is dark; the bony calvarium *(C)* and calcified pineal gland *(large arrowhead)* are white. The corticomedullary junction is easily seen *(small arrowheads)* as are the anterior and posterior limbs of the internal capsules *(dots)*. Caudate nucleus *(c)*; thalamus *(T)*. **B,** Contrast-enhanced study. Enhancing structures include arteries (middle cerebral artery *[double dots]*, anterior cerebral artery *[small single dots]*, basilar artery *[large single dot]*), the tentorial membrane *(straight arrows)*, and the midline pituitary infundibulum *(large arrow)*.

sity (darkest). Intracranially, abnormal low densities include air (pneumocephalus), fat (lipomatous lesions), and edema, caused by a wide variety of pathologic conditions (e.g., trauma, neoplasm, infection).

Normal areas of high density are well represented by calvarial bone and skull base. Multiple, high-density, physiologic calcifications also seen include the pineal gland (greater than 8 years of age), choroid plexus, falx cerebri, and, in the elderly, the basal ganglia (see Fig. 8-1, *A*). Abnormal areas of high density are associated with hemorrhage and pathologic calcifications present in certain tumors, infections, and metabolic states. In the spine, high density is represented by the bony axis. Abnormal high density includes areas of calcification, such as calcified herniated disks, calcified ligaments, osteophytes, and neoplastic calcifications.

The intravenous injection of iodinated contrast causes certain normal and abnormal areas to enhance or brighten ("contrast-enhanced" study) (Fig. 8-1, *B*). On these studies, high density is identified in major arterial and venous structures. The choroid plexus, dural membranes, pineal gland, and pituitary gland and infundibulum also normally enhance. The main advantage of contrast is that it helps identify areas of blood-brain barrier disruption, in which case pathologic processes causing this disruption enhance. Contrast-enhanced studies increase the conspicuousness of certain lesions and permit differentiation among pathologic lesions, based on varying enhancement patterns. However, contrast material is organotoxic, especially to the kidneys, and its use must be restricted in patients with impaired renal function.[19,107]

Magnetic Resonance

Magnetic resonance (MR), using an external magnetic field, is an imaging modality that permits imaging in the axial, coronal, and sagittal planes without moving the patient or gantry. The normal spinning proton in the hydrogen atom generates a small magnetic field (dipole) that, ordinarily, spins randomly.[10] When introduced to an external magnetic field, a small percentage of protons align their magnetic fields with the main MR magnetic field.[22] A radiofrequency pulse is then used to displace these dipoles off this main magnetic field alignment. When the radiofrequency pulse is stopped, the dipoles are allowed to slowly "decay" or realign with the magnet's main magnetic field. This ability to realign in turn produces a radiofrequency pulse or *resonance* that can be measured. The detected resonance frequencies are processed by a computer to produce an image that reflects the hydrogen densities of the tissues studied. In contradistinction to CT, MR does not use ionizing radiation but rather uses magnetic and radiofrequency waves. Available data indicate that current use of MR in clinical practice is free of deleterious bioeffects. However, a significant amount of preprocedural patient screening still is required. Patients with cardiac pacemakers, pre-6000-series Starr-Edwards cardiac valves, and intraocular metal-

lic fragments should not undergo MR examinations. MR evaluation is also contraindicated for patients with older cerebral aneurysm clips because some of these clips have been found to move during MR studies.[59] Newer aneurysm clips have been developed that are MR compatible and considered safe to scan. Before the study, the clip's manufacturer and the date of placement should be noted. Orthopedic prosthetic devices are considered safe for MR studies but can produce artifacts that may preclude a diagnostic study. Most middle ear prostheses are nonmagnetic, but there are still exceptions, and screening is required.[101]

Imaging personnel must also be screened and aware of magnetic field effects. Medical equipment, including stethoscopes, hemostats, scissors, and many monitoring devices must remain outside the MR suite because the magnetic field is frequently strong enough to attract these objects. This is especially true during resuscitation procedures, and the patient should be removed from the magnet room to avoid the projectile effects of equipment.

A major problem with many MR studies is inadequate sedation. Claustrophobia is a leading factor in suboptimal and incomplete studies. MR examinations may involve sequences varying from 2 to 20 minutes, and any motion produces an uninterpretable study. Certain patients require sedation and, on occasion, general anesthesia is necessary. Only monitors that are known to be MR compatible should be used.[77,102] In addition, only oxygen and nitrogen tanks composed of aluminum can enter the magnet suite.

The indications for MR are continuously increasing as techniques and pathologic appearances become well-known and availability becomes more widespread. MR is especially useful for evaluation of midline lesions; posterior fossa pathology, including the cerebellum, brainstem, and cerebellopontine angle; suspected cranial nerve lesions; congenital abnormalities; and white matter processes. In addition, all spinal abnormalities, including craniocervical junction abnormalities, benefit from MR as the imaging modality of choice.

Normal and Abnormal MR Images

The MR image is a map of the relative amounts of current received from each level of tissue and reflects the number of hydrogen protons aligned and spinning while the image is obtained.[9] Relative signals from different tissues can be manipulated to alter contrast among tissues. This is possible because aligned protons are affected by two different decay mechanisms. These mechanisms, termed T_1 and T_2 decay, are based on inherent tissue characteristics. By changing the way in which the system obtains the image, one can take advantage of these different decay mechanisms and change the contrast between soft tissues. On T_1-weighted images (T_1WI), the relative contrast differences among tissues are based primarily on differing T_1 decay values. On these images fat has a short T_1 value and appears bright; water (CSF) has a long T_1 value and appears black (Fig. 8-2, *A*). On T_2-weighted images (T_2WI), the relative

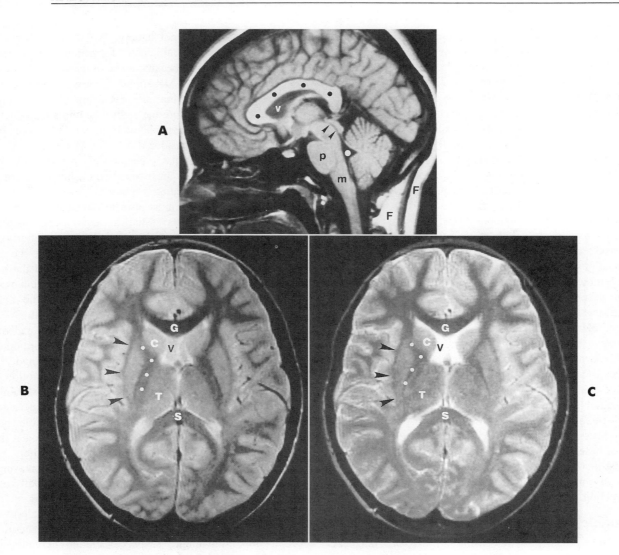

FIG. 8-2   Normal brain MR. **A,** Sagittal T_1-weighted image. CSF in ventricles *(v)* and sulci
is low intensity and fat *(F)* is high intensity. Midline anatomy is well demonstrated: corpus
callosum *(black dots)*; pons *(p)*; medulla *(m)*; aqueduct *(arrowheads)*, fourth ventricle *(white dot)*.
First- **(B)** and second-echo **(C)** axial T_2-weighted images. CSF within the ventricles becomes
increasingly bright *(V)*. Gray- and white-matter structures are more apparent: genu of corpus
callosum *(G)*; splenium of corpus callosum *(S)*; thalamus *(T)*; caudate nucleus *(C)*; internal
capsule *(dots)*; external capsule *(arrowheads)*.

contrast difference among tissues is based primarily on T_2
decay values. Sequencing parameters permit acquisition of
multiple images that are both intermediate and heavily T_2-
weighted. On heavily T_2-weighted images, fat is intermediate in signal and appears gray, and water and CSF appear bright (Fig. 8-2, *B* and *C*). Cortical bone, composed
of relatively fixed protons, does not produce a signal. Flowing blood produces no signal (a signal void) as the displaced
dipoles exit the imaging field. Similarly, tissues follow the
same T_1 and T_2 signal characteristics in MR imaging of the
spine (Fig. 8-3).

In general, pathologic processes usually contain excess

amounts of free water and therefore are dark on T_1-
weighted images and bright on T_2-weighted images. The
use of an intravenous MR contrast agent (gadolinium-
DTPA) permits increased conspicuousness of both intracranial and intraspinal pathology, manifested as areas of abnormal contrast enhancement.[12,93] Pathologic appearances
will be discussed further in this chapter.

Angiography

Percutaneous transfemoral catheterization is used to evaluate cerebral and spinal vascular anatomy and integrity. A
small diameter, soft catheter is advanced from the femoral

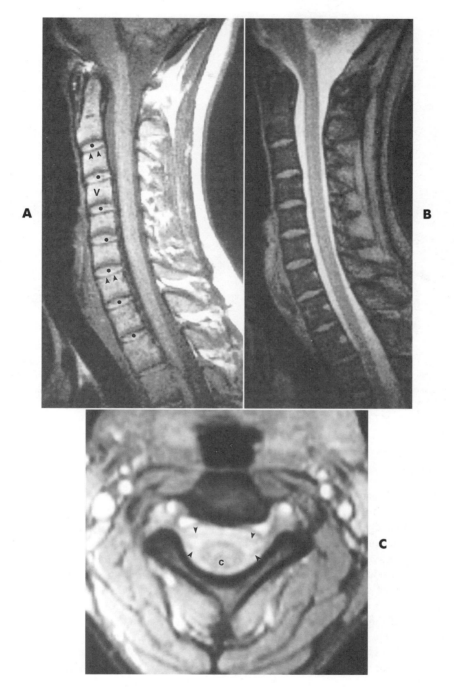

FIG. 8-3 Normal spine MR. **A,** Sagittal T$_1$-weighted image of the cervical spine. Cortical bone is low intensity *(small arrowheads)* and contrasts sharply with the high intensity of hydrated intervertebral disks *(dots)* and the fatty marrow of the vertebral bodies *(v)*. The spinal cord is isointense to muscle, and the CSF and ligaments are hypointense. **B,** Sagittal T$_2$-weighted image produces bright CSF that optimally outlines the spinal cord (myelogram effect). The disks remain slightly hyperintense while the fatty marrow of the vertebrae becomes hypointense. **C,** Axial T$_2$-weighted image of the cervical spine. The gray and white matter of the cord *(c)* can be discerned. The exiting isointense dorsal and ventral nerve roots are outlined by the bright CSF *(arrowheads)*.

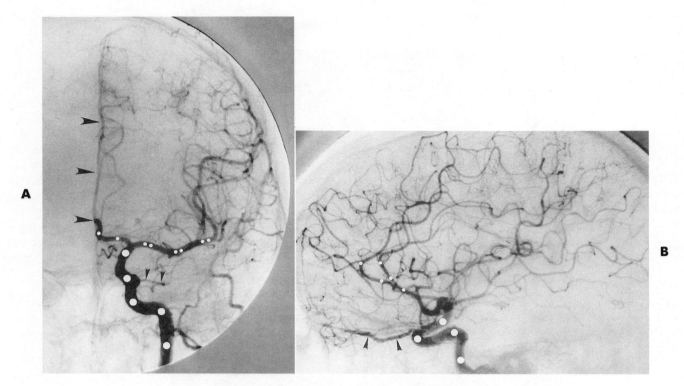

FIG. 8-4   Normal angiogram. Anteroposterior **(A)** and lateral **(B)** films of the head after selective injection into the internal carotid artery. The major arteries and the peripheral branches are well seen. Note how the vessels arborize (reduce in size) the more distal they become. ICA *(large dots)*, ACA *(small single dots)*, MCA *(double dots)*, ophthalmic artery *(small arrowheads)*, pericallosal artery *(large arrowheads)*.

artery into the aortic arch and subsequently placed into the extracranial carotid or vertebral arteries. During bolus injection of an iodinated contrast agent, biplane standard films or digital subtraction images are obtained at a predetermined rate. The contrast appears opaque on the x-ray images and mimics the flow of blood through the vessels. Eventually replaced by unopacified blood, it gradually decreases in density. Serial filming, timed to include arterial, capillary, and venous phases of circulation, is performed during the contrast injection. Two views (anteroposterior and lateral) are required for all vessels studied (Fig. 8-4). For evaluation of the extracranial circulation, additional views of the neck are obtained.

Cerebral angiography is an invasive procedure and, as such, imposes some risk. The overall complication rate is 2% to 4%.[32,52] The majority of these complications are minor and transient (groin hematomas, subintimal injections, and minor allergic reactions). However, more severe complications occasionally occur (cerebral infarction, seizure, and death). In addition, the iodinated contrast medium is organotoxic, and complications associated with its use (acute tubular necrosis, anaphylactic shock) are also a consideration.[19,107] Spinal angiography imposes the same risks

as cerebral angiography, with the added danger of cord infarction secondary to spinal artery embolus. For this reason, spinal angiography should only be performed when a vascular malformation is demonstrated by another imaging modality or the patient has a subarachnoid hemorrhage with normal pancerebral angiography and a spinal source is strongly suspected.

Cerebral angiography is still considered the "gold standard" for evaluation of cerebrovascular disease (atherosclerotic disease, vasculitis, vascular malformations, and aneurysms). In cases of trauma, angiography is frequently used to evaluate vascular integrity. MR angiography is being used in many centers for evaluation of both intracranial and extracranial vascular disease in the nonacute setting.[70,83] However, its role in the detection of subtle intracranial vascular pathology is not yet firmly established.[73,100]

Normal and Abnormal Cerebral Angiograms

The normal artery has a smooth lumen that gradually tapers the more distal it becomes (arborization). As time passes during the angiogram, smaller and more distal branches become apparent. Contrast remains intraluminal throughout the study and completes the arterial phase in 3 to 4 seconds. Capillaries, not directly identified on angiographic studies, are represented by an overall increased density (blush) on the film. Within 6 to 8 seconds from the time of the injection, venous structures opacify. Smaller veins are usually visualized first, and, as time passes, larger veins opacify. Abnormal angiographic appearances are discussed in relation to specific disease processes in subsequent sections.

Myelography

Routine myelography involves the injection of iodinated, water-soluble contrast material into the spinal subarachnoid space via a lumbar or lateral C1-C2 puncture. Plain radiographs are obtained in multiple projections while the contrast is moved cranially or caudally to evaluate multiple levels. Newer contrast agents and smaller gauge spinal needles now permit myelography to be performed on an outpatient basis. After the study, the contrast agent is left in the subarachnoid space, from which it is absorbed and excreted in the urine. Myelography is typically followed by immediate or delayed CT examination (CT myelography). The newer, nonionic contrast agents have dramatically reduced the side effects and complications associated with myelography.[42] The most common postprocedural complication is mild-to-severe headache with nausea and/or vomiting. In the past, arachnoiditis, meningitis, and CNS changes (hallucinations) occurred but are rarely associated with newer myelographic agents. Because contrast material lowers the seizure threshold, patients with a history of seizures should be studied cautiously, and patients on medications known to lower the seizure threshold (i.e., tricyclic antidepressants) are commonly instructed to stop taking the drug 3 days before myelography to allow for adequate drug clearance.[58]

As MR has become the primary modality for imaging most spinal pathology, indications for myelography are now more limited. Myelography is still indicated for patients unable to undergo MR examination (e.g., claustrophobia, metallic devices in the region of interest, pacemakers). Conventional and CT myelography are still widely used to evaluate disk disease and spinal stenosis because they are relatively safe, easy to perform, and more available than MR. For evaluation of degenerative bony changes and facet disease, CT myelography is often superior to MR because there is no signal from cortical bone on MR images. Because of phase dispersion produced by the pulsatile flow of blood, myelography is still performed when vascular lesions, such as arteriovenous malformations, are suspected.

Normal and Abnormal Conventional and CT Myelograms

Radioopaque contrast material outlines the spinal cord and nerve roots, which appear as filling defects within the contrast column (Fig. 8-5, *A* and *B*). The cord and roots have smooth margins and taper gradually. Normal fusiform enlargements occur in the lower cervical and conus regions of the spinal cord, where the upper and lower extremity nerve root plexi arise. Pathologic processes appear as abnormal filling defects in the contrast column. The filling defect location and its relationship to surrounding structures help compartmentalize the lesion and aid in differential diagnosis. This method of evaluation is detailed in the section on spinal tumors.

The CT myelogram has all the features of routine CT with the added benefit of high-density contrast replacing the normal low-density CSF (Fig. 8-5, *C*). The relationships of the cord and surrounding structures can be easily discerned. Individual nerve roots, surrounded by contrast, can be followed within the subarachnoid space, through their respective foramina. Pathologic lesions appear as abnormal filling defects within the contrast, and any cord enlargement or deviation from normal position is easily appreciated.

CERVICAL SPINE AND SPINAL CORD
Normal Gross Anatomy of the Cervical Spine

Ligaments of the cervical spine are extremely important for maintaining stability, even in the absence of fracture. The important posterior ligament complex consists of the supraspinous and interspinous ligaments, the interfacet joint capsules, the ligamentum flava, and the posterior longitudinal ligament.[53] Also important are the intervertebral disks, attaching to the vertebral endplates primarily by Sharpey's fibers, and the anterior longitudinal ligament. In addition, several smaller ligaments, specific to the cervicocranium, are of paramount importance in maintaining stability of the skull in relation to the cervical spine and contribute to the prevertebral soft tissue shadow on the lateral radiograph.[53] These ligaments are detailed in Fig. 8-6.[25,53]

Normal Radiographic Anatomy of the Cervical Spine

Routine plain film radiography remains the most effective screening technique for initial detection of cervical spine injuries.[7] A complete radiographic examination consists of direct lateral, anteroposterior, open-mouth (odontoid), and right and left posterior oblique views. Lateral views in flexion and extension, obtained under a physician's supervision, may sometimes be necessary to assess stability.[27]

Direct Lateral View

The cross-table lateral view is the first view obtained when injury to the cervical spine is suspected. It is the most important view of the routine trauma series, with 90% of significant cervical spine injuries detected on this view.[7] One should ensure that this view is truly lateral and affords adequate visualization of all cervical vertebrae, including C7. If all seven cervical vertebrae are not clearly demonstrated, one must make additional efforts to further assess this area. The swimmer's view is often helpful in this regard. CT

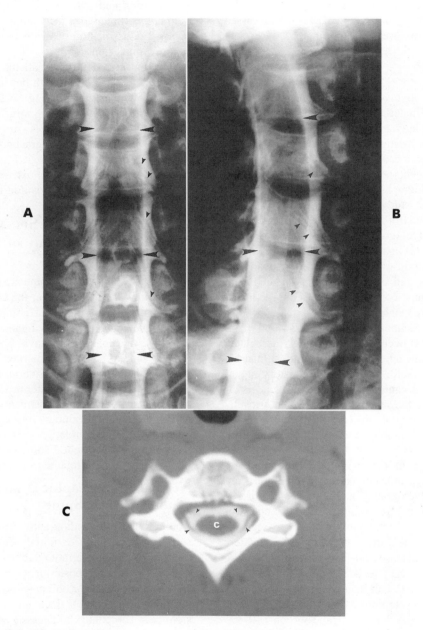

FIG. 8-5 Normal myelogram. Anteroposterior **(A)** and left oblique **(B)** views of a cervical myelogram. The cervical cord is outlined by contrast *(large arrowheads)*. The nerve roots appear as linear filling defects in the contrast-filled root sleeves *(small arrowheads)*. **C,** Axial CT with intrathecal contrast (CT myelogram) highlights the normal cord *(c)* surrounded by high-density contrast. Dorsal and ventral nerve roots are well seen *(arrowheads)*. Bony structures are dense. (Compare with Fig. 8-3, *C*).

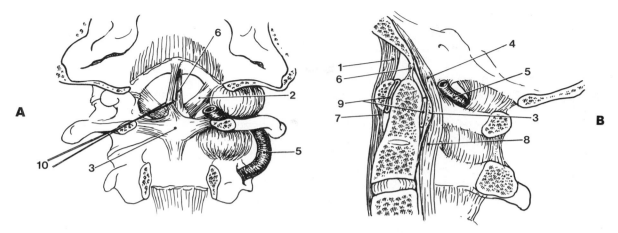

FIG. 8-6 Ligaments of the cervicocranium. Anteroposterior (**A**) and lateral (**B**) line diagrams. *1*, anterior atlantooccipital membrane; *2*, alar ("check") ligament; *3*, transverse atlantal ligament; *4*, tectorial membrane; *5*, vertebral artery; *6*, apical ligament of the dens; *7*, anterior atlantoaxial ligament; *8*, posterior atlantoaxial ligament; *9*, articular cavity (synovial joint); *10*, upper band of the transverse atlantal ligament.

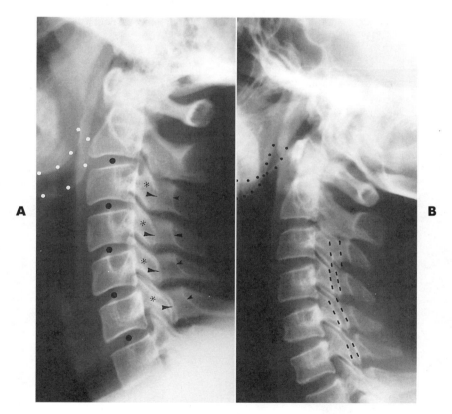

FIG. 8-7 Radiograph of the spine. **A,** Well-positioned lateral view in which the mandibular angles are almost superimposed *(white dotted lines)*. The right and left lateral masses (articular facets) *(asterisks)* are perfectly superimposed such that the paired posterior cortical surfaces appear as a single cortical density *(large arrowheads)*. The heights of the intervertebral disks are symmetric *(black dots)*, the "spaces" between the interfacet and spinolaminar lines are "clear" and uniform in density (laminar clear space, between *large* and *small arrowheads*), and the distances between adjacent laminae and spinous processes are uniform in height. **B,** "Off-lateral" lateral view reveals evidence of tilting and rotation of the head, manifested by the lack of mandible superimposition *(crossed black dotted lines)*. The articular facets are consensually offset such that two posterior cortical margins are identified *(dashed lines)*.

scanning of C6, C7, and T1 may occasionally be necessary to "clear" the lower cervical spine.

On a perfectly positioned lateral view, the articular facets, mandibular rami, and mandibular angles are superimposed (Fig. 8-7). Detailed evaluation of the lateral radiograph should include specific attention to the following nine features:

1. *Wackenheim's clivus baseline:* A line extrapolated along the posterior margin of the clivus should fall tangent to or intersect the posterior one third of the odontoid process (Fig. 8-8).[7,26] Marked deviation of this relationship may be associated with atlanto-occipital dislocations.

2. *Anterior atlantodental interval (AADI):* The distance between the posterior border of the anterior arch of the atlas and the anterior margin of the odontoid process (dens), maintained by the transverse ligament of the atlas, should not exceed 3.0 mm in adults or 5.0 mm in children (see Fig. 8-8).[56,71] Abnormal widening in a trauma patient may indicate ligament disruption, such as that associated with Jefferson fracture. However, there are a number of conditions associated with an increased AADI that are nontraumatic in origin, such as retropharyngeal infections, Down syndrome, and rheumatoid arthritis.[53]

3. *Vertebral body lines:* Lines drawn along the anterior and posterior margins of the vertebral bodies should be smooth, lordotic, and parallel (Fig. 8-9).

4. *Interfacet line:* A line drawn tangent to the superimposed posterior margins of the articular facets should be smooth and parallel to the vertebral body lines (see Fig. 8-9). When the patient is in a slightly off-lateral position, margins of both facets are seen (see Fig. 8-7, *B*). Lines drawn tangent to the posterior margins of both facets should still parallel the vertebral body lines.

5. *Spinolaminar line:* A line connecting the inner laminar cortices where they fuse to form the base of the spinous processes (posterior wall of the spinal canal) should form a smooth, lordotic curve all the way to the posterior margin of foramen magnum (see Fig. 8-9). Occasionally, the base of the spinous process of C2 is "displaced" backward in relation to the spinolaminar line. If not in excess of 2 to 3 mm, this may be a normal variant.[60]

6. *Intervertebral disk spaces:* The intervertebral disks should be uniform in height (see Fig. 8-7).

7. *Laminar clear space:* The "space" between the interfacet and spinolaminar lines should be of the same density, especially between C3 and C6 (see Fig. 8-7).

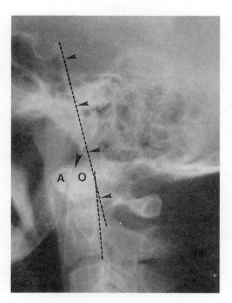

FIG. 8-8 Wackenheim's clivus baseline. A line drawn along the posterior margin of the clivus and extrapolated inferiorly *(arrowheads)* falls tangent to the posterior-superior aspect of the odontoid process *(O)*. The anterior atlantodental interval *(large arrowhead)* lies between the anterior arch of the atlas *(A)* and the anterior margin of the odontoid *(O)*.

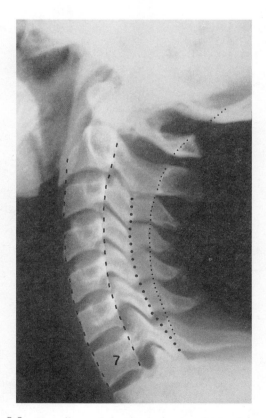

FIG. 8-9 Four lines of the cervical spine. Lines drawn tangent to the anterior and posterior margins of the vertebral bodies *(dashed lines)*, the posterior margins of the lateral masses (interfacet line, *large dotted line*), and the bases of the spinous processes (spinolaminar line, *small dotted line*) form uninterrupted, smooth, gentle, lordotic curves. "7" denotes C7.

No cortical bone should be present.[126] If an abnormal cortical fragment is identified, fracture of an articular facet (pillar fracture) or lamina should be suspected.

8. *Interspinous distance:* The interspinous distance should be approximately equal to or should decrease in height regularly from the level of C3 downward (see Fig. 8-7).[7,53] An increase in an interlaminar space, in the trauma setting, is a reliable sign of posterior ligament complex tear, such as those that occur with hyperflexion injuries.[53]

9. *Prevertebral soft tissues:* The retropharyngeal space should be 7 mm or less at C3 (average 3.4 mm) and the retrotracheal space should be no greater than 22 mm (average 14.0 mm) measured at C6.[121]

Anteroposterior View

The atlantoaxial articulation is typically obscured on the anteroposterior (AP) view (Fig. 8-10) because of superimposition of the mandible and occiput. The following four features of the AP view should be evaluated:

1. *Lateral column margins:* Because of superimposition of the articular masses, their lateral cortical margins appear as a continuous column of bone (lateral columns). They should be smooth, undulating, and symmetrically aligned.

2. *Spinous processes alignment and interspinous distance:* All spinous processes should be midline. If not, one should note whether the deviation from midline is smooth and consensual, as might be encountered in normal rotation, or is abrupt, as is seen in association with unilateral facet dislocations. In addition, the interspinous distances should be fairly equal. Focal widening at a single level may indicate a hyperflexion injury.

3. *Uncinate processes and uncovertebral joint integrity:* These should be sharp uncinate processes with symmetric joints.

4. *Vertebral body margins:* The cortical margins of the superior and inferior vertebral body endplates should be smooth, without step-offs.

Odontoid (Open-Mouth) View

It is extremely important for the odontoid view (Fig. 8-11) to be obtained with the cervicocranium aligned in a straight AP position for accurate evaluation. The following relationships should be assessed:

1. *Atlantoaxial joints:* Joints should be open, symmetrically angled, their contiguous surfaces parallel.

2. *Medial atlantodental spaces:* The odontoid process should be symmetrically situated between the lateral masses of the atlas such that the medial atlantodental spaces are the same.

3. *Lateral atlantoaxial margins:* The lateral margins of the contiguous facets of the atlas and the axis should lie on the same vertical plane, symmetrically. This

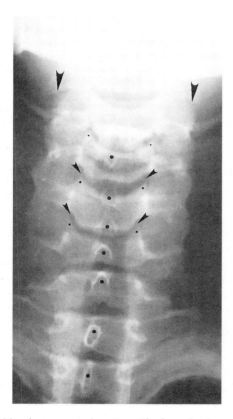

FIG. 8-10 Anteroposterior view. The lateral column margins are smooth and undulating *(large arrowheads)*, the spinous processes are midline and the interspinous distances decrease in height from above downward *(large dots)*, the uncinate processes are sharp *(small dots)*, and the uncovertebral joints are symmetric *(small arrowheads)*.

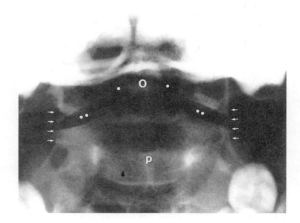

FIG. 8-11 Odontoid view. The atlantoaxial joints *(double dots)* and medial atlantodental intervals *(single dots)* are symmetric, the lateral margins of the atlas and axis facets lie on the same vertical plane *(arrows)*, the spinous process of the axis *(p)* is midline. Odontoid process *(O)*.

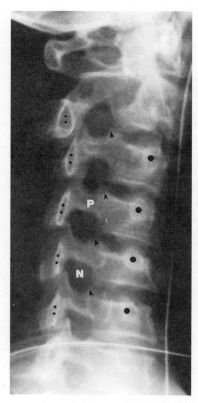

FIG. 8-12   Posterior oblique view. The left posterior oblique view demonstrates a normal shingle arrangement of the laminae *(black double dots)*, the integrity of the ipsilateral pedicles *(p)* is well-demonstrated, the contralateral pedicles project through the vertebral bodies as solid round densities that are all well aligned *(black large dots)*, the uncinate processes *(arrowheads)* are sharp, and the intervertebral foramina *(N)* are rounded, smooth, and widely patent.

lateral alignment may be "off" bilaterally, and the medial atlantodental spaces may be physiologically asymmetric in the presence of head tilt or rotation, occasionally making the diagnosis of Jefferson's fracture or atlantoaxial rotary subluxation problematic. Positioning is critical!

4. *Axis spinous process:* The typically bifid spinous process of C2 should be midline in position.

Oblique Views

Posterior oblique views (Fig. 8-12) are designed to demonstrate the integrity of the intervertebral foramina and surrounding structures (e.g., pedicles, laminae, uncinate processes, uncovertebral joints). They also offer additional views of various, previously obscured, portions of the atlas and axis.

Cervical Spine Trauma

Injuries to the cervical spine are produced by a variety of mechanisms. For the purposes of classification, it is useful

TABLE 8-1

Cervical Spine Trauma: Classification by Mechanism of Injury

Type of Injury	Classification
Hyperflexion Injuries	
Anterior subluxation (hyperflexion sprain)	Unstable
Wedge fracture (simple compression fracture)	Stable
Flexion teardrop fracture	Unstable
Clay shoveler's fracture	Stable
Bilateral facet dislocation	Unstable
Hyperflexion-Rotation Injuries	
Unilateral facet dislocation	Stable
Hyperextension Injuries	
Hyperextension dislocation	Unstable
Traumatic spondylolisthesis (hangman's fracture)	Unstable
Laminar fracture	Stable
Isolated posterior C1 arch fracture	Stable
Avulsion fracture of the anterior arch of the atlas	Stable
Extension teardrop fracture of the axis	Unstable in extension
Hyperextension-Rotation Injuries	
Hyperextension fracture-dislocation	Unstable
Pillar fracture (lateral mass fracture)	Stable
Vertical Compression Fractures	
Jefferson fracture (bursting atlas fracture)	Unstable
Lower C-spine burst fracture	Stable
Miscellaneous Injuries	
Atlantooccipital dislocation	Unstable
Atlantoaxial dislocation	Stable
Odontoid fractures	
Type I	Stable
Type II	Unstable
Type III	Stable

Modified from Anderson LD, D'Alonzo RT: *J Bone Joint Surg* 56(A):1663-1674, 1974.

to think of the various injuries according to the forces producing the injury (Table 8-1).[53] Only those injuries that are unstable or difficult to diagnose are discussed in detail here.

HYPERFLEXION INJURIES
Anterior Subluxation

Anterior subluxation (hyperflexion sprain) is the result of limited hyperflexion, producing disruption of the posterior ligament complex.[49] The traumatic force is insufficient to cause interfacet joint disruption and/or facet interlocking. This injury is, nevertheless, the most *unstable* cervical spine injury, with a 21% to 50% incidence of delayed instability caused by the failure of ligamentous healing.[16,53,95] The radiographic features of anterior subluxation may include (1) localized hyperkyphotic angulation at the level of injury, (2) anterior narrowing and posterior wid-

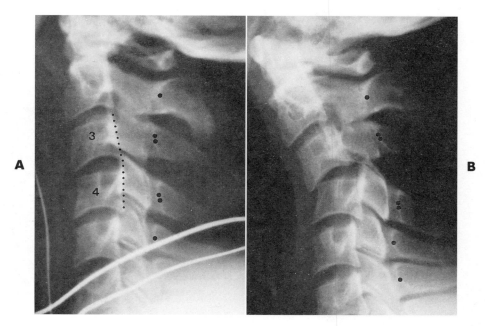

FIG. 8-13 Anterior subluxation. **A**, Initial lateral radiograph reveals subtle angulation at C3-C4 *(dotted line)*, slight fanning of the C3-C4 spinous processes *(large double dots)*, widening of the posterior aspect of the intervertebral disk space, and prevertebral soft tissue swelling. None of these findings were appreciated, and the patient was discharged, only to return 1 week later with complaints of persistent neck pain. **B**, Follow-up lateral view revealed marked anterior subluxation and angulation. Note the marked spinous process fanning at C3-C4 *(double dots)*.

ening of the intervertebral disk space, (3) anterior displacement of the inferior articular facets of the subluxed vertebra in relation to their contiguous subjacent facets, (4) widening of the interspinous space ("fanning" of the spinous processes) at the level of injury, and (5) anterior rotation or displacement of the subluxed vertebra a distance of 1 to 3 mm.[49] On the AP view, a widened interspinous space (ISS) that measures more than one and one half times the ISS above and below indicates the presence of anterior subluxation.[81] All of these findings may be extremely subtle when there is not frank rotation or anterior displacement of the involved vertebrae (Fig. 8-13). In these instances, lateral views in flexion and extension may be extremely useful.[53]

Flexion Teardrop Fracture

Flexion teardrop fracture, considered the most devastating cervical spine fracture compatible with life, is produced by the most severe of hyperflexion forces.[53] The characteristic neurologic injury associated with this fracture is acute anterior cervical cord syndrome consisting of immediate, complete quadriplegia with loss of anterior column function (pain, temperature, and touch) but preservation of posterior column function (position, motion, and vibration).[97]

Pathologically there is disruption of the intervertebral disk, the anterior and posterior longitudinal ligaments, and the posterior ligament complex, with associated subluxation or frank disruption of the interfacetal joints.[53] This injury is completely *unstable*. Radiographic features may include (1) a characteristic triangle-shaped fragment that fractures from the anteroinferior corner of the vertebral body, resembling a drop of water, (2) posterior displacement of the involved vertebral body with concomitant narrowing of the spinal canal at the level of injury and posterior displacement of the upper column of the divided cervical spine in relation to the lower column, (3) widening of the interlaminar and interspinous spaces ("fanning"), indicative of posterior ligament complex disruption, (4) subluxation or dislocation of the facet joints, and (5) kyphotic deformity of the cervical spine at the level of injury (Fig. 8-14).[53,61]

Bilateral Facet Dislocation

Bilateral facet dislocation results from complete disruption of the posterior ligament complex, the posterior longitudinal ligament, the intervertebral disks, the articular facets, and, usually, the anterior longitudinal ligament.[2] It is highly *unstable*, with a high incidence of cord damage.[53] With

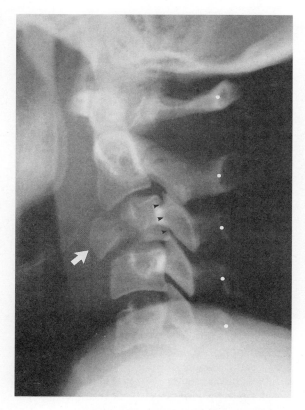

FIG. 8-14 Flexion teardrop fracture. Lateral radiograph reveals acute flexion deformity at the C3-C4 level. A large fracture fragment *(arrow)*, comprising primarily the anteroinferior aspect of C3, is evident. Prevertebral soft tissue swelling is present. There is a mild amount of retropulsion of the posterior fragment into the spinal canal *(arrowheads)*. Although the interspinous distances of the C2-C3, C3-C4, and C4-C5 spaces appear normal *(dots)*, there is an increase in the interspinous distance at C1-C2, indicative of a flexion injury.

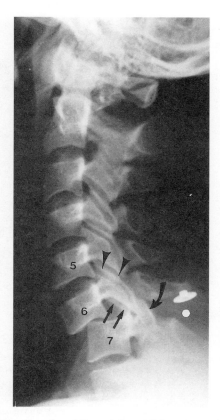

FIG. 8-15 Complete bilateral facet dislocation. The inferior facets of C5 articulate normally and are parallel to the superior facets of C6 *(arrowheads)*. However, the inferior facets *(arrows)* of C6 are completely dislocated and do not articulate at all with the superior facets of C7 *(curved arrow)*. The C6 vertebral body is displaced anteriorly a distance greater than one half the anteroposterior diameter of the C7 vertebral body. Note fanning and separation of the laminae and spinous processes at C6-C7 *(dot)*.

"complete" dislocation, the dislocated facets pass upward, forward, and over the inferior facets of the joint, coming to lie within the intervertebral foramina (Fig. 8-15). There is anterior displacement of the dislocated vertebra a distance equal to or greater than 50% of the AP diameter of the vertebral body.[6] In addition, there is hyperkyphotic angulation at the site of injury and fanning of the spinous processes (see Fig. 8-15). Because this dislocation is bilateral, the spinous processes maintain their midline position on the AP view. When the bilateral facet dislocation is "incomplete," the posterior-anterior-inferior margins of the inferior facets of the dislocated vertebra come to rest on top of the anterior-superior margins of the superior facets of the subjacent vertebra ("perched" facets) (Fig. 8-16). In this instance the dislocated vertebra is anteriorly displaced a distance somewhat less than 50% of the AP vertebral body diameter.[53]

HYPERFLEXION-ROTATION INJURIES
Unilateral Facet Dislocation

Unilateral facet dislocation, produced by simultaneous flexion and rotation, involves disruption of the posterior ligament complex, including the facet joint capsules. There is at least partial disruption of the posterior longitudinal ligament and the posterior annulus fibrosis. However, because the dislocated facet is "locked" in position and the anterior longitudinal ligament and anterior aspect of the intervertebral disk are typically intact, this is considered a *stable* injury. Despite its stability, early recognition of this injury is essential because delays make reduction extremely difficult, and root deficit recovery is impaired.[96] Essentially pathognomonic findings are present on both the lateral and AP views. Rotation of the cervical spine above the level of dislocation produces the diagnostic appearance on the lateral

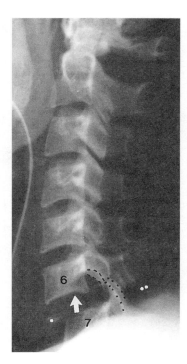

FIG. 8-16 Incomplete bilateral facet dislocation. The posterior-inferior margins of the C6 inferior facet *(dashed line)* are "perched" on the anterior-superior margins of the C7 superior facet *(dotted line)*. There is marked separation of the C6 and C7 vertebral bodies *(arrow)* and the interlaminar/interspinous distances *(double dots)*. A small fracture from the anterior-superior aspect of C7 is identified *(single dot)*.

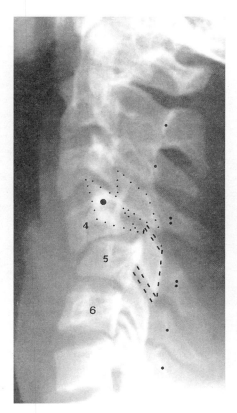

FIG. 8-17 Unilateral facet dislocation. This lined lateral radiograph demonstrates the normal relationship of the articular facets at C5-C6 and C6-C7. However, one facet is dislocated at C4 *(large dot)* such that its inferior surface does not articulate with the corresponding C5 superior articular facet. The articular facets of C5 are almost superimposed *(dashed lines)*. However, because of unilateral dislocation, the articular facets of C4 and above are completely offset and assume a butterfly or bowtie configuration *(dotted lines)*. C4 is displaced anteriorly less than one half the AP diameter of the C5 vertebra, and there is wide separation of the C4 and C5 spinous processes *(double dots)*.

view. The articular facets of the vertebra below the dislocation lie symmetrically parallel such that they are superimposed. Above the dislocation, however, a double set of articular facets are identified, resulting in a butterfly or bowtie configuration (Fig. 8-17). The dislocated facet is partially superimposed on or obscured by the vertebral body, making close scrutiny of the homogeneity of the vertebral body densities and facet lines, along with a high index of suspicion, critical to early diagnosis. The body of the dislocated vertebra is typically displaced anteriorly a distance of less than 50% of the AP diameter of the vertebra but more than the 1 to 3 mm seen in association with anterior subluxation.[53] Because the posterior ligament complex is disrupted, fanning of the spinous processes will also be present with this injury. The widened interspinous distance is usually identified on the AP view. Additionally, there is typically *abrupt* deviation of the spinous processes from the level of the dislocation cephalad, *toward* the side of the dislocated facet.

HYPEREXTENSION INJURIES
Hyperextension Dislocation

Hyperextension dislocation is an uncommon injury, most often the result of a high-velocity, abrupt-deceleration, motor-vehicle accident.[34] It is produced by a straight backward or backward-and-upward force.[53] There is rupture of the anterior longitudinal ligament and intervertebral disk and stripping of the posterior longitudinal ligament from the subjacent vertebral body. An avulsion fracture of the anteroinferior corner of the involved vertebra is reported in 65% of patients with this injury.[34] Posterior vertebral body displacement, coupled with infolding of the dura and ligamentum flavum, results in pinching of the cord.[34] With dissipation of the vector force, the dislocation reduces spontaneously and the alignment of the cervical spine reduces

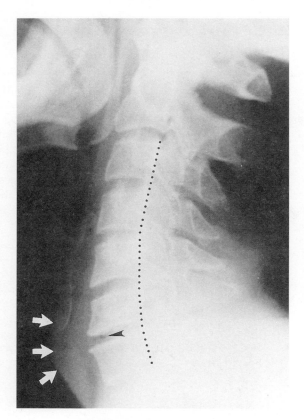

FIG. 8-18   Hyperextension dislocation. The vertebral bodies are normally aligned *(dotted line)*. There is marked focal prevertebral swelling at C6-C7 *(arrows)*. The height of the C6-C7 intervertebral disk appears normal, but air (vacuum disk) is identified within the disk *(arrowhead)*.

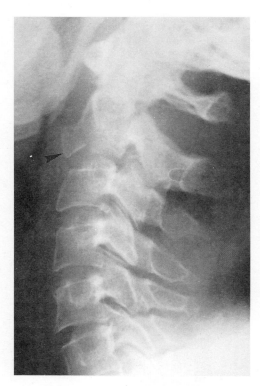

FIG. 8-19   Extension teardrop fracture. Lateral radiograph demonstrates an extension teardrop fracture in this 46-year-old woman *(arrowhead)*. Note the lack of extensive prevertebral soft tissue swelling in this patient.

to normal.[53] Pinching of the cord, albeit transient, most often produces an acute central cord syndrome.[34] Because of the disruption of the anterior ligament complex, this injury is *unstable* in extension, and uncontrolled hyperextension could severely aggravate the patient's condition.[17] Radiographic features associated with hyperextension dislocation may include (1) normal alignment of the cervical spine; (2) diffuse prevertebral soft tissue swelling; (3) avulsion of the anteroinferior corner of the involved vertebra, with the horizontal dimension of the fracture fragment greater than the vertical dimension; (4) widening of the involved disk space (15%); and (5) vacuum disk (15%), probably related to the negative pressure associated with transection of the intervertebral disk during hyperextension (Fig. 8-18).[34]

Traumatic Spondylolisthesis (Hangman's Fracture)

The mechanism responsible for the "hangman's fracture" is generally believed to be a hyperextension injury, with or without a component of initial or rebound hyperflexion.[53] In its pure form, this injury represents a bilateral fracture

through the pars interarticularis (the thin portion of the articular mass of the axis between the superior and inferior facets) with avulsion of the neural arch from the axis body and should be considered an *unstable* injury. These fractures may also occur at the junction of the articular mass and axis body, through the posterior aspect of the axis body, through the superior or inferior facets, or through the laminae.[35,69]

The classical teaching regarding the hangman's fracture emphasized the associated increased AP diameter of the spinal canal ("autodecompression") and thus the lack of spinal cord injury and severe neurologic findings. Much of the older literature supported this concept.[11,21,36,98,99] More recent reports, however, reveal that severe and/or permanent neurologic injury is not rare.[31,69,78] C2 neural arch fractures are reported to involve the transverse foramina in up to 52% of patients.[78] Significant vertebral artery injury may occur, producing a variety of symptoms, including cranial nerve involvement.[86,92,98]

Extension Teardrop Fracture of the Axis

Extension teardrop fracture consists of avulsion of a triangular fragment from the anteroinferior corner of the axis at the site of insertion of the intact anterior longitudinal ligament during hyperextension (Fig. 8-19). Because the posterior ligament complex is intact, this injury is *stable* in *flexion*. However, because the anterior longitudinal ligament is no longer attached to the bulk of the axis, the extension teardrop fracture is *unstable* in *extension*. Prevertebral swelling may be associated with this injury and is more extensive in younger patients.

HYPEREXTENSION-ROTATION INJURIES
Hyperextension Fracture-Dislocation

This complex injury results from a force delivered to the upper face or forehead, eccentrically or with the head rotated, forcing the head and upper cervical spine in a downward and posterior direction. Additional force produces anterior longitudinal ligament rupture and articular facet impaction on the side opposite the direction of rotation. With continued force the subjacent vertebra translates anteriorly and there is subluxation or dislocation of the articular mass ipsilateral to the side of rotation.[43] Radiographically there is anterior vertebral body displacement, which may be to such a degree that the vertebral bodies themselves are actually locked. The disrupted anatomy of the involved articular facets and facet joints may be so severe as to render them unidentifiable (absent facet). This fracture is completely *unstable*. It is important that this injury be recognized as a hyperextension injury, despite the anterior vertebral subluxation because extension positioning can exacerbate the injury.

VERTICAL COMPRESSION INJURIES
Jefferson Fracture (Bursting Atlas Fracture)

The classical Jefferson fracture consists of fractures involving both the anterior and posterior arches of the atlas, crossing the equator of the atlas.[67] Prevertebral soft tissue swelling is prominent with this injury and helps to distinguish it from an isolated posterior C1 arch fracture. On the lateral view, the posterior arch fracture(s) are typically visible although the anterior arch fracture is not. On the open-mouth odontoid view there is symmetric bilateral widening of the medial atlantodental intervals with offset of the lateral C1 masses in relation to C2. If the sum of the overhang of the lateral masses is greater than 6.9 mm, the transverse ligament has probably ruptured and the spine is *unstable*.[106] In this case, widening of the anterior atlantodental interval may be identified on the lateral radiograph.

If a medial lateral mass-fracture fragment is retained in normal position by an intact transverse atlantal ligament, there may be asymmetry of the medial atlantodental intervals on the open-mouth odontoid view. CT is very helpful in the evaluation of Jefferson fractures for assessing the presence of transverse ligament disruption and the extent of the fractures and for differentiating this injury from congenital C1 arch hypoplasias, rachischises, or isolated posterior arch fracture.

MISCELLANEOUS INJURIES
Atlantooccipital Dislocation (AOD)

Dislocation of the head in relation to the cervical spine is a rare, typically fatal, injury, although there are multiple reports of survival.* It is most commonly produced by extreme hyperflexion but, occasionally, by extreme hyperextension. As virtually all ligaments of the cervicocranium are disrupted, this is a highly *unstable* injury. Three radiologic types of AOD are possible: (1) longitudinal distraction with axial separation of the occiput and atlas, typically the most difficult to diagnose[8,20,44,68]; (2) anterior dislocation of the occiput with respect to the atlas; and (3) posterior dislocation of the occiput with respect to the atlas.[42] The radiographic diagnosis is usually obvious from the initial lateral radiograph although, on occasion, the findings may be extremely subtle.[85] The distance between the tip of the clivus and the tip of the dens should not exceed 4 to 5 mm in an adult on these studies. At times, however, marked distraction may be present. A number of methods for assessment of AOD have been proposed.[68,88] The X-line method appears to be the most reliable but is not useful in children less than 5 years of age.[68] On the lateral radiograph, in the majority of cases, Wackenheim's baseline is abnormal.

Atlantoaxial Rotary Subluxation

This injury results from a combination of rotation and lateral flexion that produces ligamentous injury and facet joint derangement.[53] Clinically, atlantoaxial rotary subluxation is distinguished from transient torticollis by its failure to resolve within a few weeks. It most commonly results from relatively insignificant cervical trauma or from upper respiratory infections.[64] In the presence of this condition it is impossible to get a "lateral" radiograph on which both the head and spine are lateral; when the head is lateral, the spine is oblique, and vice versa. The anterior atlantodental interval is obliterated and there is loss of the normal hemispheric configuration of the anterior atlas arch on the lateral view. On the open-mouth odontoid view, the medial atlantodental intervals are asymmetric as are the C1-C2 joint spaces. It is impossible on the plain radiographic study to differentiate transient torticollis from rotary subluxation, and functional scanning may be necessary.[64] CT and MR are extremely helpful in assessing the exact position of the atlas and in identifying any associated cord compression.

Odontoid Fractures

Three types of odontoid fractures are described, according to the classification of Anderson and D'Alonzo.[2] The type I odontoid fracture, an oblique avulsion fracture of the tip of the odontoid at the site of attachment of the alar ligament, is extremely rare. This fracture is considered *stable* and uncomplicated by nonunion.

The type II (high) dens fracture is a transverse fracture,

---

*References 8, 68, 80, 85, 115, 124.

typically through the lower portion of the odontoid process at its base, with or without displacement. This fracture, by definition, is confined to the dens and does not involve the body of C2. The type II fracture is the most common of the odontoid fractures. Although the mechanism of injury is controversial, there is universal agreement that this is an *unstable* injury. Radiographic findings may be extremely subtle, especially in the absence of fragment displacement. Prevertebral soft tissue swelling, however, is virtually universal. There may be only subtle angulation of the odontoid process, or there may be frank displacement of the odontoid-atlas complex in relation to C2. Although occasionally visible at the odontoid base, the fracture is typically obscured on the open-mouth odontoid view by superimposition of the C1 arch and/or occiput. Because the fracture line is parallel to the routine axial CT plane, it is easily missed on CT if sagittal reconstructions are not obtained. Because of the high cortical bone content of that portion of the odontoid involved in the type II fracture, nonunion is reported to occur in 64% of patients overall and in almost 100% of patients in whom more than 5 mm of posterior displacement is present.[94]

The type III (low) odontoid fracture extends into the axis body. It is usually *stable* and characteristically heals without the problem of nonunion. Depending on the plane of the fracture line, the fracture may or may not be visible on routine lateral or AP radiographs. The only finding may be the identification of a "fat C2" in relation to C3 on the lateral view, such as that seen in pure axis body fractures.[105]

SPINAL TUMORS AND TUMORLIKE CONDITIONS

It is helpful to consider spinal canal pathology according to spaces: intramedullary, extramedullary-intradural, and extradural. If a lesion can be localized to one of these spaces, the diagnostic considerations can be narrowed. In general, unless there is a specific contraindication, MR is the imaging modality of choice for the majority of these lesions. The addition of intravenous gadolinium-DTPA is particularly useful for evaluation of suspected intramedullary and extramedullary-intradural pathology.[108,109] If MR is not available, myelography followed by CT examination (CT myelogram) is the second choice of study. A CT examination without the use of intrathecal contrast is not adequate for evaluation of most lesions.

Intramedullary Lesions

Intramedullary lesions expand the spinal cord as they enlarge, gradually thinning the subarachnoid space, usually symmetrically (Fig. 8-20). If of sufficient size, intramedullary processes may produce changes of the bony spinal canal, including posterior scalloping of the vertebral bodies, flattening of the spinous processes, widening of the interpediculate distance (or flattening of the medial aspect of the pedicles), and overall widening of the canal (Fig. 8-21). In the cervical region, the AP diameter of the spinal canal is

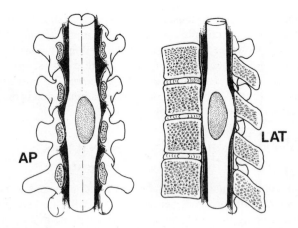

FIG. 8-20   Intramedullary lesion. AP and lateral line diagrams demonstrate the appearance of an intramedullary mass *(stippled area)*. Note the symmetric enlargement of the spinal cord in all dimensions.

less than its transverse diameter so that widening is first appreciated on the lateral view.[28] Normally, the cervical canal funnels in a gradual fashion as one progresses caudally, ranging from 17 to 32 mm at the C1 level to 14 to 23 mm at the C7 level.[28] A lack of funneling or actual enlargement over two or more levels should raise suspicion of an intramedullary process.

Conventional or CT myelography demonstrates widening of the spinal cord with symmetric attenuation of the subarachnoid space (Fig. 8-21). On occasion, the intramedullary process produces complete obstruction to the flow of contrast.

MR examination of an intramedullary lesion usually demonstrates the length of cord involvement (Fig. 8-21). The exact margins of an infiltrating tumor may be difficult to identify. The use of intravenous contrast for suspected intramedullary pathology is essential and improves visualization in most cases.[109]

Intramedullary widening of the spinal cord may be produced by a variety of tumors, including gliomas by far the most common (ependymomas, 65% [Fig. 8-21]; astrocytomas, 30%; glioblastoma multiforme, oligodendrogliomas, medulloblastomas); dermoid cysts, sarcomas, hemangioblastomas, and intramedullary metastases. Infections (transverse myelitis, granulomas [sarcoidosis, TB], and intramedullary abscesses), traumatic injuries (cord contusions and hematomas), and syringohydromyelic cavities may also present as intramedullary lesions.

Extramedullary-Intradural Lesions

By definition, these lesions are contained "within" the subarachnoid space, displacing the arachnoid layer of the meninges but leaving the dura in place. On myelography, CT, or MR, the subarachnoid space flares out to form a "cap" at its interface with the lesion (Fig. 8-22). A search for this

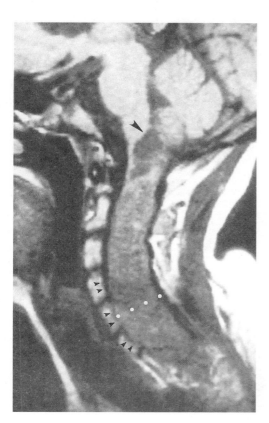

FIG. 8-21   Intramedullary lesion: ependymoma. Sagittal T$_1$-weighted MR scan demonstrates a massive tumor involving all of the cervical cord and extending to involve the distal medulla (*large arrowhead*). The cervical cord has been so greatly expanded (*dots*) that it has scalloped and eroded most of the cervical vertebral bodies (*small arrowheads*).

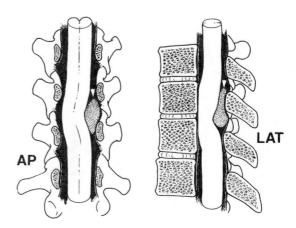

FIG. 8-22   Extramedullary-intradural lesion. Anterior-posterior and lateral line diagrams demonstrate the appearance of an extramedullary-intradural mass (*stippled area*). Because the mass lies within the dura, the CSF forms a subarachnoid "cap" outlining the lesion (*arrowheads*).

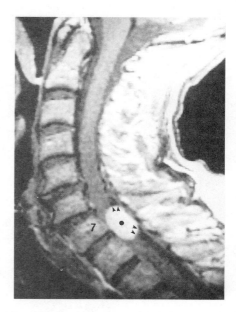

FIG. 8-23   Extramedullary-intradural lesion: schwannoma. Sagittal T$_1$-weighted image after intravenous gadolinium-DTPA demonstrates an enhancing mass (*large, single black dot*). The "cap" configuration of the CSF on the sagittal image (*arrowheads*) places the lesion in the extramedullary-intradural compartment.

cap, on at least one projection or plane, should be made on all examinations (Fig. 8-23).

Tumors in this space represent the largest number of spinal cord tumors, mostly benign. The vast majority consist of meningiomas and nerve sheath tumors (Fig. 8-23). Meningiomas occur most frequently in women (80% to 85%) and favor a thoracic location (82%). They generally occur later in life than the nerve sheath tumors and are rarely multiple. Nerve sheath tumors, on the other hand, tend to occur in younger individuals and have no location or sex predilection. They are commonly multiple in patients with neurofibromatosis. Nerve sheath tumors may protrude in a dumbbell shape from the neural foramen, being both intradural and extradural (and thereby widening the intervertebral foramen), or they may, occasionally, be entirely extradural. Other much less common pathology occurring in this space includes arachnoid cysts, drop metastasis (usually secondary to primary brain tumors, with medulloblastomas and ependymomas being most common), lymphomas, and dermoid and epidermoid lesions.

Extradural Lesions

Because these lesions, being extradural, lie outside the subarachnoid space, there is no subarachnoid cap at the interface with the lesion (Fig. 8-24). In all other respects, extradural lesions may be indistinguishable from extramedullary-intradural lesions, and, at times, compart-

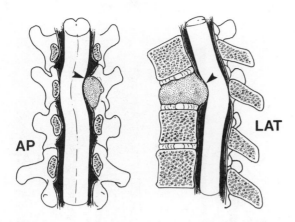

FIG. 8-24 Extradural lesion. Anterior-posterior and lateral line diagrams demonstrate the appearance of an extramedullary mass *(stippled area)*. Although the pattern of spinal cord displacement is similar to that associated with extramedullary-intradural masses, the lesion, lying outside the dura, is *not* outlined by a "cap" configuration of CSF between the arachnoid and dura *(arrowheads)*.

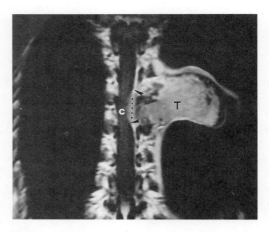

FIG. 8-25 Extradural lesion: Ewing's sarcoma. Coronal T_1-weighted MR image demonstrates a large thoracic tumor *(T)* that has crept through the intervertebral foramina into the extradural compartment *(black dots)*. The spinal cord *(c)* is compressed to the opposite side by the mass. Examination of the configuration of the CSF column outlining the tumor fails to reveal a subarachnoid "cap," clearly placing the lesion in the epidural space *(arrowheads)*.

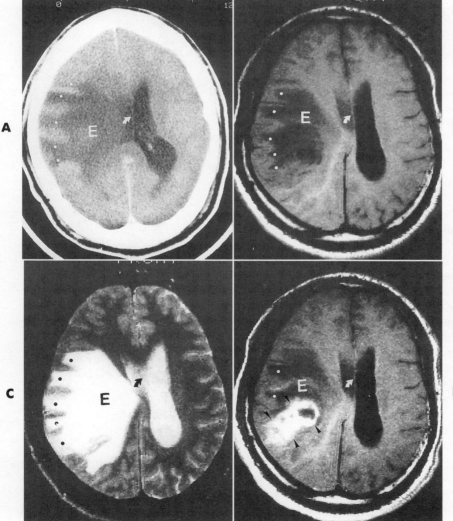

FIG. 8-26 Vasogenic edema (parietal lobe glioma). Non-contrast-enhanced CT **(A)**, T_1-weighted MR **(B)**, T_2-weighted MR **(C)**, and T_1-weighted MR **(D)** after contrast administration (Gd-DTPA). Areas of edema *(E)* are well seen on all images, extending along white-matter fibers *(dots)* with normal gray matter interposed. After contrast enhancement, the enhancing tumor nidus can be distinguished from surrounding edema **(D**, *arrowheads)*. Subfalcine herniation is demonstrated on all images *(curved arrow)*.

mentalization may not be possible. Excluding disk disease, the most common extradural pathology, metastatic disease with epidural extension accounts for the largest percentage of extradural lesions and is particularly common in carcinoma of the breast and lung. Pathologic fractures of the involved vertebrae are frequent, often associated with spinal cord compression. Primary tumors of the spine and direct extension from paraspinal neoplasms make up the other malignant lesions of the extradural compartment, including lymphoma (particularly Hodgkin's lymphoma), myeloma/plasmacytomas, sarcomas (Fig. 8-25), and vertebral body chordomas.[119]

Benign lesions in this compartment are uncommon and include extradural nerve sheath tumors, meningiomas (which have a greater tendency to be malignant in this location), lipomas, dermoid and epidermoid tumors, and primary vertebral body tumors (osteoblastoma, osteochondroma, giant cell tumors, aneurysmal bone cysts, and hemangiomas).[119]

INTRACRANIAL DISEASE
Patterns of Disease
Edema

Cerebral edema (swelling) results from an increase in brain volume caused by a localized or diffuse abnormal accumulation of water and sodium.[75] This is different from cerebral engorgement, which results from an increase in blood volume caused by vasodilation or obstructed venous outflow. Except for location, the imaging appearance of edema is essentially similar for all pathologic processes. On CT scans, any increase in water is seen as a decrease in density and appears dark. Because MR uses hydrogen proton characteristics to produce an image, an increase in water molecules is seen as an area of decreased signal (black) on T_1-weighted studies and as an area of increased signal (white) on T_2-weighted studies.

Three types of edema have been described[41,63,72]:

1. **Vasogenic edema** primarily involves the white matter and is associated predominantly with brain tumor, abscess, trauma, and hemorrhage. Vasogenic edema is seen as an area of decreased density on CT or abnormal intensity on MR that extends along the fingers of white matter, interposed between normal gray matter (Fig. 8-26). When this pattern is associated with mass effect in a nonvascular distribution, neoplasm or abscess are the most likely diagnoses.

2. **Cytotoxic edema**, involving both gray and white matter, is most commonly associated with ischemia or infarction. Hypoosmolar states (dilutional hyponatremia, acute sodium depletion, inappropriate ADH syndrome), and osmotic disequilibrium syndromes (hemodialysis, diabetic ketoacidosis), can also produce this form of edema. Because it involves both the gray and white matter, areas of cytotoxic

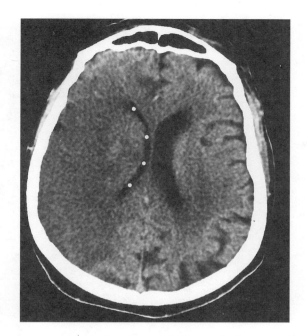

FIG. 8-27 Cytotoxic edema (middle cerebral artery infarction). Non-contrast-enhanced head CT reveals a large area of low density involving both the gray and white matter of the right hemisphere. The gyri and sulci, so well seen on the left, are obliterated by the edema and are absent on the right. The right lateral ventricle *(white dots)* is compressed, although midline shift (subfalcine herniation) is not appreciated.

edema extend to the calvarium on both CT and MR (Fig. 8-27). Because it is associated with ischemia and infarction, cytotoxic edema has a more vascular distribution and produces less mass effect.

3. **Interstitial edema** results from CSF migration into the periventricular white matter, most frequently because of conditions that impede CSF absorption. This is covered more fully in the later discussion of hydrocephalus.

Contrast enhancement may help define areas of edema and suggest an etiology. Because contrast accumulates in regions of blood-brain barrier breakdown, areas of vasogenic edema enhance. Areas of cytotoxic edema typically enhance only in later stages.

Hemorrhage

Intracranial hemorrhage may be traumatic or nontraumatic in origin. When blood is seen in the extraaxial space (epidural, subdural, subarachnoid), trauma is the most likely etiology. Subarachnoid hemorrhage is also associated with ruptured congenital aneurysms. Parenchymal hemorrhage is more likely to be nontraumatic in origin, secondary to an underlying disease such as hypertension, neoplasm, or vascular anomaly.

Regardless of location, acute hemorrhage is seen on a CT scan as an area of high density (Fig. 8-28, *A*). During

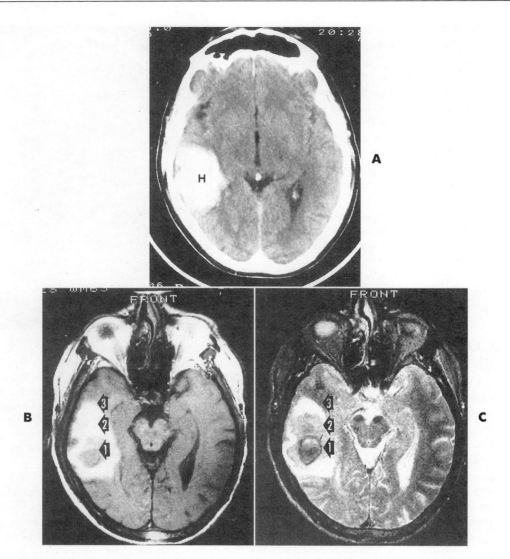

FIG. 8-28 Hemorrhage. **A,** Non-contrast-enhanced head CT demonstrates a large area of hemorrhage in the right temporal lobe *(H)*. T_1-weighted MR **(B)** and T_2-weighted MR **(C)** demonstrate the hemorrhage in various stages of breakdown. The center of the lesion is dark on the T_1-weighted and T_2-weighted images, indicating deoxyhemoglobin *(1)*. The intermediate zone is bright on the T_1-weighted image and gray on the T_2-weighted image, indicating intracellular methemoglobin *(2)*, whereas the outer rim is bright on both the T_1-weighted and T_2-weighted images, indicating extracellular methemoglobin *(3)*.

resolution, the density diminishes because of disintegration of blood components, eventually becoming isodense to brain parenchyma and resolving to an area of hypodensity. A normal CT scan does not totally exclude hemorrhage.[76] Anemic patients may present with isodense extraaxial or intraparenchymal blood collections, and only the presence of mass effect suggests the presence of hemorrhage. In addition, a small subarachnoid hemorrhage may also be isodense to brain parenchyma and only fill the cisterns and sulci.

The appearance of hemorrhage on MR is complicated because of varying paramagnetic properties of blood break-

down products. One should consider the age of hemorrhage in relation to these breakdown products.* During the first 24 hours after parenchymal hemorrhage, intact red blood cells containing oxyhemoglobin accumulate. Being diamagnetic, oxyhemoglobin is slightly hypointense to isointense on T_1-weighted images and isointense to slightly hyperintense on T_2-weighted images. Over the next 3 to 5 days, hemoglobin becomes deoxygenated. Because deoxyhemoglobin is paramagnetic, the T_2 intensity values fall (become hypointense), while the T_1 values essentially remain the

---

*References 18, 45-47, 112, 117, 118, 129.

same. With respect to brain parenchyma, the acute hematoma appears dark on T_2-weighted images and slightly dark to isointense on T_1-weighted images.

Between 3 and 7 days, intracellular methemoglobin begins to accumulate, beginning peripherally and advancing toward the center of the clot. During this stage, T_2 intensity values remain unchanged but T_1 values begin to increase, the periphery of the clot becoming hyperintense. The hematoma is black on T_2-weighted images and bright on T_1-weighted images. Between 7 days and 2 to 3 months, intracellular methemoglobin is released from erythrocytes (extracellular methemoglobin). During this stage, signal intensities on both T_1 and T_2 images increase (bright on both images). During the final stage, which may begin within the first 2 weeks and last for years, phagocytic degradation of methemoglobin to hemosiderin occurs. This process, which also begins peripherally and extends toward the center, effectively removes iron from the hematoma and deposits it at the periphery. Signal intensities again decrease, and hemosiderin appears black on both T_1- and T_2-weighted images, beginning at the periphery, as a ring, eventually replacing the entire hemorrhage. This progression represents a continuum of changing intensity values and is not an all-or-nothing phenomenon (Fig. 8-28, *B* and *C*). Most hematomas produce a surrounding area of edema that should not be misinterpreted as an additional area of hemorrhage. Edema, dark on T_1-weighted images and bright on T_2-weighted images, gradually fades.

Mass Effect, Shift, and Herniation

All lesions that increase intracerebral mass eventually cause brain herniation. This may be the direct consequence of an enlarging mass (tumor or abscess) or an indirect consequence of a lesion (edema from an infarct). The earliest abnormality noted on imaging studies is subtle effacement of adjacent cortical sulci caused by early edema. At later stages, mass effect produces compression or distortion of a ventricle.

Various dural partitions within the skull create compartments. The falx cerebri separates the cerebral hemispheres while the tentorium separates the middle from the posterior cranial fossa. Subfalcine herniation occurs when a hemispheric mass compresses the medial surface, typically the cingulate or supracingulate gyri, beneath the falx. It is easily recognized on CT or MR by deviation of the falx and extension of hemispheric structures across the midline (see Fig. 8-26). The exact location of the lesion giving rise to the herniation can also be determined.

Lying beneath the anterior free margin of the falx, the normal pericallosal branch of the anterior cerebral artery follows a straight or gently undulating midline course. Angiographically, the presence of subfalcine herniation is demonstrated by shift patterns involving this artery.[68] The term *round shift,* (the most common), applies to deviation of the pericallosal artery in a smooth rounded arc, typically from a mass in the anterior frontal lobe. *Square shift* de-

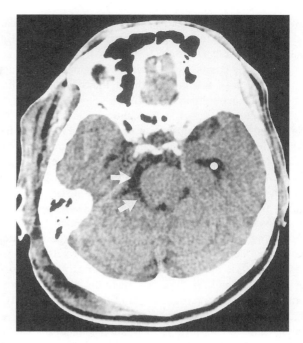

FIG. 8-29 Right descending tentorial herniation. Axial non-contrast-enhanced CT scan at the level of the midbrain in a patient with a large right subdural hematoma. The ispilateral subarachnoid cistern is widened *(arrows)*, and the contralateral subarachnoid cistern is obliterated because of brainstem rotation. The left temporal horn is dilated *(white dot)*, indicating trapping of the left lateral ventricle.

scribes an abrupt change in direction of the pericallosal artery and return to midline from a mass posterior to the genu of the corpus callosum in the posterior frontal, temporal, or parietal lobes. *Proximal shift* describes displacement of only the most proximal pericallosal artery and places the mass in the subfrontal or anterior temporal regions. *Distal shift* occurs when the pericallosal artery, in normal position proximally, gradually shifts across the midline as it courses distally. This shift places the mass in the parietal, occipital, or midposterior temporal regions.

Transtentorial herniation occurs when a mass arising on either side of the tentorium results in brain herniation through the tentorial incisura, either descending (downward) or ascending (upward). The term *transtentorial herniation* typically applies to descending herniation because it is more common, caused by a supratentorial mass displacing the medial temporal lobe through the tentorial incisura. It may be anterior (involving the uncus), posterior (involving the parahippocampal or lingual gyri), or complete. On CT or MR, the herniated uncus and/or parahippocampal gyrus produce widening of the ipsilateral subarachnoid cistern and obliteration of the contralateral subarachnoid cistern as the brainstem is displaced to the opposite side (Fig. 8-29).[40,82] Associated findings include downward pineal displacement and dilation of the ipsilateral temporal horn (trapping). Occipital lobe infarction (ipsilateral or contralateral) may also occur if the posterior cerebral artery is compressed between the temporal lobe and the crus cerebri.[120] Compression of the sylvian aqueduct may produce acute hydrocephalus.

Ascending transtentorial herniation is caused by an infratentorial mass that pushes the pons, vermis, and adjacent portions of the cerebellar hemispheres upward, through the incisura. On CT or MR, the subarachnoid cisterns are effaced symmetrically as the cerebellar vermis bulges up through the incisura.[51] The upper pons is pushed forward, against the clivus, and there is often acute hydrocephalus caused by compression of the sylvian aqueduct.

After sutural closure, there is only one large exit from the skull—the foramen magnum. A mass of sufficient size tends to extrude the cranial contents, typically the cerebellar tonsils, through the foramen magnum. Tonsillar herniation results in compression of the medulla, producing dysfunction of the vital control centers of respiration and cardiac rhythm.[75] This form of herniation is most commonly caused by hydrocephalus, an infratentorial mass, or a midline supratentorial mass. MR, with its sagittal imaging capabilities, is the primary imaging modality for demonstrating the presence of tonsillar herniation and secondary effects on the brainstem (Fig. 8-30). On CT, although partially obscured by bone artifact, the cerebellar tonsils can,

occasionally, be seen below the level of the foramen magnum.

Hydrocephalus

Hydrocephalus, increased intraventricular pressure causing adjacent brain compression, may be of two types: obstructive and nonobstructive.[54] Obstructive hydrocephalus results from obstruction to CSF flow and, depending on the site of obstruction, can be subdivided into communicating (CH) and noncommunicating (NCH). Communicating, obstructive (extraventricular) hydrocephalus results from obstruction to CSF absorption by arachnoid villi. CT and MR show symmetric enlargement of the lateral, third, and fourth ventricles with effacement of cerebral sulci. Under elevated pressure, CSF may leak from the ventricles into the brain (interstitial edema). On CT this is demonstrated by symmetric, indistinct low density in the periventricular regions that masks the normal ventricular wall and gradually fades into the surrounding white matter. On MR, this appears as low intensity on T_1-weighted images and high intensity on T_2-weighted images. Most often, communicating hydrocephalus results from remote inflammatory disease or traumatic subarachnoid hemorrhage. These processes, because they are remote, may not be identified on CT and/or MR. Occasionally, however, the etiology of communicating hydrocephalus is evident on CT or MR. Chronic subdural hematoma, venous thrombosis, or deformity of the skull vault, as seen with Hurler's syndrome or achondroplasia, can be detected on either imaging modality. Meningeal carcinomatosis and meningitis may be seen as diffuse nodular meningeal enhancement on postcontrast CT or MR.[23,110]

Noncommunicating, obstructive (intraventricular) hydrocephalus is secondary to obstruction along the CSF pathway, between the lateral ventricles and the fourth ventricular outlets. The CT and MR appearance is identical to that of communicating hydrocephalus with the exception that, in NCH, not all ventricles are enlarged. The ventricles dilate proximal, but not distal, to the obstruction (Fig. 8-30). For example, in aqueduct obstruction, the fourth ventricle remains normal as the third and lateral ventricles enlarge. The etiology of NCH often can be identified by CT or MR. MR is the preferred modality for evaluation of NCH for two reasons:

1. MR can provide coronal and sagittal images, invaluable in demonstrating obstruction at the foramen of Monro, the aqueduct, or the level of the fourth ventricle (see Fig. 8-30).[5,103] Tumors are readily seen, and webs or atresia of the aqueduct occasionally can be identified.
2. Newer techniques with CSF flow phenomena are helpful in classifying types of obstruction.[38,90,103]

Nonobstructive hydrocephalus results from excessive CSF production. Choroid plexus papillomas or benign tumors of the glomus of the lateral ventricle are common etiologies. CT and MR findings are identical to CH and NCH,

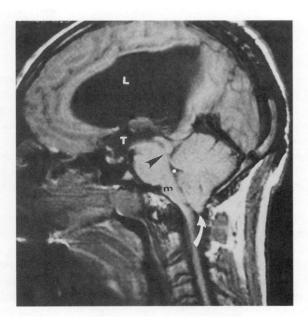

FIG. 8-30   Hydrocephalus and tonsillar herniation. Sagittal T_1-weighted image of a patient with hydrocephalus. The third (T) and lateral (L) ventricles, including the temporal horns, are dilated, but the fourth ventricle is normal in size (dot). The upper portion of the aqueduct of Sylvius is dilated, placing the level of obstruction in the lower portion of the aqueduct (arrowhead). The cerebellar tonsils (curved arrow) are displaced inferiorly through the foramen magnum, compressing the medulla (m).

and the responsible lesion can frequently be identified with either modality.

Specific Intracranial Disease Processes
Vascular Lesions

Evaluation of vascular disease of the brain typically involves multiple modalities. This holds true for occlusive disease as well as for evaluation of structural abnormalities such as arteriovenous malformations (AVM) or aneurysms.

Vascular Occlusive Disease and Infarct. Radiographic evaluation of the extracranial or intracranial vasculature is usually performed because of an acute episode of ischemic symptomatology referable to the CNS. The etiology is most often due to atherosclerotic vascular disease (ASVD), but it may also be secondary to fibromuscular dysplasia (FMD), vascular dissection, or arteritis. Angiography, considered the gold standard for evaluation of vascular disease, demonstrates the presence, location, and extent of disease, and may indicate underlying etiology.

Atherosclerosis involves intimal proliferation of smooth muscle cells and fatty plaques in the intima that progress to fibrous plaques and, in turn, to more complicated atherosclerotic lesions with vascular occlusion. The most common sites of atherosclerotic disease are the origins of the internal carotid arteries (common carotid artery bifurcations) and the carotid siphons.[29,65] Angiographic findings include (1) ulceration and subintimal hemorrhage with associated arterial narrowing; (2) stenosis, which may appear smooth or as severe eccentric irregularity; and (3) complete occlusion (Fig. 8-31, *A*).[29] The "string" sign represents the most severe degree of stenosis (99%), with only a small wisp of contrast seen in the lumen (Fig. 8-31, *B*). This, however, is important to document because these plaques are still amenable to endarterectomy.

Fibromuscular dysplasia (FMD), a nonatheromatous angiopathy of unknown etiology involving the tunica media, most commonly occurs in young adult females. It predisposes to vascular dissections and premature atherosclerosis and should be considered in the differential diagnosis of CNS ischemia in young women. In addition, patients with FMD have an increased incidence of congenital berry aneurysms, an association that should be considered when a young female presents with subarachnoid hemorrhage.[104] Angiographically, the characteristic irregularly spaced, arterial dilations and constrictions ("string of beads") are virtually pathognomonic.[84]

Arterial dissections usually result from trauma, although

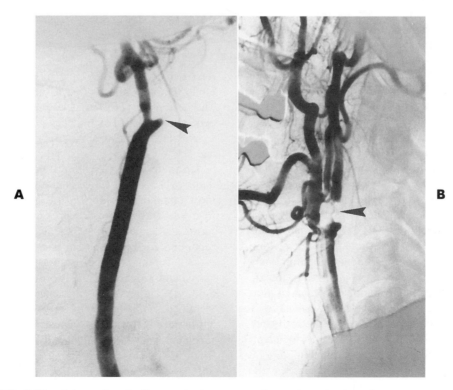

FIG. 8-31   Atherosclerotic disease. **A,** Anteroposterior neck projection of a common carotid angiogram demonstrates complete ICA occlusion, just distal to its origin *(arrowhead)*, without evidence of filling of the more distal ICA. **B,** Lateral neck projection of a common carotid angiogram demonstrating a "string" sign. High-grade stenosis *(arrowhead)* is present at the origin of the ICA although the distal ICA still fills in an antegrade fashion.

spontaneous forms and forms associated with underlying pathology (FMD, ASVD) also occur. Typically, the traumatic form is secondary to blunt, nonpenetrating neck trauma but may also be associated with rapid head turning or chiropractic manipulation.[33,39,66,74] Angiographically, an intimal tear appears as a thin, linear lucency within the opacified artery. Often there is complete occlusion of the artery at the level of dissection.[79]

Intracranial arteritis has a myriad of etiologies, all leading to progressive narrowing of one or more vessels. The vasculitis associated with the use of cocaine and methamphetamines is becoming particularly common.[116] Angiographic findings include narrowing of variable lengths of one or more vessels, progressing to complete occlusion.

An important use of angiography in the evaluation of vascular occlusive disease involves identification of collateral circulation, which plays a significant role in blood supply to ischemic areas.[29] In general, there are three collateral pathways:

1. Extracranial to intracranial, whereby branches of the external carotid artery (ECA) supply blood flow to the internal carotid artery (ICA) (e.g., internal maxillary artery to ophthalmic artery to supraclinoid ICA).
2. Transdural anastomoses, whereby meningeal branches provide flow to ICA branches (e.g., middle meningeal artery to middle cerebral artery branches).
3. Intracranial to intracranial anastomoses involving communications around the circle of Willis and parenchymal leptomeningeal anastomoses.

Although acute CNS ischemia is a clinical diagnosis, CT is the imaging modality of choice in evaluating patients with symptoms of transient ischemic attack (TIA), reversible ischemic neurologic deficit (RIND), or completed stroke.[29] Performed primarily to exclude hemorrhage before anticoagulation, CT scan also demonstrates the presence, extent, and location of the infarct. In addition, lesions that mimic stroke may also be excluded (i.e., tumor). The CT appearance depends on the age of the infarct. In the acute stage, there is vague decreased density in the territory of the occluded vessel with effacement of sulci caused by early mass effect from cytotoxic edema (Fig. 8-32). High density areas (thrombus or embolus) may occasionally be seen within the vessel lumen.[114] Within 24 to 48 hours the infarct may become very hypodense because of massive cytotoxic edema, associated with brain herniation and marked ventricular compression. The subacute stage may persist for 1 to 2 weeks, during which time the infarct gradually becomes less dense with more distinct margins and slight contrast enhancement, reflecting breakdown of the blood-brain barrier. In later stages, the density further decreases, the edema and contrast enhancement resolve, and the infarct behaves as a contracting, rather than an expanding, mass.

MR does not offer significant advantages over CT in evaluating acute ischemic disease.[14,57] However, because of its sensitivity, MR is valuable in identifying hyperacute

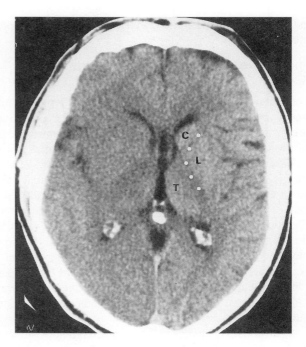

FIG. 8-32 Acute infarction. Axial non-contrast-enhanced head CT demonstrates subtle acute infarction in the right middle cerebral artery distribution. The left caudate (c) and lentiform (L) nuclei, thalamus (T), and internal capsule (dots) are all well seen. These structures are all obscured on the right because of early cytotoxic edema. Also note that the sulci and gyri, well seen on the left, are obliterated on the right.

(less than 8 hours old) infarcts[13-15,37,127] and lacunar infarcts (2 to 15 mm), often associated with hypertension. The lesions usually involve regions supplied by small penetrating arteries and appear as areas of low intensity on T_1-weighted images and high intensity on T_2-weighted images.

Congenital Aneurysm. Four kinds of aneurysms involve the CNS: Congenital (berry) aneurysms are the most common, making up 90% of all aneurysms, with fusiform/atherosclerotic, septic/mycotic, and neoplastic forms making up the remaining 10%.[29] Evaluation of a ruptured cerebral aneurysm is an emergent condition and usually begins with non-contrast-enhanced CT that typically demonstrates subarachnoid hemorrhage (SAH) (Fig. 8-33, A). Unless large, the aneurysm itself is usually not identified.[29] Contrast-enhanced CT may demonstrate the aneurysm[125]; however, the use of contrast-enhanced CT precludes immediate angiography because of contrast dose limitations. This is an important consideration if early aneurysm surgery is contemplated. Complications associated with SAH include infarction secondary to vasospasm, hydrocephalus, and rebleeding from an unclipped aneurysm. MR is not indicated for evaluation of patients with acute subarachnoid hemorrhage. However, because of flow artifact produced by a pulsating aneurysm, MR may

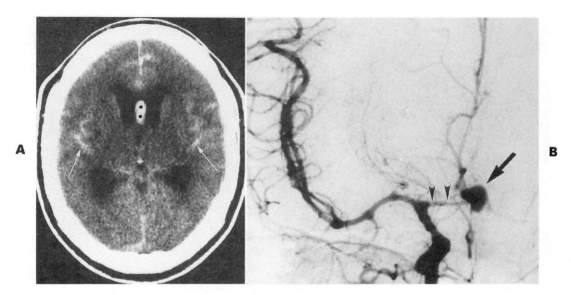

FIG. 8-33 Ruptured congenital aneurysm. **A,** Axial non-contrast-enhanced head CT demonstrates high-density subarachnoid blood, symmetrically replacing the normal low-density CSF in the sulci and sylvian fissures bilaterally *(arrows)*. Blood has also dissected into the septum pellucidum *(black dots)*. This distribution of hemorrhage is typical of a ruptured anterior communicating artery aneurysm. **B,** Anteroposterior angiogram of the head. A large, congenital anterior communicating artery aneurysm *(arrow)* is identified, associated with significant vasospasm *(arrowheads)*.

demonstrate a berry aneurysm noninvasively when CT is in question[1] and is extremely useful for evaluation of giant and fusiform aneurysms. MR angiography may prove extremely useful for screening patients at high risk for berry aneurysms, but its utility in the acute setting currently is not established. An angiogram is the second study obtained when SAH is demonstrated on CT. The goals of angiography are not only to identify the aneurysm but also to identify additional aneurysms, to determine which aneurysm ruptured when multiple aneurysms are present, and to assess the presence or absence of associated vasospasm (Fig. 8-33, *B*).

Vascular Malformations. Approximately 10% of patients presenting with SAH or an intracerebral hematoma have a vascular malformation.[29] Vascular malformations are the most common cause of nontraumatic SAH in patients under the age of 40. Four types of vascular malformations are described[29]:

1. Arterial venous malformations (AVM), the most common type, are composed of abnormal, enlarged arteries and veins that are not separated by normal capillary channels. The unruptured AVM may not be seen on non-contrast-enhanced CT or may appear as a subtle, hyperdense region (Fig. 8-34, *A*). After contrast administration, large, tortuous, high-density structures, representing the serpentine vessels, are

identified (Fig. 8-34, *B*), usually without associated mass effect or edema. On MR, these abnormal vessels are represented as areas of absent signal (flow voids) caused by rapid flow of blood through the normal vessels. Angiography is typically performed for evaluation of these lesions because it demonstrates the feeding arteries and draining veins, thereby indicating a pial, dural, or mixed origin (Fig. 8-34, *C*).[48] This information is important for treatment planning decisions. With rupture of an AVM, the imaging characteristics are those of hemorrhage, which was described previously.

2. Capillary telangiectasias, with normal interstitial neural tissue.
3. Cavernous angiomas, without normal intervening neural tissue. These last two groups of malformations are best evaluated by MR because angiography is usually normal and CT is insensitive. The MR signal characteristics are variable, because of the presence or absence of blood products.
4. Venous angiomas that are composed of dilated medullary veins leading to a single, dilated draining vein do not involve arteries. Non-contrast-enhanced CT is frequently normal, but, after contrast administration, the large transcortical vein can be identified. On MR, this vein is seen as a linear flow void. Angiography

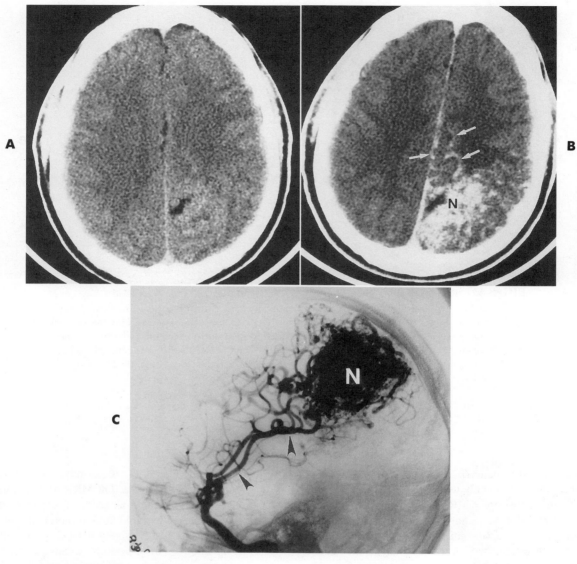

FIG. 8-34 Arteriovenous malformation. **A,** Non-contrast-enhanced axial CT scan of the head reveals a subtle area of hyperdensity in the left posterior parietal lobe. **B,** Contrast-enhanced CT scan reveals serpentine vessels *(arrows)* supplying the large nidus of an arteriovenous malformation *(N)*. **C,** Lateral projection of an internal carotid angiogram demonstrates enlarged middle cerebral artery feeding vessels *(arrowheads)* supplying the nidus *(N)*.

is not necessary for evaluation of venous angiomas because they have a classic appearance on contrast-enhanced CT or MR.[123]

Neoplasms

Many classification schemes have been proposed for tumors, the most popular being based on location or histology.[30] When one is imaging a neoplasm, the age and sex of the patient, clinical presentation, lesion location, and its imaging characteristics often suggest a specific diagnosis. With this in mind, neoplasms are typically grouped by radiologists according to location (Table 8-2).[30,122] The following discussion address-

es the imaging aspects of tumors in general.

On CT or MR, tumors may be seen as enhancing or non-enhancing masses, often surrounded by a rim of edema (see Fig. 8-26). Low-grade gliomas may appear as subtle non-enhancing masses, but higher-grade gliomas often demonstrate heterogenous enhancement with large areas of necrosis and associated edema.[97] Low-density/intensity metastatic lesions, most often secondary to lung or breast carcinomas, typically enhance. Associated calvarial metastases can easily be identified on CT studies when bone window levels are obtained. Epidermoid and dermoid tumors frequently contain areas of fat density and do not enhance. Tumors, such as pediatric cystic astrocytomas, may be

TABLE 8-2
Tumors Classifiable by Location

Location	Type of Tumor
Meninges/extracranial	Meningioma Meningeal carcinomatosis Leukemia/lymphoma Arachnoid cyst Lipoma Dermoid/epidermoid/teratoma
Supratentorial	Glioma Metastasis Primary lymphoma
Infratentorial	Astrocytoma Hemangioblastoma Medulloblastoma Ependymoma
Sella/juxtasellar	Adenoma Craniopharyngioma Meningioma Hypothalamic/chiasmatic glioma Dermoid/epidermoid/teratoma
Pineal	Germinoma Pineocytoma/pineoblastoma Glioma Dermoid/epidermoid/teratoma
Intraventricular	Choroid plexus papilloma Choroid plexus carcinoma Ependymoma Meningioma Epidermoid Colloid cyst
Cerebellopontine angle	Acoustic schwannoma Meningioma Epidermoid

composed of large CSF-density cysts.[3,50]

Some tumors demonstrate increased density on noncontrast CT, secondary to calcifications (meningioma, oligodendroglioma, craniopharyngioma), hemorrhage (hypernephroma or melanoma metastases), or the tumor cells themselves (lymphoma). These tumors frequently appear heterogenous because of associated cellular necrosis and cavity formation, in addition to calcification or hemorrhage.[3]

MR has high sensitivity but low specificity in evaluation of neoplasms, with most lesions appearing similar on MR studies; lesions have low intensity on T_1-weighted images and high intensity on T_2-weighted images. There are a few notable exceptions because the signal characteristics reflect lesion composition. For example, meningiomas, because of their homogenous cellular makeup, tend to be isointense on both T_1- and T_2-weighted images. Tumors that contain fat, such as epidermoid tumors, appear bright on T_1-weighted images and less bright on T_2-weighted images, reflecting their high fat content.[3]

The angiographic appearance of neoplasms depends on lesion vascularity.[30] Often only secondary signs (mass effect and shift) are apparent. Avascular, cystic, or hemorrhagic tumors appear as hypovascular regions ("hole in the brain"), which are especially obvious in the late arterial and capillary phases. Malignant tumor neovascularity is seen as a bizarre, irregular collection of vessels (puddling), producing an angiographic stain or blush. Early venous drainage may also be identified, secondary to arteriovenous shunting, but this is a nonspecific finding. Meningiomas have a pathognomonic appearance. Fed by ECA circulation (or dural branches of the ICA), they demonstrate a starburst pattern in the arterial phase, and a dense cloudlike blush persists very late, throughout the venous phase.

Trauma

Management decisions in acute head-injury patients must be made rapidly and depend on accurate evaluation of intracranial damage. Numerous studies have shown that plain skull radiographs and/or MR have little use in the evaluation of acute cranial trauma and CT remains the primary imaging modality.[89,113] For evaluation of chronic head injury, MR is the modality of choice because it is able to demonstrate small foci of old hemorrhage and gliosis with greater sensitivity than CT.[128] In addition, the presence and extent of white matter shear injury (diffuse axonal injury [DAI]) can best be appreciated with T_2-weighted MR sequences.

Parenchymal Lesions. Injury to brain parenchyma may result in contusion, shearing (DAI), or hematoma. Hematomas have been described previously. Contusions are caused by impact of parenchyma directly against bone and are most commonly seen in the frontal and temporal lobes. Shear injuries, secondary to rotational forces that produce tears in axonal fibers, involve white matter tracts (subcortical white matter, corpus callosum, internal capsule, and brainstem). Except for location, imaging characteristics of nonhemorrhagic contusions and shear injuries are similar. Initial studies may be normal or merely demonstrate small foci of edema. MR is more sensitive to small lesions, but, because the acute management of the patient is not typically altered by demonstration of these small foci, the long imaging times and difficulties encountered with MR imaging in the acute trauma setting preclude its use.

Extraaxial Lesions. Damage to the brain coverings may lead to hemorrhage into the intraventricular, subarachnoid, subdural, or epidural spaces. Hemorrhage into the ventricles is most easily identified as a high-density collection layering in the occipital horns of the lateral ventricles (Fig. 8-35). Traumatic subarachnoid hemorrhage, which may appear identical to that caused by a ruptured aneurysm, often occurs in association with other cerebral injuries. Subdural hematomas (SDH), secondary to rupture of bridging cortical veins, typically appear as crescentic, high-density collections between the dura and arachnoid, displacing the gray/white matter junction (Fig. 8-36). As SDH resolves, the density decreases and a fibrovascular membrane forms,

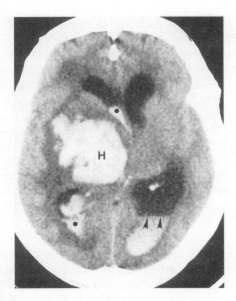

FIG. 8-35   Intraventricular hemorrhage. Axial non-contrast-enhanced CT scan demonstrates a large right basal ganglia hypertensive hemorrhage *(H)*, which has ruptured into the ventricular system. Intraventricular hemorrhage is seen layering in the occipital horn of the left lateral ventricle *(arrowheads)*. High-density hemorrhage also is identified in the frontal and occipital horns of the right lateral ventricle *(dots)*.

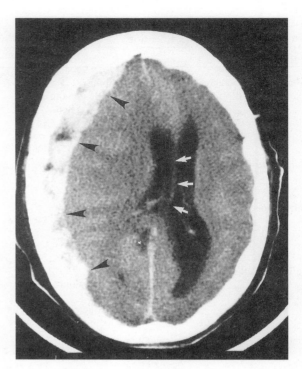

FIG. 8-36   Subdural hematoma. Non-contrast-enhanced axial CT scan demonstrates a crescentic collection of extraaxial blood *(arrowheads)*. This configuration is indicative of a subdural location. Deviation of the septum pellucidum to the left of midline *(arrows)* indicates subfalcine herniation.

separating the hematoma from brain parenchyma. The SDH becomes isodense after a few days and eventually appears as a hypodense collection with an enhancing underlying membrane at about 3 weeks of age. Epidural hematomas (EDH), secondary to laceration of meningeal arteries, are confined to the potential space between the dura and inner table of the skull (Fig. 8-37). They appear as biconvex, high-density mass lesions along the inner calvarial surface, also associated with displacement of the gray/white matter junction. Brain herniation is commonly associated with both subdural and epidural hematomas.

Calvarial Lesions.   Fractures, commonly detected on plain radiographs, are also demonstrated on CT but require wide windows. However, small linear fractures, parallel to the scan plane, can be missed on CT. The presence or absence of a fracture identified on plain radiographs does not offer any prognostic information regarding associated brain damage.[113] CT is, therefore, more useful in evaluating acute trauma patients than plain radiographs, both for detection of the fracture itself and for identification of associated brain injury or complications such as intraaxial or extraaxial hematoma, infection, CSF leak, pneumocephalus, and posttraumatic cephalocele. Depressed skull fractures are important to identify because they frequently require emergent surgical decompression.

Infection/Inflammation

Infectious and inflammatory processes may be considered according to their primary site of involvement, either pa-

renchymal or meningeal. Parenchymal infections include encephalitis, cerebritis, and abscess.

Encephalitis, diffuse inflammation of the brain, is often viral or toxic in etiology. Regardless of etiology, the imaging characteristics are similar. On CT, there are focal or multifocal areas of low density, typically involving the temporal lobes. Gyral contrast enhancement may be seen but is usually subtle. MR is more sensitive and demonstrates the lesions earlier than does CT, with the lesions appearing hypointense on T_1-weighted images and hyperintense on T_2-weighted images.

Cerebritis can be considered an early phase of abscess formation, requiring 10 to 14 days to undergo liquefactive necrosis and encapsulation. Non-contrast-enhanced CT demonstrates an irregular, poorly marginated area of low density in the white matter or basal ganglia, producing effacement of sulci and ventricles. On contrast-enhanced CT, enhancement is usually ill-defined and patchy in the early stages, becoming more ringlike in later stages. MR signal characteristics are nonspecific, usually hypointense on T_1-weighted images and hyperintense on T_2-weighted images. As with CT, contrast enhancement first is patchy, with gradual progression to a ring.

A cerebral abscess results from liquefactive necrosis in an area of untreated cerebritis, producing a localized collection of pus or caseous material in a cavity surrounded

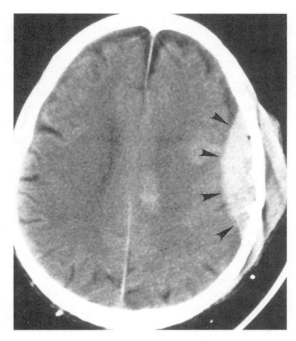

FIG. 8-37   Epidural hematoma. Non-contrast-enhanced axial CT scan demonstrates a biconvex extraaxial collection *(arrowheads)*. This configuration is indicative of an epidural location.

by a fibrous capsule. On CT scan, an abscess cavity demonstrates central hypodensity (necrotic cavity), a thin isodense ring (capsule), and a surrounding area of low density (edema). After contrast administration, there is enhancement of the capsule, which is typically smooth, well defined, and uniform in thickness, unlike the shaggy, irregular walls associated with tumors. MR findings are similar to those on CT. The capsule is isointense to hyperintense on T_1-weighted images and hypointense on T_2-weighted images. The central cavity has variable signal characteristics, depending on the contents, and surrounding edema is prominent although identical to any edematous process. Ring enhancement is also demonstrated on contrast-enhanced MR images.

Extraaxial infections include ventriculitis, meningitis, and subdural or epidural empyemas. Ventriculitis (ependymitis) is characterized by inflammation of the ependymal wall of a ventricle and usually results from rupture of an abscess into the ventricle. Intravenous contrast is necessary because the CT and MR findings consist only of enhancement of the wall of the involved ventricle(s).

Meningitis, affecting the dura mater (pachymeningitis) or piaarachnoid (leptomeningitis), is often the result of hematogenous dissemination from a distant source but may also result from direct extension of sinus or middle ear disease. The diagnosis is made clinically on the basis of physical examination and CSF analysis. Imaging is mainly performed to exclude associated abscess or empyema and to evaluate for complications (hydrocephalus, subdural effusion, vascular thrombosis, infarction). CT and MR may be normal or demonstrate diffuse enhancement of the meningeal surfaces after contrast administration.

Subdural and epidural empyemas are collections of pus in the subdural and epidural spaces, respectively, that most often occur as complications of sinusitis, otitis, surgery, or trauma. On CT, the collections frequently have a slightly higher density than CSF but a lower density than that of acute blood. In time, membrane formation occurs, similar to that associated with resolving traumatic extraaxial collections. On MR, the collections are typically hypointense to brain on T_1-weighted images and hyperintense on T_2-weighted images. Membrane enhancement is common.

CNS Manifestations of AIDS

CNS involvement is the presenting complaint in approximately 10% of AIDS patients. More than 33% eventually develop neurologic complications, with CNS involvement seen in more than 75% of cases at autopsy.[111] Most pathogens are opportunistic (*Toxoplasma gondii*, cytomegalovirus [CMV], herpes simplex type 1) or fungal (*mucormycoses, Aspergillus, Cryptococcus, Coccidioides*) infections. In addition, primary involvement by the HIV virus, producing HIV leukoencephalopathy, or by human papovavirus, producing progressive multifocal leukoencephalopathy (PML), can be seen. CNS lymphoma, primary or secondary, represents the most common tumor in AIDS. Although the imaging features of non-HIV lymphomas are characteristic, lymphomas seen in HIV patients have a variable, nonspecific appearance, making it difficult to differentiate tumor from infection. *Cryptococcus* and CMV most commonly produce a picture of meningitis. Lymphoma, toxoplasmosis, and other fungal diseases present as abscess cavities with mass effect. The viral agents produce variable patterns of white matter involvement.[4,91,111]

White-Matter Disease

White-matter diseases are classified as dysmyelinating (improper formation or maintenance of myelin) or demyelinating (normal myelin is destroyed by endogenous or exogenous agents). Dysmyelinating disorders include the leukodystrophies and storage diseases. Demyelinating disorders can be idiopathic (multiple sclerosis), postinfectious (PML), postirradiative, toxic-degenerative, or vascular.

MR imaging is much more sensitive than CT and, although nonspecific, is the study of choice for evaluation of white-matter disease. On T_1-weighted MR, these lesions appear as vague regions of low intensity. Multiecho T_2-weighted MR is the most sensitive sequence for evaluating white-matter disease. Lesions are hyperintense compared with CSF on the first echo sequence (long TR, short TE), and isointense to CSF on the second echo sequence (long TR, long TE).[24,62] Occasionally, a single white-matter lesion may be of such size that it mimics a neoplastic lesion (i.e., giant multiple sclerosis plaque). However, there may be a distinct lack of both edema and mass effect associated with even large areas of demyelination, as opposed to the edema and mass affect so commonly accompanying tumors.

S U M M A R Y

In acute spinal trauma, plain radiographs are the first studies obtained. Fractures, subluxation, and degree of stability can be rapidly confirmed on a properly performed plain film series. In general, the mechanism of damage and the treatment plan can also be inferred from the films; these are based on the type of fracture present. When questions arise concerning osseous integrity or relationships or there is difficulty in obtaining the necessary views, thin-section CT, with its reconstruction ability, is a useful secondary procedure. In the acute setting of spinal cord injury, especially with incomplete paresis, MR can readily demonstrate intrinsic cord damage or surgically amenable lesions that impinge on the cord. However, care is necessary during this procedure because of the difficulties encountered with monitors and life support systems.

In the evaluation of nontraumatic spinal pathology, MR has increasingly become the imaging modality of choice. MR can frequently place the lesion into one of the three canal spaces and can offer a reasonable differential as to the type of lesion. CT myelography, although slightly invasive, is an adequate back-up examination for patients unable to undergo MR studies. It is also particularly useful for evaluation of osseous pathology, such as degenerative disk disease and spondylosis.

When considering intracranial pathology, CT and MR are the primary imaging modalities. In the acute setting, such as traumatic brain injury or acute stroke, CT is preferred because of its ease of use, speed, and degree of accuracy. In the nonacute setting, MR is more useful because of its higher sensitivity than CT and its multiplanar capabilities. Regardless of which modality is used, evaluation of pathology should always begin with a knowledge of disease patterns and their appearance on imaging studies. Edema patterns, hemorrhage, mass effect, calcification, and enhancement characteristics may offer clues to the type of pathology present.

The radiologic armamentarium available for investigation of pathology in patients with neurologic dysfunction is extensive. A basic understanding of these radiologic modalities is essential not only for proper interpretation of radiologic images but for proper selection of the modality that will give the most useful information. How an image is generated with each modality, what the images demonstrate, and the correlation between the image and a lesion's imaging characteristics are prerequisites to proper modality choice and image interpretation.

References

1. Alvarez O, Hyman RA: Even echo MR rephasing in the diagnosis of giant intracranial aneurysms, *J Comput Assist Tomogr* 10:699-701, 1986.

2. Anderson LD, D'Alonzo RT: Fractures of the odontoid process of the axis, *J Bone Joint Surg* 56(A):1663-1674, 1974.

3. Atlas SW: Adult supratentorial tumors, *Semin Roentgenol* 25:130-154, 1990.

4. Balakrishnan J, Becker PS, Kumar AJ et al: Acquired immunodeficiency syndrome: correlation of radiologic and pathologic findings in the brain, *Radiographics* 10:201-215, 1990.

5. Barkovich AJ, Newton TH: MR of aqueductal stenosis: evidence of a broad spectrum of tectal distortion, *AJNR* 10:471-476, 1989.

6. Beatson TR: Fractures and dislocations of the cervical spine, *J Bone Joint Surg* 45(B):21-35, 1963.

7. Berquist TH: Imaging of adult cervical spine trauma. *RadioGraphics* 8:667-694, 1988.

8. Bools JC, Rose BS: Traumatic atlantooccipital dislocation: two cases with survival, *AJNR* 7:901-904, 1986.

9. Bradley WG Jr: Pathophysiologic correlates of signal alterations. In Brant-Zawadzki M, Norman D, editors: *Magnetic resonance imaging of the central nervous system,* New York, 1987, Raven Press, pp 23-43.

10. Brant-Zawadzki M: Magnetic resonance imaging principles: the bare necessities. In Brant-Zawadzki M, Norman D, editors: *Magnetic resonance imaging of the central nervous system,* New York 1987, Raven Press, pp 1-12.

11. Brashear HR, Venters GC, Preston ET: Fractures of the neural arch of the axis, *J Bone Joint Surg* 57A:879-887, 1975.

12. Breger RK, Williams AL, Daniels DL et al: Contrast enhancement in spinal MR imaging, *AJNR* 10:633-643, 1989.

13. Brown JJ, Hesselink R, Rothrock JF: MR and CT of lacunar infarcts, *AJNR* 9:477-482, 1988.

14. Bryan RN, Levy LM, Whitlow WD et al: Diagnosis of acute cerebral infarction: comparison of CT and MR imaging, *AJNR* 12:611-620, 1991.

15. Bryan RN: Imaging of acute stroke, *Radiology* 177:615-616, 1990.

16. Cheshire DJE: The stability of the cervical spine following the conservative treatment of fractures and fracture dislocations, *Paraplegia* 7:193-203, 1969.

17. Cintron E, Gilula LA, Murphy WA et al: The widened disc space: a sign of cervical hyperextension injury, *Radiology* 141:639-644, 1981.

18. Clark RA, Watanabe AT, Bradley WG et al: Acute hematomas: effects of deoxygenation, hematocrit, and fibrin-clot formation and retraction on T_2 shortening, *Radiology* 175:201-206, 1990.

19. Cohan RH, Dunnich NR: Progress in radiology. Intravascular contrast media: adverse reactions, *Am J Roentgenol* 149:655-670, 1987.

20. Collalto PM, DeMuth WW, Schwenker EP et al: Traumatic atlantooccipital dislocation. Case report, *J Bone Joint Surg* 68(A):1106-1109, 1986.

21. Cornish BL: Traumatic spondylolisthesis of the axis, *J Bone Joint Surg* 50(A):31-43, 1968.
22. Curry III TS, Dowdey JE, Murry Jr RC: *Christensen's physics of diagnostic radiology,* ed 4, Philadelphia, 1990, Lea & Febiger, pp 320-350, 470-504.
23. Davis PC, Friedman NC, Fry SM et al: Leptomeningeal metastases: MR imaging, *Radiology* 163:449-454, 1987.
24. Demaerel P, Faubert C, Wilms G et al: MR findings in leukodystrophy, *Neuroradiology* 33:368-373, 1991.
25. DeOliveira E, Rhoton Al, Peace D: Microsurgical anatomy of the region of the foramen magnum, *Surg Neurol* 24:293-352, 1985.
26. Dolan KD: Cervical spine injuries below the axis, *Radiol Clin North Am* 15:247-259, 1977.
27. Dolan KD: Cervicobasilar relationships, *Radiol Clin North Am* 15:247-259, 1977.
28. Dolan KD: Expanding lesions of the cervical spinal canal, *Radiol Clin North Am* 15:203-214, 1977.
29. Drayer BP: Diseases of the cerebral vascular system. In Rosenberg RN, editor: *The clinical neurosciences: neuroradiology,* New York, 1984, Churchill-Livingstone, pp 247-360.
30. Dubois PJ: Brain tumors. In Rosenberg RN, editor: *The clinical neurosciences: neuroradiology,* New York 1984, Churchill-Livingstone, pp 361-455.
31. Dussault RG, Effendi B, Nuy D et al: Locked facets with fracture of the neural arch of the axis, *Spine* 8:365-367, 1983.
32. Earnest IV F, Forbes G, Sandok BA et al: Complications of cerebral angiography: prospective assessment of risk, *Am J Roentgenol* 142:247-253, 1984.
33. Easton JD, Sherman DG: Cervical manipulation and stroke, *Stroke* 8:594-597, 1977.
34. Edeiken-Monroe B, Wagner LK, Harris JH: Hyperextension dislocation of the cervical spine, *AJNR* 7:135-140, 1986.
35. Effendi B, Ruy D, Cornish B et al: Fractures of the ring of the axis: a classification based on analysis of 131 cases, *J Bone Joint Surg* 63(B):319-327, 1981.
36. Elliott JM, Rogers LF, Wissinger JP et al: The hangman's fracture, *Radiology* 104:303-307, 1972.
37. Elster AD, Moody DM: Early cerebral infarction: gadopentate dimeglumine enhancement, *Radiology* 177:627-632, 1990.
38. Enzmann DR, Pelc NJ: Normal patterns of intracranial and spinal cerebrospinal fluid defined with phase-contrast cine MR imaging, *Radiology* 178:467-474, 1991.
39. Fast A, Zincola DF, Marin EL: Vertebral artery damage complicating cervical manipulation, *Spine* 12:840-842, 1987.
40. Feldman E, Gandy SE, Becker R et al: MRI demonstrates descending transtentorial herniation, *Radiology* 170:588, 1989.
41. Fishman RA: Brain edema, *N Engl J Med* 293:706-711, 1975.
42. Floras P, Deliac PH, Gross C et al: Neurotoxicity of Iohexol vs. Iopamidol in lumbar myelography: clinical, electrophysiological and brain CT scan correlations, *J Neuroradiol* 17:190-200, 1990.
43. Forsyth HF: Extension injuries of the cervical spine, *J Bone Joint Surg* 46(A):1792-1797, 1964.
44. Gerlock AJ, Mirfakhraec M, Benzel EC: Computed tomography of traumatic atlantooccipital dislocation, *Neurosurgery* 13:316-319, 1983.
45. Gomori JM, Grossman RI: Mechanisms responsible for the MR appearance and evolution of intracranial hemorrhage, *RadioGraphics* 8:427-440, 1988.
46. Gomori JM, Grossman RI, Goldberg HI et al: Intracranial hematomas: imaging by high-field MR, *Radiology* 157:87-93, 1985.
47. Gomori JM, Grossman RI, Hackney DB et al: Variable appearances of subacute intracranial hematomas on high-field spin-echo MR, *Am J Roentgenol* 150:171-178, 1988.
48. Graves VB, Duff TA: Intracranial arteriovenous malformations: current imaging and treatment, *Invest Radiol* 25:952-960, 1990.
49. Green JD, Harle TS, Harris JH: Anterior subluxation of the cervical spine: hyperflexion sprain, *AJNR* 2:243-250, 1981.
50. Gusnard DA: Cerebellar neoplasms in children, *Semin Roentgenol* 25:263-278, 1990.
51. Hahn FJ, Witte RJ: CT signs of ascending transtentorial cerebellar herniation, *J Comput Assist Tomogr* 13:1091, 1989.
52. Hankey GJ, Warlow CP, Sellar RJ: Cerebral angiographic risk in mild cerebrovascular disease, *Stroke* 21:209-222, 1990.
53. Harris JH, Edeiken-Monroe B: *The radiology of acute cervical spine trauma,* ed 2, Baltimore, 1987, Williams & Wilkins.
54. Haughton VM: Hydrocephalus and atrophy. In Williams AL, Haughton VM editors: *Cranial computed tomography: a comprehensive text,* St Louis, 1985, CV Mosby, pp 240-256.
55. Heinz ER: Techniques in imaging of the brain: computerized tomography. In Rosenberg RN, editor: *The clinical neurosciences: neuroradiology,* New York, 1984, Churchill-Livingstone, pp 51-93.
56. Hinck VC, Hopkins CE: Measurement of the atlanto-dental interval in the adult, *Am J Roentgenol* 84:945-951, 1960.
57. Imakita S, Nishimura T, Yamado N et al: Magnetic resonance imaging of cerebral infarction: time course of Gd-DTPA enhancement and CT comparison, *Neuroradiology* 30:372-378, 1988.
58. Junck L, Marshall WH: Neurotoxicity of radiological contrast agents, *Ann Neurol* 13:469-484, 1983.
59. Kanal E, Shellock FG, Talagela L: State of the art: safety considerations in MR imaging, *Radiology* 176:593-606, 1990.
60. Kattan KR: Backward "displacement" of the spinolaminal line at C2: a normal variation, *Am J Roentgenol* 129:289-290, 1977.
61. Kim KS, Chen HH, Russell EJ et al: Flexion teardrop fracture of the cervical spine: radiographic characteristics, *Am J Roentgenol* 152:319-326, 1989.
62. Kirkpatrick JB, Hayman LA: White matter lesions in MR imaging of clinical healthy brains of elderly subjects: possible pathologic basis, *Radiology* 162:509-511, 1987.
63. Klatzo I: Neuropathological aspects of brain edema, *J Neuropathol Exp Neurol* 26:1-14, 1967.
64. Kowalski HM, Cohen WA, Cooper P et al: Pitfalls in the CT diagnosis of atlantoaxial rotary subluxation, *AJNR* 8:697-702, 1987.
65. Kricheff II: State of the art: arteriosclerotic ischemic cerebrovascular disease, *Radiology* 162:101-109, 1987.

66. Krueger BR, Okazaki H: Vertebral-basilar distribution infarction following chiropractic cervical manipulation, *Mayo Clin Proc* 55:322-332, 1980.

67. Landells CD, VanPeteghem PK: Fractures of the atlas: classification, treatment and morbidity, *Spine* 13:450-452, 1988.

68. Lee C, Woodring JH, Goldstein SJ et al: Evaluation of traumatic atlantooccipital dislocations, *AJNR* 8:19-26, 1987.

69. Levine AM, Edwards CC: The management of traumatic spondylolisthesis of the axis, *J Bone Joint Surg* 67(A):217-226, 1985.

70. Litt AW, Eidelman EM, Pinto RS et al: Diagnosis of carotid artery stenosis: comparison of 2 DFT time-of-flight MR angiography with contrast angiography in 50 patients, *AJNR* 12:149-154, 1991.

71. Locke GR, Gardner JE, Van Epps EF: Atlas-dens interval (ADI) in children, *AJR* 97:135-140, 1966.

72. Manz HJ: The pathology of cerebral edema, *Human Pathol* 5:291-313, 1974.

73. Marchal G, Bosman H, Van Fraeyenhaven L et al: Intracranial vascular lesions: optimization and clinical evaluation of three-dimensional time-of-flight MR angiography, *Radiology* 175:443-448, 1990.

74. Mas JL, Bousser M-G, Hasboun D et al: Extracranial vertebral artery dissections: a review of 13 cases, *Stroke* 18:1037-1047, 1987.

75. McComb JG, Davis RL: Choroid plexus, cerebrospinal fluid, hydrocephalus, cerebral edema and herniation phenomena. In Davis RL, Robertson DM, editors: *Textbook of neuropathology,* Baltimore, 1985, Williams & Wilkins, pp 147-175.

76. Messina AV, Chernick NL: Computed tomography: the "resolving" intracerebral hemorrhage, *Radiology* 118:609-613, 1975.

77. Mirvis SE, Burg U, Belzberg H: MR imaging of ventilator-dependent patients: preliminary experience, *AJR* 179:845-846, 1987.

78. Mirvus SE, Young JMR, Lim C et al: Hangman's fracture: radiologic assessment in 27 cases, *Radiology* 163:713-717, 1987.

79. Mokri B, Piepgas DG, Houser OW: Traumatic and spontaneous extracranial internal carotid artery dissec-

tions, *J Neurosurg* 68:189-197, 1988.

80. Montane I, Eismont FJ, Green BA: Traumatic occipital-atlantal dislocation, *Spine* 16:112-116, 1991.

81. Naidich JB, Naidich TP, Gorfein C et al: The widened interspinous distance: a useful sign of anterior cervical dislocation in the supine frontal projection, *Radiology* 123:113-116, 1977.

82. Nguyen JP, Djindjian M, Brugieres P et al: Anatomy-computerized tomography correlations in transtentorial brain herniation, *J Neuroradiol* 16:181, 1989.

83. Nussel F, Wegmuller H, Huber P: Comparison of magnetic resonance angiography, magnetic resonance imaging and conventional angiography in cerebral arteriovenous malformation, *Neuroradiology* 33:56-61, 1991.

84. Osborn AG, Anderson RE: Angiographic spectrum of cervical and intracranial fibromuscular dysplasia, *Stroke* 8:617-626, 1977.

85. Papadopoulos SM, Dickman CA, Sonntag VKH et al: Traumatic altanooccipital dislocation with survival, *Neurosurgery* 28:574-579, 1991.

86. Pelker RR, Dorfman GS: Fracture of the axis associated with vertebral artery injury, *Spine* 11:621-623, 1986.

87. Perrett LV, Margolis MT: Brain herniations: angiography. In Newton TH, Potts DG, editors: *Radiology of the skull and brain,* vol 2, St Louis, 1974, CV Mosby, pp. 2671-2699.

88. Powers B, Miller MO, Kramer RS et al: Traumatic anterior atlanto-occipital dislocation, *Neurosurgery* 4:12-17, 1979.

89. Quencer RM: Neuroimaging and head injuries: where we've been—where we're going, *Am J Roentgenol* 150:13-18, 1988.

90. Quencer RM, Post MJD, Hinks RS: CINE MR in the evaluation of normal and abnormal CSF flow: intracranial and intraspinal studies, *Neuroradiology* 32:371-391, 1990.

91. Ramsey RG, Geremia GK: CNS complications of AIDS: CT and MR findings, *AJR* 151:449-454, 1988.

92. Roda JM, Castro A, Blazquez MG: Hangman's fracture with complete dislocation of C2 on C3, *J Neurosurg* 60:633-635, 1984.

93. Russell EJ, Schaible TF, Dillon W et al: Multicenter double-blind placebo-

controlled study of gadopentate dimeglumine as MR contrast agent: evaluation in patients with cerebral lesions, *AJNR* 10:53-63, 1989.

94. Schatzker J, Rorabeck CH, Waddell JP: Fractures of the dens (odontoid process): an analysis of 37 cases, *J Bone Joint Surg* 53(B):392-405, 1971.

95. Scher AT: Anterior cervical subluxation: an unstable position, *AJR* 133:275-280, 1979.

96. Scher AT: Unilateral locked facet in cervical spine injuries, *AJR* 129:45-48, 1977.

97. Schneider RC, Kahn EA: Chronic neurological trauma to the spine and spinal cord. Part 1. The significance of the acute flexion or "teardrop" fracture dislocation of the cervical spine, *J Bone Joint Surg* 38(A):985-997, 1956.

98. Schneider RC, Livingstone KE, Cave AJE et al: "Hangman's" fracture of the cervical spine, *J Neurosurg* 22:141-154, 1965.

99. Seljeskog EL, Chou SN: Spectrum of the hangman's fracture, *J Neurosurg* 45:3-8, 1976.

100. Sevick RJ, Tsuruda JS, Schmalbrock P: Three-dimensional time-of-flight MR angiography in the evaluation of cerebral aneurysms, *J Comput Assist Tomogr* 14:874-881, 1990.

101. Shellock FG, Curtis JS: MR imaging and biomedical implants, materials, and devices: an updated review, *Radiology* 180:541-550, 1991.

102. Shellock FG, Myers SM, Kimble KJ: Monitoring heart rate and oxygen saturation with a fiber-optic pulse oximeter during MR imaging, *AJR* 158:663-664, 1992.

103. Sherman JL, Citrin CM, Bowen BJ et al: MR demonstration of altered cerebrospinal fluid flow by obstructing lesions, *AJNR* 7:571-579, 1986.

104. Smoker WRK: The neuroradiology of aneurysmal subarachnoid hemorrhage, *Semin Neurol* 4:315-342, 1984.

105. Smoker WRK, Dolan KD: The "fat" C2: a sign of fracture, *AJR* 148:609-614, 1987.

106. Spence KF, Decker S, Sell KW: Bursting atlantal fracture associated with rupture of the transverse ligament, *J Bone Joint Surg* 52(A):543-549, 1970.

107. Stacul F, Carraro M, Magnaldi S et al: Contrast agent nephrotoxicity:

comparison of ionic and nonionic contrast agents, *AJR* 149:1287-1289, 1987.

108. Sze G, Abramson A, Krol G et al: Gadolinium-DTPA in the evaluation of intradural extramedullary spinal disease, *AJNR* 9:153-163, 1988.

109. Sze G, Krol G, Zimmerman RD et al: Intramedullary disease of the spine: diagnosis using gadolinium-DTPA-enhanced MR imaging, *AJNR* 9:847-858, 1988.

110. Sze G, Soletsky S, Brunen R et al: MR imaging of the cranial meninges with emphasis on contrast enhancement and meningeal carcinomatosis, *AJNR* 965-975, 1989.

111. Sze G, Brant-Zawadski MN, Norman D et al: The neuroradiology of AIDS, *Semin Roentgenol* 22:42-53, 1987.

112. Taber KH, Miglivre PJ, Pagnani JJ et al: Temporal changes in the oxidative state in vitro blood, *Invest Radiol* 25:240, 1990.

113. Thornburg JR, Campbell JA, Masters SJ et al: Skull fracture and the low risk of intracranial sequelae in minor head trauma, *AJR* 143:661-664, 1984.

114. Tomsick TA, Broh TG, Chambers AA et al: Hyperdense middle cerebral artery sign on CT, *AJNR* 11:473-477, 1990.

115. Traynelis VC, Marano GD, Dunker GO et al: Traumatic atlanto-occipital dislocation. Case report, *J Neurosurg* 65:863-870, 1986.

116. Wang A-M, Suojanen JN, Colucci VM et al: Cocaine- and methamphetamine-induced acute cerebral vasospasm, *AJNR* 11:1141-1146, 1990.

117. Weingarten K, Zimmerman RD, Cahill PT et al: Detection of acute intracerebral hemorrhage on MR imaging, *AJNR* 12:475-479, 1991.

118. Weingarten K, Zimmerman RD, Deo-Narine V et al: MR imaging of acute intracranial hemorrhage, *AJNR* 12:457-467, 1991.

119. Weinstein JN, McLain RF: Primary tumors of the spine, *Spine* 12:843-851, 1987.

120. Wernick S, Wells RG: Sequelae of temporal lobe herniation: MR imaging, *J Comput Assist Tomogr* 13:323, 1989.

121. Wholey MH, Brewer AJ, Baker HL: The lateral roentgenogram of the neck, *Radiology* 71:350-356, 1958.

122. Williams AL: Tumors. In Williams AL, Haughton VM, editors: *Cranial computed tomography: a comprehensive text,* St Louis, 1985, CV Mosby, pp 148-240.

123. Wilms G, Marchal G, Van Hecke D et al: Cerebral venous angiomas, *Neuroradiology* 32:81-85, 1990.

124. Woodring JH, Selke AC, Duff DE: Traumatic atlantooccipital dislocation with survival, *Am J Roentgenol* 137:21-24, 1981.

125. Yamamoto Y, Asari S, Sunami N et al: Computed tomography of the unruptured cerebral aneurysm, *J Comput Assist Tomogr* 10:21-27, 1987.

126. Young JWR, Nesnick CS, De Candido P et al: The laminar clear space in the diagnosis of rotational flexion injuries of the cervical spine, *AJR* 152:103-107, 1989.

127. Yuh WTC, Crain MR, Loes DJ et al: MR imaging of cerebral ischemia: findings in the first 24 hours. *AJR* 157:565-574, 1991.

128. Zimmerman RA, Bilaniuk LT, Hackney DB et al: Head injury: early results of comparing CT and high-field MR, *AJR* 147:1215-1222, 1986.

129. Zyed A, Hayman LA, Bryan RN: MR imaging of intracerebral blood: diversity in the temporal pattern of 1.5 and 1.0T, *AJNR* 12:469-474, 1991.

9

Neurophysiologic Brain Monitoring: Evoked Potentials

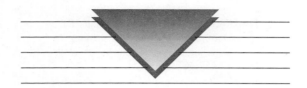

ROBERT W. MCPHERSON

MONITORING TECHNIQUES
SENSORY EVOKED POTENTIALS
   Visual evoked response (VER)
   Somatosensory evoked potentials

Brainstem auditory evoked response
   (BAER)
ELECTROMYOGRAPHY (EMG)

MOTOR EVOKED POTENTIALS
   (MEP)
   Effects of anesthetic drugs
SUMMARY

Intraoperative neurologic assessment is difficult because injury to small areas of the nervous system may result in permanent disability, other monitors are not available to confirm or refute changes in neurologic function, and equipment for neurologic monitoring is complex (computer based), expensive, and labor intensive. In addition to spontaneous electrical activity (electroencephalogram; EEG), the nervous system responds to stimuli applied to peripheral or cranial nerves with electrical activity (evoked responses) that is small compared to spontaneous activity but that can be readily identified by computer averaging techniques. Sensory evoked potentials (visual evoked response [VER], somatosensory evoked potentials [SSEP], brainstem auditory evoked response [BAER], and motor evoked potentials [MEP]) may be monitored in the operating room to assess function of parts of the nervous system.

Intraoperative evoked potential monitoring differs from nonoperative monitoring in several ways. First, monitoring is undertaken expectantly as indicated by the disease or operation rather than by symptoms. Second, the majority of patients have robust, easily obtainable waveforms. Third, comparisons are made using the patient as the control. For example, in the case of operations involving intracranial an-

eurysm clip application, preclipping waveforms can be compared with postclipping data rather than with "normative values." Fourth, anesthetics and neuromuscular blocking drugs can change waveforms compared with the waveforms in the unanesthetized state but do not prevent rapid waveform generation and analysis (at least for the sensory evoked potentials). Finally, decisions concerning waveform changes must be made rapidly to prevent permanent neurologic injury.

Transient changes in brain electrical activity that are reversed spontaneously or by therapeutic interventions create difficulty for interpreting what constitutes *true positives* and *true negatives* as well as *false positives* and *false negatives* for intraoperative monitoring. Change or lack of change in brain electrical activity that correlates with presence or absence of postoperative neurologic change is a *true positive* or a *true negative*. Transient changes in electrical activity (in response to intraoperative events) that are reversed by alteration of clinical technique (elevation of systemic blood pressure, removal of spinal distraction, or removal of a surgical retractor) are more difficult to evaluate. Strictly defined, transient changes are *false positives* because these intraoperative waveform changes are not associated with changes in postoperative neurologic function compared with preoperative function. Finally, there are *false negatives* (changes in neurologic function without changes in monitored electrical activity). For instance, postoperative neurologic changes after spinal surgery may occur without changes or with only modest changes in intraoperative SSEP waves.[18] Important in understanding *false negatives* is determining whether the neurologic monitor (SSEP, BAER, VER) should be affected by the process that alters neurologic function. Aggressive intraoperative monitoring does not guarantee prevention of neurologic injury because all parts of the brain are not assessed using currently available monitoring.

In developing a strategy for intraoperative neurophysiologic monitoring, the following guidelines are helpful:

1. VER monitors the function of the retina, optic chiasm, optic radiations, and occipital cortex.
2. SSEP assesses the sensory neural axis from peripheral nerve through brainstem to cortex.
3. BAER assesses only brainstem function (waves occurring <10 msec after stimuli) although long latency cortical waves (>20 msec after stimuli) can be assessed to evaluate cortical function.
4. MEP assesses function of the motor cortex and descending tracts. The peripheral response of the MEP is recorded by measuring the compound muscle action potential.

Monitoring Techniques

Electrical activity of the nervous system, both spontaneous and evoked, is measured using a reference electrode system that records voltage changes over time at an active electrode compared with a reference electrode (electrically quiet). The international 10-20 system of electrode placement normalizes electrode placement by controlling for variability in skull shape and size and is used for electrode placement for both EEG and evoked potential monitoring. Active electrodes are placed over the parietal cortex for median nerve SSEP, the vertex for posterior tibial SSEP, the vertex for BAER, the occiput for VER, and the hand or foot muscles for MEP. Successful monitoring requires a monitoring plan that does not exclude any possible sources of injury.

Injury may be due to factors other than direct surgical intervention. Hypotension in the presence of severe vasospasm may lead to decreased regional blood flow. Likewise an apparently adequate blood pressure may lead to decreased cerebral blood flow if the brain is being retracted (perfusion pressure equals arterial pressure minus retractor pressure). Surgical positioning may cause changes in brain electrical activity that suggest injury, but these changes can be rapidly reversed by changing position.[68]

Rapid localization of injury during SSEP monitoring is facilitated by monitoring responses over the spinal cord (second cervical vertebra) and peripheral nervous system (Erb's point, over the brachial plexus). Loss of scalp-recorded waves with retention of response over the spinal cord demonstrates an intracranial injury, whereas loss of peripheral and scalp response may be due to a peripheral injury (e.g., malposition with pressure on the brachial plexus or failure of peripheral stimulation caused by equipment failure or displacement of the stimulating electrode).

Sensory Evoked Potentials

Sensory evoked potentials occur in response to repetitive peripheral stimuli. These waves are small (1 to 2 μV) compared with the average EEG voltage (50 to 100 μV), and individual evoked responses are usually hidden in the spontaneous EEG. In addition, scalp-recorded evoked potentials are contaminated with large amounts of background noise from electroencephalogram, electrocardiogram, and electromyogram. In general, the technique of signal averaging is used to visualize these evoked potentials. Briefly stated, the averaging phenomenon reinforces electrical activity that occurs during the same interval and of the same polarity after a stimulation, whereas random electrical activity is eventually averaged to zero. The noise component diminishes during averaging in proportion to the square root of the number of stimuli, and the signal to noise ratio increases. For averaging of SSEP, a sampling rate of 1 kHz is required to prevent waveform deterioration caused by asynchronous averaging (variation in the start point of averaging).[73]

Waveforms are evaluated for *latency* (delay from stimulus to wave appearance) or *amplitude* (peak to trough voltage) of characteristic waves. These data are obtained by manually placing the cursor of the computer on the desired wave. Waveforms (SSEP and VER) are designated for polarity, negative (N) or positive (P), and nominal latency after stimulation. Generally, negative waves are shown upward in figures. This convention is followed in this chapter.

BAER waves occurring within 10 msec of stimulation are designated in order of appearance by consecutive Roman numerals (I to VII), whereas later waves are designated in a manner similar to SSEP and VER waves.

Brain electrical activity may be classified as *near field* or *far field*. *Near-field* waves are generated near the recording electrode (e.g., scalp-recorded SSEP waves), and *far-field* waves are recorded by electrodes distant from the neural generators. Brainstem auditory waves are generated in the brainstem but recorded over the vertex of the skull and are thus *far-field* waves.

Visual Evoked Response (VER)

Stimulation of the retina by light produces an evoked response of the occipital cortex, which is sensitive to changes in function of the visual apparatus caused by tumors. Thus VER might be useful as a monitor for detecting injury during surgery near the optic chiasm. For intraoperative mon-

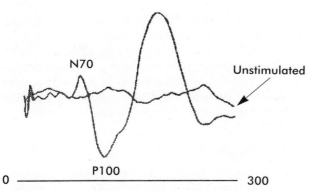

FIG. 9-1 Visual evoked response developed from stimulation using goggles containing light-emitting diodes. Negative waves are upward going in all figures. P100 is the wave usually used for intraoperative monitoring. The wave without major deflections is the result of averaging brain electrical activity in the absence of specific stimulation.

TABLE 9-1
Effects of Anesthetic Drugs on Visual Evoked Responses

Drug	Amplitude	Latency (N70, P100)
Thiopental[11]	Decreased	Increased
Etomidate (0.3 mg/kg)[12]	No change	Increased
Fentanyl (60 µg/kg)[10]	Decreased	No change
Diazepam (10 mg)[26]	Decreased	No change
Nitrous oxide[29]	Decreased	Variable
Halothane[110]	Decreased	Increased
Enflurane[13]	Decreased	Increased
Isoflurane[9]	Decreased	Increased

itoring, the retina is usually stimulated through closed eyelids using goggles containing light-emitting diodes, and potential recordings are made from over the occipital cortex (position O_1 and O_2 according to 10-20 system).

Characteristic waves of the VER are N70 (negative polarity; 70 msec latency) and P100 (positive polarity; 100 msec latency) (Fig. 9-1). The P100 is usually used for intraoperative monitoring. More complex waves may be generated using either flashes of white light or pattern reversal using a television screen. The latter two methods of stimulation are difficult to use intraoperatively because of the difficulty in placing the stimulator so that a constant level of stimulation can be achieved.

Because there is no uniformity in choice of stimulus type, reported latency for waves varies from study to study. Nominal latency of the wave appearing about 100 msec after stimulation is emphasized because that wave is generally the most resistant to anesthetic depression. Although the waves reported are similar, nominal latencies reported may vary slightly because of technique (e.g., N65; N70, or P95, P100).

Effects of Anesthetic Drugs on the VER

Anesthetic drugs generally depress VER wave amplitude and increase latency (Table 9-1). Less information is available concerning the effect of combinations of these on the VER. For example, etomidate, 0.3 mg/kg, alone does not change the amplitudes of P100 or N70 but slightly increases the latencies of P60, N70, and P100.[12] During fentanyl-nitrous oxide anesthesia, however, a similar dose of etomidate decreases the amplitude of P100 but increases the P60 and N70 latencies.

Inhaled anesthetics generally depress, in a dose-dependent fashion, the amplitude and increase the latency of the VER.[13,37] For example, with nitrous oxide the N65-

P95 wave appears to be the most sensitive, and its amplitude is depressed by as little as 10% nitrous oxide.[30] The inspired concentration of anesthetic drug that completely suppresses the response varies.[9]

Clinical Considerations

Intraoperative waveform variability limits VER utility during intracranial surgery. Cedzich et al.[6] assessed flash VER in 35 patients with tumors of the visual pathways (90% symptomatic). Of the patients with perisellar lesions, 13 had transcranial and 12 had transsphenoidal surgery. During removal of the bone flap or during the transsphenoidal approach, a reversible loss of VER was observed in 11 of 25 patients, profound alteration in waveform in 8 of 25 patients, and loss of single peaks in 15 of 25 patients. There was no correlation between intraoperative VER changes and postoperative changes in visual function. Thus instability of the waveforms is not simply a result of cranial bone flap removal. In another study, complete intraoperative VER loss, unassociated with postoperative neurologic changes, occurred in 21 of 45 patients.[7]

VER is altered by increased intracranial pressure[117] and hypothermia.[82] In patients with hydrocephalus and head injury, an early VER wave (N70 recorded from an active vertex electrode) correlates with intracranial pressure.[117] There is an inverse relationship between temperature and VER amplitude and latency.[82]

VER may be monitored during surgical procedures involving the optic nerves and optic chiasm. However, the high percentage of false positives (VER changes without injury to optic apparatus[6]) suggests that a very conservative interpretation of waves changes should be used. An anesthetic technique using low-dose volatile anesthetic and avoidance of bolus injection of sedatives and hypnotics may reduce waveform variability.

Somatosensory Evoked Potentials

Somatosensory evoked potentials, recorded at the contralateral somatosensory cortex, are the response of the neural axis from stimulation at a peripheral nerve. Function of peripheral nerve, spinal cord (posterior columns), brainstem, medial lemniscus, internal capsule, and contralateral so-matosensory cortex can be assessed. SSEP can be used for detection of localized injury to specific areas of the neural axis by assessing cortically generated waves or it can serve as a nonspecific indicator of adequacy of cerebral oxygen delivery.

Axons in the ipsilateral dorsal column, ipsilateral dorsal spinocerebellar tract, and contralateral ventrolateral tracts carry SSEP responses to lower-extremity stimulation.[80] A lesion of one half of the dorsal column causes changes in the amplitude of both early and late scalp-recorded waves produced by stimulation ipsilateral to the side of the lesion. A lesion of the dorsal spinocerebellar tract or ventrolateral tract decreases amplitude of only the later waves (latency greater that 40 msec). Thus major changes in SSEP after lower-extremity stimulation indicate injury to the posterior columns of the spinal cord.

Most commonly the median or posterior tibial nerve is used. Paired-disk electrodes may be placed over the nerve of interest. For transcutaneous stimulation, a percutaneous 23 gauge needle can be placed near the nerve. Stimulating electrodes should be placed before complete neuromuscular blockade so that correct placement can be demonstrated by motor response to stimulation. An advantage of needles for intraoperative monitoring is the provision of a constant stimulus location and intensity. Discomfort during SSEP stimulation may be reduced by minimizing current intensity and increasing the stimulus electrode surface area. Although anesthetics alter the generation and transmission of the SSEP, suppression of muscle artifact by neuromuscular blocking drugs and the ability to use a much higher stimulus intensity in the anesthetized patient allow rapid production of waves that are reproducible although they differ from those found in the awake patient. Optimizing the signal-to-noise ratio is particularly important in patients who have small waveforms because of disease, such as spinal cord stenosis or spinal cord compression from an extraaxial mass. With extremely small waves, generation of a reproducible lower-extremity SSEP waveform may require 500 to 1000 stimuli delivered at 4 per sec, so wave development time can be as long as 2 to 4 minutes.

The operating room is an extremely hostile environment for recording evoked potentials. Artifactual changes in recorded waves (i.e., recorded waves changed when actual waves are unchanged) may be caused by electrical or mechanical factors. Sources of electrical artifact are electrocautery and other electrical equipment, such as warming blankets. Another source of electrical artifact is patient contact with the surgeon's hands or with instruments that produce low-voltage slow waves that are not rejected as artifact by the computer. These waves are incorporated into the averaged wave and may cause substantial changes in the waveform. Mechanical artifact may be due to displacement of the stimulating electrodes.

The effect of electrical artifact can be recognized by observing the unprocessed EEG segments that are being av-

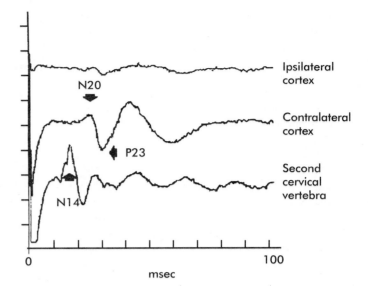

FIG. 9-2 Median nerve somatosensory evoked potential in a patient receiving fentanyl-isoflurane (0.8% end-tidal) anesthesia. The upper trace shows waves recorded ipsilateral to stimulation. The second trace shows waves recorded contralateral to stimulation. The lower trace shows waves recorded over the cervicomedullary junction. Central conduction time (cervicomedullary junction to contralateral cortex) is the N20 minus the N14 latency.

eraged. Artifact of 60 cycles appears as low-voltage, repetitive waves occurring at 60/sec. Movement artifact appears as an occasional slow wave of substantial voltage. The effect of a large-voltage slow wave on the developing average wave is a sudden decrease in amplitude and loss of waveform complexity. Alteration in effective stimulus intensity (movement of stimulating electrodes) is indicated by change in peripherally recorded waves (Erb's point over brachial plexus; second cervical vertebra) in conjunction with changes in scalp-recorded waves.

Fig. 9-2 shows a median nerve SSEP recorded from an anesthetized patient. The characteristic wave over the second cervical vertebrae is N14 (negative, 14 msec latency). Over the scalp, the characteristic waves are N20 and P23. Central conduction time (CCT) is the delay from the second cervical vertebrae to the cortex (i.e., N20 to N14). Simultaneous presentation of ascending locations allows rapid determination of the site of interruption of the signal. Attenuation of the scalp-recorded signal with maintenance of signal over the upper spinal cord suggests a brainstem site of injury, whereas attenuation of the signal at the level of the spinal cord suggests injury of a peripheral nerve or the brachial plexus.

Stimulation of the median nerve for upper extremity and the posterior tibial nerve for lower extremity is used frequently for intraoperative monitoring. Stimulation of the posterior tibial nerve results in responses that can be monitored over the popliteal fossa, lumbar spinal cord, and somatosensory cortex (P40, N50). Scalp-recorded waves after posterior tibial stimulation are frequently of highest amplitude when recorded 1 to 2 cm lateral to the midline, ipsilateral to the stimulation, because of paradoxic localization.[62]

In unanesthetized subjects, a stimulus frequency as high as 5.7 Hz does not affect amplitude or latencies. In patients with spinal cord injury, amplitude after posterior tibial nerve stimulation is attenuated by higher stimulus rates (>5.1 Hz), and good-quality waves are obtained at lower rates (1.1 or 2.1 Hz). A majority of patients (86%) who had a decrease in amplitude with increased stimulus rate had a discrete sensory level, bilateral lower-extremity weakness, or both. Only 28% of patients whose SSEP was not affected by an increased stimulus rate had similar neurologic impairment.[89]

In neonates, scalp-recorded SSEP can be recorded using a low-frequency stimulus (1.1/sec). Adequate waveforms were not obtained at a higher stimulus frequency (4.1/sec). A stimulus intensity higher than that needed in older children is required to elicit a motor response (up to 20 mA), but this intensity is well tolerated by infants. The latency of N20 decreases from 31 msec in the newborn to 21 msec by 7 to 13 weeks of age.[33]

The spinal cord SSEP may be stimulated directly by percutaneous placement of flexible epidural electrodes. Electrodes can be placed by fluoroscopic guidance and used to stimulate the spinal cord directly. This technique is useful during thoracic aortic aneurysm surgery when aortic cross-clamping produces peripheral nerve ischemia. The epidural electrode can also be used to record large-amplitude waves, which are relatively resistant to anesthetic depression.[41]

Cortical SSEP recording can be used to localize the motor cortex because of its location adjacent to the somatosensory cortex. The somatosensory cortex is identified by approximately mirror-image waveforms recorded at electrode sites on opposite sides of the central sulcus (hand area).[115]

With conventional averaging, diagnosis of waveform change may be delayed until a large number of altered waves are added to the current average. Analytic methods that emphasize changes in waveforms as they are added to the total number averaged shorten the time for recognition of a changing waveform. Several such methods for evoked potentials are available in addition to standard averaging. One method is the moving window average (MWA), which estimates, by averaging within a window containing the N most recent sweeps, when N is some specific window length. Exponentially weighted average (EWA) estimates are obtained by weighted averaging of sweeps, with the weight of older sweeps diminishing in an exponential manner. Vaz et al[112] compared Fourier series modeling (Fourier linear combined, FLC) with MWA and EWA in a circumstance of rapidly changing evoked potential waveforms (etomidate bolus). They showed that FLC follows transient evoked potential changes much faster than EWA or MWA.

Diagnostic criteria to evaluate intraoperative waveform changes have been difficult to establish. Using conventional averaging techniques, latency changes of 7% to 15% and amplitude decreases of 45% to 50% may occur without changes in postoperative neurologic function.[57,64,117] Notable in those studies was a lack of control subjects, an appreciation of the anesthetic management, or concern about the potential effects of anesthetic changes on SSEP waveforms. Avoiding changes in inhaled gas concentration and bolus injection of hypnotics during periods of risk minimizes difficulties in determining whether waveform changes are due to surgical manipulation.

Effects of Anesthetic Drugs

Early components of the SSEP (<40 msec for upper extremity nerve stimulation; <80 msec for lower-extremity nerve stimulation) are readily generated for intraoperative monitoring and are generally resistant to anesthetic depression. Table 9-2 shows the effects of anesthetic drugs on SSEP. Intravenous drugs generally have only moderate effects on early parts of the waveforms and allow generation of waveforms adequate for rapid evaluation. Barbiturates such as thiopental (5 mg/kg) cause moderate or no decrease in amplitude[22,54] and a moderate increase in latency. Diazepam depresses scalp-recorded waves,[26] whereas the effect of midazolam is unclear, with reports ranging from no effect on amplitude with a slight increase in latency[54] to a 40% amplitude depression.[96] Propofol (2.5 mg/kg) depresses waves occurring later than N20. It increases N20 latency 8% and central conduction time (N20 to N14 latency) 20%. N14 and N20 amplitudes are not affected by propofol.[86] Fentanyl has modest effects on early components of the SSEP waveform. The amplitude remains unchanged in doses of up to 75 µg/kg,[19,69,76] but latency is increased. Intrathecal morphine (15 µg/kg) does not alter scalp-recorded responses to posterior tibial nerve stimulation.[91]

A most surprising drug effect on SSEP waveform is the

TABLE 9-2

Effects of Anesthetic Drugs on Somatosensory Evoked Potential

Drug	Amplitude	Latency
Thiopental[54]	Small or no change	Increased
Etomidate[54,70]	Increased	Increased
Fentanyl[19,54,76]	Modest or no decrease	Modest or no increase
Diazepam[26]	Decreased	Increased
Midazolam[96]	Decreased	Increased
Ketamine[90]	Increased	Increased
Propofol[86]	No change	Increased
Nitrous oxide[69,78,114]	Decreased	No change
Halothane[77,79]	Decreased	Increased
Enflurane[93]	Decreased	Increased
Isoflurane[16,69]	Decreased	Increased

200% to 600% augmentation of amplitude of scalp-recorded waves caused by etomidate.[54] Etomidate increases latency and amplitude of cortical waves without changes in waves recorded in the thalamus, demonstrating that the augmentation effect occurs in the cortex.[85] Waveform augmentation has been used clinically to enhance abnormally small waves, thus allowing monitoring that otherwise would not have been possible.[95] Ketamine (2 mg/kg) also increases SSEP amplitude, with the maximum effect occurring within 2 to 10 minutes.[90]

Volatile anesthetics and nitrous oxide depress the SSEP waveform in an apparently dose-dependent manner.[76,79,93,115] With halothane, enflurane, and isoflurane, the amplitude is smaller and the latency is longer with coadministration of nitrous oxide (60%). Enflurane decreases SSEP amplitude and increases latency in patients anesthetized with intravenous drugs (fentanyl and thiopental).[69] Enflurane 0.6% and 1.7% under other circumstances may increase amplitude compared with a control.[15] Isoflurane decreases amplitude in a dose-dependent manner from 1.2 μV at 0.5 MAC (isoflurane plus nitrous oxide) to 0.3 μV at 1.5% MAC (isoflurane plus nitrous oxide). Elimination of nitrous oxide increases amplitude by 100%.[114] Isoflurane decreases amplitude and increases latency in patients anesthetized with fentanyl and thiopental.[69] The effect of isoflurane on SSEP may occur within a very few minutes.[2]

Clinical Considerations

Branston et al[3] assessed the effects of ischemia on early components of SSEP in brainstem, thalamus, and cerebral cortex and found a cephalic-to-caudal decrease in the cerebral blood flow (CBF) required to maintain normal electrical activity. In terms of blood flow, the threshold for cortical SSEP change was 15 to 20 ml/min/100 g, for thalamus it was 10 to 15 ml/min/100 g, and for medial lemniscus the threshold was 10 ml/min/100 g. With intracranial hypertension, SSEP latency is maintained at control levels until CBF falls more than 55% to 65%. Central conduction time is prolonged when CBF falls below 15 to 20 ml/min/100 g and is associated with a decrease in $CMRo_2$ of 20% to 30%.[53]

Postischemia recovery of SSEP amplitude correlates with the residual blood flow that was present during the ischemic period in both the ipsilateral middle cerebral artery territory and white matter.[67] After reperfusion, animals developing ischemic lesions of the cortex had more rapid loss and slower recovery of scalp SSEP than animals who did not subsequently develop lesions.[20]

SSEP During Cerebral Aneurysm Surgery. Central conduction time (CCT; N20 to N14) correlates with postoperative neurologic deficits in patients undergoing middle cerebral artery aneurysm clipping. If CCT increased to 10 msec (normal for anesthetized patient is 6 msec) or the scalp-recorded response disappeared, postoperative neurologic deficits were present.[106] Momma et al[71] also found that CCT changed during temporary clip application. In that study, no patient with unchanged intraoperative CCT had postoperative morbidity. In six patients, temporary arterial occlusion prolonged CCT up to 10 msec, and two of these six patients had an immediate postoperative neurologic deficit (1 recovered). The scalp-recorded response became flat in 15 patients. Of these 15, seven had hemispheric deficits in the immediate postoperative period although four recovered. A permanent postoperative deficit is unlikely if wave disappearance takes more than 3 to 4 minutes, and recovery is likely if N20 recovers within 20 minutes after reperfusion.[71]

Manninen et al.[65] assessed SSEP during temporary arterial occlusion in 97 patients. SSEP changes during vessel occlusion were found in 24% of patients (in 65% of these the SSEP normalized after release of occlusion, but 35% had persistent SSEP changes). A persistent SSEP change predicted a postoperative neurologic deficit, whereas of the 15 patients with reversible changes, only 5 had postoperative deficits. In 80% of the patients, there was no change in SSEP, and 14% of these had a new neurologic deficit postoperatively. Thus the false-positive rate was 43% and the false-negative rate was 14%. If only persistent SSEP changes are considered as predictors of neurologic deficits, the false-positive rate was 0%.

In a series of 53 patients with middle cerebral artery aneurysms, only one of 37 patients with no change in SSEP had new postoperative neurologic deficits. All four patients who had significant changes and incomplete or no return to baseline had new deficits. Only one of five patients who had significant changes with return of waves to baseline suffered injury. Improvement in SSEP in the latter group was due to clip adjustment, clip removal, or increase in mean arterial blood pressure.[32] Fig. 9-3 shows changes in median nerve SSEP with aneurysm clip application and recovery of SSEP with replacement of the clip. Fig. 9-4 shows SSEP changes that occurred with changes in mean arterial blood pressure in a patient having diffuse vasospasm.

The neurologic outcome of basilar artery surgery is not predicted by SSEP or BAER.[31] The failure of SSEP to correlate with outcome is probably caused by the vascular distribution at risk, the posterior cerebral arteries and basilar perforating vessels do not reliably include either the BAER or SSEP pathways. Studies[32] comparing amplitude and latency values at dural opening and dural closure in patients undergoing cerebral aneurysm clipping found a false-positive incidence of only 2%. There was a 6% false-negative incidence, but this false-negative rate was reduced to 4% when basilar aneurysms were excluded. SSEP changes correctly predicted a neurologic deficit in only 38% of patients with vertebrobasilar artery aneurysms, compared with 75% of patients with middle cerebral artery or carotid artery aneurysm.[65]

SSEP During Carotid Endarterectomy. SSEP changes have been measured in patients undergoing surgery for carotid artery disease. In a large series, 59 of 734 patients could not be evaluated because of technical problems.

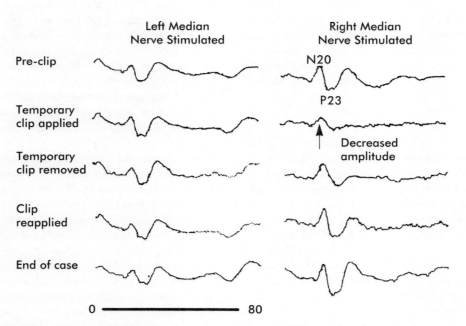

FIG. 9-3 Median nerve SSEP during clipping of a left middle cerebral artery aneurysm. Application of a temporary clip resulted in a decrease of N20 to P23 wave and a loss of later waves from stimulation of the median nerve contralateral to the aneurysm *(right)*. The depression was rapidly reversed with clip replacement *(right panel)*. Neurologic function was normal at the end of the operation.

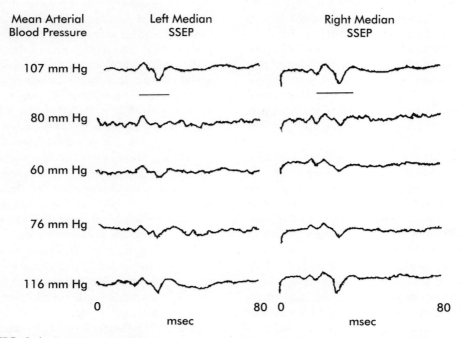

FIG. 9-4 Median nerve SSEP in a patient with diffuse vasospasm undergoing aneurysm clipping. Induced hypotension caused a bilateral decrease in the amplitude of the N20 to P23 waves *(horizontal line)*, which was reversed with an increase in mean arterial blood pressure.

Only four of 586 patients with no intraoperative change in SSEP had immediate postoperative neurologic deficits. Abnormal SSEPs were found in 89 procedures. Of these patients, 83 showed reversible changes in SSEP during surgery. Six had an irreversible change in SSEP, and all these six had permanent postoperative neurologic deficit. The incidence of SSEP abnormality increased with increasing stenosis of the contralateral carotid artery.[45]

EEG and median nerve SSEP were compared during carotid endarterectomy with shunt placement in 64 patients. SSEP amplitude decreased more than 50% in six of the 64 patients. EEG changes occurred in six patients, four of whom also had SSEP changes. Two patients had transient postoperative neurologic deficits, both of whom had SSEP changes, but only one of those patients had EEG changes.[56] This study suggests that brain-wave changes consistent with neurologic injury during carotid endarterectomy are more easily appreciated with SSEP than EEG.

In a prospective study, 3 of 400 patients undergoing carotid endarterectomy had neurologic deficits postoperatively despite the continued presence of SSEP waves during the period of cross-clamping. The SSEP was completely lost in 17 patients, and five of seven patients without shunt placement and 3 of ten with shunt insertion had postoperative neurologic deficits. Of the postoperative neurologic deficits, approximately two thirds resolved within 4 days.[92]

Intraoperative SSEP changes also correlate with neurologic function other than motor strength. Four of 14 patients who had SSEP amplitude decreases of 50% or more during carotid endarterectomy performed worse on neuropsychologic testing 7 days after operation.[4]

SSEP and the Spinal Cord. In animals, changes in spinal-cord evoked potentials measured immediately after injury correlate well with the amount of edema measured 5 hours after injury and thus have a good prognostic value in predicting neurologic outcome after traumatic spinal cord injury.[94]

Posterior tibial SSEP monitoring in 220 patients (121 with scoliosis, 41 with neoplasm, and 58 with other diseases) demonstrated that only three of seven patients who had worsening neurologic function after surgery had significant and persistent changes in intraoperative SSEP (57% false negative). In an additional 4 cases, a substantial decrease (>50%) in amplitude occurred without a change in postoperative neurologic status (2% false positive).[18] Fig. 9-5 shows normal posterior tibial SSEP to left-nerve stimulation and absent SSEP to right-nerve stimulation. Because the scalp-recorded wave returned in response to a change in operative management, this would be classified a *false positive.*

Postoperative paraplegia with intraoperative preservation of SSEP has been reported in an achondroplastic dwarf who had preservation of the scalp-recorded response to individual peroneal nerve stimulation but no response to pinprick below T12.[37] Lesser et al.[61] described six patients who had postoperative deficits despite unchanged intraoperative

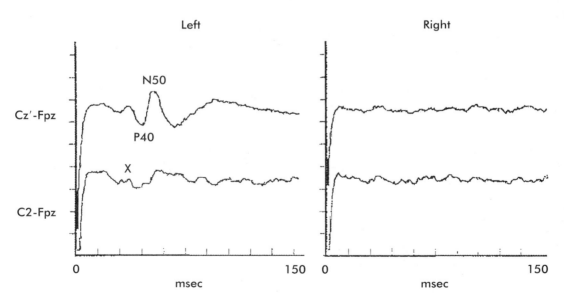

FIG. 9-5 Posterior tibial SSEP during complex instrumentation of the spine from T12 to L2. The upper trace shows scalp-recorded waves at the vertex *(Cz')* referenced to forehead *(Fpz)*. The lower trace shows waves recorded over the second cervical vertebra *(C2)*. Scalp-recorded waves were symmetric until a sponge was placed on the right side to control bleeding, which produced absent waves at the scalp and over the second cervical vertebra. With removal of the sponge, the scalp-recorded waves in response to right posterior nerve stimulation promptly returned (waves not shown).

SSEP. Autopsy has documented anterior spinal artery syndrome with retained lower-extremity SSEP.[120]

Schmid et al.[87] assessed SSEP in 28 patients with symptomatic cervical radiculopathy and found that 68% of patients had false-negative waveform changes on the side of the symptoms, and 36% of patients had false-positive changes on the side contralateral to symptoms. Veilleux et al.[113] reviewed median-nerve SSEP in patients undergoing surgery of the cervical spine who had no intradural process expanding or compressing the cervical cord. This group of patients had baseline values available. In patients with preoperative evidence of spinal injury, intraoperative scalp-recorded waves were lost without major changes in anesthesia or surgery. These data suggest that abnormal waves are more sensitive to anesthetics and temperature changes that occur during operations. Intraoperative ulnar and tibial responses should be monitored in all patients in whom baseline studies can be obtained.

During spinal cord embolization of arteriovenous malformation (AVM) under neuroleptic anesthesia (droperidol, fentanyl), SSEP amplitude decreased coincidentally with opacification of the anterior spinal artery. The amplitude usually returned within 2 to 4 minutes after catheter removal. In three patients in whom the spinal cord AVM was embolized, SSEP amplitude increased and changes were associated with immediate improvement of neurologic symptoms. In several patients, SSEP changes preceded motor weakness.[1]

Spinal cord stimulation from a percutaneously, fluoroscopically placed electrode has been used during thoracolumbar aneurysm surgery, and these waveforms were compared with waveforms generated by stimulation of the posterior tibial nerves. Without intraoperative aortic shunting, all patients lost scalp-recorded responses to posterior tibial nerve stimulation, whereas only two of eight patients lost spinal-cord SSEP. One of these two patients became paraplegic, and the other died before a neurologic examination could be performed.[75]

Median nerve SSEP has been used to diagnose brachial plexus lesions in patients with injury, cervical spondylopathic radiculopathies without myelopathy, and brachial plexopathy with systemic cancer. Median nerve SSEP was normal after injuries of the upper trunk and root avulsion confined to one or two root levels. Median nerve SSEPs were abnormal after multiple trunk lesions and multiple root avulsions. In patients with spondylopathic radiculopathies, median-nerve SSEPs were normal in all but one patient.[107] SSEPs were useful in assessing brachial plexus dysfunction caused by cancer infiltration, except for lower trunk infiltration.

Hypothermia increases SSEP latency,[104,111] with latency change correlating with nasopharyngeal temperature. The effect of hypothermia on SSEP amplitude is less clear, with reports of no change[104] or decreased amplitude with hypothermia.[104] Latency of the initial waves is prolonged, about 1.15 msec/degree C, suggesting that a decrease in temperature of 2 to 3° C increases latency about 3 msec,[111] an amount of change previously suggested to indicate neural injury. Hyperthermia (42° C) suppresses SSEP amplitude, with the amplitude being only 15% of that at normothermia.[23]

Automated long-term SSEP monitoring has been used to evaluate outcome in posttraumatic coma (overall mortality 44%). Of 14 patients with an initial absence of waves after the N20 wave or who lost this activity during monitoring, 12 died. The remaining 2 had only minimal functional activity. Of 22 patients who had preservation or enhancement of waves after N20, 18 had a functional survival (3 months). SSEP deterioration was not directly associated with elevated intracranial pressure.[72]

Trigeminal Evoked Potentials

Reproducible, very-short-latency waves of the trigeminal system are produced by stimulation of the lip at 2 to 4 Hz (512 stimuli). Waves occur from 0.8 to 7.2 msec after the stimulus, with the main response being a large-amplitude (4 μV) positive wave with a latency of 2.9 msec.[38] This modality of evoked potential is abnormal in patients with posterior fossa masses in the region of the fifth cranial nerve or in symptomatic hydrocephalus.[103] In 23 patients with skull base tumors (perisellar or cerebellopontine angle), all patients who had clinical signs or symptoms in the trigeminal area and seven of 12 patients without signs or symptoms had abnormalities of the trigeminal evoked potential generated by stimulation of the infraorbital nerve.[59] This modality of evoked potential monitoring may be useful in patients with large posterior fossa tumors that cause severe eighth cranial nerve dysfunction and make BAER monitoring impossible.

Brainstem Auditory Evoked Response (BAER)

Auditory nerve stimulation (clicks) produces both brainstem components and cortical components although the latter have received only modest interest for intraoperative monitoring. The BAER has been used extensively in patients at risk of brain injury during intracranial surgery and after head injury. Widespread use has occurred despite the extremely small amount of neural tissue assessed and the resistance of BAER to oxygen deprivation when compared with other neural monitors such as the EEG or cortical SSEP waves.[100]

The BAER is generated by delivering pure-tone clicks individually to each ear (1000 to 2000 at 11.9/sec). After stimulation, a series of waves occur within 10 msec of stimulation and are designated in sequence using Roman numerals according to wave origin: wave I (auditory nerve), wave II (pontomedullary junction), wave III (caudal pons), wave IV (rostral pons), wave V (midbrain) and wave VI (thalamus). Because of some brainstem crossover, the contralateral ear is usually masked with white noise. For intraoperative monitoring, small ear inserts that are easily se-

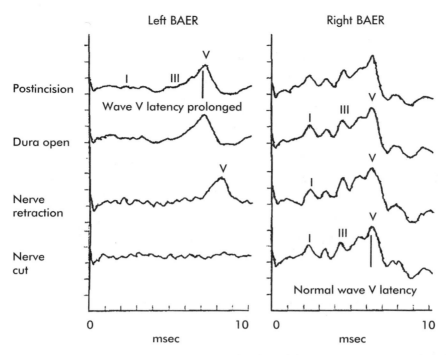

Left BAER   Right BAER

Postincision

Wave V latency prolonged

Dura open

Nerve
retraction

Nerve
cut

Normal wave V latency

0   10   0   10
msec   msec

FIG. 9-6   Intraoperative BAER in a patient with a large left acoustic neuroma. Right-sided
BAER shows normal morphology with wave latencies slightly greater than normal because of
isoflurane anesthesia. The left-sided BAER is abnormal with ill-defined waves (the patient had
nonfunctional hearing on left). Nerve retraction caused a reversible increase in wave V latency,
and all waves were subsequently lost when the nerve was sacrificed to remove the tumor.

cured work well. Technical difficulties may make intraoperative BAER interpretation difficult. For example, factors that decrease the effective stimulus intensity alter the waveform. Thus partial obstruction of the external auditory canal by cerumen or fluid decreases the stimulus intensity, and increases in latency occur that mimic neural injury. Similar waveform changes occur with partial dislodgment of the stimulator from the external auditory canal.

BAER monitoring should be undertaken in all patients at risk of brainstem injury, even if the primary disease causes hearing on the affected side to decrease below the functional level. Fig. 9-6 shows a patient with a large cerebellopontine angle with greatly diminished hearing ipsilateral to the tumor. Unilateral BAER changes occurred with nerve retraction, and the BAER was lost completely with nerve transection.

In addition to the brainstem response to auditory stimulation, longer latency responses also occur. The P300 (positive; 300 msec) is a late auditory wave that appears to be an electrophysiologic correlate of complex processes such as directed attention, stimulus detection, sequential information processing, short-term memory, and decision-making.[81] The amplitude of P300 varies with stimulus probability (relative frequency and sequential structure), meaning (stimulus complexity, stimulus value), and infor-

mation transmission (discrimination difficulty, allocation of attendance).[47] Middle latency auditory responses (10 to 40 msec) are generated intracortically in neural elements of the primary auditory cortex and may be used when this area is a risk of injury.[52]

Effects of Anesthetic Drugs

BAER waveforms are resistant to both intravenous and inhalational drugs. Table 9-3 shows anesthetic effects on BAER. Increasing blood levels of barbiturates and ketamine increase BAER interpeak latency.[14,102] Propofol (2 mg/kg, IV, followed by an infusion) increases the latency of I, III, and V waves without a change in the amplitudes, but it completely suppresses middle-latency auditory waves.[8] Fentanyl in large doses does not alter the BAER.[84]

Houston et al.[46] found a linear decrease in BAER amplitude with an increase in nitrous oxide concentration (10% to 40%) and an increase in hearing threshold that was of sufficient magnitude to explain BAER changes caused by nitrous oxide. Nitrous oxide (33%) reduces the amplitude of auditory (long-latency) evoked potentials without altering latency.[29,44] The effect of halothane on BAER is unclear, with reports ranging from no effect[25] to drug-induced increases in latency.[109] In the latter study, the increase in wave V latency at 1% (end expired concentration of halo-

TABLE 9-3
Effects of Anesthetic Drugs on Brainstem Auditory
Evoked Responses

Drug	Latency
Thiopental[102]	Increased
Fentanyl[84]	No change
Propofol[8]	Increased
Ketamine[14]	Increased
Nitrous oxide[46]	Increased
Halothane[108]	Increased
Enflurane[24,108]	Increased

thane) was slightly less than 1 msec. Slight increases in BAER latency occur in a dose-dependent manner during enflurane anesthesia.[23,109]

Clinical Considerations

In humans, hypercapnia (7.5% to 10% end tidal CO_2) does not change BAER. In anesthetized cats, hypercapnia affects BAER less than it affects the EEG. Hypercapnia increases latency slightly and is associated with a small decrease in amplitude. At a $Paco_2$ of 90 mm Hg, the EEG is isoelectric while the BAER is essentially normal in experimental animals.[97]

Sohmer et al.[99] found that the EEG became isoelectric at a cerebral perfusion pressure (CPP) of 24 mm Hg, whereas the BAER became isoelectric at 7 mm Hg. In most animals, a stage of decreased CPP was reached (14 mm Hg) in which wave I was preserved but brainstem waves were absent.[99] Sohmer et al.[98] assessed BAER in cats during decreased CPP and found that, at CPP of 26 mm Hg, EEG and BAER rapidly decreased, with EEG changes occurring before significant changes in BAER. Goitein et al.,[39] assessed BAER in 25 children with reduced CPP and found that BAER became abnormal when CPP decreased to less than 30 mm Hg.

Sohmer et al.[101] compared the effect of severe hypoxia (Pao_2 20 to 30 mm Hg) on BAER, SSEP, and VER. If MABP was maintained during severe hypoxia, there was no effect on SSEP or VER, but BAER and long-latency auditory EP waves were depressed. However, if MABP was allowed to decrease during hypoxia, all evoked potentials became severely depressed or isoelectric. These results suggest that the early changes in BAER during hypoxia are not due to failure of brainstem conduction, but rather occur because the cochlear microphonic is sensitive to hypoxia. These data suggest that the mechanism of changes of BAER with decreased cerebral perfusion (decreased cerebral blood flow) is different from changes that occur during hypoxia with high cerebral blood flow and low arterial oxygen content.

Kalmarchey et al.[48] studied BAER during surgery for unilateral cerebellopontine angle (CPA) tumors and found BAER changes with lumbar drainage and tumor dissection in all patients. Bilateral latency prolongation occurred in

five of nine patients, and ipsilateral latency increase occurred in six of nine patients, suggesting that the intraoperative BAER is too sensitive for intraoperative monitoring. Patients with small CPA tumors may have normal BAER at high stimulus intensity, but, at a lower intensity, abnormal latencies of wave V compared with the unaffected side can be demonstrated.[60,74]

Lam et al.[55] reported BAER measurements in three patients undergoing clipping of a basilar artery aneurysm. In two patients, ligation of the basilar artery and a vertebral artery produced deterioration of BAER that correlated with postoperative neurologic injury. In the third patient, transient postoperative neurologic changes correlated with intraoperative BAER changes.

An exponential increase in BAER latency occurs as temperature is decreased to 19° C in both primates[21] and rodents.[88] The increase in latency appears to be greater for the later waves. Waves are easily identifiable at more frequently used levels of hypothermia (29° C) although latencies are delayed by about 33%.[66] BAER latency is inversely related to temperature over the range of 36° to 42° C, with a decrease in amplitude as temperature increases.[40]

The BAER appears to be a sensitive monitor of the auditory apparatus in response to direct injury. Thus BAER monitoring accurately assesses brainstem function during events that may contribute to brainstem injury, such as brainstem retraction. It appears to be much less sensitive to diffuse insults such as hypoxia or intracranial hypertension than the EEG or SSEP.

ELECTROMYOGRAPHY (EMG)

Electromyography (EMG) is the response of the muscle to stimulation of the motor nerve. Facial nerve stimulation with EMG monitoring is frequently used to decrease the risk of facial nerve injury during surgery for removal of cerebellopontine angle tumors. Because the response is generated by contraction of muscle, the use of neuromuscular blocking drugs is restricted.

Kartush[49] reviewed electromyography and intraoperative facial nerve monitoring. He emphasized that a monopolar stimulator with insulated tip be used because CSF can disperse the stimulus, leading to false negatives. Typical stimulus parameters include a constant current of 2 mA at 5 c/s and a 200 μsec duration. EMG recording electrodes are placed near the orbicularis oris and orbicularis oculi muscles, with a ground electrode on the forehead.

Anesthetic management, particularly the use of neuromuscular blocking drugs, has been inadequately studied. Clearly the neuromuscular junction must be functional for an EMG response to occur when the nerve is stimulated. The degree of neuromuscular blockade should be maintained at a light level until response of the respective muscles (orbicularis oris and orbicularis oculi) is verified. Whether a nerve that has been stretched by a tumor or otherwise injured will respond to a normal level of stimulation is unclear.

MOTOR EVOKED POTENTIALS (MEP)

Limitations in SSEP for monitoring the spinal cord have produced interest in directly monitoring the motor system. The motor cortex has been stimulated through transcranial electrical stimulation (MEP-E) and more recently by magnetic stimulation (MEP-M). Electrical stimulation produces discomfort and is poorly tolerated by the awake subject. Although a less precise stimulus, magnetic stimulation offers the advantages of producing less discomfort and better tolerance by awake subjects. Magnetic stimulation penetrates whole body structures, including skull, without creating large electrical fields at the surface; thus there is little pain during stimulation of cortex or peripheral nerves. The corticospinal response to direct stimulation of the motor cortex (magnetic or electric) can be recorded from the lateral column of the spinal cord or spinal epidural space using percutaneous needles.[50] However, monitoring of MEP from these locations is difficult because of the efficiency of the central nervous system in conducting impulses via the spinal cord and peripheral nerves to muscle groups. These extremely small electrical impulses from spinal cord or peripheral nerve are difficult to record. The muscle response to stimulation of the motor cortex is much larger than the neural response and is, therefore, easier to record. Thus most MEP studies are done by measuring compound muscle action potential responses despite the fact that both volatile anesthetic and neuromuscular blocking drugs obtund these responses. Magnetic compared with electrical generation of the MEP has a longer latency. Less stimulus artifact is produced with magnetic stimulation than with electrical stimulation. With magnetic stimulation, the stimulus artifact ceases at termination of stimulus, whereas, with electrical stimulation, artifact persists for a short time.[17] Electrical stimulation theoretically can cause seizures. However, stimuli typically necessary to cause seizures are of greater duration than those required for MEP, and kindling is not produced at a stimulus rate less than 3/sec. Implanted metallic devices such as aneurysm clips pose risks with magnetic stimulation because of the potential for clip movement.

MEP-M is produced by discharging an electromagnet near the skull over the motor cortex. Currently both circular and butterfly shaped coils are being investigated in an attempt to better focus the magnetic field. In addition, coil characteristics and orientation are under intense investigation. The technique for MEP-E is to place the anode 8 cm from the midline, immediately posterior to the coronal suture, with the cathode placed at the bregma for hand area stimulation. For foot stimulation, the anode is placed in the bregma and the cathode is placed 6 cm posterior in the midline.

Effects of Anesthetic Drugs

Table 9-4 shows anesthetic effects on MEP. Ghaly et al[35] studied the effect of incremental doses of ketamine on MEP-M in the monkey and found no depression (compared with basal ketamine anesthesia) at doses of <20 mg/kg. At

TABLE 9-4

Effects of Anesthetic Drugs on Motor Evoked Potentials

Drug	Amplitude	Latency
Etomidate[34]	No change	Increased
Fentanyl[118]	No change(?)	No change(?)
Diazepam[34]	Decreased	Increased
Ketamine[35]	Decreased	Increased
Nitrous oxide[35,119]	Decreased	Increased
Halothane[43]	Decreased	Increased
Isoflurane (0.5-1.5%)[42]	Decreased	Increased

higher doses, amplitude depression ranged from 14% to 45% with adductor pollicis brevis muscle (APB) response and 57% to 82% with adductor hallucis muscle (AH) response. Latency increased 12% to 18%, and the stimulus threshold was increased.

In primates, etomidate causes only moderate depression of amplitude and increase in latency in doses sufficient to produce anesthesia.[36]

Nitrous oxide appears to depress both MEP-M and MEP-E. In humans, the addition of nitrous oxide to thiopental-fentanyl anesthesia depresses the upper extremity response to 11% of baseline and the lower extremity response to 7% of baseline.[118] A similar depression is seen in human volunteers breathing 60% nitrous oxide.[118]

Loughman et al.[63] studied the effects of halothane added to nitrous oxide narcotic anesthesia using epidurally recorded MEP-E and found that halothane did not alter either amplitude or latency compared with waves recorded during nitrous narcotic anesthesia. Isoflurane (0.5% to 1.5%) increases latency and decreases amplitude of the MEP-E, with changes occurring within 2 minutes of anesthesia induction.[42]

Fig. 9-7 shows the effect of isoflurane on compound motor action potential (cMAP) after electrical stimulation of the motor cortex. Isoflurane causes a rapid (within 2 minutes) and profound decrease in the amplitude of the cMAP. Although small compared with preanesthetic amplitudes, the amplitudes of the waves are much larger than scalp-recorded SSEP waves and thus should be easily monitored using conventional averaging techniques.

Haghighi et al.[43] compared volatile anesthetics to basal fentanyl-droperidol anesthesia on the MEP-E in rats and found a dose-dependent amplitude suppression with halothane to be more depressant than with either isoflurane or enflurane.

In eight patients receiving nitrous oxide narcotic anesthesia and partial neuromuscular blockade with vecuronium, the effect of addition of isoflurane was assessed by MEP-E every 20 seconds. During basal anesthesia, reproducible responses were demonstrated. Addition of isoflurane (<0.5% end tidal) attenuated MEP-E amplitude within 5 minutes.[5] Edmonds et al.[27] assessed bilateral anterior tibialis muscle responses to MEP-M and found that preopera-

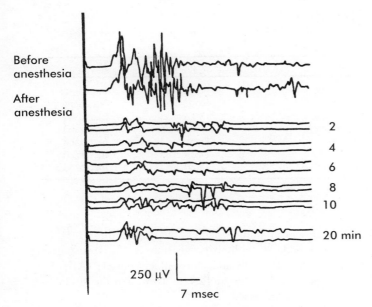

Before anesthesia

After anesthesia

2
4
6
8
10
20 min

250 μV

7 msec

FIG. 9-7 Effect of isoflurane on motor evoked potentials. The response is measured by electromyogram.

tively 11 of 11 patients had recordable waves, whereas, during nitrous oxide narcotic anesthesia using a nondepolarizing muscle relaxant, only 9 of 11 had MEP-M waves. Anesthesia decreased average amplitude to 25% of control. MEP is very sensitive to anesthetics when the response is evaluated by recording an electromyographic response in a single twitch. Averaging of multiple responses may allow monitoring during volatile anesthesia. Thus nitrous narcotic anesthesia and a stable level of neuromuscular blockade such as that provided by an infusion of neuromuscular blocking agent should be used to provide a stable response.

Clinical Considerations

The proposed utility of MEP is for situations in which monitoring of SSEP has been found to be inadequate. For example, concern about the use of SSEP during spinal cord surgery exists because of the high incidence of false negatives (injury without change in SSEP).[61] However, in some patients at risk, MEP may not be sufficiently robust to allow measurement. For instance, in unanesthetized patients with cervical spondylitic myelopathy, eight of eleven patients had MEP (abductor digiti minimi muscle) abnormalities, with prolongation of central conduction time in seven of the patients and absence of MEP in another patient. Five of the eleven patients had normal SSEP.[116]

MEPs have been investigated in unanesthetized humans with space-occupying lesions of the brainstem or spinal cord. Transcranial electrical stimulation and recording EMG from contralateral thenar or anterior tibial muscle was used.[119] A correct correlation of MEP and clinical motor status occurred in 77% of thenar muscles and 84% of anterior tibial muscles, with 23% false positive in thenar re-

cording and 16% in anterior tibial recording. There were no false negatives.

The reliability of delivering stimuli to the motor cortex has led to evaluation of MEP-E in patients at risk of injury during spinal surgery.[51,118] Zentner[118] found that MEP-E could be elicited in all 50 patients studied preoperatively but, during neuroleptic anesthesia, waveforms were absent in 12% of thenar muscles and 14% of anterior tibial muscles tested. A 50% change in amplitude was used as a criterion for change. Amplitude changes correlated with postoperative neurologic status in 81% of patients with anterior tibial muscle changes (19% false negative) and 76% with thenar muscle changes (24% false positive). In another study,[51] 25% of patients had transient amplitude decreases of 50% recovered completely and had normal postoperative neurologic function. One patient, however, had complete intraoperative loss of MEP and awoke quadriplegic. Two patients had increased amplitude that was associated with improved motor function in the immediate postoperative period.

MEP Monitoring During Thoracic Aneurysm Surgery. Electrical MEP has been assessed in animal studies of spinal cord ischemia using thoracic aorta cross-clamping.[58] Aortic cross-clamping produces a characteristic deterioration and loss of MEP that is time and spinal level dependent. Ischemic cord dysfunction (as evidenced by change in MEP) progressed from a distal to proximal cord location with changes at the L4 level occurring after 11 minutes and at T10 level after 17 minutes. In that study,[58] reperfusion resulted in MEP return that progressed from proximal to distal.

Neurologic function 24 hours after spinal ischemia has been compared with MEP waves recorded by translaminar electrodes at T13 and scalp-recorded SSEP. MEP was lost at the time of cross-clamp in only nine of 20 animals that developed paraplegia; MEP was not lost at the time of cross-clamp in the seven animals that remained neurologically normal. All animals that lost MEP at time of cross-clamp became paraplegic. However, MEP persisted in three of eleven paraplegic animals, so that the sensitivity was 46%, specificity was 100%, and overall accuracy was 59% for the ability to predict neurologic injury. At the time of cross-clamp, SSEP responses were lost in 19 of 20 animals that developed paraplegia, but they were also lost in three of seven animals that did not develop paraplegia. Loss of SSEP correlated with neurologic injury (P < .01). SSEP had a sensitivity of 95%, a specificity of 67%, and an overall accuracy of 89%. Spinal-cord blood flow was lower in animals developing neurologic deficits.[28]

Injection of hydrogen-containing solutions while one monitors current generated over discrete parts of the spinal cord has been used to localize important feeding vessels to the spinal cord originating from the aorta.[105] With reversible clamping of arteries known to supply the cord, there was a reversible loss or 80% decrease of spinal cord MEP amplitude and no postoperative paralysis.[105] Sacrifice of arteries known to perfuse the cord caused at minimum, a permanent decrease in spinal MEP amplitude of 50%, whereas, with artery preservation, amplitude was maintained.[105]

Intraoperative SSEP, blinded neurologic examinations after 2 weeks, and histopathologic and neurochemical measurements have been used to compare the effects of direct spinal cord stimulation (silver ball electrodes) with transvertebral stimulation to generate MEP. Compound MEP of quadriceps muscle was measured. Stimuli were delivered over 1 hour, and each animal received approximately 5000 stimuli with a stimulus intensity of 1 mA. Epidural stimulation produced more interanimal variability in wave morphology than translaminar stimulation. All animals that received translaminar stimulation were neurologically normal at the 2-week evaluation, whereas 72% of animals receiving epidural stimulation manifested mild-to-moderate postoperative defects, with full recovery in only five of 18 cases. The deficit severity did not appear related to stimulus intensity. Loss of SSEP preceded neurologic damage in only two cases; both animals suffered severe neurologic deficits. Neurologic changes were accompanied by histologic changes.[83]

Intraoperative MEP is not as widespread as SSEP for several reasons. First, reproducible delivery of stimuli is more difficult than with SSEP. Second, profound sensitivity to commonly used anesthetic techniques has made definition of the optimal anesthetic technique difficult. Third, low and consistent level of neuromuscular blockade is required. All these problems are under active investigation and should be resolved.

▼
SUMMARY

The intraoperative monitoring of nervous system function should be a routine component of the operative management of patients at risk for neurologic injury. Although anesthetics alter the various monitoring modalities (EEG, sensory evoked potentials, motor evoked potentials), all modalities can be successfully monitored during a stable anesthesic that has been selected to minimize waveform depression. The optimal monitor depends on the neural tissue and risk and must be determined for each patient. An experienced monitoring team capable of using all techniques in conjunction with an anesthesia team capable of optimizing this anesthetic management to minimize depression of the neural wave generators used minimizes the risk of neural injury. Evoked potentials have an advantage over spontaneous potentials (EEG) in that the pathways are known so that the relationship between anatomic trespass and waveform changes are better correlated. Evoked potentials have a disadvantage in that the potential of the waveforms tend to be smaller than for spontaneous potentials, signal averaging is required, and thus there is a delay between neurologic changes and their recognition. The most commonly used evoked potentials are the SSEPs, which are used for spinal cord surgery as well as determining ischemic changes in the brain (the use of EEG vs. SSEP for monitoring of intraoperative brain ischemia is still a topic of debate). The ability to monitor motor tracks during spinal cord surgery has sustained an interest in MEPs, but their role has not, as yet, been determined.

References

1. Berenstein A, Young W, Ransohoff J et al: Somatosensory evoked potentials during spinal angiography and therapeutic transvascular embolization, *J Neurosurg* 0:777-785, 1984.
2. Boston JR, Davis PJ, Brandon BW et al: Rate of change of somatosensory evoked potentials during isoflurane anesthesia in newborn piglets, *Anesth Analg* 70:275-283, 1990.
3. Branston NM, Ladds A, Symon L et al: Comparison of the effects of ischaemia on early components of the somatosensory evoked potential in brainstem, thalamus, and cerebral cortex, *J Cereb Blood Flow Metab* 4:68-81, 1984.
4. Brinkman SD, Braun P, Ganji S et al: Neuropsychological performance one week after carotid endarterectomy reflects intraoperative ischemia, *Stroke* 15:497-503, 1984.
5. Calancie B, Klose KJ, Baier S et al: Isoflurane-induced attenuation of motor evoked potentials caused by electrical motor cortex stimulation during surgery, *J Neurosurg* 74:897-904, 1991.
6. Cedzich C, Schramm J, Fahbusch R: Are flash-evoked visual potentials useful for intraoperative monitoring of visual pathway function? *Neurosurgery* 21:709-715, 1987.
7. Cedzich C, Schramm J, Mengedoht CF et al: Factors that limit the use of flash visual evoked potentials for surgical monitoring, *Electroencephalogr Clin Neurophysiol* 71:142-145, 1988.
8. Chassard D, Joubaub A, Colson A et al: Auditory evoked potentials during propofol anaesthesia in man, *Br J Anaesth* 62:522-526, l989.
9. Chi OZ, Field C: Effects of isoflurane on visual evoked potentials in humans, *Anesthesiology* 65:328-330, 1986.
10. Chi OZ, McCoy CL, Field C: Effects of fentanyl anesthesia on visual evoked potentials in humans, *Anesthesiology* 67:827-830, 1987.
11. Chi OZ, Ryterband S, Field C: Visual evoked potentials during thiopentone–fentanyl–nitrous oxide anaesthesia in humans, *Can J Anesth* 36:637-640, 1989.
12. Chi OZ, Subramoni J, Jasaitis D: Visual evoked potentials during etomidate administration in humans, *Can J Anesth* 37:452-456, 1990.
13. Chi OZ, Field C: Effects of enflurane on visual evoked potentials in humans, *Br J Anaesth* 64:163-166, 1990.
14. Church MW, Gritzke R: Effects of ketamine anesthesia on the rat brainstem auditory evoked potential as a function of dose and stimulus intensity, *Electroencephalogr Clin Neurophysiol* 67:570-583, 1987.
15. Clark DL, Hosick EC, Rosner BS: Neurophysiological effects of differ-

ent anesthetics in unconscious man, *J Appl Physiol* 31:884-891, 1971.

16. Clark DL, Hosick EC, Adam N et al: Neural effects of isoflurane (Forane) in man, *Anesthesiology* 39:261-270, 1973.

17. Cracco RQ: Evaluation of conduction in central motor pathways: techniques, pathophysiology, and clinical interpretation, *Neurosurgery* 20:199-203, 1987.

18. Dinner DS, Luders H, Lesser RP et al: Intraoperative spinal somatosensory evoked potential monitoring, *J Neurosurg* 65:807-814, 1986.

19. Dolman J, Silvay G, Zappulla R et al: The effect of temperature, mean arterial pressure, and cardiopulmonary bypass flows on somatosensory evoked potential latency in man, *Thorac Cardiovasc Surgeon* 34:217-222, 1986.

20. Dowman R, Boisvert DP, Gelb AW et al: Changes in the somatosensory evoked potential during and immediately following temporary middle cerebral artery occlusion predict somatosensory cortex ischemic lesions in monkeys, *J Clin Neurophysiol* 7:269-281, 1990.

21. Doyle WJ, Fria TJ: The effects of hypothermia on the latencies of the auditory brain-stem response (ABR) in the rhesus monkey, *Electroencepha Clin Neurophysiol* 60:258-266, 1985.

22. Drummond, JC, Todd MM, Hoi Sang U: The effect of high dose sodium pentothal on brainstem auditory and median nerve evoked responses in humans, *Anesthesiology* 63:249-254, 1985.

23. Dubois M, Coppola R, Buchsbaum MS: Somatosensory evoked potential during whole body hyperthermia in humans, *Electroencephalogr Clin Neurophysiol* 52:157-162, 1981.

24. Dubois MY, Sato S, Chassy J: Effects of enflurane on brainstem auditory evoked response in humans, *Anesth Analg* 61:898-902. 1982.

25. Duncan PG, Sanders RA, McCullough DW: Preservation of auditory-evoked brainstem responses in anesthetized children, *Can Anaesth Soc J* 26:492-495, 1979.

26. Ebe M, Meier-Ewert KH, Broughton R: Effects of intravenous diazepam (Valium) upon evoked potentials of photosensitive epileptic and normal subjects, *Electroencephalogr Clin Neurophysiol* 27:429-435, 1969.

27. Edmonds HL Jr, Paloheimo MP, Backman MH et al: Transcranial magnetic motor evoked potentials (tcMMEP) for functional monitoring of motor pathways during scoliosis surgery, *Spine* 14:683-686, 1989.

28. Elmore JR, Gloviczki P, Harper CM et al: Failure of motor evoked potentials to predict neurologic outcome in experimental thoracic aortic occlusion, *J Vasc Surg* 14:131-139, 1991.

29. Fenwick P, Bushman J, Howard R et al: Contingent negative variation and evoked potential amplitude as a function of inspired nitrous oxide concentration, *Electroencephalogr Clin Neurophysiol* 47:473-482, 1979.

30. Fenwick P, Stone SA, Bushman J: Changes in the pattern reversal visual evoked potential as a function of inspired nitrous oxide concentration, *Electroencephalogr Clin Neurophysiol* 57:178-183, 1984.

31. Friedman WA, Kaplan BL, Day AL et al: Evoked potential monitoring during aneurysm operation: observations after fifty cases, *Neurosurgery* 20:678-687, 1987.

32. Friedman WA, Chadwick GM, Verhoeven FJ et al: Monitoring of somatosensory evoked potentials during surgery for middle cerebral artery aneurysms, *Neurosurgery* 29:83-88, 1991.

33. George SR, Taylor J: Somatosensory evoked potentials in neonates and infants: developmental and normative data, *Electroencephalogr Clin Neurophysiol* 80:94-102, 1991.

34. Ghaly RF et al: The effect of etomidate on transcranial magnetic-induced motor evoked potentials in primates, *Anesthesiology* 73:3A, 1990.

35. Ghaly RF, Stone JL, Aldrete A et al: Effects of incremental ketamine hydrochloride doses on motor evoked potentials (MEPs) following transcranial magnetic stimulation: a primate study, *J Neurosurg Anesthesiology* 2:79-85, 1990.

36. Ghaly RF, Stone JL, Levy WJ et al: The effect of etomidate on motor evoked potentials induced by transcranial magnetic stimulation in the monkey, *Neurosurgery* 27:936-942, 1990.

37. Ginsburg HH, Shetter AG, Raudzens PA: Postoperative paraplegia with preserved intraoperative somatosensory evoked potentials, *J Neurosurg* 63:296-300, 1985.

38. Godfrey RM, Mitchell KW: Somatosensory evoked potentials to electrical stimulation of the mental nerve, *Br J Oral Maxillofac Surg* 25:300-307, 1987.

39. Goitein KJ, Fainmesser P, Sohmer H: Cerebral perfusion pressure and auditory brain-stem responses in childhood CNS diseases, *Am J Dis Child* 137:777-781, 1983.

40. Gold S, Cahani M, Sohmer H et al: Effects of body temperature elevation on auditory nerve brain-stem evoked responses and EEGs in rats, *Electroencephalogr Clin Neurophysiol* 60:146-153, 1985.

41. Grossi EA, Laschinger JC, Krieger KH et al: Epidural-evoked potentials: a more specific indicator of spinal cord ischemia, *J Surg Res* 44:224-228, 1988.

42. Haghighi SS, Green KD, Oro JJ et al: Depressive effect of isoflurane anesthesia on motor evoked potentials, *Neurosurgery* 26:993-997, 1990.

43. Haghighi SS, Madsen R, Green DG et al: Suppression of motor evoked potentials by inhalation anesthetics, *J Neurosurg Anesth* 2:73-78, 1990.

44. Harkins SW, Benedetti C, Colpitts YH et al: Effects of nitrous oxide inhalation on brain potentials evoked by auditory and noxious dental stimulation, *Prog Neuropsychopharmacol Biol Psychiatry* 6:167-174, 1982.

45. Horsch S, DeVleeschauwer P, Ktenidis K: Intraoperative assessment of cerebral ischemia during carotid surgery, *J Cardiovasc Surg* 31:599-602, 1990.

46. Houston HG, McClelland RJ, Fenwick PBC: Effects of nitrous oxide on auditory cortical evoked potentials and subjective thresholds, *Br J Anaesth* 61:606-610, 1988.

47. Johnson R Jr: A triarchic model of P300 amplitude, *Psychophysiology* 23:367-384, 1986.

48. Kalmarchey R, Avila A, Symon L: The use of brainstem auditory evoked potentials during posterior fossa surgery as a monitor of brainstem function, *Acta Neurochir* 82:128-136, 1986.

49. Kartush JM: Electroneurography and intraoperative facial monitoring in contemporary neurotology, *Otolaryngol Head Neck Surg* 101:496-503, 1989.

50. Katayama Y, Tsubokawalt T, Maejima S: Corticospinal direct response in humans: identification of the motor cortex during intracranial surgery under general anaesthesia, *J Neurol Neurosurg Psychiatry* 51:50-59, 1988.

51. Kitagawa H, Itoh T, Takano H et al: Motor evoked potential monitoring during upper cervical spine surgery, *Spine* 14:1078-1083, 1989.

52. Knight RT, Brailowsky S: Auditory evoked potentials from the primary auditory cortex of the cat: topographic and pharmacological studies, *Electroencephalogr Clin Neurophysiol* 77:225-232, 1990.

53. Koehler RC, Backofen JE, McPherson RW et al: Cerebral blood flow and evoked potentials during Cushing response in sheep, *Am J Physiol* 256:H779-H788, 1989.

54. Koht A, Schutz W, Schmidt G et al: Effects of etomidate, midazolam, and thiopental on median nerve somatosensory evoked potentials and the additive effects of fentanyl and nitrous oxide, *Anesth Analg* 67:435-41, 1988.

55. Lam AM, Keane JF, Manninen PH: Monitoring of brainstem auditory evoked potentials during basilar artery occlusion in man, *Br J Anaesth* 57:924-928, 1985.

56. Lam AM, Manninen PH, Ferguson GG et al: Monitoring of electrophysiologic function during carotid endarterectomy: a comparison of somatosensory evoked potentials and conventional electroencephalogram, *Anesthesiology* 75:15-21, 1991.

57. LaMont RL, Wasson SL, Green MA: Spinal cord monitoring during spinal surgery using somatosensory spinal evoked potentials, *J Pediatr Orthop* 3:31-36, 1983.

58. Laschinger JC, Owen J, Rosenbloom M et al: Direct noninvasive monitoring of spinal cord motor function during thoracic aortic occlusion: use of motor evoked potentials, *J Vasc Surg* 7:161-171, 1988.

59. Leandri M, Parodi CI, Faval E: Early trigeminal evoked potentials in tumors of the base of the skull and trigeminal neuralgia, *Electroencephalogr Clin Neurophysiol* 71:114-124, 1988.

60. Legatt AD, Pedley TA, Emerson RG et al: Normal brain-stem auditory evoked potentials with abnormal latency-intensity studies in patients with acoustic neuromas, *Arch Neurol* 45:1326-1330, 1988.

61. Lesser RP, Raudzens P, Luders H et al: Postoperative neurological deficits may occur despite unchanged intraoperative somatosensory evoked potentials, *Ann Neurol* 19:22-25, 1986.

62. Lesser RP, Luders H, Dinner DS et al: The source of paradoxical lateralization of cortical evoked potentials to posterior tibial nerve stimulation, *Neurology* 37:82-88, 1987.

63. Loughman BA, Anderson SK, Hetreed MA et al: Effects of halothane on motor evoked potential recorded in the extradural space, *Br J Anaesth* 63:561-564, 1989.

64. Lubicky JP, Spadaro JA, Yuan HA et al: Variability of somatosensory cortical evoked potential monitoring during spinal surgery, *Spine* 14:790-798, 1989.

65. Manninen PH, Lam AM, Nantau WE: Monitoring of somatosensory evoked potentials during temporary arterial occlusion in cerebral aneurysm surgery, *J Neurosurg Anesth* 2:97-104, 1990.

66. Markland ON, Warren CH, Moorthy SS et al: Monitoring of multimodality evoked potentials during open heart surgery under hypothermia, *Electroencephalogr Clin Neurophysiol* 59:432-440, 1984.

67. Matsumiya N, Koehler RC, Traystman RJ: Consistency of cerebral blood flow and evoked potential alterations with reversible focal ischemia in cats, *Stroke* 21:908-916, 1990.

68. McPherson RW, Szymanski J, Rogers MC: Somatosensory evoked potential changes in position-related brainstem ischemia, *Anesthesiology* 61:88-90, 1984.

69. McPherson RW, Mahla M, Johnson R et al: Effects of enflurane, isoflurane and nitrous oxide on somatosensory evoked potentials during fentanyl anesthesia, *Anesthesiology* 62:626-633, 1985.

70. McPherson RW, Sell B, Traystman RJ: Effects of thiopental, fentanyl, and etomidate on upper extremity somatosensory evoked potentials in humans, *Anesthesiology* 65:584-589, 1986.

71. Momma F, Wang AD, Symon L: Effects of temporary arterial occlusion on somatosensory evoked responses in aneurysm surgery, *Surg Neurol* 27:343-352, 1987.

72. Moulton R, Kresta P, Ramirez M et al: Continuous automated monitoring of somatosensory evoked potentials in posttraumatic coma, *J Trauma* 31:676-685, 1991.

73. Nakamura M, Nishida S, Shibasaki H: Deterioration of average evoked potential waveform due to asynchronous averaging and its compensation, *IEEE Trans Biomed Eng* 38:309-312, 1991.

74. Nataloni S, Gentili M, Pagni R et al: Prognostic value of brainstem auditory evoked potentials in pediatric patients with traumatic coma, *Resuscitation* 16:127-131, 1988.

75. North RB, Drenger B, Beattie C et al: Monitoring of spinal cord stimulation evoked potentials during thoracoabdominal aneurysm surgery, *Neurosurgery* 28:325-330, 1991.

76. Pathak KS, Brown RH, Cascorbi HF et al: Effect of fentanyl and morphine on intraoperative somatosensory evoked potentials, *Anesth Analg* 63:833-837, 1984.

77. Pathak KS, Ammadio M, Kalamchi A et al: Effects of halothane, enflurane, and isoflurane on somatosensory evoked potentials during nitrous oxide anesthesia, *Anesthesiology* 66:753-757, 1987.

78. Persson A, Peterson E, Wahlin A: EEG changes during general anaesthesia with enflurane (Ethrane^R) in comparison with ether, *Acta Anaesth Scand* 22:339-348, 1978.

79. Peterson DO, Drummond JC, Todd MM: Effects of halothane, enflurane, isoflurane, and nitrous oxide on somatosensory evoked potentials in humans, *Anesthesiology* 65:35-40, 1986.

80. Powers SK, Bolger CA, Edwards MS: Spinal cord pathways mediating somatosensory evoked potentials, *J Neurosurg* 57:472-482, 1982.

81. Pritchard WS: Psychophysiology of P300, *Psychol Bull* 89:506-540, 1981.

82. Russ W, Kling D, Loesevitz A et al: Effect of hypothermia on visual evoked potentials (VEP) in humans, *Anesthesiology* 61:207-210, 1984.

83. Sabato S, Agresta CA, Freeman GM et al: Safety versus efficacy of spinal cord stimulation for the generation of

motor-evoked potentials in the rat, *J Neurotrauma* 8:27-44, 1991.

84. Samra SK, Lilly DJ, Rush NL et al: Fentanyl anesthesia and human brainstem auditory evoked potentials, *Anesthesiology* 61:261-265, 1984.

85. Samra SK, Sorkin LS: Enhancement of somatosensory evoked potentials by etomidate in cats: an investigation of its site of action, *Anesthesiology* 74:499-503, 1991.

86. Scheepstra GL, de Lange JJ, Booij LH et al: Median nerve evoked potentials during propofol anaesthesia, *Br J Anaesth* 62:92-94, 1989.

87. Schmid UD, Hess CW, Ludin HP: Somatosensory evoked potentials following nerve and segmental stimulation do not confirm cervical radiculopathy with sensory deficit, *J Neurol Neurosurg Psychiatry* 51:182-187, 1988.

88. Schorn V, Lennon V, Bickford R: Temperature effects on the brainstem evoked responses (BAERS) of the rat, *Proc San Diego Biomed Symp* 16:313-318, 1977.

89. Schubert A, Drummond JC, Garfin SR: The influence of stimulus presentation rate on the cortical amplitude and latency of intraoperative somatosensory-evoked potential recordings in patients with varying degrees of spinal cord injury, *Spine* 12:969-973, 1987.

90. Schubert A, Licina MG, Lineberry PJ: The effect of ketamine on human somatosensory evoked potentials and its modification by nitrous oxide, *Anesthesiology* 72:33-39, l990.

91. Schubert A, Licina MG, Lineberry PJ et al: The effect of intrathecal morphine on somatosensory evoked potentials in awake humans, *Anesthesiology* 75:401-405, 1991.

92. Schweiger H, Kamp HD, Dinkel M: Somatosensory evoked potentials during carotid artery surgery: experience in 400 operations, *Surgery* 109:602-609, 1991.

93. Sebel, PS, Erwin, CW, Neville WK: Effects of halothane and enflurane on far and near field somatosensory evoked potentials, *Br J Anaesth* 59:l492-l496, 1987.

94. Sharma HS, Winkler T, Stalberg E et al: Evaluation of traumatic spinal cord edema using evoked potentials recorded from the spinal epidural space. An experimental study in the rat, *J Neurol Sci* 102:150-162, 1991.

95. Sloan TB, Ronai AK, Toleikis JR et al: Improvement of intraoperative somatosensory evoked potentials by etomidate, *Anesth Analg* 67:582-585, 1988.

96. Sloan TB, Fugina ML, Toleikis JR: Effects of midazolam on median nerve somatosensory evoked potentials, *Br J Anaesth* 64:590-593, 1990.

97. Sohmer H, Gafni M, Chisin R: Auditory nerve–brainstem potentials in man and cat under hypoxic and hypercapnic conditions, *Electroencephalogr Clin Neurophysiol* 53:506-512, 1982.

98. Sohmer H, Gafni M, Goitein K et al: Auditory nerve brainstem evoked potentials in cats during manipulation of the cerebral perfusion pressure, *Electroencephalogr Clin Neurophysiol* 55:198-202, 1983.

99. Sohmer H, Gafni M, Havatselet G: Persistence of auditory nerve response and absence of brain-stem response in severe cerebral ischaemia, *Electroencephalogr Clin Neurophysiol* 58:65-72, 1984.

100. Sohmer H, Freeman S, Malachi S: Multi-modality evoked potentials in hypoxemia, *Electroencephalogr Clin Neurophysiol* 64:328-333, 1986.

101. Sohmer H, Freeman S, Gafni M et al: The depression of the auditory nerve brain-stem evoked response in hypoxemia—mechanism and site of effect, *Electroencephalogr Clin Neurophysiol* 64:334-338, 1986.

102. Sohmer H, Goitein K: Auditory brain-stem (ABP) and somatosensory evoked potentials (SEP) in an animal model of a synaptic lesion: elevated plasma barbiturate levels, *Electroencephalogr Clin Neurophysiol* 71:382-388, 1988.

103. Soustiel JF, Feinsod M, Hafner H: Short latency trigeminal evoked potentials: normative data and clinical correlations, *Electroencephalogr Clin Neurophysiol* 80:119-125, 1991.

104. Stejskal L, Travnicek V, Sourek K et al: Somatosensory evoked potentials in deep hypothermia, *Appl Neurophysiol* 43:1-7, 1980.

105. Svensson LG, Patel V, Robinson MF et al: Influence of preservation of perfusion of intraoperatively identified spinal cord blood supply on spinal motor evoked potentials and paraple-

gia after aortic surgery, *J Vasc Surg* 13:355-365, 1991.

106. Symon L, Wang AD, Costa De Silva IE et al: Perioperative use of somatosensory evoked responses in aneurysm surgery, *J Neurosurg* 6:269-275, 1984.

107. Synek VM: Validity of median nerve somatosensory evoked potentials in the diagnosis of supraclavicular brachial plexus lesions, *Electroencephalogr Clin Neurophysiol* 65:27-35, 1986.

108. Thornton C, Catley DM, Jordan C et al: Enflurane anaesthesia causes graded changes in the brainstem and early cortical auditory evoked response in man, *Br J Anaesth* 55:479-486, 1983.

109. Thornton C, Heneghan CP, James MF et al: Effects of halothane or enflurane with controlled ventilation on auditory evoked potentials, *Br J Anaesth* 56:315-323, 1984.

110. Uhl RR, Squires KC, Bruce DL et al: Effect of halothane anesthesia on the human cortical visual evoked response, *Anesthesiology* 53:273-276, 1980.

111. Van-Rheineck-Leyssius AT, Kalkman CJ, Bovil JG: Influence of moderate hypothermia on posterior tibial nerve, *Anesth Analg* 65:475-480, 1986.

112. Vaz CA, McPherson RW, Thakor NV: Adaptive fourier series modeling of time-varying evoked potentials: study of human somatosensory evoked response to etomidate anesthetic, *Electroencephalogr Clin Neurophysiol* 80:108-118, 1991.

113. Veilleux M, Daube JR, Cucchiara RF: Monitoring of cortical evoked potentials during surgical procedures, *Mayo Clin Proc* 62:256-264, 1987.

114. Wolfe DE, Drummond JC: Differential effects of isoflurane/nitrous oxide on posterior tibial somatosensory evoked responses of cortical and subcortical origin, *Anesth Analg* 67:852-859, 1988.

115. Wood CC, Spencer DD, Allison T et al: Localization of human sensorimotor cortex during surgery by cortical surface recording of somatosensory evoked potentials, *J Neurosurg* 68:99-111, 1988.

116. Xiao T, Zu-yuan R: Magnetic transcranial motor and somatosensory evoked potentials in cervical spondy-

litic myelopathy, *Chin Med J* 104:409-415, 1991.

117. York DH, Chabot RJ, Gaines RW: Response variability of somatosensory evoked potentials during scoliosis surgery, *Spine* 12:864-876, 1987.

118. Zenter J, Kiss I, Ebner A: Influence of anesthetics—nitrous oxide in particular—on electromyographic response evoked by transcranial electrical stimulation of the cortex, *Neurosurgery* 24:253-256, 1989.

119. Zentner J, Rieder G: Diagnostic significance of motor evoked potentials in space-occupying lesions of the brainstem and spinal cord, *Eur Arch Psychiatr Neurol Sci* 289:285-289, 1990.

120. Zornow MH, Grafe MD, Tybor C et al: Preservation of evoked potentials in a case of anterior spinal artery syndrome, *Electroencephalogr Clin Neurophysiol* 77:137-139, 1990.

10

Neurophysiologic Brain Monitoring: Electroencephalography

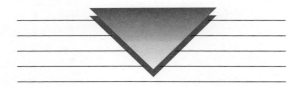

WARREN J. LEVY

For many years, electroencephalography—the recording of the spontaneous electrical activity of the brain—was the only noninvasive technique available for monitoring the central nervous system. As a result it was often applied injudiciously, and failures, misunderstandings, and erroneous conclusions litter the historical electroencephalogram (EEG) monitoring literature. Periodically, technological advances—such as the application of computerized analysis techniques—have rejuvenated interest in the EEG. Unfortunately, many of the early misconceptions about the EEG persist, and, to the extent that they do, the proper role for perioperative EEG monitoring will be misunderstood. Only by understanding the source of the EEG and the effect of external factors on the generation of the EEG can the appropriate role for EEG monitoring be derived. Satisfactory use of the EEG in this role necessitates a thorough understanding of technologic issues, a complex area that continually diversifies as researchers develop more alternatives to decipher the hidden implication of the tracings. Finally, in

practical terms, the application of EEG to clinical care will be discussed.

Although commonly referred to as a recording of "brain waves," the EEG is not generated by the brain as a whole. Only one specific portion of cortex—the superficial layer of pyramidal cells—generates this activity and then only as a result of the postsynaptic potentials that occur on the dendrites that are oriented perpendicular to the cortical surface.[12] Action potentials make no direct contributions to the signal eventually measured as the EEG. In addition, in the absence of a relatively uniform anatomic pattern, the electrical charges (dipole moments) produced by the dendritic postsynaptic potentials would offset each other. However, the parallel structure of these dendrites allows the dipole moments to summate to a measurable extent, producing electrical activity that can be recorded on the surface of the brain.[50]

This electrocorticogram differs in several important aspects from the EEG, which is recorded on the scalp. The

228

cortical electrogram is a more localized phenomenon, often differing markedly from activity recorded only millimeters away. The EEG, by comparison, shows regional differences only over much larger distances because the electric fields generated by nearby (but electrically isolated) brain tissue summate widely in the more conductive bone and soft tissues of the head. Thus very focal differences are blurred and extraneous factors, such as bone thickness and density (or absence) and soft tissue abnormalities, may produce small but definable differences in the EEG.[20]

The formation of the EEG by summation of cortical activity in the overlying tissues is also different from the formation of electrocardiogram (ECG). The ECG is generated by the organized conduction of a single impulse through the entire mass of tissue. Because such a discrete impulse has a single vector, all recording electrodes reflect the same electrical activity, modified only by the three-dimensional geometry of the vectors of the recording electrodes and the cardiac electrical wave. By comparison, the summation of the many cortical potentials into EEG is strongly influenced by the relative distances of those cortical generators from the recording electrode, as well as the geometry of the vectors of the individual potentials and the electrodes.[20] Because the contribution of a dipole to the sum decreases as the square of the distance to the measurement electrode, the EEG reflects almost exclusively nearby electrical activity. In fact, cortical activity more than 2 cm from the recording electrode represents less than 10% of the observed activity and thus is easily masked by nearby activity, even if such activity is actually lower in amplitude.[17]

There are several important implications for EEG monitoring that may be inferred from this discussion. First, because the EEG is derived from only cortical tissue, severe injury to subcortical structures can produce disastrous neurologic consequences with little, if any, change in the EEG. Second, multichannel recordings from many electrodes will be necessary to adequately survey electrical activity. Finally, areas of low activity will appear smaller than they actually are because of electrical spread from adjacent areas; conversely, high activity areas will appear larger. In the extreme case, very small lesions producing little EEG activity (e.g., lacunar infarcts) may not be definable at all.

RECORDING TECHNOLOGY

Anyone familiar with ECG monitoring in the operating room knows how difficult it is to obtain a baseline that is sufficiently flat to allow accurate measurement of S-T segment abnormalities. Now consider that essentially all of the EEG activity of importance occurs in less than the smallest significant S-T change, and the complexity of perioperative EEG monitoring becomes apparent. Technical considerations take on enhanced importance; short-cuts acceptable for the measurement of high-amplitude signals are no longer good enough. Contamination of the EEG with electrical artifact can destroy its usefulness and seriously mislead the

unwary, particularly when the EEG is being monitored for the loss of activity and the observed "activity" is actually artifact. No amount of filtration, computerized processing, or other manipulation will remove artifact once it has been incorporated into the signal. Only careful attention to the technical details will provide data suitable for interpretation.

The skin, by virtue of its cornified layers and oils, is a major impediment to the passage of an electrical signal. To record the EEG it is necessary to reduce this obstruction (known as the impedance) to acceptable values. Needle electrodes provide one approach, simply bypassing the high-impedance layers of the skin, and placing the electrode just beneath the surface. Unfortunately, needle electrodes have a small surface area, and impedance is increased by a small surface. Because of this, needle electrodes can never provide as high quality a recording as a well-applied surface electrode. In addition, needle electrodes are traumatic to both nerve endings and blood vessels, the former commonly producing a pain response during electrode placement, while the latter—whose perforation is likely in the highly vascular tissues of the scalp—may produce a significant hematoma, which itself interferes with recording. Needles are inherently unstable, coming out of the skin as easily as they enter it and moving within the skin whenever the tension on the wire changes. Their need to be sterilized between uses and placed in an aseptic fashion further complicates their placement, but their ease of placement within a sterile field can be most advantageous. Thus they have a niche in the intraoperative monitoring of the EEG, albeit a limited one.

Surface electrodes have numerous potential advantages over needles but require attention to detail to realize this potential. Because the skin impedance will not be bypassed by piercing, it must be reduced by removal of oils and abrasion to remove some of the cornified cells. A commercial preparation, Omniprep, is most useful for this process, although other solvents and abrasives are also satisfactory. Once the impedance has been reduced, an ionic medium can conduct the electrical current between the skin and the electrode wire. Such a conductive substance may be a jelly or a paste. The latter dries more quickly and may lose its conductivity when doing so but has the advantage of providing sufficient support for the electrode, so that additional adhesives are unnecessary. Electrode jelly provides no such support, necessitating the additional step of gluing the electrode to the scalp.

It is this final process, fixing the electrode in position, that separates the functional performance of stick-on and standard disk EEG electrodes. The conventional disk electrodes are secured with gauze soaked in collodion, which clings tightly to the scalp and adjacent hair despite the lack of a smooth surface for adhesion. Stick-on electrodes rarely form an equally stable connection, unless the subject is bald or the head is shaved. This weaker mechanical contact predisposes to electrode movement, which—in turn—

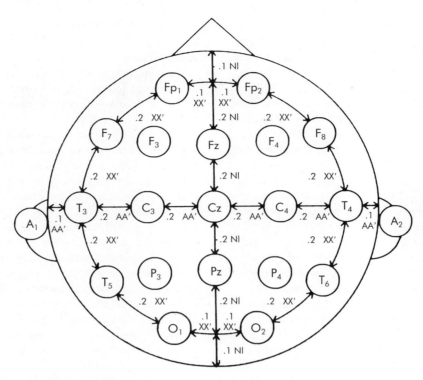

FIG. 10-1 International 10-20 system. Twenty-one electrode positions are defined by 10% or 20% of three measurements: the nasion-inion *(NI)* distance, the preauricular *(AA')* distance, and the hemicircumference *(XX')*. *(From Kaplan JA, editor:* Cardiac anesthesia, *ed 2, Philadelphia, 1987, WB Saunders, p 322.)*

changes electrode impedance. Changes in electrode impedance is very undesirable because it adversely affects the EEG recording. Although the details of this process are beyond the scope of this chapter, the need to ensure low electrode impedances throughout the monitoring process is a major consideration that cannot be taken lightly. Depending on the design of the EEG amplifiers and the technique used to measure it, electrode impedances up to 3000 ohms may be acceptable. Values over 10,000 ohms will rarely allow adequate intraoperative recordings to be obtained.

Previously in this chapter, the considerations of the formation of the EEG were discussed and the limited spread of the electrical activity emphasized. The natural corollary is the need for many electrodes to allow examination of the electrical activity of different areas of the brain. It is most useful if the electrodes can be positioned on the basis of easily obtained surface measurements that place electrodes in fairly constant relationships to the known cortical anatomy, thus simplifying clinical inference from the recording. The International 10-20 system is one such formula for electrode positioning (Fig. 10-1).[30] Even though it is not exhaustive in its coverage of cortical activity, much intraoperative monitoring is done with only a subset of this montage. Regardless of the number of electrodes used, careful electrode positioning is important to ensure that compari-

sons among patients refer to comparable neurologic structures.

There are numerous ways of combining these electrodes to record cortical activity; to some extent the pattern of activity is influenced by the pattern of electrode interconnections. There are two major classifications of linkage: bipolar (Fig. 10-2) and referential (Fig. 10-3). Referential montages may be subdivided into common reference and average reference techniques.

It is important to remember that all recordings are bipolar in nature (i.e., the measurement is made between two active electrodes with a third serving as the neutral or ground). A bipolar montage is a pattern of connecting individual electrodes so that both of the active electrodes lie over cortex, and the recording represents the difference of this activity. Changes occurring near both electrodes, such as diffuse synchronous activity, are not amplified because there is only a small difference in the voltage at adjacent electrodes. Bipolar recordings are quite useful for locating focal phenomena, particularly when displayed as an analog multichannel recording.[42] In such a recording, a focal phenomenon creates a higher voltage in nearby channels. In addition, because each electrode in a bipolar chain functions as the negative for one channel and the positive for the next, the direction of the pen deflection for a specific

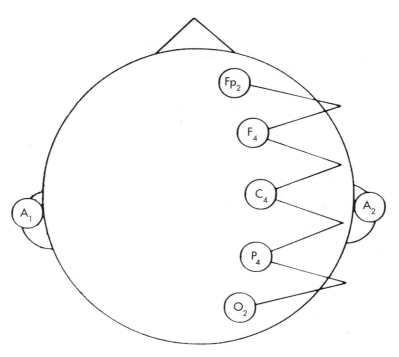

FIG. 10-2   Bipolar montage. The right parasagittal electrodes are connected in a bipolar chain generating four recorded channels: Fp_2-F_4, F_4-C_4, C_4-P_4, P_4-O_2. *(From Lake C, editor:* Clinical monitoring, *Philadelphia, 1988, WB Saunders, p 692.)*

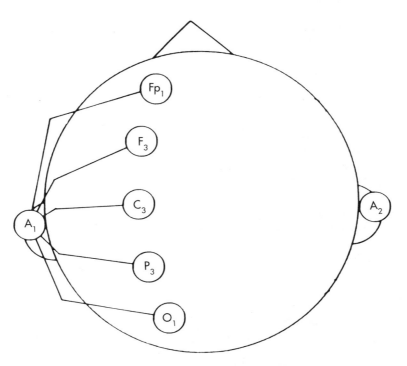

FIG. 10-3   Referential montage. Left parasagittal electrodes are connected in a common reference montage using the ear *(A₁)* as one of the active electrodes for each recorded pair. Five channels, Fp_1-A_1, F_3-A_1, C_3-A_1, P_3-A_1, O_1-A_1, are recorded. *(From Lake C, editor:* Clinical monitoring, *Philadelphia, 1988, WB Saunders, p 693.)*

event is opposite in channels on opposite sides of the lesion.

Referential montages record activity between pairs of electrodes, all of which have one electrode (the reference electrode) in common. One consequence of this arrangement is that the interelectrode distances are large and variable. Thus diffuse activity is more easily observed in this type of montage. Another consequence is that any activity in the area of the reference electrode is displayed in all of the channels recorded. Not only does this imply that the reference electrode should be placed over a quiescent area, but this places exceptional demands on the quality of the signal recorded at the reference electrode. Any artifact occurring at the referential electrode can obliterate the entire recording. On the other hand, if this reference electrode contains no cortical electrical signal, the recorded activity represents only the electrical activity generated in proximity to the other electrode. This explains the common, albeit incorrect, terminology of "unipolar" electrodes for referential montages.

Common reference montages contain a single electrode (usually the mastoid or earlobe) that serves as the reference for all ipsilateral channels. Often both ears are connected, providing a channel that may be used as the reference for both sides of the head. Carried to the extreme, this linkage of electrodes evolves into the average reference montage, in which the reference "electrode" is the average of all the active electrodes linked together.

All referential montages share the characteristic that any activity present at the reference electrode is seen in all channels of the recording. If the reference electrode of a common reference montage is technically unsatisfactory, the entire recording will suffer. This extreme sensitivity to the quality of the reference electrode poses potential problems for intraoperative recordings. The problem is, in some respects, even worse for average reference montages because any noise from any electrode contributes to noise in all channels. If a full 21-electrode montage is used, the contribution of a single channel's artifact is only 5%. Unfortunately, artifact is often many times the amplitude of the actual EEG and, with a less extensive montage, artifact from a single electrode can seriously interfere with the entire montage. The sensitivity of the referential montages to electrical noise is the primary reason for suggesting the use of the bipolar montages for intraoperative recordings. The relative robustness of linked bipolar chains allows the identification of electrodes that may generate artifact and prevents contamination of other data.

Modern EEG equipment may allow "post-montaging," a process in which the EEG that would have been recorded using a bipolar montage is derived from a stored, referentially recorded signal. This process can be very useful for the neurologist who is examining an infrequent phenomenon because the localizing attributes of the bipolar chain can be explored at will, and uncommon linkages, such as coronal or diagonal chains, can be examined. For purposes

of perioperative monitoring, however, this capability would seem to be less important because a clinical decision needs to be rendered quickly on the basis of readily identifiable changes in the EEG when recorded under notably adverse conditions of electrical and mechanical artifact. For this, the bipolar montage appears well suited.

Because of the difficult monitoring conditions present in the operating room, artifact can be problematic, even though proper electrode application and recording techniques have been used. Both low- and high-frequency artifact can occur, and, in the proper circumstances, judicious use of filters may improve recording quality with minimal impairment of the record. More frequently, however, excessive filtration is employed in lieu of adequate recording technique, and the resultant recording is seriously inadequate.

The standard band width for EEG recording extends from 0.3 to 70 Hz. This means that the amplifier gain at 0.3 and 70 Hz is 50% (or 3 db lower than) the gain at frequencies in the middle of this range. This band width results in very constant amplification of activity between 1 and 35 Hz. Filters (which are also described by their 3 db points) may be used to remove a modest amount of high- or low-frequency noise, (e.g., by adding a 1 Hz low-frequency or 30 Hz high-frequency filter). Unfortunately, such filtration often does not eliminate the artifact, and more aggressive filtration with 2 or 4 Hz low-frequency or 15 to 20 Hz high-frequency cut-offs seriously distorts the EEG. There is a very important role for filtering in all digital signal processing: the prevention of aliasing. Aliasing is a phenomenon that occurs when a high frequency signal is sampled at an inadequate rate (Fig. 10-4). When the analog signal is only sampled once per cycle, the sampled points also describe a lower-frequency signal as well. Thus the high-frequency signal is "aliased" down to a lower frequency. By filtering high-frequency signals that are out of the range of interest for the EEG, it is possible to ensure that aliasing does not occur. This is particularly important for some of the automated processing techniques whose

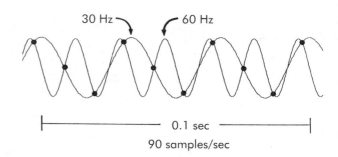

FIG. 10-4   Aliasing. Illustration demonstrates aliasing of a high-frequency signal resulting from an inadequate digitization rate. At the points where digitization occurs, the 30 and 60 Hz signals have the same amplitude. *(From Lake C, editor:* Clinical monitoring, *Philadelphia, 1988, WB Saunders, p 704.)*

computational complexity increases dramatically as the number of samples increases. Such filtering, however, is designed into the system by the design engineers; supplemental filtering of the signal should not be necessary and a band width of 1 to 35 Hz is the most limited range of frequencies suitable for routine intraoperative monitoring.

It is also worth emphasizing that the foregoing discussion is limited to artifact at the extremes of the frequencies of interest in the EEG. Artifact can also occur within the frequencies of interest. No amount of filtering or processing can eliminate such artifact, and any attempt to use filtering to rectify technical problems of this type can only reduce the recorded signal to rubbish. The very best that one can hope to do when such artifact occurs is to recognize it and attempt to visually interpret the EEG while mentally removing the offending signal.

Such visual identification of artifact is a skill that is acquired only with repeated experience. There are few guidelines, except perhaps that the observed activity does not look like an EEG recording—a somewhat useless suggestion if one is inexperienced in EEG interpretation. Among the more recognizable artifacts exemplified in Fig. 10-5 are 60-Hz line noise; ECG, whose identification is simplified by a concurrent ECG; and muscle artifact, which is rarely

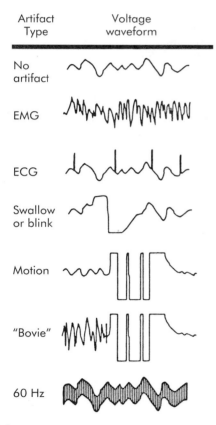

FIG. 10-5 Artifact. Examples of a variety of forms of artifact are shown. In most cases, the original EEG is obliterated. *(From Rampil I: Anesthesiol Clin North Am 10:3,692, 1992.)*

a problem during general anesthesia although it can obliterate the baseline EEG when the patient is shivering before induction of anesthesia. Other sources of artifact include electrocautery, movement, optic and oral muscles, sweating, and roller head perfusion devices.

The Analog Recording

As has already been implied, the EEG is the measurement of an electrical voltage that varies with time. By recording this voltage as a vertical displacement on horizontally moving paper, a conventional or strip chart recording can be produced. Paper speeds of 60 mm/sec may be used when high fidelity is required; slower ones may suffice for some aspects of intraoperative monitoring that do not demand the recognition of discrete waveforms. Even at slow speeds, long periods of monitoring generate large amounts of paper, and finding relevant sections for comparison may be difficult. Electronic recording and playback can reduce the amount of paper required. Unfortunately, even when stored electronically, the analog tracing is an inefficient display form at best, and electronic data retrieval is almost as cumbersome as a large pile of paper tracings.

Despite these shortcomings, high-speed (30 mm/sec) paper tracings of the EEG are the standard display technique. Regardless of what computerized analysis and display may be performed on this data, the individual using EEG monitoring intraoperatively must be familiar with the EEG presented in this fashion. Most forms of artifact (cardiac electrical activity is one of the most common) are more recognizable in the strip chart than after further processing. The presence of synchronous spikelike waves in the EEG and an audible pulse indicator identify this form of electrical contamination immediately. The strip chart also forms the basis for conventional EEG interpretation.

Conventional interpretation of the EEG is performed by the inspection of the tracing for characteristic wave patterns that have been identified as indicative of either normal or abnormal cortical activity. Waves are defined not only by their frequency but by their topography, shape, and association with other waves. All of these characteristics may be important and should be considered when describing EEG activity. Nowhere is this distinction as important as when distinguishing between the alpha rhythm and other EEG activity in the alpha-frequency range. The alpha band of frequencies extends from 8 to 12 Hz. Alpha waves (Fig. 10-6) are patterns of waves predominating in occipital regions that are seen in normal individuals who are resting with eyes closed and that are obliterated by mental activity, especially visual attention.[52] Typically, these waves have frequencies in the alpha band; however, the alpha rhythm slows with age and an alpha variant with frequencies in the range of 7 to 8 Hz can be seen.[49] Another characteristic of the alpha rhythm is bilateral synchrony. Activity from symmetric regions of occipital cortex tends to occur simultaneously and is therefore coherent.[19] Such coherence is not seen in another characteristic alpha-frequency waveform, the mu

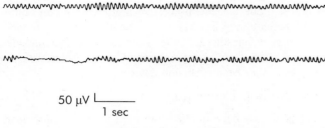

50 μV
1 sec

FIG. 10-6 Alpha rhythm. This example of alpha rhythm shows the amplitude and frequency characteristics of this pattern. The sample was obtained from electrodes in the P_3 and O_1 locations in an awake subject with his eyes closed. The lower segment follows continuously after the upper one. *(From Lake C, editor: Clinical monitoring, Philadelphia, 1988, WB Saunders, p 696.)*

rhythm.[67] The mu rhythm also differs in location from the alpha rhythm, being located centrally rather than occipitally. The mu rhythm is attenuated by manual, not visual, activity.

Other characteristic patterns of activity include spike or spike and wave activity, commonly associated with seizures and often occurring about three times a second. "Sharp waves" have a similar shape to spikes but are slower, with a duration of 80 to 200 msec (5 to 12 Hz), compared with spikes, which have durations of 1 to 80 msec (125 to 1000 Hz).

Sleep spindles are fusiform bursts of electrical activity seen during certain stages of natural sleep. Commonly occurring at about 14 Hz, this pattern is rarely seen during anesthesia, emphasizing the distinction between normal sleep and drug-induced anesthesia.

Burst-suppression activity (Fig. 10-7) is another pattern of activity that would be highly abnormal in an unanesthetized (or undrugged) individual. It is, however, commonly produced by a large number of anesthetic agents—including barbiturates, isoflurane, and desflurane—and may be

seen with almost any anesthetic when hypothermia is added.

Distinct from these identifiable patterns, and composing the vast majority of the EEG activity recorded during anesthesia, are waves that are not specifically associated with recognizable entities or specific patterns. Such activity is commonly described by its location and frequency. The classical frequency bands are delta (below 4 Hz), theta (4 to 8 Hz), alpha (8 to 12 Hz) and beta (above 12 Hz). Beta activity is sometimes divided into beta 1 (12 to 20 Hz) and beta 2 (20 Hz and above) classes although it is not clear that this is either necessary, useful, or desirable. In fact, in some situations, the entire process of describing EEG activity in fixed, classical bands is misleading and seriously distorts the representation of the EEG activity.

Fig. 10-8 exemplifies the type of EEG behavior most seriously misrepresented by this process. There is both slow- and fast-wave activity present, a low-frequency component at 1 to 2 Hz, and a high-frequency component that slows from 15 to 20 Hz to about 8 Hz during the roughly 5 minutes separating each of the three samples. Samples of EEG activity recorded between those shown would also show intermediate frequencies, confirming the gradual slowing of a constant band of activity.

The effect of interpreting activity in arbitrary bands is seen most clearly in Fig. 10-9, in which the previous tracing is simplified to a single Gaussian distribution of frequencies centered in the alpha band. As this activity is shifted linearly (in Hz) the activity changes in a markedly nonlinear fashion, emphasizing the misrepresentation produced by lumping activity into defined bands and consequently implying that changes across the edges of bands are somehow more important than those within the band.

The major problem that occurs when using the unprocessed EEG for intraoperative monitoring is its inconvenience. It is impractical to watch the recording continuously, yet after a minute or less the EEG pattern disappears from the CRT or chart recorder into an electronic or paper morass from which it can be extracted only with great ef-

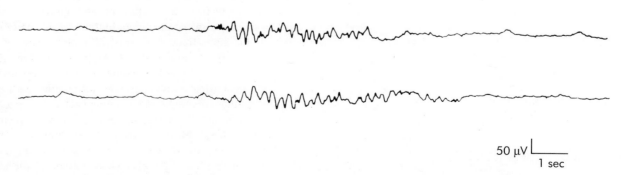

50 μV
1 sec

FIG. 10-7 Burst suppression. This example of burst-suppression activity was recorded during hypothermic cardiopulmonary bypass while the patient was under isoflurane-induced anesthesia. The lower segment follows continuously after the upper one. *(From Lake C, editor: Clinical monitoring, Philadelphia, 1988, WB Saunders, p 705.)*

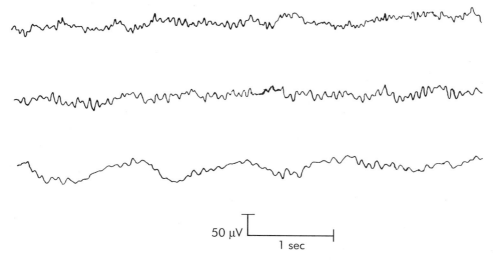

FIG. 10-8   Mixed-frequency EEG. Three segments of EEG recorded from the same individual at 5-minute intervals show mixtures of low-frequency oscillations at 1 to 2 Hz and higher frequency components at 8 to 20 Hz. The slowing of the higher-frequency activity was gradual through this recording period and would be misrepresented by presentation of the data as power in specific fixed bands. *(From Levy WJ:* Anesthesiology *55:254, 1980.)*

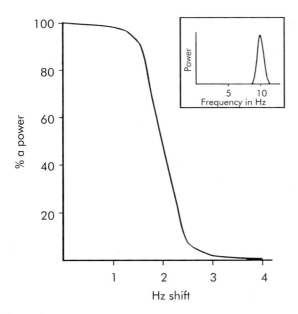

FIG. 10-9   Effect of banding. When EEG activity *(shown by the hypothetical distribution graphed in the inset)* slows, the percent of power in a band changes very slowly until the edge of the distribution reaches the edge of the band. Then the percentage of power changes precipitously, showing the distortion produced by artificially banding the data. *(From Lake C, editor:* Clinical monitoring, *Philadelphia, 1988, WB Saunders, p 700.)*

fort. In large measure, this problem can be traced to the disparity between the time course of intraoperative events (minutes) and the time course of EEG waves (fractions of seconds). The obvious solution to this problem is to develop a system that automatically analyzes the waveform activity and displays it at a rate more like that of intraoperative events.

Automated EEG Processing

Perhaps one would expect that such a straightforward goal, the display of EEG waveform information at a slower rate, could be easily and simply achieved. If, as is the case with the ECG, it were known exactly which components or waveforms were to be extracted from the EEG and displayed for monitoring, it would be easy to design an automated EEG system. Unfortunately, it is not clear which components of the EEG (if any) are unimportant. Because the EEG may demonstrate aspects of both random and non-random behavior, there is even disagreement about the suitability of some numeric analysis techniques for EEG analysis. Such issues have resulted in the development of numerous approaches to EEG analysis.

One of the simplest approaches to EEG analysis is known as period-amplitude analysis. This technique analyzes the underlying waveform by detecting the duration (period) of a wave, from which its frequency is easily calculated. The size (amplitude) of the wave is then calculated as well. The process is repeated for each individual wave. At least two different detection algorithms are commonly used to identify waves, and several alternative approaches exist for measuring amplitude as well. Because these dif-

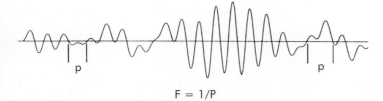

F = 1/P

FIG. 10-10 Zero-crossing analysis. This example of period analysis shows how the frequency of waves may be computed by measuring the amount of time before the waveform changes polarity (crosses the axis). For any wave the equation F = 1/P gives the equivalent frequency. *(From Lake C, editor:* Clinical monitoring, *Philadelphia, 1988, WB Saunders, p 699.)*

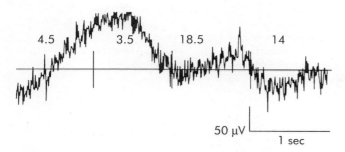

FIG. 10-11 Variability of zero-crossing analysis. A combination of high-amplitude slow-wave activity (about 0.5 Hz) and high-frequency activity produces a highly variable zero-crossing frequency. The numbers are the zero-crossing frequency of each 1-second segment of EEG. In this 4-second strip, a fivefold range of values is observed despite little actual change in the EEG. *(From Kaplan JA, editor:* Cardiac anesthesia, *ed 2, Philadelphia, 1987, WB Saunders, p 328.)*

ferences may markedly alter the results of the analysis, each technique will be discussed in some detail.

Zero-crossing analysis (Fig. 10-10) is the simplest of the period-analysis techniques.[33] The period of a wave is measured as the time that the polarity of the EEG signal remains constant, either positive or negative. Alternatively, the period could be defined as the time for a cycle of polarity, (i.e., positive and negative waves), but this distinction is trivial. One of the major advantages of this approach is the extreme simplicity of such a circuit: merely count the number of changes of polarity each second and divide by two. The result is the frequency. With simplicity, however, comes a problem that is related to the underlying problem of recording the intraoperative EEG—namely baseline drift. Because zero-crossing analysis relies on a change in polarity to measure the period of a wave, any movement of the baseline resulting from very low-frequency artifact may seriously distort the results. Even the combination of low-frequency and high-frequency EEG activity can cause this distortion, as shown in Fig. 10-11.

An alternative approach, aperiodic analysis, circumvents

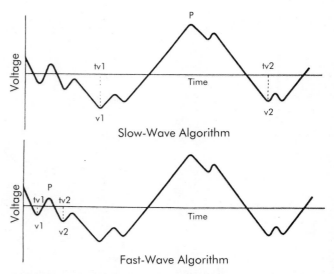

FIG. 10-12 Aperiodic analysis. In order to minimize the effect of low-frequency activity on period-amplitude analysis, this technique uses two algorithms. Note that local maxima that do not cross the isoelectric line are not detected as peak on the slow-wave algorithm. All peaks are detected on the fast-wave algorithm whether or not they are associated with a change in polarity. (For simplicity no filtration has been applied to the waveform for the slow-wave algorithm.) *(From Gregory TK: J Clin Monitor 2:192, 1986.)*

this problem by using two wave-detection algorithms.[21,27] The slow-wave algorithm, which processes a heavily filtered version of the original signal, measures the period of a wave as the time between successive negative minima that have an intervening positive maximum. The fast-wave algorithm determines the period as the time between successive minima without regard to the polarity and is applied to an essentially unfiltered signal (Fig. 10-12). Although the developer of this technique claimed increased validity compared with other (mainly power spectral) techniques, comparative studies were never published.

As might be expected, each of these period-analysis techniques uses a different amplitude measure to determine the size of the wave. Zero-crossing analyses typically employ a zero-referenced measure, such as the peak, average, or root-mean-square voltage. Aperiodic analysis measures the wave amplitude from its peak to a voltage halfway between the voltages of the two minima defining the wave.

Power-Spectrum Analysis

One of the major disadvantages of period-amplitude analyses is their lack of mathematical rigor (i.e., there is no specific theoretic basis for these techniques and, therefore, they do not evolve into more complex or sophisticated analyses). However, such benefits do derive from power-spectrum analysis, an all-purpose technique for describing the amplitudes of the components of a complex waveform.

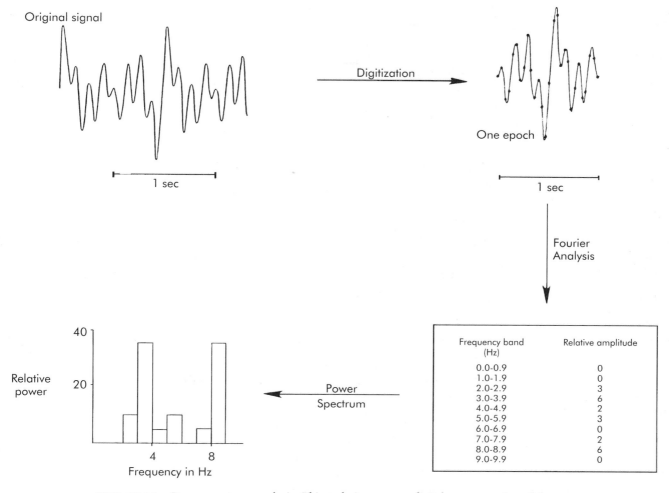

Original signal

Digitization

One epoch

1 sec

1 sec

Fourier
Analysis

Frequency band (Hz)	Relative amplitude
0.0-0.9	0
1.0-1.9	0
2.0-2.9	3
3.0-3.9	6
4.0-4.9	2
5.0-5.9	3
6.0-6.9	0
7.0-7.9	2
8.0-8.9	6
9.0-9.9	0

Power
Spectrum

Relative
power

40

20

4   8

Frequency in Hz

FIG. 10-13   Power spectrum analysis. This technique uses a digital representation of the analog signal, which is subjected to Fourier analysis. The power at each frequency component is then computed. *(From Levy WJ:* Anesthesiology *53:226, 1980.)*

As a result, power-spectrum analysis has become a common technique for quantifying the EEG.

The heart of power-spectrum analysis is Fourier transformation, a mathematical manipulation that converts data from the time domain to the frequency domain.[7] This simply means that, in the original EEG, time was measured explicitly and the frequency of activity was implicit in the changes in amplitude over time. In the Fourier-transformed signal, frequency is explicit and the changes with time are now implicit in the phase angles computed for each frequency component. After Fourier transformation, power-spectrum analysis further simplifies the data by computing an amplitude measure (power) at each frequency component (Fig. 10-13).

There are many advantages to power-spectrum analysis that derive from its strict mathematical basis. Different spectra can be compared numerically, and statistical manipulations may be performed. As a result, power spectra have become an intermediate step in EEG analysis, and many additional manipulations are commonly performed on spectra as if they were the original signal. Unfortunately, there are at least a few ways in which the EEG is not, strictly speaking, suitable for power-spectral analysis.

The mathematical assumptions on which Fourier analysis is based require that the signal analyzed by Fourier techniques be periodic and stationary (i.e., not evolving over time).[10] Although the EEG is not a stationary signal nor periodic, because sequential segments (epochs) of data are not identical, with one notable exception (i.e., during burst-suppression activity), EEG activity appears to be sufficiently stationary and periodic that the application of power-spectrum techniques is appropriate. These techniques are appropriate during burst-suppression activity if the analysis is performed using epochs of greater duration than the repeat cycle of the burst-suppression activity. However, because this is not the normal approach to power-spectrum analysis of the EEG, problems can arise.[35]

The frequency resolution of the Fourier transformation,

and thus the power spectrum, is determined by the duration of the epoch. Thus, a 1-second epoch generates frequency components at 1-Hz intervals, whereas 2-second epochs yield 0.5-Hz intervals, 4-second epochs produce 0.25-Hz intervals, and so on. Because computational requirements increase nonlinearly as the epoch is lengthened and because identification of rapid changes is easier with short epochs, it is useful to limit the epoch length to the shortest that provides adequate frequency resolution of the power spectrum. Typically a 2-second epoch is used.[37]

The frequency of digitization of the analog EEG determines the highest frequency that can be resolved by the Fourier transformation. Very high data sampling rates present problems when there is the need to transform an excessively large mass of data, whereas inadequate sampling predisposes to aliasing, discussed earlier. Because Fourier transformation is most convenient (mathematically) if the data set is a power of two, a sampling rate of 128 Hz is often used. This allows the resolution of 64 Hz signals before aliasing occurs and even permits the recognition of EEG signal in the presence of modest amounts of 60 Hz artifact. (This elimination of 60 Hz artifact is not an excuse for sloppy electrode placement or high impedances; it is just a small benefit that derives from the use of a sampling rate in excess of 128 Hz.) Data sampling rates of 64 Hz only resolve to 32 Hz, and, even worse, 60 Hz noise appears as a constant band of 4 Hz activity—an obviously undesirable situation.

Other Analyses

As has already been noted, computing the power spectrum requires an additional step after Fourier transformation. Other computations can be performed as well, and these provide further information about the EEG. Coherence analysis[4,62] is one such technique that has only recently been applied to the EEG during anesthesia.

Coherence analysis is the complement to power-spectral analysis, in that the former analyzes phasic relationships and does not consider amplitude at all, whereas the latter considers only amplitude and ignores the phasic relationship. Coherence analysis differs from power-spectral analysis in another way as well. Coherence analysis is a frequency-dependent correlation function that is derived from two channels of data, whereas power spectrum analysis is a function of only a single channel of EEG. There has been little use of coherence analysis to examine the behavior of the EEG during anesthesia, but what has been done suggests that anesthesics cause profound changes in the interhemispheric coherences.[38] Whether these changes are common to all anesthetics and thus tell us something about anesthesia in general, or whether these changes are agent-specific, remains to be demonstrated.

Another mathematical approach to the analysis of the processed EEG is neural network analysis.[69] This technique begins with a spectrum, such as the power spectrum, and attempts to define the differences between spectra that dis-

tinguish different states. The analysis defines three layers of nodes: input, intermediate, and output. The relationships between input to a node and its output are not dictated *a priori* but are "learned" by "training" the network with a training data set. Also, the relationships need not be linear, resulting in unique potentials for this type of analysis. For example, given a learning set of EEG power spectra, it is possible to demonstrate that only certain portions of the spectrum are needed to discriminate the states in the training set. Training is not limited to binary situations, and the analysis can discriminate among as many states as exist in the training set.[68] Unfortunately, the training does not necessarily yield a general algorithm, and small changes in state or the addition of another state necessitates complete retraining. In addition, networks may (like any student) fail to train, either because of inadequacies in the training set or the training algorithm. The usefulness of this approach to analyzing the EEG remains to be demonstrated.

Processed EEG Display

Once the EEG has been processed, it must be displayed in an intelligible way. This is not a trivial issue, because the data are essentially three-dimensional: frequency, amplitude (or coherence), and time, the latter arising because the period-amplitude or power-spectral analysis is repeated as new EEG data are recorded from the patient. One approach to resolving this dilemma is to perform additional processing on the data to yield a very simple univariate descriptor that can then be trended. Although simple, this approach destroys a huge amount of information that may be contained in the processed EEG. As a result, a large number of descriptors have been proposed[11,13,29,43] The spectral edge frequency is probably the best known univariate descriptor and has been evaluated as a monitor of cerebral ischemia. Originally defined as the upper limit of the power spectra, determined using an instrument-specific algorithm, it is often represented as the frequency below which 95% of the power is found. Other univariate frequency descriptors include the peak-power frequency, the median-power frequency, and the average (mean) frequency. Other descriptors use the classical bands of the EEG as the basis for analysis, either as absolute or relative power or a ratio of band powers. Thus descriptors, such as relative theta power or alpha/theta quotient (the ratio of alpha power to theta power), can be developed. In general, these descriptors have been developed through "fishing expeditions," in which many descriptors are examined and the one is selected that most closely parallels the desired observation. Perhaps with sufficient studies, it will be possible to define some single variable that can be used as a monitor for a specific condition, but for now no such "magic number" exists and univariate descriptors are commonly selected to enhance the desired phenomenon.[16,60] For general usage, complex three-dimensional graphics techniques are needed.

The oldest of these, the compressed-spectral array (CSA) graphs individual epochs of data on an amplitude-frequency plane and moves the origin vertically to specify the passage of time[5] (Fig. 10-14). When the new data are graphed at the largest vertical displacement, there is a tendency for old data to obscure newer data, particularly if the new data are of lesser amplitude. This can be eliminated by reversing the movement of the origin with time, so that new data are plotted at the bottom of the graph (Fig. 10-15). Al-

though this is an improvement, the presence of time and amplitude on the same axis can be confusing.

One alternative approach is to use a traditional three-dimensional graphic representation in which the z axis (usually time) is portrayed as perpendicular to the x-y plane by visualizing it at an angle (Fig. 10-16). Of necessity some data must be hidden, and interaction between the data and

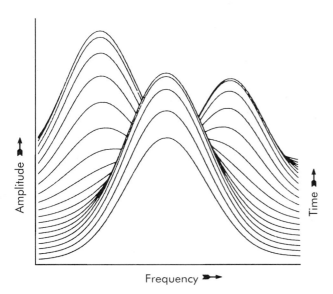

FIG. 10-14 Compressed spectral array (CSA). This display of three variables places time and amplitude on the same axis. As a result, new data tends to be hidden behind old data. *(From Kaplan JA, editor:* Cardiac anesthesia, *ed 2, Philadelphia, 1987, WB Saunders, p 325.)*

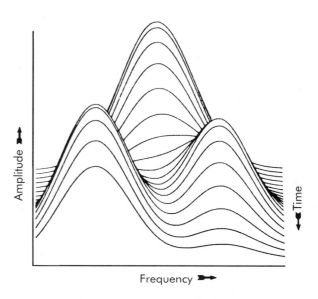

FIG. 10-15 Inverted CSA. In this display, time progresses downward so that new data are placed at the bottom of the plot. Legibility for new data is improved even though confusion of time and amplitude changes can still occur. *(From Kaplan JA, editor:* Cardiac anesthesia, *ed 2, Philadelphia, 1987, WB Saunders, p 322.)*

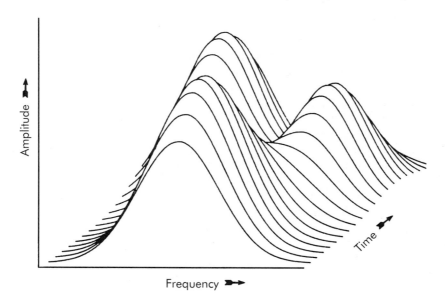

FIG. 10-16 Three-dimensional display. This three-dimensional display shows the classic position of the z axis (time) angularly displaced from both x and y axis. *(From Kaplan JA, editor:* Cardiac anesthesia, *ed 2, Philadelphia, 1987, WB Saunders, p 322.)*

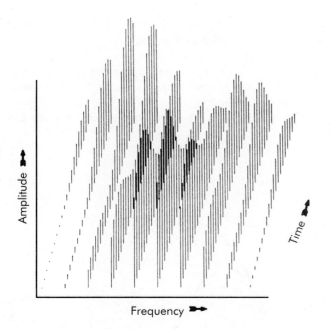

FIG. 10-17   Three-dimensional histogram. The same data as in Figs. 10-13 and 10-15 are displayed in histogram form. Even though only one fourth as much data is displayed, legibility is poor without the addition of color. *(From Kaplan JA, editor: Cardiac anesthesia, ed 2, Philadelphia, 1987, WB Saunders, p 326.)*

the perspective make some perspectives better than others. Unfortunately, this problem cannot be predicted, and thus there is no guarantee that the problem will not occur with any preselected perspective.

Another alternative displays the data as a three-dimensional histogram[64] (Fig. 10-17). This approach is inherently somewhat less readable, particularly in a monochrome figure, so that color has also been used (along with x-axis displacement) to signify frequency. Such redundancy may improve legibility but suggests that a more efficient display may be developed if color is used effectively.

Such a display is the density-spectral array (DSA).[25] The transformation from three-dimensional graph to two dimensions (Fig. 10-18) is quite analogous to the technique cartographers use to signify the altitude of mountains or the depth of the oceans on a map. The height (land) or amplitude (EEG) is quantified, and each step is assigned a color value. The remaining axes (frequency and time) are then oriented in the most convenient arrangement. Because most forms of monitoring, from the anesthesia record to a strip-chart recorder, display time on the x axis, it is most reasonable to do so with the DSA as well. In fact, the placement of time on the abscissa is unique to this display and greatly improves the legibility when integrated with other physiologic monitors.[40]

Thus far, this discussion has emphasized the three-dimensional aspect of one channel of EEG. In fact, one can consider the EEG to be four-dimensional, with the fourth

dimension representing the topographic position of the area being recorded. Although this regionality is often ignored by anesthesiologists, it is important. A variety of graphic representations have been developed in an attempt to present all of this data, but none is entirely satisfactory. Most commonly, small DSA or pie chart displays are superimposed over the appropriate portions of a schematic of the head or brain. The resultant diminution in size of the individual DSA often renders them illegible, while the pie chart approach sacrifices the temporal trends.

THE EEG DURING ANESTHESIA

Describing the EEG during anesthesia is a bit like describing a tree. It is relatively easy to know a particular plant is a tree and even to tell that it is alive and growing although it may be very difficult to generalize the description to suit all trees. Similarly, the EEG waves may vary greatly, depending on the drugs administered. Mixtures of anesthetics may produce unexpected patterns of EEG activity that differ from those of the individual agents when used separately. Other factors—including temperature[37] and CO_2[31]—may modify the EEG pattern, and surgical stimulation can also produce effects.[6] Clearly, the EEG is not the analog output of a biologic device for the measurement of the concentration of anesthetic agents, and precise relationships between anesthetic agents and the intraoperative EEG do not exist.

Barbiturates produce a wide spectrum of EEG effects, depending on the dose.[32] At the lowest levels, EEG activation is observed, with an increase in high-frequency activity. Progressive increases in concentration then produce slowing, with the amplitude of the activity tending to increase as the frequency falls. Eventually burst-suppression occurs, and ultimately even this activity may be suppressed to produce an isoelectric tracing. Such suppression is associated with a significant reduction in the cerebral metabolism, and thus titrating the EEG to burst suppression is often used to control the infusion of barbiturates being administered to reduce cerebral metabolism.

Propofol is another intravenous agent that causes marked EEG slowing. Although activation may be the first EEG change observed, high-amplitude slow-wave activity is characteristic of this agent, and burst suppression is seen.[28,59] Studies of EEG changes during induction have suggested an extrapyramidal source for the seizurelike movement that occasionally occurs.[8]

Induction of anesthesia with etomidate produces EEG effects that are grossly similar to those observed with the barbiturates. A burst of beta activity is followed by progressive slowing until a burst-suppression pattern is observed.[26] EEG activity is not related to the clonic muscle activity commonly seen with etomidate.[44] As with other intravenous agents, the pattern of EEG change during wakening is generally the reverse of that seen following rapid induction.

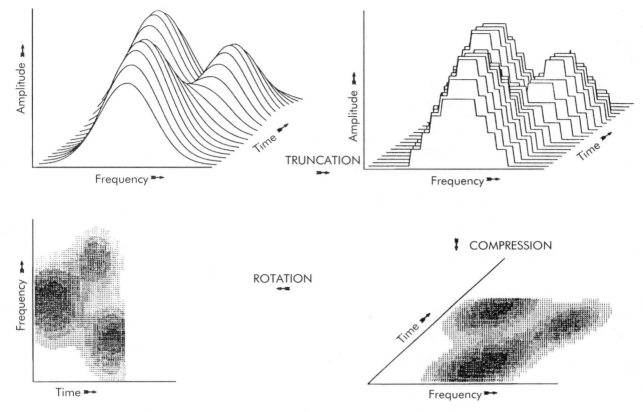

FIG. 10-18 Density spectral array (DSA). This display reduces amplitude to color (or gray scale) and compresses the three dimensions onto the frequency-time plane. Rotation of the axis places time on the x axis. *(From Kaplan JA, editor:* Cardiac anesthesia, *ed 2, Philadelphia, 1987, WB Saunders, p 327.)*

In the doses commonly used for analgesia, the narcotics produce little change in the EEG. In anesthetic doses (50 to 100 µg/kg of fentanyl), high-amplitude slow-wave activity is observed.[9,52,61] Burst suppression is not seen, and there appears to be a plateau in the EEG response to the drug.[60] There are anecdotal reports of seizure activity after the administration of large doses of narcotics;[54] however, unlike the response of animals in which narcotics clearly produce seizures,[71] the sporadic and unpredictable nature of these events in humans has made it difficult to determine whether this is true seizure activity, movement dictated by extrapyramidal activity, or myotonic/myoclonic activity that is independent of the CNS.[46,65]

Ketamine produces a different pattern of EEG changes, showing both desynchonization (higher frequencies and lower amplitudes) at low doses and synchronization (lower frequencies and higher amplitudes) at higher doses. Low-amplitude high-frequency activity (20 to 40 Hz) is often seen superimposed on the 4- to 6-Hz activity that is characteristic of the anesthetized state.[58] Interestingly, ketamine is a racemic mixture whose optical isomers differ in potency. EEG studies reflect this difference, demonstrating greater slowing of the median power frequency by the (+) isomer than by the (-) isomer.[57]

The acute administration of diazepam produces prominent changes in the EEG. The alpha rhythm disappears and is largely replaced by beta activity, which is more prominent frontally.[51] The effect does not appear to be particularly dose-dependent because the pattern is seen after 1 to 2 mg used for sedation or 20 mg, which produces sleep in a number of subjects. Other benzodiazepines, especially midazolam, produce essentially similar patterns. Patients receiving these drugs on a chronic basis do not necessarily demonstrate this beta-active pattern. The beta-activation of the EEG is common in states of sedation, and attempts have been made to correlate the EEG changes with sedation and amnesia, especially for use during long-term ventilator therapy in intensive care settings.[68] Such studies have shown modest correlations; however, the clinical usefulness of these findings appears minimal, primarily because of the complexity of the monitoring and the variability of the patients.

Isoflurane[23] and desflurane[53] also produce suppression of the EEG at clinically useful concentrations. For isoflurane, burst suppression is often seen at about 1.75% end-tidal and may occur at MAC (1.25%). Although only limited human experience with desflurane is available, it too produces prominent burst suppression at concentrations near the MAC. The addition of nitrous oxide does not appear to have an effect on this activity, provided that the concentration of the isoflurane or desflurane is not concomitantly reduced.

Alone among the potent inhaled agents, enflurane is known for its potential to cause seizure activity.[14] Such activity is increased by rhythmic stimulation, high concentrations of the agent, and hypocarbia.[47] Although much discussion has focused on the clinical significance of electrical seizures with adequate oxygenation, little evidence of neurologic injury was ever produced. The conditions necessary to induce this behavior in normal patients are sufficiently excessive that the entire issue is not of major importance; for a patient with a seizure disorder, other effective inhaled anesthetics make the question moot.

Halothane does not produce either seizures, burst suppression, or an isoelectric EEG in clinically useful concentrations.[2] Like the other inhaled agents, there is a tendency toward increased slow-wave activity as anesthesia is deepened.

The effect of nitrous oxide on the EEG is difficult to assess because as an anesthetic it is always used in conjunction with other agents. When combined with narcotics in a classic "balanced" technique, an EEG containing large amounts of alpha- and beta-frequency components is commonly observed. Very high-frequency components have also been reported.[70] When nitrous oxide is added to potent inhalational agents, EEG changes may be seen. When nitrous oxide is added to halothane and isoflurane, slowing occurs; however, it is unclear whether this difference results from changes in anesthetic depth or is an independent effect of the nitrous oxide. By comparison Rampil has shown that the addition of nitrous oxide to desflurane changes the burst-suppression activity in a way that suggests a limited EEG effect for the observed deepening of anesthesia.[53]

INDICATIONS FOR EEG MONITORING

It is clear that many factors influence EEG activity. Their mere existence, however, does not provide sufficient justification for expending the time and effort necessary to monitor the EEG. The justification for this effort arises when clinical decisions that change therapy are made based on information obtained from the EEG and are available through no other monitoring modality. One such application is for the detection of central nervous system ischemia. Such ischemia may arise during cerebrovascular surgery, such as carotid endarterectomy; during altered physiologic states, such as extracorporeal perfusion; or during misadventures, such as ventilator disconnection or hypoxic respiratory mixtures. The usefulness of the EEG as a monitor varies rather remarkably among these conditions.

For the detection of ventilatory problems, whether of gas mixture or supply, the EEG is not nearly as valuable as exhaled gas volume, inspired oxygen concentration, airway pressure, pulse oximetry, and end-tidal CO_2 tracings. Indeed, these provide earlier warning of a malfunction, may identify the problem in a very specific fashion (e.g., inadequate inspired oxygen), and are less likely to produce false alarms resulting from anesthetic effects than is the EEG.

During extracorporeal circulation or deliberate hypotension, a stronger case for EEG monitoring can be advanced. The failure of oxygenation appears to be primarily a circulatory one, so that a monitor of end-organ function is desirable. However, most studies of EEG during cardiopulmonary bypass have failed to demonstrate a significant role for EEG monitoring,[3,36,39] although a few suggest otherwise.[1,22] This may be because of confounding influences, such as hypothermia,[56] that make the identification of ischemia difficult or because of technical factors, including artifact produced by the bypass pumps, that interfere with EEG recording.[41] Finally, most neurologic injury during extracorporeal circulation is believed to be embolic in origin,[41,48,55,63] necessitating an extensive montage for identification and reducing the likelihood that such therapies as changing perfusion pressure will be of value. The one exception to this limited role may be the application of the EEG to ensure cerebral electrical silence before beginning circulatory arrest. Because increases in electrical activity are associated with increases in metabolic needs, it seems reasonable to ensure electrical silence before interrupting the cerebral circulation for an extended period.[18,45] Despite the infrequency of such procedures, they appear to be the only cases using extracorporeal circulation that warrant EEG monitoring.

This role for EEG stands in contrast to the situation during carotid endarterectomy, when both surgical and anesthetic management may be modified by EEG monitoring and the resultant changes in treatment may reduce morbidity. The interruption of carotid artery blood flow during carotid endarterectomy carries a modest (15% to 20%) risk of producing cerebral ischemia, and some percentage of these patients (perhaps 10%) will go on to stroke if no steps are taken to improve cerebral perfusion. Placement of an intravascular shunt can eliminate ischemia resulting from hypoperfusion but may increase the risk of emboli and postoperative thrombosis resulting from mechanical abrasion of the vessel. Studies in which all patients undergoing carotid endarterectomy have received shunts have reported about a 2% incidence of stroke, presumably caused by emboli, thrombosis after the repair, and other such complications.[24] Obviously, if these risks could be restricted to those patients in whom a shunt was necessary to treat ischemia during carotid occlusion, the cerebral morbidity would be reduced. The magnitude of the reduction in morbidity depends upon the relative risks of infarction in the absence of shunting and complications caused by shunt placement. The percentage reduction in stroke rate may be as much as 50%;

however, the actual numbers—from 2% to 1%—mandate a study of many thousand patients to confirm these predictions. Thus the EEG is commonly used to make this decision in the absence of controlled studies demonstrating its efficacy.[66]

Under the conditions of a stable anesthetic, a stable active EEG, and acute interruption of cerebral perfusion, *any* EEG change may represent cerebral ischemia. The classic changes characteristic of hypoxia are slowing, flattening, and progression to an isoelectric signal. Studies in a different clinical situation (cardiac arrest during testing of implanted defibrillators) have suggested that loss of low-frequency activity or increased rhythmicity can be the first sign of ischemia.[15] Seizure activity is also compatible with a diagnosis of ischemia although in the most common scenario this may represent a postanoxic phenomenon.

EEG monitoring has been extensively investigated as a measure of level of consciousness in situations ranging from ICU sedation to head injury to routine anesthesia. Many of these investigations suffered from methodologic flaws, whereas others have substituted complex technical procedures for simple clinical assessment—a process that adds nothing to patient care except expense. A major problem in assessing sedation or head injury is the lack of an objective measure; cardiovascular responsiveness is commonly used even though such reactivity is commonly seen during entirely satisfactory levels of surgical anesthesia. The ob-

servation that EEG changes occur between, for example, MAC and twice that concentration is useless for determining the level of consciousness of a patient, and sufficient studies have not been performed at or near the occurrence of awareness to demonstrate reproducible EEG indicators of consciousness. Thus, while the EEG changes in response to drugs that change level of consciousness, its usefulness as a monitor of consciousness (or sedation) remains to be demonstrated.

SUMMARY

Despite considerable emotional appeal, the EEG has limited usefulness as a monitor. It is technically difficult to use in the intraoperative and intensive care settings and many confounding influences make the interpretation of even high-quality recordings difficult. However, during the carefully controlled setting of carotid endarterectomy, the EEG can assist in the decision to place a vascular shunt or to proceed without it, an option that may have consequences for the patient's well-being. Further understanding of anesthesia, cognitive function, and cerebral neurophysiology may yet extend the indications for this intraoperative EEG monitoring.

References

1. Arom K, Cohen D, Strobl FT: Effect of intraoperative intervention on neurological outcome based on electroencephalographic monitoring during cardiopulmonary bypass, *Ann Thorac Surg* 48:476-483, 1989.
2. Backman LE, Löfström B, Widen L: Electroencephalography in halothane anaesthesia, *Acta Anaesthesiol Scand* 8:115-130, 1964.
3. Bashein G, Nessly ML, Bledsoe SW et al: Electroencephalography during surgery with cardiopulmonary bypass and hypothermia, *Anesthesiology* 76:878-891, 1992.
4. Benignus VA: Estimation of the coherence spectrum and its confidence interval using the fast Fourier transform, *IEEE Trans Audio Electroacoustics* 2:145-150, 1969.
5. Bickford RG, Billinger TW, Fleming NI et al: The compressed spectral array (CSA)—a pictorial EEG, *Proc San Diego Biomed Symp* 11:365-370, 1972.
6. Bimar J, Bellville JW: Arousal reactions during anesthesia in man, *Anesthesiology* 47:449-454, 1977.
7. Blackman RB, Tukey JW: *The measurement of power spectra,* New York, 1958, Dover.
8. Borgeat A, Dessibourg C, Popvic V et al: Propofol and spontaneous movements: an EEG study, *Anesthesiology* 74:24-27, 1991.
9. Bovill JG, Sebel PS, Wauquier A et al: Electroencephalographic effects of sufentanil anaesthesia in man, *Br J Anaesth* 54:45-54, 1982.
10. Brazier MAB, Walter DO, editors: *Handbook of electroencephalography and clinical neurophysiology,* vol 5-A, Amsterdam, 1974, Elsevier.
11. Burrows FA, Volgyesi GA, James PD: Clinical evaluation of the augmented delta quotient monitor for intraoperative electroencephalographic monitoring of children during surgery and cardiopulmonary bypass for repair of congenital cardiac defects, *Br J Anaesth* 53:565-573, 1989.
12. Calvet J, Calvet MC, Scherrer J: Etude stratigraphique corticale de l'activité EEG spontanée, *Electroenceph Clin Neurophysiol* 17:109-125, 1964.
13. Chotas HG, Bourne JR, Teschan PE: Heuristic techniques in the quantification of the electroencephalogram in renal failure, *Comput Biomed Res* 12:299-312, 1979.
14. Clark DL, Hosick EC, Rosner BS: Neurophysiological effects of different anesthetics in unconscious man, *J Appl Physiol* 31:884-891, 1971.
15. Clute HL, Levy WJ: Electroencephalographic changes during brief cardiac arrest in humans, *Anesthesiology* 73:821-825, 1990.
16. Cooke JE, Scott JC: Theta ratio—a better correlate of anesthetic depth, *Anesthesiology* 65:A541, 1986.
17. Cooper R, Osselton JW, Shaw JC: *EEG technology,* Boston, 1980, Butterworths.
18. Coselli JS, Crawford ES, Beall AC et al: Determination of brain temperatures for safe circulatory arrest during cardiovascular operation, *Ann Thorac Surg* 45:738-642, 1988.
19. Da Silva FHL, van Lierop THMT, Schrijer CF et al: Organization of thalamic and cortical alpha rhythms: spectra and coherences, *Electroenceph*

Clin Neurophysiol 35:627-639, 1973.

20. Delucchi MR, Garoutte B, Aird RB: The scalp as an electroencephalographic averager, *Electroenceph Clin Neurophysiol* 14:191-196, 1962.

21. Demetrescu TM: The aperiodic character of the electroencephalogram (EEG), new approach to data analysis and condensation, *Physiologist* 18: 189, 1975.

22. Edmonds HL, Griffths L, van der Laken J et al: Quantitative electroencephalographic monitoring during myocardial revascularization predicts postoperative disorientation and improves outcome, *J Thorac Cardiovas Surg* 103:555-563, 1992.

23. Eger EI, Stevens WC, Cromwell TH: The electroencephalogram in man anesthetized with Forane, *Anesthesiology* 35:504-508, 1971.

24. Ferguson GG: Intra-operative monitoring and internal shunts: are they necessary in carotid endarterectomy? *Stroke* 13:287-289, 1983.

25. Fleming RA, Smith NT: Density modulation, a technique for the display of three-variable data in patient monitoring, *Anesthesiology* 50:543-546, 1979.

26. Ghoneim MM, Yamada T: Etomidate: a clinical and electroencephalographic comparison with thiopental, *Anesth Analg* 56:479-485, 1977.

27. Gregory TK, Pettus DC: An electroencephalographic processing algorithm specifically intended for analysis of cerebral electrical activity, *J Clin Monit* 2:190-197, 1986.

28. Hemelrijck JV, Tempelhoff R, White PF et al: EEG-assisted titration of propofol infusion during neuroanesthesia: effect of nitrous oxide, *J Neurosurgical Anesth* 4:11-20, 1992.

29. Holzer JA, Quest DO et al: Prognostic value of computerized EEG analysis during carotid endarterectomy, *Anesth Analg* 62:186-192, 1983.

30. Jasper HH: The ten-twenty electrode system of the International Federation, *Electroenceph Clin Neurophysiol* 10:372-5, 1958.

31. Kalkman CJ, Boezeman EH, Ribberink AA et al: Influence of changes in arterial carbon dioxide tension on the electroencephalogram and posterior tibial nerve somatosensory cortical evoked potentials during alfentanil/nitrous oxide anesthesia, *Anesthesiology* 75:68-74, 1991.

32. Kiersey DK, Bickford RG, Faulconer A Jr: Electroencephalographic patterns produced by thiopental sodium during surgical operations: description and classification, *Br J Anaesth* 23:141-152, 1951.

33. Klein FF: A waveform analyzer applied to the human EEG, *IEEE Trans Biomed Eng* 23:246-252, 1976.

34. Levy WJ: Effect of epoch length on power spectrum analysis of the EEG, *Anesthesiology* 66:489-495, 1987.

35. Levy WJ: Intraoperative EEG patterns: implications for EEG monitoring, *Anesthesiology* 60:430-434, 1984.

36. Levy WJ: Monitoring of the electroencephalogram during cardiopulmonary bypass: know when to say when, *Anesthesiology* 76:876-877, 1992.

37. Levy WJ: Quantitative analysis of EEG changes during hypothermia, *Anesthesiology* 60:291-297, 1984.

38. Levy WJ, Canals-Curtis: Coherence analysis of the EEG during isoflurane anesthesia, *Anesthesiology* 75:A178, 1991.

39. Levy WJ, Parcella PA: Electroencephalographic evidence of cerebral ischemia during acute extracorporeal hypoperfusion, *J Cardiothorac Anesth* 1:300-304, 1987.

40. Levy WJ, Shapiro HM, Maruchak G et al: Automated EEG processing for intraoperative monitoring, *Anesthesiology* 53:223-236, 1980.

41. Levy WJ, Shapiro HM, Meathe E: The identification of rhythmic EEG artifacts by power-spectrum analysis, *Anesthesiology* 53:505-507, 1980.

42. MacGillivray BB: *Handbook of EEG and clinical neurophysiology,* vol 3-C, Amsterdam, 1974, Elsevier.

43. Matteo RS, Ornstein E, Schwartz AE et al: Effects of low-dose sufentanil on the EEG: elderly vs young, *Anesthesiology* 65:A553, 1986.

44. Meinck HM, Möhlenhof O, Kettler D: Neurophysiological effects of etomidate, a new short-acting hypnotic, *Electroenceph Clin Neurophysiol* 50:515-522, 1980.

45. Mizrahi EM, Patel VM, Crawford ES et al: Hypothermic-induced electrocerebral silence, prolonged circulatory arrest, and cerebral protection during cardiovascular surgery, *Electroenceph Clin Neurophysiol* 72:81-85, 1989.

46. Murkin JM, Moldenhauer CC, Hug CC Jr et al: Absence of seizures during induction of anesthesia with high-dose fentanyl, *Anesth Analg* 63:489-494, 1984.

47. Neigh JL, Garman JK, Harp JR: The electroencephalographic pattern during anesthesia with Ethrane, *Anesthesiology* 35:482-487, 1971.

48. Nussmeier NA, Arlund CA, Slogoff S: Neuropsychiatric complications after cardiopulmonary bypass: cerebral protection by a barbiturate, *Anesthesiology* 64:165-170, 1986.

49. Obrist WD: The electroencephalogram of normal aged adults, *Electroenceph Clin Neurophysiol* 6:235-244, 1954.

50. Peronnet F, Sindon M, Laviron A et al: Human cortical electrogenesis: stratigraphy and spectral analysis. In Petsche H, Brazier MAB, editors: *Synchronization of EEG activity in epilepsies,* New York, 1972, Springer-Verlag.

51. Pichlmayr I, Lips U: Diazepameffekte im elektroenzephalogramm, *Anaesthesist* 29:317-327, 1980.

52. Picklmayr I, Lips U, Kunkel H: *The electroencephalogram in anesthesia,* New York, 1984, Springer-Verlag.

53. Rampil IJ, Lockhart SH, Eger EI et al: The electroencephalographic effects of desflurane in humans, *Anesthesiology* 74:434-439, 1991.

54. Rao TLK, El-Etr AA: Fentanyl and convulsions, *Anesth Analg* 62:859, 1983 (letter).

55. Reed GL, Singer DE, Picard EH et al: Stroke following coronary-artery bypass surgery: a case-control estimate of the risk from carotid bruits, *N Engl J Med* 319:1246-1250, 1988.

56. Russ W, Kling D, Sauerwein G et al: Spectral analysis of the EEG during hypothermic cardiopulmonary bypass, *Acta Anaesthesiol Scand* 31:111-116, 1987.

57. Schüttler J, Stanski DR, White PF et al: Pharmacodynamic modeling of the EEG effects of ketamine and its enantiomers in man, *J Pharmacol Biopharmacol* 15:241-253, 1987.

58. Schwartz MS, Virden S, Scott DF: Effects of ketamine on the electroencephalograph, *Anaesthesia* 29:135-140, 1974.

59. Schwilden H, Stoeckel H, Schüttler J: Closed-loop feedback control of propofol anaesthesia by quantitative EEG analysis in humans, *Br J Anaesth* 62:290-296, 1989.

60. Scott JC, Ponganis KV, Stanski DR: EEG quantitation of narcotic effect. The comparative pharmacodynamics of fentanyl and alfentanil, *Anesthesiology* 62:234-241, 1985.

61. Sebel PS, Bovill JG, Wauquier A et al: Effects of high-dose fentanyl anesthesia on the electroencephalogram, *Anesthesiology* 55:203-211, 1981.

62. Shaw JC: An introduction to the coherence function and its use in EEG signal analysis, *J Med Eng Tech* 6:279-288, 1981.

63. Slogoff S, Reul GJ, Keats AS et al: Role of perfusion pressure and flow in major organ dysfunction after cardiopulmonary bypass, *Ann Thorac Surg* 50:911-8, 1990.

64. Smith NT: Monitoring the electroencephalogram in the operating room. In Gravenstein JS, Newbower RS, Ream AK et al, editors: *Monitoring surgical patients in the operating room,* Springfield, Ill, 1979, Charles C Thomas, p 134.

65. Smith NT, Benthuysen JL, Bickford RG et al: Seizures during opioid anesthetic induction—are they opioid-induced rigidity? *Anesthesiology* 71:852-862, 1989.

66. Sundt Jr TM: The ischemic tolerance of neural tissue and the need for monitoring and selective shunting during carotid endarterectomy, *Stroke* 14:93-98, 1983.

67. Van Leeuwen WS, Wieneke G, Spoelstra P et al: Lack of bilateral coherence of mu rhythm, *Electroenceph Clin Neurophysiol* 44:140-146, 1978.

68. Veselis RA, Reinsel R, Sommer S et al: Use of neural network analysis to classify electroencephalographic patterns against depth of midazolam sedation in intensive care unit patients, *J Clin Monit* 7:259-267, 1991.

69. Wasserman PD: *Neural computing: theory and practice,* New York, 1989, Van Nostrand Reinhold 1989.

70. Yamamura T, Fukuda M, Takeya H et al: Fast oscillatory EEG activity induced by analgesic concentrations of nitrous oxide in man, *Anesth Analg* 60:283-288, 1981.

71. Young ML, Smith DS, Greenberg J et al: Effects of sufentanil on regional cerebral glucose utilization in rats, *Anesthesiology* 61:564-568, 1984.

11

Intraoperative Fluid Management During Craniotomy

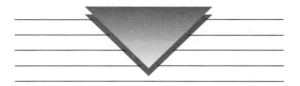

MARK H. ZORNOW
MARK S. SCHELLER

The intraoperative fluid management of neurosurgical patients presents special challenges for the anesthesiologist. Neurosurgical patients often experience rapid changes in intravascular volume caused by hemorrhage, the administration of potent diuretics, or the onset of diabetes insipidus. During surgery, the administration of volatile anesthetics and potent vasodilators may further decrease cardiac filling pressures without actual changes in intravascular volume. In the midst of this dynamic situation, the anesthesiologist often faces the additional concern of minimizing increases in cerebral water content and thus intracranial pressure. Intracranial hypertension secondary to cerebral edema is now known to be one of the most common causes of morbidity and mortality in the intraoperative and postoperative periods.

In this chapter, we will first examine some of the physical determinants of water movement between the intravascular space and the central nervous system. Subsequent sections will address specific clinical situations with suggestions for the types and volumes of fluids to be administered.

OSMOLALITY, ONCOTIC PRESSURE, AND INTRAVASCULAR VOLUME
Osmolality

Osmolality is one of the four colligative properties of a solution (the others being vapor pressure, freezing point depression, and boiling point elevation). The addition of 1 osm of any solute to 1 kg of water causes the vapor pressure to fall by 0.3 mm Hg, the freezing point to decrease by 1.85° C, and the boiling point to increase by 0.52° C.[3] The colligative properties are determined solely by the *number* of particles in solution and are independent of the chemical structure of the solute. The solute may exist in either an ionized or a nonionized state, and the size (molecular weight) of the solute is of no import. Although it may seem counterintuitive, equimolar concentrations of glucose, urea, or mannitol have the same effect on the colligative properties of a solution. Osmolality is strictly a function of the number of particles in solution.

For physiologic solutions, *osmolality* is commonly ex-

TABLE 11-1
Osmolarity of Commonly Used Intravenous Fluids

Fluid	Osmolarity (mOsm/L)	Oncotic Pressure (mm Hg)
Lactated Ringer's solution	273	0
D5 lactated Ringer's solution	525	0
0.9% Saline	308	0
D5 0.45% Saline	406	0
0.45% Saline	154	0
20% Mannitol	1098	0
Hetastarch (6%)	310	31[16]
Dextran 40 (10%)	≈300	169[26]
Dextran 70 (6%)	≈300	19[26]
Albumin (5%)	290	19
Plasma	295	21

EXAMPLE 1.
Calculate the Osmolarity of a 0.9% Solution of Saline.

FACT: The molecular weight of NaCl is 58.43 g/mole. Calculator
FACT: A 0.9% solution of NaCl contains 9 g of NaCl per 1000 ml of solution.

The first step is to calculate the molarity of the 0.9% solution. To do this we divide 9 g/L by 58.43 g/mole, which is equal to 0.154 mole/L, or a 154 μM solution of NaCl. Because each molecule of NaCl disassociates in water into a Na^+ and a Cl^- ion, we multiply the molar value by 2 to get an osmolarity of 308 mOsm/L. This value can be verified by examining the listed osmolarity of any container of 0.9% saline.

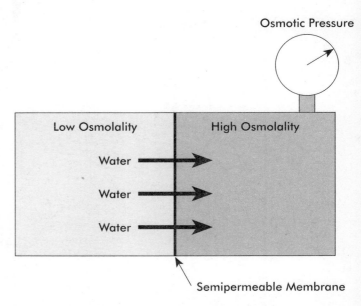

FIG. 11-1   When solutions of unequal osmolality are separated by a semipermeable membrane, water moves from the solution of lower osmolality through the membrane and into the more concentrated solution. This process continues until the solutions are of equal osmolality or the osmotic pressure reaches the point that there can be no further net flux of water across the membrane.

---

pressed as milliosmoles (mOsm) *per kilogram of solvent,* whereas the units of measure for *osmolarity* are milliosmoles *per liter of solution.* For dilute solutions (including most of physiologic importance), the two terms may be used interchangeably. Osmolarity can be calculated if the molecular weight of the solute and its tendency to disassociate in solution are known (Example 1). The osmolarities of some commonly used intravenous fluids are shown in Table 11-1.

Osmolarity is important in determining fluid movement between various physiologic compartments because of the osmotic pressure that is generated when solutions of unequal osmolarity are separated by a membrane permeable to water but not the solutes. According to the second law of thermodynamics, which states that all systems spontaneously change in a manner to maximize entropy, there will be a tendency for water to move from the solution of lower osmolality, across the membrane, and into the solution of higher osmolality (Fig. 11-1).

This process continues until the solutions are of equal osmolality or the hydrostatic pressure is sufficient to preclude any further net flow of water across the membrane. The hydrostatic pressure that can be generated by osmolar differences is formidable and may be calculated by the following equation:

$$\pi = CRT$$

where

π = osmotic pressure in atmospheres
C = concentration of the solution in moles per liter
R = gas constant (0.08206 liter-atm/mole-degree)
T = temperature in degrees Kelvin

Using this equation, we can calculate the osmotic pressure exerted by a 1 mOsm solution at body temperature (Example 2). Using this formula, one can calculate that for each milliosmole difference across a semipermeable membrane, a pressure of more than 19 mm Hg is generated. Thus osmolar differences can provide a potent driving force for the movement of water between the intracellular and extracellular spaces, and, as we will see later, across the blood-brain barrier. Although transient osmolar gradients can be produced by the administration of hypoosmolar or hyperosmolar fluids, these gradients are fleeting, and water moves from one compartment to another so that all body fluids again are of equal osmolarity.

EXAMPLE 2.
Calculation of Osmotic Pressure

Calculate the osmotic pressure generated by a 1 mOsm solution at body temperature and express the results in mm Hg.

Formula for calculation of osmotic pressure is

$$\pi = CRT$$

where

    C = 0.001 mol (i.e., 1 mOsm)
    R = 0.08206
    T = 273° + 36° = 309° (body temperature in degrees Kelvin)

Therefore $\pi = 0.001 \times 0.08206 \times 309° = 0.02535$ atm or 19.27 mm Hg.

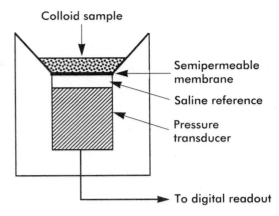

FIG. 11-2 The oncotic pressure of various fluids can be measured using a simple device constructed from a pressure transducer and a semipermeable membrane. A chamber containing a saline reference is positioned above the pressure transducer and is separated from the sample well by a semipermeable membrane. The colloidal fluid being tested is placed in the sample well. The oncotic pressure of the colloidal fluid draws a small volume of saline across the semipermeable membrane, thereby creating a negative pressure above the pressure transducer. This pressure is digitally displayed and represents the colloid oncotic pressure of the sample.

Oncotic Pressure

Oncotic pressure is nothing more than the osmotic pressure generated by solutes larger than an arbitrary limit (usually 30,000 molecular weight). Albumin (approximate molecular weight, 69,000), hetastarch (mean molecular weight, 480,000), dextran 40 (mean molecular weight, 40,000) and dextran 70 (mean molecular weight, 70,000) are compounds of clinical interest that are capable of exerting oncotic pressure. Reported values for the oncotic pressures of plasma, mannitol, albumin, and hetastarch are shown in Table 11-1. The oncotic pressure produced by all plasma proteins (e.g., albumin, globulins, fibrinogen) accounts for less than 0.5% of total plasma osmotic pressure. The oncotic pressure of various solutions can be easily measured using an electronic pressure transducer and a membrane freely permeable to low-molecular-weight solutes but that prevents the passage of particles greater than 30,000 molecular weight (Fig. 11-2).

Determinants of Fluid Movement between Vasculature and Tissues

Nearly 100 years ago, Ernest Starling described those forces that determine the movement of water between the tissues and the intravascular space.[41] This description was subsequently formalized in what is now known as the Starling equation[31]:

$$Q_f = K_f S \left[(P_c\text{-}P_t) - \sigma(\pi_c - \pi_t) \right]$$

where

    Q_f = net amount of fluid that moves between the capillary lumen and the surrounding extracellular space
    K_f = filtration coefficient for the membrane
    S = surface area of the capillary membrane
    P_c = hydrostatic pressure in the capillary lumen
    P_t = hydrostatic pressure (usually negative) in the extracellular space of the surrounding tissue
    σ = coefficient of reflection (this number, which can range from 0 [no movement of the solute across the membrane] to 1 [free diffusion of the solute across the membrane] quantitates the "leakiness" of the capillary and is different for vessels in the brain than those in peripheral tissues)
    π_c = oncotic pressure of the plasma
    π_t = oncotic pressure of the fluid in the extracellular space[31]

Capillary pressure, tissue pressure (which has been shown to be negative in nonedematous tissues), and tissue oncotic pressure all act to draw fluid from the capillaries and into the extracellular space of the tissue (Fig. 11-3). The only factor that serves to maintain intravascular volume is the plasma oncotic pressure, which is produced predominantly by albumin and to a lesser extent by immunoglobulins, fibrinogen, and other high-molecular-weight plasma proteins (Fig. 11-3).

Under most circumstances, the summation of the forces results in a value for Q_f that is slightly greater than zero, indicating a net outward flux of fluid from the vessels and into the tissue extracellular space. This fluid is cleared from the tissue by the lymphatic system, thereby preventing the development of edema (Fig. 11-4).

The clinical effects of altering one or more of the variables in the Starling equation may frequently be observed in the operating room. Many patients who have been resuscitated from hemorrhagic hypovolemia with large volumes of crystalloid solutions develop pitting edema caused by a dilution of plasma proteins. This results in a decrease

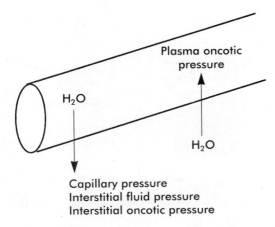

FIG. 11-3 There are four forces acting on intravascular water. Capillary hydrostatic pressure, interstitial fluid pressure (which is negative in most tissues), and interstitial oncotic pressure (pressure exerted by proteins in the interstitial space) act to draw water from the intravascular space into the interstitium. The only force that acts to maintain intravascular volume is plasma oncotic pressure. This force is produced by the presence in plasma of high-molecular-weight proteins that cannot cross the capillary wall.

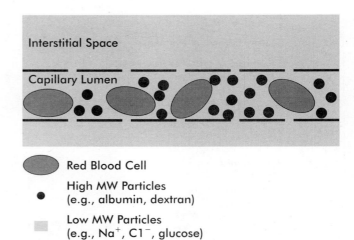

FIG. 11-4 In peripheral capillaries, there is free movement of most low-molecular-weight particles (including sodium, chloride, glucose, and mannitol) between the capillary lumen and the interstitial space. Intravenous administration of low-molecular-weight solutes cannot affect the movement of water between the interstitium and the vasculature because no osmotic gradient can be established. In contrast, raising the plasma oncotic pressure by administering concentrated albumin, hetastarch, or dextran may draw water from the interstitium into the vessel because these high-molecular-weight particles are precluded from passing through the capillary wall.

in intravascular oncotic pressure (π_c). In the face of relatively unchanged capillary hydrostatic pressure, there is an increased movement of fluid from the vasculature into the tissues. When this fluid flux exceeds the drainage capacity of the lymphatics, clinically apparent edema is the result.

Another example of the Starling equation in action is the facial edema that is frequently seen in patients who have been placed in the Trendelenburg position for prolonged periods. In this case, the edema is not due to a decrease in plasma oncotic pressure but rather to an increase in the capillary hydrostatic pressure (P_c), favoring an increased transudation of fluid into the tissue.

Fluid Movement Between Capillaries and the Brain

The Starling equation describes those factors that govern fluid movement between the intravascular and peripheral extracellular spaces (e.g., the interstitium of lung, bowel, and muscle). However, the brain and spinal cord are unlike most other tissues in the body in that they are isolated from the intravascular compartment by the blood-brain barrier. Morphologically, this barrier is now thought to be composed of endothelial cells that form tight junctions in the capillaries supplying the brain and spinal cord. In normal brain, these tight junctions severely limit the diffusion of molecules between the intravascular space and the brain. By measuring the movement of water out of the central nervous system after abrupt changes in plasma osmolality, Fenstermacher calculated the effective pore radius for the

blood brain barrier to be only 7 to 9 Å.[9] This small pore size of the blood-brain barrier prevents the movement not only of plasma proteins but also of sodium, chloride, and potassium ions between the intravascular compartment and the brain's extracellular space (Fig. 11-5). In effect, the blood-brain barrier acts like the semipermeable membrane of an osmometer, and movement of water across this membrane is determined by the relative concentrations of impermeable solutes. This situation is markedly different from that in peripheral tissues, where endothelial cells do not form tight junctions. In the capillaries of peripheral tissues, the pore sizes may be as much as several orders of magnitude greater. Although these pores are small enough to preclude the movement of most protein components of plasma, electrolytes pass freely from the capillary lumen into the extracellular space. Thus, in peripheral tissues, movement of water is governed by the plasma concentration of large macromolecules (oncotic gradient) as defined by the Starling equation. In contrast, fluid movement in and out of the central nervous system is determined by the *osmolar* gradient (which is determined by relative concentrations of all osmotically active particles, including most electrolytes) between the plasma and the extracellular fluid. This difference in the determinants of fluid flux explains why the administration of large volumes of isoosmolar crystalloid results in peripheral edema caused by dilutional reduction of

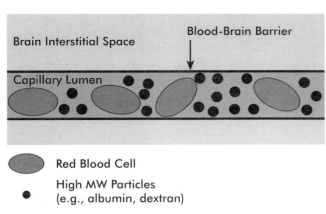

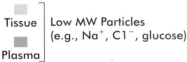

FIG. 11-5 In cerebral capillaries, the presence of the blood-brain barrier (estimated pore size of 7 to 9 Å) prevents the movement of even very small particles between the capillary lumen and the brain's interstitial space. Increasing plasma osmolality by the intravenous infusion of mannitol or hypertonic saline can therefore establish an osmotic gradient between the brain and the intravascular space that acts to move water from the brain into the capillaries.

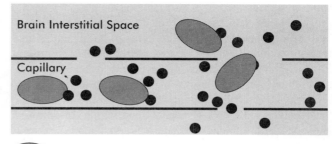

FIG. 11-6 After any of a variety of brain injuries (e.g., ischemia, contusion), there may be a breakdown of the blood-brain barrier that allows the escape from the capillary lumen of both low- and high-molecular-weight particles (i.e., the capillaries become "leaky"). In severe cases, there may even be extravasation of red blood cells into the interstitium. In this situation, the administration of neither hyperosmolar nor hyperoncotic solutions is of benefit in reducing edema formation *in the area of the injury.* Hyperosmolar solutions may be still be of benefit in areas remote from the injury where the blood-brain barrier remains intact.

plasma protein content but does not increase brain water content or intracranial pressure.

There can be little doubt that osmolarity is the primary determinant of water movement across the intact blood-brain barrier.[52] The administration of excess free water (either iatrogenically or as a result of psychogenic polydipsia) can result in an increased ICP and an edematous brain.[7] Conversely, the intravenous administration of markedly hyperosmolar crystalloids (e.g., mannitol) to increase plasma osmolarity results in a decrease in brain water content and ICP. Use of hyperosmolar solutions is a daily occurrence in operating rooms throughout the world and represents a standard therapeutic maneuver for the treatment of intracranial hypertension.

In the presence of an intact blood-brain barrier, plasma osmolarity is the key determinant of water movement between the central nervous system and the intravascular space. But what occurs when there has been injury to the brain with disruption of the barrier? If the blood-brain barrier is partially disrupted, will blood vessels in the brain start to act more like peripheral capillaries? Although experimental evidence is not conclusive, it appears that if the injury is of sufficient severity to allow the extravasation of plasma proteins into the interstitial space (i.e., capillaries have become "leaky"), plasma oncotic pressure will not have any effect on water movement because no oncotic gradient between the plasma and the brain interstial space can be produced (i.e., the proteins leak out of the capillaries

and into the brain tissue) (Fig. 11-6). In an acute animal study using a cryogenic lesion as a model of brain injury, a 50% decrease in plasma oncotic pressure had no effect on regional water content or ICP.[50] These results were confirmed in a subsequent study that demonstrated that decreasing the plasma oncotic pressure from approximately 21 mm Hg to 10 mm Hg for 8 hours had no effect on ICP or brain water content in animals with a cryogenic brain injury despite the fact that the anticipated increase in water content was documented in peripheral tissues (muscle and jejunum).[18]

Despite a lack of convincing experimental evidence that isoosmolar crystalloids are detrimental, the neurosurgical literature is filled with admonishments to restrict the use of crystalloids in patients at risk for intracranial hypertension.[38] The infusion of colloids is often recommended to maintain intravascular volume in such patients, with the implication that maintaining or increasing plasma oncotic pressure decreases cerebral edema. In the case of the intact blood-brain barrier, neither theoretic nor experimental evidence suggests a benefit of colloids over crystalloids in terms of brain water content or intracranial pressure. More recently, the crystalloid/colloid question has been addressed in animal models of cerebral injury, with varying and sometimes conflicting results. Warner et al.[45] studied the effects of hemodilution with either saline or 6% hetastarch in rats subjected to 10 minutes of severe forebrain ischemia. Despite an approximately 50% reduction in plasma oncotic pressure in the saline group (from 17.2 ± 0.8 to 9.0 ± 0.6 mm Hg), no beneficial effect in terms of decreased edema formation could be demonstrated for the hetastarch group. Similarly, in a study that used a cryogenic lesion as a model of cerebral injury, Zornow et al.[50] found no differences in regional water content or intracranial pressure in animals that received saline, 6% hetastarch, or albumin. In contrast, Korosue et al.[20] found a smaller infarct volume and improved neurologic status in dogs who were hemodiluted with a colloid (low-molecular-weight dextran) compared with animals hemodiluted with lactated Ringer's solution after ligation of the middle cerebral artery. The authors speculated (but did not provide evidence) that this beneficial effect was due to decreased edema formation in the ischemic zone. They further speculated that in this model of moderate ischemic injury, the blood-brain barrier may become selectively permeable to ions with preservation of its impermeability to high-molecular-weight compounds (e.g., dextran and proteins). If this is the case, then the brain tissue in the ischemic region may act very much like tissues in the periphery (i.e., decreases in plasma oncotic pressure result in increased water movement into the tissue). Unfortunately, the true nature of alterations in the blood-brain barrier during ischemia remains in question because a number of other studies using animal models of stroke have failed to show a benefit of colloid infusions.[23]

Beneficial effects of hypertonic solutions in cases of localized brain injury with disruption of the blood-brain barrier appear to be primarily derived from the ability of hypertonic solutions to cause a fluid flux out of brain tissue where the blood-brain barrier remains intact. In effect, normal brain is dehydrated to compensate for the edema that forms in the vicinity of the lesion. Once again, using a cryogenic lesion to model brain injury in the laboratory, it has been demonstrated that, although the infusion of a hypertonic solution attenuates the increase in ICP associated with this lesion, the hypertonic solution did not have any significant effect on the water content of brain tissue at the lesion site or in its immediate vicinity.[51] The most likely mechanism for this beneficial effect is a decrease in brain water content in regions remote from the lesion.

SOLUTIONS FOR INTRAVENOUS USE

The anesthesiologist may choose among a variety of fluids suitable for intravenous administration. These fluids may be categorized conveniently on the basis of their osmolality, oncotic pressure, and whether they contain dextrose. Crystalloid is the term commonly applied to solutions that do not contain any high-molecular-weight compounds and thus have an oncotic pressure of zero. Crystalloids may be hyperosmolar, hypoosmolar, or isoosmolar and may or may not contain dextrose. Some examples of commonly used crystalloid solutions are shown in Table 11-1. Crystalloids may be made hyperosmolar by the inclusion of electrolytes

(e.g., Na^+ and Cl^-, as in hypertonic saline), or low-molecular-weight solutes, such as mannitol (molecular weight, 182), glycerol (molecular weight, 92), glucose (molecular weight, 180), or urea (molecular weight, 60). Urea and glycerol are now rarely used because over time they penetrate the blood-brain barrier and may result in a worsening of intracranial hypertension hours after their initial beneficial effect.[39]

Colloid is the term used to denote solutions that have an oncotic pressure similar to that of plasma. Some commonly administered colloids include 6% hetastarch (Hespan), 5% and 25% albumin, the dextrans (40 and 70), and plasma. Dextran and hetastarch are dissolved in normal saline, so the osmolarity of the solution is approximately 290 to 310 mOsm/L with a sodium and chloride content of about 145 mEq/L.

Hyperosmolar Solutions

There is renewed interest in the use of hyperosmotic fluids for the resuscitation of patients with hemorrhagic hypovolemia. The reputed advantages of such solutions include a more rapid resuscitation with smaller infused volumes, improved cardiac output, decreased peripheral resistance, and lower intracranial pressures.[19] Benefits of a variety of hypertonic solutions in terms of intracranial pressure and cerebral blood flow have been demonstrated by a number of authors using a variety of animal models.[13,14,37,44,51] Clearly, these solutions exert at least part of their beneficial effects by osmotically shifting water from the central nervous system's interstitial and intracellular spaces to the intravascular space. Additional benefit may be derived from a reported decrease in CSF production.[33]

Although an acute beneficial effect has been demonstrated, the longer term (24 to 48 hours) effect of such hyperosmotic fluid therapy remains unknown. One primary area of concern is the hypernatremia that results from many of these solutions. Although survival has been reported with serum sodium levels as high as 202 mEq/L, acute increases to values much greater than 170 mEq/L are likely to result in a depressed level of consciousness and/or seizures.[40] Even with the administration of relatively small volumes (4.5 L) of moderately hypertonic saline (Na, 250 mEq/L; osmolarity, 514), serum sodium levels peaked at over 155 mEq/L in the postoperative period.[35,36] Currently, none of these compounds are commercially available for use in the United States.

An anecdotal report showed a beneficial effect of hypertonic saline solutions in patients with intracranial hypertension. In two patients, the administration of small volumes of markedly hypertonic saline resulted in a striking and sustained decrease in intracranial pressure. Both patients had suffered closed head injuries that resulted in ICPs in the range of 30 to 50 mm Hg. After conventional therapy with repeated doses of mannitol and hyperventilation had failed, 100 to 250 mMol of hypertonic saline was administered, resulting in prompt control of the intracranial hypertension.[48] In a subsequent animal study designed to directly compare in a controlled fashion the cerebral effects of mannitol (20%) and hypertonic saline (3.2%), rabbits were randomized to receive an equiosmolar load of either of these two solutions (10 ml/kg). Plasma osmolality increased to a similar degree in both groups, and no differences could be identified in ICP reduction or regional water contents (Fig. 11-7).[34]

A prospective controlled trial of hypertonic saline in pediatric head trauma was recently completed. In this study, patients received a bolus (approximately 10 ml/kg) of either 0.9% or 3% saline. Baseline ICP was similar in both groups (20 mm Hg). There was no significant change in ICP in those patients who received 0.9% saline. In contrast, after a bolus of 3% saline, ICP decreased significantly and averaged 15.8 mm Hg for the succeeding 2 hours. In those patients who received 3% saline, serum sodium concentrations increased from a mean of 147 mEq/L to 151 mEq/L.[10]

In summary, it appears that hypertonic saline solutions can exert a beneficial effect on intracranial hypertension while providing rapid volume resuscitation. The sodium load and consequent hypernatremia may be a concern in patients with neurologic injury who are at risk for seizures and who may have an altered mental status caused by their underlying injury. Whether hyperosmolar saline solutions will prove to provide significant advantages over the more conventional mannitol awaits further investigation.

Dextrose Solutions and Hyperglycemia

It has now been fairly well established that hyperglycemia before or during an episode of ischemia worsens neurologic outcome. Several independent investigators using a variety of animal models have reached this conclusion. Worsened neurologic outcome has been repeatedly demonstrated after global ischemia of either the brain or spinal cord. The elevations in plasma glucose do not need to be marked to produce a significant worsening of neurologic outcome. In one of the early studies to demonstrate this effect, Lanier et al., using a primate model, showed that dextrose infusions (50 ml of dextrose 5% in 0.45% saline) markedly worsened the neurologic score after 17 minutes of global cerebral ischemia. Although plasma glucose levels were slightly higher in those animals who received the dextrose infusion (181 ± 19 mg/dl vs. 140 ± 6 mg/dl), this elevation did not even reach statistical significance.[21] More recently, Drummond et al. demonstrated a similar detrimental effect of hyperglycemia on spinal cord function after transient ischemia. Elevation of plasma glucose by either the infusion of D5W or bolus administration of D50 resulted in substantially worsened outcome. In those animals who received dextrose by infusion before the ischemic event, plasma glucose was only mildly elevated (177 vs. 137 mg/dl). Nonetheless, 9 out of 10 of these animals were rendered paraplegic vs. 3 out of 10 in the control group.[8]

Although there appears to be a consensus that hyperglycemia during transient global ischemia is detrimental, both beneficial and adverse effects of glucose have been shown in models of focal ischemia. Ginsberg et al. have demonstrated a decrease in infarct volume in rats from 12.5 ± 4.0 mm³ (normoglycemic controls) to 9.3 ± 3.3 mm³ in rats made hyperglycemic before the ischemic event.[12] Even greater beneficial effects (approximately 50% reduction in ischemic area) have been reported in an acute study of hyperglycemic cats after ligation of the middle cerebral artery.[49] The significance of these findings is of some question because in a chronic cat study (survival time of 14

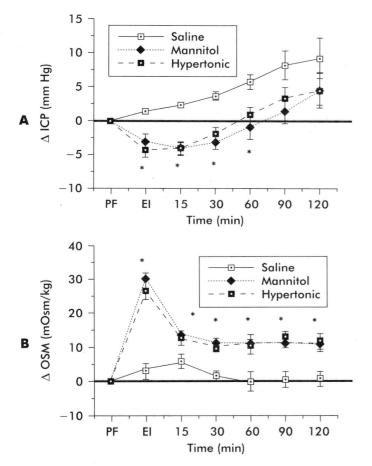

FIG 11-7 **A,** Changes in plasma osmolality after intravenous administration of 0.9% saline, or 11 mOsm/kg of either 20% mannitol or 3.2% NaCl. Note the prompt and equal increase (approximately 29 mOsm/kg) in plasma osmolality after the administration of either of these two osmotic agents. There were no differences in plasma osmolality between the hypertonic saline and mannitol groups at any time during the study. **B,** Effect of hypertonic saline and mannitol on intracranial pressure. Both of these osmotic agents produced transient decreases in intracranial pressure when compared with an equal volume of 0.9% saline. (*PF,* 45 minutes after production of cryogenic brain lesion; *EI,* end of infusion of 0.9% saline, mannitol, or hypertonic saline; °, p < 0.05 mannitol and hypertonic saline groups vs. 0.9% saline group.)

days), the hyperglycemic animals sustained infarcts twice the size of normoglycemic controls.[6]

The mechanism by which hyperglycemia worsens neurologic outcome is not clear. It has been repeatedly hypothesized that the glucose loading of central nervous system tissue that occurs during periods of hyperglycemia provides additional substrate for the production of lactic acid during the ischemic period. This increase in intracellular lactate is postulated to have a neurotoxic effect resulting in neuronal death. Although there is little doubt that there is increased lactate production in brains of hyperglycemic animals, the neurotoxic effect of this lactate is less firmly established. Indeed, in neuronal cell cultures, the production of a lactic acidosis has recently been shown to be neuroprotective.[4,11]

The clinical implication of these studies is simple: hyperglycemia should be avoided in patients who are at risk for an ischemic event. Dextrose solutions should not be infused in patients undergoing neurosurgical procedures unless they are needed for the treatment or prevention of hypoglycemia. A more complex question is how to proceed when confronted with a patient who presents to the operating room with hyperglycemia. Although it may be tempting to normalize this patient's plasma glucose by insulin infusion, whether this intervention reduces the risk of adverse outcome is not clear. It is possible that such therapy may only serve to increase intracellular stores of glucose.

FLUID ADMINISTRATION DURING CRANIOTOMY
Preoperative Deficits

The preoperative intravascular volume deficit of neurosurgical patients may be estimated in a manner similar to that used for patients undergoing other types of surgical procedures. For the nonfebrile adult patient, daily water loss averages approximately 100 ml/hr (Box 11-1). This loss of water occurs as evaporative loss from the skin and airways (insensible losses) and in urine, sweat, and feces.[15]

In addition to these obligatory losses, fluid loss caused by nasogastric suction, diarrhea, emesis, and phlebotomy must be considered. Patients who have undergone angiographic studies using intravenous contrast agents have excessive urinary losses caused by the diuresis produced by

---

BOX 11-1
DAILY WATER LOSS FOR ADULT

Insensible loss	
Skin	350
Lungs	350
Urine	1400
Sweat	100
Feces	200
Total	2400 ml/day

---

these hyperosmotic agents. Respiratory and insensible losses are increased in those patients who are febrile from any cause in the preoperative period. To arrive at the net deficit, one must add whatever fluids have been administered to the patient. These usually consist of IV or PO intake. Consideration of these values gives an estimate of the net volume deficit for a given patient. Confirmation of this calculated deficit should be sought through an examination of the patient (skin turgor, heart rate, blood pressure). Should a discrepancy appear between the calculated volume deficit and the appearance of the patient, additional investigation may be indicated, including a reexamination of the recorded input and outputs for the previous 24 hours, performance of a "tilt test" to search for evidence of hemodynamically significant hypovolemia, and in some cases the preoperative insertion of a central venous or pulmonary artery catheter.

Intraoperative Fluids: Crystalloids

Intraoperative maintenance fluid administration usually consists of lactated Ringer's or normal saline solution. As stated previously, these fluids are crystalloids and are approximately equiosmolar to normal plasma. As a general rule, hypoosmolar solutions and dextrose-containing solutions should be avoided. Isoosmolar crystalloids are given at a rate sufficient to replace the patient's urine output and insensible losses milliliter for milliliter. Blood loss is replaced at approximately a 3:1 ratio (crystalloid:blood) down to a hematocrit of approximately 25% to 30%, depending on the rate of hemorrhage and the patient's physical status. During procedures in which there is marked brain swelling, there are often requests made to keep the patient "dry" in the false belief that fluid restriction lessens brain edema formation. Complete water restriction in dogs for 72 hours results in an 8% loss of body weight, but only a 1% decrease in brain water content.[17] Given the severe physiologic stress such severe water restriction imposes, the benefit to be gained by the minimal decrease in brain water content is unwarranted. Under no circumstances should isoosmolar fluids be withheld to the point that the patient manifests hemodynamic instability caused by hypovolemia.

Mannitol

Mannitol is a 6-carbon sugar with a molecular weight of 182. Mannitol is the most commonly administered hyperosmolar solution and is available as either 20% or 25% solutions with osmolalities of 1098 and 1372 respectively. Mannitol is often administered whenever significant brain swelling occurs or when it becomes necessary to decrease brain volume to facilitate exposure and thereby reduce brain retractor ischemia. Mannitol should be given only after other potential causes of increased brain volume have been considered (e.g., hypercapnia, administration of vasodilators, obstruction to venous outflow). Mannitol is commonly given as 0.5 to 1.0 g/kg doses administered as a rapid IV infusion. The effects of 1 and 2 g/kg doses of mannitol on serum electrolytes and plasma osmolality have been examined by Manninen et al.[25] In addition to the anticipated transient increase in plasma osmolality, there was an associated decrease in serum sodium and bicarbonate concentrations, probably caused by osmotic-induced expansion of the extracellular volume. Those patients who received the high-dose mannitol (i.e., 2 g/kg) also manifested a marked increase in serum potassium concentration (maximum mean increase of 1.5 mMol/L). Possible explanations include solvent drag (as water leaves the intracellular compartment, potassium is carried with it) and hemolysis of red cells near the tip of the infusion catheter caused by the locally high concentration of mannitol. Although transient, the associated hyperkalemia has been reported to be associated with characteristic electrocardiographic changes.[28]

Mannitol may have a biphasic effect on intracranial pressure. Concomitant with the infusion, intracranial pressure may transiently increase, presumably because of vasodilation of cerebral vessels in response to the acute increase in plasma osmolality.[39] Subsequent reduction in intracranial pressure is achieved by the movement of water from the brain's interstitial and intracellular spaces into the vasculature.

Intraoperative Fluids: Colloids
Hetastarch

The commonly used non–blood-derived colloids available for infusion are hetastarch, dextran 40, and dextran 70. Hetastarch (Hespan) is a 6% solution of enzymatically hydrolyzed amylopectin (a waxy starch) in a solution of normal (0.9%) saline. These polymerized glucose molecules are nonuniform in size, with 80% of them falling within a molecular weight range of 30,000 to 2,400,000. The mean molecular weight for hetastarch is approximately 480,000. The smaller molecules (less than 50,000 molecular weight) are rapidly filtered by the kidneys so that approximately 30% of the administered dose is excreted into the urine within the first 24 hours. Hetastarch, unlike dextran, has had an extremely low reported incidence of anaphylactic reactions and is useful when rapid intravascular volume expansion is required. The volume expansion produced by hetastarch is approximately equal to that of an equal volume of 5% albumin. Use of hetastarch is contraindicated in patients with coagulopathies because administration of large volumes of this colloid may result in prolongation of prothrombin and partial thromboplastin times. These adverse effects on the ability of the blood to clot have limited the use of hetastarch in neurosurgery. Sporadic case reports of cerebral hemorrhage after hetastarch infusion have made some anesthesiologists and neurosurgeons reluctant to use this compound. In 1987, Cully and Larson[5] reported the occurrence of a subdural hematoma in a craniotomy patient who developed a moderately prolonged partial thromboplastin time after the infusion of 2000 ml of 6% hetastarch. Although the authors admit that they could not conclusively link this coagulopathy to the hetastarch administration, they thought that there were no other obvious explanations for

this event. The PTT failed to correct even after the administration of three units of fresh frozen plasma, with the subsequent development in the patient of a subdural hematoma.

Pentastarch

Recently, a new formulation of hydrolyzed amylopectin called pentastarch (Pentaspan) has been made available for leukopheresis and is currently under investigation as a volume expander. This colloidal solution differs from hetastarch primarily in its lower molecular weight (mean of 264,000 vs. 480,000 for hetastarch). The smaller size of the pentastarch molecules results in more rapid renal excretion (approximately 70% of administered dose within the first 24 hours). Whether this compound will prove useful for volume replacement in neurosurgical patients depends on results of ongoing investigations into its effects on hemostasis and brain water content. Preliminary studies suggest that pentastarch may have less of an effect on clotting parameters than hetastarch. Infusion of pentastarch did not prolong the bleeding time, had little effect on factor VIII, and did not change the urokinase-activated clot lysis time.[43]

Dextrans

Dextran solutions are colloids composed of glucose polymers with predominantly 1-6 glucosidic linkages. Although dextran 70 has an oncotic pressure similar to plasma, the oncotic pressure of dextran 40 is significantly greater, thus infusion of dextran 40 can actually draw water from the interstitial space into the intravascular compartment. Effective volume expansion may therefore be greater than the volume of dextran infused. This volume expansion lasts approximately 3 to 4 hours for low-molecular-weight preparations (Dextran 40, 10% solution, mean molecular weight of 40,000) and approximately 6 to 8 hours for the high-molecular-weight form (Dextran 70, 6% solution, mean molecular weight of 70,000). Within 24 hours of intravenous injection, 60% of dextran 40 and 35% of dextran 70 are cleared from the intravascular space, predominantly by renal excretion of the lower molecular weight fractions of these compounds.[29]

Dextrans are known to be associated with a variety of adverse effects that have limited their clinical use. Dextrans, in a manner analogous to hetastarch, interfere with normal blood coagulation. This may be due, in part, to the hemodilution of the various clotting factors caused by the volume-expanding properties of dextran but is also thought to be caused by a "coating" of cellular elements and the vascular endothelium that reduces their efficiency in propagating the coagulation cascade. Because of these effects, it has been recommended that dextran infusions not exceed 2 g of dextran per kilogram of body weight.[2] Dextrans also are associated with pseudoallergic reactions in approximately 0.032% of patients who receive these solutions. In severe cases, patients may develop bronchospasm and circulatory collapse. To prevent such occurrences, it is now recommended that immediately before one starts the infusion of dextran 40 or 70, 20 ml of very-low-molecular-weight dextran (dextran 1, 15% solution) should be administered intravenously. The dextran 1 binds to circulating IgG, which mediates most of the allergic reactions, thereby preventing it from cross-linking with the much larger dextran molecules when they are infused for volume expansion.

Another problem associated with dextran administration is that it may interfere with blood typing and crossmatching. When more than 20% of the blood volume has been replaced by dextran, it may be difficult to determine the ABO type. With smaller volumes, Rh and various minor antigenic markers may be difficult to identify.[24] In addition, the presence of circulating dextrans can interfere with a number of clinical laboratory tests, including blood sugar, bilirubin, and protein assays. Finally, there has been a case report of acute renal failure caused by the overzealous administration of dextran 40 with the resultant production of a hyperoncotic state (plasma oncotic pressure of 33.1 mm Hg).[27]

Albumin

Human albumin is available for infusion in either 5% or 25% solutions. These solutions do not contain any of the clotting factors found in fresh whole blood or fresh plasma. Because all of the isoagglutinins also are removed in the processing, albumin may be given without regard to the patient's blood type. The albumin is derived from the plasma of volunteer donors, pooled, heat treated at 60° C for 10 hours to inactivate possible viral contamination, and finally sterilized by ultrafiltration. Albumin has a molecular weight of approximately 69,000 and constitutes 50% of the total plasma proteins by weight. Intravenously infused albumin has a plasma half-life of 16 hours in nonedematous patients. Although albumin is useful as a volume expander, it is expensive. At our institution, the current cost to the patient of 500 ml of 5% albumin is $195, whereas an equal volume of hetastarch is only $76.

Plasma and Red Blood Cells

The increased professional and public awareness of the hazards associated with the infusion of blood products has markedly curtailed their use. Currently, red blood cells should be given only to maintain hematocrit at a "safe" level. What this level is will vary from patient to patient, and, even in a specific circumstance, it may be difficult to objectively define what constitutes "safe." Thus, no specific recommendation can be made as to how far the hematocrit may fall before initiation of transfusion. In general, however, healthy individuals easily tolerate hematocrits in the 20% to 25% range. In vitro studies have shown that oxygen delivery to the tissues is maximal at a hematocrit of approximately 30%. At higher hematocrits, oxygen delivery is compromised by the increased viscosity of the blood, whereas at hematocrits much below 25%,

delivery falls off because of decreased carrying capacity of the hemoglobin.

Plasma should be administered only in an attempt to correct a coagulation defect caused by a deficiency of one or more of the coagulation factors. Volume expansion is no longer considered an appropriate use of this blood product. Coagulation defects may arise in neurosurgical patients for a variety of reasons. An abnormality in the prothrombin time, partial thromboplastin time, or platelet count at admission was shown to be present in 55% of head-injured patients who had evidence of new or progressive lesions on CT scans.[42] Victims of traumatic injury may require massive fluid resuscitation because of hemorrhagic hypovolemia. If this initial fluid resuscitation is achieved with asanguinous fluids, a dilutional coagulopathy may aggravate a preexisting clotting disorder.

Specific Neurosurgical Challenges
Fluid Management of Patients with Cerebral Aneurysms

Patients who present for surgery after rupture of a cerebral aneurysm pose additional problems in fluid management. Cerebral vasospasm is a leading cause of morbidity in these patients, producing death or severe disability in approximately 14% of patients who survive rupture of their aneurysm. Angiographic evidence of vasospasm occurs in as many as 60% to 80% of patients after subarachnoid hemorrhage. The mediators by which blood in the subarachnoid space provokes large cerebral arteries to spasm is the subject of intense investigation and debate. We know that vasospasm after aneurysm rupture can be so severe that it causes cerebral ischemia and infarction. The incidence of vasospasm reaches a peak at 4 to 10 days after the rupture of the aneurysm. There are currently two accepted therapeutic interventions that may decrease the incidence and/or severity of vasospasm. The first of these is hypervolemic/hyperdynamic therapy. Studies have shown that volume loading of patients suffering from neurologic impairment secondary to vasospasm in conjunction with inotropic support can reverse or reduce the neurologic morbidity. This approach can only be used in those patients in whom the aneurysm already has been secured and is no longer at risk of rerupture. Institution of hypervolemic/hyperdynamic therapy should be guided by hemodynamic data provided by a pulmonary artery catheter. In previously healthy individuals, maximum cardiac performance is obtained at a pulmonary capillary wedge pressure of 14 mm Hg. Volume expansion beyond this point results in increased wedge pressures but no further increase in cardiac index.[22] Volume loading may be accomplished by infusion of isoosmolar crystalloids, colloids, or red blood cells with the goal of hemodiluting the patient to a hematocrit of approximately 30%. Frequent assessment of pulmonary function with arterial blood gases, chest films, and physical examination is essential because onset of pulmonary edema with hypoxia will negate any possible beneficial effects of increased flow to ischemic brain tissue.

The second therapy for vasospasm is use of the calcium channel blocker nimodipine (Nimotop). Nimodipine has been shown to decrease the incidence of severe neurologic impairment caused by vasospasm. Nimodipine has an advantage over hypervolemic/hyperdynamic therapy because it can be administered before clipping of the aneurysm; it has no adverse hemodynamic effects that may provoke re-rupture.[1,30,32]

Fluid Management of Diabetes Insipidus

Neurogenic diabetes insipidus may occur in patients with lesions in the vicinity of the hypothalamus, after pituitary surgery, or after traumatic head injury. This syndrome is characterized by a failure of the neurons located in the supraoptic nuclei of the hypothalamus to release sufficient quantities of vasopressin into the systemic circulation. Diabetes insipidus is characterized by the production of large volumes of dilute urine in the face of a normal or elevated plasma osmolality. In severe cases, urinary output can be as great as a liter per hour. Left untreated or unrecognized, diabetes insipidus can quickly result in severe dehydration, hypovolemia, and hypotension.[46] To promptly diagnose diabetes insipidus, one must have a high index of suspicion when dealing with patients who are at risk. Confirmation may be obtained by documenting elevated serum osmolality and sodium concentration in conjunction with a low urine specific gravity or osmolality. Vigorous rehydration of the patient should be carried out with 0.45% saline until euvolemia is established. Because of the preexisting hyperosmolar/hypernatremic state, normal saline should *not* routinely be used for the initial rehydration of these patients. Concomitantly, replacement therapy should be initiated with either aqueous vasopressin (5 to 10 units by intravenous or intramuscular injection) or desmopressin (1 to 4 μg subcutaneously).

Fluid Management of the Head-Injured Trauma Patient

Victims of traumatic injury often have associated closed head injuries. Some of these patients present in hemorrhagic shock and require immediate volume resuscitation. For such a patient, the anesthesiologist is confronted by a variety of concerns, including the question of how to rapidly restore intravascular volume and organ perfusion while minimizing cerebral edema formation. Although a variety of hypertonic, hyperoncotic solutions appear ideally suited for this purpose based on animal studies, none are commercially available, and their use in humans is not presently considered the standard of care. Currently, the ideal resuscitation fluid for patients who are hypovolemic with ongoing blood loss is fresh whole blood. Because whole blood is a colloid rather than a crystalloid, smaller volumes of whole blood are required to restore intravascular volume, thus producing a more rapid resuscitation. Whole blood re-

places those clotting factors and platelets that have been lost and may therefore prevent the emergence of a dilutional coagulopathy. Finally, use of fresh whole blood may reduce the infectious risk to the trauma patient because the patient is exposed to a smaller donor pool than are patients who are resuscitated with red blood cells from one donor, platelets from another, and plasma from a third. Unfortunately, because blood banks have embraced the concept of fractionating all donor units and because of the need to test donor units for infectious agents, there are few, if any, institutions in the United States where fresh whole blood is available. Hetastarch is not widely used because of its potential to induce a coagulopathy when given in large volumes. Dextrans have also been implicated in causing increased bleeding and carry the risk (although slight) of an anaphylactoid reaction. Albumin is expensive and does not reduce cerebral edema or intracranial pressure when compared with isotonic crystalloids during the initial resuscitative efforts.[47] In pragmatic terms, this leaves isotonic crystalloid solutions as the first choice for volume resuscitation of the head-injured trauma patient. Normal saline is a good choice because it is inexpensive, can be given with packed cells when they become available, has a long shelf life, and is mildly hyperosmolar in comparison with normal plasma. Fluids to be avoided include hypotonic solutions (i.e., 0.45% saline) and any solution containing dextrose.

▼

SUMMARY

The movement of water between the vasculature and the brain's extracellular space is driven primarily by the presence of osmotic gradients. Clinically, these gradients can be established by administration of either hyperosmolar (e.g., mannitol) or hypoosmolar (e.g., D5W) solutions. In the brain (unlike peripheral tissues), plasma oncotic pressure has little impact on cerebral edema formation. Attempts to minimize cerebral edema formation by fluid restriction are unlikely to be successful and, if overzealously pursued, may lead to hemodynamic instability. Although no single intravenous solution is best suited for the neurosurgical patient who is at risk for intracranial hypertension, the use of isoosmolar crystalloids is widely accepted and can be justified on a scientific basis.

Acknowledgement

The authors wish to thank Dr. Michael M. Todd for his review of this chapter and for the inspiration for Figs. 11-4 to 11-6.

References

1. Allen GS, Ahn HS, Preziosi TJ et al: Cerebral arterial spasm—a controlled trial of nimodipine in patients with subarachnoid hemorrhage, *N Engl J Med* 308:619-624, 1983.
2. Alexander B, Odake K, Lawlor D et al: Coagulation, hemostasis, and plasma expanders: a quarter century enigma, *Fed Proc* 34:1429-1440, 1975.
3. Bevan DR: Osmometry. 1. Terminology and principles of measurement, *Anaesthesia* 33:794-800, 1978.
4. Choi DW, Monyer H, Giffard RG et al: Acute brain injury, NMDA receptors, and hydrogen ions: observations in cortical cell cultures, *Adv Exp Med Biol* 268:501-504, 1990.
5. Cully MD, Larson CP, Silverberg GD: Hetastarch coagulopathy in a neurosurgical patient, *Anesthesiology* 66:706-707, 1987.
6. De Courten-Meyers G, Myers RE, Schoolfield L: Hyperglycemia enlarges infarct size in cerebrovascular occlusion in cats, *Stroke* 19:623-630, 1988.
7. Dodge PR, Crawford JD, Probst JH: Studies in experimental water intoxication, *Arch Neurol* 5:513-529, 1960.
8. Drummond J, Moore S: The influence of dextrose administration on neurologic outcome after temporary spinal cord ischemia in the rabbit, *Anesthesiology* 70:64-70, 1989.
9. Fenstermacher JD, Johnson JA: Filtration and reflection coefficients of the rabbit blood-brain barrier, *Am J Physiol* 211:341-346, 1966.
10. Fisher B, Thomas D, Peterson B: Hypertonic saline lowers raised intracranial pressure in children after head trauma, *J Neurosurg Anesth* 4:4-10, 1992.
11. Giffard RG, Monyer H, Christine CW et al: Acidosis reduces NMDA receptor activation, glutamate neurotoxicity, and oxygen-glucose deprivation neuronal injury in cortical cultures, *Brain Res* 506:339-342, 1990.
12. Ginsberg MD, Prado R, Dietrich WD et al: Hyperglycemia reduces the extent of cerebral infarction in rats, *Stroke* 18:570-574, 1987.
13. Gunnar W, Jonasson O, Merlotti G et al: Head injury and hemorrhagic shock: studies of the blood brain barrier and intracranial pressure after resuscitation with normal saline solution, 3% saline solution, and dextran-40, *Surgery* 103:398-407, 1988.
14. Gunnar WP, Merlotti GJ, Jonasson O et al: Resuscitation from hemorrhagic shock: alterations of the intracranial pressure after normal saline, 3% saline and Dextran-40, *Ann Surg* 204:686-692, 1986.
15. Guyton AC: *Textbook of medical physiology,* Philadelphia, 1976, WB Saunders, pp 424-437.
16. Haupt MT, Rackow EC: Colloid osmotic pressure and fluid resuscitation with hetastarch, albumin, and saline solutions, *Crit Care Med* 10:159-162, 1982.
17. Jelsma LF, McQueen JD: Effect of experimental water restriction on brain water, *J Neurosurg* 26:35-40, 1967.
18. Kaieda R, Todd MM, Warner DS: Prolonged reduction in colloid oncotic pressure does not increase brain edema following cryogenic injury in rabbits, *Anesthesiology* 71:554-560, 1989.
19. Kien ND, Kramer GC, White DA: Acute hypotension caused by rapid hypertonic saline infusion in anesthetized dogs, *Anesth Analg* 73:597-602, 1991.
20. Korosue K, Heros RC, Ogilvy CS et al: Comparison of crystalloids and colloids for hemodilution in a model of focal cerebral ischemia, *J Neurosurg* 73:576-584, 1990.
21. Lanier WL, Stangland KJ, Scheithauer BW et al: The effects of dextrose infusion and head position on neurologic outcome after complete cerebral ischemia in primates: examination of a model, *Anesthesiology* 66:39-48, 1987.
22. Levy ML, Giannotta SL: Cardiac performance indices during hypervolemic therapy for cerebral vasospasm, *J Neurosurg* 75:27-31, 1991.
23. Little JR, Slugg RM, Latchaw JP et al: Treatment of acute focal cerebral ischemia with concentrated albumin, *Neurosurgery* 9:552-558, 1981.
24. Lutz H, Georgieff M: Effects and side effects of colloid plasma substitutes as compared to albumin, *Curr Stud Hematol Blood Transf* 53:145-154, 1986.
25. Manninen PH, Lam AM, Gelb AW et al: The effect of high-dose mannitol on serum and urine electrolytes and osmolality in neurosurgical patients, *Can J Anaesth* 34:442-446, 1987.
26. Marty AT, Zweifach BW: The high oncotic pressure effects of dextrans, *Arch Surg* 101:421-424, 1970.
27. Moran M, Kapsner C: Acute renal failure associated with elevated plasma oncotic pressure, *N Engl J Med* 317:150-153, 1987.
28. Moreno M, Murphy C, Goldsmith C: Increase in serum potassium resulting from the administration of hypertonic mannitol and other solutions, *J Lab Clin Med* 73:291-298, 1969.
29. Nearman HS, Herman ML: Toxic effects of colloids in the intensive care unit, *Crit Care Clin* 7:713-723, 1991.
30. Ohman J, Heiskanen O: Effect of nimodipine on the outcome of patients after aneurysmal subarachnoid hemorrhage and surgery, *J Neurosurg* 69:683-686, 1988.
31. Peters RM, Hargens AR: Protein vs electrolytes and all of the Starling forces, *Arch Surg* 116:1293-1298, 1981.
32. Petruk KC, West M, Mohr G et al: Nimodipine treatment in poor-grade aneurysm patients, *J Neurosurg* 68:505-517, 1988.
33. Sahar A, Tsiptstein E: Effects of mannitol and furosemide on the rate of formation of cerebrospinal fluid, *Exp Neurol* 60:584-591, 1978.
34. Scheller MS, Zornow MH, Oh YS: A comparison of the cerebral and hemodynamic effects of mannitol and hypertonic saline in a rabbit model of acute cryogenic brain injury, *J Neurosurg Anesth* 3:291-296, 1991.
35. Shackford SR, Fortlage DA, Peters RM et al: Serum osmolar and electrolyte changes associated with large infusions of hypertonic sodium lactate for intravascular volume expansion of patients undergoing aortic reconstruction, *Surg Gyn Obstet* 164:127-136, 1987.
36. Shackford SR, Sise MJ, Fridlund PH et al: Hypertonic sodium lactate versus lactated Ringer's solution for intravenous fluid therapy in operations on the abdominal aorta, *Surgery* 94:41-51, 1983.
37. Shackford SR, Zhuang J, Schmoker J: Intravenous fluid tonicity: effect on intracranial pressure, cerebral blood flow, and cerebral oxygen delivery in focal brain injury, *J Neurosurg* 76:91-98, 1992.
38. Shenkin HA, Bezier HS, F.Bouzarth W: Restricted fluid intake: rational management of the neurosurgical patient, *J Neurosurg* 45:432-436, 1976.

39. Shenkin HA, Goluboff B, Haft H: Further observations on the effects of abruptly increased osmotic pressure of plasma on cerebrospinal-fluid pressure in man, *J Neurosurg* 22:563-568, 1964.

40. Sotos JF, Dodge PR, Meara P et al: Studies in experimental hypertonicity. I. Pathogenesis of the clinical syndrome, biochemical abnormalities and cause of death, *Pediatrics* 26:925-938, 1960.

41. Starling EH: On the absorption of fluids from the connective tissue spaces, *J Physiol* 19:312-326, 1896.

42. Stein SC, Young GS, Talucci RC et al: Delayed brain injury after head trauma: significance of coagulopathy, *Neurosurgery* 30:160-165, 1992.

43. Strauss RG, Stansfield C, Henriksen RA: Pentastarch may cause fewer effects on coagulation than hetastarch, *Transfusion* 28:257-260, 1988.

44. Todd MM, Tommasino C, Moore S: Cerebral effects of isovolemic hemodilution with a hypertonic saline solution, *J Neurosurg* 63:944-948, 1985.

45. Warner DS, Boehland LA: Effects of iso-osmolal intravenous fluid therapy on post-ischemic brain water content in the rat, *Anesthesiology* 68:86-91, 1988.

46. Wilson JD, Braunwald E, Isselbacher KJ et al: *Harrison's principles of internal medicine*, New York, 1991, McGraw-Hill, pp 1684-1689.

47. Wisner D, Busche F, Sturn J et al: Traumatic shock and head injury: effects of fluid resuscitation on the brain, *J Surg Res* 46:49-59, 1989.

48. Worthley LIG, Cooper DJ, Jones N: Treatment of resistant intracranial hypertension with hypertonic saline, *J Neurosurg* 68:478-481, 1988.

49. Zasslow MA, Pearl RG, Shuer LM et al: Hyperglycemia decreases acute neuronal ischemic changes after middle cerebral artery occlusion in cats, *Stroke* 20:519-523, 1989.

50. Zornow MH, Scheller MS, Todd MM et al: Acute cerebral effects of isotonic crystalloid and colloid solutions following cryogenic brain injury in the rabbit, *Anesthesiology* 69:180-184, 1988.

51. Zornow MH, Scheller MS, Shackford SR: Effect of a hypertonic lactated Ringer's solution on intracranial pressure and cerebral water content in a model of traumatic brain injury, *J Trauma* 29:484-488, 1989.

52. Zornow MH, Todd MM, Moore SS: The acute cerebral effects of changes in plasma osmolality and oncotic pressure, *Anesthesiology* 67:936-941, 1987.

12

Care of the Acutely Unstable Patient

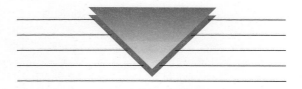

KAREN B. DOMINO

BRAIN INJURY
  Neurologic evaluation
  Radiologic evaluation
  Evaluation of other organ systems
  Airway management of the brain-injured
    patient

Aims in the acute care of the brain-
  injured patient
SPINAL CORD INJURY
  Neurologic evaluation
  Radiologic evaluation
  Evaluation of other organ systems

Airway management of the patient with
  suspected cervical spine injury
Aims in the acute care of the spinal cord–
  injured patient
SUMMARY

Most neurologic emergencies that require the acute care of an anesthesiologist are caused by head and spinal cord trauma. On occasion, patients with ruptured cerebral aneurysms or arteriovenous malformations, acute hydrocephalus, intracerebral hematomas, and intracranial tumors present with impending brain herniation. Likewise, masses (tumors or hematomas) compressing the spinal cord may cause acute spinal cord injury. This chapter will focus on the acute care of the neurologically unstable patient with brain and spinal cord injuries, regardless of etiology. It will focus on the initial neurologic evaluation, the evaluation of other organ systems, the management of the airway, and the aims in the acute care of the unstable patient.

BRAIN INJURY
Neurologic Evaluation

The Glasgow Coma Scale[183] is used to quickly evaluate the neurologic status of patients with a brain injury (Box 12-

1). It evaluates the best verbal response, best motor response, and presence of eye opening using a scale from 3 to 15. The scaling system is useful because it is easy to use, it has good interobserver reliability, it helps guide diagnosis and therapy, and it has prognostic significance. Morbidity and mortality are closely related to the initial Glasgow Coma Scale irrespective of the etiology of the head injury.[22,85] Another factor that predicts the severity of the head injury is age, with a better prognosis noted among pediatric patients.[22,103,106]

Respiratory pattern, pulse, blood pressure, pupillary responses, and gag reflexes are also evaluated in the initial neurologic examination. If the patient is comatose (e.g., no eye opening, verbal response, or ability to follow commands), evaluation of midbrain and brainstem reflexes (e.g., pupillary response, corneal reflexes, oculomotor movements, and the gag reflex) may aid in localization of the lesion. In the acute setting, examination of the size and reactivity of the pupils is particularly important. A dilated,

BOX 12-1
NEUROLOGIC EVALUATION OF THE BRAIN-INJURED PATIENT

A. Glasgow Coma Scale
  1. Eye Opening
    Spontaneous 4
    To speech 3
    To pain 2
    None 1
  2. Best verbal response
    Oriented 5
    Confused 4
    Inappropriate 3
    Incomprehensible 2
    None 1
  3. Best motor response
    Obeys commands 6
    Localizes pain 5
    Withdraws 4
    Flexion to pain 3
    Extension to pain 2
    None 1
B. Pupillary size and reactivity
  1. Uncal herniation — dilated, unresponsive pupil
C. CT Scan
  1. Mass lesion
  2. Cerebral edema
  3. Midline shift/absent basal cisterns

unresponsive ("blown") pupil may be a sign of ipsilateral uncal herniation, in which the medial aspect of the temporal lobe (uncus) herniates through the tentorium, thereby compressing the midbrain and nucleus of the third cranial nerve.[84] Anisocoria is also associated with mechanical brain compensation.[4] Bilateral pupillary dilation may be due to bilateral uncal herniation or injury (such as ischemic or metabolic) to the midbrain. Local eye trauma or third nerve compression may cause a dilated, unreactive pupil in the absence of a brain injury. In head-injured patients with systolic blood pressures greater than 60 mm Hg, clinical signs of tentorial herniation or upper brainstem dysfunction are valid indicators of possible mechanical compression.[4] However, in patients with systolic blood pressure of less than 60 mm Hg or a cardiac arrest, pupillary signs are unreliable indicators of mechanical compression.[4]

Radiologic Evaluation

After neurologic evaluation and initial stabilization, radiologic evaluation with a CT scan is performed to diagnose the underlying disease process. If the patient is hemodynamically unstable with intraabdominal or intrathoracic bleeding, the CT scan is delayed until the life-threatening surgical bleeding is stopped. If the physical examination indicates high likelihood of a brain injury, an intracranial

pressure (ICP) monitor and/or burr holes may be placed concurrently with the laparotomy or thoracotomy. Intracranial mass lesions that require rapid surgical treatment, such as epidural, subdural, or large intracerebral hemorrhages, are readily identified on CT scan (Figs. 12-1 and 12-2). Nonsurgical lesions, such as cerebral edema and hemorrhagic contusion, are also identified (Fig. 12-3). Diffuse cerebral swelling may develop after head trauma, especially in children.[16] The severity of the brain injury can be correlated with the magnitude of the midline shift (Fig. 12-2)[103] and compression of the basal cisterns (Fig. 12-3).[187] Patients with Glasgow Coma Scale scores of 6 to 8 who had absent or compressed basal cisterns on initial CT scan had a fourfold additional risk of poor outcome compared with those with normal cisterns.[187] As patients may often have a delayed neurologic deterioration,[24,103] a repeat CT scan is indicated after any deterioration in neurologic status. Of patients who deteriorated after a mild head injury, 80% had a mass lesion that potentially required surgery.[103] In contrast, cerebral swelling is more likely to be the cause of deterioration in patients with severe head injury.[24] Occasionally, intracerebral hematomas have a delayed presentation after head trauma.[176]

Evaluation of Other Organ Systems

In addition to the neurologic evaluation, a quick evaluation of other organ systems should be performed (Box 12-2).

Respiratory System

A chest x-ray should be performed soon after the patient arrives in the emergency room. Many patients are hypoxemic after head trauma, and an increased degree of pulmonary shunting is associated with a worsened neurologic outcome.[63,173] Hypoxemia may be due to airway obstruction, hypoventilation from the brain injury, atelectasis, aspiration, pneumothorax, or pulmonary contusion. On rare occasions, neurogenic pulmonary edema may occur, often in the more devastating injuries. Neurogenic pulmonary edema has been reported after a variety of central nervous system insults, including subarachnoid hemorrhage, intracranial hemorrhage, head trauma, spinal cord trauma, acute hydrocephalus, colloid cyst of the third ventricle, seizures, and hypothalamic lesions.[28] An acute rise in intracranial pressure often, but not always, accompanies the development of pulmonary edema. Increases in intracranial pressure may only elicit the sympathetic activation and cardiopulmonary responses that are essential for the development of edema. The mechanism of neurogenic pulmonary edema is not completely understood.[110] Marked sympathetic activation at the time of the injury may damage the pulmonary capillary endothelium by both hydrostatic and increased permeability mechanisms.[110,115] Increased pulmonary shunting may also be observed in patients with head trauma in the absence of distinct pulmonary edema or pathology.[138,160] The increased alveolar-arterial oxygen tension

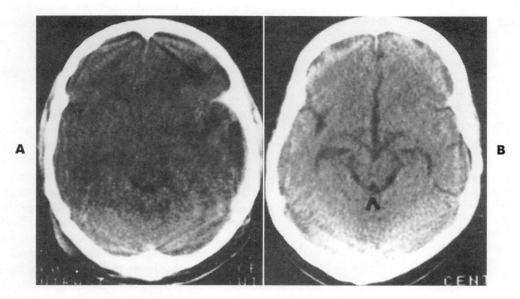

FIG. 12-1   Computed tomography (CT) scan of an epidural hematoma. **A,** Plain CT scan shows parietal epidural hematoma. **B,** Contrast-enhanced CT scan shows enhancing dural rim *(arrow).* *(From Haaga JR, Alfidi RJ, editors:* Computed tomography of the whole body, *vol 1, St Louis, 1983, CV Mosby, p 185.)*

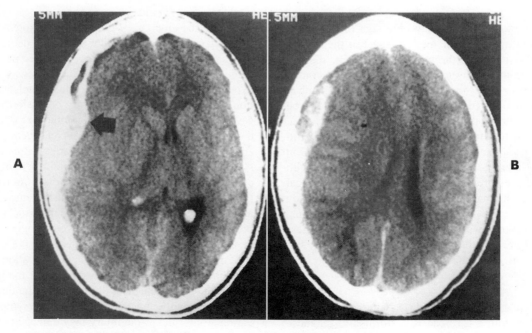

FIG. 12-2   **A,** CT scan revealing an acute subdural hematoma *(arrow).* **B,** Note the marked midline shift, with displacement of the lateral ventricles toward the left. *(From Haaga JR, Alfidi RJ, editors:* Computed tomography of the whole body, *vol 1, St Louis, 1983, CV Mosby, p.187).*

BOX 12-2
BRAIN INJURY: EFFECTS ON OTHER ORGAN SYSTEMS

Respiratory System

Increased pulmonary shunting
Neurogenic pulmonary edema
Associated pulmonary injuries: atelectasis, aspiration, pneumothorax, pulmonary contusion

Cardiovascular System

Sympathetic nervous system overactivity
Cushing response (hypertension, bradycardia)
Hypotension (look for another cause)

Musculoskeletal System

Cervical spine injury in 10% of cases
Long bone or pelvic fractures

Gastrointestinal System — "Full Stomach"

"Full stomach"
Alcohol use
Possible intraabdominal injury

Other Systems

Disseminated intravascular coagulation
Hypokalemia
Hyperglycemia
Diabetes insipidus
Hyponatremia

gradient in these patients may be related to airway closure caused by a decreased functional residual capacity in a comatose patient[29] or by neurogenic alterations in ventilation-perfusion matching.[53]

Cardiovascular System

Severe brain injury activates the autonomic nervous system and causes a hyperdynamic cardiovascular response consisting of hypertension, tachycardia, increased cardiac output, and ECG changes that may mimic myocardial ischemia.[25,26,37,122] A Cushing response in which bradycardia accompanies the hypertension may occur.[41] This response is thought to occur because marked intracranial hypertension causes medullary ischemia because of decreased cerebral perfusion pressure and brainstem distortion,[149] resulting in activation of medullary sympathetic and vagal centers.[41] Although bradycardia accompanies the hypertension in a classic Cushing response, the presence of a relative tachycardia in a patient with a "blown" pupil may indicate that the patient is hypovolemic. If the patient is outright hypotensive, other sources of blood loss (e.g., pelvic, thoracic, abdominal) should be sought. An isolated head injury is not generally associated with hypotension because the blood loss from the head wound is usually insufficient to cause hypotension in adults.

Musculoskeletal System

A lateral cervical spine x-ray should be performed immediately because approximately 10% of patients with head injuries have associated cervical spine injuries. The lateral

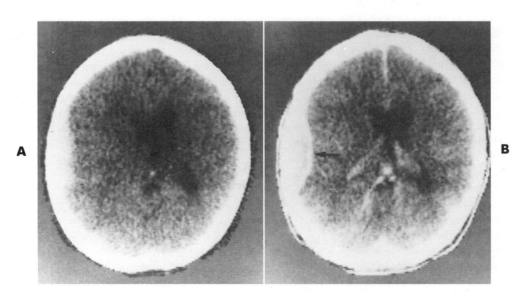

FIG. 12-3 CT scan showing compressed basal cisterns (**A**) and normal basal cisterns (**B**, *arrow*). The presence of compressed basal cisterns after head trauma increases the risk of poor outcome. *(From Toutant SM, Klauber MR, Marshall LF et al: J Neurosurg 61:691, 1984.)*

cervical spine x-ray picks up approximately 80% of cervical spine fractures[157,181] and can display lethal injuries such as atlantooccipital separation. The remainder of the spine series that is required to "clear the neck" should be completed later after complete evaluation of the head injury. Many head-trauma patients also have long-bone or pelvic fractures that may cause significant blood loss or fat emboli.

Gastrointestinal System

All patients with a neurosurgical emergency should be assumed to have a full stomach and to be at risk for aspiration. Patients with acute head trauma may also have intraabdominal injuries. Delayed gastric emptying may persist for several weeks after severe head injury.[125] Significant blood alcohol levels have been found in more than 50% of head-injured patients.[90]

Other Systems

Patients with head trauma may also develop disseminated intravascular coagulation, possibly caused by release of brain thromboplastin into the systemic circulation.[9,23,48,186] Outcome is poorer in patients who develop disseminated intravascular coagulation.[9] An increase in fibrin split products may identify patients with head injury who are at high risk for adult respiratory distress syndrome.[35] Coagulation factors need to be checked in the emergency room, and aggressive replacement of platelets and clotting factors may be required.

The patient may develop hypokalemia and hyperglycemia in response to stress and trauma.[172] Beta-adrenergic stimulation from epinephrine causes a decrease in serum potassium by driving potassium into the cells.[154] Similarly, when pH is elevated, as is common in the brain-injured patient in whom hyperventilation is used to reduce intracranial pressure, potassium is driven into cells as hydrogen ions are released. Decreases in serum potassium associated with acute hyperventilation and stress do not need to be treated because total body potassium is unchanged. However, diuretic-induced renal losses of potassium do require replacement to avoid complications of acute intracellular potassium depletion, including potentiation of neuromuscular blockade and cardiac dysrhythmias. Often, in the acutely brain-injured patient, the etiology of hypokalemia is multifactorial. Initiation of treatment depends on the predominate clinical circumstances.

Diabetes insipidus may occur in patients with basilar skull fractures or severe head injuries involving the hypothalamus or posterior pituitary. Antidiuretic hormone (ADH) is synthesized in the hypothalamus and secreted by the posterior pituitary.[76] ADH enhances the permeability of free H_2O in the distal convoluted tubule and collecting duct of the kidney. Patients with diabetes insipidus can lose large volumes (25 L/day) of dilute urine, resulting in marked increases in serum sodium and osmolality.

Diabetes insipidus should be considered in the differential diagnosis of polyuria in any patient with head trauma or pituitary and hypothalamic lesions. The differential diagnosis of intraoperative polyuria includes excessive fluid administration, osmotic agents (e.g., hyperglycemia with glucose > 180 mg/dl, mannitol), diuretics, paradoxic diuresis in brain-tumor patients, and nephrogenic and central diabetes insipidus. Diabetes insipidus is diagnosed intraoperatively by ruling out iatrogenic causes and hyperglycemia and by demonstrating marked increases in serum sodium and osmolality with low urine osmolality.

Treatment of diabetes insipidus involves adequate fluid replacement with 5% dextrose in water and administration of ADH. Aqueous vasopressin may be given intramuscularly (5 to 10 U) or as a slow intravenous infusion (3 U/hr) for rapid control of intraoperative or postoperative diabetes insipidus.[76] Larger doses may cause hypertension. For less frequent dosage, DDAVP (desmopressin) 1 to 2 μg intravenously or subcutaneously every 6 to 12 hours may be administered. DDAVP may be given more frequently if the diabetes insipidus is not controlled. DDAVP has less vasopressor activity than aqueous vasopressin and is preferable to vasopressin in patients with coronary artery disease and hypertension.

Hyponatremia may also occur in the acutely brain-injured patient. Hyponatremia may be associated with diminished (e.g., diuretic usage, adrenal insufficiency, salt-losing nephritis), expanded (e.g., congestive heart failure, renal failure), or normal (e.g., hypothyroidism, syndrome of inappropriate ADH [SIADH]) extracellular fluid volumes. Rapid reduction of serum sodium to less than 125 to 130 mEq/L may cause changes in mental status and seizures. The first step in diagnosis is to establish the category to which the patient belongs. Although many clinicians are quick to suggest SIADH in patients with brain pathology, this diagnosis should be made only after excluding other etiologies. In neurosurgical patients, hyponatremia is most commonly associated with intravascular volume depletion caused by diuretic administration or a loss of sodium by the kidney. After subarachnoid hemorrhage, patients may have a primary natriuresis ("cerebral salt wasting"), which, unlike SIADH, is associated with a decreased intravascular volume.[124] Aggressive fluid therapy is required in subarachnoid hemorrhage patients to maintain a normal intravascular volume.

Airway Management of the Brain-Injured Patient

Patients with a Glasgow Coma Scale score of 8 or less or with impending herniation generally require endotracheal intubation in the emergency room. Uncooperative patients who require sedation for CT scan and other radiologic studies also require intubation because patients with suspected head injury should not be sedated without an endotracheal tube in place and control of ventilation assured. Trauma patients should be assumed to have a cervical spine injury until proved otherwise. Nasal intubation should be avoided in patients with suspected basilar skull fractures and sinus injuries.

The patient's airway and hemodynamic status should be quickly assessed before choosing a plan for endotracheal intubation (Fig. 12-4). If the airway is difficult, hypnotic drugs and muscle relaxants are contraindicated unless the ability to ventilate has been established. Direct laryngoscopy is usually used with minimal sedation. If time permits, fiberoptic laryngoscopy or retrograde insertion of an endotracheal tube may be used. In some cases, a cricothyroidotomy may be required.

If the airway appears normal, a muscle relaxant should be given to reduce coughing and increases in ICP that may occur with endotracheal intubation.[19,60,170,197] In fact, the prevention of the cough by the prior administration of a muscle relaxant appears to be most important in preventing marked increases in ICP with endotracheal intubation. White et al.[197] found that succinylcholine, but not thiopental, fentanyl, or lidocaine, prevented marked increases in ICP with endotracheal suctioning in comatose head-injured patients because of the greater reduction in coughing after succinylcholine. However, barbiturates and lidocaine were effective in attenuating the increase in ICP caused by tracheal stimulation in patients who also received a muscle re-

laxant.* These drugs and narcotics may also be necessary to prevent increases in mean arterial pressure and ICP with endotracheal intubation.

One should assess the patient's hemodynamic status to choose an anesthetic induction agent that reduces the increase in ICP that accompanies endotracheal intubation. The primary goal is to maintain an adequate cerebral perfusion pressure by ensuring hemodynamic stability while decreasing ICP. Severe hypotension from the inappropriate administration of a large dose of thiopental in a hypovolemic patient may be worse for the patient than the transient rise in ICP that accompanies endotracheal intubation. If the patient is hypertensive or hemodynamically stable, a rapid-sequence induction with head and neck stabilization, defasciculation, cricoid pressure, thiopental, lidocaine, and succinylcholine can be used. To avoid hypoxemia and excessive increases in $Paco_2$, the patient is manually hyperventilated while cricoid pressure is maintained before intubation. If the patient is hypertensive, administration of narcotics (such as fentanyl 4 to 6 μg/kg) and/or antihypertensive agents may be necessary to prevent severe hypertension and increases in ICP with endotracheal intubation.

*References 10, 46, 74, 168, 170, 190.

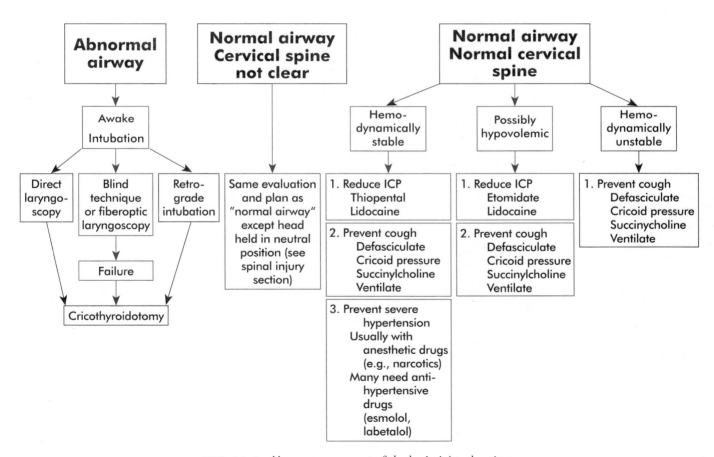

FIG. 12-4 Airway management of the brain-injured patient.

Esmolol and labetalol have less potential to raise ICP than sodium nitroprusside, which is a marked cerebrovasodilator.[33,113,191] If the patient is somewhat hypovolemic (as is common in the multiply injured patient), etomidate (0.1 to 0.2 μg/kg) should be used as an alternative to thiopental because it is effective in reducing cerebral blood flow and ICP.[123] If the patient is severely hypovolemic, a hypnotic agent is contraindicated, and defasciculation followed by succinylcholine should be used. Ketamine should be avoided because it increases ICP.[171]

The use of succinylcholine as the muscle relaxant of choice in endotracheal intubation of the acutely head-injured patient is somewhat controversial. Succinylcholine may transiently increase ICP because of increased CO_2 production or cerebral stimulation from the fasciculations.[95] Defasciculation with metocurine appears to prevent succinylcholine-induced increases in ICP.[179] In addition, thiopental, etomidate, and lidocaine reduce intracranial pressure and minimize the succinylcholine effect.[114] Therefore the benefits of rapid intubation and hyperventilation outweigh the disadvantages in the acutely injured patient. In contrast, succinylcholine is contraindicated for reintubation in patients with a significant closed head injury of greater than 48 hours' duration because of risks of succinylcholine-induced hyperkalemia, even in the absence of paresis.[58] A high-dose vecuronium (0.25 to 0.4 mg/kg) technique[100] should be chosen in this circum-

stance, assuming the airway is not difficult and the patient can be ventilated.

Aims in the Acute Care of the Brain-Injured Patient

The aim in the acute medical management of the head-injured patient is to prevent secondary neurologic injury. Factors contributing to secondary neurologic injury include hypoxia, hypercapnia, hypotension, intracranial hypertension, and transtentorial or cerebellar herniation.[8] Many of these factors are potentially treatable. Rose et al.[155] found that an avoidable factor (such as hypoxia, hypotension, and delay in the treatment of an intracranial hematoma) was identified in 54% of 116 "talk before dying" patients. Both cerebral perfusion pressure greater than 90 mm Hg and higher Glasgow Coma Scale scores correlated with better neurologic outcome.[20] Low cerebral perfusion pressures were independently associated with poor outcome after head trauma. Box 12-3 summarizes the aims in the acute care of the patient with head injuries.

High-dose steroids do not reduce ICP in head trauma.[68] In contrast to acute spinal cord injury, steroids do not affect outcome from severe head injury.[44] However, they are useful in reducing edema in the rare patient who presents with impending brain herniation from a brain tumor.[93,121] In these patients, clinical improvement occurs within hours of starting steroid therapy.

Reduction in Intracranial Pressure (ICP)

A major goal in the acute treatment of the head-injured patient is to reduce ICP, which may be accomplished through head position, hyperventilation, mannitol or furosemide, barbiturates, and surgical treatment.

Head Position. A slightly head-up position (10- to 20-degree head-up tilt) with the neck in neutral position promotes cerebral venous drainage and reduces ICP if the cerebral spinal fluid (CSF) pathways are still patent.[88,170] Lateral turning of the head, tight endotracheal or tracheostomy tube ties around the neck, or the Trendelenburg position may dramatically increase ICP because venous return from the brain is restricted.[102] The patient should be paralyzed to prevent coughing and bucking on the endotracheal tube, which also increases ICP. On the other hand, marked elevation of the head in a hypovolemic patient, if it causes a decrease in mean arterial pressure, may cause decreased brain perfusion and cerebral ischemia.[156]

Hyperventilation. Hyperventilation is a rapid and effective way to acutely lower ICP.[40,170] Hyperventilation causes an extracellular alkalosis, which constricts cerebral arterioles.[97] A $Paco_2$ of 25 to 30 mm Hg is commonly chosen as the optimal level of $Paco_2$ to decrease ICP. This level reduces cerebral blood flow (CBF) to levels that probably do not cause cerebral ischemia and therefore are appropriate in the acute setting.[75] However, in the intensive care unit, the amount of hyperventilation should be chosen by balancing the need to reduce ICP with the possibility of cre-

▼

BOX 12-3
AIMS IN THE ACUTE CARE OF THE BRAIN-INJURED PATIENT

A. Reduction in intracranial pressure
  1. Head position
  2. Hyperventilation
  3. Mannitol and furosemide
  4. Barbiturates
  5. Surgical procedures: drainage of cerebrospinal fluid and evacuation of hematoma
B. Maintenance of blood pressure
  1. Treat hypertension
    a. Sympathetic nervous system overactivity
    b. Increased intracranial pressure
    c. Light anesthesia
  2. Prevent hypotension
    a. Avoid glucose-containing solutions
    b. Intravascular volume status — aim for euvolemia
C. Treatment of hypoxemia
  1. Increase inspired oxygen tension
  2. Treat pulmonary pathology
  3. Positive end-expiratory pressure (10 cm H_2O or less)

ating cerebral ischemia. This can be gauged by inserting a jugular venous catheter and optimizing jugular venous bulb oxygen content.[38] Mechanical hyperventilation may have significant adverse cardiopulmonary effects. It may lower systemic blood pressure by reducing venous return, sympathetic stimulation, and cardiac output. It results in a leftward shift of the oxyhemoglobin dissociation curve, resulting in lower mixed venous and arterial oxygen tensions for any given oxygen saturation. Hypocapnia inhibits hypoxic pulmonary vasoconstriction[15] and causes bronchoconstriction.[165] Increases in pulmonary shunt may occur in hyperventilated patients.[120]

Mannitol and Furosemide. Mannitol decreases brain water content and ICP primarily by increasing plasma osmolality, thereby creating an osmotic gradient across the intact blood-brain barrier. The amount of water that can be withdrawn from the brain depends on the magnitude of the osmotic gradient, the total time the gradient exists, and the integrity of the blood-brain barrier. Mannitol is less effective with larger lesions because, with damaged blood-brain barriers, mannitol moves down its concentration gradient into the brain. This may account for a rebound increase in ICP occasionally seen after mannitol.

Administration of mannitol may cause a triphasic hemodynamic response. Transient (1 to 2 minutes) hypotension may occur after rapid administration of mannitol.[31] Mannitol then increases blood volume, cardiac index, and pulmonary capillary wedge pressure, with a maximum increase shortly after termination of infusion.[158] ICP may increase transiently because of increases in cerebral blood volume[144] and CBF.[82] ICP increases are attenuated by slowly infusing mannitol, which tends to naturally occur when a bag of 20% mannitol is administered by gravity, as opposed to more concentrated solutions being administered under pressure. Transient increases in ICP are uncommon in the patient with elevated ICP.[1,143] At 30 minutes after mannitol administration, blood volume returns to normal and pulmonary capillary wedge pressure and cardiac index drop to below normal levels because of peripheral vascular pooling.[158]

Mannitol decreases blood viscosity and red blood cell rigidity, which may enhance perfusion of the brain microcirculation. Mannitol transiently reduces hematocrit, and it increases serum osmolality. It also causes hyponatremia, hyperkalemia, and decreases in pH caused by HCO_3 dilution.[111] Prolonged and marked hyperosmolity with hyponatremia can occur in patients with acute and chronic renal failure.[11]

Doses of mannitol from 0.25 to 2 g/kg are usually administered; a typical dose is 1 g/kg. Lower doses are effective in reducing ICP acutely and cause fewer electrolyte abnormalities; however, they need to be given more frequently. Rapid administration of mannitol causes a more profound reduction in ICP but may transiently cause hypotension and more marked increases in intravascular and cerebral blood volumes. The benefits and disadvantages of a particular dose and speed of administration need to be weighed carefully in any patient. It is seldom effective to give more mannitol when the patient's serum osmolality is above 330 mOsm/L.

Furosemide has been reported to lower ICP and brain water content when used alone in large (1 mg/kg) doses[34] or in combination with mannitol in smaller doses.[136,151,159] In contrast to mannitol, there are some studies in which furosemide alone did not reduce ICP. Clinical impressions are that mannitol produces a better reduction of brain bulk than does furosemide. However, furosemide may be advantageous to patients with heart and renal diseases because it does not increase blood volume, or ICP, or cause as severe electrolyte abnormalities as does mannitol.

The mechanism of furosemide's action on reducing ICP is unknown. It is not related to its diuretic effect. Furosemide may reduce CSF formation and water and ion penetration across the blood-brain barrier. Furosemide also potentiates mannitol by sustaining the increase in serum osmolality induced by mannitol. Therefore reductions in ICP and brain shrinkage are consistently greater and longer in duration with mannitol plus furosemide than with either agent alone.[136,159] However, hyponatremia, hypokalemia, hypochloremia, hyperosmolality, and a significantly greater rate of water and electrolyte excretion occur with this combination of diuretics. Water excretions of up to 42 ml/min have been reported with the combination of drugs, compared with 17 ml/min with mannitol alone.

Low doses of furosemide (5 to 20 mg) added to mannitol (0.25 to 1 g/kg) are very effective in reducing brain bulk. Larger doses of furosemide may be required in the patient who chronically takes diuretics to produce the same effect. Mannitol-induced increases in blood volume and ICP may also be attenuated when furosemide is administered before mannitol. However, with administration of combined diuretics, vigorous intravascular fluid and electrolyte replacement are required. A urine loss of 2 to 3 L over 2 hours is common with combined diuretic therapy.

Barbiturates. Barbiturates reduce cerebral metabolism, CBF, cerebral blood volume, and ICP.[132] In the acute management of the brain-injured patient, barbiturates are useful to reduce the intracranial response to noxious stimuli, such as endotracheal intubation, tracheal suctioning, or surgical stimulation.[167,168,170,190] They may also acutely reduce intraoperative brain swelling. Barbiturates have also been used successfully to reduce ICP in patients with head trauma refractory to other treatments.[145,153] However, long-term barbiturate therapy probably does not affect long-term outcome after head trauma.[112,161,196]

While barbiturates may aid in the acute control of ICP, their use is limited by the fact that they may reduce mean arterial blood pressure and cerebral perfusion pressure. Because hypotension is a definite risk factor for worsened neurologic outcome, it is particularly important to maintain a normal blood pressure in the brain-injured patient. Thus barbiturates should be carefully titrated (e.g., thiopental in

1 to 4 mg/kg doses) and blood pressure supported with vasopressors as necessary. Barbiturates should not be administered to hypovolemic or hypotensive patients. Likewise, high doses of barbiturates (e.g., greater than 8 to 10 mg/kg of thiopental) are contraindicated before the surgical evacuation of an intracranial mass because the blood pressure may severely decrease with the reduction in sympathetic tone that accompanies brain decompression. Given the instability of the acutely injured patient, high doses of barbiturates are best reserved for use in the intensive care unit.

Surgical Treatment. Surgical treatment may be required to acutely lower ICP. If hydrocephalus is present, as commonly occurs after a subarachnoid hemorrhage, a ventriculostomy with drainage of CSF is indicated to reduce ICP. Ventriculostomies are seldom helpful in patients with head trauma because the degree of brain swelling may prevent localization of the ventricles.

Prompt removal of an acute subdural, epidural, or large solitary intracerebral hematoma is indicated. Mortality and morbidity are reduced by prompt diagnosis and surgical treatment of an epidural hematoma, especially if done before signs of tentorial herniation occur.[8] In addition, mortality from an acute subdural hematoma is reduced by rapid diagnosis and surgical treatment.[163] Patients who underwent surgery within 4 hours of injury had a 30% mortality rate, compared with a 90% mortality in those who had surgery after 4 hours.[163]

Maintenance of Blood Pressure

Patients are often hypertensive after an isolated brain injury because of an increase in catecholamines from stress-induced activation of the sympathetic nervous system.[25,26] Because autoregulation may be impaired after head trauma,[52,101] hypertension may cause brain hyperemia, promote the development of vasogenic edema, and further increase ICP. However, before immediately treating the blood pressure elevation with an antihypertensive agent, other causes of hypertension (such as increased ICP or inadequate anesthesia) should be first eliminated. Assuring adequate oxygenation and ventilation, placing the head up slightly in neutral position, preventing coughing, or administering barbiturates alone or together with narcotics may help reduce ICP and/or provide greater anesthesia. Usually these measures are effective to control blood pressure in the acute management of the brain-injured patient. However, in the patient with preexisting hypertension or the severely hyperdynamic patient, control of hypertension with beta-adrenergic antagonists (e.g., propranolol, labetalol, esmolol) or trimethaphan may also be indicated.[55,189] These drugs specifically treat the cause of hypertension (e.g., sympathetic overactivity), and they are not cerebral vasodilators.[191] Prophylactic beta-adrenergic receptor blockade may also have utility in reducing supraventricular tachycardia, ST-segment and T-wave changes, and myocardial necrosis associated with severe head injury.[37] Systemic vasodilators, such as sodium nitroprusside, nitro-

glycerin, and hydralazine may increase ICP and should be avoided.[32,33,83,113,189] A significant disadvantage of infusions of trimethaphan is that it may interfere with the pupillary examination because it may cause pupillary dilation and anisocoria, and block pupillary reflexes. However, small (1 to 2 mg IV) bolus doses cause little problem.

In contrast to the patient with isolated brain injury, the most common hemodynamic problem in the multiply-injured patient with head trauma is hypovolemia caused by blood loss, profound diuresis from mannitol, and inappropriate attempts to restrict fluid intake. Because the damaged brain tolerates hypotension poorly, intravenous fluids should be administered in sufficient quantities to rapidly restore intravascular volume and cerebral blood flow. Intraoperative blood loss may be severe in vascular injuries and skull fractures. Massive volume replacement may be required intraoperatively if a dural sinus is injured. In addition, blood loss may be difficult to quantify because it spills on the drapes and on the floor. Patients with large intracranial hemorrhages, with normal blood pressures in the lower range (systolic blood pressure of 100 to 120 mm Hg), and with a relative tachycardia (greater than 100 beats per minute) should be considered to be hypovolemic unless proved otherwise. The hypovolemia may become manifest by severe hypotension when the brain is decompressed. With the acute reduction of ICP, sympathetic tone and systemic vascular resistance are reduced, revealing profound intravascular volume depletion. Vasopressors may be helpful in restoring blood pressure while fluid is being given to restore intravascular volume to normal. However, overzealous fluid administration that elevates cerebral venous pressure may exacerbate brain edema.

The presence of hypovolemia is best assessed by clinical signs such as hypotension, tachycardia, inability to tolerate anesthetic agents, and inspiratory-expiratory variation in blood pressure with positive pressure ventilation. A decrease in systolic pressure of greater than 10 mm Hg with positive pressure ventilation is a sensitive indicator of a 10% reduction in blood volume (Fig. 12-5).[130] This decrease in systolic pressure is a significantly better indicator than the central venous pressure. The variation in systolic pressure correlates well with the degree of hemorrhage in dogs. However, a central line may be helpful in the acute setting, especially to prevent overhydration, and should be ultimately inserted to help guide fluid replacement. Timely evacuation of the brain mass must be first accomplished, with placement of central line performed later after surgery has begun and the patient has been stabilized.

Glucose-containing solutions should not be administered acutely to the brain-injured patient because they may exacerbate neurologic damage. Numerous animal studies provide convincing evidence that glucose administration, with or without marked hyperglycemia, augments neurologic damage from global and regional cerebral ischemia.[42,96,142] The mechanisms for the enhanced neurologic damage are unclear. How glucose administration affects outcome after

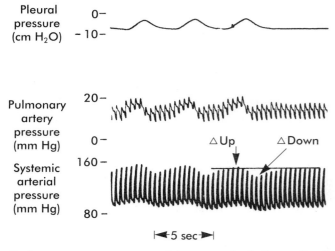

FIG. 12-5   Continuous record from a mechanically ventilated dog after hemorrhage of 10% of blood volume. Pleural, pulmonary arterial, and systemic pressures are shown. Note the fluctuation in systolic blood pressure with positive-pressure ventilation. The difference between maximum and minimum systolic blood pressure is divided into the Δ up component and Δ down component. The Δ up component is the difference between the maximum systolic and the end-expiratory systolic blood pressure during a 5-second period of apnea. The Δ down component is the difference between the end-expiratory and the minimum systolic blood pressure. The systolic pressure variation and Δ up and Δ down components correlate better than central venous pressure to the degree of hypovolemia *(From Perel A, Pizov R, Cotev S:* Anesthesiology 67:498, 1987.*)*

brain injury also is not known. In a rat model of head trauma, glucose administration did not alter neurologic outcome or formation of brain edema.[166] However, increased blood glucose is correlated with increased neurologic damage in people after stroke,[141] cardiac arrest,[104] and head trauma.[94] In these human studies, it is unclear whether the hyperglycemia is the cause or the result of the increased severity of the neurologic damage.

The threshold level of blood glucose above which ischemic neurologic damage is increased is also not known; however, it appears to be less than 200 mg/dl. Administration of relatively small amounts of glucose, which caused only modest increases in blood glucose, exacerbated neurologic damage in animals. Lanier et al.[96] demonstrated that monkeys given 50 ml intravenously of 5% glucose in 0.45% normal saline solution (equivalent to 1.1 ml per 70 kg patient; blood glucose equalled 180 mg/dl), before global cerebral ischemia had a significantly greater neurologic deficit than monkeys who had received lactated Ringer's solution (glucose equalled 140 mg/dl).

Part of the difficulty in determining a "safe" level of blood glucose in patients is that blood glucose levels may not accurately reflect brain glucose levels during periods of transient hyperglycemia. Brain glucose remains elevated af-

ter glucose infusion while blood glucose decreases in response to insulin. Recent experimental evidence has suggested that postischemic treatment of acute hyperglycemia with insulin reduces neurologic damage.[192] Rats that received low doses of insulin to lower blood glucose to 67 mg/dl after an ischemic brain insult had a reduced seizure incidence, cortical infarction size, and mortality compared with control animals that remained hyperglycemic (212 mg/dl). This data suggests that at least acute elevations (as associated with stress caused by the neurologic injury) in blood glucose should be treated. Chronic elevations in blood glucose presumably also should be treated. However, the actual benefits and risks of acute reductions of blood glucose in patients with chronic hyperglycemia are unclear from current experimental evidence.

Isoosmolar crystalloid and/or colloid solutions should be used to replace intravascular volume. These include Plasma-Lyte, Normosol-R, Ringer's solution, 0.9% normal saline, hetastarch, and albumin. Although use of any of these solutions may markedly increase ICP after resuscitation from shock,[70,71] ICP would be higher after inadequate resuscitation because of the development of cytotoxic edema from cerebral ischemia.[175] The blood-brain barrier may be damaged by head trauma, allowing all fluids to cross the blood-brain barrier. Thus overhydration, causing increases in central venous pressure, should be avoided. Therefore the aim of fluid management is to maintain a euvolemic patient. Likewise, bloody, less urgent procedures (e.g., many orthopedic procedures) should be delayed several days until the brain injury has stabilized, because of the potential for exacerbation of cerebral edema.

The choice of colloid vs. crystalloid for fluid replacement remains controversial. Most recent experimental evidence suggests brain water content and ICP are not different when a colloid or crystalloid solution is administered, as long as the solution is not hypotonic.[202] Water movement across the blood-brain barrier depends primarily on the difference in osmolality between plasma and brain. Decreases in oncotic pressure generally do not affect brain water content because oncotic pressure makes only a small contribution to total plasma osmolality. However, because of the uncertainties of the current research and the tradition of using colloids in neurosurgery, most neuroanesthesiologists prefer to avoid marked reductions in colloid oncotic pressure. Often some colloid is added after several liters of crystalloid are administered. Large quantities (over 1 to 2 L) of lactated Ringer's solution should be avoided because it is relatively hypoosmolar. Therefore administration of lactated Ringer's solution increases ICP and brain water content.[137,185] Large volumes (> 500 ml) of 6% hetastarch should also not be administered because it may cause a coagulopathy that may be manifest by an intracranial hematoma.[39] Hetastarch prolongs the partial thromboplastin time (PTT) through a decrease in factor VIII coagulant activity and in von Willebrand factor.

In the future, hypertonic saline solutions may have utility in the resuscitation of brain-injured patients. Experimental studies have demonstrated consistent reductions in brain water content and ICP with hypertonic saline, in contrast to marked increases in brain water and ICP when normal saline or colloids are used for fluid resuscitation in animals with and without brain injury.* A 3% sodium chloride solution has an osmolarity similar to 20% mannitol. However, the long-term effects of the sodium load are of concern and have delayed rapid movement of these fluids into routine clinical use. Use of hypertonic saline in the fluid resuscitation of human patients is currently under investigation.

Treatment of Hypoxemia

Prompt and aggressive treatment of hypoxemia in head-injured patients is imperative because hypoxemia is associated with a worsening of neurologic outcome.[63] Positive end-expiratory pressure (PEEP) may increase ICP in the brain-injured patient because PEEP may increase cerebral venous volume by reducing cerebral venous outflow.[169] However, most recent studies suggest that 10 cm H_2O PEEP improves oxygenation and usually causes clinically inconsequential increases in ICP in patients with severe head trauma.[18,30,62] PEEP may affect ICP less in patients with the stiffest lungs, who are presumably the ones who need PEEP the most.[18,30]

SPINAL CORD INJURY

Spinal injuries occur in 5% to 10% of major trauma cases, with cervical spine injuries occurring in 1.5% to 3%.[17] Most victims of spinal cord injuries are males (82%) in the age range of 15 to 35 years.[180] Motor vehicle accidents are the most common cause of injury, followed by falls, sports injuries, and gunshot/stab wounds. People with head-first falls or unrestrained drivers or passengers in high-speed, front-end motor-vehicle accidents are at particularly high risk (6% to 10%) for cervical spine injury.[150] At moderate risk (1% to 3%) are people in lower speed motor-vehicle accidents, with blunt head trauma, or with side or foot-first falls. Totally alert patients without any neck pain or tenderness are generally not at risk for spinal injury[91] because there is a significant association between neck pain or tenderness and cervical injury. However, if the patient has even minimal spinal tenderness, has other painful injuries, or is intoxicated, the cervical spine should be considered unstable and should be fully evaluated.

Only about 5% of all spinal cord injuries are observed in children. In childhood, fractures are less common because spine mobility is greater compared with adults because of ligamentous laxity and incompletely ossified wedge-shaped vertebrae.[56] However, these anatomic features make children prone to extremely high cervical lesions and increase the incidence of spinal cord injury without radiographic abnormality.[73,129,135]

---

*References 70, 71, 139, 140, 184, 200.

Neurologic Evaluation
Evaluation of the Extent of Spinal Cord Injury

A convenient way to visualize the structure of the vertebral column uses the three-column concept.[45] The anterior column contains the anterior longitudinal ligament and the anterior two thirds of the vertebral body and annulus fibrosus. The middle column contains the posterior one third of the vertebral body, annulus fibrosus, and posterior longitudinal ligament. The posterior column consists of the posterior neural arch, spinous processes, articular facet processes, and their corresponding posterior ligamentous column. The three-column concept is useful in localizing spinal injury, depending on the mechanism of injury.

Injuries to the spine may be classified as extension, flexion, compression, rotation, or some combination of these four basic mechanisms (Fig. 12-6).[59] Extension injuries, such as those from blows under the chin or whiplash,

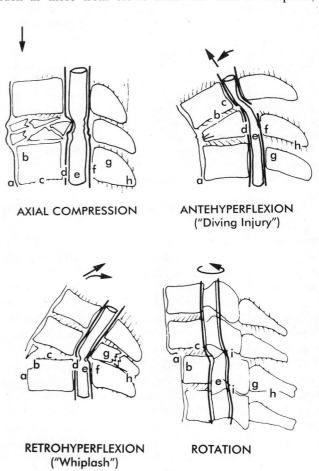

FIG. 12-6 Mechanisms of spinal cord injury: axial compression, antehyperflexion (flexion injury), retrohyperflexion (extension injury), and rotation. a, Anterior spinal ligament; b, vertebral body; c, intervertebral disk; d, posterior spinal ligament; e, spinal cord; f, ligamentum flavum; g, spinal process; h, interspinous ligaments; i, intervertebral facet joint. Note compression of anterior elements in flexion injury and compression of posterior elements in extension injuries. (From Fraser A, Edmonds-Seal J: Anaesthesia 37:1084, 1982.)

mostly disrupt the posterior column. Flexion injuries, such as a diving injury, mostly disrupt the anterior column. The degree of stability of the spine is variable and ranges from stable (e.g., burst fracture or wedge of a vertebral body) to very unstable (e.g., hangman's fracture).[188] The primary factor that determines the stability of the injury is the integrity of the ligaments, intervertebral disks, and osseous articulators.[36] In addition, the spinal cord may be uninjured or injured. With a complete injury there is loss of all motor or sensory function below the level of the injury. With incomplete injuries there is some preservation of function. Incomplete lesions may result in one of several syndromes: central cord syndrome, Brown-Séquard syndrome, and anterior cord or posterior cord syndrome (Table 12-1). Of patients with a significant spinal injury, 30% to 70% have neurologic deficits.[78] Fracture dislocations or bony injuries from C5 to C7 are most likely to result in injury. However, the degree of spinal cord injury cannot be correlated with the stability of the spine.[148]

Extension injuries are twice as common as flexion injuries.[36] One third of extension injuries involve the atlantoaxial joint. Hyperextension with compression may cause fracture dislocation disruption of both anterior and posterior columns and is highly unstable. A hangman's fracture, which occurs with violent hyperextension, fractures the pedicles of C2 and causes anterior subluxation of C2 or C3, and is also highly unstable, with a variable degree of spinal cord damage.[188] Flexion injuries may result in wedge fractures of the vertebral body without ligamentous injuries.[36] These are often stable, except in severe injures in which greater disruption of the anterior and posterior columns may occur. The most severe flexion injury is a teardrop fracture, which is highly unstable.[188] Compression injuries may cause burst fractures, and posterior displacement of vertebral body fragments may cause spinal cord injury, despite the relative stability of the fracture.[188]

Spine Immobilization

Because high-speed multiple-trauma and head-injured patients are at increased risk for spinal cord injury, their cervical spine should be immobilized and they should be moved using the logroll technique until the evaluation reveals no injury. The best way to immobilize the neck in the acute setting is by use of a rigid collar, sandbags on either side of the neck, and tape across the forehead.[133] Soft collars do not effectively limit neck motion, as they permit 96% of normal flexion and 73% of normal extension,[27] and they do not restrict motion in the lateral or rotational directions.[77,133] Thus soft collars serve only as a reminder of the possibility of cervical spine injury. Rigid collars (e.g., Philadelphia collars or the extrication collar), still allow about 30% of neck extension and flexion and about 45% of normal rotation or lateral movement.[133] The Philadelphia collar is preferred because it is a two-piece collar that is easy to place without significantly moving the patient.[133] In contrast, lateral sandbags and forehead tape effectively prevent flexion, reducing lateral or rotary motions to 5% of normal and extension to 35% of normal.[133] After the initial diagnosis and workup are completed, tong or halo fixation can be applied. These fixation devices dramatically reduce neck motion, allowing only 4% of flexion/extension and 1% of normal rotation.[77]

Radiologic Evaluation

The standard radiologic evaluation of the cervical spine involves obtaining cross-table lateral, anteroposterior, and odontoid (open-mouth) x-rays of the cervical spine. Because 7% to 14% of all spinal fractures occur at C7,[107] all seven cervical vertebrae must be evident on the lateral spine film.[198] The cross-table lateral x-ray (Fig. 12-7) allows evaluation of the alignment of the vertebrae, the bony structure of each vertebra, and the width of the prevertebral and intervertebral spaces.[198] A lordotic alignment should be present on each of the four anatomic lines on the cervical spine, (i.e., along the anterior and posterior margins of the vertebral border, the spinolaminar line, and the posterior margins of the spinous process) (Fig. 12-8). The bony structure of each vertebra is examined for the structure of the vertebral body and spinous processes, the size of the intervertebral disk space, the relationship of the articular face and joints, and the interspinous process distance.[198] Widening of the prevertebral space may indicate the presence of a severe and unstable spine injury, even with an otherwise normal C-spine x-ray,[65] or it may be associated with airway obstruction (Fig. 12-9).[12,81,118] The cross-table lateral x-ray misses about 15% to 20% of cervical spine fractures.[157,181] Therefore, if a lateral film alone has been

TABLE 12-1
Spinal Cord Injury Syndromes

Syndrome	Signs
Complete neurologic injury	Loss of all motor and sensory innervation below the level of injury
Incomplete neurologic injury	
Central cord	Motor loss (arms greater than legs)
	Bladder dysfunction
	Variable sensory loss
Brown-Séquard syndrome	Ipsilateral paralysis
	Ipsilateral loss of proprioception, touch, and vibration
	Contralateral loss of pain and temperature
Anterior cord	Bilateral motor loss
	Bilateral loss of pain and temperature
	Preserved proprioception, touch, and vibration
Posterior cord	Loss of touch and temperature
	Motor function intact
	Proprioception and vibration intact

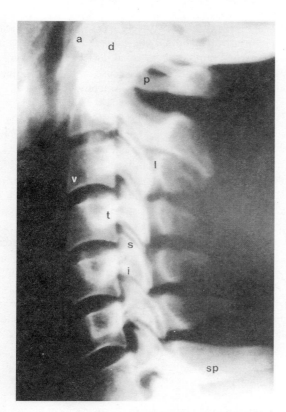

FIG. 12-7   Cross-table lateral radiograph of the normal cervical spine. *a,* Anterior arch of C1; *∂,* posterior arch of C1; *v,* vertebral body of C3; *l,* lamina of C3; *t,* transverse process of C4; *ſ,* superior articulating facet of C5; *i,* inferior articulating facet of C5; *ſp,* spinous process of C7. *(From Ovaſſapian A:* Fiberoptic airway endoscopy in anesthesia and critical care, *New York, 1990, Raven Preſſ.)*

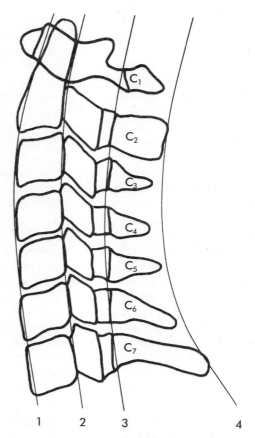

FIG. 12-8   Diagram of the lateral view of the cervical spine demonstrating normal alignment. The "ABCs" of interpretation involve alignment, bones, cartilage, and soft-tissue spaces. There are four smooth, lordotic curves drawn along the anterior margins of the vertebral border *(1),* the posterior margins *(2),* the junction between the lamina and spinous processes *(3),* and the tips of the spinous processes *(4).* Lines *2* and *3* are the approximate borders of the spinal canal. *(From Williams CF, Bernstein TW, Jelenko C:* Ann Emerg Med 10:198, 1981.)

taken, the neck in a high-risk patient should continue to be treated as injured and potentially unstable. The sensitivity of the x-rays can be increased to 93% by adding an anteroposterior view and an odontoid view.[157] The anteroposterior view (Fig. 12-10) demonstrates the vertical alignment of the spinous and articular process and abnormalities in disk and joint spaces, such as disk space enlargement, which may indicate a severe ligamentous injury.[36] The open mouth or odontoid view (Fig. 12-11) visualizes the atlantooccipital and atlantoaxial joints and the odontoid process. Supplemental films, such as oblique or flexion-extension views, may be required for further detail.

CT scanning may be used to rule out cervical spine injury when the plain films are suspicious, equivocal, or negative in the face of clinical spinal cord injury.[107] It is also used to evaluate the cervical spine in patients who cannot open their mouths (such as intubated patients). It is superior to the plain radiographs in diagnosing cervical spine trauma, especially at C1 or C2[107]; however, ligamentous injuries may be missed.[78] In rare cases, magnetic resonance

imaging or myelography may be required to dilineate the extent of spine injury.

Evaluation of Other Organ Systems
Respiratory System

Forced vital capacity and functional residual capacity are reduced in patients with spinal cord injuries, with the greatest degree of respiratory impairment observed with cervical lesions (Box 12-4, Table 12-2).[98,117] The diaphragm, which contributes 60% to normal vital capacity, is innervated by the phrenic nerve (C3 to C5). Lesions above this level cause total diaphragmatic paralysis and inability to ventilate (see Table 12-2). Patients with lesions below C6 have an intact diaphragm but variable loss of intercostal and abdominal muscle function. Patients with C6 lesions have a marked decrease in vital capacity to 30% of predicted,

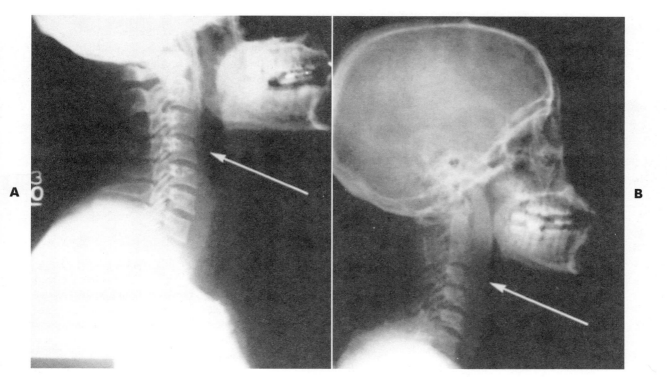

FIG. 12-9 Example of severe prevertebral soft tissue swelling secondary to a whiplash injury. **A,** Radiograph illustrates the lateral cervical spine in a normal patient. The arrow points to the prevertebral plane, which has a width of 3.2 mm at C2. **B,** Radiograph illustrates a patient with marked widening of the prevertebral plane, which measures 11 mm at C2. The patient presented with airway obstruction, requiring endotracheal intubation using a fiberoptic technique. *(From Biby L, Santora AH:* Anesth Analg *70:112, 1990.)*

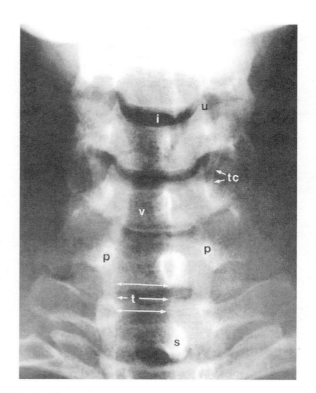

FIG. 12-10 Anteroposterior radiograph of the normal cervical spine. *i,* Intervertebral foramen of C3-4; *u,* uncinate process of C4; *tc,* thyroid cartilage; *v,* vertebral body of C5; *p,* pedicle of C6; *s,* spinous process of C7; *t,* trachea *(arrows). (From Ovassapian A:* Fiberoptic airway endoscopy in anesthesia and critical care, *New York, 1990, Raven Press, p 37.)*

associated with a reduction in functional residual capacity, caused primarily by loss of expiratory reserve volume. Paradoxical ventilation (chest retraction on inspiration and chest expansion during expiration), relaxation of the abdominal wall that interferes with the normal position and movement of the diaphragm, loss of cough, reduced ability to handle secretions, and associated chest injuries also contribute to respiratory compromise.[105] Vital capacity is higher in the supine than in the head-up or prone position because of diaphragmatic mechanics. Postural hypoxemia may develop. In addition to impaired ventilation, other pulmonary injuries, such as atelectasis, aspiration, pulmonary contusion, hemothorax, pneumothorax, and neurogenic or nonneurogenic pulmonary edema, may also contribute to respiratory failure in the acute setting. Like patients with head injury, patients with spinal cord trauma are at a particular risk for the development of neurogenic pulmonary edema.[2,3,105,134]

Although the patient's ventilation may be adequate on initial presentation in the emergency room, progressive at-

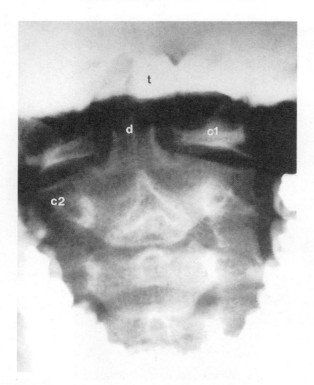

FIG. 12-11 Open-mouth or odontoid radiograph of the normal cervical spine. *d*, Dens of axis (C2); *c1*, anterior arch of C1; *c2*, body of C2; *t*, teeth. *(From Ovassapian A: Fiberoptic airway endoscopy in anesthesia and critical care, New York, 1990, Raven Press, p 37.)*

electasis and pneumonia caused by inability to cough and clear secretions, sedative and narcotic administration, gastric atony and dilation, and spinal cord edema may contribute to the patient's subsequent development of respiratory failure. Ledsome and Sharp[98] found that five patients with an injury at the C4 to C5 level had a vital capacity of 25% of predicted on admission, and all required ventilatory support 1 to 5 days after injury.

Cardiovascular System

At the time of primary injury, intense sympathetic nervous system activation causes a brief period of severe hypertension.[54,131] The excessive sympathetic discharge may increase ICP and cause ST segment and T wave changes that may mimic myocardial ischemia or dysrhythmias, or it may result in neurogenic pulmonary edema.

Spinal shock occurs subsequently, and it may last up to several weeks after the injury.[2,99,105,131] It is characterized by gastric dilation and atony, bowel and bladder distension, flaccid paralysis, vasodilation, absence of tendon and plantar reflexes below the level of the lesion, hypotension, and bradycardia. The loss of sympathetic tone results in a decrease in systemic vascular resistance, an increase in venous capacitance with venous pooling, a reduced ability to vasoconstrict in response to changes in position and hypovolemia, and a poor hemodynamic response to surgical stimulation. Unopposed vagal tone with loss of cardioaccelerator fibers (T2 to T5) contributes to the bradycardia. Severe reflex bradycardia and asystole may occur in response to airway instrumentation, which may be prevented by prophylactic atropine. A relative tachycardia in a quadriplegic patient may indicate hypovolemia.

▼
BOX 12-4
SPINAL CORD INJURY: EFFECTS ON OTHER ORGAN SYSTEMS

Respiratory System

Decreased ability to ventilate, dependent on level of injury

Associated pulmonary injuries: atelectasis, aspiration, pulmonary contusion, pneumothorax, neurogenic or nonneurogenic pulmonary edema

Cardiovascular System

Initial sympathetic nervous system overactivity

Spinal shock: hypotension, bradycardia

Severe bradycardia (or asystole) with airway instrumentation

Temperature Control

Poikilothermia

Other Systems

Possible orthopedic, intrathoracic, intraabdominal, or head injuries

---

TABLE 12-2
Effects of Spinal Cord Injury on Respiratory Function

Damaged Cord Segment	Degree of Respiratory Compromise
C3-C5	Decrease in vital capacity to 20% to 25% of normal or lower
	Paradoxical respiration
	Use of accessory muscles
	Variable loss of phrenic nerve function and paralysis of diaphragm
	Loss of intercostal and abdominal muscles
	Need for ventilatory support
C5-C8	Decrease in vital capacity to 30% of normal
	Paradoxical respiration
	Use of accessory muscles
	No cough
	Ventilation improved when supine
	Loss of intercostal and abdominal muscles
T1-T6	Variable intercostal muscle functions
	Partial loss of diaphragm effectiveness
	Weak cough
T6-T12	Weak cough
	Variable abdominal muscle strength

Treatment of spinal shock involves the careful administration of isotonic fluids and possibly vasopressors to maintain spinal cord perfusion pressure.[105] Some authors suggest using pulmonary artery catheters to gauge fluid requirements in all quadriplegic patients because even previously healthly patients may be susceptible to pulmonary edema and myocardial dysfunction.[108] In most patients, judicious fluid replacement alone is adequate to moderately raise blood pressure to improve spinal cord perfusion. Pulmonary artery catheters should be placed in the patient who requires large volumes of fluid and/or vasopressors. Ephedrine, phenylephrine, and dopamine are commonly used as vasopressors, with the exact choice of drug dependent on heart rate, cardiac output, and vascular resistance as measured by a pulmonary artery catheter.

Temperature Control

There is a loss of thermoregulatory ability below the level of the lesion. Patients with injury above T6 tend to become poikilothermic, assuming the temperature of their surroundings. Careful monitoring of temperature and warming efforts are required.

Associated Injuries

As with head trauma, multiple organ systems (e.g., orthopedic, intrathoracic, intraabdominal, head) may be affected by the injury. Patients are assumed to have a "full stomach." Intravenous access, Foley catheters, and nasal gastric tube should be placed. Long-bone fractures should be immobilized.

Airway Management of the Patient with Suspected Cervical Spine Injury

In the airway management of a patient with a potentially unstable cervical spine, the goal of the anesthesiologist is to establish endotracheal intubation without causing further injury to the spinal cord. Unfortunately, the safety of the various airway maneuvers and intubation techniques is not known (see Crosby and Lui,[36] Hastings and Marks,[78] and Wood and Lawler[199] for excellent reviews of the subject). Unrestricted neck motion associated with excessive traction during spine fixation[61] or the failure to detect a cervical spine fracture on initial workup[146] has been associated with new neurologic deficits. For instance, a secondary neurologic defect occurred in 10.5% of patients with a missed diagnosis of cervical spine fracture, compared with 1.4% of those correctly diagnosed.[146] Laryngoscopy without neck stabilization has resulted in quadriplegia or death in two reported patients.[78] However, there are no studies or case reports that elucidate the actual risk of airway management techniques in patients with cervical spine injuries, when standard "cervical spine" precautions are used.[78] Because of the lack of outcome studies, there is no consensus regarding which technique for endotracheal intubation is safest in patients with suspected cervical spine injuries.[36,78,199] Therefore the optimal technique must be chosen by the an

esthesiologist, depending on the particular patient's medical condition, the urgency with which the airway must be secured, the patient's level of cooperation, and the anesthesiologist's skills.

Effects of Various Airway Maneuvers on Cervical Spine Mobility

Basic Airway Maneuvers. There is impressive radiologic evidence that many airway maneuvers may increase distraction and subluxation at the site of a cervical spine injury.[5,13] Aprahamian et al.[5] found that chin lift and jaw thrust in a cadaver model with an unstable C5 to C6 ligamentous injury caused a greater than 5 mm widening of the disk space, which was not prevented by a Philadelphia collar. Insertion of an esophageal obturator airway caused a 3 to 4 mm increase in disk space.[5] Anterior neck pressure (similar to cricoid pressure) used to stabilize the larynx for nasal tracheal intubation caused greater than 5 mm posterior subluxation. In contrast, head tilt, insertion of an oral airway, or insertion of a nasopharyngeal airway resulted in only a minimal change in the disk space. Although the data suggests that chin lift, jaw thrust, cricoid pressure, and esophageal obturator airway placement may be hazardous to the patient with an unstable cervical spine injury, the study was performed in only one cadaver, and there are no outcome studies to determine whether these maneuvers are, in fact, dangerous to living patients.[78]

There is also concern that the use of "manual in-line traction" to stabilize the neck, depending on the force of the traction and integrity of the surrounding tissues, may by itself result in significant subluxation and distraction of the disk space.[13,87] Cervical traction increases distraction of the vertebra, especially at the C5 to C6 level.[6,13] Whether traction may cause neurologic damage is not clear; however, deterioration of neurologic function has been reported with excessive traction during cervical spine stabilization procedures.[61] Therefore "manual in-line traction" should involve neck stabilization only, and traction should not be performed.

Techniques for Urgent Airway Control. The following sections discuss techniques for urgent airway control.

Direct laryngoscopy. To secure the airway quickly, a rapid-sequence induction with direct laryngoscopy may be needed. Unfortunately, direct laryngoscopy is associated with cervical spine movement in normal anesthetized volunteers[109] as well as cadavers with unstable spines.[5,13] Horton et al.[80] found that direct laryngoscopy progressively increased extension from C4 to C1. Atlantoaxial (C1 to C2) extension was near the upper limit of normal, while the lower cervical spine was relatively straight. Laryngoscopy with either a straight or curved blade caused a 3 to 4 mm widening of the C5 to C6 disk space in the cadaver model of an unstable C5 to C6 injury.[5] The cervical spine movement was not prevented by a Philadelphia collar; however, it was reduced 60% using in-line stabilization by an assistant.[5,109]

Although direct laryngoscopy does result in motion of the cervical spine, especially at C1 to C2, the actual risk of exacerbating neurologic damage associated with laryngoscopy is not known. There are no large outcome studies on the safety of direct laryngoscopy in patients with unstable cervical spines. The available evidence suggests that neurologic deterioration after oral intubation with neck stabilization is rare.* A retrospective analysis of four papers dealing with laryngoscopy with neck stabilization in 62 patients with known cervical spine injury did not detect an exacerbation of neurologic damage. Unfortunately, the number of patients is small, many had stable injuries (such as 6 of 18 patients in Rhee et al.[147]), and few had C1 or C2 injuries, which may be associated with greater risk for damage during oral laryngoscopy.[78] In a recent review article on cervical spine injury and airway management, Hastings and Marks[78] suggested that the 95% confidence limits of the pooled outcome data places the risk of neurologic deterioration with direct laryngoscopy at 0% to 7%, a relatively wide interval because of the small size of the available series.

In addition to the risks of causing secondary neurologic injury during endotracheal intubation, direct laryngoscopy may be difficult in the patient who is obese, has facial fractures, has blood in pharynx, or has oral soft tissue injuries. Prevertebral swelling may occur with cervical spine fractures, which may cause airway compromise and distort the larynx, causing difficult visualization.[12,81,118]

Cricothyroidotomy. Cricothyroidotomy has been suggested as an alternative to direct laryngoscopy for rapidly securing the airway in the patient with suspected or actual cervical spine injury.[86,92,194] In theory, with cricothyroidotomy, the trachea might be intubated without causing neck motion. In reality, lack of spinal motion has not been documented because x-ray studies on the risk of cervical spine motion during cricothyroidotomy and neurologic outcome studies have not been performed.[78] In addition, the complication rate of cricothyroidotomy is fairly high. When performed in the field or the emergency department, cricothyroidotomy has a very high immediate complication rate (32%),[116,177] including an execution time greater than 3 minutes (10%), incorrect (13%) or unsuccessful tracheostomy tube placement (8% to 25%), significant hemorrhage (5%), or subcutaneous emphysema. Long-term complications, such as infection and damage to the larynx, may also occur (2%).[92] Cricothyroidotomy may also make definitive repair of the cervical spine by an anterior approach difficult or impossible because of the presence of the contaminated wound in the surgical field. Many of the complications can be attributed to the inexperience of the physician performing the procedure. However, the lack of documentation of any beneficial effect on neurologic outcome; the relative inexperience of most anesthesiologists, emergency

room physicians, and surgeons in using the technique; and the usually high complication rate suggest that use of cricothyroidotomy should be reserved to secure the airway quickly in selected patients in whom direct laryngoscopy has or is anticipated to fail.

Transtracheal jet ventilation. Transtracheal jet ventilation may be used to temporarily oxygenate the patient during difficult direct laryngoscopy, cricothyroidotomy, or fiberoptic laryngoscopy.[174] Use of a 14-gauge catheter placed through the cricothyroid membrane and a high pressure source of oxygen may provide adequate oxygenation and ventilation.[201] However, it does not protect against aspiration, and it may be associated with barotrauma (10%) and catheter dislodgment.[174] As such, it should only be used as a temporary measure to oxygenate a patient while definitive airway control is achieved.

Techniques for Elective Airway Control. The following sections discuss techniques for elective airway control.

Awake intubation (blind nasal, light wand, or fiberoptic laryngoscopy). Awake nasotracheal or orotracheal intubation has been advocated as a safer technique for endotracheal intubation in the patient with an unstable cervical spine.[36,43,89,195] Meschino et al.[119] reported their institutional experience using awake tracheal intubation in patients with cervical spine injuries. They found that neurologic outcome with cervical spine injury was not different in the 136 patients who required endotracheal intubation compared with 233 patients who did not require intubation. Awake intubation was used; however, details of how the intubations were performed, how the neurologic examination was assessed, and the location and degree of instability of the injury were not reported. Hastings and Marks[78] suggested that the risk of secondary neurologic damage caused by intubation was probably less than 4% with 95% confidence intervals. Although the neurologic risk may appear to be less with awake intubation, the smaller confidence interval may only reflect the larger size of the series.

Although awake intubation is often appropriate, especially for an elective intubation, it may not secure the airway quickly enough if rapid intubation is required, as in the hypoxemic, hemodynamically unstable, or head-injured patient. Nasal intubation should be avoided in the patient with a midface or basilar skull fracture because bacteria and foreign materials may enter the cranial cavity.[162] It also may induce a nose bleed, aggravated in the multiple trauma victim by dilutional coagulopathy, and, with long-term intubation, it may cause sinusitis and sepsis. Uncooperative, inebriated, or head-injured patients may thrash about and cause even greater neck motion (and potential cervical spine damage) than if direct laryngoscopy were performed under general anesthesia. Although blind nasotracheal intubation is often successful, it may be slower and may require multiple attempts. Ovassapian et al.[127] found that blind nasotracheal intubation required multiple attempts in 70% to 90% of patients.

Fiberoptic laryngoscopy has often been recommended

*References 21, 47, 66, 78, 147, 178, 182, 199.

for intubation in the patient with an unstable cervical spine because it allows intubation under direct vision without much neck motion.[36,78,195] It has a high rate of success under elective conditions with an anesthesiologist knowledgeable with the technique.[126,128] However, in practice, fiberoptic laryngoscopy may be difficult to use in the acutely injured patient because of excessive salivation, airway bleeding, and edema in the pharyngeal space. It may be time-consuming because it requires a cooperative patient and adequate topical anesthesia of the supraglottic and infraglottic regions to prevent gagging. Anesthetizing the area below the vocal cords is controversial. Although it may prevent severe coughing and bucking (which potentially may exacerbate neurologic damage), it might increase the likelihood of aspiration. Ovassapian et al.,[127] however, found no evidence of aspiration 24 hours after fiberoptic intubation after laryngeal anesthesia in 105 patients at risk for aspiration. There is also no evidence that coughing increases neurologic risk to the spinal cord.

Retrograde tracheal intubation. Another possible technique advocated to minimize neck motion in the trauma patient is retrograde tracheal intubation over a wire passed through the cricothyroid membrane. Barriot and Riou[7] found retrograde orotracheal intubation was easily and quickly (less than 5 minutes) performed in 19 trauma patients in whom conventional techniques failed or were expected to fail. However, large-scale assessment of the reli-

ability and safety of this technique as the primary means to secure the airway has not been performed.

Management of Endotracheal Intubation

Because of the lack of outcome studies, there is no consensus regarding the relative safety of the various techniques to achieve endotracheal intubation.[36,78,199] Many techniques are feasible, and the exact choice often depends on the particular anesthesiologist's skills. However, the possible risk of secondary damage to the spinal cord with laryngoscopy (which varies with stable vs. unstable injuries) must be balanced by other considerations, such as the degree of urgency in achieving intubation, associated medical conditions (head trauma, airway trauma or pathology, hypoxemia, and cardiovascular instability), and level of cooperation.

The first step of the airway management plan involves determination of the degree of urgency for securing the airway (Fig. 12-12). Immediate endotracheal intubation is required in patients with cardiovascular instability, hypoxemia, or elevated intracranial pressure. Oxygenation and ventilation initially are provided by bag and mask, with an airway or jaw thrust as required to open the airway. If the patient has an anatomically normal airway (i.e., one in which endotracheal intubation is expected to be easily achieved with the head and neck secured in neutral position), a modified rapid-sequence induction should be per-

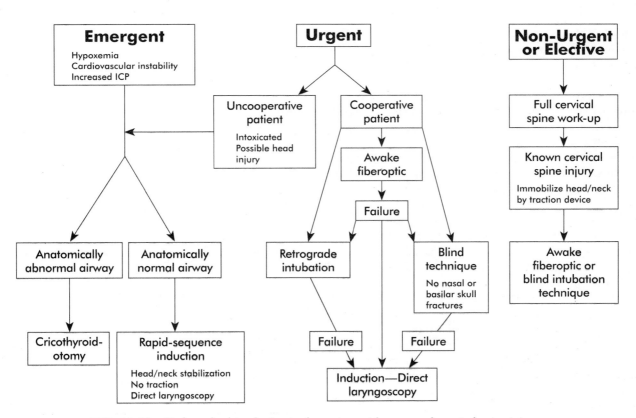

FIG. 12-12 Endotracheal intubation in the patient with suspected cervical spine injury.

formed. The front half of the Philadelphia collar should be removed before laryngoscopy because it interferes with mouth opening. To prevent aspiration, cricoid pressure should be applied. Although it may cause a posterior subluxation of the cervical cord, adverse effects have not been documented (especially when the posterior portion of the neck is stabilized by the Philadelphia collar). Succinylcholine is the muscle relaxant of choice if the injury is less than 48 hours old because hyperkalemia does not occur until later.[67] Patients should continue to be ventilated with cricoid pressure in place until the intubation is complete. During laryngoscopy, an assistant should stabilize the head in a neutral position without applying traction. Neck flexion should be avoided, and the minimum of neck extension needed to visualize the glottis should be used.

If immediate control of the airway is required and the airway is anatomically abnormal, a cricothyroidotomy should be performed to secure the airway. Ventilation using a laryngeal mask or transtracheal jet ventilation may be required as a temporary measure if ventilation by bag and mask is difficult. Patients with severe facial fractures, soft tissue swelling or injuries, marked obesity, or airway obstruction caused by massive prevertebral hematoma in whom endotracheal intubation appears to be or is impossible should be managed by cricothyroidotomy.

If the airway needs to be secured urgently, but not immediately, the other techniques for endotracheal intubation may be useful. Examples of such cases include the patient with a known or suspected cervical spine injury who is hemodynamically stable but has a ruptured spleen, or a patient who is beginning to show signs of respiratory insufficiency but is not in extremis and is not hypoxic. The key point in the decision for urgent endotracheal intubation is whether the patient is cooperative (Fig. 12-12). If the patient is uncooperative or inebriated, or has a possible significant head injury, the steps listed under emergent intubation, namely, a rapid-sequence induction, should be performed. In a cooperative patient, a retrograde intubation, awake fiberoptic intubation, or a blind technique may be chosen. Fiberoptic intubations may seem desirable but may be difficult in patients with edema, blood, secretions, or emesis in the airway. Theoretically, these methods minimize cervical spine movement because they minimize atlantooccipital extension. However, the safety of these techniques over direct laryngoscopy has not been unequivocally proved.[78]

In the nonurgent elective setting, such as requiring anesthesia for the repair of orthopedic or facial injuries, the patient should first undergo a full evaluation of the cervical spine. In the patient with a known cervical spine injury, the head and neck should be immobilized first by a traction device, such as tongs or halo traction, before endotracheal intubation. Awake fiberoptic or a blind intubation technique may then follow. Direct laryngoscopy is seldom useful because visualization of the glottis is difficult with the traction devices in place.

Aims in the Acute Care of the Spinal Cord–Injured Patient

As with head trauma, the primary aim in the management of patients with spinal cord injury is to prevent secondary cord injury (Box 12-5). The principal way to prevent additional injury is by immobilization of the spine. Treatment, therefore, has consisted of anatomic realignment and stabilization with or without surgery for decompression and stabilization. The aim of medical care is primarily supportive, and, while in the past, although morbidity and mortality was reduced little was done to improve neurologic function.[2,105]

However, prevention of secondary neurologic damage by treating hypoxemia and maintaining spinal cord perfusion is also important in the acute management of these patients. Spinal cord blood flow is autoregulated in a fashion similar to bloodflow in the brain,[79] and autoregulation may be impaired several hours after injury.[164] Maintenance of spinal cord perfusion pressure at > 60 mm Hg is advised to improve spinal cord blood flow after injury.[69] In an experimental model of spinal injury, spinal cord blood flow was increased by infusion of phenylephrine but not mannitol or hetastarch although neurologic function was not improved.[51] However, the control blood pressure was 80 mm Hg, which suggests that elevation of blood pressure beyond a minimum of 60 mm Hg is not helpful. Additionally, hypertension may cause hemorrhage and increase edema formation.[69] There is no evidence that hyperventilation to reduce Pa_{CO_2} (and theoretically to decompress the spinal cord) improves outcome with experimentally induced spinal cord injury.[57]

Hyperglycemia should be avoided immediately after spinal cord injury. Minimally increased blood glucose levels (177 mg/dl), associated with intravenous infusions of glucose before experimentally induced spinal cord ischemia, worsened neurologic outcome.[49] Nine out of ten animals that received 5% glucose in water were paraplegic compared with only three out ten control animals. Reduction of blood glucose by insulin improved recovery of electrophysiologic function after experimentally induced spinal

---

BOX 12-5
AIMS IN ACUTE CARE OF SPINAL CORD INJURY

Immobilize the spine
Prevent subsequent damage associated with hypoxemia and decreased spinal cord perfusion pressure
Treat hyperglycemia and avoid glucose-containing solutions in first 24 hours of the injury
Administer methylprednisolone (30 mg/kg load then 5.4 mg/kg/hr for 23 hours) starting within 8 hours of injury
Possibly administer GM-1 ganglioside within 72 hours of injury for 3 to 4 weeks

cord ischemia.[152] These results suggest that infusion of glucose-containing solutions within the first 24 hours of injury should be avoided. In addition, hyperglycemia should be promptly treated.

Until recently, no medical treatment improved the recovery of the initial neurologic deficit. High-dose steroids now appear to be useful in improving neurologic outcome after spinal cord injury.[14] Large doses of methylprednisolone (30 mg/kg followed by a continuous infusion of 5.4 mg/kg/hr for 23 hours) improved neurologic outcome in patients with complete and incomplete lesions. Significant improvement in motor function and sensation to pin and touch were noted at both 6 weeks and 6 months. To be effective, the methylprednisolone must be administered within 8 hours of injury. Complications of steroids, such as wound infection and gastrointestinal hemorrhage, were slightly, but not significantly, increased in the patients receiving steroids. The improvement in neurologic outcome was small but clinically relevant. For instance, a patient with complete quadriplegia might gain enough upper-body strength to transfer from bed to chair and become more self-sufficient.[50]

Another medical therapy that appears promising in improving recovery of function after spinal cord injury is GM-1 ganglioside.[64,193] Gangliosides are complex acidic glycolipids found in central nervous system cells that may stimulate the regeneration and sprouting of neurons. GM-1 ganglioside improved recovery of motor function in a small study of spinal-cord-injured patients[64] when started within 72 hours after injury and administered for 3 to 4 weeks. Although a larger study is needed to definitively demonstrate the safety and efficacy of GM-1 ganglioside, the results are promising and suggest that there may soon be more medical therapies to ameliorate neurologic damage in the acute setting.

SUMMARY

The care of the acutely unstable patient involves neurologic and radiologic examination, evaluation of other organ systems, appropriate airway management, and treatment of associated problems. Brain and spinal cord injuries are both accompanied by physiologic derangements in other bodily functions, challenges in airway control, and a primary management goal of prevention of secondary injury and further neurologic damage. In head injury, this involves a reduction in intracranial pressure and treatment of hypoxemia. In spinal cord injury, immobilization of the spine, supportive care, and early administration of methylprednisolone are of paramount importance.

References

1. Abou-Madi M, Trop D, Abou-Madi N et al: Does a bolus of mannitol initially aggravate intracranial hypertension. A study at various Paco$_2$ tensions in dogs, *Br J Anaesth* 59:630, 1987.
2. Albin MS: Resuscitation of the spinal cord, *Crit Care Med* 6:270, 1978.
3. Albin MS, Bunegin L, Wolf S: Brain and lungs at risk after cervical spine cord transection: intracranial pressure, brain water, blood-brain barrier permeability, cerebral blood flow, and extravascular lung water changes, *Surg Neurol* 24:191, 1985.
4. Andrews BT, Levy ML, Pitts LH: Implications of systemic hypotension for the neurological examination in patients with severe head injury, *Surg Neurol* 28:419, 1987.
5. Aprahamian C, Thompson BM, Finger WA et al: Experimental cervical spine injury model: evaluation of airway management and splinting techniques, *Ann Emerg Med* 13:584, 1984.
6. Bard G, Jones MD: Cineradiographic recording of traction of the cervical spine, *Arch Phys Med Rehabil* 45:403, 1964.
7. Barriot P, Riou B: Retrograde technique for tracheal intubation in trauma patients, *Crit Care Med* 16:712, 1988.
8. Becker DP, Miller JD, Ward JD et al: The outcome from severe head injury with early diagnosis and intensive management, *J Neurosurg* 47:491, 1977.
9. Becker DP, Zieger S, Rother U et al: Complement activation following severe head injury, *Anaesthetist* 36:301, 1987.
10. Bedford RF, Persing JS, Poberskin L et al: Lidocaine or thiopental for rapid control of intracranial hypertension? *Anesth Analg* 58:435, 1980.
11. Berry AJ, Peterson ML: Hyponatremia after mannitol administration in the presence of renal failure, *Anesth Analg* 60:165, 1987.
12. Biby L, Santora AH: Prevertebral hematoma secondary to whiplash injury necessitating emergency intubation, *Anesth Analg* 70:112, 1990.
13. Bivins HG, Ford S, Bezmalinovic Z et al: The effect of axial traction during orotracheal intubation of the trauma victim with an unstable cervical spine, *Ann Emerg Med* 17:25, 1988.
14. Bracken MB, Shepard MJ, Collins WF et al: A randomized, controlled trial of methylprednisolone or naloxone in the treatment of acute spinal-cord injury, *N Engl J Med* 322:1405, 1990.
15. Brimioulle S, Lejeune P, Vachiery J et al: Effect of acidosis and alkalosis on hypoxic pulmonary vasoconstriction in dogs, *Am J Physiol* 258:H347, 1990.
16. Bruce DA, Alavi A, Bilaniuk L et al: Diffuse cerebral swelling following head injuries in children: the syndrome of "malignant brain edema," *J Neurosurg* 54:170, 1981.
17. Bryson BL, Mulkey M, Mumford B et al: Cervical spine injury: incidence and diagnosis, *J Trauma* 26:669, 1986.
18. Burchiel K, Steege TD, Wyler AR: Intracranial pressure changes in brain-injured patients requiring positive end-expiratory pressure ventilation, *Neurosurgery* 8:443, 1981.
19. Burnay RG, Winn R: Increased cerebrospinal fluid pressure during

larygoscopy and intubation for induction of anesthesia, *Anesth Analg* 54:687, 1975.

20. Changaris DG, McGraw CP, Richardson JD et al: Correlation of cerebral perfusion pressure and Glascow coma scale to outcome, *J Trauma* 27:1007, 1987.

21. Chekan E, Weber S: Intubation with or without neuromuscular blockade in trauma patients with cervical spine injury, *Anesth Analg* 70:S54, 1990.

22. Choi SC, Muizelaar JP, Barnes TY et al: Prediction tree for severely head-injured patients, *J Neurosurg* 75:251, 1991.

23. Clark JA, Finelli RE, Netsky MG: Disseminated intravascular coagulation following cranial trauma: case report, *J Neurosurg* 52:266, 1980.

24. Clifton GL, Grossman RG, Makela ME et al: Neurological cause and correlated computerized tomography findings after severe closed head injury, *J Neurosurg* 52:611, 1980.

25. Clifton GL, Robertson CS, Kyper K et al: Cardiovascular response to severe head injury, *J Neurosurg* 59:447, 1983.

26. Clifton GL, Ziegler MG, Grossman RG: Circulating catecholamines and sympathetic activity after head injury, *Neurosurgery* 8:10, 1981.

27. Colachis S, Strohm B, Ganter E: Cervical spine motion in normal women: radiographic study of effect of cervical collars, *Arch Phys Med Rehabil* 54:161, 1973.

28. Colice GL, Matthay MA, Bass E et al: Neurogenic pulmonary edema, *Am Rev Respir Dis* 13:941, 1984.

29. Cooper KR, Boswell PA: Reduced functional residual capacity and abnormal oxygenation in patients with severe head injury, *Chest* 84:29, 1983.

30. Cooper KR, Boswell PA, Choi SC: Safe use of PEEP in patients with severe head injury, *J Neurosurg* 63:552, 1985.

31. Cote CJ, Greenhow DE, Marshall BE: The hypotensive response to rapid intravenous administration of hypertonic solutions in man and rabbit, *Anesthesiology* 50:30, 1979.

32. Cottrell JE, Gupta B, Rappaport H et al: Intracranial pressure during nitroglycerin-induced hypotension, *J Neurosurg* 53:309, 1980.

33. Cottrell JE, Patel K, Turndorf H et al: Intracranial pressure changes induced by sodium nitroprusside in patients with intracranial mass lesions, *J Neurosurg* 53:309, 1980.

34. Cottrell JE, Robustelli A, Post K et al: Furosemide- and mannitol-induced changes in intracranial pressure and serum osmolarity and electrolytes, *Anesthesiology* 47:28, 1977.

35. Crone KR, Lee KS, Kelly DL: Correlation of admission fibrin degradation products with outcome and respiratory failure in patients with severe head injury, *Neurosurgery* 21:532, 1987.

36. Crosby ET, Lui A: The adult cervical spine: implications of airway management, *Can J Anaesth* 37:77, 1990.

37. Cruickshank JM, Neil-Dwyer G, Hayes Y et al: Stress/catecholamine induced cardiac necrosis: reduction by beta$_1$-selective blockade, *Postgrad Med* 83:140, 1988.

38. Cruz J, Miner ME, Allen SJ et al: Continuous monitoring of cerebral oxygenation in acute brain injury: injection of mannitol during hyperventilation, *J Neurosurg* 73:725, 1990.

39. Cully MD, Larson CP, Silverberg GD: Hetastarch coagulopathy in the neurosurgical patient, *Anesthesiology* 66:706, 1987.

40. Cunitz G, Soerensen N: Control of intracranial pressure during pediatric neurosurgery anesthesia, *Child's Brain* 4:205, 1978.

41. Cushing H: Concerning a definite regulatory mechanism of the vasomotor center which controls blood pressure during cerebral compression, *Johns Hopkins Hosp Bull* 12:290, 1901.

42. D'Alecy LG, Lundy EF, Barton KJ et al: Dextrose containing intravenous fluid impairs outcome and increases death after eight minutes of cardiac arrest and resuscitation in dogs, *Surgery* 100:505, 1986.

43. Danzl D, Thomas D: Nasotracheal intubation in the emergency department, *Crit Care Med* 8:677, 1980.

44. Deardon NM, Gibson JS, McDowall DG: Effect of high-dose dexamethasone on outcome from severe head injury, *J Neurosurg* 64:81, 1986.

45. Denis F: The three column spine and its significance in the classification of acute thoracolumbar spinal injuries, *Spine* 8:817, 1983.

46. Donegan MF, Bedford RF: Intravenously administered lidocaine prevents intracranial hypertension during endotracheal suctioning, *Anesthesiology* 52:516, 1980.

47. Doolan LA, O'Brian JF: Safe intubation in cervical spine injury, *Anaesth Intens Care* 13:319, 1985.

48. Drayer BP, Poser CM: Disseminated intravascular coagulation and head trauma: two case studies, *JAMA* 231:174, 1975.

49. Drummond JC, Moore SS: The influence of dextrose administration on neurologic outcome after temporary spinal cord ischemia in the rabbit, *Anesthesiology* 70:64, 1989.

50. Ducker TB: Treatment of spinal-cord injury (editorial), *N Engl J Med* 322:1459, 1990.

51. Dyste GN, Hitchon PW, Girton RA et al: Effect of hetastarch, mannitol, and phenylephrine on spinal cord blood flow following experimental spinal injury, *Neurosurgery* 24:228, 1989.

52. Enevoldsen EM, Jensen FT: Autoregulation and CO$_2$ responses of cerebral blood flow in patients with acute severe head injury, *J Neurosurg* 48:689, 1978.

53. Epstein FM, Cooper KR, Ward JD: Profound pulmonary shunting without edema following stereotactic biopsy of hypothalamic germinoma, *J Neurosurg* 68:303, 1988.

54. Evans DE, Kobrine AI, Rizzoli HV: Cardiac arrhythmias accompanying acute compression of the spinal cord, *J Neurosurg* 52:52, 1980.

55. Feibel JH, Baldwin CA, Joynt RJ: Catecholamine associated refractory hypertension following acute intracranial hemorrhage: control with propranolol, *Ann Neurol* 9:340, 1981.

56. Fesmire FM, Luten RC: The pediatric cervical spine: developmental anatomy and clinical aspects, *J Emerg Med* 7:133, 1989.

57. Ford RWJ, Malm DN: Therapeutic trial of hypercarbia and hypocarbia in acute experimental spinal cord injury, *J Neurosurg* 61:925, 1984.

58. Frankville DD, Drummond JC: Hyperkalemia after succinylcholine administration in a patient with a closed head injury without paresis, *Anesthesiology* 67:264, 1987.

59. Fraser A, Edmonds-Seal J: Spinal cord injuries: a review of the problems facing the anesthetist, *Anaesthesia* 37:1084, 1982.

60. Friesen RH, Honda AT, Thieme RE:

Changes in anterior fontanel pressure in preterm neonates during tracheal intubation, *Anesth Analg* 66:874, 1987.

61. Fried L: Cervical spinal cord injury during skeletal traction, *JAMA* 229:181, 1974.

62. Frost EAM: Effects of positive end-expiratory pressure on intracranial pressure and compliance in brain-injured patients, *J Neurosurg* 47:195, 1977.

63. Frost EAM, Arancibia CU, Shulman K: Pulmonary shunt as a prognostic indicator in head injury, *J Neurosurg* 50:768, 1979.

64. Geisler FH, Dorsey FC, Coleman WP: Recovery of motor function after spinal-cord injury—a randomized, placebo-controlled trial with GM-1 ganglioside, *N Engl J Med* 324:1829, 1991.

65. Gopalakrishnan KC, El Masri W: Prevertebral soft tissue shadow widening—an important sign of cervical spinal injury, *Br J Accid Surg* 17:125, 1986.

66. Grande CM, Barton CR, Steve JK: Appropriate techniques for airway management of emergency patients with suspected spinal cord injury (letter), *Anesth Analg* 67:710, 1988.

67. Gronert GA, Theye R: Pathophysiology of hyperkalemia induced by succinylcholine, *Anesthesiology* 43:89, 1975.

68. Gudeman SK, Miller JD, Becker DP: Failure of high-dose steroid therapy to influence intracranial pressure in patients with severe head injury, *J Neurosurg* 51:301, 1979.

69. Guha A, Tator CH, Rochon J: Spinal cord blood flow and systemic blood pressure after experimental spinal cord injury in rats, *Stroke* 20:372, 1989.

70. Gunnar WP, Jonasson O, Merlotti G et al: Head injury and hemorrhagic shock: studies of the blood brain barrier and intracranial pressure after resuscitation with normal saline solution, 3% saline solution, and dextran-40, *Surgery* 103:398, 1988.

71. Gunnar WP, Merlotti GJ, Barrett J et al: Resuscitation from hemorrhagic shock: alterations of the intracranial pressure after normal saline, 3% saline, and dextran-40, *Ann Surg* 204:686, 1986.

72. Haaga JR, Alfidi RJ, editors: *Computed tomography of the whole body,* vol 1, St Louis, 1983, CV Mosby.

73. Hadley MN, Zabramski JM, Browner CM et al: Pediatric spinal trauma—review of 122 cases of spinal cord and vertebral column injuries, *J Neurosurg* 68:18, 1988.

74. Hamill JF, Bedford RF, Weaver DC et al: Lidocaine before endotracheal intubation—intravenous or laryngotracheal? *Anesthesiology* 55:578, 1981.

75. Harp JR, Wollman H: Cerebral metabolic effects of hyperventilation and deliberate hypotension, *Br J Anaesth* 45:256, 1973.

76. Harris AS: Clinical experience with desmopressin: efficacy and safety in central diabetes insipidus and other conditions, *J Pediatr* 114:711, 1989.

77. Hartman JT, Palumbo F, Hill BJ: Cineradiography of the braced normal cervical spine: a comparative study of five commonly used cervical orthoses, *Clin Orthop* 109:97, 1975.

78. Hastings RH, Marks JD: Airway management for trauma patients with potential cervical spine injuries, *Anesth Analg* 73:471, 1991.

79. Hickley R, Albin M, Bunegin L et al: Autoregulation of spinal cord blood flow: is the cord a microcosm of the brain? *Stroke* 17:1183, 1986.

80. Horton WA, Fahy L, Charters P: Disposition of cervical vertebrae, atlanto-axial joint, hyoid and mandible during x-ray laryngoscopy, *Br J Anaesth* 63:435, 1989.

81. Howcroft AJ, Jenkins DHR: Potentially fatal asphyxia following a minor injury of the cervical spine, *J Bone Joint Surg* 59:93, 1977.

82. Jafar JJ, Johns LM, Mullan SF: The effect of mannitol on cerebral blood flow, *J Neurosurg* 64:754, 1986.

83. James DJ, Bedford, RF: Hydralazine for controlled hypotension during neurosurgical operations, *Anesth Analg* 61:1016, 1982.

84. Jennett WB, Stern WE: Tentorial herniation, the midbrain and the pupil: experimental studies in brain compression, *J Neurosurg* 17:598, 1960.

85. Jennett B, Teasdale G, Gulbraith S: Severe head injuries in three countries, *J Neurol Neurosurg Psychiatry* 40:291, 1977.

86. Kapp JP: Endotracheal intubation in patients with fractures of the cervical spine, *J Neurosurg* 42, 731, 1975.

87. Kauffman HH, Harris JH, Spencer JA et al: Danger of traction during radiography for cervical trauma (letter), *JAMA* 247:2369, 1982.

88. Kenning JA, Toutant SM, Saunders RL: Upright patient positioning in the management of intracranial hypertension, *Surg Neurol* 15:148, 1981.

89. Knopp RK: The safety of orotracheal intubation in patients with suspected cervical-spine injury (editorial), *Ann Emerg Med* 603:157, 1990.

90. Kraus JF, Morganstern H, Fife D et al: Blood alcohol tests: prevalence of involvement and early outcome following brain injury, *Am J Public Health* 79:294, 1989.

91. Kreipke DL, Gillespie KR, McCarthy MC et al: Reliability of indications for cervical spine films in trauma patients, *J Trauma* 29:1438, 1989.

92. Kress TD, Balasubramanian S: Cricothyroidotomy, *Ann Emerg Med* 11:197, 1982.

93. Kullberg G, West KA: Influence of corticosteroids on the ventricular fluid pressure, *Acta Neurol Scand* 41(suppl 13):445, 1965.

94. Lam AM, Winn HR, Cullen BF et al: Hyperglycemia and neurologic outcome in patients with head injury, *J Neurosurg* 75:545, 1991.

95. Lanier WL, Milde JH, Michenfelder JD: Cerebral stimulation following succinylcholine in dogs, *Anesthesiology* 64:551, 1986.

96. Lanier WL, Strangland KL, Scheithauer BW et al: The effects of dextrose and head position on neurologic outcome after complete cerebral ischemia in primates: examination of a model, *Anesthesiology* 66:39, 1987.

97. Lassen NA: Brain extracellular pH: the main factor controlling cerebral blood flow, *Scan J Clin Lab Invest* 30:113, 1972.

98. Ledsome JR, Sharp JM: Pulmonary function in acute cervical cord injury, *Am Rev Respir Dis* 124:41, 1981.

99. Lehmann KG, Lane JG, Piepmeier JM et al: Cardiovascular abnormalities accompanying acute spinal cord injury in humans: incidence, time course and severity, *J Am Coll Cardiol* 10:46, 1987.

100. Lennon RL, Olson RA, Gronert GA: Atracurium or vecuronium for rapid sequence endotracheal intubation, *Anesthesiology* 64:510, 1986.

101. Lewelt W, Jenkins LW, Miller JD:

Effects of experimental fluid-percussion injury of the brain on cerebrovascular reactivity to hypoxia and to hypercapnia, *J Neurosurg* 56:332, 1982.

102. Lipe HP, Mitchell PH: Positioning the patient with intracranial hypertension: how turning and head rotation affect the internal jugular vein, *Heart Lung* 9:1031, 1980.

103. Lobato RD, Rivas JJ, Gomez PA et al: Head-injured patients who talk and deteriorate into coma: analysis of 211 cases studied with computerized tomography, *J Neurosurg* 75:256, 1991.

104. Longstreth WT, Inui TS: High blood glucose level on hospital admission and poor neurological recovery after cardiac arrest, *Ann Neurol* 15:59, 1984.

105. Luce JM: Medical management of spinal cord injury, *Crit Care Med* 13:126, 1985.

106. Luerssen TG, Klauber MR, Marshall LF: Outcome from head injury related to patient's age, *J Neurosurg* 68:409, 1988.

107. Mace SE: Emergency evaluation of cervical spine injuries: CT versus plain radiographs, *Ann Emerg Med* 14:973, 1985.

108. Mackenzie CF, Shin B, Krishnaprasad D et al: Assessment of cardiac and respiratory function during surgery on patients with acute quadriplegia, *J Neurosurg* 62:843, 1985.

109. Majernick TG, Bieniek R, Houston JB et al: Cervical spine movement during orotracheal intubation, *Ann Emerg Med* 15:417, 1986.

110. Malik AB: Mechanisms of neurogenic pulmonary edema, *Circ Res* 57:1, 1985.

111. Manninen PH, Lam AM Gelb AW, et al: The effect of high-dose mannitol on serum and urine electrolytes and osmolality in neurosurgical patients, *Can J Anaesth* 34:442, 1987.

112. Marshall LF, Smith RW, Shapiro HM: The outcome with aggressive treatment in severe head injuries: part II: acute and chronic barbiturate administration in the management of head injury, *J Neurosurg* 50:26, 1979.

113. Marsh ML, Shapiro HM, Smith RW et al: Changes in neurologic status and intracranial pressure associated with sodium nitroprusside administration, *Anesthesiology* 51:538, 1979.

114. Marsh ML, Dunclop BJ, Shapiro HM et al: Succinylcholine-intracranial pressure in neurosurgical patients, *Anesth Analg* 59:550, 1980.

115. McClellan MD, Dauber IM, Weil JV: Elevated intracranial pressure increases pulmonary vascular permeability to protein, *J Appl Physiol* 67:1185, 1989.

116. McGill J, Clinton JE, Ruiz E: Cricothyrotomy in the emergency department, *Ann Emerg Med* 11:361, 1982.

117. McMichan JC, Michel L, Westbrook PR: Pulmonary dysfunction following traumatic quadriplegia, *JAMA* 243:528, 1980.

118. Meakem TD, Meakem TJ, Rappaport W: Airway compromise from prevertebral soft tissue swelling during placement of halo-traction for C-spine injury, *Anesthesiology* 73:775, 1990.

119. Meschino A, Devitt JH, Schwartz ML et al: The safety of awake tracheal intubation in cervical spine injury, *Can J Anaesth* 35:131, 1988.

120. Michenfelder JD, Fowler WS, Theye RA: CO_2 levels and pulmonary shunting in anesthetized man, *J Appl Physiol* 21:1471, 1966.

121. Miller JD, Sakalas R, Ward JD et al: Methylprednisolone treatment in patients with brain tumors, *Neurosurgery* 1:114, 1977.

122. Miner ME, Allen SJ: Cardiovascular effects of severe head injury. In Frost, E, editor: *Clinical anesthesia in neurosurgery*, Stoneham, MA, 1991, Butterworth, pp 439.

123. Moss E, Powell D, Gibson RM et al: Effect of etomidate on intracranial pressure and cerebral perfusion pressure, *Br J Anesth* 51:347, 1979.

124. Nelson PB, Seif S, Gutai J et al: Hyponatremia and natriuresis following subarachnoid hemorrhage in a monkey model, *J Neurosurg* 60:233, 1984.

125. Ott L, Young B, Phillips R et al: Altered gastric emptying in the head-injured patient: relationship to feeding intolerance, *J Neurosurg* 74:738, 1991.

126. Ovassapian A: *Fiberoptic airway endoscopy in anesthesia and critical care,* New York, 1990, Raven Press.

127. Ovassapian A, Krejcie TC, Yelich SJ et al: Awake fibreoptic intubation in the patient at high risk of aspiration, *Br J Anaesth* 62:13, 1989.

128. Ovassapian A, Yelich SJ, Dykes MHM et al: Fiberoptic nasotracheal intubation. Incidence and causes of failure, *Anesth Analg* 62:692, 1983.

129. Pang D, Wilberger JE: Spinal cord injury without radiographic abnormalities in children, *J Neurosurg* 57:114, 1982.

130. Perel A, Pizov R, Cotev S: Systolic blood pressure variation is a sensitive indicator of hypovolemia in ventilated dogs subjected to graded hemorrhage, *Anesthesiology* 67:498, 1987.

131. Piepmeier JM, Lehman KB, Lane JG: Cardiovascular instability following acute cervical spine cord trauma, *Cent Nerv Syst Trauma* 2:153,1985.

132. Pierce EC Jr, Lambertsen CJ, Deutsch S et al: Cerebral circulation and metabolism during thiopental anesthesia and hyperventilation in man, *J Clin Invest* 41:1664, 1962.

133. Podolsky S, Baraff LJ, Simon RR et al: Efficacy of cervical spine immobilization methods, *J Trauma* 23:461, 1983.

134. Poe RH, Reisman JL, Rodenhouse TG: Pulmonary edema in cervical spinal cord injury, *J Trauma* 18:71, 1978.

135. Pollack IF, Pang D, Sclabassi R: Recurrent spinal cord injury without radiographic abnormalities in children, *J Neurosurg* 69:177, 1988.

136. Pollay M, Fullenwider C, Roberts PA et al: Effect of mannitol and furosemide on blood-brain osmotic gradient and intracranial pressure, *J Neurosurg* 59:945, 1983.

137. Poole GV, Prough DS, Johnson JC et al: Effects of resuscitation from hemorrhage shock on cerebral hemodynamics in the presence of an intracranial mass, *J Trauma* 27:18, 1987.

138. Popp AJ, Shah DM, Berman RA et al: Delayed pulmonary dysfunction in head-injured patients, *J Neurosurg* 57:784, 1982.

139. Prough DS, Johnson JC, Poole GV et al: Effects of intracranial pressure on resuscitation from hemorrhagic shock with hypertonic saline versus lactated Ringer's solution, *Crit Care Med* 13:407, 1985.

140. Prough DS, Johnson JC, Stump DA et al: Effects of hypertonic saline ver-

sus lactated Ringer's solution on cerebral oxygen transport during resuscitation from hemorrhagic shock, *J Neurosurg* 64:627, 1986.

141. Pulsinelli WA, Levy DE, Sigsbee B et al: Increased damage after ischemic stroke in patients with hyperglycemia with or without established diabetes mellitus, *Am J Med* 74:540, 1983.

142. Pulsinelli WA, Waldman S, Rawlinson D et al: Moderate hyperglycemia augments ischemic brain damage: a neuropathologic study in the rat, *Neurology* 32:1239, 1982.

143. Ravussin P, Abou-Madi M, Archer D et al: Changes in CSF pressure after mannitol in patients with and without elevated CSF pressure, *J Neurosurg* 69:869, 1988.

144. Ravussin P, Archer DP, Tyler JL et al: Effects of rapid mannitol infusion on cerebral blood volume, *J Neurosurg* 64:104, 1986.

145. Rea GL, Rockswold GL: Barbiturate therapy in uncontrolled intracranial hypertension, *Neurosurgery* 12:401, 1983.

146. Reid DC, Henderson R, Saboe L et al: Etiology and clinical course of missed spine fractures, *J Trauma* 27:980,1987.

147. Rhee KJ, Green W, Holcroft JW et al: Oral intubation in the multiply injured patient: the risk of exacerbating spinal cord damage, *Ann Emerg Med* 19:511, 1990.

148. Riggins RS, Kraus JF: The risk of neurologic damage with fractures of the vertebrae, *J Trauma* 17:126, 1977.

149. Robard S, Saiki H: Mechanism of the pressure response to increased intracranial pressure, *Am J Physiol* 168:234, 1952.

150. Roberge R, Wears R, Kelley M et al: Selective application of cervical spine radiography in alert victims of blunt trauma: a prospective study, *J Trauma* 28:784, 1988.

151. Roberts PA, Pollay M, Engles C et al: Effect on intracranial pressure of furosemide combined with varying doses and administration rates of mannitol, *J Neurosurg* 66:440, 1987.

152. Robertson CS, Grossman RG: Protection against spinal cord ischemia with insulin-induced hypoglycemia, *J Neurosurg* 67:739, 1987.

153. Rockoff MA, Marshall LF, Shapiro HM: High-dose barbiturate therapy in humans: a clinical review of 60 patients, *Ann Neurol* 6:194, 1979.

154. Rosa RM, Silva P, Young JB et al: Adrenergic modulation of extrarenal potassium disposal, *N Engl J Med* 302:431, 1980.

155. Rose J, Valtonen S, Jennett B: Avoidable factors contributing to death after head injury, *Br Med J* 2:615, 1977.

156. Rosner MJ, Coley IB: Cerebral perfusion pressure, intracranial pressure, and head elevation, *J Neurosurg* 65:636, 1986.

157. Ross SE, Schwab CW, ET David et al: Clearing the cervical spine: initial radiologic evaluation, *J Trauma* 27:1055, 1987.

158. Rudehill A, Lagerkranser M, Lindquist C et al: Effects of mannitol on blood volume and central hemodynamics in patients undergoing cerebral aneurysm surgery, *Anesth Analg* 62:875, 1983.

159. Schettini A, Stahurski B, Young HF: Osmotic and osmotic-loop diuresis in brain surgery. Effects on plasma and CSF electrolytes and ion excretion, *J Neurosurg* 56:579, 1983.

160. Schumaker PT, Rhodes GR, Newell JC et al: Ventilation-perfusion imbalance after head trauma, *Am Rev Respir Dis* 119:33, 1979.

161. Schwartz ML, Tator CH, Rowed DW et al: The University of Toronto Head Injury Treatment Study: a prospective randomized comparison of pentobarbital and mannitol, *Can J Neurol Sci* 11:434, 1984.

162. Seebacher J, Nozik D, Mathieu A: Inadvertent intracranial introduction of a nasogastric tube, a complication of severe maxillofacial trauma, *Anesthesiology* 42:100, 1975.

163. Seelig JM, Becker DP, Miller JD et al: Traumatic acute subdural hematoma: major mortality reduction in comatose patients treated within four hours, *N Engl J Med* 304:1511, 1981.

164. Senter HJ, Venes JL: Loss of autoregulation and posttraumatic ischemia following experimental spinal cord trauma, *J Neurosurg* 50:198, 1976.

165. Severinghaus JW, Swenson EW, Finley TN et al: Unilateral hypoventilation produced in dogs by occluding one pulmonary artery, *J Appl Physiol* 16:53, 1961.

166. Shapira Y, Artru AA, Cotev S et al: Brain edema and neurologic status following head trauma in the rat, *Anesthesiology* 77:79, 1992.

167. Shapiro HM, Galindo A, Loyte DR et al: Acute intracranial hypertension during anesthetic induction. Partial control with thiopental, *Eur Neurol* 8:188, 1972.

168. Shapiro HM, Galindo A, Wyte SR et al: Rapid intraoperative reduction of intracranial pressure with thiopentone, *Brit J Anaesth* 45:1057, 1973.

169. Shapiro HM, Marshall LF: Intracranial pressure responses to PEEP in head-injured patients, *J Trauma* 18:254, 1978.

170. Shapiro HM, Wyte SR, Harris AB et al: Acute intraoperative intracranial hypertension in neurosurgical patients: mechanical and pharmacological factors, *Anesthesiology* 37:399, 1972.

171. Shapiro HM, Wyte SR, Harris AB: Ketamine anesthesia in patients with intracranial pathology, *Br J Anaesth* 44:1200, 1972.

172. Shin B, Mackenzie CF, Helrich M: Hypokalemia in trauma patients, *Anesthesiology* 65:90, 1986.

173. Sinha RP, Ducker TB, Perot PL: Arterial oxygenation. Findings and its significance in central nervous system trauma patients, *JAMA* 224:1258, 1973.

174. Smith RB, Schaer WB, Pfaeffle H: Percutaneous transtracheal ventilation for anaesthesia and resuscitation: a review and report of complications, *Can Anaesth Soc J* 22:607, 1975.

175. Smith SD, Cone JB, Bowser BH et al: Cerebral edema following acute hemorrhage in a murine model: the role of crystalloid resuscitation, *J Trauma* 22:588, 1982.

176. Solonick D, Pitts LH, Lovely M et al: Traumatic intracerebral hematomas: timing of appearance and indicators for operative removal, *J Trauma* 26:787, 1986.

177. Spaite DW, Maralee J: Prehospital cricothyrotomy: an investigation of indications, technique, complications, and patient outcome, *Ann Emerg Med* 19:279, 1990.

178. Stellin GP, Barker S, Murdock M et al: Orotracheal intubation in trauma patients with cervical fractures, *Crit Care Med* 17:537, 1989.

179. Stirt JA, Grosslight KR, Bedford RF et al: "Defasciculation" with metocurine prevents succinylcholine-induced increases in intracranial pressure, *Anesthesiology* 67:50, 1987.

180. Stover SL, Fine PR: The epidemiology and economics of spinal cord injury, *Paraplegia* 25:225, 1987.

181. Streitwieser DR, Knopp R, Wales LR et al: Accuracy of standard radiographic views in detecting cervical spine fractures, *Ann Emerg Med* 12:538, 1983.

182. Talucci RC, Shaikh KA, Schwab CW: Rapid sequence induction with oral endotracheal intubation in the multiply injured patient, *Am Surg* 54:185, 1988.

183. Teasdale G, Jennett B: Assessment of coma and impaired consciousness. A practical scale, *Lancet* 2:81, 1974.

184. Todd MM, Tommasino C, Moore S: Cerebral effects of isovolemic hemodilution with a hypertonic saline solution, *J Neurosurg* 63:944, 1985.

185. Tommasino C, Moore S, Todd MM: Cerebral effects of isovolemic hemodilution with crystalloid or colloid solutions, *Crit Care Med* 16:862, 1988.

186. Touho H, Hirakawa K, Hiro A et al: Relationship between abnormalities of coagulation and fibrinolysis and postoperative intracranial hemorrhage in head injury, *Neurosurgery* 19:523, 1986.

187. Toutant SM, Klauber MR, Marshall LF et al: Absent or compressed basal cisterns on first CT scan: ominous predictors of outcome in severe head injury, *J Neurosurg* 61:691, 1984.

188. Trafton PG: Spinal cord injuries, *Surg Clin North Am* 62:61, 1982.

189. Turner JM, Powell D, Gibson RM et al: Intracranial pressure changes in neurosurgical patients during hypotension induced with sodium nitroprusside or trimethaphan, *Br J Anesth* 49:419, 1977.

190. Unni VKN, Johnston RA, Young HSA et al: Prevention of intracranial hypertension during laryngoscopy and endotracheal intubation: use of a second dose of thiopentone, *Br J Anesth* 56:1219, 1984.

191. VanAken H, Puchstein C, Schweppe ML et al: Effect of labetal on intracranial pressure in dogs with or without intracranial hypertension, *Acta Anaesth Scand* 26:615, 1982.

192. Voll CL, Auer RN: The effect of postischemic blood glucose levels on ischemic brain damage in the rat, *Ann Neurol* 24:638, 1988.

193. Walker MD: Acute spinal-cord injury (editorial), *N Engl J Med* 324:1885, 1991.

194. Walls RM: Orotracheal intubation and potential cervical spine injury (letter), *Ann Emerg Med* 16:373, 1987.

195. Wang JF, Reves JG, Gutierrez FA: Awake fiberoptic laryngoscopic tracheal intubation for anterior cervical spinal fusion in patient with cervical cord trauma, *Intl Surg* 64:69, 1979.

196. Ward JD, Becker DP, Miller JD et al: Failure of prophylactic barbiturate coma in the treatment of severe head injury, *J Neurosurg* 62:383, 1985.

197. White PF, Schlobohm RM, Pitts LH et al: A randomized study of drugs for preventing increases in intracranial pressure during endotracheal suctioning, *Anesthesiology* 57:242, 1982.

198. Williams CF, Bernstein TW, Jelenko C: Essentiality of the lateral cervical spine radiograph, *Ann Emerg Med* 10:198, 1981.

199. Wood PR, Lawler PGP: Managing the airway in cervical spine injury. A review of the Advanced Trauma Life Support protocol, *Anaesthesia* 47:792, 1992.

200. Zornow MH, Oh YS, Scheller MS: A comparison of the cerebral and haemodynamic effects of mannitol and hypertonic saline in an animal model of brain injury, *Acta Neurochir Suppl (Wien)* 51:324, 1990.

201. Zornow MH, Thomas TC, Scheller MS: The efficacy of three different methods of transtracheal ventilation, *Can J Anaesth* 36:624, 1989.

202. Zornow MH, Todd MM, Ward DM: The acute cerebral effects of changes in plasma osmolality and oncotic pressure, *Anesthesiology* 67:936, 1987.

13

Supratentorial Masses: Surgical Considerations

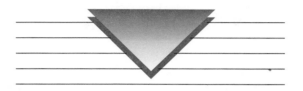

DANIEL K. O'ROURKE
EDWARD H. OLDFIELD

BASIC PHYSIOLOGIC PRINCIPLES
  UNDERLYING SURGICAL
  MANAGEMENT
  Intracranial pressure
  Autoregulation and chemoregulation of
    cerebral blood flow
  The herniation syndromes
  Local disruption of function by
    supratentorial masses
NEOPLASMS

Classification
Primary central nervous system
  neoplasms
Metastatic tumors
Presentation of patients with
  supratentorial masses
Perioperative evaluation
HEMATOMAS
Trauma
Spontaneous hematomas

SURGICAL APPROACHES
  Craniotomy
  Image-guided stereotactic surgery
  Transphenoidal approach
  Intracranial imaging
NEW FRONTIERS
  Brain imaging
  Regional treatment of malignant tumors
SUMMARY

The supratentorial space contains the portion of the brain that lies superior to the taut transverse fold of dura known as the tentorium cerebelli (Fig. 13-1). Surgical procedures in the supratentorial space comprise the majority of intracranial surgeries performed by neurosurgeons. Numerous and diverse pathologies occur in this space (Box 13-1).[3,7,30,42] In this chapter, we review the major categories of and the surgical considerations for supratentorial masses, including the pertinent pathophysiology, diagnostic and surgical approaches, and principles of management. Certain physiologic principles underlie perioperative management of all patients requiring supratentorial surgery. Although these principles are covered in greater detail in other chapters in this text, because of their importance in the surgical management of these patients, they are briefly reviewed here.

BASIC PHYSIOLOGIC PRINCIPLES UNDERLYING SURGICAL MANAGEMENT
Intracranial Pressure

The Monroe-Kelly doctrine describes homeostasis of intracranial pressure (ICP) during changes in the volume of the principal space-occupying intracranial constituents: intravascular blood, cerebrospinal fluid (CSF), and brain.[1,5] Because the principal space-occupying intracranial constituents are noncompressible and the adult skull is unyielding, an increase in the mass of one of these normal elements or the addition of an abnormal mass, such as a tumor, must be accompanied by a reduction in the volume of one or more of the three normal components. Thus, to varying degrees, these three tissues, particularly CSF and blood, serve as potential buffers to increasing ICP with increasing size of a supratentorial mass.[39,56]

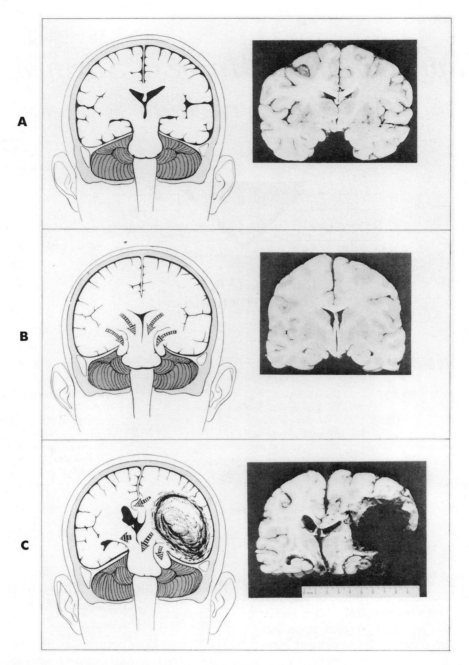

FIG. 13-1 Schematic representation of the brain in coronal section at the level of the brainstem. The tentorium separates the supratentorial and infratentorial compartments. **A,** Normal anatomy. **B,** Transtentorial herniation, a bilateral shift of the supratentorial contents through the tentorial notch, which is usually caused by a bilateral or a global process. **C,** Subfalcine, transtentorial, and uncal herniation in a patient who died from a large hemorrhagic cerebral infarction. Subfalcine herniation is a shift of the medial portion of the frontal and parietal lobes of the brain beneath the falx. Uncal herniation is a shift of the uncus, a medial temporal lobe structure, through the tentorial notch. *(From Plum F, Posner JB:* Diagnosis of stupor and coma, *ed 3, Philadelphia, 1980, FA Davis.)*

BOX 13-1

SUPRATENTORIAL MASSES

I. Neoplasms
  A. Primary
    1. Intraaxial
      a. Brain parenchyma
        (1) Neuroectodermal tumors
          (a) Astrocytoma
          (b) Oligodendroglioma
          (c) Ependymoma
          (d) Primitive neuroectodermal tumor
          (e) Ganglioglioma
          (f) Pinealoma
      b. Intraventricular
        (1) Ependymoma
        (2) Choroid plexus papilloma
        (3) Meningioma
    2. Extraaxial
      a. Meningioma
      b. Schwannoma
      c. Dermoid and epidermoid
      d. Craniopharyngioma
      e. Pituitary adenoma
      f. Chordoma
  B. Metastatic

II. Blood and Blood Vessels
  A. Hematomas
    1. Epidural
    2. Subdural
      a. Acute
      b. Subacute
      c. Chronic
    3. Intracerebral
      a. Traumatic
        (1) Hematoma
        (2) Contusion
      b. Idiopathic
      c. Hemorrhagic cerebral infarction

      d. Ruptured aneurysm
      e. Ruptured arteriovenous malformation
      f. Hemorrhagic tumor
      g. Amyloid angiopathy
    4. Intraventricular
      a. Ruptured aneurysm
      b. Trauma
  B. Blood vessel
    1. Aneurysm (saccular, micotic, atherosclerotic)
    2. Arteriovenous malformation
    3. Cavernous angioma

III. Infection
  A. Bacterial abscess
    1. Intracerebral
    2. Subdural
    3. Epidural
  B. Paracytic (cyst)
  C. Viral
    1. AIDS
    2. Toxoplasmosis
    3. Cytomegalovirus
    4. Other

IV. Hydrocephalus
  A. High pressure
    1. Communicating
    2. Noncommunicating
  B. Normal pressure

V. Other
  A. Cerebral infarction
  B. Cerebral edema
  C. Pneumocephalus
  D. Arachnoid cyst
  E. Radiation necrosis

Two factors limit the effectiveness of this homeostatic mechanism. Because maintenance of normal ICP in the face of an expanding intracranial mass requires sufficient time for displacement of the normal contents to occur, the rapidity with which a mass expands may exceed the rate of the compensatory process. When the rate at which these volume shifts can occur is exceeded, ICP rises rapidly, even with small increases in the abnormal mass.[5] For example, a rapidly expanding epidural hematoma may increase the ICP sufficiently to displace brain from the skull and cause death, whereas a more slowly expanding mass of similar size may be accommodated such that the ICP does not rise significantly and the clinical effects are minimal. Thus, for rapidly expanding masses, the volume-pressure curve is shifted to the left. The second limitation to ICP homeosta-

sis occurs when the compensatory mechanisms are exhausted; then ICP rises rapidly with small changes in volume.[1]

The initial compensation for a rapidly expanding mass is a decrease in the volume of the intracranial venous blood. Although this occurs relatively early, its buffering capacity is limited. The second important component in the homeostasis of ICP is the cerebrospinal fluid (CSF), the displacement of which provides much of the compensation for intracranial masses. However, displacement of CSF may not occur if the flow of CSF is obstructed by blood or by a mass, such as a tumor, which distorts the normal route of CSF flow.[56] Thus, in the presence of obstructive hydrocephalus, the mechanisms for compensation for an expanding intracranial mass are compromised, clinical deterioration occurs earlier and faster, and the urgency for treatment is greater.

Because the brain is largely incompressible, very little space is provided by a reduction in supratentorial brain volume. A reduction in brain water may help to accommodate mass lesions that accrue mass slowly, such as meningiomas, but the space that this furnishes is limited and this means of compensation is ineffective in the short term.[1] Displacement of brain underlies the herniation syndromes and represents the end stage of the compensatory processes.

Autoregulation and Chemoregulation of Cerebral Blood Flow

The homeostatic processes of the central nervous system serve to preserve adequate blood flow to meet metabolic demand. Maintenance of cerebral blood flow (CBF) is tightly controlled. Homeostatic mechanisms for maintenance of CBF are given priority over those for ICP.[1,35,36,55]

Autoregulation of cerebral vasomotor tone maintains CBF within a narrow range in the face of a changing mean arterial pressure (MAP) or changing cerebral perfusion pressure (CPP).[39] CPP is the difference in the MAP and the ICP (normally ICP is similar to central venous pressure, CVP). Autoregulation occurs at the level of the cerebral arteriole, which dilates in response to diminished CPP (increased ICP or reduced MAP). The relationship of CBF, CPP, and cerebral vascular resistance (CVR) is expressed as:

$$CBF = \frac{CPP}{CVR} \text{ or } CBF = \frac{MAP - ICP}{CVR} \quad (1)$$

During surgery, CVR and CBF are not routinely measured.

Autoregulation of arteriole diameter depends on the pressure gradient across the vessel wall (CPP). With increased ICP, CPP diminishes, arterioles relax, and CBF is maintained to meet cerebral metabolic demand. Furthermore, the systemic autonomic response to inadequate CPP is to increase the MAP.[5,35,36,39] Autoregulation is effective when CPP is between about 50 and 180 mm Hg. Thus, with MAP < 50 mm Hg, in circumstances with high ICP and CPP of less than 50 mm Hg, or in conditions in which autoregulation is impaired (e.g. trauma), cerebral ischemia will occur unless steps are taken to increase CPP by increasing MAP, decreasing ICP, or reducing cerebral metabolic demand.

Cerebral blood flow is also regulated by chemoregulation. Alterations in plasma $Paco_2$ affect the cerebral vascular tone (CVR). Chemoregulation, as with autoregulation, occurs at the level of the cerebral arteriole. Because hypocarbia associated with hyperventilation immediately induces vasoconstriction,[36] which reduces CBF and cerebral blood volume,[55] the most rapid technique available to lower ICP in a patient with an intracranial mass is controlled hyperventilation. Hypercarbia induces dilation of the cerebral arterioles, increasing CBF and cerebral blood volume, and

can rapidly increase ICP, particularly if the patient has an intracranial mass and is at, or beyond, the compensatory portion of the intracranial volume-pressure relationship.

The Herniation Syndromes

Three types of brain herniation, a shift of brain tissue out of the compartment in which it normally resides, occur in the supratentorial compartment: displacement of brain within the supratentorial compartment across the midline beneath the falx, protrusion of brain from the supratentorial compartment through the tentorial incisura and into the posterior fossa, and protrusion of brain through an opening in the cranial vault produced by surgery or trauma.[42]

Subfalcine herniation occurs with asymmetrically located supratentorial masses (Fig. 13-1, C). The appearance of this process on diagnostic imaging studies is referred to as a "midline shift." The midportion of the anterior cerebral arteries, which supply areas of the brain critical to movement and sensation of the lower extremities, may be compressed and occluded during subfalcine herniation.

The tentorium serves as a shelf upon which the posterior half of each cerebral hemisphere rests (Fig. 13-1, A). When the physiologic systems previously described are no longer able to compensate for an expanding supratentorial mass, the central portion of the brain is forced out of the supratentorial compartment into the infratentorial compartment, a process known as transtentorial herniation (Fig. 13-1, B). As this process occurs, stretching and shearing of the perforating arteries of the brainstem may produce small hemorrhages in the brainstem known as "Duret's hemorrhages." Transtentorial herniation produces impairment of level of consciousness, paralysis of eye movement, respiratory irregularity, and abnormal posturing of the extremities.

When a space-occupying mass shifts the anterior medial portion of the temporal lobe (the uncus) medially and downward against the tentorial edge, the uncus may be cut, sheared, and/or contused (Fig. 13-1, C). In this type of transtentorial herniation, uncal herniation, uncal compression of the third cranial nerve (the occulomotor nerve, which controls pupil size, elevates the eyelid, and moves the eye medially) may occur early, producing a dilated pupil, ptosis, and lateral deviation of the eye. Anisocoria is the most important early sign of this process and mandates immediate action toward reversing the responsible space-occupying supratentorial process.

Local Disruption of Function by Supratentorial Masses

The local effects of intracranial masses on the brain are conveyed mechanically and chemically. A mass may compress a functional area of brain and impair its function. Swelling of the cerebral tissue contiguous to a mass (i.e., cerebral edema) increases the mass effect of the tumor, impairing

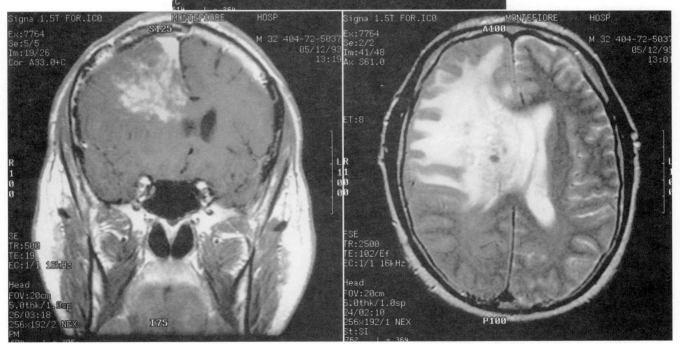

FIG. 13-2   MR image of a patient with a glioblastoma multiforme diagnosed histologically by stereotactic biopsy. **A,** Gadolinium contrast-enhanced T_1-weighted axial image. Note the shift and distortion of the ventricles, which are black in this sequence (very low signal intensity). **B,** T_1-weighted contrast-enhanced coronal image in the same patient. Subfalcine herniation in this view is readily apparent (compare with Fig. 13-1, *C*). **C,** T_2-weighted axial image. With this sequence, water density is bright. The ventricles appear white because of the cerebrospinal fluid. Note the tumor-associated cerebral edema that outlines the cortical border laterally.

brain function further. Vasogenic cerebral edema, the form of cerebral edema that responds to glucocorticoid treatment, surrounds most tumors (Fig. 13-2). Because cerebral swelling increases the pressure on nearby brain it reduces regional CBF or by contributing to intracranial volume it increases ICP. Tumor infiltration of the brain, most often seen with glial tumors, or hemorrhage can also mechanically disrupt cerebral tissue and cause potentially irreversible functional loss of the affected region. These latter processes are most notable with glial tumors.[42]

Tumors may also impair local or regional brain metabolism. Positron emission tomography (PET) scanning has been used to identify and map changes in brain metabolism in vivo, such as diminished glucose utilization, in the region surrounding tumor. Similarly, magnetic resonance spectroscopy (MRS), which permits measurement of the concentration of certain metabolites (e.g., lactate, pH, and certain phosphorus-containing compounds involved with energy metabolism) in vivo, reveals abnormalities in the brain chemistry adjacent to a tumor.

Optimal perioperative management of the patient with an intracranial mass neccesitates consideration of the following: the influence of elevated ICP and regional pressure differentials within the cranial vault, the effects of supratentorial masses on local and regional CBF and metabolism, and the mechanical distortion of cerebral tissue by the effects of the mass.

NEOPLASMS
Classification

The utility of a tumor classification system is a function of its accuracy in predicting the natural history of the tumor, patient outcome, and response to treatment. Supratentorial neoplasms are classified by the cell of origin, the degree of anaplasia, and the site of occurrence, all of which influence prognosis and treatment strategy.[46,51,54,64] Although

several general histologic classification schemes have been used in the past, such as the four-stage grading system of Kernohan for gliomas, many of the histologic features that were once considered important are now known to have little or no relationship to tumor behavior or prognosis.[45,63,64] Furthermore, the prognosis associated with a specific tumor type and the potential efficacy of therapy, surgical or nonsurgical, available for that tumor dictate whether aggressive therapy is or is not appropriate. The location of the tumor often influences its surgical accessibility and therefore influences the prognosis and location and may also limit treatment options. For instance, brainstem gliomas are often histologically benign but are usually not surgically resectable because of their location and thus may be rapidly lethal. The patient's age may adversely affect the prognosis associated with some types of central nervous system tumors, particularly the glial tumors (Fig. 13-3). Fig. 13-4 summarizes the relative incidence of the principal types of supratentorial tumors.

Primary Central Nervous System Neoplasms

Primary brain tumors account for 55% to 60% of all supratentorial tumors. Most primary brain tumors are comprised of neuroepithelial tumors, meningiomas, and pituitary adenomas. Glial tumors, which comprise over 90% of the neuroepithelial tumors, include the tumors of astrocytic lineage, such as oligodendrogliomas, ependymomas, and pilocytic astrocytomas.[3,34,45]

Tumors That Originate From Astrocytes

Well-differentiated astrocytomas, anaplastic astrocytomas, and glioblastoma multiforme are the principal astrocytic tumors. The less malignant tumors often exhibit over time more aggressive clinical behavior and become malignant. A supratentorial tumor that is biopsied and diagnosed as a well-differentiated astrocytoma or an oligodendroglioma often later demonstrates rapid growth and develops the histo-

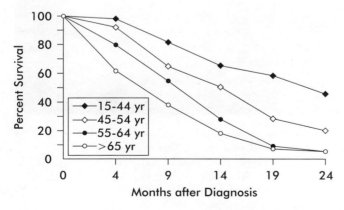

FIG. 13-3 Age-related survival of patients with glioblastoma multiforme after surgery and chemotherapy. *(From Deutsch M, Green SB, Strike TA et al:* Int J Radiation Oncol Biol Phys *16:1389-1396, 1989.)*

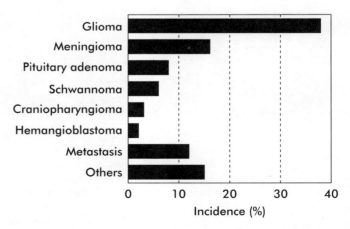

FIG. 13-4 Relative incidence of the principal types of brain tumors. *(Data from Zimmerman, HM:* Ann Acad Sci *159:337-359, 1969.)*

logic features of a more malignant tumor.[3,25,47,59] These tumors extend fingerlike, microscopic projections into the surrounding brain. These infiltrating extensions of tumor, which are not visible at surgery or with current imaging techniques, extend for several centimeters into the ipsilateral or contralateral hemisphere and often reach the brainstem by the time of death. Complete, curative surgical removal of infiltrating gliomas is not possible.[18]

Well-Differentiated Astrocytoma. The least aggressive of the fibrillary astrocytic neoplasms is the well-differentiated or nonanaplastic (also called "low-grade") astrocytoma, which accounts for only about 3% of primary brain tumors. These tumors generally do not enhance or enhance minimally on computed tomography (CT) and magnetic resonance imaging (MR). Patients may have surgical excision and/or radiation therapy or be followed conservatively and live symptom-free for five years or longer without evidence of recurrence. When a low-grade tumor will recur or evolve into a malignant tumor varies greatly and cannot be accurately predicted in individual patients.[3] Depending on tumor location, surgery, either biopsy or debulking via craniotomy, is performed to establish the diagnosis or to debulk the tumor. Whether radiation treatment should be used in these patients at diagnosis or when tumor growth recurs after surgery is controversial and is the subject of a current prospective study.

Anaplastic Astrocytoma. Anaplastic astrocytomas, which comprise 20% of primary brain tumors, usually have abnormal blood vessels with disruption of the blood-brain barrier (BBB). This disruption of BBB is routinely identified on CT and MR as an area of contrast enhancement. These tumors often evolve into glioblastoma multiforme, the type of glial tumor exhibiting the greatest malignant behavior.[55] The median survival after diagnosis of patients with an anaplastic astrocytoma is intermediate between low-grade astrocytomas and glioblastoma. Surgical excision of accessible tumors and irradiation therapy provide a median survival of 2 to 3 years. Chemotherapy with Carmustine (1,3-*bis*[2-chloroethyl]-1-nitrosourea; BCNU) enhances survival for several months in patients less than 40 years old.[25,46]

Glioblastoma Multiforme. This, the most common primary brain tumor, accounts for about 30% of all primary brain tumors. On CT and MR it is characterized by an irregular ring or a heterogeneous mass of contrast enhancement surrounded by cerebral edema and mass effect (see Fig. 13-2).[6] The center of the contrast-enhancing ring often represents the necrotic portion of the tumor. The median survival of patients with untreated glioblastoma multiforme is only 8 to 16 weeks.[41] Treatment with surgical resection followed by radiation extends mean survival to 36 to 50 weeks (see Fig. 13-3).* The prognosis of patients with

a glioblastoma with the same histologic features and site in the brain varies significantly with age. Because of the dismal prognosis for patients with glioblastoma and the high incidence of glioblastoma in patients with primary brain tumors, many experimental treatments are in development.* In young patients (less than 40 years old) with a glioblastoma, BCNU combined with irradiation therapy and surgery extends mean survival a few months compared with patients who receive irradiation without BCNU.[22]

Pilocytic Astrocytoma. The pilocytic astrocytoma is less common than other astrocytic tumors, accounting for only 1% of all primary brain tumors. This tumor is more common in children and young adults. It usually arises in the cerebellum, the cerebral hemispheres, the hypothalamus, or the optic pathways. The well-demarcated, densely enhancing tumor mass is almost always associated with a contiguous cyst. The growth of this tumor, in contrast to the other types of astrocytic tumors, is as a well-defined mass rather than by infiltration of adjacent brain. Because of the noninvasive growth by this histologically benign tumor, the prognosis for total surgical resection is quite good. Long-term survival without additional therapy is common.[3]

Oligodendroglioma

Oligodendrogliomas, which arise from oligodendrocytes, the glial cells that myelinate the central nervous system, are infiltrating glial tumors. They comprise 6% of primary intracranial neoplasms. They often contain areas of calcification that can be detected with imaging studies, particularly CT. Patients with oligodendrogliomas often present with seizures, which may predate the occurrence of other symptoms and the diagnosis of the tumor by 5 to 10 years.[3,45] Even after diagnosis the natural history of these tumors is usually a protracted interval of 8 to 20 years, during which their presence is rather silent clinically. Because they are comprised of oligodendrocytes mixed with a smaller fibrillary astrocytic component, ultimately the astrocytic component becomes malignant and the tumor behaves like an anaplastic astrocytoma or glioblastoma. The initial treatment is surgical removal although surgical cure is rare. Radiation therapy is not recommended during the stage of the tumor that is predominantly oligodendroglial with uniform benign-appearing oligodendrocytes or while the tumor remains clinically indolent because this stage is characterized by very slow growth and radioresistance. With oligodendrogliomas that contain necrosis, neovascularity, or pleomorphic cells, irradiation may lengthen survival and should be considered. The prognosis of the mixed oligodendroglioma-astrocytoma depends on the histologic features of the astrocytic component of the tumor. The decision to irradiate is based on the nature of that component of the tumor.

---

*References 3, 12, 16, 47, 50, 58, 60.

*References 4, 11, 13-15, 20, 23, 27, 28, 32, 33, 40, 43, 44, 48, 57, 61, 62.

Meningioma

Meningiomas are thought to arise from the arachnoidal cap cells (cells forming the outer lining of the arachnoid membrane).[45] Meninges or their stem cells, the meningothelial cap cell.[45] The common type of meningioma originates from, and is directly attached to, the meninges on the brain surface. Rarely meningiomas may arise within the brain or the ventricles, presumably caused by the embryonic distribution of the stem cells. Most meningiomas can be cured with surgical excision alone, especially when the location permits complete excision of the tumor and its dural attachment. The incidence of recurrence after surgery is related to the extent of resection[2,8,47,53] (Fig. 13-5). Reoperation and radiation therapy are often necessary for the two subtypes of meningiomas that exhibit more invasive growth, angioblastic (hemangiopericytomas) and papillary meningiomas, because these tumors commonly recur after surgery, invade the brain and contiguous structures, and may metastasize outside the central nervous system.[8,53,63,64]

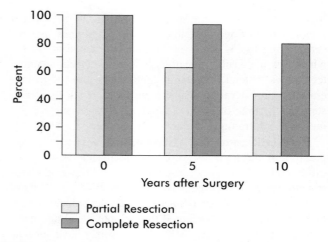

FIG. 13-5   The rate of recurrence of meningioma after surgery is related to the extent of resection. (*Modified from Chan RC, Thompson GB:* J Neurosurg *60:52-60, 1984, and Simpson D:* J Neurol Neurosurg Psychiatry *20:22-39, 1957.*)

Pituitary Adenomas

These benign tumors (Table 13-1), which arise within the sella turcica, present with endocrine disturbances caused by

TABLE 13-1
Pituitary Adenomas

	Normal Function				Pituitary Adenoma
	Pituitary		Endorgan		Adenoma
Hypothalamus	Pituitary Cell	Pituitary Hormone	Organ/Hormone	Primary Functions	Tumor/Clinical Syndrome
Releasing Factors					
Corticotropin releasing hormone (CRH)	Corticotroph	Adrenocorticotropin (corticotropin, ACTH)	Adrenals; cortisol	General metabolism; required for physiologic adaptation to stress	ACTH-secreting adenoma (corticotropinoma); Cushing's disease
	Thyrotroph	Thyroid-stimulating hormone (TSH)	Thyroid; thyroid hormones (T_3, T_4)	General metabolism; influences pace of metabolism	TSH-secreting adenoma (thyrotropinoma); hyperthyroidism
Gonadotropin releasing hormone (GnRH)	Gonadotroph	Follicle-stimulating hormone (FSH)	Ovaries; estradiol progesterone	Required for normal female sexual development and fertility	FSH-secreting adenoma; endocrine-inactive macroadenoma
		Luteinizing hormone (LH)	Testes; testosterone	Required for normal male sexual development and fertility	LH-secreting adenoma; endocrine-inactive macroadenoma
Growth hormone releasing hormone (GHRH)	Somatotroph	Growth hormone (somatotropin, GH)	Liver and other tissues; somatomedin (insulin-like growth factor-I) (IGF-I)	Growth, glucose regulation	GH-secreting adenoma (somatotropinoma); acromegaly (in children, gigantism)
Inhibiting Factors					
Dopamine (PIF)	Lactotroph	Prolactin (PRL)	Breast, gonads	Lactation	PRL-secreting adenoma (prolactinoma); amenorrhea-galactorrhea
Somatostatin	Somatotroph	Growth hormone (GH)	Liver and other tissues; somatomedin (insulin-like growth factor-I) (IGF-I)	Growth, glucose regulation	None

excess hormone secretion or by symptoms produced by local compression of adjacent structures, most commonly the optic chiasm, producing loss of visual acuity and visual field deficits, and the pituitary gland, causing hypopituitarism. Other adjacent structures, such as the cavernous venous sinuses, venous channels through which course several cranial nerves (the occulomotor, trochlear, and the abducens nerve, and the ophthalmic and maxillary divisions of the trigeminal nerve) as well as the carotid artery may be compressed or invaded by lateral extension of a pituitary tumor. Rarely large pituitary tumors (macroadenomas, tumors greater than 1 cm in diameter) extend so far superiorly that they occlude the foramen of Monro and cause obstructive hydrocephalus.

The amplification of the hormonal product of the target organs in response to the trophic pituitary hormones underlies the capacity of very small pituitary tumors (microadenomas, tumors less than 1 cm in diameter) to produce disfiguring and life-threatening endocrinopathies. Adrenocorticotropin (ACTH)-secreting tumors cause Cushing's disease, which is commonly associated with osteoporosis, proximal myopathy, hypertension, diabetes mellitus, and accelerated atherosclerosis. Growth hormone secreting tumors lead to acromegaly with macroglossia and obstructive sleep apnea, arthritis, diabetes mellitus, hypertension, and accelerated atherosclerosis. Prolactinomas secrete excess prolactin, which leads to amenorrhea, infertility, and galactorrhea in women and loss of libido in women and men. Hypopituitarism associated with larger tumors often includes hypothyroidism and hypocortisolism, which must be treated before surgery. Pituitary adenomas may occur as part of one of the multiple endocrine neoplasia (MEN) syndromes, familial syndromes in which pheochromocytoma, pancreatic islet cell tumors, parathyroid tumors, and thyroid carcinoma may also occur.

The initial therapy of pituitary tumors is contingent on the specific tumor type, its size, and the patient's symptoms. The treatment of choice for prolactinomas, the most common type of pituitary adenoma, is bromocriptine, a dopaminergic agonist that inhibits prolactin secretion and production. The latter effect is responsible for shrinkage of the tumor cells and a significant reduction of tumor size in most patients. Surgery for prolactinomas is reserved for patients whose tumors do not respond to bromocriptine or for those patients intolerant of the medication. The initial treatment of choice for the other types of pituitary tumors is transsphenoidal surgery, which cures most patients. The use of sellar irradiation therapy postoperatively depends on the extent of resection and the patient's age. Most patients with pituitary tumors are cured with surgery alone or surgery combined with irradiation therapy.

Metastatic Tumors

Metastatic tumors to the central nervous system (CNS) now affect at least one fourth of the 500,000 patients in the United States with cancer each year.[3,17,24,47] Although they

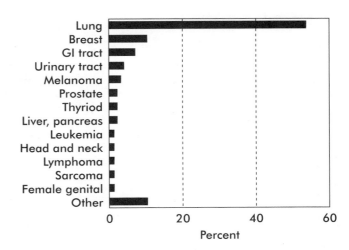

FIG. 13-6 Most metastatic tumors to the brain (approximately 70%) arise from the lung, breast, or gastrointestinal tract. *(Modified from Galicich JH, Arbit E: Metastatic brain tumors. In Youmans JR, editor:* Neurological surgery. A comprehensive reference guide to the diagnosis and management of neurosurgical problems, *ed 3, 1990, Philadelphia, WB Saunders.)*

are the most common type of supratentorial tumor, autopsy studies suggest that many patients with metastatic neoplasms in the CNS never receive treatment.[45] Fig. 13-6 summarizes the relative incidence of brain metastases from the tissues of origin in one large series. Over 70% of metastatic brain tumors arise from the lung, breast, or gastrointestinal tract.[17] The brain is a sanctuary from chemotherapy and other systemic therapies, including immunotherapy, for metastases. Patients whose systemic tumors respond to anticancer therapies often have isolated progression of CNS disease. Thus, as more successful palliative, but noncurative, therapy permits patients with systemic cancer to live longer, the incidence of patients with symptomatic metastatic tumors is expected to increase.[17,34]

The location and number of metastases, as well as the overall condition and prognosis of the patient, are important factors that must be considered before selecting appropriate treatment for these patients. Excision of a solitary brain metastasis in a surgically accessible area benefits patients whose systemic disease is being controlled.

Presentation of Patients with Supratentorial Masses

Neoplasms of the CNS may provoke generalized or focal neurologic symptoms. Patients with tumors producing increased ICP complain of headache, nausea and vomiting, ataxia, syncope, and changes in vision or cognition. Focal neurologic signs in a patient with intracerebral tumor are produced by effects of the tumor on adjacent functional areas. Fig. 13-7 illustrates the location of the motor and sensory functions of the cortical surface of the posterior frontal and anterior parietal lobes, respectively. Tumors affecting these areas or their axonal projections elicit weakness

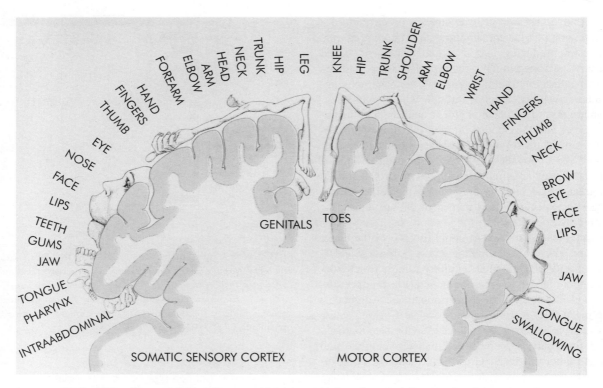

FIG. 13-7 Sensory *(left)* and motor *(right)* homunculus of cortical function for the precentral and postcentral gyri in the posterior aspect of the frontal and the anterior aspect of the parietal lobes, respectively. *(From Geschwind N:* Scientific American *241:182, 1979.)*

or sensory loss on the opposite side of the body. Visual field abnormalities occur in predictable patterns depending on the position of the mass in relation to the optic nerves, optic tracts, optic radiations, and cortical visual areas.[19]

Seizures result from alteration of the normal neuronal function produced, most likely by changes in the metabolic milieu surrounding neurons or by a permanent alteration in neuronal structure. An epileptic focus sporadically controls the electrical activity of other brain areas by synchronizing electrical activities and inhibiting the spontaneous function of other brain areas. Loss of spontaneous activity in regions of the brain produces a magnification of the epileptic activity, causing the clinical signs and symptoms of a seizure. The onset of seizures in an adult is often the initial indication of a supratentorial tumor. Patients with tumors that are associated with a high risk of seizures receive prophylactic anticonvulsant treatment, usually diphenylhydantoin (Dilantin), perioperatively.[47]

Perioperative Evaluation

The evaluation of patients having or suspected of having intracranial neoplasms begins with the clinical history and neurologic examination. A brief, directed history provides essential information for all medical personnel engaged in the treatment of the patient. Thyroid storm, bleeding disorders, adrenal insufficiency, hyperthermia, and hemodynamic instability from an unsuspected pheochromocytoma are among the many situations that are best discovered from the patient's history, rather than during surgery. The neurologic examination evaluates the functional status of the brain. Most information about the patient's progress before, during, and after treatment is derived from sequential examination of mental status, cranial nerve function, and motor and sensory function of the extremities.

Diagnostic Studies

Imaging studies of the brain are essential for preoperative diagnosis and localization and for postoperative assessment of patients with a supratentorial mass. The selection of the necessary investigations depends on the level of urgency, the availability of the imaging device, and the suspected pathology. More than one type of study may be required for optimal evaluation.

Computed axial tomography is based on computerized modification of the conventional radiograph. The x-ray emitter travels in a circular path with an x-ray collector 180 degrees in opposition. The collector receives the energy that has been emitted less that deflected or absorbed by the brain and skull. The transmission energy data is integrated and plotted in a two-dimensional format. The images produced by cranial CT are images of the radiographic density of the skull and its contents. CT scanning has several advantages over MR: It can be performed more rapidly and with convenient and immediate access to the patient, it demonstrates bony and tissue (tumor) calcification, and it has relatively few medical contraindications. CT is the study of choice for certain emergencies, such as head trauma, because it clearly and precisely demonstrates acute hemorrhage. Iodinated contrast agents are used to highlight lesions that alter the blood-brain barrier, as do most tumors, and to provide information critical for the differential diagnosis of intracranial masses.

Magnetic resonance imaging provides superior definition of soft tissue anatomy in any plane. The signal detected during MR is created by manipulating the magnetic axis of the protons of water in the brain. A background magnetic axis of fixed magnitude is produced by an electromagnet. A second magnetic field, the pulsed field, pulls the magnetic spin axis of the protons out of the alignment of the background magnetic field and toward the direction of the pulsed axis. The image is produced by the energy given off by the protons as each returns to its background axis. The image is created by an entirely different signal than is CT, which permits distinguishing certain tissue characteristics that cannot be detected using any other current technique. Both MR and CT are used in some patients.[49] Paramagnetic contrast agents, such as gadolinium-DTPA, which demonstrate areas of altered blood-brain barrier, are used to delineate tumors, abscesses, and areas of infarction.[6] Furthermore, MR angiography is now available for noninvasive demonstration of the relationship of mass lesions with intracerebral arteries and veins.

Cerebral arteriography is used for high-resolution delineation of the cerebral vessels and tumor vasculature. Arteriography is used to plan surgery on vascular tumors encasing or contiguous to major intracranial arteries, vascular malformations, and aneurysms. It is sometimes possible to anticipate surgical blood loss based on a tumor's arteriographic appearance. Embolization, selective intraarterial injection of particulate materials or polymerizing glues into vessels that supply highly vascular lesions to occlude the blood flow, is occasionally used during cerebral arteriography. Although embolization can be used alone to treat certain lesions, with tumors it is an adjunct to surgery.

Although analysis of CSF aids in the differential diagnosis of certain intracranial mass lesions, it rarely provides critical information and generally is contraindicated in patients with a supratentorial mass. Removing CSF relatively rapidly or removing more than a few milliliters of CSF from the lumbar sac in these patients may reduce the intraspinal CSF pressure, disrupt the pressure equilibrium between the infratentorial and supratentorial spaces, and lead to transtentorial or tonsillar herniation with rapid, potentially irreversible neurologic deterioration as the brain shifts downward.[42]

HEMATOMAS
Trauma

Operative trauma presents unique problems to the anesthesiologist and surgeon. Many physiologic systems may be simultaneously disturbed. Neurologic outcome with closed head injury is related to the presence and severity of other, non-CNS injuries, multiple brain injuries, size of the hematoma, and the amount of time that the brain is exposed to the pressure of a mass, as well as the presenting neurologic status of the patient. The Glasgow Coma Scale score is useful for predicting outcome and for sequentially evaluating the neurologic status of the patient.

The classification of trauma-induced hematomas is based on (1) the anatomic location of the hematoma in relation to the membranes covering the brain (epidural hematomas lie between the skull and the dura, subdural hematomas arise between the dura and the pia-arachnoid covering the brain, and intracerebral hematomas occur within the brain) and (2) the pace of development of symptoms (acute—within 24 hours after trauma, subacute—within 2 weeks of injury, and chronic—more than 2 weeks after injury).[42]

Epidural hematomas often are associated with a skull fracture and tearing of a meningeal artery. The most frequent location is the temporal area, associated with tearing of the middle meningeal artery. Immediate craniotomy or craniectomy is almost always required to evacuate the hematoma and to identify and coagulate the source of bleeding. The prognosis associated with an epidural hematoma is related to the neurologic status at treatment and varies greatly.

Subdural hematomas are produced either by tearing of "bridging" veins, which span the subdural space, or by injury to cortical vessels. The high incidence of an extremely poor outcome in young patients with acute subdural hematoma results from the associated and extensive direct brain injury produced by the severe impact, usually a motor vehicle accident. In the elderly, in whom brain atrophy associated with aging makes the bridging veins more susceptible to disruption by shearing forces during movement of the brain within the skull, acute subdural hematomas may occur after only minor trauma. Treatment of an acute subdural hematoma is usually by immediate craniotomy and evacuation of the hematoma. Uncontrollable cerebral swelling accompanied by increased ICP that is refractory to treatment, commonly causes death in patients with acute subdural hematomas. On the other hand, chronic subdural hematomas, which are generally not associated with direct, impact-related brain injury, can usually be evacuated via burr-hole drainage if the blood has accumulated slowly, permitting the intracranial contents to accommodate the mass with sufficient time for conversion of the blood to a proteinaceous fluid. Although surgical drainage is indicated in most symptomatic patients, those with minimal neurologic disturbance occasionally can be safely and effectively managed with careful monitoring and glucocorticoid therapy while the hematoma is being resorbed.

Traumatic acute and subacute hematomas require surgery if they cause progressive neurologic deterioration or if they produce a life-threatening mass effect. Many of these hematomas do not require surgery. The outcome is usually established by the extent of associated direct brain injury and extracranial injuries.

BOX 13-2
MAJOR CAUSES OF INTRACRANIAL HEMORRHAGE

Trauma
Hypertension
Tumor
Sacular aneurysm
Cerebral infarction
Arteriovenous malformation
Coagulopathy
Cerebral angiopathy

Spontaneous Hematomas

The spontaneous (nontraumatic) occurrence of an intracerebral hemorrhage should raise suspicion of the presence of underlying abnormalities of blood vessel integrity or coagulopathy. Box 13-2 lists the important causes of spontaneous intracerebral hemorrhage in the adult. In addition to patient management for the effects of the acute hemorrhage, identification and correction of the underlying cause of a spontaneous intracranial hemorrhage is required. When the hematoma has been caused by an abnormality of vessel anatomy that is likely to bleed again, such as an intracerebral arteriovenous malformation or an aneurysm, surgery is performed to eliminate further hemorrhage. Surgery solely to evacuate a spontaneous intracerebral hematoma is usually reserved for those hematomas that cause progressive, or life-threatening, neurologic deficits by mass effect.

SURGICAL APPROACHES

Several general principles of management must be integrated to decide whether to operate and, if surgery is indicated, to develop a surgical plan. In patients with tumors, the concepts of curable vs incurable and operable vs inoperable are separate issues. To classify a tumor as operable and as appropriate for surgery, the surgeon must decide that the likely benefits of surgery outweigh the risks. Surgical removal of the tumor accomplishes maximum reduction of tumor mass, provides adequate tissue sampling for diagnosis, relieves elevated ICP, and permits time for the effects of further therapy, such as irradiation and chemotherapy, to occur. With malignant tumors, among the factors to be considered in reaching a decision to operate are the specific neurologic deficits, their severity, and the likelihood of useful recovery. Many patients with an incurable tumor receive surgery to increase survival time and/or to increase their quality of life. Consideration of these issues is also critical during surgery. If cure is not possible, aggressive attempts at complete tumor removal are inappropriate if they are likely to cause or increase neurologic impairment. However, a nondisabling neurologic deficit after surgery may be acceptable in certain tumors, such as an ependy-

moma or a meningioma, if a curative resection is contingent on it. In contrast, a similar deficit might be unacceptable if it occurred during an overly aggressive attempt to remove completely the visible component of a malignant tumor that cannot be cured by surgery, particularly if the additional increment of tumor removal would only marginally influence survival, if at all.[47]

The development of the surgical plan requires consideration of the patient's overall condition. Certain genetic diseases, such as Von Hippel–Lindau syndrome, tuberous sclerosis, and neurofibromatosis type 1, are associated with development of multiple intracerebral tumors. These patients may require surgery for the same type of tumor on multiple occasions. The decision to recommend surgical treatment of the patient with a metastatic brain tumor requires a contemporary assessment of the extent of extracranial disease. The presence of an overall treatment plan and philosophy is clearly important when addressing these types of patients, as is the development and coordination of a team experienced in the management of all aspects of the disease. The members of the team must consider the patient in terms of the entire syndrome, as well as the existing, immediate problems and the specific interests of each specialist.

Preoperative treatment, in addition to the common administration of steroids and anticonvulsants, is now commonplace in the surgical plan for treatment of certain tumors. Embolization of vascular tumors, such as highly vascular meningiomas of the skull base that are supplied by branches of the external carotid artery, often makes subsequent surgical excision safer and technically easier. Staged resections are sometimes incorporated into the surgical plan to permit separate operative approaches to different portions of a tumor that cannot be adequately exposed and excised using either approach alone, to allow for redistribution of the blood supply to the brain, or to avoid excess fatigue of the surgeon in procedures that may require long, tedious dissections of over 14 to 18 hours.

Optimal positioning of the patient for surgery requires integration of the objectives and concerns of the neurosurgeon and the neuroanesthesiologist. Positioning of the head to avoid jugular venous compression (by avoiding extreme rotation or flexion of the neck), which can exacerbate elevated ICP, and slight elevation of the head in reference to the heart, which facilitates venous drainage, are achieved before surgical draping. Because modern neurosurgery is often performed through narrow, long, confined channels, nuances of patient positioning often dictate the ease or difficulty and the success or failure of the operation. The groin, breasts, axillary regions, and pressure points are checked by the surgeon and the anesthesiologist before draping, and, if necessary, by the anesthesiologist periodically during surgery. Headrests and skull fixation devices are checked for stability. For certain operations, such as transsphenoidal surgery and operations of the anterior skull base, responsibility for the position and function of the endotracheal tube is shared by the surgeon and anesthesiologist. Generally, one person is designated to protect the endotracheal tube during removal of the drapes. Many new types of drapes incorporate adhesives that may stick to the endotracheal tube, mandating extra caution so as to avoid accidental extubation while removing the drapes. Application of the head dressing flexes and extends the neck, which may induce coughing and inadvertent dislodgment of an endotracheal tube that is positioned high in the larynx.

The final patient position depends on the location of the tumor, the operative route to the supratentorial mass, the size and location of the required operative field, and the preferences of the surgeon and anesthesiologist. Other features that are specific for the operation, such as the use of the operating microscope, the laser, or intraoperative ultrasound, fluoroscopy, or arteriography need to be taken into account. Knowledge of these positions facilitates the place-

ment of venous and arterial lines so as to permit optimal access to them during surgery. The design of the operating room, patient positioning, and the use of other equipment, such as C-arm fluoroscopy or intraoperative arteriography, dictate the location of personnel and equipment in relation to the patient. Figs. 13-8 to 13-12 show the typical distribution of the personnel and equipment during some of the most common neurosurgical approaches to supratentorial masses.

The surgical approach to a lesion is based on the location and extent of the lesion and on the goals of the surgery. For all intracranial surgery, but particularly for lesions that arise within the brain, such as gliomas, the surgeon integrates the results of the preoperative radiographic imaging studies to create a three-dimensional mental image of the lesion in relation to the brain and the skull topography. The scalp incision for a craniotomy is shaped to ex-

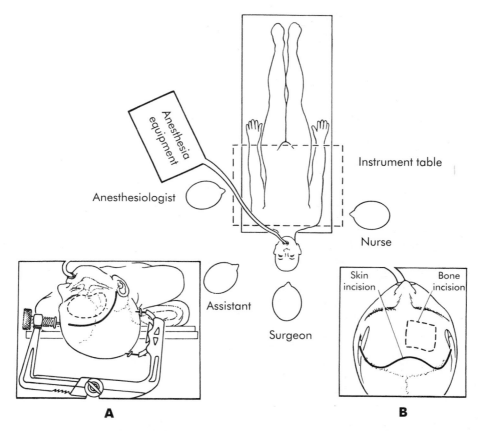

FIG. 13-8 Commonly used surgical approaches for removal of mass lesions in the anterior and temporal cranial fossae, including lesions of the frontal lobe, anterior aspect of the temporal lobe, along the sphenoid wing, or at the base of the anterior cranial fossa. The patient is supine with the head straight up (for frontal lesions) or turned to one side (for the pterional approach). For lesions in the tip of the temporal lobe and along the sphenoid wing and for transcranial exposure of the region of the sella and parasellar area, a pterional approach (**A**) is used, whereas, for lesions in the frontal lobes and at the base of the anterior fossa, a frontal craniotomy (**B**) is performed. For all procedures, the personnel and equipment are distributed so that the surgeon has optimal exposure; the anesthesiologist has access to the patient, the airway, and the arterial and venous lines; and the nurse can hand instruments to the surgeon unimpeded by the operating microscope or the assistant surgeon.

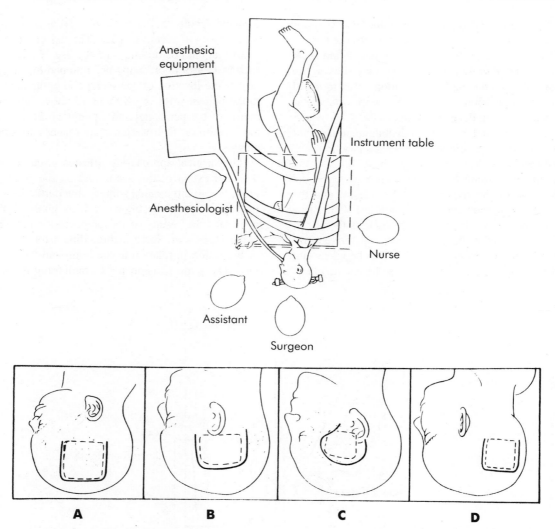

FIG. 13-9 Surgical approaches to lesions of the cerebral convexity. For lesions of the calvarium and intracerebral masses of the posterior portion of the frontal lobes and the parietal and occipital lobes, a free bone flap, centered over the route used to reach the lesion, is removed from the cerebral convexity. A lateral decubitus patient position is used, with the sagittal plane of the patient's head parallel to the floor. **A,** With lesions high in the cerebral hemispheres, the vertex of the head is elevated. **B,** To approach lesions in the posterior two thirds of the temporal lobe, the craniotomy is centered above the ear. **C,** For large lesions in the anterior aspect of the temporal lobe or for temporal lobe seizure surgery, the craniotomy is extended to include the temporal bone superior to the zygoma and anterior to the external auditory meatus. **D,** For posterior parietal and occipital lesions, more rotation of the head, with the nose down about 15 to 30 degrees, is required so that the point of entry is the uppermost point of the skull.

pose the area of the bone flap, preserve the vascular supply to the scalp, and retain the innervation of the muscles that move the face. The line of the incision is marked on the scalp before draping the patient, while superficial landmarks are visible. The operative personnel are positioned so that (1) the surgeon and the assistant surgeon have optimal and comfortable access for the approach to the lesion, (2) the anesthesiologist can provide optimal patient monitoring and has access to the airway and intravenous and intraarterial lines, and (3) the scrub nurse can hand instruments directly to the surgeon without crossing the assistant, the operative field, or the field of the operating microscope.

During surgery for mass lesions, optimal results require the space provided by a relaxed brain. To this end, hyperventilation (to $Paco_2$ of 25 to 30 mm Hg) is used and 20% mannitol (0.25 to .50 mg/kg body weight, administered as an IV bolus) and furosemide (0.7 mg/kg IV), which provide maximum reduction in ICP 60 to 90 min after administration, are administered about 60 min before the dural opening is expected.

Craniotomy

Most craniotomies for surgery anterior to the coronal suture are performed with the patient supine with the head

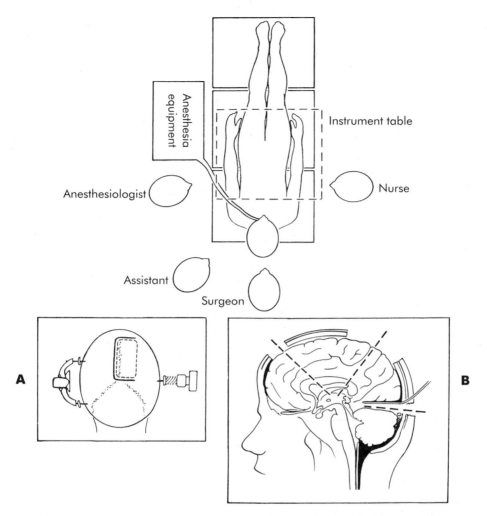

FIG. 13-10 A parasagittal route is used to reach lesions of the falx or the corpus callosum and to enter the ventricular system, particularly the third ventricle. The skull is fixed with a three-point skeletal fixation device and a craniotomy is performed that extends across the midline by 1.5 to 2.0 cm **(A).** The medial portion of the cerebral hemisphere is gently retracted from the midline. To avoid injury to the cerebral veins, surgical entry is always via the anterior or posterior one third of the distance from the nasion to the external occipital protuberance **(B).** The middle third of this midsagittal line is avoided because of the number and importance of the cerebral veins in that segment. The cerebral veins must be left intact to avoid cerebral venous infarction and serious neurologic impairment. For anterior lesions the neck is neutral, but, for the posterior parasagittal approaches, the neck is gently flexed or the patient is placed in a semisitting position.

slightly elevated. The pterional, frontal, and parasagittal approaches are the most common. The pterional craniotomy (Fig. 13-8, *A*) is probably the most common approach for supratentorial surgery. It provides access along the sphenoid wing and sylvian fissure to the anterior and medial portions of the temporal lobe, the parasellar and suprasellar space, and the upper portion of the clivus. Thus it is commonly used for clipping aneurysms of the anterior circulation, for excision of tumors in the anterior aspect of the temporal lobe, for transcranial removal of pituitary tumors and craniopharyngiomas, and for basal tumors in the parasellar area and along the sphenoid wing.

A curvilinear incision is made posteriorly and laterally from the frontal area just behind the hairline to end 1 cm anterior to the tragus of the ear at the level of the zygomatic arch (Fig. 13-8, *A*).

The frontal craniotomy provides access to the frontal lobes and to the anterior horn of the lateral ventricle and the foramen of Monro (Fig. 13-8, *B*). The scalp is incised just behind the hairline parallel to the coronal suture bilaterally. For a unilateral approach, a bone flap is removed just above the superior orbital rim to the midline near the nasion. A bifrontal bone flap is used for bilateral lesions, such as large bifrontal meningiomas.

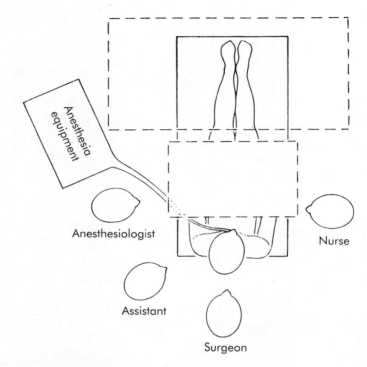

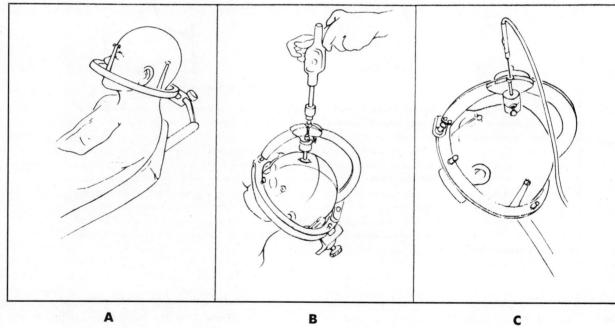

A   **B**   **C**

FIG. 13-11   **A,** Coordinates of the target for CT- and MR-guided stereotactic surgery are obtained by using a head frame fixed to the patient's skull by a base ring. The CT or MR is performed with a localizing frame (not shown) in place on the base ring. **B,** For surgery, the localizing frame is replaced with a surgical frame. For stereotactic biopsy, a small opening is drilled in the skull **(B),** and a biopsy needle is guided to the target **(C).**

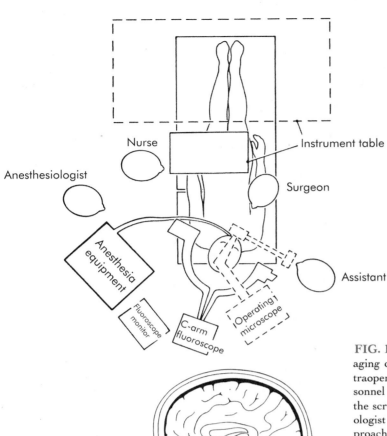

FIG. 13-12   Transsphenoidal pituitary surgery uses lateral imaging of the skull with the **C**-arm fluoroscope to guide the intraoperative route to the sella turcica. The positioning of the personnel shown here provides optimal ease of interaction between the scrub nurse and the surgeon and still permits the anesthesiologist access to the patient. The midsagittal route of the approach is shown in the lower portion of the figure.

For access to lesions beneath the cranial convexity in the parietal lobe, occipital lobe, the posterior aspect of the temporal lobe, or high within the cranial vault, a free rectangular-shaped bone flap centered over the intracranial entry point (Fig. 13-9) is removed to provide the most direct path to the lesion in convexity craniotomy. For intracerebral masses, the route to the lesion through a region of the brain that is least likely to produce a functionally significant neurologic deficit is selected. The craniotomy is performed after incising the scalp in an inverted U-shape centered over the route to the lesion. For lateral masses the patient is either (1) supine with the torso rotated 20 to 30 degrees by elevating the shoulder and pelvis on the side of the lesion with rolls or folded sheets or (2) in the lateral decubitus position with the head rotated away from the side of the mass so that the craniotomy site is the most superior portion of the skull and is parallel to the floor. Lesions in the posterior temporal lobe can be resected by using a bone flap, as outlined in Fig. 13-9, *B*, but temporal lobectomy, which requires exposure from the anterior to the posterior portions of the temporal lobe and visualization of the anterior surface of the middle fossa along the sphenoid wing,

is performed via a larger flap. For paramedian lesions behind the coronal suture, the patient is placed in a semisitting position or a lateral decubitus position with the vertex elevated. Parietal lesions require the patient to be in the lateral decubitus position with the face rotated below the horizontal plane of the operating table or in a semisitting position.

For the parasagittal approach to lesions in the falx, the third ventricle, or the corpus callosum, a horseshoe-shaped incision, based laterally, is extended 2 cm over the midline to expose the sagittal sinus and to provide a line of surgery parallel to the falx (Fig. 13-10). Because of the presence of cerebral veins passing from the cortical surface to the sagittal sinus in the middle one third of the sinus and the importance of preserving them, the route is usually via the anterior or the posterior one third of the length of a line extending from the nasion to the inion.

Image-Guided Stereotactic Surgery

With the refinement of computer-based imaging and the development of stereotactic systems that provide integration of the three-dimensional information from CT or MR with the coordinates of stereotactic frames, stereotactically guided surgery has become convenient and is now being used to precisely guide the surgeon to deep lesions in the brain for resection as well as, by needle biopsy, to provide small amounts of tissue for establishing the pathologic diagnosis (Fig. 13-11). Depending on the procedure to be performed and the preferences of the surgeon and patient, stereotactic surgery can be performed under local or general anesthesia. When general anesthesia is used, the localizing frame is placed on the patient after induction of anesthesia and tracheal intubation. The patient receives a CT or MR scan with the localizing frame in place, and the patient is transported to the operating room, where the surgical procedure is performed.[31] The systems that are now in use provide reliable surgical localization, with a resolution of a millimeter or so, of a lesion defined by CT or MR. Biopsies are obtained through a small circular opening, either a twist-drill hole or a burr hole, by passing a special biopsy needle to the precise site of the target and obtaining small cores of tissue. Stereotactic localization and guidance is now also commonly performed during open surgery via a craniotomy. For this, a catheter may initially be placed to the target to provide the surgeon a path to the lesion, or a low-energy laser beam (the source is attached to a stereotactic arc on the head ring) may be positioned and followed to the target. The capability for accurate registration of the three-dimensional information from CT and MR scans with the images from arteriography and PET and the ability to convey the geometric aspects of the information with precision to the intracranial space during surgery underlie the significant advances in accuracy and safety with which surgery now can be performed deep within the brain.

Transphenoidal Approach

The transphenoidal approach is used for surgery of the pituitary gland and for other types of sellar and suprasellar tumors (Fig. 13-12). The endotracheal tube is placed at the angle of the mouth away from the surgeon, and the oropharynx is packed with gauze to prevent pooling of blood there. The patient is placed in a supine, semisitting position with the head in gentle flexion, tilted toward the left shoulder (right-handed surgeon), and fixed with a three-point skull fixation device. To facilitate intraoperative orientation in the sagittal plane, the C-arm fluoroscope is used for lateral imaging of the sella. After entering the nasal cavity via a sublabial or a transnasal path, one continues dissection submucosally to the posterior aspect of the nasal cavity so as to expose the anterior surface of the sphenoid sinus. Creation of a 1.5 to 2.0 cm opening in the anterior wall of the sphenoid sinus exposes the anterior and inferior surface of the sella turcica, the pituitary fossa, and, after the dura is opened, the pituitary gland.

Intracranial Imaging

Intraoperative imaging is used much more commonly than previously. Intraoperative transcranial Doppler examination

of the basal vessels permits real-time estimates of blood flow, and intraoperative ultrasound can be integrated with Doppler imaging to yield a two-dimensional anatomic image in association with flow imaging. Intraoperative anatomic ultrasound imaging localizes and defines the limits of intracerebral mass lesions that are deep to the brain surface and not obvious from inspection of the cortical surface.[26] X-ray fluoroscopy also is used routinely in certain procedures, such as transsphenoidal pituitary surgery and percutaneous stimulation and lesioning of the trigeminal nerve for trigeminal neuralgia.

New Frontiers
Brain Imaging

The advances in imaging of the past decade underlie a revolution that has occurred and is occurring in neurosurgery with the evolution of precise three-dimensional imaging modalities. The rapidly advancing technology of MR has produced a new standard for image resolution. This same technology is now used to provide much more information than is available using the standard imaging techniques. Surgery for a cerebral aneurysm, vascular malformation, or vascular tumor requires an imaging study of the vasculature, currently a cerebral arteriogram. However, risks of stroke attend cerebral angiography; there are also problems with allergic reactions to the iodinated contrast agents that are used. Magnetic resonance angiography is noninvasive, safe, and much less uncomfortable. Although the fine detail of MR angiography is not yet equal to that of an angiogram and the position of small vessels that are critical to successful surgery are not imaged with current techniques of MR angiography, the carotid bifurcation can be imaged and the presence of occlusive disease and the degree of carotid stenosis can be estimated. The resolution of this imaging modality is rapidly improving, and the technique is expected to have increased clinical application, particularly for such functions as noninvasive evaluation of the carotid bifurcation for screening patients with occlusive cerebrovascular disease.

Magnetic resonance spectroscopy, another imaging study based on magnetic resonance, is used to quantify the concentration of certain chemicals, such as the phosphorylated metabolic products of glucose metabolism, at targeted sites in the brain. If the various types of mass lesions have unique, identifying chemical constituents, magnetic resonance spectroscopy may become an important diagnostic technique, but it remains in an early phase of development.

Positron emission tomography (PET) permits in vivo assessment of brain physiology and biochemistry. PET scanning makes use of the physical principle that positrons emitted from decaying isotopes undergo an annihilation reaction when they collide with electrons in nearby tissues. The two photons generated by this reaction travel from the site of reaction in opposite directions. Sensors in the PET scanner detect the photons, permitting construction of a computerized image of brain metabolism and physiology, depending on the positron-emitting isotope selected. Attaching an isotope to a glucose or oxygen molecule allows imaging of the distribution and utilization of these compounds, thus yielding quantitative spatial and temporal measurements of regional glucose or oxygen use. The spatial resolution of PET currently is inferior to that of CT and MR. However, PET distinguishes recurrent tumor from radiation-induced necrosis, which often appear similar on MR and CT scans. Further, the rate of glucose consumption by tumor correlates with the histologic grading of the tumor, a relationship that can be used to predict the biologic aggressiveness of tumors based on flouro-deoxyglucose PET imaging.

Regional Treatment of Malignant Tumors

Antineoplastic treatments can be characterized in terms of their differential effects on neoplastic and nonneoplastic cells and in their ability to reach the tumor cells. Treatments fail when they are either not potent enough (i.e., tumor cells survive) or when the therapy is not specific, (i.e., when toxicity to normal tissues arises before all tumor cells are destroyed). For brain tumors, efficacy also may be restricted by inadequate exposure of the tumor to the agent because of limited delivery of the drug imposed by the blood-brain barrier. One strategy to overcome the latter problem is regional delivery. Because brain tumors cause disability and death by local and regional growth and rarely metastasize, several forms of regional treatment have been developed to treat them.

Because brain tumors have a steep radiation dose–tumor response relationship and because the adult brain is relatively resistant to irradiation-induced injury,[52] one approach for enhancing tumor control is by regional delivery of a high dose of irradiation. This can be achieved with external or internal sources of radiation. For solid tumors, internal delivery requires stereotactic intratumoral placement of radioactive seeds.[9,12,21,37] For cystic tumors, such as some craniopharyngiomas, ^{32}P is placed into the cyst, or for other types of tumors, into the cavity after tumor resection. The mechanism of action of these two approaches is similar; greater exposure to the irradiation occurs in those tissues close to the radioactive material, and more distant areas receive a lower dose. Special techniques required for safely handling radioactive compounds in the operating room must be used during these procedures. With certain tumors and with appropriate patient selection, internal irradiation enhances tumor control and prolongs survival, but it is not curative. In patients with solid tumors treated with implanted radioactive seeds, repeated craniotomies for excision of necrotic tissue often are required. Whether this can be justified with a palliative treatment remains controversial.

External delivery of stereotactically focused radiotherapy, either from multiple sources of radioactivity (the "gamma knife") or from a single, rotating source of high-energy radiation (a specially adapted linear accelerator), precisely focuses the ionizing radiation on the target.[10,29] The advantage of this approach compared with standard de-

livery techniques is that the irradiation reaches the target by passing through a much larger area of normal tissue, reducing the risk of injury to normal brain by distributing the total dose over many separate paths on its way to the target and permitting very high doses to be delivered to the target site. The individual beams of energy coalesce at the target, where the cumulative energy is of sufficient magnitude to be destructive. This type of treatment is effective for small vascular malformations (less than 2 cm maximum diameter) and certain types of small, benign tumors (pituitary tumors, vestibular schwannomas). Other devices now are becoming available that use different energy sources, such as neutrons, but that are focused in much the same manner. The principal limitation of this therapy is its relatively low specificity for tumor.

Regional intratumoral chemotherapy with chemotherapeutic agents imbedded in polymers (to control the rate of drug release) that are placed into the tumor stereotactically or into the tumor bed after excision of the tumor by craniotomy is a new approach that may prove efficacious for the delivery of a range of chemotherapeutic agents. Placing the drug into the tumor greatly increases the exposure of the tumor to the drug, circumvents the blood-brain barrier, and avoids systemic toxicity. However, this delivery technique depends on diffusion to carry the drug into the tumor and into the brain that has been infiltrated by tumor. Whether the diffusion distances will permit active drug to reach all tumor sites before the drug is metabolized, inactivated by nonspecific or specific binding in the tissue, or cleared by the blood flow in the tumor and brain, will depend on the drug used and has not yet been thoroughly studied.

Hyperthermia selectively kills tumor cells and may also make them more susceptible to other types of treatment, such as ionizing radiation. Various procedures have been developed to heat tumor selectively. Most require stereotatic placement of the thermal source and other specialized equipment.

The extremely high potency and specificity of immunotoxins—conjugates of peptide toxins with monoclonal antibodies or other ligands that bind specifically to tumor-associated cell surface antigens—have made them attractive for refinement and antitumor treatment.[32,38] The immunoglobulin directs its attached antitumor agent to antigen targets expressed only on, or to a greater extent on, neoplastic cells. The immunoglobulins are conjugated to a substance that is toxic to the cell or a compound that makes the cell susceptible to adjuvant therapy. Despite early optimism, it has not been possible to identify purely tumor-specific antigens. In addition, because tumor-specific antigens may be unique for each tumor, and because tumors are quite heterogeneous, the approach would demand that each neoplasm be addressed individually, making progress slow, expensive, and perhaps futile. An alternative approach is one that targets more universally expressed cell surface antigens that are more prevalent in tumors, such as the transferrin receptor or receptors for tumor-associated growth factors. The brain is an ideal organ for these agents, because it is essentially a nondividing tissue and does not express many of these antigens. Treatments using this latter approach are now underway in the clinic for solid brain tumors and for leptomeningeal carcinomatosis.

Differentiating agents induce maturation (differentiation) of cells. Highly differentiated cells in the brain lose their ability to replicate and therefore lose their neoplastic features. The differentiating agent can be administered directly or can be a drug that stimulates the tumor cells to produce excess endogenous differentiating compounds. Theoretically, these agents are less apt to produce toxicity to the nonneoplastic tissues, which are already maximally differentiated. Several of these compounds have been investigated and are now in preclinical and clinical trials.

Genetic therapy is one of the most recent advances in medicine. Genetic antitumor therapy is designed to alter the genome or the genetic transcription or translation in the replicating, but not the nonreplicating, cells. Current directions include in vivo transduction (genetic alteration by a noninfectious genetic vector) of the tumor cells with viral vectors or with infection with replication-competent, attenuated, tissue-specific viruses to induce production of antisense oligonucleotides to bind the mRNA of essential growth factors and the use of replication-incompetent vectors to transduce tumor cells. The latter approach, using genetic transduction of tumors with the thymidine kinase gene of the herpes simplex virus, is currently being investigated in humans. The basis of this approach is that the retroviral vector carrying the thymidine kinase gene will be integrated into only the genome of replicating cells and the gene will

be expressed only if it is integrated. The herpes simplex type of thymidine kinase, but not mammalian-type thymidine kinase, converts a nontoxic drug, ganciclovir, into a toxic product that destroys the cell. Furthermore, nearby tumor cells are also killed by a mechanism that is still poorly understood. Thus it is hoped that the advancements in molecular biology and the recently acquired capacity to easily and efficiently alter or synthesize genetic material will provide a route to control tumor growth or to selectively destroy tumors with minimal, if any, effects on the normal tissues.

SUMMARY

Masses in the supratentorial space are common and comprise a great variety of different types of malignant and benign lesions. Basic understanding of the pathophysiology produced by these processes is necessary to deliver appropriate and optimal care. In the past few years great strides have been made in the development of techniques to establish the diagnosis, noninvasively or with minimal invasion, and to treat these entities, and many of them are commonly cured by surgery. Many types of supratentorial tumors still challenge the team caring for those afflicted. The clinical application of advances in neuroscience and tumor biology offers the possibility of exciting new solutions.

References

1. Avezaat JH, Van Eijndhoven JH, Wyper DJ: Cerebrospinal fluid pulse pressure and intracranial volume-pressure relationships, *J Neurol Neurosurg Psychiatry* 42:687-700, 1979.
2. Beks JW, de Windt HL: The recurrence of supratentorial meningiomas after surgery, *Acta Neurochir* 95:3-5, 1988.
3. Black PMcL: Brain tumors, *N Engl J Med* 324:1471-1476, 1555-1564, 1991.
4. Bobo H, Kapp JP, Vance R: Effect of intra-arterial cisplatin and 1,3-bis (2chloroethyl)-1-nitrosourea (BCNU) dosage on radiographic response and regional toxicity in malignant glioma patients: proposal of a new method of intra-arterial dosage calculation, *J Neurooncol* 13:291-299, 1992.
5. Bouma GJ, Muizelaar JP, Bandoh K et al: Blood pressure and intracranial pressure-volume dynamics in severe head injury: relationship with cerebral blood flow, *J Neurosurg* 77:15-19, 1992.
6. Brant-Zawadzki M, Berry I, Osaki L et al: Gd-DTPA in clinical MR of the brain: 1. Intraaxial lesions, *Am J of Roentgenol* 147:1223-1230, 1986.
7. Buetow PC, Smirniotopoulos JG, Done S: Congenital brain tumors: a review of 45 cases, *Am J Roentgenol* 155:587-593, 1990.
8. Chan RC, Thompson GB: Morbidity, mortality, and quality of life following surgery for intracranial meningiomas: a retrospective study in 257 cases, *J Neurosurg* 60:52-60, 1984.
9. Chun M, McKeough P, Wu A et al: Interstitial iridium-192 implantation for malignant brain tumours. Part II: clinical experience, *Br J Radiol* 62:158-162, 1989.
10. Coffey RJ, Lunsford LD, Flickinger JC: The role of radiosurgery in the treatment of malignant brain tumors, *Neurosurg Clin North Am* 3:231-244, 1992.
11. Deutsch M, Green SB, Strike TA et al: Results of a randomized trial comparing BCNU plus radiotherapy, streptozotocin plus radiotherapy, BCNU plus hyperfractionated radiotherapy, and BCNU following misonidazole plus radiotherapy in the postoperative treatment of malignant glioma, *Int J Radiat Oncol Biol Phys* 16:1389-1396, 1989.
12. Duncan GG, Goodman GB, Ludgate CM et al: The treatment of adult supratentorial high grade astrocytomas, *J Neurooncol* 13:63-72, 1992.
13. Eagan RT, Dinapoli RP, Hermann RC Jr et al: Carmustine and Baker's antifol combination chemotherapy for primary brain tumors progressive after irradiation and chemotherapy, *Cancer Treat Reports* 68:431-433, 1984.
14. Evans RG, Kimler BF, Morantz RA et al: A phase I/II study of the use of Fluosol as an adjuvant to radiation therapy in the treatment of primary high-grade brain tumors, *Int J Radiat Oncol Biol Phys* 19:415-420, 1990.

15. Feun LG, Yung WK, Leavens ME et al: A phase II trial of 2,5,-diaziridinyl 3,6-bis (carboethoxy amino) 1,4-benzoquinone (AZQ, NSC 182986) in recurrent primary brain tumors, *J Neurooncol* 2:13-17, 1984.

16. Fried H, Feyer P: Combined treatment with neurosurgery-radiotherapy of malignant brain tumors, *Zentralblatt Fur Neurochirurgie* 51:208-211, 1990.

17. Galicich JH, Arbit E: Metastatic brain tumors. In Youmans JR, editor: *Neurological surgery. A comprehensive reference guide to the diagnosis and management of neurosurgical problems,* ed 3, Philadelphia, 1990, WB Saunders.

18. Garfield J: Present status and future role of surgery for malignant supratentorial gliomas, *Neurosurg Rev* 9:23-25, 1986.

19. Geschwind: Specializations of the human brain, *Scientific American* 241:182, 1979.

20. Greenberg HS, Ensminger WD, Layton PB et al: Phase I-II evaluation of intra-arterial diaziquone for recurrent malignant astrocytomas, *Cancer Treat Reports* 70:353-357, 1986.

21. Gutin PH, Leibel SA: Stereotaxic interstitial irradiation of malignant brain tumors, *Neurol Clin* 3:883-893, 1985.

22. Hollerhage HG, Zumkeller M, Becker M et al: Influence of type and extent of surgery on early results and survival time in glioblastoma multiforme, *Acta Neurochir* 113:31-37, 1991.

23. Jackson D, Kinsella T, Rowland J et al: Halogenated pyrimidines as radiosensitizers in the treatment of glioblastoma multiforme, *Am J Clin Oncol* 10:437-443, 1987.

24. Kryk H, Blenkhorn F, Carney A et al: Grand rounds on brain tumors, *Can Nurse* 71:42-46, 1975.

25. Laramore GE, Martz KL, Nelson JS et al: Radiation Therapy Oncology Group (RTOG) survival data on anaplastic astrocytomas of the brain: does a more aggressive form of treatment adversely impact survival? [see comments], *Int J Radiat Oncol Biol Phys* 17:1351-1356, 1989.

26. Le Roux PD, Berger MS, Wang K et al: Low grade gliomas: comparison of intraoperative ultrasound characteristics with preoperative imaging studies, *J Neurooncol* 13:189-198, 1992.

27. Levin VA, Crafts DC, Wilson CB et al: BCNU (NSC-409962) and procarbazine (NSC-77213) treatment for ma-

lignant brain tumors, *Cancer Treat Reports* 60:243-249, 1976.

28. Levin VA: Chemoradiation in brain tumors: assets vs. adverse effects [editorial; comment], *Int J Radiat Oncol Biol Phys* 17:1357-1358, 1989.

29. Loeffler JS, Alexander E III, Shea WM et al: Radiosurgery as part of the initial management of patients with malignant gliomas [see comments], *J Clin Oncol* 10:1379-1385, 1992.

30. Lohle PN, Verhagen IT, Teelken AW et al: The pathogenesis of cerebral gliomatous cysts, *Neurosurgery* 30:180-185, 1992.

31. Lunsford LD, Parrish R, Albright L: Intraoperative imaging with a therapeutic computed tomographic scanner, *Neurosurgery* 15:559-561, 1984.

32. Mahaley MS Jr., Urso MB, Whaley RA et al: Immunobiology of primary intracranial tumors: IX. Phase I study of human lymphoblastoid interferon, *J Biol Response Modifiers* 3:19-25, 1984.

33. Malkin MG, Shapiro WR: Brain tumors, *Cancer chemother & biol response modifiers,* 9:377-389, 1987.

34. Mao Y, Desmeules M, Semenciw RM et al: Increasing brain cancer rates in Canada, *Can Med Assoc J* 145:1583-1591, 1991.

35. Muizelaar JP, Marmarou A, DeSalles AA et al: Cerebral blood flow and metabolism in severely head-injured children. Part 1: relationship with GCS score, outcome, ICP, and PVI, *J Neurosurg* 71:63-71, 1989.

36. Muizelaar JP, Ward JD, Marmarou A et al: Cerebral blood flow and metabolism in severely head-injured children. Part 2: autoregulation, *J Neurosurg* 71:72-76, 1989.

37. Mundinger F, Braus DF, Krauss JK et al: Long-term outcome of 89 low-grade brainstem gliomas after interstitial radiation therapy, *J Neurosurg* 75:740-746, 1991.

38. Obbens EA, Feun LG, Leavens ME et al: Phase I clinical trial of intralesional or intraventricular leukocyte interferon for intracranial malignancies, *J Neurooncology* 3:61-67, 1985.

39. Paulson OB, Strandgaard S, Edvinsson L: Cerebral autoregulation, *Cerebrovasc Brain Metab Rev* 2:161-192, 1990.

40. Philipov P, Tzatchev K: Selenium in the treatment of patients with brain gliomas. A pilot study, *Zentralblatt Fur Neurochirurgie* 51:145-146, 1990.

41. Pigott TJ, Lowe JS, Palmer J: Statis-

tical modelling in analysis of prognosis in glioblastoma multiforme: a study of clinical variables and Ki-67 index [see comments], *Br J Neurosurg* 5:61-66, 1991.

42. Plum F, Posner JB: *Diagnosis of stupor and coma,* ed 3, Philadelphia, 1980, FA Davis.

43. Recht L, Fram RJ, Strauss G et al: Preirradiation chemotherapy of supratentorial malignant primary brain tumors with intracarotid cis-platinum (CDDP) and IV BCNU. A phase II trial, *Am J Clin Oncol* 13:125-131, 1990.

44. Roberts JT, Bleehen NM, Walton MI et al: A clinical phase I toxicity study of Ro 03-8799: plasma, urine, tumour and normal brain pharmacokinetics, *Br J Radiol* 59:107-116, 1986.

45. Rubenstein LJ: Tumors of the central nervous system. In *Atlas of tumor pathology,* second series, Fasicle 6, Armed Forces of Pathology, Washington, DC 1972.

46. Sachsenheimer W, Piotrowski W, Bimmler T: Quality of life in patients with intracranial tumors on the basis of Karnofsky's performance status, *J Neurooncology* 13:177-181, 1992.

47. Salcman M: The morbidity and mortality of brain tumors. A perspective on recent advances in therapy, *Neurol Clin* 3:229-257, 1985.

48. Sandberg-Wollheim M, Malmstrom P, Stromblad LG et al: A randomized study of chemotherapy with procarbazine, vincristine, and lomustine with and without radiation therapy for astrocytoma grades 3 and/or 4, *Cancer* 68:22-29, 1991.

49. Schwartz RB, Mantello MT: Primary brain tumors in adults, *Semin Ultrasound CT MR* 13:449-472, 1992.

50. Shapiro WR: Therapy of adult malignant brain tumors: what have the clinical trials taught us? *Semin Oncol* 13:38-45, 1986.

51. Shepherd CW, Scheithauer BW, Gomez MR et al: Subependymal giant cell astrocytoma: a clinical, pathological, and flow cytometric study, *Neurosurgery* 28:864-868, 1991.

52. Shibamoto Y, Yamashita J, Takahashi M et al: Supratentorial malignant glioma: an analysis of radiation therapy in 178 cases, *Radiother Oncol* 18:9-17, 1990.

53. Simpson D: The recurrence of intracranial meningiomas after surgical treatment, *J Neurol Neurosurg Psychiatry* 20:22-39, 1957.

54. Sorensen FB, Braendgaard H, Chistiansen AO et al: Stereological estimates of nuclear volume and other quantitative variables in supratentorial brain tumors. Practical technique and use in prognostic evaluation, *J Neurooncol* 10:253-262, 1991.

55. Strandgaard S, Paulson OB: Regulation of cerebral blood flow in health and disease, *J Cardiovasc Pharmacol* 19 Suppl 6:S89-S93, 1992.

56. Tans JT, Poortvliet DC: Relationship between compliance and resistance to outflow of CSF in adult hydrocephalus, *J Neurosurg* 71:59-62, 1989.

57. Tirelli U, D'Incalci M, Canetta R et al: Etoposide (VP-16-213) in malignant brain tumors: a phase II study, *J Clin Oncol* 2:432-437, 1984.

58. Vecht CJ, Avezaat CJ, van Putten WL et al: The influence of the extent of surgery on the neurological function and survival in malignant glioma. A retrospective analysis in 243 patients, *J Neurol Neurosurg Psychiatry* 53:466-471, 1990.

59. Vertosick FT Jr, Selker RG, Arena VC: Survival of patients with well-differentiated astrocytomas diagnosed in the era of computed tomography, *Neurosurgery* 28:496-501, 1991.

60. Victor S, Lausberg G: Malignant brain glioma—a catamnestic study of 100 operated patients, *Zentralblatt Fur Neurochirurgie* 52:59-68, 1991.

61. Watne K, Hannisdal E, Nome O et al: Combined intra-arterial and systemic chemotherapy for recurrent malignant brain tumors, *Neurosurgery* 30:223-227, 1992.

62. Weir B, Band P, Urtasun R et al: Radiotherapy and CCNU in the treatment of high-grade supratentorial astrocytomas, *J Neurosurg* 45:129-134, 1976.

63. Weller RO: Grading of brain tumours. The British experience, *Neurosurg Rev* 15:7-11, 1992.

64. Yates AJ: An overview of principles for classifying brain tumors, *Mol Chem Neuropathol* 17:103-120, 1992.

65. Zimmerman HM: Brain tumors: their incidence and classification in man and their experimental production, *Ann Acad Sci* 159:337-359, 1969.

14

Supratentorial Masses: Anesthetic Considerations

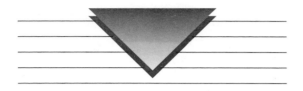

ROBERT BEDFORD

SUPRATENTORIAL TUMORS
Preoperative Considerations

Approximately 35,000 adult Americans develop brain tumors each year as either primary or metastatic lesions.[40,73] Most of these lesions require a tissue diagnosis to initiate appropriate therapy, which varies depending on tumor location and cell type and may range from surgical extirpation to radiation or chemotherapy. Furthermore, other lesions that are radiologically similar to tumors, such as brain abscess or radiation necrosis, can, at this time, be positively identified only under a microscope. Indeed, approximately 11% of suspected tumor biopsies reveal unexpected, non-neoplastic findings such as inflammation or degenerative disease.[21] Accordingly, tumor biopsy and/or excision are integral to the diagnosis and treatment of brain tumors, and optimal neuroanesthetic management is required to minimize neuronal injury during craniotomy.

Primary brain tumors are generally classified as either benign or malignant. Meningiomas are benign lesions that account for approximately 15% of all primary brain tumors.

They tend to be highly vascular lesions that enhance markedly with intravenous (IV) contrast solutions on computed tomographic (CT) or magnetic resonance imaging (MR) scans.[43] Typically, meningiomas located near the falx, convexity dura, lateral sphenoid wing, or frontal base of the skull are amenable to total resection. By contrast, those close to the sagittal sinus, ventricles, tentorial notch, or optic nerve sheath are more difficult to remove entirely.[55] Because total resection of the meningioma is essentially curative, with a recurrence rate of only 9% at 10 years,[34] the anesthesiologist should anticipate an operation with the goal of complete excision whenever a meningioma is suspected preoperatively. In addition, because meningiomas tend to be slow-growing, they may achieve a relatively large size, particularly in the "silent" frontal region. In this circumstance, the neurosurgeon may confront a difficult dissection that requires extraordinary measures to reduce brain bulk sufficiently to achieve total tumor resection.

Among the other benign tumors, colloid cysts of the third ventricle and epidermoid tumors arising in the basal

307

cisterns are the most common nonpituitary supratentorial lesions. The former usually present with symptoms of obstructive hydrocephalus and may present the anesthesiologist with a patient having high intracranial pressure (ICP) at the time of anesthetic induction. Colloid cysts may be treated by transventricular or transcallosal excision, by stereotaxic aspiration, or simply by ventricular shunting.[28] In contrast, epidermoid tumors are more commonly heralded by seizures and only occasionally cause symptoms of obstructive hydrocephalus.[8] Intraoperative considerations tend to focus on maximizing brain relaxation to facilitate exposure to the base of the skull.

Malignant brain tumors may be either primary or metastatic in origin. The brain edema surrounding these tumors is a common characteristic seen on preoperative CT or MR scans. It apparently results from secretory factors that increase vascular permeability in the nearby brain.[12] The most common primary brain tumor is the malignant astrocytoma. Virtually all of the malignant tumors present with headaches, seizures, or progressive neurologic deficit. The appearance on enhanced CT or MR scanning is varied although high-grade lesions tend to display a contrast-enhanced border representing rapidly dividing cells and a border of edematous brain (Fig. 14-1). Before the development of the CT scanner, these tumors often became large

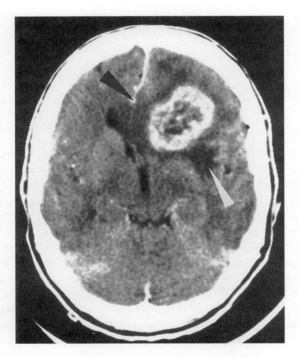

FIG. 14-1   Typical CT appearance of a high-grade malignant astrocytoma of the frontal lobe. Note the enhancing "rim" of rapidly dividing malignant cells surrounding the necrotic core of the tumor, which in turn is surrounded by edematous brain *(white arrow)*. The tumor/edema mass has obliterated the anterior horn of the ipsilateral ventricle and is compressing and laterally displacing the falx *(black arrow)*.

before a surgical procedure was contemplated. Accordingly, the anesthesiologist often confronted a patient who had a huge lesion with considerable evidence of compromised intracranial compliance. In contemporary practice, however, most of these lesions tend to measure 3 to 4 cm in diameter and patients rarely present with acutely elevated ICP. Preoperative treatment with dexamethasone usually results in dramatic decreases in surrounding brain edema,[44] and ICP in these patients tends to be normal or only slightly elevated. In dealing with primary malignant brain tumors, the cell type is of minimal consequence in planning or executing an anesthesic. If an unexpected diagnosis such as brain abscess or radiation necrosis results from microscopic examination of the lesion biopsy, there is essentially no difference in planning the patient's anesthetic maintenance or emergence.

Secondary brain tumors may present a variety of anesthetic challenges over and above those of the patient's neuropathology. Forty percent of metastatic brain tumors originate in the lung,[9] and it is not unusual to confront a patient who has severe chronic obstructive pulmonary disease and possibly a lung resection. In addition, the patient may have received chemotherapy with a toxic agent such as bleomycin, which may result in pulmonary tissue injury during exposure to high oxygen concentrations. Other well-recognized complications of chemotherapeutic agents include cardiomyopathy from adriamycin and inhibition of plasma cholinesterase activity after cytoxan therapy.[31] Finally, one must suspect the presence of HIV infection if a lymphoma is diagnosed on tumor biopsy. Universal precautions should be an integral part of every anesthetic.

Preoperative Preparation

The neuroanesthesiologist should examine the patient's head CT and/or MR scans to gain an understanding of the potential problems that might be encountered during the perioperative period. It is not difficult for a physician to learn to discern the location and size of a brain tumor on an enhanced scan. Small superficial lesions tend to cause minimal difficulty in surgical exposure and require modest efforts to maintain brain laxity during excision. Larger and deeper lesions, in contrast, usually require vigorous measures to reduce brain bulk to facilitate surgical exposure. Large lesions also have the potential for massive intraoperative hemorrhage.

The extent of peritumor brain edema is usually obvious, particularly with an appropriately weighted MR scan; thus it is possible to estimate the mass effect of the tumor-edema unit. In general, the greater the edema surrounding the tumor, the greater the chance of elevation in ICP before the cranium is opened.[7] If the mass effect is large enough to cause lateral shift of midline structures such as the falx or the third ventricle, vigorous efforts should be directed at ICP reduction during anesthesia[27] (Fig. 14-2).

Because the CSF compartment is compressible, it constitutes one of the major compensatory mechanisms for in-

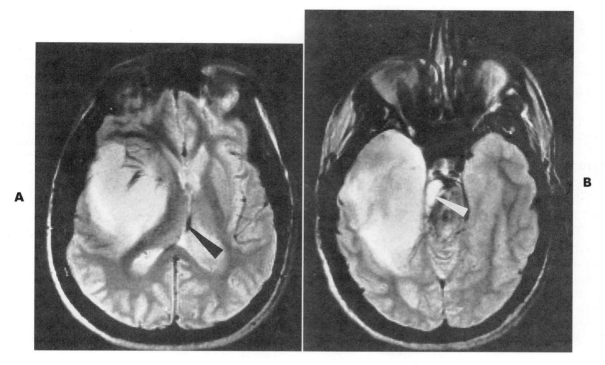

FIG. 14-2 **A,** MR scan of low-grade astrocytoma of temporal lobe showing marked lateral displacement of midline structures *(black arrow).* **B,** Lower level cut of same low-grade astrocytoma as in **A.** There is transtentorial herniation of tumor, which is compressing the brainstem *(white arrow).* Acute elevation of ICP in this situation may result in further tumor herniation, with subsequent brainstem injury.

tracranial compliance. Thus the lateral ventricles should be examined for evidence of effacement by tumor mass or for expansion of the ventricles caused by obstructive hydrocephalus. Both of these conditions indicate that the intracranial pressure-volume curve is at the "knee" of its hyperbolic relationship and that any maneuver resulting in an increase in ICP volume will cause a disproportionate increase in ICP and/or brain swelling.[66]

Many patients with brain tumors present with complaints of headache, decreased level of consciousness, or visual disturbances that suggest the presence of elevated ICP. Usually, however, dexamethasone treatment is initiated shortly after hospital admission, with the result that brain edema and signs of intracranial hypertension will have abated considerably by the time the patient is examined by the anesthesiologist.[44] The patient's near normal neurologic examination may lull the neuroanesthesiologist into believing that the patient is not at risk for perioperative intracranial hypertension. In general, one should assume that any patient who presents to the hospital with signs or symptoms of elevated ICP is still at risk for perioperative intracranial hypertension and should be treated as such even though the presenting symptoms no longer exist.

Seizures are often the presenting sign of a supratentorial brain tumor. In fact, brain tumor should be presumed in any adult patient presenting with a first seizure; CT and MR scanning should be performed shortly thereafter.[12] Treatment with phenytoin and other antiseizure medications is initiated before surgery in an attempt to prevent both preoperative and postoperative seizures.[54] Because phenytoin markedly stimulates enzymatic pathways responsible for metabolism of a variety of drugs, not the least of which are barbiturates and neuromuscular blocking agents, the neuroanesthesiologist must be aware of the possibility that typical dosages of these agents may not have the anticipated intensity or duration of effect.[56]

Craniotomy for supratentorial tumor presents several unique challenges related to control of brain bulk and ICP. Hyperventilation tends to impair venous return and decrease cardiac output as do diuretics that inhibit sodium reuptake at the loop of Henle. Hypocarbia also causes a linear reduction in coronary artery blood flow. Osmotic diuretic agents create a temporary hypervolemia. Because of these stresses, it is important to assure that myocardial performance is maximized with appropriate inotropic and antianginal medications before surgery. Because respiratory alkalosis induces hypokalemia, it is likewise advisable to optimize potassium levels before craniotomy, particularly for patients who are being treated with digitalis and diuretics.

Because hypocarbia is often crucial to reducing brain bulk, it is important to optimize pulmonary function preoperatively. In particular, it is important that bronchospastic disease be appropriately treated with aminophylline, steroids, antibiotics, and beta$_2$-adrenergic drugs. If chronic obstructive pulmonary disease (COPD) is nonreversible, it is advisable to consult with the neurosurgeon preoperatively to select methods of reducing brain bulk that do not rely on high levels of alveolar ventilation.

Preoperative Medication

In brain tumor patients who have a marked mass effect and intracranial hypertension, preoperative sedation is contraindicated. The sedative-induced blunting of the ventilatory response to carbon dioxide may produce hypercarbia, further elevation of ICP, and the potential for brain herniation. However, in current practice most brain tumors are relatively small lesions and preoperative brain edema and ICP are reduced with dexamethasone.[44] These advances have made it practical and safe to administer sedative medication to many brain tumor patients before induction of general anesthesia. Given the current tendency toward placement of invasive cardiovascular monitoring catheters in the operating room while patients are awake, a small amount of opioid analgesic and appropriate sedative seems to be entirely reasonable, particularly because patient anxiety and pain perception are recognized causes of elevated ICP[66] as well as myocardial ischemia.[39] The majority of neuroanesthesiologists currently tend to titrate judicious doses of intravenous sedatives to effect, only after the patient is in the operating room and under the direct observation of an anesthesiologist. Typical anxiolysis in this setting might consist of midazolam, in a dose range of 1 to 3 mg IV, perhaps in combination with fentanyl, 25 to 100 μg IV. Only an occasional patient might require premedication before coming to the operating room.

Perioperative Monitoring

Invasive cardiovascular monitoring has become a mainstay of contemporary neuroanesthetic practice primarily because of the desire to monitor cerebral perfusion and physiologic parameters such as arterial CO_2 tension ($PaCCO_2$) and plasma levels of glucose and potassium. Cannulation of a peripheral artery, usually the radial, and transduction of the mean arterial pressure at midhead level (usually the external auditory meatus) affords a close approximation of mean arterial pressure at the level of the Circle of Willis. When MAP is combined with direct ICP monitoring, the mean cerebral perfusion pressure (CPP) can be approximated using the formula: CPP = MAP − ICP. When the cranium is open and ICP is equal to atmospheric pressure, then CPP = MAP, except in regions where retractors may be compressing brain and preventing perfusion.

Because end-tidal CO_2 tension ($PETCO_2$) may have only a poor correlation with $PaCO_2$, particularly in elderly patients or those with poor ventilation-perfusion matching,[76] an arterial cannula also permits verification of the adequacy of hyperventilation. It is not unusual to see a 10 to 15 mm Hg $PETCO_2$-to-$PaCO_2$ gradient in patients with COPD. If the patient has preoperative evidence of compromised intracranial compliance, it is then necessary to titrate hyperventilation against $PaCO_2$ rather than against $PETCO_2$ data acquired from a capnometer.

Most neuroanesthesiologists also opt for a central venous cannula for cardiovascular monitoring during supratentorial tumor resection. Although it is widely recognized that CVP is a relatively poor reflection of cardiovascular performance, a central venous cannula ensures rapid access to the central circulation for administration of vasoactive agents and/or blood volume expanders, as needed. In addition, a central venous cannula can be both diagnostic and therapeutic if an air embolism occurs. Air embolism is relatively unusual during craniotomy for supratentorial tumor because the horizontal position is typically used. However, the head is often elevated several centimeters above heart level to minimize venous and CSF pressure at the incision, and air embolism may occur if the superior sagittal sinus or some other noncollapsible venous structure is entered.[3] Because of the slight risk of venous air embolism whenever the head is slightly elevated, many clinicians also place a precordial Doppler monitor to expedite detection of air bubbles in the venous circulation.

Intraoperative blood glucose level is a significant concern because of evidence that hyperglycemia tends to promote neuronal lactic acidosis and worsens cellular injury during cerebral ischemia.[29] Because brain retraction may cause temporary focal ischemia during dissection for supratentorial tumors,[2] it is considered prudent to monitor blood glucose levels during craniotomy, particularly because preoperative dexamethasone treatment tends to elevate resting glucose levels. General anesthesia likewise promotes gluconeogenesis,[70] and this situation is further aggravated by infusion of glucose-containing intravenous solutions.[68]

Monitoring of patient temperature is now regarded as a standard of care during general anesthesia. Unlike most operative interventions, where normothermia is thought desirable, most contemporary neuroanesthesiologists tend to allow the patient's temperature to spontaneously decrease to approximately 34° C. The rationale for this is based on evidence that a modest degree of hypothermia confers a measurable degree of neuronal protection during focal ischemia.[10] The risks of this level of hypothermia are relatively minimal in patients with reasonably normal cardiorespiratory status, and the potential for protection of valuable neuronal function appears to be significant, particularly when surgery of the dominant hemisphere is concerned. Monitoring of temperature allows for fine-tuning of the degree of hypothermia by altering of the temperature of the operating room, the intravenous solutions, or the inspired gas mixture. Only rarely is it necessary to actively cool the patient with a cooling blanket or ice packs placed in the groin or axilla.

Monitoring neuromuscular function is also a standard of anesthetic care but should be pursued with caution in patients with supratentorial tumors, particularly those with signs of hemiparesis. Increased acetylcholine receptor density has been documented at the motor endplate region of lower motor units innervated by dysfunctional or nonfunctioning upper motor neurons[25] and is thought to be due to loss of motoneuron function in the face of impaired or absent upper motor neuron function.[45] Placement of a neuromuscular stimulator on a limb contralateral to a supratentorial tumor may thus reflect resistance to nondepolarizing muscle relaxants, which, in turn, may result in a relative overdose of a drug and prolonged postoperative neuromuscular blockade.[67] To avoid this problem, care should be taken to monitor neuromuscular transmission in a limb ipsilateral to the supratentorial tumor.

A corollary to the phenomenon of increased acetylcholine receptor density in hemiparetic motor units is the hypothetic concern that hyperkalemia might ensue in response to succinylcholine, as has been reported in paraplegic and burn patients.[26] To date, however, succinylcholine probably has been administered to more than a million patients with supratentorial tumors, and only one instance of hyperkalemic cardiac arrest has been reported.[33] Indeed, when serum potassium levels were measured after succinylcholine administration to a series of patients with supratentorial tumors, no significant increase in potassium level was found.[50]

ICP monitoring is one of the more controversial aspects of care for patients with supratentorial tumors. A great deal of useful, albeit anecdotal, information can be gleaned by monitoring ICP before opening the dura.[6] In particular, the effect of proper (or improper) head positioning, the efficacy of hyperventilation and/or diuretics in reducing brain bulk, and the effect of anesthetic agents on ICP can be quantitated and corrected, if necessary, before the time that the craniotomy flap is turned. These problems are unlikely, however, if the patient has already received meticulous positioning and neuroanesthetic care. Thus few neurosurgeons are willing to take the time to place ICP monitors before the initiation of craniotomy for supratentorial tumor resection.

Postoperative ICP monitoring, however, appears to be gaining advocates, particularly with the ready availability of catheter tip transducers that are simple to insert and have an extremely low complication rate. Apparently up to 20% of patients undergoing supratentorial tumor resection will develop intracranial hypertension during emergence from anesthesia, while CO_2 tension is allowed to normalize, or in the immediate postoperative period when brain swelling or hematoma formation occurs.[15] Given the safety of contemporary ICP monitoring technology, compared with the risks of waiting for a patient to "fail to emerge from anesthesia," postoperative ICP monitoring will continue to be an increasingly popular postoperative monitoring modality after supratentorial tumor resection.

Brain Relaxation

A brain tumor and its surrounding brain edema form a mass that creates pressure on adjacent intracranial structures, including nearby normal brain, meninges, blood vessels, and CSF-containing ventricles. When the cranium is closed, this tension can be quantified as ICP. When the cranium is open, it has been quantified as "brain protrusion pressure."[19] When ICP is elevated to supranormal levels, brain contents tend to protrude, forcing the dura mater through the craniotomy incision. The neurosurgeon will not open the dura under such circumstances because herniation of the cortex will invariably lead to neuronal injury. Furthermore, it is impossible to manipulate the brain without causing undue damage to the cortex when it protrudes through the craniotomy. In contrast, under optimal conditions, the brain collapses inward after craniotomy, and the brain is said to be relaxed or "slack." In this situation, it is possible for the neurosurgeon to proceed with dissection toward the lesion while exerting only minimal retraction pressure on adjacent structures.

When an ICP monitor has been placed preoperatively, an ICP reading above 10 mm Hg tends to be followed by a complaint from the surgeon that the brain is "too tight" for optimal operating conditions. In most circumstances, simply increasing alveolar ventilation such that Pa_{CO_2} is approximately 25 mm Hg will result in sufficient reduction of intracranial blood volume to decrease ICP and permit dural incision and brain dissection. This assumes that the patient's head is slightly elevated and that the neck is neither flexed nor rotated enough to obstruct cerebral venous outflow.

Before craniotomy, examination of the patient's head CT scan can assist in identifying patients at risk for brain protrusion. Evidence of intracranial mass effect large enough to displace midline structures by 10 mm is often associated with intraoperative increased ICP despite hyperventilation.[27] In addition, patients with evidence of peritumor edema spread throughout the ipsilateral hemisphere can be expected to require additional interventional measures beyond hyperventilation to assure satisfactory brain relaxation.[5,70a]

Osmotic diuretics form the next line of drugs for brain relaxation and ICP control. These drugs increase the osmolality of blood relative to brain, thus pulling water across an intact blood-brain barrier from brain to blood so as to restore osmolar balance between brain and blood. Currently, the only agent widely used for this purpose is mannitol. Urea, with its propensity for causing rebound brain swelling, is only of historic interest.[24] Most practitioners empirically administer an IV infusion of mannitol in a dose of approximately 0.5 to 1 g/kg before opening the skull. Although earlier studies in patients with normal ICP suggested that the increase in intravascular and cerebral blood volume induced by mannitol infusion might result in worsening of intracranial hypertension, more recent work in patients with elevated ICP has demonstrated that mannitol infusion results in a prompt ICP reduction in this circumstance.[61] Quantitative measurement of brain water using CT scanning technology in brain tumor patients has shown that mannitol, 1 to 2 g/kg IV, reduces brain water content by approximately 90 ml at a peak serum osmolarity increase of approximately 18 mOsm/l.[13] The observable effect on ICP lasts approximately 2 to 3 hours. Some groups therefore administer one half the dose of mannitol before performing the craniotomy, with the other half administered slowly during surgery until brain dissection is completed.

The renal loop diuretic furosemide has also been advocated for reduction of ICP before craniotomy.[15] Unlike mannitol, furosemide does not cause a decrease in brain water content,[13] but rather it induces an isosmotic contraction of the extracerebral-extracellular space, which may be caused by a reduction in cerebral blood volume, CSF formation, or brain sodium transport. Although the reported decreases in ICP are small, electrolyte disturbances are less with furosemide than after mannitol. This may be important in patients receiving digitalis because hyperventilation causes hypokalemia, which may induce digitalis-toxic cardiac rhythms during surgery. Although mannitol is by far the more commonly used diuretic for ICP control during craniotomy, it is contraindicated for patients with congestive heart failure, in whom furosemide is probably a better agent.

Another mechanism for reducing intracranial pressure and/or brain bulk is to remove CSF from the neuraxis. This may be accomplished after craniotomy by piercing the lateral ventricle with a ventriculostomy tube and removing enough CSF to cause the cerebral mantle to relax inward. Although this maneuver injures some neuronal tissue, it has the advantage of allowing the neurosurgeon to create as much brain relaxation as is desired. If supratentorial tumors have obliterated the ipsilateral ventricle or if the craniotomy is performed over a critical area of cortex, however, lateral ventricular drainage is not practical. A spinal needle or catheter placed in the lumbar subarachnoid space also permits CSF drainage from the lateral ventricles if there is no obstruction to CSF outflow in the third ventricle or posterior fossa. Although this technique carries the possibility of inducing rostrocaudal herniation of brain contents if a large amount of CSF rapidly escapes from a patient with elevated ICP, it remains an effective method of decompressing the intracranial compartment in well-compensated patients who are hyperventilated at the time CSF drainage occurs and have no preoperative signs or symptoms of intracranial hypertension. Typically, removal of only 10 to 20 ml of CSF will markedly improve operating conditions, although in more severe circumstances, more than 50 ml may be removed. An additional advantage of a lumbar subarachnoid catheter is that it can be attached to a strain gauge before the opening of the cranium and thus can be used to measure CSF pressure responses to anesthetic agents or other drugs.

One final method for inducing brain relaxation is the use of anesthetic drugs that increase cerebrovascular resistance and thus lower cerebral blood volume and ICP. Virtually all inhalational anesthetics cause increases in CBF although this effect usually can be successfully opposed by the cerebral vasoconstriction induced by hypocarbia. When brain protrusion is problematic despite the use of hyperventilation, osmotic diuretics, head-up positioning, and CSF drainage, the next logical step is to change to an anesthetic that increases cerebrovascular resistance. Barbiturates, opioids, benzodiazepines, propofol, and etomidate are the currently available options. The classic approach to this was introduced by Hunter, with the use of a continuous thiopental infusion,[32] but the prolonged postoperative somnolence that may be induced by thiopental or other long-acting agents is generally considered undesirable for elective tumor resection. Propofol, usually supplemented with small amounts of fentanyl, may become the anesthetic drug of choice for continuous intravenous anesthesia.[72]

Anesthetic Approaches
Before Induction

As indicated previously, most clinicians prefer to use direct monitoring of both arterial and central venous pressures via percutaneously placed cannula. Although radial arterial cannulation is only a little more uncomfortable than cannulation of a peripheral vein, central venous cannulation is more problematic. Central venous cannulation can be performed from an antecubital vein with little discomfort or risk.[60] By contrast, the jugular venous route requires head-down positioning, neck rotation, and some element of discomfort, all of which may elevate ICP. The added risks of pneumothorax or carotid artery injury and the remote possibility of jugular venous thrombosis[57] make this a less favorable route unless it is necessary. Although some might advocate insertion of monitoring lines after induction of general anesthesia, in general, I believe the value of the information obtained during the awake "control" state is worth the time and minimal discomfort invested.

Induction Sequence

Currently, most clinicians probably induce anesthesia with a sleep-dose of thiopental (3 to 5 mg/kg) supplemented with fentanyl (up to 10 μg/kg), intravenous lidocaine (1.5 mg/kg) and perhaps a beta-sympatholytic such as esmolol, 100 mg, to suppress the hemodynamic and ICP increases anticipated with endotracheal intubation.[5,70a] After gentle hyperventilation has been established with 100% oxygen by face mask, endotracheal intubation is usually facilitated by a dose of nondepolarizing neuromuscular blocker, ordinarily vecuronium, 0.1 mg/kg. Endotracheal intubation can then be performed in 2 to 3 minutes. Assuming the patient's cardiovascular parameters have been stable up to this time, an additional 2 to 3 mg/kg dose of thiopental can be administered to deepen anesthesia just before endotracheal intubation.[71]

I pretreat all craniotomy patients with metocurine, 2 mg IV, before inducing general anesthesia. This benign dose of muscle relaxant performs two functions: (1) it speeds the onset and prolongs the duration of vecuronium-induced neuromuscular blockade, and (2) it counteracts the adverse ICP consequences of succinylcholine in the event that it is needed for a more rapid onset of muscle relaxation in the midst of anesthetic induction.[49] Whether other benzylisoquinolinium-derived muscle relaxants (mivacurium, atracurium) are as effective as metocurine in this regard remains to be studied as of this writing. Although the ICP increases induced by succinylcholine are minimal in well-compensated brain tumor patients, this issue becomes more acute when dealing with the semiconscious patient with an intracranial hematoma.

Maintenance

There has been a longstanding debate regarding the optimal anesthetic maintenance regimen for craniotomy. Those in favor of relying on volatile anesthetic agents, such as isoflurane, point to their long history of safe use and minimal ICP consequences in brain tumor patients (as long as hyperventilation is maintained).[47] Those in favor of using primarily intravenous drugs, such as barbiturates, opioids, benzodiazepines, and propofol, point to the ability to increase cerebrovascular resistance and reduce ICP. Both approaches have their disadvantages. Virtually every inhalational anesthetic increases cerebral blood flow and will increase ICP and/or brain bulk if hyperventilation cannot overcome the induced increase in cerebral blood volume. On the other hand, excessive doses of intravenous anesthetics could result in prolonged postoperative somnolence, respiratory depression, and inability to assess neurologic status. This, in turn, causes concern that a surgical complication has occurred, resulting in emergent CT scans to rule out brain swelling or hematoma formation.

An additional issue in the inhalational vs. intravenous agent controversy has been the recent findings that the synthetic opioids may have adverse cerebrovascular effects for some neurosurgical patients. Sufentanil has been shown to increase cerebral blood flow in dogs.[48] Although this has not been seen in humans, both sufentanil and alfentanil cause increases in CSF pressure in brain tumor patients anesthetized with nitrous oxide.[42,35]

In an effort to minimize either the total dose of intravenous agent or the required concentration of volatile agent used, nitrous oxide, 50% to 70% in oxygen, is typically administered in the belief that its cerebrovascular and ICP effects are relatively minimal.[69] This belief has been called into question recently by studies suggesting that, at equipotent doses, isoflurane has a less adverse effect than nitrous oxide on ICP[36] and CBF.[38]

These controversies regarding optimal anesthetic agents for neurosurgery have relatively little bearing for the well-compensated brain tumor patient who has received preoperative corticosteroids and intraoperative diuretic agents.

Assuming proper head positioning, hyperventilation to a $Paco_2$ of approximately 25 mm Hg, and avoidance of arterial hypertension by judicious use of adrenergic blockade, the available evidence suggests that synthetic opioids administered either with 60% to 70% nitrous oxide in oxygen[22] or with 0.5% to 1.5% isoflurane in oxygen[30] result in satisfactory operating conditions for supratentorial tumor excision or biopsy. Indeed, most clinicians probably use a combination of nitrous oxide, isoflurane, and synthetic opioid for anesthetic maintenance, assuming that operating conditions appear satisfactory at the time the craniotomy flap is turned.

The results of an extensive outcome study tend to support this impression. Todd et al.[70a] randomized 121 patients to receive one of three anesthetic maintenance techniques: propofol/fentanyl infusions, isoflurane/nitrous oxide, or fentanyl/nitrous oxide. They were unable to show any significant difference in outcome or recovery between the techniques although more patients in the isoflurane/nitrous oxide group had ICPs greater than 24 mm Hg at the time the initial craniotomy burr hole was produced, and more of these patients tended to be relatively slow to awaken from anesthesia (Todd, MM, personal communication).

If brain protrusion appears to be a problem despite optimal positioning, hyperventilation, blood pressure control, and diuretic treatment, then discontinuation of agents known to increase cerebral blood volume appear to be appropriate. Brain protrusion may persist, however, and the method used to further decompress the brain then becomes a matter of the surgeon's discretion: CSF drainage via a lateral ventriculostomy or amputation of temporal or frontal lobe tissue are maneuvers that occasionally must be employed. This problem is more often confronted after head injury surgery than during elective tumor resection.

Emergence

Emergence from anesthesia after elective craniotomy has specific considerations. Coughing and straining before the endotracheal tube is removed may cause severe elevations of intracranial venous and arterial pressure, which, in turn, may produce bleeding into the tumor bed. Residual respiratory depression may cause hypercarbia and lead to intracranial hypertension if the brain has not been well-decompressed before closure. Neurosurgeons appreciate having a patient who awakens promptly at the end of surgery so that neurologic status can be evaluated. The patient who remains somnolent postoperatively is often exposed to the risks of transport to the radiology department for emergent head CT scanning to rule out occult brain swelling or an intracranial hematoma.

In facilitating emergence from anesthesia, one prevalent approach is to discontinue all volatile anesthetic agents approximately 30 minutes before antagonism of muscle relaxation. After completion of surgery, nitrous oxide and/or intravenous agent infusions are discontinued and the patient is allowed to awaken while respiration is assisted via the endotracheal tube. Although coughing may occur with this approach, this can be obviated by prophylactic administration of lidocaine, 1.5 mg/kg IV, or a small dose of an opioid such as fentanyl, 25 to 50 μg IV. After the patient can open his/her eyes on command, extubation is accomplished as swiftly as possible. This approach facilitates early documentation of neurologic status such as eye opening and the following of simple commands. This technique may also avoid hypercarbia because the patient should awaken promptly, but it risks creating an intracranial catastrophe if vigorous coughing produces an intracranial hematoma.

The alternative approach is to extubate the patient after reversal of neuromuscular blockade but while the patient is sufficiently anesthetized with a volatile agent to avoid coughing. The patient is then allowed to return to spontaneous ventilation before extubation. With this technique, $Paco_2$ tends to be near 50 mm Hg, which may elevate ICP. Although this approach avoids the problems of coughing and straining on the endotracheal tube, it often results in delayed postoperative awakening because of residual anesthetic effect and lack of stimulation. The approach is facilitated if an ICP monitor is in place because temporary elevations in ICP caused by hypercarbia can be recognized and promptly treated with assisted ventilation. Delayed emergence from anesthesia seems to be less likely to provoke anxiety if ICP is near normal because the risk of severe brain swelling or hematoma formation is relatively low in this situation.[55]

Arterial hypertension is a frequent occurrence after craniotomy[53] and has been associated with postoperative intracerebral hemorrhage.[4] Although the genesis of the hypertension is related to elevated catecholamine levels,[74] the pathophysiology is poorly understood. In any event, either combined alpha and beta blockade with labetalol or titration of the beta-sympatholytic agent esmolol are standard approaches for controlling hypertension in the immediate postoperative period.

Intraoperative Management of the Awake Patient

Given the multiple problems associated with induction of, maintenance of, and emergence from general anesthesia, it is not difficult to understand the interest in performing diagnostic and therapeutic supratentorial tumor surgery while patients are conscious. This is particularly applicable for small lesions near the motor and speech centers in the dominant hemisphere and for tumors amenable to biopsy using stereotaxic technology. In general, this requires a favorably disposed surgeon and a motivated patient who is willing to tolerate the moderate discomfort of local anesthetic infiltration of the scalp and meninges. Because there are no pain receptors in brain substance, a considerable amount of tumor manipulation and/or brain penetration can be tolerated after the meninges have been incised.

Sedation, however, is virtually always an integral part of the procedure because these operations can be time-consuming and tedious for all involved. Although each neurosurgical center seems to have evolved its own preferred sedation regimen, virtually all rely on some combination of a short-acting opioid and a nonnarcotic sedative. The goal is to render the patient responsive to verbal commands while also affording sufficient analgesia both to tolerate local anesthetic infiltration and to comply with the need to remain still for a significant period of time. Preferred drug combinations include careful titration of small doses of fentanyl, sufentanil, or alfentanil for analgesia along with midazolam, droperidol, or propofol for sedation. The risk of the patient losing consciousness and becoming apneic is of paramount concern; accordingly, opioid antagonists should be readily at hand. In addition to directly observing chest excursion and respiratory sounds and monitoring hemoglobin-oxygen saturation with a pulse oximeter, some clinicians monitor end-tidal CO_2 concentration by placing a small catheter in the nares and connecting it to a capnometer. Full preparation for immediate control of the patient's airway and intravascular volume status needs to be immediately available during such procedures, in the event that the operation does not go as planned.

Stereotaxic brain biopsy is made possible by placement of a halo cast, which is affixed to the skull. Under CT scan control, the coordinates of the intracranial mass can be determined relative to the halo. The halo then orients the biopsy needle in three dimensions so that tissue can be obtained with no more brain dissection than that caused by passage of the needle. If general anesthesia is required, however, it can be complicated by the presence of the halo directly in front of the patient's face. This not only renders mask ventilation impossible but often seriously compromises endotracheal intubation. Stereotaxic biopsies can be performed under local anesthesia, as they are little more than a scalp incision, a twist-drill burr hole, and a dural nick. However, the risks of sudden neurologic deterioration caused by inadvertent hemorrhage or brain swelling tend to sway the conservative clinician toward protecting the airway. The means by which this is done varies widely among centers. Some place the halo under local anesthesia, and the awake patient returns for surgery after the preoperative CT scan. In most circumstances, this requires fiberoptically guided endotracheal tube placement under excellent topical anesthesia and superior laryngeal nerve blocks. Although modestly uncomfortable for the patient, this is considerably safer than the risk of a neurorespiratory emergency at a time when the airway is unprotected.

An alternative approach is to induce general anesthesia before placement of the halo and then to maintain anesthesia during transport to and from the CT scanner as well as during stereotaxic surgery. Although this results in a prolonged anesthetic and is demanding of anesthesia resources, it does obviate the problems the stereotaxic halo creates for airway control. This may not be necessary in the near future, however, as new halo designs have managed to leave the face relatively accessible for induction of anesthesia.

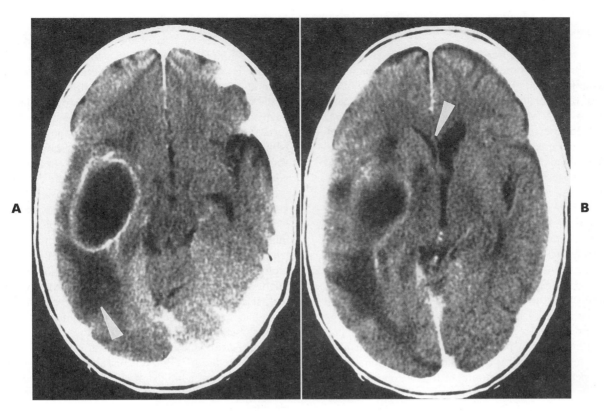

FIG. 14-3   **A,** Supratentorial brain abscess with the classic enhancing "ring" surrounding the abscess cavity. Note the widespread edema *(arrow),* which contributes to the mass effect of this lesion. **B,** Higher level cut of same abscess as in **A.** Note the nearly complete obliteration of the lateral ventricle and shift of midline structures *(arrow)* in response to the mass effect created by the abscess/edema complex.

Patients with Infectious Conditions

Brain abscess is a condition that can mimic supratentorial tumor in its effects on neural structures and ICP. The primary threat to the patient's well-being is the mass effect created by the abscess core and the surrounding edematous brain tissue (Fig. 14-3). Although there may be a recognizable cause for the abscess, such as a contiguous sinus or ear infection, brain abscess is also a well-recognized hazard whenever there is the possibility of a right-to-left cardiac shunt, particularly in intravenous drug abusers or immunocompromised patients.[23] Whenever low-grade fever and neurologic deterioration occur together, CT scanning for brain abscess is warranted.[11] Initial treatment is with broad-spectrum antibiotics; diuretics and corticosteroids are also administered in an attempt to control brain edema before surgical intervention.

Treatment for well-demarcated brain abscess invariably involves craniotomy and aspiration of the necrotic abscess core. In many cases this can be performed stereotaxically, as previously described, with the patient conscious throughout the procedure. If the patient is unable to cooperate, gen-

eral anesthesia must be used, with all the ICP precautions previously enumerated. After a bacteriologic diagnosis has been made, definitive antibiotic therapy can be initiated.[60]

Severely immunocompromised patients infected with human immunodeficiency virus often present with non-Hodgkin's lymphomas affecting the central nervous system. These may present as single or multiple supratentorial lesions that require biopsy and/or definitive resection. For the most part, the surgical and anesthetic considerations outlined previously apply to these patients as well. However, given their immunocompromised status, it is of paramount importance that sterile technique and the universal precautions recommended by the Centers for Disease Control be followed *meticulously,* both to protect the patient and to protect the patient's caregivers.[14] Current data suggest a 36% exposure rate to patients' blood and bodily fluids during routine anesthesia care.[37] It is crucial that compliance with the CDC recommendations be 100% when caring for these patients. A compliance rate of less than 50%, as reported recently,[17] is entirely unsatisfactory.

INTRACRANIAL HEMATOMAS
Preoperative Considerations

Most intracranial hematomas large enough to cause signs of neurologic deterioration require surgical extirpation to minimize injury to adjacent brain tissue. The rapidity of expansion of the hematoma and its size at the time of operation can vary widely, however. At one extreme are chronic subdural hematomas, where the brain usually has accommodated to the gradual expansion of the lesion and the patient often is wide awake and demonstrates only subtle neurologic signs preoperatively. These patients can be anesthetized as if they were undergoing an elective tumor resection.

By contrast, the patient who has sustained either an acute epidural or subdural hematoma (Figs. 14-4 and 14-5) or an intraparenchymal hemorrhage that results in deformation of basal cisterns is usually unconscious and hypertensive, with Cheyne-Stokes respirations if ventilation is not controlled. In this situation, the decreased level of consciousness and CT scan evidence of mass effect, midline shift, basal cistern compression, etc. all indicate that control of intracranial hypertension is of paramount importance.[63,64] Unlike anesthetic management for elective tumor resection, where avoiding increases in ICP optimizes surgical conditions, anesthesia for intracranial hematoma requires aggressive reduction of preexisting intracranial hypertension.

Preoperative Preparation

Preoperative preparation of the patient with elevated ICP resulting from an intracranial hematoma begins with securing the airway and initiating hyperventilation to a Pa_{CO_2} of 20 to 25 mm Hg with 100% oxygen. If there is a history of head trauma and the patient appears to be ventilating adequately, a lateral X-ray of the cervical spine should be performed to rule out a vertebral fracture before tracheal intubation. If ventilation is compromised, tracheal intubation should be performed as expeditiously and atraumatically as possible. Because this procedure may initiate coughing and profound arterial and intracranial hypertension, many advocate a standard anesthetic induction as described for tumor surgery before intubation. In a flaccid, comatose, multiple-trauma victim, where a full stomach and hypovolemia are major considerations, the hazards of massive aspiration of gastric contents or profound arterial hypotension might sway one toward performing intubation with minimal, if any, additional medication. If the patient is struggling and semiconscious, however, use of muscle relaxant in combination with etomidate, 0.25 to 0.5 mg/kg IV, may be required to minimize straining and coughing. Some recommend the use of a defasciculating dose of nondepolarizing agent before administration of succinylcholine[49]; others might opt for a "priming" dose of nondepolarizing muscle relaxant 3 minutes before a larger, intubating dose[46] al-

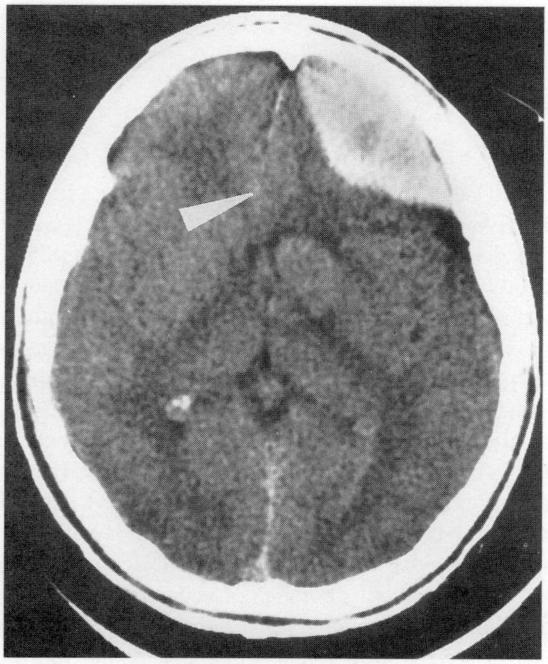

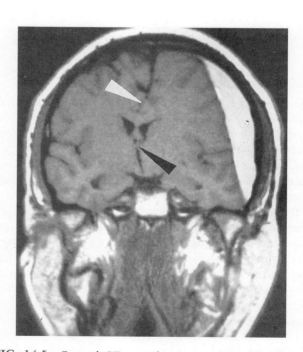

FIG. 14-4   Acute epidural hematoma with frontal dissection of blood forward of the lacerated middle meningeal artery. The shift of midline structures *(arrow)* again reflects elevated ICP in response to a rapidly expanding hematoma.

FIG. 14-5   Coronal CT scan showing a subdural hematoma causing massive distortion of lateral and third ventricles *(black arrow)* and herniation of cingulate gyrus below the falx *(white arrow).*

though this has been associated with the occasional episode of pulmonary aspiration.[52a] Alternatively, a single large bolus (1.5 times the intubating dose) of vecuronium [38a] or mivacurium[59a] will permit satisfactory intubating conditions in approximately 1 minute.

After the airway is secured and hyperventilation established, the patient can undergo additional diagnostic tests as needed. Time is of the essence for intracranial hematoma surgery, but it is also important that, in the case of a multiple-trauma patient, possible concurrent intraabdominal, vascular, and other critical injuries be identified before craniotomy. Sedation for the semistuporous or comatose patient during preoperative workup is usually a matter of titrating intravenous agents, including opioids, benzodiazepines, barbiturate, or etomidate, as the patient's cardiovascular status dictates. In this situation, long-acting nondepolarizing muscle relaxants can facilitate hyperventilation until definitive surgery can be performed.

It is also appropriate to administer diuretic agents early to reduce brain swelling. Mannitol and furosemide act synergistically and can be given safely in combination if the patient is normovolemic.[16,61] Alternatively, in a hypovolemic patient, mannitol and a hypertonic solution such as hetastarch should be administered.[59] Unlike the situation with supratentorial tumors and abscesses, corticosteroids have been shown not to improve outcome in patients with either traumatic[18] or primary[58] intracranial hematomas.

Perioperative Monitoring

As discussed previously, an arterial cannula is useful for repeated measurement of blood gas tensions and pH status. In addition, direct arterial pressure monitoring is usually necessary because patients with intracranial hematomas either require antihypertensive agents or are hypotensive from blood loss associated with concurrent injuries. In a hypovolemic multiple trauma patient, I attempt to place an arterial cannula before induction of anesthesia because occasionally it is the last chance to palpate a bounding pulse. In a normovolemic patient with an isolated head injury, a noninvasive blood pressure monitor is entirely satisfactory for prompt management of anesthetic induction and surgical skin preparation; the arterial cannula can be placed at leisure later.

Electrocardiographic monitoring may be deceptive in patients with head trauma, particularly those with crushed-chest injuries. T-wave inversion occurring in a patient with an isolated head injury probably reflects blood entering the ventricular system or basal cisterns.[14a] By contrast, cardiac dysrhythmias, conduction disorders, or elevated ST segments in the precordial leads are more likely to reflect cardiac contusion, whereas loss of ECG voltage may be an early sign of cardiac tamponade.[44a]

Because the patient will be receiving maximal ICP reduction measures before and during surgery, there is no advantage to placing an ICP monitor until after the hematoma has been evacuated.

Elevated blood glucose levels appear to adversely influence outcome from ischemic brain injury.[12a,38b] Because hematomas cause ischemia in adjacent brain tissue, it seems reasonable to monitor blood glucose levels at the same time that blood gas tensions are being determined. Glucose-containing resuscitation fluids should be administered only in response to documented hypoglycemia, and glucose levels above 150 to 200 mg/dl probably should be avoided. Finally, the patient's hematocrit and coagulation status (as determined by activated partial thromboplastin time) should be monitored. Brain tissue is a rich source of thromboplastin, which may enter the circulation during hematoma evacuation or tumor resection and lead to disseminated intravascular coagulopathy.[75]

Anesthetic Approaches

Because the first goal of anesthetic management for intracranial hematoma surgery is maximal control of ICP, drugs that are known to increase cerebral blood flow should not be considered as first-choice anesthetics. Although drugs such as nitrous oxide and isoflurane are not normally associated with increases in ICP during hypocarbia, a severe brain injury is not the circumstance in which to test whether the drug-induced increase in CBF can be overcome by the cerebral vasoconstriction caused by hypocarbia.[51] I have observed acute transtentorial herniation in response to isoflurane administration in this setting.

Available anesthetic drugs that increase cerebral vascular resistance and decrease cerebral metabolic rate for oxygen include barbiturates,[32] propofol,[72] and etomidate.[62,52] Because these drugs are cardiovascular depressants, they must be titrated according to the patient's individual response. Avoidance of arterial hypotension is a primary concern until the hematoma is evacuated so that brain ischemia near the hematoma can be minimized.

Control of arterial hypertension in the face of intracranial pathology is controversial. Some think that an elevated arterial blood pressure may help maintain perfusion to ischemic brain compressed by hematoma; others believe it may contribute to brain edema by increasing permeability of the blood-brain barrier. For those who believe in avoiding marked arterial hypertension, this can be accomplished in many instances by simply supplementing the intravenous anesthetic agent with an opioid. However, both fentanyl and sufentanil may produce increases in ICP in severely head-injured patients despite hyperventilation[1,69a] although the mechanism of this action has not been elucidated and many studies in non–head-injured patients support the use of these two drugs. Given the current state of controversy surrounding the effect of fentanyl derivatives on ICP, perhaps morphine or meperidine should be considered if an opioid is deemed necessary during intracranial hematoma surgery. Ordinarily, relatively small doses, equivalent to 10 to 20 mg of morphine sulfate IV, are all that is required to control or prevent arterial hypertension during general anesthesia for emergent craniotomy.

Vasoactive agents may also be required for control of arterial hypertension. Currently the weight of evidence supports use of either labetalol or esmolol for this purpose because neither drug has appreciable effect on ICP.[53] By contrast, direct vasodilating agents such as sodium nitroprusside[41] and hydralazine[65] can be associated with marked increases in ICP, thus impairing cerebral perfusion pressure even as they lower arterial pressure. In a patient with hypertension and severe bradycardia, I would administer enalapril at 1.25 mg IV over several minutes.

Brain Relaxation

In the face of an intracranial hematoma and/or severe brain edema, every effort should be directed toward maximizing relaxation of the normal brain to minimize ICP until the skull flap is turned and the dura incised. This should include use of head-up tilt and avoidance of excessive neck rotation or flexion. If the brain appears adequately relaxed under direct visualization, the anesthesiologist has the latitude to modify the anesthetic technique as seems appropriate: reduce the dosage of intravenous anesthetic, introduce inhalational anesthetic, allow the Paco$_2$ to increase, or slow diuretic therapy.

Occasionally acute, severe brain swelling occurs, often coincident with decompression of brain tissue by removal of a supratentorial hematoma, although it may also follow extirpation of a brain tumor or other supratentorial lesion. Although the pathophysiology of acute brain edema is poorly understood, it appears to be related to sudden decompression of brain tissue adjacent to a mass lesion. Frequently the brain swelling may be so severe that it is impossible for the neurosurgeon to close the dura and craniotomy despite complete removal of hematoma, tumor, or abscess. In this situation it is imperative that the anesthesiologist avoid maneuvers that tend to promote brain edema. One of the few studies examining the effect of anesthetic agents on brain edema formation compared the effects of barbiturate infusion vs. halothane anesthesia on blood-brain barrier function in rabbits made hypertensive with phenylephrine infusions.[20] Not surprisingly, halothane was associated with far more brain edema formation in this model than was thiopental infusion, presumably because halothane relaxed cerebral resistance vessels and exposed the blood-brain barrier to the elevated blood pressure. This study supports the concept that maintenance of cerebral vasoconstriction is an important element in minimizing brain edema when hypertension occurs during anesthesia for intracranial hematoma surgery or, for that matter, whenever brain swelling is of concern.

Emergence Sequence

If the patient was unconscious before surgery, one should expect that the patient will be transported to the neurointensive care unit intubated, under an extended anesthetic, and with full neuromuscular blockade and appropriate dosages of sedative/anesthetic agents. While neurointensive care management is beyond the scope of this chapter, I believe that after supratentorial hematoma surgery, emergence from anesthesia should be undertaken in the ICU after gradual respiratory weaning and only with concomitant ICP monitoring.[15] In summary, patients with rapidly expanding supratentorial hematomas present far different pathophysiology and anesthetic management needs than do those with slowly expanding lesions such as brain tumors or brain abscesses. Acute intracranial hematomas require maximal therapy directed toward reduction of ICP and cerebral protection; failure to deliver this level of care can result in unnecessary neurologic compromise.

SUMMARY

Patients with rapidly expanding supratentorial hematomas present far different pathophysiology and anesthetic management needs than do those with slowly expanding lesions, such as brain tumors or brain abscesses. Acute intracranial hematomas require maximal therapy directed toward reduction of ICP and cerebral protection; failure to deliver this level of care can result in unnecessary neurologic compromise. By contrast, extirpation of slowly growing lesions requires optimal surgical conditions and rapid emergence from anesthesia. These goals can be achieved by a variety of anesthetic approaches, including use of mild cerebral vasodilating agents, as long as brain bulk is controlled by judicious use of hyperventilation, diuretic agents, and CSF drainage, where appropriate. Throughout administration of the anesthetic, it is important to consider the impact of anesthetic drugs on the neuropathologic process and to be prepared to respond promptly to potential complications.

References

1. Albanese J, Durbec O, Viviand X et al: Sufentanil increases intracranial pressure in patients with head trauma, *Anesthesiology* 79:493, 1993.
2. Albin MS, Bunegin L, Bennett MH et al: Clinical and experimental brain retraction pressure monitoring, *Acta Neurol Scand* 56:522, 1977.
3. Albin MS, Carroll RG, Maroon JC: Clinical considerations concerning detection of venous air embolism, *Neurosurgery* 3:380, 1978.
4. Asiddao CB, Donegan JH, Whitesell RC et al: Factors associated with perioperative complications during carotid endarterectomy, *Anesth Analg* 61:631, 1982.
5. Bedford RF: Circulatory responses to tracheal intubation, *Probl Anesthesia* 2:201, 1988
6. Bedford RF, Colley PS: Intracranial tumors: supratentorial and infratentorial. In Matjasko MJ, Katz J, editors: *Clinical controversies in neuroanesthesia and neurosugery,* Orlando, Fla, 1986, Grune & Stratton, pp 135-179.
7. Bedford RF, Morris L, Jane JA: Intracranial hypertension during surgery for supratentorial tumor: correlation with preoperative computed tomography scans. *Anesth Analg* 61:430, 1982.
8. Berger MS, Wilson CB: Epidermoid cysts of the posterior fossa, *J Neurosurg* 62:214, 1985.
9. Black PM: Brain tumors: part 1, *N Engl J Med* 324:1471, 1991.
10. Boris-Moller F, Smith ML, Siesjo BK: Effects of hypothermia on ischemic brain damage: a comparison between pre-ischemic and post-ischemic cooling, *Neurosci Res Comm* 5:87, 1989.
11. Britt RH, Enzmann DR: Clinical stages of human brain abcesses on serial CT scans after contrast infusion. Computerized tomographic, neuropathological and clinical correlations, *J Neurosurg* 59:972, 1983.
12. Bruce JN, Crisculo GR, Merrill MJ et al: Vascular permeability induced by protein product of malignant brain tumors: inhibition by dexamethasone, *J Neurosurg* 67:880, 1987.
12a. Candelise L, Landi G, Orazio EN et al: Prognostic significance of hyperglycemia in acute stroke, *Arch Neurol* 42:661, 1985.
13. Cascino T, Baglivo J, Conti J et al: Quantitative CT assessment of furosemide- and mannitol-induced changes in brain water content, *Neurology* 33:898, 1983.
14. Centers for Disease Control: Update: universal precautions for prevention of transmission of human immunodeficiency virus, hepatitis B virus and other blood-born pathogens in health care settings, *MMWR* 37:377, 1988.
14a. Clifton GL, Robertson CS, Kyper K et al: Cardiovascular responses to severe head injury, *J Neurosurg* 59:447, 1983.
15. Constantini S, Cotev S, Rappaport ZH et al: Intracranial pressure monitoring after elective intracranial surgery, *J Neurosurg* 69:540, 1988.
16. Cottrell JE, Robustelli A, Post K et al: Furosemide- and mannitol-induced changes in intracranial pressure and serum osmolality and electrolytes, *Anesthesiology* 47:28, 1977.
17. Courington KR, Patterson SL, Howard RJ: Universal precautions are not universally followed, *Arch Surg* 126:93, 1991.
18. Dearden NM, Gibson JS, McDowell DG et al: Effect of high-dose dexamethasone on outcome from severe head injury, *J Neurosurg* 64:81, 1986.
19. Drummond JC, Todd MM, Toutant SM et al: Brain surface protrusion during enflurane, halothane and isoflurane anesthesia in cats, *Anesthesiology* 59:28, 1983.
20. Forster AF, Van Horn K, Marshall LF et al: Anesthetic effects on blood-brain barrier function during acute arterial hypertension, *Anesthesiology* 49:26, 1978.
21. Friedman WA, Sceats DJ Jr, Nestok BR et al: The incidence of unexpected pathological findings in an image-guided biopsy series: a review of 100 cases, *Neurosurgery* 25:180, 1989.
22. From RP, Warner DS, Todd MM et al: Anesthesia for craniotomy: a double-blind comparison of alfentanil, fentanyl and sufentanil, *Anesthesiology* 73:896, 1991.
23. Garvey G: Current concepts of bacterial infections of the central nervous system, *J Neurosurg* 59:735, 1983.
24. Goluboff B, Shenkin HA, Haft H: The effects of mannitol and urea on cerebral hemodynamics and cerebrospinal fluid pressure, *Neurology* 14:891, 1964.
25. Graham DH: Monitoring neuromuscular block may be unreliable in patients with upper motor neuron lesions, *Anesthesiology* 52:74, 1980.
26. Gronert GA, Theye RA: Pathophysiology of hyperkalemia after succinylcholine, *Anesthesiology* 43:89, 1975.
27. Grosslight K, Foster R, Colohan AR et al: Isoflurane for neuroanesthesia: risk factors for increases in ICP, *Anesthesiology* 63:533, 1985.
28. Hall WA, Lunsford LD: Changing concepts in the treatment of colloid cysts: an 11-year experience in the CT era, *J Neurosurg* 66:186, 1987.
29. Helgason CM: Blood glucose and stroke, *Stroke* 19:1049, 1988.
30. Herrick IA, Gelb AW, Manninen PH et al: Effects of fentanyl, sufentanil and alfentanil on brain retractor pressure, *Anesth Analg* 72:359, 1991.
31. Howland WS, Rooney SM, Goldiner PL: Complications of chemotherapy. In *Manual of anesthesia in cancer care,* New York, 1986, Churchill-Livingstone, pp 73-90.
32. Hunter AR: Thiopentone supplemented anaesthesia for neurosurgery, *Br J Anaesth* 44:506, 1972.
33. Iwatsuki N, Akaishi T, Amaha K: Upper motor neuron lesion and succinylcholine-induced hyperkalemia, *Masui* 29:1509, 1980.
34. Jaaskelainen J: Seemingly complete removal of histologically benign intracranial meningioma: late recurrence rate and facts predicting recurrence in 657 patients, *Surg Neurol* 26:461, 1986.
35. Jung R, Shoh N, Reinsel R et al: CSF Pressure in patients with brain tumors: impact of fentanyl versus alfentanil during nitrous oxide–oxygen anesthesia, *Anesth Analg* 71:419, 1990.
36. Jung RS, Reinsel R, Marx W et al: Isoflurane and nitrous oxide: comparative impact on cerebrospinal fluid pressure in patients with brain tumors, *Anesth Analg* 75:724, 1992.
37. Kristensen M, Sloth E, Jensen T: Relationship between anesthetic procedure and contact of anesthesia personnel with patient bodily fluids, *Anesthesiology* 73:619, 1990.
38. Lam AM, Slee TA, Cooper JO et al: Nitrous oxide is a more potent cerebrovasodilator than isoflurane in humans, *Anesthesiology* 75:A168, 1991.
38a. Lennon RL, Olson RA, Gronert GA:

Atracurium or vecuronium for rapid sequence endotracheal intubation, *Anesthesiology* 64:510, 1986.

38b. Longstreth WT Jr, Inui TS: High blood glucose level on hospital admission and poor neurologic recovery after cardiac arrest, *Ann Neurol* 15:59, 1984.

39. Lunn JK, Stanley TH, Webster LR et al: Arterial blood-pressure and pulse rate responses to pulmonary and radial arterial catheterization prior to cardiac and major vascular operations, *Anesthesiology* 51:265, 1979.

40. Mahaley MS Jr, Mettlin C, Natarajan N et al: National survey of patterns of care for brain-tumor patients, *J Neurosurg* 71:826, 1989.

41. Marsh ML, Shapiro HM, Smith RW et al: Changes in neurologic status and intracranial pressure associated with sodium nitroprusside administration, *Anesthesiology* 51:336, 1979.

42. Marx W, Shah NK, Long C et al: Sufentanil, alfentanil and fentanyl: impact on CSF pressure in patients with brain tumors, *J Neurosurg Anesth* 1:3, 1989

43. Maxwell RE, Chou SN: Preoperative evaluation and management of meningiomas. In Schmidek HH, Sweet WH, editors: *Operative neurosurgical techniques,* ed 2, vol 1, New York, 1988, Grune & Stratton, pp 547-554.

44. Maxwell RE, Long DM, French LA: The clinical effects of a synthetic glucocorticoid used for brain edema in the practice of neurosurgery. In Reulen HJ, Schurmann K, editors: *Steroids and brain edema,* Berlin, 1972, Springer-Verlag, pp 219-232.

44a. Mayfield W, Hurley EJ: Blunt cardiac trauma, *Am J Surg* 148:162, 1984.

45. McComas AJ: Functional changes in motoneurones of hemiparetic patients, *J Neurol Neurosurg Psychiatry* 36:183, 1973.

46. Mehta MP, Choi WW, Gergis SD et al: Facilitation of rapid endotracheal intubations with divided doses of nondepolarizing neuromuscular blocking drugs, *Anesthesiology* 62:392, 1985.

47. Michenfelder JD: The 27th Rovenstine Lecture: neuroanesthesia and the achievement of professional respect, *Anesthesiology* 70:695, 1989.

48. Milde LN, Milde JH, Gallagher WJ: Effects of sufentanil on cerebral circulation and metabolism in dogs, *Anesth Analg* 70:138, 1990.

49. Minton MD, Grosslight K, Stirt JA et al: Increases in ICP from succinylcholine: prevention by prior nondepolarizing blockade, *Anesthesiology* 65:165, 1986.

50. Minton MD, Stirt JA, Bedford RF: Serum potassium following succinylcholine in patients with brain tumors, *Can Anaesth Soc J* 33:328-31, 1986.

51. Moss E, McDowall DG: ICP increases with 50% nitrous oxide in oxygen in severe head injuries during controlled ventilation, *Br J Anaesth* 51:347, 1979.

52. Moss E, Powell D, Gibson RM: Effect of etomidate on intracranial pressure and cerebral perfusion pressure, *Br J Anaesth* 51:757, 1979.

52a. Musich J, Walts LF: Pulmonary aspiration after a priming dose of vecuronium, *Anesthesiology* 64:517, 1986.

53. Muzzi DA, Black S, Losasso T et al: Labetalol and esmolol in the control of hypertension after intracranial surgery, *Anesth Analg* 70:68, 1990.

54. North JB, Penhall RK, Hanieh A et al: Phenytoin and postoperative epilepsy: a double-blind study, *J Neurosurg* 58:672,1983.

55. Ojemann RG: Meningiomas: clinical features and surgical management. In Wilkins RH, Rengacharry SS, editors: *Neurosurgery,* vol 1, New York, 1985, McGraw-Hill, pp 635-654.

56. Ornstein E, Matteo RS, Schwartz AE et al: The effect of phenytoin on the magnitude and duration of neuromuscular block following atracurium and vecuronium, *Anesthesiology* 67:191, 1987.

57. Perkins NA, Cail WS, Bedford RF et al: Internal jugular vein function after Swan-Ganz catheterization, *Anesthesiology* 61:456, 1984.

58. Poungvarin N, Bhoopat W, Viriyavejakul A et al: Effects of dexamethasone in primary supratentorial intracerebral hemorrhage, *N Engl J Med* 316:1229, 1987.

59. Prough DS, Johnson JC, Poole GV Jr et al: Effects on intracranial pressure of resuscitation from hemorrhagic shock with hypertonic saline versus lactated Ringer's solution, *Crit Care Med* 13:407, 1985.

59a. Pühringer FK, Khuenl-Brady KS, Koller J et al: Evaluation of the endotracheal intubating conditions of rocuronium (ORG 9426) and succinylcholine in outpatient surgery, *Anesth Analg* 75:37, 1992.

60. Ragasa J, Shah N, Watson RC: Where antecubital catheters go: a study under fluoroscopic control, *Anesthesiology* 71:378, 1989.

61. Ravussion P, Abou-Madi M, Archer D et al: Changes in CSF pressure after mannitol in patients with and without elevated CSF pressure, *J Neurosurg* 69:869, 1988.

62. Renou AM, Vernhiet J, Macrez P et al: Cerebral blood flow and metabolism during etomidate anaesthesia in man, *Br J Anaesth* 50:1047, 1978.

63. Ropper AH: Lateral displacement of the brain and level of consciousness in patients with an acute hemispheral mass, *N Engl J Med* 314:953, 1986.

64. Ross DA, Olsen WL, Ross AM et al: Brain shift, level of consciousness and restoration of consciousness in patients with acute intracranial hematoma, *J Neurosurg* 71:498, 1989.

65. Schroeder T, Sillesen H: Dihydralazine induces marked cerebral vasodilation in man, *Eur J Clin Invest* 17:214, 1987.

66. Shapiro HM: Intracranial hypertension: therapeutic and anesthetic considerations, *Anesthesiology* 43:445, 1975.

67. Shayevitz JR, Matteo RS: Decreased sensitivity to metocurine in patients with upper motoneuron disease, *Anesth Analg* 64:767, 1985.

68. Sieber F, Smith DS, Kupferberg J et al: Effects of intraoperative glucose on protein catabolism and plasma glucose levels in patients with supratentorial tumors, *Anesthesiology* 64:453, 1986.

69a. Smith AL, Wollman H: Cerebral blood flow and metabolism: effects of anesthetic drugs and techniques, *Anesthesiology* 36:378, 1972.

69. Sperry RJ, Bailey PL, Reichman MV et al: Fentanyl and sufentanil increase ICP significantly in resuscitated head trauma patients, *Anesthesiology* 77:416, 1992.

70. Stevens WC, Eger EI, Joas TA et al: Comparative toxicity of isoflurane, halothane, fluoroxene and diethyl ether in human volunteers, *Can Anaesth Soc J* 20:357, 1973.

70a. Todd MM, Warner DS, Sokol MD et al: A prospective comparative trial of three anesthetics for elective supratentorial craniotomy: propofol/fentanyl, isoflurane/nitrous oxide, and fentanyl/nitrous oxide, *Anesthesiology* 78:1005, 1993.

71. Unni VKN, Johnston RA, Young HSA: Prevention of intracranial hypertension during laryngoscopy and endotracheal intubation: use of second dose of thiopentone, *Br J Anaesth* 56:1219, 1984.

72. Vandesteene A, Trempont V, Engelman E et al: Effect of propofol on cerebral blood flow and metabolism in man, *Anaesthesia* 43(suppl):42, 1988.

73. Walker AE, Robins M, Weinfeld FD: Epidemiology of brain tumors: the national survey of intracranial neoplasms, *Neurology* 35:219, 1985.

74. Wallach R, Karp RB, Reues JG et al: Pathogenesis of paroxysmal hypertension developing during and after coronary bypass surgery: a study of hemodynamic and humoral factors, *Am J Cardiol* 46:559, 1980.

75. Weinberg S, Phillips L, Twersky R et al: Hypercoaguability in a patient with a brain tumor, *Anesthesiology* 61:200, 1984.

76. Whitesell R, Asiddao C, Gullman D et al: Relationship between arterial and peak expired carbon dioxide pressure during anesthesia and factors influencing the difference, *Anesth Analg* 60:508, 1981.

15

Posterior Fossa: Surgical Considerations

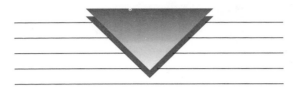

DENNIS Y. WEN
STEPHEN J. HAINES

The anatomy of the posterior fossa results in some unique considerations when undertaking surgery in this region. The close proximity of large venous sinuses (transverse, sigmoid, and the torcula), a thick anterior bony wall (basiocciput and petrous bone), an irregularly surfaced occipital squamosa posteriorly, the firm tentorium cerebelli superiorly and bony foramen magnum inferiorly enclose the contents of the posterior fossa. Every efferent pathway from the brain passes through the posterior fossa. The presence of so many critical structures in such a small rigid compartment results in rapid and severe effects from pathology affecting the cerebellum and adjacent structures, such as the cranial nerves and blood vessels. Obstructive hydrocephalus is an important feature of many disorders of the posterior fossa because of the critical outflow of CSF through the aqueduct of Sylvius to the fourth ventricle and then through the foramen of Magendie and Luschka into the basal cisterns. The intricate anatomy of the brainstem, cranial nerves, and vertebrobasilar arteries and the problems of gaining adequate surgical exposure in such a small confined space where only minimal retraction of adjacent structures is possible have made posterior fossa surgery a challenge for decades.

The bony surroundings of the posterior fossa limit the

ability to adequately visualize structures within it. Even computed tomography (CT) is hampered by significant bone artifact. Fortunately, the development of magnetic resonance imaging (MR) has allowed clinicians to make many diagnoses at a far earlier stage of the disease process while gaining exquisite anatomic definition of the posterior fossa structures.

Location of a lesion within the posterior fossa is the primary determinant of the patient's symptoms. A wide spectrum of disease processes may occur in the posterior fossa, including neoplastic, developmental, and vascular processes that may require surgical intervention. Such intervention has become possible not only through advances in imaging and microsurgical techniques but also through advances in the perioperative care of the patient and the excellent anesthetic techniques now available.

TUMORS

Tumors in the posterior fossa are not uncommon. The frequency and type of intracranial tumors in the posterior fossa show a marked age discrepancy (Table 15-1). In children, primary central nervous system tumors are the commonest solid tumor and the second commonest pediatric malignancy (after leukemia).[50,58] Almost two thirds of intracranial tumors in children occur in the posterior fossa and comprise medulloblastoma/primitive neuroectodermal tumors (PNET), cerebellar astrocytomas, brainstem gliomas, and ependymomas.[39]

In adults, both benign and malignant tumors may occur. Acoustic neurilemomas, meningiomas, and metastases occur along with the neuroepithelial tumors (glioblastomas) common in the supratentorial location. The cerebellum is the primary site of hemangioblastomas. Epidermoids are usually found in the cerebellopontine angle, and dermoids

TABLE 15-1
Distribution of Posterior Fossa Brain Tumors by Age

Tumor Type	Percentage of Total*
0-20 yr	
Astrocytoma	20
Medulloblastoma	20
Brainstem glioma	10
Ependymoma	5
20-60 yr	
Metastases	5
Acoustic	3
Meningioma	1
More than 60 yr	
Acoustic	20
Metastases	5
Meningioma	5

*Percentage of all (supratentorial and infratentorial) brain tumors for that age group.
Modified from Butler AB, Netsky MG: Classification and biology of brain tumors. In Youmans JR, editor: *Neurological surgery*, Philadelphia, 1973, WB Saunders.

in the vermis. Although any intracranial tumor found in the supratentorial region may be present in the posterior fossa, the tumors discussed here account for the vast majority of primary tumors found in the posterior fossa. Metastases probably account for up to two thirds of all cerebellar masses in adults.

The primary intraaxial lesions (astrocytoma, medulloblastoma/PNET, ependymoma) tend to be malignant (except for hemangioblastoma), but the extraaxial lesions tend to be benign (acoustic neurilemoma, epidermoid). Box 15-1 shows the tumors commonly found at various topographic regions of the posterior fossa.

BOX 15-1
LOCATION OF TUMORS OF THE POSTERIOR FOSSA

Cerebellar Hemisphere
Hemangioblastoma
Astrocytoma/glioblastoma
Metastasis

Cerebellopontine Angle
Neurilemoma
  Acoustic
  Trigeminal
  Facial
Meningioma
Epidermoid
Arachnoid cyst

Fourth Ventricle
Medulloblastoma/PNET
Ependymoma
Choroid plexus papilloma/carcinoma
Meningioma

Cerebellar Vermis
Astrocytoma
Dermoid

Clivus
Meningioma
Chordoma

Foramen Magnum
Meningioma
Neurilemoma

Brainstem
Glioma

Pineal Region
Pineocytoma/blastoma
Germ cell tumors
Gliomas
Tentorial meningioma

Presentation

The presence of the cerebellum, midbrain, pons, medulla, and multiple cranial nerves in the posterior fossa provides lesions in this area with a multitude of possible signs and symptoms. Patients may present with signs and symptoms of elevated intracranial pressure, which may occur as a result of local mass effect or hydrocephalus secondary to obstruction of CSF flow either through the aqueduct or out of the fourth ventricle. The initial presenting symptom can be nonspecific, and false localizing signs are especially common with medulloblastomas, fourth ventricular ependymomas, and hemangioblastomas. Early symptoms may be very nonspecific: listlessness, headache, fatigue, vomiting, anorexia, and personality changes. As lesions increase in size, signs of brainstem and cerebellar involvement appear. More specific clinical syndromes may occur with tumors that early on involve neural structures, such as acoustic neurilemomas, other cerebellopontine angle tumors, brainstem gliomas, and carotid body tumors. Five symptom complexes will be discussed.

Elevated Intracranial Pressure

As the lesion progresses and elevated intracranial pressure develops, headache (which may be nocturnal or worse on awakening and relieved by vomiting), vomiting, nausea, drowsiness, diplopia, unsteady gait, urinary incontinence, and mental status changes may occur. The unsteady gait, urinary incontinence, and mental status changes may result from hydrocephalus. Hydrocephalus is most likely to occur in midline lesions and at an early stage. In infants an enlarging head or tense fontanelle may indicate underlying hydrocephalus. Hydrocephalus also can reduce visual acuity because of an enlarging blind spot, and patients may present with visual problems. Headache may occur well before the development of any neurologic signs. Early neurologic signs may be vague: gait ataxia or a head tilt (from a trochlear nerve [IV] paresis or tonsillar herniation) or be falsely localizing, such as a unilateral or bilateral abducens nerve (VI) palsy. Unlike supratentorial lesions, oculomotor nerve (III) problems are uncommon and are usually a late manifestation unless associated with an internuclear ophthalmoplegia. Failure of upgaze indicates pressure on the midbrain.

Midline Cerebellar Lesions

Midline and fourth ventricular tumors tend to result in truncal ataxia, wide-based gait, nystagmus, extraocular movement abnormalities, and truncal titubation. Hydrocephalus is common and occurs early, and papilledema is frequent. As the lesion increases in size, the brainstem becomes compressed.

Lateral Cerebellar Hemispheric Lesions

With more lateral lesions in the cerebellar hemisphere, other signs may occur, including hypotonia, intention tremor, limb ataxia, dysmetria, dysdiadochokinesia, and dysarthria. Ocular abnormalities include nystagmus, gaze paresis, and skew deviation. Hydrocephalus is less frequent, later in appearance, and is characterized by hemispheric lesions.

Tonsillar Herniation

Meningismus, head tilt, muscle spasm, and opisthotonos may result from herniation of the cerebellar tonsils through the foramen magnum, especially in children. Vomiting, skew deviation of the eyes, and downbeat nystagmus may be present. Posturing from tonsillar herniation may be mistaken for "cerebellar fits." Long-tract signs indicate involvement of the brainstem. Bulbar palsies with vocal cord paralysis and swallowing and gag dysfunction may occur. Occipital headaches and neck pain are common. Coughing may induce paroxysms of increased symptomatology, including loss of consciousness, as the tonsils are impacted further into the foramen magnum. As further herniation compresses the medulla, respiration becomes irregular and death may result.

Brainstem Syndromes

A variety of ocular problems (pupil size, ocular motility, nystagmus) and sensory or motor deficits may occur. Respiratory changes vary depending on the level of brainstem compression (hyperventilation changing to apneustic and ataxic breathing as the compression passes caudally).[42] Multiple cranial nerve problems, including bulbar palsies, are common. Cranial nerve problems ipsilateral to the lesion and extremity motor/sensory deficits contralateral to the lesion are characteristic of brainstem lesions. With progressive external compression of the brainstem from midline/fourth ventricular lesions, gaze and facial palsies develop with rapid loss of consciousness, respiratory changes, bradycardia, and hypertension.

Distant Symptoms

Leptomeningeal spread of tumors (medulloblastoma, ependymoma, glioblastoma) may produce spinal cord or nerve root symptoms. Involvement of the cerebral cortex may result in seizures.

SPECIFIC TUMOR TYPES WITHIN THE POSTERIOR FOSSA
Medulloblastoma/PNET

Medulloblastomas are believed by some to be the fourth ventricular manifestation of primitive neuroectodermal tumors (PNET).[44] They occur primarily in 4- to 8-year olds, and there is an equal sex distribution. Medulloblastoma accounts for 4% to 10% of all brain tumors and a fifth of pediatric brain tumors.[48] Patients present with a short history (1 to 5 months)[5] because of the aggressiveness of the tumor and its midline location, which results in obstructive hydrocephalus. Elevated intracranial pressure, therefore, occurs early with truncal ataxia.

Cerebellar Astrocytoma

Cerebellar astrocytoma is a lesion that develops in the first two decades and is usually not anaplastic, unlike the adult glial cerebellar tumors. It is also usually circumscribed and frequently cystic. Symptoms are present for longer periods than with the more aggressive PNETs and may even be present for 1 or 2 years. As the lesion is usually hemispheric, limb ataxia predominates although unsteadiness is still common. Headaches and vomiting are a later manifestation.[23,54]

Ependymoma

Ependymomas are twice as common in children and adolescents (10% of all brain tumors) than adults and tend to occur in the first decade. The majority of posterior fossa ependymomas arise from the floor of the fourth ventricle, which is also the commonest site for ependymomas in children.[45] They may extend laterally through the foramen of Magendie and Luschka, interrupting CSF flow, or they may invade the medulla. Symptoms tend to be like those in medulloblastoma but with a longer time course and with few early cerebellar signs. Lower cranial nerve involvement and long-tract signs may occur in addition to the signs of elevated intracranial pressure.[11]

Choroid Plexus Papilloma

Choroid plexus papilloma of the fourth ventricle occurs primarily in the first decade. Symptoms are primarily that of hydrocephalus. Lateral extension out of the foramen of Luschka may result in cerebellopontine angle symptoms.[29]

Hemangioblastoma

Hemangioblastoma may occur as part of the von Hippel–Lindau syndrome, which may be inherited as an autosomal dominant trait or may be isolated. It is the commonest adult primary cerebellar tumor (7% of adult posterior fossa tumors)[45] and is located in the cerebellar hemisphere. Dizziness and gait and limb ataxia develop along with signs of intracranial hypertension. Polycythemia secondary to erythropoietin secretion is not uncommon.

Acoustic Neurilemoma

Acoustic neurilemomas are benign tumors usually occurring in the fifth to sixth decade with an equal sex distribution. They are usually solitary, but bilateral tumors may occur as part of type II neurofibromatosis. Such tumors usually occur early, bilaterally, and with multiple meningiomas. The tumor arises from the vestibular division of the cochlear nerve (VIII) within the internal auditory canal and then grows out into the posterior fossa in the cerebellopontine angle. Here the facial (VII) and trigeminal (V) nerves may be compressed. The lower cranial nerves are rarely involved although displacement of the pons and lateral medulla may occur along with hydrocephalus if the tumor is large enough.

Hearing loss is the commonest symptom. Headaches, altered balance, unsteady gait, tinnitus, and, rarely, facial pain or weakness may be initial complaints.[38] Vertigo, nausea, and vomiting may also be present. Variable involvement of the VIII nerve is present on examination. Some facial weakness or facial sensory loss (especially a reduced corneal reflex) may be found on examination. Gait abnormalities and unilateral limb ataxia may be present.

Meningioma

Posterior fossa meningiomas account for 10% of all meningiomas and are found at the cerebellopontine angle, posterior surface of the petrous ridge, tentorium cerebelli, clivus, foramen magnum, fourth ventricle, and occipital squamosa. Cerebellar symptoms predominate, with lesions arising from the occipital squamosa, the tentorium, and the petrous ridge. Clival lesions produce brainstem and lower cranial nerve problems, but obstructive hydrocephalus occurs early from fourth ventricular tumors. The rare foramen magnum tumors present with occipital and neck pain and extremity dysesthesia followed by upper extremity weakness and gait and urinary problems. Cranial nerve involvement is likely with the cerebellopontine angle and tentorial meningiomas. The trigeminal and facial nerve are most likely to be involved.

Other Cerebellopontine Angle Tumors

Trigeminal nerve neurilemomas may present in a way similar to acoustic nerve neurilemomas although facial numbness is seen earlier and deafness and tinnitus later in the former cases. Other lesions include epidermoids, glomus jugulare tumors, metastases, arachnoid cysts, and vascular malformations. In this latter group, lower cranial nerve involvement is more common and the time course is different from that of acoustic nerve involvement. Rarely, fourth ventricular tumors may grow laterally into the cerebellopontine angle and mimic an acoustic nerve tumor. Vertigo may be present with lesions in this area.

Brainstem Glioma

Brainstem gliomas tend to occur in childhood and adolescence although cases in older adults are not unknown.[32] The majority arise in the pons and are usually slow growing and diffusely infiltrating although focal, cystic, cervicomedullary, and exophytic lesions occur.[9] Anaplastic changes can occur. Symptoms are variable and often insidious.[40] Most patients present with some form of cranial nerve involvement, which is initially unilateral and often involves nerves VI and VII. Long-tract signs with hemiparesis or paraparesis, hemisensory syndromes, unilateral ataxia, gait ataxia, and gaze palsies then develop. Headaches and vomiting are late manifestations. Symptoms usually progress over several years unless there is a malignant transformation to glioblastoma.

Clival Tumors

Clival tumors are rare and usually comprise meningiomas and chordomas with early involvement of the lower cranial nerves. Such tumors are frequently inoperable. If surgery is indicated, tumors of the lower clivus can be treated through a cerebellopontine angle or transfacial or far lateral transcondylar approach. Midclival tumors can also be treated from a transfacial, transpetrosal, or lateral infratemporal approach. Above the midportion of the clivus, a supratentorial exposure is often used although transfacial, subfrontal transbasal, and lateral approaches are also possible.

Preoperative Evaluation
Radiology

With the advent of computed tomography in the 1970s and magnetic resonance imaging in the 1980s, neurodiagnostic studies of posterior fossa lesions have been revolutionized. Magnetic resonance (MR) is the imaging modality of choice whenever a lesion in the brainstem, posterior fossa, or craniocervical junction is suspected. The more recent use of gadolinium enhancement has added even more sensitivity to this diagnostic procedure. The lack of artifacts from the surrounding bony structures, the ability to image in multiple planes, and the excellent contrast resolution give MR a clear superiority over CT for many lesions. This is especially true for small acoustic neurilemomas and other cerebellopontine angle lesions, brainstem lesions, and skull base tumors, and for the assessment of tonsillar herniation.

CT is still a useful technique, and when conducted with contrast and carried out on high-resolution equipment can detect nearly all posterior fossa tumors. It allows visualization of hydrocephalus and mass effect. Its greatest value, however, is high-resolution determination of detailed bony anatomy. Air or dye cisternograms with high-resolution CT are now rarely indicated except in cases of equivocal CT or MR studies for small acoustic neurilemomas. Advances in MR technology should soon make these techniques redundant.

Imaging allows intraaxial and extraaxial lesions to be differentiated, allows visualization of the surrounding anatomic structures, and may provide information on the pathology of the lesion itself. All these factors are useful in the surgeon's deliberations on the need for surgery and the most optimal approach. The displacement of parenchymal structures, presence of bone erosion, well-delineated margins, and contiguity with surrounding dural or bony structures are characteristic of extraaxial lesions. Intraaxial lesions do not erode bone and often have indistinct margins (except for cerebellar astrocytomas and hemangioblastomas).[55] Nonneoplastic lesions, such as abscess, hematoma, or infarct, are usually easily distinguished although the thin enhancing rim of abscesses may sometimes be indistinguishable from the shaggy rim usually found with metastases.

The main differential diagnosis of a lesion in the cerebellopontine angle is that of meningioma vs. acoustic neurilemoma. The meningioma usually enhances more evenly on CT, has a broader base, may extend into the middle fossa, and rarely erodes the internal auditory canal.[28]

Vascular lesions may be visible on CT or MR imaging. The indications for MR angiography remain to be determined. Formal cerebral angiography remains the procedure of choice in diagnosing aneurysms and vascular malformations. The so-called angiographically occult vascular malformations are readily visualized with MR, where they have a classic appearance and where the multiplanar images of MR allow excellent visualization of their exact location. MR also allows, in most cases, inflammatory/demyelinating lesions, such as occur with multiple sclerosis, to be clearly differentiated from brainstem neoplasms.

Neurophysiologic Studies

Brainstem auditory evoked responses and electronystagmography are rarely required for diagnosis. They may still be of some use for acoustic neurilemomas and multiple sclerosis if MR is not available. Auditory evoked responses and facial nerve stimulation intraoperatively are of some value in reducing complications from surgical manipulation. Audiology preoperatively and postoperatively for acoustic neurilemomas is useful for follow-up.

Treatment
Surgical

The aim of any surgical procedure for a tumor in the posterior fossa, as for a tumor anywhere else in the central nervous system, is to obtain a pathologic diagnosis, reduce any mass effect, and, if possible, undertake a curative resection. With the exception of extraaxial lesions in the cerebellopontine angle, dermoids, epidermoids, and some hemangioblastomas, most tumors are unlikely to be cured by surgery alone. Certain lesions such as brainstem gliomas may only require biopsy for diagnosis. With infiltrative pontine gliomas, the diagnosis is usually obvious from the clinical and radiographic findings, and biopsy usually is not indicated. If deemed necessary, biopsy is usually carried out using a stereotactic needle biopsy technique although exophytic lesions may lend themselves to open biopsy and even debulking. Other lesions should be resected only to the extent possible without significant harm to the patient. Hemispheric lesions are more likely to be completely resectable than those involving the fourth ventricle or brainstem. The operating microscope, ultrasonic aspirator, and laser now enable surgeons to remove many tumors previously thought to be unresectable.

Patients with obstructive hydrocephalus may require some form of CSF diversion, usually a temporary ventriculostomy. Preoperative shunting is rarely done. The degree of hydrocephalus and the likelihood of resolution with removal of the mass determine whether preoperative CSF diversion is required. In cases where preoperative shunting is not mandated by patient condition to relieve raised intracranial pressure, perioperative ventriculostomy may be sufficient, and a permanent shunt is avoided. The use of filters in shunt systems to prevent systemic spread of tumors such as medulloblastomas is not thought to be useful because of the high shunt failure rates caused by blockage of the filters and the low incidence of shunt-induced tumor dissemination.[3]

Nonsurgical

Radiotherapy is useful both as primary and adjuvant therapy.[30] In brainstem gliomas and with other tumors deemed nonsurgical (multiple metastases with known primary lesion or poor patient condition), radiotherapy is the mainstay of treatment. After resection of malignant tumors such as medulloblastomas, ependymomas, and glioblastomas, radiation is useful. It may also be helpful in recurrences of "benign" tumors such as cerebellopontine angle and petrous ridge meningiomas or clival chordomas, where further resection is not possible. Radiation therapy after subtotal resection of astrocytomas. may also have some benefit. Tumors with a propensity for leptomeningeal spread (medulloblastoma and ependymoma) may require craniospinal radiation.[46] This has severe intellectual and endocrinologic effects in young children in addition to the neurotoxicity from radiation found in any age group. Prophylactic craniospinal radiation prevents recurrences and prolongs survival in patients with medulloblastoma and possibly ependymoma. Lymphomas in the posterior fossa, as elsewhere, respond well to radiation.

The role of stereotactic radiosurgery in the treatment of posterior fossa tumors remains to be determined. Acoustic neurilemomas have been treated and the disease stabilized.[31] Facial nerve dysfunction still occurs, although in a delayed fashion, and there has been a considerable rate of trigeminal nerve dysfunction after such therapy.[4] Patients with malignant tumors of the posterior fossa that have recurred or where no further external beam radiation is possible may be potential candidates for radiosurgery. Brainstem lesions cannot be treated with this modality because of the sensitivity of the brainstem to such high doses of radiation.

Chemotherapy for medulloblastoma appears to be useful, especially in younger patients in whom radiation is best avoided.[1] Chemotherapy has not been shown to be clearly beneficial in ependymoma. As with supratentorial glioblastomas, lesions in the posterior fossa may show some response to chemotherapy. Steroids (dexamethasone) remain vitally important in both preoperative and postoperative management of patients with tumors, especially if significant edema is present. The role of hormonal therapy for meningiomas and newer therapies such as hyperthermia, immunotherapy, immunotoxins, and photodynamic therapy remains to be determined.

Prognosis

Hemangioblastomas, acoustic neurilemomas, meningiomas, epidermoids, and choroid plexus papillomas are potentially curable if completely resected. The cystic nature, the presence of a mural nodule in many hemangioblastomas, and their hemispheric location make them especially amenable to surgical cure although recurrences and distant tumors after subtotal resection occur.[45]

Glioblastoma, even after surgery, radiation, and chemotherapy, is associated with a median survival of little more than a year.[47] The well-circumscribed cystic astrocytoma of the cerebellum in patients under 20 years of age is associated with an excellent prognosis of 80% at 20 years.[14] However, anaplastic change and even distant CSF metastases are not unknown.[45] Survival rates for children with medulloblastoma are variable; those who had a total resection and no distal spread, who were over 3 years of age, and who had undifferentiated tumors had 5-year survival rates of 60% to 75% after treatment.[10] Ependymoma survival rates are also variable (with children doing worse) with a 5-year survival of 20% to 30%.[19] Diffusely infiltrating brainstem gliomas are associated with survival rates of less than 10% at 3 years.[32]

TUMORS OUTSIDE THE POSTERIOR FOSSA
Pineal Tumors

Although pineal tumors are not strictly posterior fossa tumors, they are discussed in this chapter because many of the surgical approaches traverse the posterior fossa. Tumors may arise from pineal parenchymal cells (pineoblastomas, pineocytomas), germ cells (germinomas, teratomas, yolk sac carcinomas) and support cells (astrocytomas, glioblastomas, meningiomas). These tumors tend to occur in children or young adults. Patients frequently present with elevated intracranial pressure from hydrocephalus resulting from aqueductal compression. The classic Parinaud's syndrome (failure of upgaze, slightly large pupil with light-near dissociation, convergence-retraction nystagmus) or a variation may be present. Cerebellar symptoms may result from superior cerebellar compression. Hypothalamic extension may cause endocrine problems.

CT and MR are the diagnostic procedures of choice. Angiography is now less useful given the ability of MR to show large vessels (such as the internal cerebral vein), although it is necessary if a vein of Galen anomaly is suspected.

Hydrocephalus may require shunting, and this may be the only treatment necessary. This was especially so in the past, when surgery of this region was associated with a significant morbidity. Histologic diagnosis is now undertaken in most cases and has acceptable morbidity with either an open or stereotactic percutaneous biopsy. Benign tumors may be curable surgically; some, such as germinomas, are very responsive to radiation.

The supracerebellar subtentorial approach is especially suited for pineal lesions that do not extend above the incisura or laterally into the trigone of the lateral ventricle. This approach avoids the problems of cerebral hemispheric retraction that occur with occipital transtentorial or transcallosal approaches and avoids the large venous structures lying over the pineal region.[51] Some neurosurgeons believe it is the only approach requiring a sitting position.

MICROVASCULAR DECOMPRESSION

The concept of vascular compression of a cranial nerve has been recognized for more than 80 years.[6,52] Compression of the trigeminal nerve at its entry zone into the pons was first suggested by Dandy.[7] Over the last 15 years, there has been an increasing trend for neurosurgeons to undertake microvascular decompressive surgery for a variety of cranial nerve disorders previously considered to be idiopathic. Jannetta[26,27] has championed these vascular decompression procedures to alleviate vascular compression at the root entry zone, which he believed to be the cause of various hyperactive cranial nerve dysfunctions causing trigeminal neuralgia, hemifacial spasm, acoustic nerve dysfunction, and glossopharyngeal neuralgia. Although the presence of small vessels impinging on the root entry zone of many cranial nerves is well documented clinically and pathologically[16,18] and the procedure is associated with good results in two thirds of patients with trigeminal neuralgia[2] and is even more successful in patients with hemifacial spasm,[33] the exact pathophysiologic mechanism remains controversial.

The procedure in essence comprises a small retromastoid craniectomy with either a superolateral cerebellar approach to the trigeminal nerve or an inferolateral approach to the facial, acoustic, and glossopharyngeal nerves. Compression of the dorsal root entry zone of the nerve in question by an arterial loop or less frequently, a venous one, is relieved by mobilizing the loop and keeping it in its new position away from the nerve with a foreign body (usually Teflon felt, muscle, silicone, or plastic sponge). Small veins may be coagulated and divided rather than displaced with a cushion of material, but larger veins are best left uncoagulated for fear of vascular impairment of the brainstem. Frequently more than one vessel may be involved. Previously unidentified mass lesions are usually extraaxial and benign and may be resectable.

Adequate imaging studies (MR) are necessary to ensure that no mass lesions are responsible for these syndromes and that other medical causes, such as multiple sclerosis, are not involved. Preoperative facial, temporal, and masseter muscle electromyography and otovestibular assessment may be useful.

Trigeminal Neuralgia

Patients with medically refractory tic douloureux, who have not responded to other procedures such as percutaneous rhizotomy and who are in good medical condition with an anticipated long survival, are candidates for microvascular decompression. Pain relief is often immediate, especially if the nerve has been manipulated during surgery. Otherwise, pain relief may come slowly over several weeks. Recurrences in 16% to 30% of patients[2,26] may be seen, depending on the follow-up and the careful selection of patients with classic tic douloureux as opposed to atypical syndromes. This procedure is less successful in patients who have had previous pain relief procedures. A descending loop of the superior cerebellar artery is usually responsible for the nerve compression although an ascending loop of the anterior-inferior cerebellar artery may be responsible, especially for pain involving the ophthalmic division of the trigeminal nerve.[26] Unlike destructive procedures for this condition, anesthesia dolorosa, numbness, and dysesthesia are avoided.

Hemifacial Spasm

Distortion of the facial nerve by the vertebral artery or the posterior inferior or anterior inferior cerebellar artery may cause hemifacial spasm. Jannetta[27] reported complete response to surgery in 89% of 366 cases followed for a mean of 5½ years. Brainstem auditory evoked potentials, direct auditory nerve compound action potentials, and facial nerve electromyography are useful adjuncts in reducing operative complications such as hearing loss[35] and assessing the completeness of decompression.[17]

Acoustic Nerve Dysfunction

Disabling positional vertigo distinct from Ménière's disease, vestibular neuritis, and benign positional vertigo has been successfully relieved in many patients by microvascular decompression.[24,36] This is especially so for those cases with vestibular involvement as opposed to those with a combination of cochlear and vestibular involvement or cochlear nerve compression only (86% success). The vertebral artery is the usual culprit.[27] Tinnitus associated with the vestibular dysfunction may be relieved as well, especially if it is mild. Postoperative deafness may occur, and, despite the use of intraoperative brainstem auditory evoked potential and direct auditory compound action potential monitoring, this still occurs in 4% of patients.

Glossopharyngeal Neuralgia

This is a rare condition, and there is little published research on treating this by microvascular decompression.[27] The vertebral artery or the posterior-inferior cerebellar artery may cause compression of the glossopharyngeal and vagal nerve root entry zones. Many surgeons continue to section the nerve because manipulation in this region may produce sudden and severe hypertension. Jannetta[25] has noted an association between left vagal nerve stretching and medullary compression after glossopharyngeal microvascular decompression and postoperative hypertension and has operated on a series of patients with "essential" hypertension to decompress the vagus nerve and anterolateral medulla.

DEVELOPMENTAL ANOMALIES
Chiari Malformation

Various types of Chiari malformation have been categorized. The commonest are the Chiari type I, where there is descent of the cerebellar tonsils into the cervical spinal canal, and the classic Arnold-Chiari or Chiari type II, where the inferior vermis is herniated through the foramen magnum along with additional anomalies including beaking of the quadrigeminal plate, elongation of the fourth ventricle, and kinking of the medulla. Various other anomalies of the brain, skull, and meninges are associated with this condition.[12] Chiari type II is nearly always associated with spina bifida aperta. Chiari type III is essentially a hindbrain hernia into an occipital encephalocele. Hydromyelia/syringomyelia is a common accompaniment of Chiari type I and type II. Hydrocephalus is nearly always present in Chiari type II but is less common in Chiari type I. Because of this association and the fact that increased intracranial pressure can exacerbate symptoms that resemble those of Chiari malformation or hydromyelia/syringomyelia, the surgeon must be sure that hydrocephalus, if present, is well controlled before embarking on the treatment of Chiari malformations or hydromyelia/syringomyelia.

Chiari type I usually presents in late childhood or young adulthood, but type II manifests itself in the neonate. Symptoms of elevated intracranial pressure, a classic downbeat nystagmus (vertical nytagmus in a downward direction), cerebellar ataxia, bulbar dysfunction, and signs and symptoms of syringomyelia (capelike sensory loss extending to the face, back of the head, and onto the trunk, long-tract signs, and upper extremity atrophy) may be present in patients with Chiari type I. Headaches may be related to craniocervical pressure dissociation across the foramen magnum and to hydrocephalus. Chiari type II infants have progressive hydrocephalus and lower cranial nerve problems with stridor and swallowing problems in addition to their spina bifida.

The use of MR has increased the diagnosis of "hindbrain hernias" tremendously. Syringomyelias are also easily recognized with MR, and surgeons have had an increasing problem in deciding whether the lesions seen are in fact symptomatic. Without doubt, many patients with this problem are being diagnosed with increasing frequency at a far earlier stage of their disease, and the exact indications for surgical treatment of asymptomatic or minimally symptomatic patients remain to be determined.

Surgical therapy is indicated when brainstem or long-tract signs are present or the patient suffers from intractable headaches. A suboccipital craniectomy with an upper cervical laminectomy and some form of dural augmentation is the standard treatment. Adequate bone decompression down to the caudal extent of the cerebellar herniation is necessary. In neonates and young children, care must be taken when opening the dura because the torcula Herophili and transverse sinuses may be caudally displaced. Unrestricted flow of CSF out of the fourth ventricle must be obtained, and lysis of dense arachnoidal adhesions or even placement of a stent may be required. Care must be taken to ensure that the entire herniated cerebellar tissue is well decompressed. Some surgeons resect the herniated cerebellar tonsils to help achieve this, but we have not found this to be necessary. Associated cervical syrinxes may require some form of syringo-subarachnoid, pleural, or peritoneal shunt. Gardner's classic plugging of the obex is less frequently conducted today.[13] Modern neurosurgical techniques allow symptomatic improvement in 86% of patients with Chiari malformations.[8]

Craniovertebral Junction Anomalies

A wide variety of developmental and acquired craniovertebral junction anomalies exist. These include Klippel-Feil syndrome, basilar invagination, and various traumatic, inflammatory (especially rheumatoid), and metabolic (Paget's disease, Morquio's disease, Hurler's syndrome) causes of odontoid problems. Foramen magnum stenosis from achondroplasia and rickets as well as atlantooccipital and atlantoaxial instability (as in Down syndrome) also occur. In addition to an attempt to realign the craniospinal axis in reducible lesions, some form of posterior fossa decompressive craniectomy with or without occipitocervical fusion, may be necessary if the principal component of brainstem compromise is from the dorsal aspect. Lesions with a primary ventral compressive effect are more effectively treated through an anterior transoral approach. Traction to correct alignment preoperatively must be maintained during surgery and may need to be continued postoperatively.[34]

VASCULAR LESIONS

Posterior circulation aneurysms account for 15% of all aneurysms. Half of these occur at the basilar bifurcation and require a supratentorial approach. Although aneurysms of the vertebral and vertebrobasilar artery are rare, they are best treated through a suboccipital approach. Lesions of the basilar trunk and anterior inferior cerebellar artery may be approached from either a suboccipital or subtemporal transtentorial approach, and the direction of projection of the aneurysmal dome determines the approach that will allow early visualization of the neck of the aneurysm.[41] The transoral transclival approach for basilar trunk lesions has been tried, but there is a high risk of meningitis. The far lateral transcondylar approach is useful for some aneurysms of the vertebral arteries, posterior inferior cerebellar artery, or vertebrobasilar junction.[21]

Arteriovenous malformations of the lateral and sigmoid dural sinuses are probably acquired lesions following some form of sinus thrombosis and usually present with pulsatile tinnitus and headache. Other manifestations of elevated intracranial pressure and focal neurologic findings secondary to arterialized cortical venous drainage may occur. A bruit is not uncommon over the mastoid area. Interventional neuroradiologic techniques with preoperative embolization are extremely useful in reducing the blood flow through these lesions, which may then be excised through a combined supratentorial and infratentorial approach exposing the transverse sinus. The medial aspect of the transverse sinus and the lower aspect of the sagittal sinus and torcula are then skeletonized and the abnormal vascular connection interrupted.[53]

Cerebellar arteriovenous malformations may present with mass effects, hemorrhage, or hydrocephalus caused by arterialized veins obstructing the aqueduct of Sylvius. A wide bilateral suboccipital craniectomy and C1 laminectomy allow exposure of the superior cerebellar artery (supracerebellar infratentorial approach), the anterior inferior cerebellar artery (cerebellopontine angle approach), and the posterior inferior cerebellar artery (approaching from under the tonsils) to ensure control of all three major posterior fossa arterial supplies.[37]

Cavernous malformations of the brainstem are becoming increasingly recognized, especially with the advent of MR. Both compressive and hemorrhagic symptoms occur. Lesions that come close to the surface, either on the floor of the fourth ventricle or the lateral pontomedullary junction, may be excised with acceptable morbidity through a suboccipital or retromastoid approach.[59]

Stereotactic radiosurgery may be of use in the treatment of small "inoperable" vascular malformations outside the brainstem. Patients are not protected from hemorrhage until the lesion is completely obliterated, a process that may take up to several years. The long-term prognosis of patients with lesions no longer angiographically visible remains to be determined, as these lesions may have been merely converted to angiographically occult malformations.[22]

Cerebellar infarction is usually due to atherosclerotic disease although embolism and trauma to the vertebral arteries may also occur. The vertebral and posterior inferior cerebellar artery are the vascular territories usually involved, and swelling of the posterior inferior half of the cerebellum may cause brainstem compression. Initial symptoms may consist of nystagmus, nausea, vomiting, ataxia, and neck stiffness. This progresses to an ipsilateral nuclear gaze palsy followed by a peripheral facial palsy. Drowsiness and coma supervene, but pupils remain small, and hemiplegia is rare. Severe hypertension is frequent. Rapid progression to decerebrate posturing and death may occur. This is a neurosurgical emergency and may be one of the few remaining indications for urgent decompression without first obtaining a scan because the clinical diagnosis is frequently obvious, an early infarct may not be seen on a CT scan, and the window of opportunity is limited.[20]

Spontaneous hypertensive hemorrhages in the cerebellar hemisphere and pons are not uncommon. Hemispheric hematomas with significant distortion of the brainstem or fourth ventricle may be evacuated, but the results of surgery on lesions involving the brainstem are usually poor. Obstructive hydrocephalus may require emergency ventriculostomy, but this should not be undertaken without subsequent evacuation of the hematoma because local pressure on the brainstem continues until the clot resolves.

POSITIONING FOR POSTERIOR FOSSA APPROACHES
Sitting Position

The sitting position (Fig. 15-1) has many advantages, but careful positioning is required to prevent complications, and the risk of air embolism and hypotension is real. The use of three-point skull-fixation devices has made positioning much easier. Proponents believe strongly that gravity-assisted blood and CSF drainage away from the operative site allows better visualization of the surgical field. The cerebellar hemispheres also fall down with gravity, allowing a supracerebellar approach without retraction on the cerebellum. This position is ideally suited for supracerebellar infratentorial approaches to the pineal region and approaches to midline/fourth ventricular lesions and the cerebellopontine angle. Some consider the former indication to be the only one for a sitting position in posterior fossa surgery. The sitting position is also suitable for microvascular decompression of the trigeminal nerve via a superolateral approach but not for decompression of the lower cranial nerves because upward retraction on the cerebellum is then necessary. Approaches under the cerebellar hemisphere requiring upward retraction on the cerebellum are best done in another position although removal of the arch of the atlas helps improve the approach from a more inferior direction under the cerebellar tonsils and reduces the amount of medial retraction of the cerebellar hemisphere that is required.

In addition to the risks of air embolism and hypotension, many other problems are associated with the sitting position, to the extent that it has fallen somewhat out of favor with many surgeons. The patient must be positioned such that the surgeon's neck is not extended and that the surgeon's arms are resting at a comfortable level below his/her eyes or arm and neck fatigue and discomfort rapidly ensue. Another problem is that of the highly angled tentorium. This may be such that, despite maximal neck flexion, the angle is too steep for the surgeon to work comfortably, with the result that the surgeon is peering up under the tentorium toward the ceiling throughout the entire case. Care must also be taken to ensure that sciatic and ulnar neuropraxias are prevented by careful flexing of the knees and padding of the elbows. The (well-padded) arms should be crossed across the chest and the weight of the arms supported. In patients with a large trunk and thick arms, it is not always possible to place the arms within the frame holding the head holder; the arms should then be placed on padded supports with the arms supported as in an armchair to prevent downward traction on the shoulder.

Cases of quadriplegia have been reported after sitting-position procedures and may be related to stretching of the spinal cord by excessive neck flexion with resultant loss of vascular autoregulation coupled with intraoperative hypotension, causing a vascular insult.[56] This is especially likely to happen in patients with a spondylitic spine, such as the elderly who may already have some stenosis of the central canal.

Some surgeons place a burr hole in the parietooccipital region at the start of the case if there is an element of hydrocephalus that has not been treated preoperatively. This is especially so for the midline lesions. This "Dandy" hole allows the surgeon to drain the ventricles quickly if necessary either during the case or in the postoperative period should postoperative swelling, causing more obstructive hydrocephalus, occur. A frontally placed ventricular drain may also be used and has the advantage of being further from the main incision and, compared with a parietooccipital catheter, there is less chance of occlusion of the catheter by choroid plexus lying in the body of the lateral ventricle.

A perioperative ventriculostomy may allow sufficient drainage until the underlying problem is surgically treated and postoperative swelling has subsided. The problems of malfunction and infection of a permanent shunt system are thus avoided. It is absolutely essential that the drainage from any CSF drainage system be well controlled during surgery. Careful placement of the drainage chamber relative to the patient's head and controlled drainage during the surgery are vital. This is especially so in the sitting position, where excessive drainage may cause major brain shifts and initiate subdural hematomas supratentorially from a collapsing brain. If a permanent system has already been placed, consideration should be given to temporarily occluding it during the surgery. This is one reason why placement of a shunt before craniotomy for treatment of the underlying problem is avoided, if possible, by using a temporary ventriculostomy if preoperative drainage is essential. It is generally considered prudent to delay placement of a permanent shunt system until after any intradural procedure in which CSF loss is likely.

There have also been a handful of cases of supratentorial hemorrhage in the subcortical white matter after posterior fossa surgery in the sitting position.[15,49] The exact mechanism is not known but may involve either altered intracranial pressure dynamics with resultant venous disruption or positional effects on the carotid or vertebral vessels leading to a hemorrhagic infarction. The initial hemorrhage may be partly mitigated by the lower pressure in the cerebral veins in the sitting position. With repositioning and increase in the venous pressure or some minor subsequent trauma from coughing or vomiting, further hemorrhage may occur, resulting in the late deterioration of some of the patients reported.

Prone Position

The prone position (Fig. 15-2) avoids somewhat the problems of air embolism and hypotension seen with the sitting

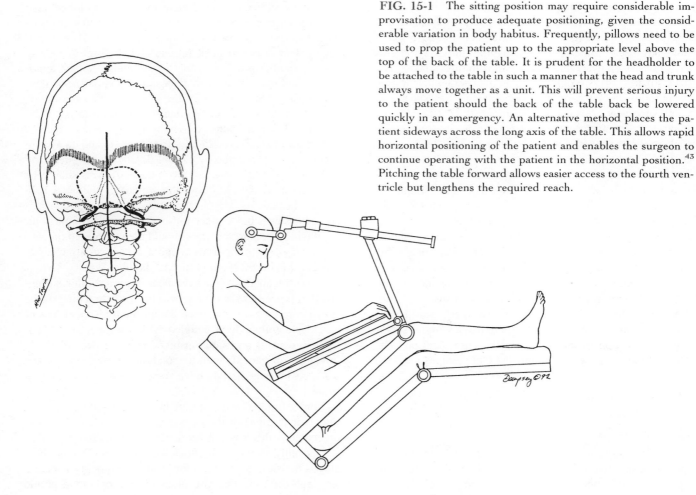

FIG. 15-1   The sitting position may require considerable improvisation to produce adequate positioning, given the considerable variation in body habitus. Frequently, pillows need to be used to prop the patient up to the appropriate level above the top of the back of the table. It is prudent for the headholder to be attached to the table in such a manner that the head and trunk always move together as a unit. This will prevent serious injury to the patient should the back of the table back be lowered quickly in an emergency. An alternative method places the patient sideways across the long axis of the table. This allows rapid horizontal positioning of the patient and enables the surgeon to continue operating with the patient in the horizontal position.[43] Pitching the table forward allows easier access to the fourth ventricle but lengthens the required reach.

position. However, because the head is usually elevated a little above the heart to help with gravity drainage of fluids from the surgical field, these problems are not totally ameliorated. The prone position is especially useful for lesions in the midline, medial hemisphere, and fourth ventricle. Exposure of the cerebellopontine angle is possible but requires rotation of the head. The position is more commonly used in children because of the ease of positioning a child in the prone position. In large adults obtaining an adequate prone position is sometimes almost impossible. There are also potential ventilation problems, whether the patient is on a frame or chest rolls, and airway access is difficult. The head should be held in position with a three-point skull-fixation device and not on a horseshoe frame because permanent damage from prolonged pressure on the eyes and forehead may occur. This has happened even if precautions were taken because the head can slip, producing pressure on the eye. Pressure necrosis of the skin can develop even if the weight of the head on the horseshoe frame is frequently relieved during the procedure. If a horseshoe headrest is used (e.g., in infants), covering the face with 3 cm thick soft foam padding is effective in lessening the risk of pressure necrosis. In some patients with a marked cervicothoracic kyphosis, the prone position does not allow sufficient flexion of the craniocervical junction to allow adequate exposure of the occiput and upper cervical area. As with the sit-

ting position, the prone position may cause problems with a highly angled tentorium and insufficient neck flexion to allow the most anterosuperior aspect of the cerebellum to be reached by the surgeon at a comfortable angle. In such cases, if the lesion is superficial in the cerebellum, an infraoccipital transtentorial approach may be necessary.

Lateral Position

Problems associated with air embolism are nearly absent in the lateral position, and this position (Fig. 15-3, *A*) lends itself well to approaches to the cerebellopontine angle and other lateral lesions as well as lesions of the clivus and lateral foramen magnum and other lesions requiring an infracerebellar approach. Gravity-assisted retraction of the cerebellum is especially useful for exposure of the cerebellopontine angle for acoustic neurilemoma and microvascular decompression procedures. The margins of the transverse and sigmoid sinus should always be uncovered by the craniectomy to ensure adequate room for approaching the cerebellopontine angle without excessive cerebellar retraction. There is, therefore, a risk of excessive bleeding and air embolism at the point of the procedure when the craniectomy is incomplete and there is still inadequate visualization of the sinus. There is nearly always a significant superior petrosal vein passing to the superior petrosal sinus, which may require division to gain adequate exposure to the cer-

FIG. 15-2 In the prone position, the head is distracted, and slightly flexed, and held in position with a three-point skull-fixation device. The space from the foramen magnum to C1 is opened up to allow better visualization of the inferior cerebellar contents.

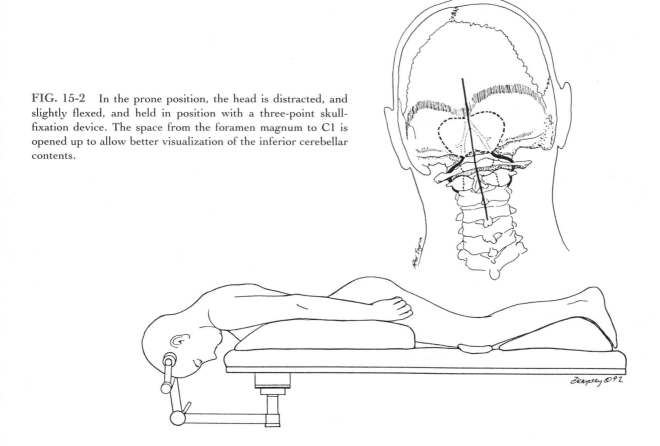

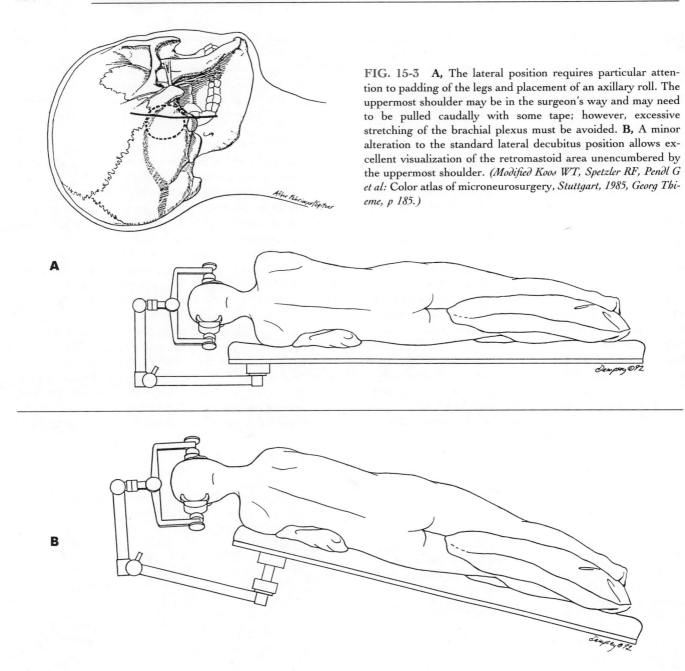

FIG. 15-3 **A,** The lateral position requires particular attention to padding of the legs and placement of an axillary roll. The uppermost shoulder may be in the surgeon's way and may need to be pulled caudally with some tape; however, excessive stretching of the brachial plexus must be avoided. **B,** A minor alteration to the standard lateral decubitus position allows excellent visualization of the retromastoid area unencumbered by the uppermost shoulder. (*Modified Koos WT, Spetzler RF, Pendl G et al: Color atlas of microneurosurgery, Stuttgart, 1985, Georg Thieme, p 185.*)

ebellopontine angle, especially so for more superior lateral problems such as with trigeminal microvascular decompressions. This vein may cause major bleeding if injudicious downward retraction on the cerebellum at the start of exposure occurs or if it is not adequately coagulated before being divided. Its short course and drainage into a major sinus make attempts to control hemorrhage difficult.

Disadvantages of the lateral position include problems with the patient's shoulders and a potential for lateral popliteal nerve palsy from inadequate padding of the fibula on the dependent leg. The superior shoulder, especially in broad-shouldered patients, may hinder the surgeon's line of

sight and require the surgeon's arms to operate in an uncomfortable position. A modification of the standard lateral decubitus position overcomes the problem of visualization of the retromastoid area and obstruction of the surgeon's arms by the uppermost shoulder. This is done by raising the head of the bed while maintaining the axis of the head parallel to the floor and allowing the uppermost shoulder to roll slightly away from the surgeon (Fig. 15-3, *B*). In any form of the lateral position, proper placement of an axillary roll is necessary to protect the inferior shoulder and axillary neurovascular structures.

A far lateral bone exposure (Fig. 15-4) using the lateral

FIG. 15-4 This modification of the position allows the exposure of far lateral structures to gain access to the vertebrobasilar junction, lower clivus, and anterior foramen magnum. It requires an extensive lateral craniectomy. Visualization is improved by tilting the head up compared with the straight lateral position. (*Modified from Heros RC: J Neurosurg 64:555-562, 1986.*)

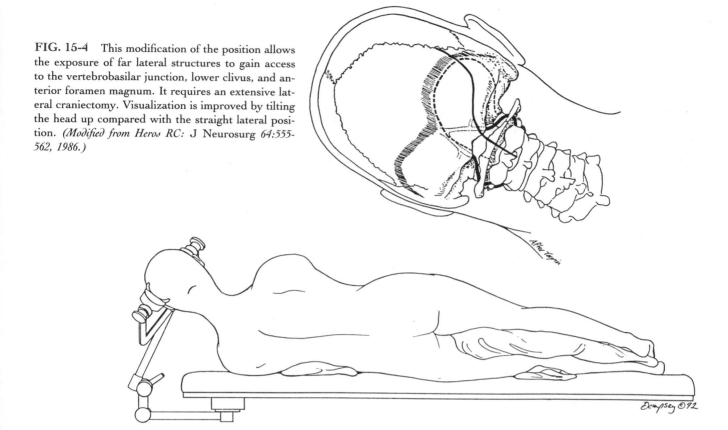

decubitus position but with the head tilted up somewhat allows excellent exposure of vertebrobasilar aneurysms, tumors of the lower clivus, and anterior meningiomas of the foramen magnum.[21]

Supine Position

The supine position (Fig. 15-5) with the head maximally laterally rotated and flexed overcomes problems in the lateral position of the superior shoulder getting in the way of the surgeon. A similar approach is possible as with the lateral position, but the surgeon does not have to peer over the patient's shoulder. The supine position also allows distribution of the patient's weight over a larger area. Nevertheless, careful elbow padding is necessary. The neck positioning required, however, is not always possible, especially in the elderly with a spondylitic spine, and careful positioning of the neck in the anesthetized patient is necessary. There is also a potential for impaired jugular venous drainage and increased brain swelling.

Park-Bench (Semiprone) Position

Compared with the prone position, the park-bench position (Fig. 15-6) allows much easier and more rapid positioning. This is useful in emergency cases where rapid access to the cerebellar hemispheres is required, such as with hematomas or infarcts. This position is usually used for parasag-

ittal approaches to hemispheric lesions. It can also be used for lateral approaches. If the patient is allowed to fall into a more prone position, the upper shoulder is also moved out of the surgeon's way, but then there is a higher risk of neck twisting and venous obstruction. Unlike the other positions, where the midsagittal plane of the head is in the true vertical or horizontal plane, the tilting of the head often makes orientation to external and internal landmarks difficult for surgeons not familiar with this head position. The dependent arm should ideally be placed at the level of the heart, but, in patients with a large body habitus, this may not be possible; therefore, it may be necessary to place the dependent arm over the edge of the head of the bed but with its weight supported.

OTHER APPROACHES
Combined Supratentorial and Infratentorial Approach

A combined lateral supratentorial and infratentorial approach is useful for many lesions that may extend through the tentorial hiatus from the anterior and superior cerebellum, from the hiatus itself, or from the cerebellopontine angle. Such an approach may require division of the transverse sinus, and a preoperative angiogram is necessary to determine the dominance of that sinus.

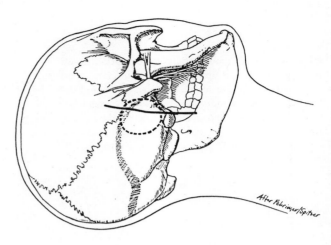

FIG. 15-5 In the supine position, careful distraction, rotation, and flexion of the neck is necessary to obtain correct head positioning. This position overcomes the problems of an obstructive shoulder often seen with the lateral position for cerebellopontine angle approaches.

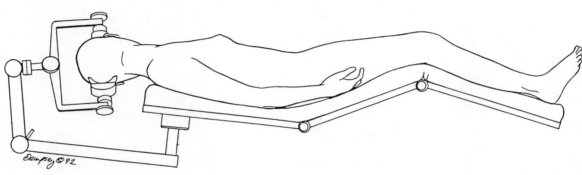

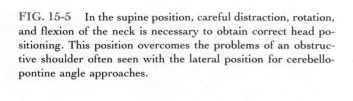

FIG. 15-6 The park-bench position is easily obtained compared with the prone position and allows lateral approaches to the cerebellar hemispheres and cerebellopontine angle.

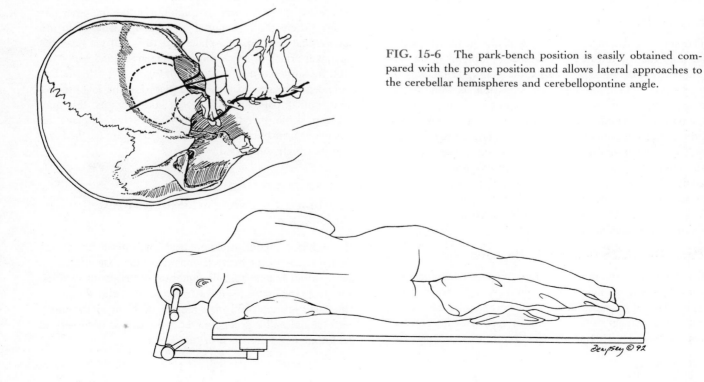

Transtentorial Approach

Lesions of the superior cerebellum, such as vascular malformations, may be treated at times more optimally via an infraoccipital transtentorial approach. Trigeminal nerve neurilemomas may be treated via a transpetrosal-transtentorial approach, which minimizes temporal lobe and cerebellar retraction. This approach also allows access to cerebellopontine angle lesions and clival lesions. An orbitozygomatic infratemporal approach for trigeminal neuromas is also possible.[57] These two approaches allow a single operation for removal of these neurilemomas, which are often dumbbell-shaped and extend into both the posterior and middle fossa. Such techniques sometimes allow one to reach as far inferiorly as the level of the facial nerve on the brainstem.

Transtemporal Approach

In addition to the standard retromastoid suboccipital approach to the cerebellopontine angle, the translabyrinthine, middle fossa, and retrolabyrinthine approaches have been used. Such approaches are usually conducted by neurosurgeons in conjunction with a neuro-otologist for the removal of acoustic neurilemomas. The translabyrinthine approach allows less cerebellar retraction and superior exposure of the lateral end of the facial nerve; the middle fossa approach allows removal of tumors limited to the internal auditory canal. The retrolabyrinthine approach requires less cerebellar retraction and is also useful for trigeminal and vestibular nerve sectioning.

Advances in skull-base surgery techniques have allowed neurosurgeons to gain access to skull-base lesions with acceptable morbidity. Such techniques may be suitable in special circumstances for approaching lesions within the posterior fossa. The majority of the transtentorial, transtemporal approaches are carried out in the lateral, supine, or semiprone position.

SUMMARY

A wide variety of pathologic conditions may require surgical intervention in the posterior cranial fossa. The commonest lesions and their typical clinical presentations have been presented. Clinical findings such as hydrocephalus and cranial nerve and cerebellar dysfunction have been discussed, and the use of a variety of diagnostic techniques, primarily radiographic studies such as CT and MR scans, to allow diagnosis and so allow the surgeon to formulate a therapeutic management plan, has been outlined.

The various patient-positioning techniques used for posterior fossa surgery have been reviewed, along with their advantages and disadvantages to the surgeon in terms of access to lesions, potential complications, and alternatives. Although the sitting position is now less commonly used than in the past, there is still a place for it in present day neurosurgery. This chapter also discussed the various decision-making processes that allow the neurosurgeon to choose the most appropriate patient position for posterior fossa surgery.

References

1. Allen J: Childhood brain tumors. Current status of clinical trials in newly diagnosed and recurrent disease, *Pediatr Clin North Am* 32:633-654, 1985.
2. Apfelbaum R: Surgery for tic douloureux, *Clin Neurosurg* 31:351-368, 1984.
3. Berger M, Baumeister B, Geyer J et al: The risks of metastases from shunting in children with primary central nervous system tumors, *J Neurosurg* 74:872-877, 1991.
4. Camarata P, Haines S, Lunsford L et al: Cranial nerve preservation after treatment of acoustic neurilemmomas: A comparison of microsurgical excision and radiosurgery, *J Neurosurg* 74:347A, 1991.
5. Choux M, Lena G: Le medulloblastome, *Neurochirurgie* 28(suppl 1), 1982.
6. Cushing H: Strangulation of the nervi abducentes by lateral branches of the basilar artery in cases of brain tumor, *Brain* 33:204-235, 1911.
7. Dandy W: Concerning the cause of trigeminal neuralgia, *Am J Surg* 24:447-455, 1934.
8. Dyste G, Menezes A, VanGilder J: Symptomatic Chiari malformation. An analysis of presentation and management and long term outcome, *J Neurosurg* 71:159-168, 1989.
9. Epstein F, Wisoff J: Brainstem tumors in childhood: surgical indications. In McLaurin R, Venes J, Schut L et al, editors: *Pediatric neurosurgery,* Philadelphia, 1989, WB Saunders, pp 357-365.
10. Evans A, Jenkin R Sposto R et al: The treatment of medulloblastoma. Results of a prospective randomized trial of radiation therapy with and without CCNU, vincristine and prednisone, *J Neurosurg* 72:572-582, 1990.
11. Fokes E, Earle K: Ependymomas: clinical and pathological aspects, *J Neurosurg* 30:585-594, 1969.
12. French B: Midline fusion defects and defects of formation. In Youmans J, editor: *Neurological surgery,* Philadelphia, 1990, WB Saunders, pp 1081-1235.
13. Gardner W, Angel J: The mechanism of syringomyelia and its surgical correction, *Clin Neurosurg* 6:131-140, 1959.
14. Gjerris F, Klinken L: Long term prognosis in children with benign cerebellar astrocytoma, *J Neurosurg* 49:179-184, 1978.
15. Haines S, Maroon J, Jannetta P: Supratentorial intracerebral hemorrhage following posterior fossa surgery, *J Neurosurg* 49:881-886, 1978.
16. Haines S, Jannetta P, Zorub D: Microvascular relations of the trigeminal nerve. An anatomical study with clinical correlation, *J Neurosurg* 52:381-386, 1980.
17. Haines S, Torres F: Intraoperative monitoring of the facial nerve during decompressive surgery for hemifacial spasm, *J Neurosurg* 74:254-257, 1991.
18. Hardy D, Rhoton A: Microsurgical relationship of the superior cerebellar artery and the trigeminal nerve, *J Neurosurg* 49:669-678, 1978.

19. Hendrik E, Raffel C: Tumors of the fourth ventricle: ependymomas, choroid plexus papillomas and dermoid cysts. In McLaurin R, Venes J, Schut L et al, editors: *Pediatric neurosurgery,* Philadelphia, 1989, WB Saunders, pp 366-372.

20. Heros R: Cerebellar hemorrhage and infarction, *Curr Concepts Cerebrovasc Dis* 16:17-22, 1981.

21. Heros R: Lateral suboccipital approach for vertebral and vertebrobasilar artery lesions, *J Neurosurg* 64:555-562, 1986.

22. Heros R, Korosue K: Radiation treatment of cerebral arteriovenous malformations (editorial), *N Engl J Med* 323:127-129, 1990.

23. Ilgren E, Stiller C: Cerebellar astrocytomas. Clinical characteristics and prognostic indices, *J Neurooncol* 4:293-308, 1987.

24. Jannetta P, Moeller M, Moeller A: Neurosurgical treatment of vertigo by microvascular decompression of the eighth cranial nerve, *Clin Neurosurg* 33:645-665, 1983.

25. Jannetta P, Segal R, Wolfson S: Neurogenic hypertension: etiology and surgical treatment I. Observations in 53 patients, *Ann Surg* 201:391-398, 1985.

26. Jannetta P: Treatment of trigeminal neuralgia by micro-operative decompression. In Youmans J, editor: *Neurological surgery,* Philadelphia, 1990, WB Saunders, pp 3928-3942.

27. Jannetta P: Cranial rhizopathies. In Youmans J, editor: *Neurological surgery,* Philadelphia, 1990, WB Saunders, pp 4169-4182.

28. Latchaw R, Johnson D, Kanal E: Primary intracranial tumors. Extra axial masses and tumors of the skull and calvarium. In Latchaw R, editor: *MR and CT imaging of the head, neck and spine,* St. Louis, 1991, Mosby–Year Book, pp 509-560.

29. Laurence K: The biology of the choroid plexus papilloma in infancy and childhood, *Acta Neurochirurgica* 50:79-90, 1979.

30. Leibel S, Sheline G: Radiation therapy for neoplasms of the brain, *J Neurosurg* 66:1-22, 1987.

31. Linskey M, Lunsford L, Flickinger J: Radiosurgery for acoustic neurinomas: early experience, *Neurosurgery* 26:736-745, 1990.

32. Littman P, Jarrett P, Bilaniuk L: Pediatric brain stem gliomas, *Cancer* 45:2787-2792, 1980.

33. Loeser J, Chen J: Hemifacial spasm: treatment by microsurgical facial nerve decompression, *Neurosurgery* 13:141-145, 1983.

34. Menezes A, VanGilder J: Anomalies of the craniovertebral junction. In Youmans J, editor: *Neurological surgery,* Philadelphia, 1990, WB Saunders, pp 1359-1420.

35. Moeller A, Jannetta P: Microvascular decompression in hemifacial spasm. Intraoperative electrophysiological observations, *Neurosurgery* 16:612-618, 1985.

36. Moeller M, Moeller A, Jannetta P et al: Diagnosis and surgical treatment of disabling positional vertigo, *J Neurosurg* 64:21-28, 1986.

37. Ojemann R, Heros R, Crowell R: Arteriovenous malformations of the brain. In: *Surgical management of cerebrovascular disease,* Baltimore, 1988, Williams & Wilkins, pp 347-414.

38. Ojemann R, Martuza R: Acoustic neuroma. In Youmans J, editor: *Neurological surgery,* Philadelphia, 1990, WB Saunders, pp 3316-3350.

39. Packer R, Schut L, Sutton L et al: Brain tumors of the posterior fossa in infants and children. In Youmans J, editor: *Neurological surgery,* Philadelphia, 1990, WB Saunders, pp 3017-3039.

40. Panitch M, Berg B: Brainstem tumors of childhood and adolescence, *Am J Dis Child* 119:465-472, 1970.

41. Peerless S, Drake C: Surgical techniques of posterior fossa aneurysms. In Schmidek H, Sweet W, editor: *Operative neurosurgical techniques. Indications, methods and results,* Orlando, 1988, Grune & Stratton, pp 973-989.

42. Plum F, Posner J: The pathologic physiology of signs and symptoms of coma. In Plum F, Posner J, editors: *The diagnosis of stupor and coma,* Philadelphia, 1980, FA Davis, pp 1-86.

43. Raimondi A: Positioning. In Raimondi A, editor: *Pediatric neurosurgery. Theoretical principles and art of surgical techniques,* New York, 1987, Springer-Verlag, pp 1-38.

44. Rorke L: The cerebellar medulloblastoma and its relationship to PNET, *J Neuropathol Exp Neurol* 42:1-15, 1983.

45. Russell D, Rubenstein L: *Pathology of tumors of the nervous system,* Baltimore, 1989, Williams & Wilkins.

46. Salazar O, Casto-Vita M, Houtte D et al: Improved survival in cases of intracranial ependymomas after radiation therapy. Late report and recommendations, *J Neurosurg* 59:652-659, 1983.

47. Salcman M: Survival in glioblastoma: historical perspective, *Neurosurgery* 7:435-439, 1980.

48. Schut L, Bruce D, Sutton L: Medulloblastoma. In Wilkins R, Rengachary S, editors: *Neurosurgery,* New York, 1985, McGraw-Hill, pp 758-762.

49. Seiler R, Zurbrugg H: Supratentorial intracerebral hemorrhage after posterior fossa operation, *Neurosurgery* 18:472-474, 1986.

50. Silverberg E: Cancer statistics, *CA* 33:9-25, 1983.

51. Stein B: Supracerebellar approach for pineal region neoplasms. In Schmidek H, Sweet W, editors: *Operative neurosurgical techniques. Indications, methods and results,* Orlando, 1988, Grune & Stratton, pp 401-409.

52. Stopford J: The arteries of the pons and medulla oblongata. Part III, *J Anat Physiol* 51:250-277, 1917.

53. Sundt T, Piepgras D, Forbes G: The surgical approach to arteriovenous malformations of the lateral and sigmoid sinuses. In Schmidek H, Sweet W, editors: *Operative neurosurgical techniques. Indications, methods and results,* Orlando, 1988, Grune & Stratton, pp 855-862.

54. Sutton L, Schut L: Cerebellar astrocytomas. In McLaurin R, Venes J, Schut L et al, editors: *Pediatric neurosurgery,* Philadelphia, 1989, WB Saunders, pp 338-346.

55. Weisberg L, Nice C: Localization of lesions. In: *Cerebral computed tomography: a text-atlas,* Philadelphia, 1989, WB Saunders, pp 37-63.

56. Wilder B: Hypothesis: the etiology of midcervical quadriplegia after operation with the patient in the sitting position, *Neurosurgery* 11:530-531, 1982.

57. Yasui T, Hakuba A, Kim S et al: Trigeminal neurinomas: operative approach in eight cases, *J Neurosurg* 71:506-511, 1989.

58. Yates A, Becker L, Sachs L et al: Brain tumors in childhood, *Childs Brain* 5:31-39, 1979.

59. Zimmerman R, Spetzler R, Lee K et al: Cavernous malformations of the brainstem, *J Neurosurg* 75:32-39, 1991.

16

Posterior Fossa: Anesthetic Considerations

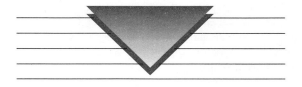

MARIE L. YOUNG

The confines of the posterior fossa and with the myriad of neuronal and vascular structures that traverse it create a challenge to the anesthesiologist, whose intraoperative goals are to facilitate surgical access, minimize nervous tissue trauma, and maintain respiratory and cardiovascular stability. The infratentorial region of the brain encloses a variety of tissue types and neuronal structures; the cerebellum, pons, and medulla are housed here, and cranial nerves V to XII originate here. Structural abnormalities in the posterior fossa requiring surgical procedures include benign and malignant tumors, aneurysms and arteriovenous malformations (AVMs), hematomas, syringomyelia, Arnold-Chiari malformation, tics, and neuralgias. This discussion will focus on the anesthetic considerations for posterior fossa surgery in adult patients; preoperative evaluation, preparation, and premedication; general monitoring considerations; choice of position for surgery; anesthetic consid-

erations; risks, prevention, detection, treatment, and complications of air embolism; and special monitoring issues.

PREOPERATIVE EVALUATION AND PREPARATION

Patient physical status, particularly regarding cardiovascular and pulmonary stability and airway manageability, has a unique effect on posterior fossa surgery because it is a determinant of the choice of patient position. Although patient position is typically decided by the operating surgeon based on an assessment of the technical demands of the surgical approach, the efforts to obtain optimal operating conditions and maintain a stable perioperative course may sometimes be at cross purposes. For example, a morbidly obese patient initially may not be considered suitable for an operation in the sitting position, but surgical access and maintenance of adequate ventilation may actually favor the sitting position over alternatives such as the prone position. On the other hand, patients with previous cerebrospinal fluid (CSF) shunting procedures may be at greater risk for subdural pneumocephalus with surgery in the sitting position.[55,84] Thus a thorough evaluation of previous operations and cardiopulmonary problems, current cardiac and respiratory status, evidence of cerebrovascular compromise, and suitability of vascular access for right-atrial catheter placement are of particular importance in the posterior fossa patient.

Patients with a history of hypertension, cardiovascular disease, cerebrovascular insufficiency or previous carotid endarterectomy may have altered limits of cerebral autoregulation, impaired cerebral perfusion, or abnormal baroreceptor function.[5,23,203] Thus the occurrence of hypotension during anesthesia in the sitting position may be especially detrimental. Placement of these patients in a more horizontal position may facilitate maintenance of adequate cerebral perfusion pressure (CPP).[66,139,185,187] However, there are no strong clinical data to support the benefits of alternative horizontal positions over the sitting position in these situations.

Intravascular volume depletion may result from decreased oral intake, supine diuresis, vomiting, and intravenous contrast administration for diagnostic studies. Incremental administration of intravenous fluids before induction may help limit hypotension during anesthetic induction and positioning. Application of thigh-high compression stockings to the legs is a routine practice in many institutions; its theoretic benefit includes limitation of venous pooling in the lower extremities,[109,180] but little clinical data support this belief.

Mental status may be influenced by several factors. Tumors or cysts of the posterior fossa may obstruct CSF outflow at the level of the fourth ventricle, producing hydrocephalus, increased intracranial pressure (ICP), and altered levels of consciousness. The resulting clinical spectrum may range from unilateral pupillary dilation, papilledema, cranial nerve palsies, and impairment of protective airway reflexes, to fatal brainstem compression.

Assessment of vascular access for right-atrial catheter placement is helpful in determining the most promising route. The right-atrial catheter is rarely, if ever, needed before induction of anesthesia, and catheterization via the upper extremity is aided by the vasodilation produced by general anesthesia. However, obese patients, those with poor vasculature caused by disease or chronic intravenous cannulation, or patients with short, thick necks should be identified early so that necessary time may be allotted for catheter placement. Subclavian vein catheterization is less popular than other routes because of the possibilities of pneumothorax and air entrainment during the sitting position.[2,103] However, if the preoperative evaluation determines that this is the most promising site for catheterization, a sheath should be placed and x-rays taken to detect a pneumothorax before patient transport to the operating room.

Screening echocardiography to detect patent foramen ovale in patients scheduled for surgery in the sitting position has been advocated by some. The use of an alternative position for those with a positive finding might reduce the occurrence of paradoxic air embolism.[48,85] A detection rate of 10% to 30% is comparable to the 20% to 30% incidence reported in autopsy findings.[86] Its noninvasive nature makes it attractive for screening purposes; its specificity is reported to be 64% to 100%.[9,105,118] However, preoperative screening echocardiography currently is costly and lacks sensitivity, (i.e., nondetection of patent foramen ovale does not guarantee its absence).[18,46] Use of transesophageal echocardiography (TEE) after induction of anesthesia may be more promising.[104,115]

GENERAL MONITORING ISSUES

The goals of monitoring during posterior fossa surgery are to assure adequate central nervous system (CNS) perfusion, maintain cardiorespiratory stability, and detect and treat air embolism. Box 16-1 lists the monitors used, regardless of patient position. Monitors that are not in routine use but that provide specialized information during certain procedures are noted with an asterisk. Not every "routine" monitor listed is always used for every posterior fossa procedure (e.g., a urinary catheter or central venous catheter may not be required for limited cervical cord decompression). The placement of central venous catheters for certain posterior fossa procedures, such as acoustic neuroma resection, is not routine in many institutions when surgery is not conducted in the sitting position.

BOX 16-1
MONITORS FOR POSTERIOR FOSSA SURGERY

Preinduction/Induction
5-Lead electrocardiogram
Blood pressure monitoring
Pulse oximetry
Precordial stethoscope
Capnography
Electrophysiologic monitoring*

Postinduction
Central venous (right atrial, pulmonary artery) catheter
Precordial Doppler probe
Esophageal stethoscope
Esophageal or nasopharyngeal temperature probe
$ETco_2$, ETn_2 monitoring*
Transesophageal ECHO*

---

*Not routine but provide specialized information during certain procedures.

When working on the head or neck, many clinicians prefer placement of central venous catheters in the forearm or the antecubital fossa, preferably via the basilic vein after induction of anesthesia. The success rate for such catheter placement is reported to range from 76% to 97%.[35,45] In patients with small veins, a modified Seldinger technique can be used for specialized right atrial catheters or pulmonary angiography catheters.[89] Others prefer the internal or external jugular vein for cannulation. The duration of the head-down position and head rotation for catheter placement should be minimized because these maneuvers may reduce cerebral blood flow by increasing intracranial blood volume and ICP. A specialized Doppler ultrasound transducer (Dymax Corp.) can be used to localize the jugular vein before needle insertion.[52,195] Whenever catheters are placed via the neck or subclavian routes, the insertion sites should be sealed with bacteriostatic ointment and dressing to minimize air entrainment, especially for patients in head-elevated positions.[103]

CHOICE OF PATIENT POSITION

Surgical access to the posterior fossa can be obtained through various patient positions, namely, the sitting position and variants of the horizontal position, which include supine, prone, three-quarter prone, and lateral positions. The "park-bench" position, a modification of the combined sitting and lateral positions, is also used.

Supine Position

Access to the lateral aspects of the posterior fossa can be achieved in the supine patient with the head turned (Fig. 16-1, *A*). Acoustic neuroma resection and microvascular decompression can often be accomplished in this manner. A small roll may be placed under the ipsilateral shoulder to facilitate exposure. Careful attention should be paid to head and neck position to avoid impairment of jugular venous drainage.

Sitting Position

This sitting position describes the posture of a patient whose back is elevated toward the vertical between 60 and 90 degrees, with thighs flexed on the trunk, legs flexed on the thighs, and the feet at or near heart level (Fig. 16-1, *B*). To establish the sitting position, the patient's skull should be secured in a three-pin head holder; infiltration of the scalp and periosteum at the pin sites reduces the hypertensive response to pin insertion into the outer table of the skull.[38] The operating table should be flexed fully and the foot section lowered approximately 30 degrees to flex the knees. The back section is elevated slowly and the table placed in slight reverse Trendelenburg position so that there is some margin for lowering the head if necessary for resuscitation.[172] The arterial-pressure transducer is zeroed at the skull base during positioning and throughout surgery to make maintenance of adequate cerebral perfusion pressure

easier. Bony prominences should be well padded, the legs placed in thigh-high compression stockings to limit pooling of blood, elbows supported by pillows or pads to avoid contact with the table or stretch on the brachial plexus, and the legs freed of pressure at the level of the common peroneal nerve just distal and lateral to the head of the fibula. Efforts to prevent cervical cord stretching and obstruction of venous drainage from the face and tongue include maintenance of at least a 1-inch space between the chin and chest, avoidance of large airways and bite blocks in the pharynx, and avoidance of excessive neck rotation, especially in elderly patients.[65,131,190] Abdominal compression, lower-extremity ischemia, and sciatic nerve injury[100] are prevented by avoiding excessive flexion of the knees toward the chest. Careful attention should be paid to the placement of compression stockings because, although they are more likely to provide uniform compression than elastic bandages, careless application can lead to a tourniquet effect and ischemic injury to the leg.

A "lounge chair" modification of the sitting position, with the thoracic cage raised between 30 and 45 degrees, may be used for lateral lesions of the posterior fossa.[200] However, access to more midline structures may be impeded by the degree of neck flexion required.

Modification of a conventional operating table has been described in which the patient is in a lateral sitting position.[73] This allows rapid head lowering to the left lateral decubitus position and continuation of surgery in the event of hypotension or persistent venous air embolism. However, the position as described does not elevate the legs to the level of the heart, which may increase venous pooling and decrease venous return. A study of one patient placed in six different positions concluded that the lateral sitting position (45 degrees) minimizes the possibility of air embolism but optimizes central venous and intracranial pressures.[32]

The sitting position provides several possible advantages to the surgeon and anesthesiologist alike. For the surgeon, advantages include improved surgical exposure and anatomic orientation to midline structures and the cerebellopontine angle; greater torsion and flexion of the neck without impairing jugular venous drainage; reduced bleeding because of lower intrathoracic airway pressures; improved CSF and blood drainage; elimination of the hazard of eyeball compression through use of the three-pin head holder; and access to the anterior chest wall for resuscitation in case of cardiovascular collapse.[74] For the anesthesiologist, advantages include: lower airway pressures and ease of diaphragmatic excursion; improved ability for hyperventilation; improved access to the endotracheal tube and thorax for monitoring; access to the extremities for monitoring, fluid or blood administration and blood sampling; and visualization of the face for observation of motor responses during cranial nerve stimulation.

Relative contraindications to the sitting position include known intracardiac defects, known pulmonary arteriove-

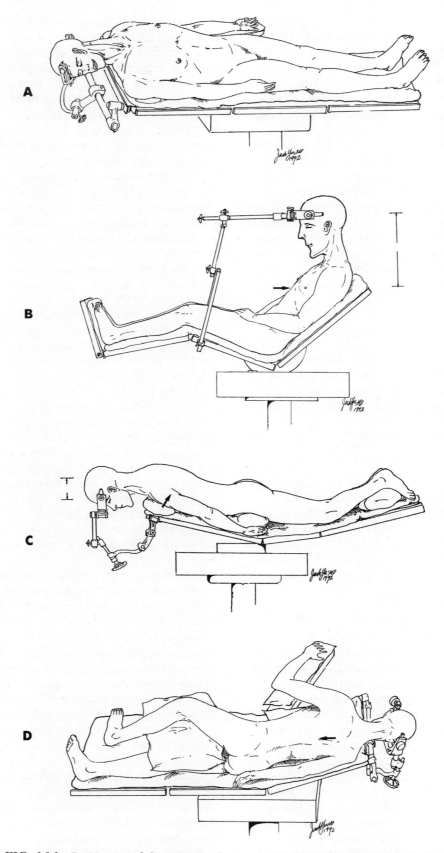

FIG. 16-1 Positions used for posterior fossa surgery. **A,** Supine. **B,** Sitting. **C,** Prone. **D,** Three-quarter prone.

nous malformations,[27] severe hypovolemia or cachexia, severe hydrocephalus, and lesion vascularity. Beta-adrenergic blockade, however, is not a contraindication to the sitting position.[143,181]

Physiologic Changes in the Sitting Position

Elevation of the head above the right atrium produces a decrease in dural sinus pressure, which decreases venous bleeding and increases the risk of venous air embolism. A study of dural sinus pressure measurements in various patient positions was conducted in 25 patients (20 adults and 5 children).[96] Head elevation to the 90 degree sitting position produced decreases in dural sinus pressure of up to 10 mm Hg. Jugular bulb venous pressure, measured in six cases, was not a reliable indicator of dural sinus pressure.

Cardiovascular effects secondary to this position include increases in pulmonary and systemic vascular resistance and decreases in cardiac output, venous return, and cerebral perfusion pressure[41,49] (for each 1.25 cm above the level of the head, local arterial pressure is reduced by approximately 1 mm Hg[66]). Dysrhythmias, such as bradycardia, tachycardia, premature ventricular contractions, or asystole, may result from manipulation or retraction of cranial nerves or the brainstem regardless of patient position.[2,106,139,209] However, their negative effects on cardiac output may be more pronounced in the sitting position as compared with horizontal positions. Albin observed that patients with ASA physical status III to IV had a higher incidence of hypotension after positioning than patients with ASA physical status I.[2] However, Black et al. detected no difference in the incidence of hypotension with sitting vs. horizontal positions in patients, regardless of the presence of cardiac disease.[19] These factors should be considered when assessing the elderly or those with impaired cardiac function for placement in the sitting position. Some have advocated use of the antigravity suit, or G-suit, for treatment of acute hypotension in the sitting position[73,126]; however, its long-term effectiveness for maintenance of normotension is questionable.[1,126,189]

Pulmonary vital capacity and functional residual capacity are improved in the sitting position. However, relative hypovolemia may result in decreased perfusion of the upper zones of the pulmonary parenchyma; this may lead to ventilation or perfusion abnormalities and hypoxemia. Data from animal models of air embolism suggest that use of inhalational anesthetics may increase the likelihood of transpulmonary passage of air in a dose-dependent manner.[30,214,215] This effect may influence choice of anesthetic in the sitting position.

The use of N_2O in the sitting position continues to be controversial. Some neuroanesthesiologists avoid its use because it increases the size of intravascular air bubbles if air embolism occurs. Others have described its usefulness in detecting residual intravascular pulmonary gas after venous air embolism.[124,173] N_2O is more soluble in blood than nitrogen, and animal studies have demonstrated a twofold reduction in the median lethal volume of venous air embolism with 50% N_2O and a greater than threefold reduction with 72% to 76% N_2O.[144] However, N_2O was not determined to be a factor in perioperative morbidity in several large series of patients undergoing posterior fossa surgery at different institutions, regardless of patient position or occurrence of venous air embolism.*

Because N_2O increases pressure in a closed air space, some neuroanesthetists have recommended discontinuation of its use before the dura is completely closed to prevent the build-up of gas pressure and possible neurologic deficit from tension pneumocephalus.[6,7,117] Others have demonstrated in an animal model that continued use of N_2O until the end of the case actually promotes removal of the gas after the N_2O is discontinued because of the gradient created between gas space and blood, provided the circulation to that area is intact.[176] Discontinuation of N_2O has not been demonstrated to be effective in preventing pneumocephalus.[70]

An investigation of 100 consecutive patients in various positions for posterior fossa surgery and another study of 30 patients in the sitting position demonstrated a high incidence of pneumocephalus and intraventricular air, but no complications from either condition.[54,192] The incidence of pneumocephalus was reported to be 100% in sitting intracranial procedures, 72% in the park-bench position, and 57% in the prone position. Pneumocephalus is usually asymptomatic and resolves spontaneously. However, tension pneumocephalus may produce postoperative neurologic deficits.[101,102,119] The diagnosis of pneumocephalus can be made intraoperatively on the basis of decreased somatosensory evoked potentials, if they are being monitored,[132,168,207] and postoperatively on CT scan.[16,149] Treatment consists of 100% O_2 administration and, in some cases, removal of gas by aspiration or reopening of the dura.

Prone Position

The prone position is a common alternative to the sitting position because it is associated with a lower incidence of venous air embolism (Fig. 16-1, *C*).[3,19] However, the patient's head is usually elevated above the heart to decrease venous bleeding; thus the risk of air embolism is not eliminated, and resuscitative efforts, if needed, are hampered. Access to superior posterior fossa structures and ease of head manipulation are not as favorable as they are in the sitting position; the sitting position may also offer better operating conditions for high cervical decompression, in which neck flexion and weight-bearing on the head are detrimental.[161]

When the patient is placed in the head-elevated prone position, it is especially important to have the shoulders at or above the edge of the operating table back. This pre-

---

*References 3, 19, 128, 183, 200, 217.

vents the patient's face from becoming compressed against the cephalad edge of the table when it is inclined.

Eye compression can produce blindness from retinal artery thrombosis; this risk is greater in prone and lateral positions, particularly when a padded facial headrest is used. For this reason, most surgeons now prefer the three-pin head holder for positioning. Confirmation of a secure grip of the head holder minimizes the risk of pin slippage and facial or eye injury. Conjunctival edema is a benign consequence of the prone position that resolves quickly.

Venous pooling sufficient to impair venous return can occur in the lower extremities when they are below the right atrium. Elderly, debilitated patients may not tolerate even a brief discontinuation of monitoring during the turn to the prone position without suffering severe hypotension. In these patients, monitoring cables and transducers should be oriented to allow uninterrupted ECG and arterial blood pressure measurements throughout the turn to the prone position and positioning adjustments.

A modification of the prone position has been described as the "sea lion" position.[94] The upper and lower halves of the body are elevated 20 degrees, and the neck is hyperextended, allowing good access to the posterior sagittal sinus area, falcotentorial junction, and pineal region. In addition, dural sinus pressure remains above zero, which minimizes the risk of air embolism from the surgical site. This position offers theoretic advantages over the alternative use of the prone position with elevation of the patient's upper body, which may result in elevated dural sinus pressures and venous bleeding. However, the position may be awkward for the operating surgeon.

Lateral and Three-Quarter Prone Positions

The lateral position is used for unilateral neurosurgical procedures in the upper posterior fossa. The three-quarter prone position, a modification of the prone and lateral positions, is used for similar procedures, but it permits greater head rotation and access to more axial structures. The operating table can be tilted head-up in these positions to allow drainage of blood and CSF. In the lateral position, the head is supported by an appropriate headrest that does not compress the downside ear. A roll is placed immediately caudal to the axilla to support the chest and to avoid axillary neurovascular compression. For the three-quarter prone position, the three-pin head holder is used for head positioning. The dependent arm is positioned along the patient's side, and a longitudinal roll is placed under the thorax on the contralateral side. The patient's legs are positioned with the dependent leg straight and the upper leg flexed on pillows (Fig. 16-1, D). An alternative position for the dependent arm is flexion under the head such that it is cradled by the head-holder support. The dependent arm can also be placed in a sling and suspended over the head of the table, an approach that works well with a large patient. Compression injuries to the brachial plexus are the most common types of nerve injuries in the lateral position; a misplaced chest roll is a frequent cause.[109] Compression on the down-

side eye can cause blindness from retinal artery thrombosis.

Park-Bench Position

This is another modification of the lateral position, with the patient's back elevated to 45 degrees, providing the surgeon with nearly the same access to midline and lateral posterior fossa structures as obtained in the sitting position. An advantage of this position over the sitting position is that the patient can be brought to a more horizontal position in the event of intraoperative air embolism.[32]

Risk-Benefit Analysis of Sitting Position Compared to Other Positions

No other subject has sparked as much controversy among neurosurgeons and neuroanesthesiologists as the usefulness or appropriateness of the sitting surgical position as compared with horizontal positions for access to the posterior fossa. Perhaps this is because there are alternative positions for posterior fossa access. Moreover, the occurrence of venous air embolism is more common and severe in sitting posterior fossa procedures than in alternative positions. There are arguments both for and against its use in certain patients and operations; however, litigation and the large monetary sums awarded in a few cases of suboptimal operative outcome with the sitting position have made some physicians reluctant to use it, despite its potential for improving operating conditions.

Complications associated with the various positions used for posterior fossa surgery are presented in detail in Table 16-1. One study[19] reported a series of 579 patients in a 4-year period, 333 of whom were in the sitting position and 246 of whom were in various horizontal positions. On average, patients in the horizontal position were 7 years older than patients in the sitting position. The incidence of hypotension was comparable in both groups (Table 16-2). There was no significant difference in the incidence of perioperative myocardial infarction or postoperative respiratory or cardiovascular complications, but the number of patients experiencing adverse effects was small.

Investigators from different institutions have reported their experience with the sitting position, with particular emphasis on complications and outcome.* These studies have generally been retrospective. Some of the reported complications might have been prevented or reduced if the sitting position had not been used; however, other complications might have replaced them. A review of 3827 cervical or occipital procedures performed in the sitting position between 1966 and 1983 at the Mayo Clinic had no intraoperative deaths resulting from venous air embolism.[43] The only intraoperative death resulting from air embolism occurred in a patient in the three-quarter prone position.[81] At the University of Pennsylvania, the only instance in which the arterial pressure waveform, capnography wave-

TABLE 16-1

Complications Associated with Surgical Position[19,128,183,200,217]

Complication	Sitting Position	Prone Position	Lateral, Three-Quarter Prone Position	Park Bench, "Lounge" Position
Nervous System				
Cerebral ischemia	++	+	0	+
Cervical spine ischemia	++	+	0	+
Palsies				
Cranial nerve	+	++	++	
Brachial plexus	+		++	++
Sciatic nerve	+	0	0	0
Peroneal nerve	+	0	?	
Airway				
Edema of face, tongue, neck (postoperative obstruction)	++	++	+	0
Endotracheal tube migration	++	++	+	+
Pulmonary				
Ventilation/perfusion abnormalities	+	+	+	+
Increased airway pressures	0	++	0-+	0
Tension pneumocephalus	++	0	0	?
Cardiovascular				
Hypotension	++	++	0	+
Dysrhythmias	++	++	±	++
Need for blood transfusion	+	++	±	+
Miscellaneous				
Eye compression	0	+++	++	+
"Compartment syndrome"	+	0	0	0
Venous air embolism	+++	++	+	++
Paradoxical air embolism	++	+	?	?

0, +, ++, +++ indicate relative probability from no risk to high risk.

TABLE 16-2

Posterior Fossa Craniotomy: Intraoperative Surgical Problems

Problem	Sitting Position (n = 333) Number of Patients (% of Total)	Horizontal Position (n = 246) Number of Patients (% of Total)
Hypotension		
With positioning	63 (19%)	60 (24%)
During procedure	86 (26%)	54 (22%)
Entire anesthetic	121 (36%)	94 (38%)
Without cardiac disease	101/297 (34%)	130/197 (34%)
With cardiac disease	30/36 (56%)	27/49 (55%)
Transfusion >2 units	3%	13%*
Average blood replacement	359 ml	507 ml†
Postoperative cranial nerve function		
Improved	41 (12%)	50 (20%)‡
Unchanged	218 (65%)	112 (45%)
Deteriorated	74 (22%)	84 (34%)

*p < 0.01 (Chi square).

†p < 0.05 (Student's t test).

‡26% of horizontal patients had decompression for tic douloureux.

From Black S, Ockert DB, Oliver WC et al: *Anesthesiology* 69:49-56, 1988.

form, and pulse oximeter trace were lost simultaneously was in a patient undergoing an occipital tumor resection in the prone position (personal communication).

Researchers have reviewed 14 documented cases of supratentorial intracerebral hemorrhage after posterior fossa surgery in the sitting position for possible causes and other related problems.[24] Different clinical circumstances for the reported cases led the authors to conclude that a variety of mechanisms were possible but that the sitting position contributed to the occurrence of morbidity.

Cases of cervical cord injury, presumably resulting from excessive retraction or neck flexion or impaired cervical spine perfusion in the sitting position, have been reported.[128,183,211,217] Advances in electrophysiologic monitoring are making such occurrences easier to detect so that appropriate therapy can be instituted early (see later section on special monitoring issues in this chapter).

There is no one best surgical position for all patients requiring exploration of the posterior fossa. As demonstrated by the considerable controversy surrounding this issue, there are significant advantages and disadvantages to both sitting and horizontal positions. Appropriate management of the patient requiring posterior fossa craniectomy, selection of the most appropriate position for that patient and the physician-provided care require consideration of advantages and disadvantages as they apply to that individual patient.[134] The available data suggest that both the sitting and horizontal positions can be used safely in appropriate patients.

ANESTHETIC CONSIDERATIONS

There are some theoretic considerations regarding the choice of anesthetic drugs for patients who undergo posterior fossa exploration. The clinical significance of these considerations remains to be determined. First is the question of the effect of inhalational vs. intravenous anesthetic drugs on the lungs' ability to retain air that enters the venous circulation, preventing its passage to the arterial circulation. The likelihood of transpulmonary air passage in humans is a subject of continuing debate. Individual case reports of cerebral air embolism in the absence of an intracardiac defect[15] as well as detection of left-heart air on echocardiogram without demonstration of an intracardiac defect[105] have been used to support the occurrence of transpulmonary air. In addition, pulmonary arteriovenous malformations, although rare, have been documented in humans.[27] Studies in animals suggest that the intravenous anesthetics, pentobarbital, fentanyl, and ketamine, maintain a higher threshold for trapping air bubbles in the pulmonary circulation than halothane.[30,214,215] Propofol, thiopental, isoflurane, and other inhalational anesthetics have not been investigated in the same manner. Therefore the clinical significance of these findings has not yet been defined.

A second consideration is the goal of maintenance of adequate CPP. Before surgical incision, administration of in-

travenous anesthetic drugs has been demonstrated to have less effect on cardiovascular function than inhalational anesthetics in patients placed in the sitting position.[125] Whether this relationship continues after the start of surgery has not been investigated.

A third issue is the potential benefit of preservation of cardiovascular responsiveness to surgical manipulation of brainstem structures. In such instances, the avoidance of anticholinergic drugs or long-acting beta-adrenergic blockers that would mask the cardiovascular response may provide useful information to surgeon and anesthesiologist alike.

An additional consideration surrounds the use of N_2O in cases where the risk of venous air embolism is increased. A prospective, randomized study of 110 patients for posterior fossa exploration and 190 patients for cervical spine surgery demonstrated that 50% N_2O had no significant effect on the incidence or severity of venous air embolism if the N_2O was discontinued when air was detected by Doppler ultrasound.[115] Studies in isoflurane-anesthetized dogs of venous air embolism in the presence of N_2O suggest that N_2O improves the sensitivity of $ETco_2$ and pulmonary artery pressure monitoring in the detection of air embolism but not that of transesophageal echocardiography or precordial Doppler.[112] The common alternatives to N_2O are 100% O_2 and nitrogen/O_2 mixtures.

Arguments for the use of N_2O in neurosurgical patients are its analgesic effect, rapid elimination and emergence, and facilitation of the postoperative neurologic assessment. However, in a study of patients who received fentanyl-based anesthesia with supplemental isoflurane, no difference in time to emergence from anesthesia was noted between patients who received 50% N_2O and those who did not.[115] The doses of fentanyl were comparable between groups, and the average end-tidal isoflurane concentrations were slightly higher (0.65% vs. 0.52%) in the no-N_2O group. Whether newer intravenous anesthetics such as propofol or inhalational anesthetics such as desflurane will offer advantages in neurosurgical patients remains to be determined.

Premedication

Administration of preoperative premedication should be individualized based on the patient's physical status, presence of evidence of increased ICP, and level of patient anxiety. Chronic antihypertensive medication is continued; preoperative corticosteroids and antibiotics are usually administered by the surgeon. Narcotic premedication is avoided in patients with space-occupying lesions or hydrocephalus from fourth ventricle occlusion because the resultant hypoventilation and CO_2 retention may increase ICP. Oral benzodiazepines given 60 to 90 minutes before arrival in the operating room are effective in reducing anxiety and do not have significant effects on ICP.[186] For neurologically intact patients with aneurysms but no intracranial mass lesions, a heavy premedication combining intramuscular morphine and scopolamine may be given to decrease the possibility of preinduction hypertension and aneurysm rupture. The addition of a barbiturate to this premedication has also been advocated for greater sedation.

Induction of Anesthesia

Direct arterial blood pressure monitoring established before induction of anesthesia allows tighter control of blood pressure and cerebral perfusion pressure during induction and intubation, especially in patients at risk for increased ICP. The use of a low-dose (4 to 6 μg/kg fentanyl), narcotic-based, N_2O/O_2, relaxant technique with supplemental volatile inhalational anesthetic after intravenous induction with thiopental or propofol affords adequate analgesia and amnesia, preservation of autonomic nervous system activity, and rapid awakening after discontinuation of the inhalational anesthetics; thus an early postsurgical neurologic examination if desired is facilitated. Advocates of the avoidance of N_2O often use higher doses of narcotic (up to 10 μg/kg fentanyl). In a series of 97 patients for posterior fossa surgery who received average fentanyl doses of 6.8 ± 3.8 μg/kg (mean ± sd), 10% of patients required naloxone postoperatively.[115]

Drugs that may be used alone or in combination to treat rises in blood pressure include beta-adrenergic blocking drugs and direct-acting vasodilators. Use of long-acting antihypertensive drugs should be avoided until the patient has been placed in the operating position. The need for vasopressor administration may arise after induction of anesthesia or positioning, especially in chronically hypertensive or debilitated patients. Short-acting drugs, such as small boluses of ephedrine or phenylephrine, are usually effective. Rarely, inotrope infusions may be required throughout the surgical procedure.

Verification of appropriate endotracheal tube position after final positioning but before surgical incision is of utmost importance, regardless of the position employed. Intraoperative access to the airway is limited by virtue of the proximity of the operative site, and neck flexion or extension can produce caudad or cephalad displacement of the endotracheal tube, respectively, by as much as 2 cm.[191] Palpation of the endotracheal tube cuff above the sternal notch is a useful maneuver to assure that the tip of the endotracheal tube is above the carina.

Maintenance of Anesthesia

Use of spontaneous ventilation during posterior fossa surgery was advocated in the past by some surgeons. It was based on the impression that changes in respiratory patterns, such as sighing or gasping, would warn of impingement on medullary respiratory structures or of the presence of air.[106,162,205] A recent clinical investigation of 50 surgical procedures advocated the use of spontaneous ventilation during vertebral basilar aneurysm surgery for early, rapid detection of brainstem ischemia.[120] However, spontaneous

ventilation produces a larger negative-pressure gradient than controlled positive-pressure ventilation, and the chances of air entry in the event of venous air embolism are increased. Thus the use of spontaneous ventilation should be reserved for patients who are supine with the operative site at heart level. Controlled positive-pressure ventilation with paralysis allows: maintenance of lighter levels of anesthesia; hyperventilation, which decreases $Paco_2$, producing a decreased sympathetic stimulation and decreased blood pressure at any given depth of anesthesia; cerebral vasoconstriction[187]; less bleeding; decreased ICP; less cardiovascular depression because of decreased anesthetic depth; and decreased likelihood of patient movement.[139]

Severe intraoperative hypothermia ($<32°$ C) should be avoided. However, a 2 to $3°$ C intraoperative fall in patient temperature may provide a measure of cerebral protection because of decreased metabolic demand without placing undue demands on the cardiovascular system secondary to postoperative shivering.[14,138]

More liberal administration of intravenous fluids may be required during sitting or head-elevated prone procedures because of relaxation of the lower extremity capacitance vessels and resultant venous pooling. This may be offset to some extent by preoperative application of compression stockings,[109] but some loss of intravascular fluid to the extravascular space will occur over time. If large volumes of fluid are administered during surgery, a small prophylactic dose (5 to 10 mg) of furosemide will promote postoperative diuresis of excess fluids reabsorbed from the extravascular space. Glucose-containing solutions are generally avoided because of the possible detrimental effects of hyperglycemia on areas of the brain at risk for cerebral ischemia.[174]

The administration of osmotic and loop diuretics for tumor resection and vascular procedures may predispose sitting patients to electrolyte disturbances and/or cardiovascular instability caused by hypovolemia.[42] In addition, the severity of pneumocephalus may be increased.[192] Simultaneous administration of intravenous colloid is appropriate to maintain cerebral perfusion pressure and should have minimal effect on the cerebral-dehydrating effect of the diuretic. The dose of diuretic should probably be limited to decrease the amount of intracranial air space remaining after the surgical dissection.

Emergence From Anesthesia

The anesthetic goals are to prevent abrupt rises in blood pressure, effect rapid awakening and return of motor strength, and minimize coughing and straining on the endotracheal tube. The feasibility of immediate postoperative extubation is determined by the nature and extent of surgery (e.g., extensive brainstem manipulation with a greater likelihood of postoperative brainstem edema or brainstem injury caused by a difficult tumor resection).[8,91,216] If extensive manipulation of the medullary structures or significant edema are factors, a secured airway should be maintained until the patient is awake, following commands, and demonstrating return of protective airway reflexes.[8,91] Additional sedation may be required until this point of recovery is reached. Persistent postoperative hypertension in a previously normotensive patient should alert the anesthesiologist to possible brainstem compression or hematoma.

VENOUS AIR EMBOLISM

A potential hazard exists whenever the operative site is above heart level. Documentation of this phenomenon has existed for more than 100 years (Table 16-3). Venous air embolism is associated most frequently with posterior fossa procedures in the sitting position because of facilitation of air entry by subatmospheric pressure in an opened vein and the presence of noncollapsible venous channels, such as diploic veins and dural sinuses. Cases in which air entered the venous circulation via burr holes or wounds from the skull head holder have also been reported, particularly when the head was elevated.[31,62,212]

Pathophysiology

A recent review of the pathophysiologic effects of gas bubbles on the vascular endothelium suggests that a form of ischemia-reperfusion injury occurs that is common to all organs involved.[147] The endothelium's key role in the inflammatory response to injury is most likely a central component of the manifestations of organ injury caused by air embolism.[142] During slow, continuous entrainment, air is dissipated into the peripheral pulmonary circulation, producing sympathetic reflex vasoconstriction resulting from mechanical obstruction or local hypoxemia. It is believed that mi-

crovascular bubbles activate the release of endothelial mediators, resulting in complement production, cytokine release, and production of reactive O_2 molecules. Pulmonary manifestations include pulmonary hypertension, impaired gas exchange and hypoxemia,[156] CO_2 retention, increased pulmonary dead space, and decreased end tidal CO_2 (ET_{CO_2}). Bronchoconstriction results in increased airway pressures. Decreased venous return leads to decreased cardiac output and decreased systemic arterial blood pressure.[1] Myocardial and cerebral ischemia may result from severe, persistent hypoxemia and/or hypotension.

If a bolus of air is entrained rapidly, it may result in air lock within the right heart or a cumulative gas volume that exceeds pulmonary arterial capacity (estimated to be 5 ml/kg from animal studies)[28,67]; this leads to blockage of right ventricular outflow tract, air/blood layer formation with obstructed venous return, decreased cardiac output, acute right-ventricular dilation and failure, myocardial and cerebral ischemia, dysrhythmias, and cardiovascular collapse.[1,50,57]

Morbidity and mortality are directly related to amount and rate of air entry.[1,57] The "symptomatic dose" of venous air is not well documented in humans, but in a review of the clinical manifestations of air embolism,[79] more than 50 ml have been retrieved in patients manifesting clinical changes such as decreases in blood pressure, dysrhythmias, or ECG changes. This same review summarized a collection of 93 early case reports in which 37 of 40 (93%) untreated patients died, and the lethal dose of intravascular air in humans is estimated to be greater than 300 ml. Early investigations in dogs reported tolerance of as much as 1000 ml of air infused over 50 to 100 minutes, but fatality with a 100 ml bolus.[57]

Factors contributing to the occurrence and severity of ve-

TABLE 16-3
Early Historical Perspective on Air Embolism[11,108,170,210]

Date	Finding	Discoverer
1667	Death in animals when air enters vein	Redi
1681	Characteristic noise of air entrainment	Hardner
1683-1686	Right-heart dilation from air insufflation; mortality is rate and dose-dependent	Camerarius, de Heyde
~1800	First recorded case of air embolism during excision of a neck tumor (not realized until 30 years later)	Barlow
1811	Small air dose well tolerated, right ventricular distention is cause of death	Nysten
1818	Sudden death associated with hissing noise in young patient having clavicular tumor resection in sitting position	Bauchene
1821	Development of experimental surgery to investigate clinical findings	Magendie
1823	Treatment of air embolism during tumor resection by closing vein wound when hissing noise occurred	Wattmann
1832	Treatment for traumatic air embolism published (but overlooked)	Wattmann
1839	Establishment of conditions, treatment for venous air embolism in humans, including air aspiration	Amussat
1843	Approximately 40 cases of air embolism described	Various scientists
1845	Wattmann's work recognized	
1846	Concept and term "embolism" created	Virchow
1877	Paradoxical embolism associated with patent foramen ovale	Cohnheim
1885	Importance of head position in air entrainment	Senn

nous air embolism include the surgical site, such as the posterior fossa, where venous channels are stented open by surrounding structures, and the degree of head elevation and negative pressure between the right atrium and the surgical site. A higher incidence and severity of venous air embolism has been reported with posterior fossa craniotomies than laminectomies.[19,124,128,183,217] Children experience greater hemodynamic derangements from venous air embolism than adults[44,128,200]; in addition, air entrainment is more difficult to treat. The incidence is decreased by careful surgical dissection, hemostasis, and liberal use of bone wax. Hypovolemia lowers central venous pressure and increases the negative pressure gradient between the elevated head and the right heart.

Incidence

Estimates of the incidence of venous air embolism range from a low of 5% to a high of 100% in patients in the sitting position[78](Table 16-4). A major determinant of the incidence in a given series is the method of detection; a lower incidence is associated when only clinical signs are the end point, and a higher incidence is associated with the use of mechanical monitoring devices.

Risks of Air Embolism

The greater the gradient between cerebral veins and the right atrium, the greater is the tendency for air to enter venous openings at the craniotomy site. Cerebral venous pressure varies with the degree of head elevation, and, in the sitting position, it can be as low as -10 mm Hg.[96] The risk of catastrophic air embolism has been reduced dramatically by improved detection and prompt treatment of venous air embolism.[12,134,135] Recently, more attention has

been directed toward recognition and treatment of paradoxic air embolism.

Risk of Paradoxical Air Embolism

Clinical evidence of paradoxical air embolism in the perioperative period is considerably less frequent than calculated estimates based on the incidence of venous air embolism and the prevalence of patent foramen ovale.[116] However, complications, such as myocardial or cerebral ischemia resulting from paradoxical air embolism, may be devastating. Thus efforts to improve its detection or prevent its occurrence constitute areas of active clinical investigation.

The most likely mechanism of systemic air embolism in humans is by right-to-left shunting through an intracardiac defect. A patent foramen ovale is reported to exist in 20% to 30% of the population.[86] Some investigators have suggested that the likelihood of right-to-left shunt is increased if right-atrial pressure exceeds left and that up to 50% of patients may experience reversal of an existing left-to-right atrial pressure gradient and thus have the potential for paradoxical air embolism after 1 hour in the sitting position.[152]

The calculated risk of paradoxical air embolism is 5% to 10%, but not all patients with a patent foramen ovale will have paradoxical air embolism. One study of precordial contrast two-dimensional echocardiography during Valsalva maneuver in healthy volunteers revealed an 18% incidence of right-to-left shunting at the atrial level.[118] A recent study of 45 anesthetized patients scheduled for surgery in the sitting position used transesophageal echocardiography, positive end-expiratory pressure (PEEP), and injection of dissolved microbubbles simultaneously with the

TABLE 16-4
Incidence of Venous Air Embolism

Investigator	Year Reported	Position	Incidence	Percentage of Patients	Method of Detection
Michenfelder et al.	1969	Sitting	37/751	5%	Right-atrial catheter, aspiration
Michenfelder et al.	1972	Sitting	26/69	42%	Right-atrial catheter, Doppler
Albin et al.	1987	Sitting	100/400	25%	Doppler, right-atrial catheter
		Horizontal	13/118	11%	Right-atrial catheter, Doppler
Marshall, Bedford	1980	Sitting	20/52	38%	Doppler only
			13/52	25%	Doppler, ↑ PAP, ↓ ETco$_2$
Voorhies et al.	1983	Sitting	41/81	50%	Doppler, PEEP (no right-atrial catheter)
Standefer et al.	1984	Sitting	22/382	6%	Right-atrial catheter, Doppler
Matjasko et al.	1985	Sitting	130/554	23.5%	Right-atrial catheter, Doppler (ETco$_2$ in 94 pts)
Young et al.	1986	Sitting	70/255	30%	Right-atrial catheter, Doppler
Black et al.*	1988	Sitting	150/333	45%	Right-atrial catheter, Doppler
		Horizontal	30/246	12%	Right-atrial catheter (33%), Doppler (30%)
Von Gossein et al.	1991	30- to 45-degree head elevation	46/704	6.5%	Right-atrial catheter, Doppler, ETco$_2$

*Mass spectroscopy after 1982.
PAP, pulmonary artery pressure; *Doppler*, precordial Doppler; *PEEP*, positive end expiratory pressure; *ETco$_2$*, end-tidal CO$_2$.

release of PEEP to elicit evidence of a right-to-left shunt.[116] A shunt was demonstrated in 10 of 45 patients, and 8 of 10 underwent surgery in the sitting position. Venous air embolism occurred in 7 of 8 patients, and paradoxical air embolism occurred in 1 of these patients although without sequelae. Nine of the 35 patients without shunts experienced venous air embolism, but there were no episodes of paradoxical air embolism. The investigators concluded that paradoxical air embolism is an infrequent occurrence, provided that the volume of air entrained is small. However, it is possible to miss an existing patent foramen ovale.

The conditions under which paradoxical embolization of air can occur through the pulmonary vascular bed in humans have not been well defined. However, echocardiographic studies[78] and anecdotal reports describe its likely occurrence.[15,93,123,160] Findings regarding the occurrence and threshold for transpulmonary air passage differ in awake vs. anesthetized animal models, and the type of anesthetic appears to influence the threshold.[214,215] There also appears to be species variation in thresholds for transpulmonary passage of air.[199] Some investigators have suggested a lack of major transpulmonary air passage in sheep and dogs,[198] but significant air passage in the presence of a patent foramen ovale.[50] However, in other studies, air doses greater than 0.30 ml/kg/min in dogs as well as pretreatment with pulmonary vasodilators have been associated with systemic passage of air.[28,29] Although the true incidence of paradoxical air embolism is unknown, it may occur without producing postoperative sequelae, depending on both the volume and ultimate destination of air that enters the arterial circulation. Paradoxical air embolism to the cerebral circulation should be suspected in any patient who manifests an unexpected neurologic deficit after a surgical procedure known to be associated with a risk of air embolism.

Hypovolemia has been proposed as a predisposing factor to the occurrence of paradoxical as well as venous air embolism.[155] Likewise, intravenous fluid loading has been recommended to decrease the likelihood of right-to-left shunting and paradoxical air embolism in the sitting position.[40]

Use of Positive End Expiratory Pressure (PEEP)

Venous air embolism and PEEP may both increase right atrial pressure. PEEP (20 cm H_2O) may increase cerebral venous pressure. Voorhies reported prophylactic use of 20 cm H_2O PEEP without complications.[202] A large, retrospective study of 670 adults and 34 children undergoing posterior fossa surgery in the head-elevated position (back raised 30 to 45 degrees) reported use of PEEP (10 to 20 cm H_2O) to the end point of venous bleeding without complications.[200] PEEP of greater than 10 cm H_2O did not raise dural sinus pressure above zero in a small series of patients in the sitting position.[95,96] In another study of 11 patients, PEEP caused significant reductions in cardiac output, stroke volume, and mean arterial blood pressure along with in-

creases in pulmonary vascular resistance and right atrial pressure.[151] A study of superior sagittal sinus pressure in pediatric patients concluded that PEEP does not reliably raise superior sagittal sinus pressure.[80] Thus the value of PEEP as a prophylactic measure against venous air embolism is unclear. Further, it may impair surgical conditions, decrease venous return, and increase the chance of right atrial pressure exceeding left atrial pressure, thus predisposing an at-risk patient to paradoxic air embolism. Although some investigators have demonstrated a lack of right-to-left shunt from use of PEEP,[150,218] data from an animal model of an intracardiac defect indicate that increases in right-to-left shunt potential occurs when PEEP is discontinued.[17] The evidence of risks from use of PEEP for prophylaxis or treatment of venous air embolism currently outweighs evidence supporting its use. Jugular venous compression has been demonstrated to be effective in reducing air entry.[80,193,194]

Monitoring for Venous Air Embolism (Table 16-5)

Doppler Ultrasound Transducer

The precordial Doppler ultrasound transducer is the most sensitive device commonly available for the detection of air in the right atrium,[63,64,76] and it should be used in every sitting case. Some authorities have recommended its use in conjunction with Doppler ultrasound for all posterior fossa procedures regardless of position[3]; however, patient position influences air detection and retrieval.[26] In addition, correctly positioning the Doppler probe over the right heart may be difficult in positions other than sitting. Crystallized mannitol may produce Doppler changes similar to those of air embolism.[114] Recent clinical investigations have described greater sensitivity with transesophageal Doppler monitoring and avoidance of difficulties with external positioning of the probe.[127,146]

The Doppler probe generates a 2.5 MHz continuous ultrasonic signal, which is reflected by moving blood and cardiac structures.[121,136] The signal is electronically converted into a readily detectable audible sound. The frequency shift produced by reflection of the signal by air produces a characteristic change in the baseline sound. Small volumes of air are detected easily because air is a good acoustic reflector.[122] The precordial probe should be placed just to the right of the sternum and a few inches above the xiphoid, as the maximal signal is detected in this location. Position of the probe is confirmed by injecting 0.25 to 0.5 ml CO_2 or 5 ml heparinized saline[39,121,188] through a right-atrial catheter and listening for the characteristic change in the Doppler tones.

Right-Atrial Catheter

The right-atrial catheter (RAC) is used to aspirate air entering the right heart; air aspiration is therapeutic during episodes of air embolism. It is useful in confirming the diagnosis of air embolism, particularly during electrocautery use, when the Doppler signal is obscured.[1,4,133] The right

TABLE 16-5
Monitors for Detection of Venous Air Embolism

Monitor	Advantages	Disadvantages
Precordial Doppler	Noninvasive Most sensitive noninvasive monitor Earliest detector (before air enters pulmonary circulation)	Not quantitative May be difficult to place in obese patients, patients with chest wall deformity, or those in the prone/lateral positions False negative if air does not pass beneath ultrasonic beam (about 10% of cases); useless during electrocautery IV mannitol may mimic intravascular air
Pulmonary artery (PA) catheter	Quantitative, slightly more sensitive than ET_{CO_2} Widely available Placed with minimal difficulty in experienced hands Can detect right-atrial pressure greater than pulmonary capillary wedge pressure	Small lumen, less air aspirated than with right-atrial catheter Placement for optimal air aspiration may not allow pulmonary capillary wedge pressure measurement Nonspecific for air
Capnography (ET_{CO_2})	Noninvasive Sensitive Quantitative Widely available	Nonspecific for air Less sensitive than Doppler, PA catheter Accuracy affected by tachypnea, low cardiac output, chronic obstructive pulmonary disease
End-tidal nitrogen (ET_{N_2})	Specific for air Detects air earlier than ET_{CO_2}	May not detect subclinical air embolism May indicate air clearance from pulmonary circulation prematurely Accuracy affected by hypotension
Transesophageal echocardiography (TEE)	Most sensitive detector of air Can detect air in left heart, aorta	Invasive, cumbersome Expensive Must be observed continuously Not quantitative May interfere with Doppler

atrium may be catheterized by any of the routes discussed in the section on general monitoring issues. Optimal catheter placement requires that the orifice(s) being placed in or near air-blood interface for best air capture.[25,26,53]

The RAC is placed with a minimum of difficulty (usually <15 minutes[45]), and most neuroanesthetists believe that efforts to place an RAC are worth the time spent. Large-diameter catheters can retrieve large quantities of air, and aspiration of air has been demonstrated to be therapeutic when larger quantities have been entrained.[36,37,137] Disadvantages are that the catheter's position can change (especially after patient repositioning),[107] it is invasive, and it may not retrieve all intravascular air.

Multiorifice RACs have been demonstrated to be more effective than single-orifice catheters in aspirating air from the circulation.[3] There is greater air recovery (80%) with the tip at or 2 cm below the sinoatrial (SA) node with 80-degree atrial tilt that is, proximal port 1 to 3 cm above SA node (in vitro)[26]; a greater zone of negative pressure exists for air capture; less impairment of function occurs if a clot forms; and there is decreased suction adhesion to the heart chamber wall.

Questions regarding positioning of the multiorifice catheter and its optimal location for air recovery in humans are under investigation. Factors that influence air retrieval include catheter length and diameter, degree of patient inclination (retrieval is most efficient at 80 degrees; retrieval at 60 degrees is equal to that at 90 degrees), number and size of orifices, and distance between orifices[20,35,89,98,204] (Table 16-6). A 25-cm modified pulmonary artery (PA) cathetersheath has also been developed, which allows air aspiration through the multi-orifice end and simultaneous placement of a PA catheter.[20] These are 9 Fr sheaths, however.

RAC positioning for optimal air aspiration can be accomplished with intravascular electrocardiography.[21,35] A method for ECG-guided catheter placement is as follows:

- For the arm or neck, venipuncture is performed aseptically using a modified Seldinger technique.
- Advance the catheter at least 20 cm via the arm or 15 cm via the neck.
- Place a specially adapted conductive connector for ECG attachment (Arrow-Johans ECG adapter, Arrow International, Inc.) in the right atrial line next to the standard stopcock. Flushing the catheter with $NaHCO_3$ will decrease electrical impedance and improve the signal.[35]
- Set the ECG monitor for lead II and attach the right arm lead to the conductive connector. Some centers use lead V, which results in deflection of the P wave in the opposite direction.

TABLE 16-6
Characteristics of Catheters Used for Venous Air Aspiration

Catheter (Manufacturer)	Length (cm)	Diameter (Fr)	Distance from Proximal-to-Distal Orifice (cm)
Multiorificed			
Bunegin-Albin multiorifice (Cook)	80 (arm)	5.8	4.2
	30 (neck)	5.8	
Flow-directed angiography (Baxter)	110	7	1.0
8 Fr multiorifice angiography (Edwards)	110	8	4.9
PAC multiorifice sheath (Cook)	25	9	4.2
Single Orificed			
Swan-Ganz thermodilution (Baxter) (single distal orifice and CVP port)	110	7	NA
Swan-Ganz pulmonary artery (Edwards) (single distal orifice and CVP port)	110	~7	NA
Single orifice CVP (Sorenson)	23.5	~5.5	NA
Single orifice drum cartridge (Abbott)	71	5	NA

• Observe the ECG trace and pressure waveform on the monitor and manipulate the catheter until the tip is in the right ventricle, then withdraw into the mid-right atrium to detect a biphasic P wave.
• Withdraw the catheter until the P wave is approximately the height of the QRS complex (Fig. 16-2). Withdraw an additional centimeter, at which point the P wave should be slightly smaller than the QRS complex, then secure the catheter.

The intracardiac ECG should be rechecked after the patient has been placed in the final position because sitting as well as movement of the neck or the catheterized arm may move the catheter.[35,107,111,191] Although a high incidence of catheter migration has been reported,[107] the conductive connector should be removed after the patient is sitting and the catheter position has been reconfirmed to eliminate its electrical microshock hazard. In addition, the catheter tip should be withdrawn from the right atrium at the end of surgery to avoid atrial perforation.

Observation of the ECG configuration to confirm proper catheter placement in the right atrium is more precise than chest x-ray. However, a recent description of pressure-wave transduction for catheter placement reported that changes in the pressure wave form are as accurate as changes in the ECG waveform.[141] If this conclusion is confirmed by others, the technique may be of greatest benefit in rechecking catheter position periodically throughout surgery.

Pulmonary Artery (PA) Catheter

Passage of air into the pulmonary circulation leads to mechanical obstruction and reflex vasoconstriction from local hypoxemia. The PA catheter detects the resultant pulmonary hypertension.[13,124,145] PA pressure measurement is slightly more sensitive than capnography for detection of venous air embolism, but it is more invasive, and the PA catheter's lumen makes air aspiration more difficult than with larger catheters.[13,20] In addition, the fixed distance between the PA catheter tip and the right-atrial port makes simultaneous optimal positioning for PCWP measurements and air aspiration difficult. Use of the pulmonary capillary wedge pressure (PCWP) to determine when left atrial pressure exceeds right atrial pressure has been advocated, but PCWP may not be a reliable estimate of left atrial pressure at higher pulmonary pressures.[17]

Exhaled Gas Analysis

Exhaled gas monitoring in the operating room makes use of infrared analysis, mass spectroscopy, Raman light-scattering spectroscopy, or some combination of these techniques. Improvements in technology have made individual use (as opposed to shared use) monitors more practical and affordable. Spectroscopy techniques can measure concentrations of volatile inhalational anesthetics in addition to O_2, N_2O, CO_2, and N_2.

Capnography ($ETco_2$)

The capnograph is a critical monitoring device for neurosurgical procedures. Not only is it useful for obtaining reliable estimates of arterial $Paco_2$ (decreasing blood gas sampling frequency), but it also gives information regarding endotracheal tube disconnects, apnea, esophageal intubation, patient efforts to breathe despite mechanical ventilation, and air embolism.[22,67,92,179] Capnography has a specific role for air embolism detection in enabling detection of the increased arterial-to-end-tidal CO_2 gradient associated with its occurrence. Factors that may influence the capnograph's accuracy include rapid respiratory rate, low cardiac output, and chronic obstructive pulmonary disease.

End Tidal Nitrogen (ET_{N_2})[56,129,130,165]

Advantages of end-tidal N_2 monitoring over capnography are its specificity for air and earlier detection than $ETco_2$

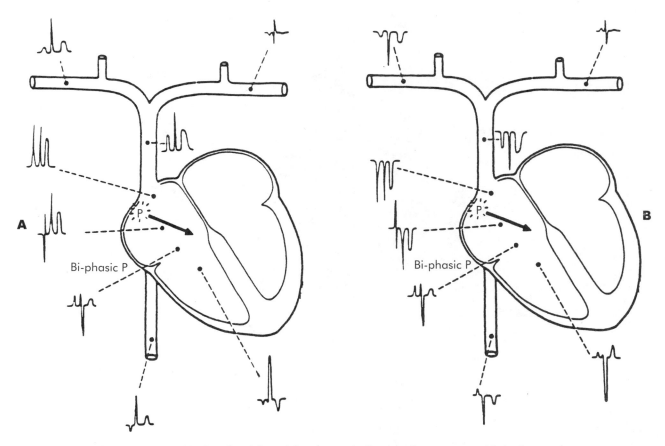

FIG. 16-2 Positioning the right-atrial catheter. **A,** P wave changes seen with lead II as the sensing lead. **B,** P wave changes seen with lead V as the sensing lead.

when air enters the pulmonary circulation.[129] However, the sensitivity of current N_2 monitoring technology available for clinical use may not be sufficient to detect subclinical venous air embolism. In addition, ET_{N_2} decreases with hypotension, and it may indicate prematurely that N_2 has been eliminated from the pulmonary circulation.[56,129]

Transesophageal Echocardiography (TEE)

Intraoperative use of TEE is increasing in cardiac anesthesia and surgery. Its use in neurosurgery is still in clinical investigative stages. TEE detects air bubbles with a 3.5 to 5.0 MHz echocardiographic probe placed behind the heart; a visual image is produced with two-dimensional TEE[77,166] (Fig. 16-3).

TEE is slightly more sensitive than precordial Doppler. In animal studies, bolus injection of 0.02 ml/kg air via the right external jugular vein was reliably detected on contrast ECHO.[72] Pulmonary artery pressure and ET_{CO_2} did not change with air injections up to 0.1 ml/kg. Doppler changes occurred consistently at 0.05 ml/kg. With continuous air infusion, Doppler and contrast ECHO showed changes 100% of the time at 0.05 ml/kg/min. Pulmonary artery pressure and ET_{CO_2} changed at an air infusion rate of 0.1 ml/kg/min in only 75% of cases.

TEE, like Doppler ultrasound, detects air when it is still in the right heart.[47,146] TEE and Doppler transducers may interfere with each other, but it is possible to use them simultaneously in patients because the TEE transducer can be directed at the right ventricular outflow tract and the Doppler probe is over the right atrium. A major advantage of TEE over other monitors currently available is that air can be detected in the left heart and aorta. A disadvantage is that detection of air bubbles is qualitative, not quantitative; thus microbubbles can generate a dramatic image.

Other Monitoring Methods
Doppler Monitoring of Carotid, Middle Cerebral Arteries

Doppler monitoring of the cerebral circulation uses the same technology currently in use for venous air embolism detection. Routine carotid Doppler monitoring may not be specific for paradoxical air embolism because air in the adjacent internal jugular veins would also be detected. However, transcranial Doppler monitoring of the middle cerebral artery may become a feasible alternative. Animal studies[163] and data from patients during carotid endarterectomy[182] demonstrate its ability to detect air-bubble emboli.

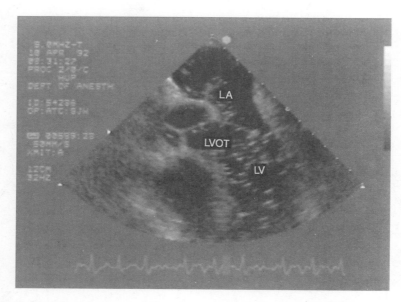

FIG. 16-3 Visualization of intracardiac air by TEE. Long-axis view of the heart at the level of the left atrium and left ventricle; left-ventricular outflow tract is shown. Microbubbles represented by the high-intensity echoes are noted in all three structures. *LA*, left atrium; *LV*, left ventricle; *LVOT*, left ventricular outflow tract.

Further investigations to determine the clinical significance of its measurements and efforts to make the equipment less cumbersome are needed.

Emission Spectroscopy

This technology offers the potential advantage of greater sensitivity for ET_{N_2} detection and lower cost than mass spectroscopy.[164] However, halogenated anesthetics and hemodynamic changes have significant effect on the accuracy of current technology. Thus its use is still in investigational stages.

Complications Resulting from Venous Air Embolism

Intraoperative Complications

Cardiovascular instability caused by venous air embolism (Table 16-7) may be manifested in a number of ways. The most common form of dysrhythmia is premature ventricular contractions, but murmurs, tachycardia, bradycardia, and ventricular tachycardia may occur.[1,4,113,135] Hypertension and tachycardia may occur initially in response to air entry into the pulmonary microcirculation. Marked alterations in blood pressure and the characteristic changes in heart sounds usually do not appear until large emboli are present. Hypotension is most likely due to decreases in cardiac output associated with larger volumes of intravascular air.[1] Hypertension has been noted in animals with cerebral air emboli.[69] With an increasing volume of air, changes in heart tones include increases in the second heart sound, S_2, a harsh systolic murmur, and the classic "mill wheel" mur-

mur.[99,210] However, the duration of these signs may be brief (i.e., less than 5 minutes) although air is still present.[67] ECG changes are generally too late to be useful diagnostically; however, evidence of transmural myocardial ischemia may indicate air flow into the coronary arteries.[58] Right-ventricular failure results from acute dilation and pulmonary outflow obstruction.[1] Rapid accumulation of large volumes of air may overwhelm the pulmonary circulation or produce air lock in the right-heart chambers, leading to cardiac arrest.

Animal studies of intracoronary air have reported ECG changes resulting from as little as 0.025 ml air injected into the anterior descending coronary artery of the dog, and 0.05 ml in the same model has resulted in death. In studies of the effects of intracerebral air embolism, acute hypertension and severe cardiac dysrhythmias after infusion of 2.0 ml/kg of air into the vertebral arteries of cats have been described.[69] Similar findings have been reported in dogs with carotid injections of air.[71]

A "gasp" has been described as a classic clinical finding when air embolism occurs.[1,108] The likelihood of this occurrence is greater in an unparalyzed patient. The extent of pulmonary dysfunction depends on the amount of air that reaches the pulmonary circulation. Hypercarbia, hypoxemia, and pulmonary hypertension may be mild, moderate, or severe.

Pulmonary edema may follow large air emboli; its development is believed to involve mechanisms similar to clot emboli as opposed to neurogenic pulmonary edema.[178] Its association with elevations in pulmonary

TABLE 16-7
Complications of Venous Air Embolism

Complications	Intraoperative	Postoperative
Cardiovascular	Dysrhythmias	Myocardial ischemia
	Hypotension/hypertension	Right-ventricular failure
	Changes in heart sounds, murmurs	
	ECG evidence of ischemia	
	Acute right-ventricular failure	
	Cardiac arrest	
Pulmonary	Hypercarbia	Perfusion defects
	Hypoxemia	Pulmonary edema
	Pulmonary hypertension	
	Pulmonary edema	
Central nervous system	Hyperemia	Neurologic deficits, stroke, coma
	Brain swelling	

capillary wedge pressure can be used to distinguish it from neurogenic pulmonary edema, which is associated with a normal wedge pressure.[33,154] Damage to the pulmonary vascular endothelium may result from repeated bouts of pulmonary hypertension.[142,148] Perfusion defects similar to those found in instances of clot pulmonary emboli have been described after pulmonary air embolism[171]; their distinguishing feature is the rapid resolution of the defect (often within 24 hours).

Intraoperative brain swelling and hyperemia are theoretic complications that may result from air embolism. The possible mechanisms include hypoxemia from impaired pulmonary gas exchange and intracerebral air embolism, which may produce derangements in cerebral blood flow and increased ICP.[51,87,88] These phenomena have been described in animal studies,[58,69,71,175] and in cases of emergency surgery for traumatic brain injury; however, they have not been described as such during intraoperative episodes of air embolism.

Postoperative Complications

Complications arising from air embolism primarily involve the central nervous, cardiovascular, and pulmonary systems. Neurologic deficits, stroke, and coma may result from surgical manipulation, hypoxic/ischemic injury, or cerebral air embolism. There are varying reports from animal studies regarding complications from intracerebral air. Dose and rate of air entrainment appear to influence the clinical findings.[51] Increases in ICP appear to be associated with more severe injury.[51,175] Rapid intracarotid injection of 1.5 to 3 ml air/kg in 16 dogs produced immediate nystagmus, loss of lid reflexes, dilation of pupils, flaccidity, opisthotonos, extensor rigidity, and convulsions.[71] Only 2 of 16 dogs survived for 3 months, and neurologic deficits persisted in both. With slow intracarotid injection of air (0.3 to 2 ml air/kg/hr) in 29 dogs, immediate physical changes were not marked; however, prolonged awakening, varying degrees of paresis,

and blindness were some of the late manifestations. Of the 29 dogs, 20 died within 24 hours. Neurologic deficits receded considerably in 9 of 29 dogs who survived for more than 3 days, but they did not resolve completely by the time of animal sacrifice (up to 3 months).

Available studies in humans have been unable to correlate morbidity and mortality with the volume of cerebral arterial air introduced. However, there is clear laboratory and clinical evidence that cerebral air can produce brain injury. In 12 patients with massive arterial air embolism during cardiopulmonary bypass, four patients experienced immediate death, three patients experienced transient neurologic deficits consisting of prolonged awakening to deep coma, and five patients had no sequelae.[140] Other studies have reported altered sensorium, convulsions, hemiplegia, monoplegia, hemianesthesia, hemianopsia, nystagmus, strabismus, and respiratory disturbances.[81,99,160] A case report described suspected arterial air embolism from an indeterminate volume of air flushed retrograde through a radial artery catheter; further investigation of this phenomenon in a primate model using ^{133}Xe cerebral scanning concluded that 5 ml of air could produce scintigraphic evidence of cerebral air embolism.[34]

Potential postoperative cardiovascular complications resulting from venous air embolism include right-ventricular failure (from pulmonary hypertension) and myocardial ischemia (from coronary air embolism or right-heart strain). Postoperative pulmonary edema may produce chest X-ray abnormalities and perfusion defects, but it is usually self-limited and responsive to conservative therapy, such as supplemental O_2 or small doses of furosemide.[153,171,178,184]

Prevention of Air Embolism

No maneuver is 100% effective in preventing the occurrence of venous air embolism if there is a gradient between the operative site and the right atrium. However, the incidence and severity can be decreased by the use of controlled positive pressure, rather than spontaneous, ventilation, adequate hydration, proper wrapping of the lower extremities, positioning such that head elevation is the lowest it can be and still provide good surgical exposure, meticulous surgical technique with careful dissection and liberal use of bone wax, avoidance of N_2O in patients with known intracardiac defects, and avoidance of drugs that may increase venous capacitance (e.g., nitroglycerin).

Application of lower-body positive pressure with an antigravity suit (G-suit) or military antishock trousers (MAST) has been advocated by some to prevent or treat venous air embolism or the hypotension that occurs during the sitting position.[75,125] Such maneuvers increase right atrial pressure via reduction of systemic venous compliance and peripheral venous pooling[61] and abdominal compression.[213] However, one study concluded that the G-suit is not consistently effective in maintaining venous pressure in normovolemic patients if inflated to 30 mm Hg for longer than 30 minutes; thus it is of minimal value as prophylaxis against venous air embolism.[126] Tinker and Vandam's review of clinical experience with the G-suit concluded that there was no benefit to its use.[189] However, lower-body positive pressure may provide a beneficial effect from the generalized decrease in capacitance and increase in central venous pressure produced by venous compression.[61] If the G-suit is used, adequate padding of the fibular head is necessary to prevent peroneal nerve compression. Placement of the G-suit or MAST may interfere with application of inflatable intermittent compression stockings, which have been used with increased frequency to decrease the risk of lower extremity deep-vein thrombosis.[196]

Treatment of Venous Air Embolism
Intraoperative Period

The intraoperative goals in the treatment of venous air embolism (Box 16-2) are to stop further air entry, remove air already present, and correct hypotension, hypoxemia, and hypercarbia. If Doppler changes occur or $ETCO_2$ decreases more than 2 mm Hg, the surgeon should be informed immediately.

Jugular compression has been shown to be effective in raising dural sinus pressure in patients in both supine and sitting positions.[80,95,96,194] However, there are potential clinical concerns about the technique of jugular venous compression. It may cause (1) cerebral venous outflow obstruction with a resulting decrease in cerebral blood flow, (2) carotid artery compression or dislodgement of atherosclerotic plaques, (3) venous engorgement, leading to brain swelling and cerebral edema, and (4) carotid sinus compression and bradycardia. Maintenance of cerebral perfusion pressure greater than 60 mm Hg in normotensive patients should minimize the risk of cerebral hypoperfusion. Higher perfusion pressures should be maintained in chronic hypertensive patients.

Aspiration of the right-atrial catheter should be initiated as quickly as possible after Doppler or TEE detection of intravascular air. This maneuver has been demonstrated ef-

▼

BOX 16-2
TREATMENT OF VENOUS AIR EMBOLISM

Intraoperative Rx
1. Inform surgeon immediately
2. Discontinue N_2O, increase O_2 flows
3. Have surgeon flood surgical field with fluids
4. Provide jugular vein compression
5. Aspirate right-atrial catheter
6. Provide cardiovascular support
7. Modify the anesthetic
8. Change patient position

Postoperative Rx
1. Provide supplemental O_2
2. Perform ECG, chest x-ray
3. Measure serial arterial blood gases
4. Provide hyperbaric compression if arterial air emboli are suspected

fective in reducing morbidity from venous air embolism.[1,4,37,135]

Patient position should be changed to lower the head to heart level when feasible. Other measures include increased intravenous fluid administration, vasopressors if hypotension occurs, antirhythmics (intravenous lidocaine is effective for premature ventricular contractions), and modification of the anesthetic in the absence of N_2O with more isoflurane, narcotic, barbiturate, scopolamine, or lidocaine. External cardiac massage has been shown to be effective in disrupting a large air lock in the event of cardiovascular collapse.[68] Changing the patient's position to left lateral decubitus to limit airflow through the pulmonary outflow tract is of limited benefit in the presence of a continuous stream of air. PEEP or Valsalva may increase likelihood of paradoxical embolus after venous air embolism has occurred and should therefore be avoided or discontinued.*

Postoperative Period

Postoperative goals include prevention of hypoxemia or other respiratory compromise, detection and treatment of myocardial ischemia, and treatment of clinical evidence of paradoxical air embolism. Useful diagnostic studies include arterial blood gas measurements, ECG, and electrophysiologic monitoring. Air bubbles in the retinal vessels, seen through fundoscopic examination, have been described as a diagnostic sign for cerebral air embolism.[10] In patients with suspected cerebral air embolism, a CT scan may aid in the diagnosis.[93,149,201] However, radiographic evidence of cerebral air may vary among patients, initial scans may be negative, and the findings may change over time.[90,97] The role of magnetic resonance imaging (MR) in the diag-

---

*References 17, 48, 82, 104, 105, 118.

nosis of air embolism remains to be determined. Although MR has been described as more sensitive than CT scan in detecting ischemic cerebral and spinal diving-related injuries,[206] technical constraints may limit its use in critically ill patients.

There is considerable controversy over the use of hyperbaric oxygen therapy (HBO) for the treatment of suspected cerebral air embolism. Rapid application of very high pressure reduces air bubble volume, which should speed elimination of dissolved gas and reduce cerebral edema.[59,165] Numerous reports, some dramatic, describe the benefits of HBO therapy for decompression sickness and arterial gas embolism.[60] However, its effects on pulmonary elimination of intravascular air and reversal of pathophysiologic changes in end organs have not been well documented. Further, HBO therapy does not always result in an improved neurologic picture. A National Heart, Lung, and Blood Institute Workshop reported that there is a significant lack of data currently available regarding the efficacy of HBO therapy.[147] More aggressive basic research and controlled clinical trials are needed before the purported beneficial effects HBO can be applied to human disease.

ELECTROPHYSIOLOGIC MONITORING

Various forms of monitoring, such as raw or processed electroencephalogram, brainstem auditory evoked potentials, and somatosensory and motor nerve stimulation are being investigated for their usefulness in determining the integrity of cerebral function during posterior fossa surgery. Such monitoring is used in selected intracranial, spinal, and cerebrovascular procedures and is generally handled by experienced electrophysiologists. Bimodal or multimodal measurement of EEG, brainstem auditory evoked potentials (BAEPs), and somatosensory evoked potentials (SSEPs) has been advocated as a more effective means of monitoring CNS function for posterior fossa surgery than single-modality monitoring.[157,167]

Brainstem Auditory Evoked Potentials (BAEPs)

BAEPs are robust signals that are minimally influenced by the type or depth of anesthesia. Cranial nerve VIII monitoring during acoustic neuroma resection or microvascular decompression has been advocated to help preserve nerve VIII function.[110,159,208] Bilateral changes in BAEP are indicative of brainstem compromise.[83,158] Normalization of BAEPs during emergency posterior fossa decompression

has been used to guide postoperative management and timing of extubation.[169]

Somatosensory Evoked Potentials (SSEPS)

SSEPs may be of use in detecting spinal cord ischemia caused by hypotension or stretch of the cord caused by excessive neck flexion. Monitoring of short-latency SSEPs, which monitor subcortical components of central sensory pathways, has been advocated for surgery on the cervical cord and posterior fossa.[197] Long-latency components of SSEPs may be difficult to evaluate because of greater variability in both latency and amplitude. The use of SSEPs may preclude the administration of high concentrations of volatile anesthetics or N_2O; thus higher doses of narcotics or intravenous sedatives may be needed.

Electroencephalogram (EEG)

EEG signals provide information regarding depth of anesthesia because they are sensitive to both inhalational and intravenous anesthetics. Intraoperative EEG monitoring during posterior fossa surgery can detect decreased cortical responses resulting from deep anesthesia or ischemia. The cortical components of SSEPs give similar information to EEG signals.

Facial Nerve Monitoring

Monitoring of facial nerve (VII) function may help reduce complications of surgical dissection and manipulation for resection of acoustic neuromas and microvascular decompression.[110] Muscle paralysis, which can interfere with the signal, should be avoided when muscle stimulation is required.

> ## SUMMARY
>
> The patient for posterior fossa surgery poses challenges to the anesthesiologist in terms of preoperative evaluation, positioning, choice of anesthetic agents, and monitoring, particularly for prevention of air embolism and preservation of neurologic function. The goals of monitoring are maintenance of hemodynamic stability and early detection of air embolism. Active clinical and basic science investigations continue to improve the means by which these challenges may be met in optimal fashion.

References

1. Adornato DC, Gildenberg PL, Ferrario CM et al: Pathophysiology of intravenous air embolism in dogs, *Anesthesiology* 49:120-127, 1978.
2. Albin MS, Babinski M, Maroon JC et al: Anesthetic management of posterior fossa surgery in the sitting position, *Acta Anaesth Scand* 20:117-128, 1976.
3. Albin MS, Carroll RG, Maroon JC: Clinical considerations concerning detection of venous air embolism, *Neurosurgery* 3:380-384, 1978.
4. Alvaran SB, Toung JK, Graff TE et al: Venous air embolism: compara-

tive merits of external cardiac massage, intracardiac aspiration, and left lateral decubitus position, *Anesth Analg* 57:166-170, 1978.

5. Appenzeller O, Descarries L: Circulatory reflexes in patients with cerebrovascular disease, *New Eng J Med* 271:820-823, 1964.

6. Artru AA: Nitrous oxide plays a direct role in the development of tension pneumocephalus intraoperatively, *Anesthesiology* 57:59-61, 1982.

7. Artru AA: Breathing nitrous oxide during closure of the dura and cranium is not indicated, *Anesthesiology* 66:719, 1987.

8. Artru AA, Cucchiara RF, Messick JM: Cardiorespiratory and cranial-nerve sequelae of surgical procedures involving the posterior fossa, *Anesthesiology* 52:83-86, 1980.

9. Banas JS, Meister SG, Gazzaniga AB et al: A simple technique for detecting small defects in the atrial septum, *Am J Cardiol* 28:467-471, 1971.

10. Barkan H: Air embolism in retinal vessels, *Arch Ophthalmol* 7:402-411, 1928.

11. Bedford RF: Venous air embolism: a historical perspective, *Semin Anesth* 2:169-176, 1983.

12. Bedford RF: Perioperative venous air embolism, *Semin Anesth* 6:163-170, 1987.

13. Bedford RF, Marshall WK, Butler A et al: Cardiac catheters for diagnosis and treatment of venous air embolism. A prospective study in man, *J Neurosurg* 55:610-614, 1981.

14. Berntman L, Welsh FA, Harp JR: Cerebral protective effect of low-grade hypothermia, *Anesthesiology* 55:495-498, 1981.

15. Black M, Calvin J, Chan KL et al: Paradoxic air embolism in the absence of an intracardiac defect, *Chest* 99:754-755, 1991.

16. Black PM, Davis JM, Kjellberg RN et al: Tension pneumocephalus of the cranial subdural space: a case report, *Neurosurgery* 5:368-370, 1979.

17. Black S, Cucchiara RF, Nishimura RA et al: Parameters affecting occurrence of paradoxical air embolism, *Anesthesiology* 71:235-241, 1989.

18. Black S, Muzzi DA, Nishimura RA et al: Preoperative and intraoperative echocardiography to detect right-to-left shunt in patients undergoing neu-

rosurgical procedures in the sitting position, *Anesthesiology* 72:436-438, 1990.

19. Black S, Ockert DB, Oliver WC et al: Outcome following posterior fossa craniotomy in patients in the sitting or horizontal positions, *Anesthesiology* 69:49-56, 1988.

20. Bowdle TA, Artru AA: Treatment of air embolism with a special pulmonary artery catheter introducer sheath in sitting dogs, *Anesthesiology* 68:107-110, 1988.

21. Bowdle TA, Artru AA: Positioning the air aspiration pulmonary artery catheter introducer sheath by intravascular electrocardiography, *Anesthesiology* 69:276-279, 1988.

22. Brechner VL, Bethune RWM: Recent advances in monitoring pulmonary air embolism, *Anesth Analg* 50:255-261, 1971.

23. Bristow JD, Honour AJ, Pickering GW et al: Diminished baroreflex sensitivity in high blood pressure, *Circulation* 39:48-54, 1969.

24. Bucciero A, Quaglietta P, Vizioli L: Supratentorial intracerebral hemorrhage after posterior fossa surgery, *J Neurosurg Sci* 35:221-224, 1991.

25. Bunegin L, Albin MS: Balloon catheter increases air capture, *Anesthesiology* 57:66-67, 1982.

26. Bunegin L, Albin MS, Helsel PE et al: Positioning the right atrial catheter—a model for reappraisal, *Anesthesiology* 55:343-348, 1981.

27. Burke CM, Safai C, Nelson DP et al: Pulmonary arteriovenous malformations: a critical update, *Am Rev Respir Dis* 134:334-339, 1986.

28. Butler BD, Hills BA: The lung as a filter for microbubbles, *J Appl Physiol* 47:537-541, 1979.

29. Butler BD, Hills BA: Transpulmonary passage of venous air emboli, *J Appl Physiol* 59:543-547, 1985.

30. Butler BD, Leiman BC, Katz J: Arterial air embolism of venous origin in dogs: effect of nitrous oxide in combination with halothane and pentobarbitone, *Can J Anaesth* 34:570-576, 1987.

31. Cabezudo JM, Gilsanz F, Vaquero J et al: Air embolism from wounds from a pin-type head-holder as a complication of posterior fossa surgery in the sitting position, *J Neurosurg* 55:147-148, 1981.

32. Calliauw L, Van Aken J, Rolly G et

al: The position of the patient during neurosurgical procedures on the posterior fossa, *Acta Neurochir (Wien)* 85:154-158, 1987.

33. Chandler WF, Dimsheff DG, Taren JA: Acute pulmonary edema following venous air embolism during a neurosurgical procedure, *J Neurosurg* 40:400-404, 1974.

34. Chang C, Dughi J, Shitabata P et al: Air embolism and the radial arterial line, *Crit Care Med* 16:141-143, 1988.

35. Colley PS, Artru AA: ECG-guided placement of Sorenson CVP catheters via arm veins, *Anesth Analg* 63:953-956, 1984.

36. Colley PS, Artru AA: Bunegin-Albin catheter improves air retrieval and resuscitation from lethal venous air embolism in dogs, *Anesth Analg* 66:991-994, 1987.

37. Colley PS, Artru AA: Bunegin-Albin catheter improves air retrieval and resuscitation from lethal venous air embolism in upright dogs, *Anesth Analg* 68:298-301, 1989.

38. Colley PS, Dunn R: Prevention of blood pressure response to skull-pin head holder by local anesthesia, *Anesth Analg* 58:241-243, 1979.

39. Colley PS, Pavlin EG, Groepper J: Assessment of a saline injection test for location of a right atrial catheter, *Anesthesiology* 50:258, 1979.

40. Colohan ART, Perkins NAK, Bedford RF et al: Intravenous fluid loading as prophylaxis for paradoxical air embolism, *J Neurosurg* 62:839-842, 1985.

41. Coonan TJ, Hope CE: Cardiorespiratory effects of change of body position, *Can Anaesth Soc J* 30:424-437, 1983.

42. Cottrell JE, Robustelli A, Post K et al: Furosemide and mannitol-induced changes in intracranial pressure and serum osmolarity and electrolytes, *Anesthesiology* 47:28-30, 1977.

43. Cucchiara RF: Safety of the sitting position, *Anesthesiology* 61:790, 1984.

44. Cucchiara RF, Bowers B: Air embolism in children undergoing suboccipital craniotomy, *Anesthesiology* 57:338-339, 1982.

45. Cucchiara RF, Messick JM, Gronert GA et al: Time required and success rate of percutaneous right atrial catheterization: description of a tech-

nique, *Can Anaesth Soc J* 27:572-573, 1980.

46. Cucchiara RF, Nishimura RA, Black S: Failure of preoperative echo testing to prevent paradoxical air embolism: report of two cases, *Anesthesiology* 71:604-607, 1989.

47. Cucchiara RF, Nugent M, Seward JD et al: Air embolism in upright neurosurgical patients: detection and localization by 2-dimensional transesophageal echocardiography, *Anesthesiology* 60:353-355, 1984.

48. Cucchiara RF, Seward JB, Nishimura RA et al: Identification of patent foramen ovale during sitting position craniotomy by transesophageal echocardiography with positive airway pressure, *Anesthesiology* 63:107-109, 1985.

49. Darymple DG, MacGowan SW, MacLeod GF: Cardiorespiratory effects of the sitting position in neurosurgery, *Br J Anaesth* 51:1079-1081, 1979.

50. Deal CW, Fielden BP, Monk I: Hemodynamic effects of pulmonary air embolism, *J Surg Res* 11:533-538, 1971.

51. De La Torre E, Meredith J, Netsky MG: Cerebral air embolism in the dog, *Arch Neurol* 6:67-76, 1962.

52. Denys BG, Breishlatt WM, Reddy PS et al: An ultrasound method for safe and rapid central venous access, *N Engl J Med* 324:566, 1991.

53. Diaz PM: Balloon catheter should increase recovery of embolized air, *Anesthesiology* 57:66, 1982.

54. Di Lorenzo N, Caruso R, Floris R et al: Pneumocephalus and tension pneumocephalus after posterior fossa surgery in the sitting position: a prospective study, *Acta Neurochir (Wien)* 83:112-115, 1986.

55. Drummond JC: Tension pneumocephalus and intermittent drainage of ventricular CSF, *Anesthesiology* 60:609-610, 1984.

56. Drummond JC, Prutow RJ, Scheller MS: A comparison of the sensitivity of pulmonary artery pressure, end-tidal carbon dioxide, and end-tidal nitrogen in the detection of venous air embolism in the dog, *Anesth Analg* 64:688-692, 1985.

57. Durant TM, Long J, Oppenheimer MJ: Pulmonary (venous) air embolism, *Am Heart J* 33:269-281, 1947.

58. Durant TM, Oppenheimer MJ, Webster MR et al: Arterial air embolism, *Am Heart J* 38:481-500, 1949.

59. Dutka AJ: A review of the pathophysiology and potential application of experimental therapies for cerebral ischemia to the treatment of cerebral arterial gas embolism, *Undersea Biomed Res* 12:403-421, 1985.

60. Dutka AJ: Air or gas embolism. In Camporesi EM, Barker AC, editors: Hyperbaric oxygen therapy: a critical review, Bethesda, Md, 1991, Undersea and Hyperbaric Medical Society, pp 1-10.

61. Echt M, Duweling J, Gauer OH et al: Effective compliance of the total vascular bed and the intrathoracic compartment derived from changes in central venous pressure induced by volume changes in man, *Circ Res* 34:61-68, 1974.

62. Edelman JD, Wingard DW: Air embolism arising from burrholes, *Anesthesiology* 53:167-168, 1980.

63. Edmonds-Seal J, Maroon JC: Air embolism diagnosed with ultrasound, *Anaesthesia* 24:438-440, 1969.

64. Edmonds-Seal J, Prys-Roberts C, Adams AP: Air embolism. A comparison of various methods of detection, *Anaesthesia* 26:202-208, 1971.

65. Ellis SC, Bryan-Brown CW, Hyderally H: Massive swelling of the head and neck, *Anesthesiology* 42:102-103, 1975.

66. Enderby GEH: Postural ischaemia and blood pressure, *Lancet* 1:185, 1954.

67. English JB, Westenskow D, Hodges MR et al: Comparison of venous air embolism monitoring methods in supine dogs, *Anesthesiology* 48:425-429, 1978.

68. Ericsson JA, Gottlieb JD, Sweet RB: Closed-chest cardiac massage in the treatment of venous air embolism, *N Engl J Med* 270:1353-1354, 1964.

69. Evans DE, Kobrine AI, Weathersby PK et al: Cardiovascular effects of cerebral air embolism, *Stroke* 12:338-344, 1981.

70. Friedman GA, Norfleet EA, Bedford RF: Discontinuance of nitrous oxide does not prevent pneumocephalus, *Anesth Analg* 60:57-58, 1981.

71. Fries CC, Lenowitz B, Adler S et al: Experimental cerebral gas embolism, *Ann Surg* 145:461-470, 1957.

72. Furuya H, Suzuki T, Okumura F et al: Detection of air embolism by transesophageal echocardiography, *Anesthesiology* 58:124-129, 1983.

73. Garcia-Bengochea F, Fernandez JC: The lateral sitting position: for operations in the posterior fossa and in the cervical and upper thoracic regions of the spine, *J Neurosurg* 13:520-522, 1956.

74. Gardner WJ: Intracranial operations in the sitting position, *Ann Surg* 101:138-145, 1935.

75. Gardner WJ, Dohn DF: The antigravity suit (G-suit) in surgery: control of blood pressure in the sitting position and in hypotensive anesthesia, *JAMA* 162:274, 1956.

76. Gildenberg PL, O'Brien RP, Britt WJ et al: The efficacy of Doppler monitoring for the detection of venous air embolism, *J Neurosurg* 54:75-78, 1981.

77. Glenski JA, Cucchiara RF, Michenfelder JD: Transesophageal echocardiography and transcutaneous O_2 and CO_2 monitoring for detection of venous air embolism, *Anesthesiology* 64:541-545, 1986.

78. Gottdiener JS, Papademetriou V, Notargiacomo A et al: Incidence and cardiac effects of systemic venous air embolism. Echocardiographic evidence of arterial embolization via noncardiac shunt, *Arch Intern Med* 148:795-800, 1988.

79. Gottlieb JD, Ericsson JA, Sweet RB: Venous air embolism: a review, *Anesth Analg* 44:773-778, 1963.

80. Grady MS, Bedford RF, Park TS: Changes in superior sagittal sinus pressure in children with head elevation, jugular venous compression and PEEP, *J Neurosurg* 65:199-202, 1986.

81. Gronert GA, Messick JM, Cucchiara RF et al: Paradoxical air embolism from a patent foramen ovale, *Anesthesiology* 50:548-549, 1979.

82. Gross CM, Wann S, Johnson G: Valsalva maneuver contrast echocardiography, a new technique for improved detection of right to left shunting in patients with systemic embolism, *Am J Cardiol* 49:995-999, 1982.

83. Grundy BL, Linda A, Procopio PT et al: Reversible evoked potential changes with retraction of the eighth cranial nerve, *Anesth Analg* 60:835-838, 1981.

84. Grundy BL, Spetzler RF: Subdural

pneumocephalus resulting from drainage of cerebrospinal fluid during craniotomy, *Anesthesiology* 52:269-271, 1980.

85. Guggiari M, Lechat Ph, Garen-Colonne C et al: Early detection of patent foramen ovale by two-dimensional contrast echocardiography for prevention of paradoxical air embolism during sitting position, *Anesth Analg* 67:192-194, 1988.

86. Hagen PT, Scholz DG, Edwards WD: Incidence and size of patent foramen ovale during the first 10 decades of life: an autopsy study of 965 normal hearts, *Mayo Clin Proc* 59:17-23, 1984.

87. Helps SC, Meyer-Witting M, Reilly PL et al: Increasing doses of intracarotid air and cerebral blood flow in rabbits, *Stroke* 21:1340-1345, 1990.

88. Helps SC, Parsons DW, Reilly PL et al: The effect of gas emboli on rabbit cerebral blood flow, *Stroke* 21:94-99, 1990.

89. Hicks HC, Hummel JC: A new catheter for detection and treatment of venous air embolism, *J Neurosurg* 52:595-598, 1980.

90. Hirabuki N, Miura T, Mitomo M et al: Changes of cerebral air embolism shown by computed tomography, *Br J Radiol* 61:252-255, 1988.

91. Howard R, Mahoney A, Thurlow AC: Respiratory obstruction after posterior fossa surgery, *Anaesthesia* 45:222-224, 1990.

92. Hurter D, Sebel PS: Detection of venous air embolism, *Anaesthesia* 34:578-582, 1979.

93. Hwang T, Fremavx R, Sears ES et al: Confirmation of cerebral air embolism with computerized tomography, *Ann Neurol* 13:214-215, 1983.

94. Iwabuchi T, Ishii M, Julow J: Biparietal-occipital craniotomy with hyperextended neck, "sea lion" position, *Acta Neurochir (Wien)* 51:113-117, 1979.

95. Iwabuchi T, Sobata E, Ebina K et al: Dural sinus pressure: various aspects in human brain surgery in children and adults, *Am J Physiol* 250:389-396, 1986.

96. Iwabuchi T, Sobata E, Suzuki M et al: Dural sinus pressure as related to neurosurgical positions, *Neurosurgery* 12:203-207, 1983.

97. Jensen ME, Lipper MH: CT in iatrogenic cerebral air embolism, *AJNR* 7:823-827, 1986.

98. Johans TG: Multi-orificed catheter placement with an intravascular electrocardiographic technique, *Anesthesiology* 64:411-413, 1986.

99. Kent EM, Blades B: Experimental observations upon certain intracranial complications of particular interest to the thoracic surgeon, *J Thorac Surg* 11:434-445, 1941.

100. Keykhah MM, Rosenberg H: Bilateral footdrop after craniotomy in the sitting position, *Anesthesiology* 51:163-164, 1979.

101. Kishan A, Naidu MR, Muralidhar K: Tension pneumocephalus following posterior fossa surgery in sitting position. A report of 2 cases, *Clin Neurol Neurosurg* 92:245-248, 1990.

102. Kitahata LM, Katz JD: Tension pneumocephalus after posteriorfossa craniotomy: a complication of the sitting position, *Anesthesiology* 45:578, 1976.

103. Kloosterboer TB, Springman SR, Coursin DB: Subclavian vein catheter as a source of air emboli in the sitting position, *Anesthesiology* 64:411, 1986.

104. Kondstadt SN, Louie EK, Black S et al: Intraoperative detection of patent foramen ovale by transesophageal echocardiography, *Anesthesiology* 74:212-216, 1991.

105. Kronik G, Mosslacher H: Positive contrast echocardiography in patients with patent foramen ovale and normal right heart hemodynamics, *Am J Cardiol* 49:1806-1809, 1982.

106. Lall NG, Jain AP: Circulatory and respiratory disturbances during posterior fossa surgery, *Br J Anaesth* 41:447-449, 1969.

107. Lee DS, Kuhn J, Shaffer MJ et al: Migration of tips of central venous catheters in seated patients, *Anesth Analg* 63:949-952, 1984.

108. Lesky E: Notes on the history of air embolism, *German Med Monthly* 6:159-161, 1961.

109. Lincoln JR, Sawyer HP: Complications related to body positions during surgical procedures, *Anesthesiology* 22:800-809, 1961.

110. Linden RD, Tator CH, Benedict D et al: Electrophysiological monitoring during acoustic neuroma and other posterior fossa surgery, *Can J Neurol Sci* 15:73-81, 1988.

111. Lingenfelter AL, Guskiewicz RA, Munson ES: Displacement of right atrial and endotracheal catheters with neck flexion, *Anesth Analg* 57:371, 1978.

112. Losasso TJ, Black S, Muzzi DA et al: Detection and hemodynamic consequences of venous air embolism: does nitrous oxide make a difference? *Anesthesiology* 77:148-152, 1992.

113. Losasso TJ, Martino JD, Muzzi DA: Venous air embolism in the recovery room producing unexplained cardiac dysrhythmias: a case report, *Anesthesiology* 72:203-205, 1990.

114. Losasso TJ, Muzzi DA, Cucchiara RF: Doppler detection of intravenous mannitol crystals mimics venous air embolism, *Anesth Analg* 71:568-569, 1990.

115. Losasso TJ, Muzzi DA, Dietz NM et al: Fifty percent nitrous oxide does not increase the risk of venous air embolism in neurosurgical patients operated upon in the sitting position, *Anesthesiology* 77:21-30, 1992.

116. Losasso TJ, Muzzi DA, Weglinski MR: The risk of paradoxical air embolism (PAE) in sitting neurosurgical patients with and without a demonstrable right-to-left (R→L) shunt, *Anesthesiology* 77:a198, 1992.

117. Lunsford LD, Maroon JC, Sheptak PE et al: Subdural tension pneumocephalus. Report of two cases, *J Neurosurg* 50:525-527, 1979.

118. Lynch JJ, Schuchard GH, Gross CM et al: Prevalence of right-to-left atrial shunting in a healthy population: detection by Valsalva maneuver contrast echocardiography, *Am J Cardiol* 53:1478-1480, 1984.

119. MacGillivray RG: Pneumocephalus as a complication of posterior fossa surgery in the sitting position, *Anaesthesia* 37:722-725, 1982.

120. Manninen PH, Cuillerier DJ, Nantau WE et al: Monitoring of brainstem function during vertebral basilar aneurysm surgery: the use of spontaneous ventilation, *Anesthesiology* 77:681-685, 1992.

121. Maroon JC, Albin MS: Air embolism diagnosed by Doppler ultrasound, *Anesth Analg* 53:399-402, 1974.

122. Maroon JC, Goodman JM, Horner TG et al: Detection of minute venous air emboli with ultrasound, *Surg Gynecol Obstet* 127:1236-1238, 1968.

123. Marquez J, Sladen A, Gendell H et al: Paradoxical cerebral air embolism without an intracardiac septal defect, *J Neurosurg* 55:997-999, 1981.

124. Marshall WK, Bedford RF: Use of pulmonary-artery catheter for detection and treatment of venous air embolism: a prospective study in man, *Anesthesiology* 52:131-134, 1980.

125. Marshall WK, Bedford RF, Miller ED: Cardiovascular responses in the seated position—impact of four anesthetic techniques, *Anesth Analg* 62:648-653, 1983.

126. Martin JT: Neuroanesthetic adjuncts for surgery in the sitting position. II. The antigravity suit, *Anesth Analg* 49:588, 1970.

127. Martin RW, Colley PS: Evaluation of transesophageal Doppler detection of air embolism in dogs, *Anesthesiology* 58:117-123, 1983.

128. Matjasko J, Petrozza P, Cohen M et al: Anesthesia and surgery in the seated position: analysis of 554 cases, *Neurosurgery* 17:695-702, 1985.

129. Matjasko J, Petrozza P, Mackenzie CF: Sensitivity of end-tidal nitrogen in venous air embolism detection in dogs, *Anesthesiology* 63:418-423, 1985.

130. Matjasko MJ, Hellman J, Mackenzie CF: Venous air embolism, hypotension and end-tidal nitrogen, *Neurosurgery* 21:378-382, 1987.

131. McAllister RG: Macroglossia—a positional complication, *Anesthesiology* 40:199-200, 1974.

132. McPherson RW, Toung TJK, Johnson RM et al: Intracranial subdural gas: a cause of false-positive change of intraoperative somatosensory evoked potential, *Anesthesiology* 62:816-819, 1985.

133. Michenfelder JD: Neuroanesthesia, *Anesthesiology* 30:65-100, 1969.

134. Michenfelder JD: The 27th Rovenstine Lecture: neuroanesthesia and the achievement of professional respect, *Anesthesiology* 70:695-701, 1989.

135. Michenfelder JD, Martin JT, Altenburg BM et al: Air embolism during neurosurgery. An evaluation of right-atrial catheters for diagnosis and treatment, *JAMA* 208:1353, 1358, 1969.

136. Michenfelder JD, Miller RH, Gronert GA: Evaluation of an ultrasonic device (Doppler) for the diagnosis of venous air embolism, *Anesthesiology* 36:164-168, 1972.

137. Michenfelder JD, Terry HR, Daw EF et al: Air embolism during neurosurgery: a new method of treatment, *Anesth Analg* 45:390-396, 1966.

138. Milde LN: Clinical use of mild hypothermia for brain protection: a dream revisited, *J Neurosurg Anesth* 4:211-215, 1992.

139. Millar RA: Neuroanesthesia in the sitting position, *Br J Anaesth* 44:495, 1972.

140. Mills NL, Ochsner JL: Massive air embolism during cardiopulmonary bypass. Causes, prevention, and management, *J Thorac Cardiovasc Surg* 80:708-717, 1980.

141. Mongan P, Peterson RE, Culling RD: Pressure monitoring can accurately position catheters for air embolism aspiration, *J Clin Monitor* 8:121-125, 1992.

142. Moosavi H, Utell MJ, Hyde RW et al: Lung ultrastructure in noncardiogenic pulmonary edema induced by air embolization in dogs, *Lab Invest* 45:456-464, 1981.

143. Morrison SC, Kumana CR, Rudnick KV et al: Selective and non-selective beta adrenoreceptor blockade in hypertension. Responses to change in posture, cold and exercise, *Circulation* 65:1171-1177, 1982.

144. Munson ES, Merrick HC: Effects of nitrous-oxide on venous air embolism, *Anesthesiology* 27:783-787, 1986.

145. Munson ES, Paul WC, Perry JC et al: Early detection of venous air embolism using a Swan-Ganz catheter, *Anesthesiology* 42:223-226, 1975.

146. Muzzi DA, Losasso TJ, Black S et al: Comparison of a transesophageal and precordial ultrasonic Doppler sensor in the detection of venous air embolism, *Anesth Analg* 70:103-104, 1990.

147. NHLBI workshop summary: hyperbaric oxygenation therapy, *Am Rev Respir Dis* 144:1414-1421, 1991.

148. Ohkuda K, Nakahara K, Binder A et al: Venous air emboli in sheep: reversible increase in lung microvascular permeability, *J Appl Physiol* 51:887-894, 1981.

149. Osborn AG, Daines JH, Wing SD et al: Intracranial air on computerized tomography, *J Neurosurg* 48:355-359, 1978.

150. Pearl RG, Larson CP Jr: Hemodynamic effects of positive end-expiratory pressure during continuous venous air embolism in the dog, *Anesthesiology* 64:724-729, 1986.

151. Perkins NAK, Bedford RF: Hemodynamic consequences of PEEP in seated neurosurgical patients—implications for paradoxical air embolism, *Anesth Analg* 63:429-432, 1984.

152. Perkins-Pearson NAK, Marshall WK, Bedford RF: Atrial pressures in the seated position: implications for paradoxical air embolism, *Anesthesiology* 57:493-498, 1982.

153. Perschau RA, Munson ES, Chapin JC: Pulmonary interstitial edema after multiple venous air emboli, *Anesthesiology* 45:364-366, 1976.

154. Peterson BT, Petrini MF, Hyde RW et al: Pulmonary tissue volume in dogs during pulmonary edema, *J Appl Physiol* 44:782-795, 1978.

155. Pfitzner J, McLean AG: Venous air embolism and active lung inflation at high and low CVP: a study in upright anesthetized sheep, *Anesth Analg* 66:1127-1134, 1987.

156. Pfitzner J, Petito SP, McLean AG: Hypoxaemia following sustained low-volume venous air embolism in sheep, *Anaesth Inten Care* 16:164-170, 1988.

157. Pfurtscheller G, Schwartz G, Schroettner O et al: Continuous and simultaneous monitoring of EEG spectra and brainstem auditory and somatosensory evoked potentials in the intensive care unit and the operating room, *J Clin Neurophysiol* 4:389-396, 1987.

158. Radtke RA, Erwin CW: Intraoperative monitoring of auditory and brain-stem function, *Neurol Clin* 6:899-915, 1988.

159. Radtke RA, Erwin CW, Wilkins RH: Intraoperative brainstem auditory evoked potentials: significant decrease in postoperative morbidity, *Neurology* 39:187-191, 1989.

160. Rangell L: Cerebral air embolism, *J Nerv Ment Dis* 96:542-555, 1942.

161. Rayport M: The head-elevated positions. Neurosurgical aspects: approaches to the occiput and cervical spine. In Martin JT, editor: *Positioning in anesthesia and surgery*, ed 2, Philadelphia, 1987, WB Saunders.

162. Rosomoff HL: Adjunct to neurosurgical anaesthesia, *Br J Anaesth* 37:246-261, 1965.

163. Russell D, Madden KP, Clark WM et al: Detection of arterial emboli using Doppler ultrasound in rabbits, *Stroke* 22:253-258, 1991.

164. Russell GB, Richard RB, Snider MT: Detection of venous air embolism in dogs by emission spectrometry, *J Clin Monit* 6:18-23, 1990.

165. Russell GB, Snider MT, Richard RB et al: Venous air emboli with $^{15}N_2$: pulmonary excretion and physiologic responses in dogs, *Undersea Biomed Res* 18:37-45, 1991.

166. Sato S, Toya S, Ohira T et al: Echocardiographic detection and treatment of intraoperative air embolism, *J Neurosurg* 64:440-444, 1986.

167. Schramm J, Watanabe E, Strauss C et al: Neurophysiologic monitoring in posterior fossa surgery. I. Technical principles, applicability and limitations, *Acta Neurochir (Wien)* 98:9-18, 1989.

168. Schubert A, Zornow MH, Drummond JC et al: Loss of cortical evoked responses due to intracranial gas during posterior fossa craniectomy in the seated position, *Anesth Analg* 65:203-206, 1986.

169. Schwartz D, Gennarelli TA, Young ML et al: Intraoperative monitoring of auditory brainstem responses following emergency evaluation of a cerebellar AVM, *J Clin Monit* 5:116-118, 1988.

170. Senn N: An experimental and clinical study of air-embolism, *Ann Surg* 3:197-302, 1885.

171. Sessler CN, Kiser PE, Raval V: Transient pulmonary perfusion scintigraphic abnormalities in pulmonary air embolism, *Chest* 95:910-912, 1989.

172. Shapiro HM: Neurosurgical anesthesia and intracranial hypertension. In Miller RD, editor: *Anesthesia*, ed 2, New York, 1986, Churchill-Livingstone.

173. Shapiro HM, Yoachim J, Marshall LF: Nitrous oxide challenge for detection of intravascular pulmonary gas following venous air embolism, *Anesth Analg* 61:304-306, 1982.

174. Sieber FE, Smith DS, Traystman RJ et al: Glucose: a reevaluation of its intraoperative use, *Anesthesiology* 67:72-81, 1987.

175. Simms NM, Kush GS, Long DM et al: Increase in regional cerebral blood flow following experimental arterial air embolism, *J Neurosurg* 34:665-671, 1971.

176. Skahen S, Shapiro HM, Drummond JC et al: Nitrous oxide withdrawal reduces intracranial pressure in the presence of pneumocephalus, *Anesthesiology* 65:192-196, 1986.

177. Sloan TB, Kimovec MA: Detection of venous air embolism by airway pressure monitoring, *Anesthesiology* 64:645-647, 1986.

178. Smelt WL, Baerts WD, de Langhe JJ et al: Pulmonary edema following air embolism, *Acta Anaesthesiol Belg* 38:201-205, 1987.

179. Smelt WL, de Lange JJ, Baerts WD et al: The capnograph, a reliable non-invasive monitor for the detection of pulmonary embolism of various origin, *Acta Anaesthesiol Belg* 38:217-224, 1987.

180. Smith PDC, Hasty JH, Scurr JH: Deep vein thrombosis: effect of graduated compression stockings on distension of the deep veins of the calf, *Br J Surg* 78:724-726, 1991.

181. Sonkodi S, Agabiti-Rosei E, Fraser R et al: Response of the renin-angiotensin-aldosterone system to upright tilting and to intravenous furosemide: effect of prior metoprolol and propranolol, *Br J Clin Pharmacol* 13:341-350, 1982.

182. Spencer MP, Thomas GI, Nicholls SC et al: Detection of middle cerebral artery emboli during carotid endarterectomy using transcranial Doppler ultrasonography, *Stroke* 21:415-423, 1990.

183. Standefer M, Bay JW, Trusso R: The sitting position in neurosurgery: a retrospective analysis of 488 cases, *Neurosurgery* 14:649-659, 1984.

184. Still JA, Lederman DS, Renn WH: Pulmonary edema following air embolism, *Anesthesiology* 40:194-196, 1974.

185. Strandgaard S, Skinhoj E, Lassen NA: Autoregulation of brain circulation in severe arterial hypertension, *Br Med J* 1:507-510, 1973.

186. Tateishi A, Maekawa T, Takeshita H et al: Diazepam and intracranial pressure, *Anesthesiology* 54:335-337, 1981.

187. Tindall GT, Craddock A, Greenfield JC: Effects of the sitting position on blood flow in the internal carotid artery of man during general anesthesia, *J Neurosurg* 26:383-389,1967.

188. Tinker JH, Gronert GA, Messick JM et al: Detection of air embolism. A test for positioning of right atrial catheter and Doppler probe, *Anesthesiology* 43:104-105, 1975.

189. Tinker JH, Vandam LD: How effective is the G-suit in neurosurgical operations? *Anesthesiology* 36:609,1972.

190. Toole JF: Effects of change on head, limb and body position on cephalic circulation, *N Engl J Med* 279:307, 1968.

191. Toung TJK, Grayson R, Saklad J et al: Movement of the distal end of the endotracheal tube during flexion and extension of the neck, *Anesth Analg* 64:1030, 1985.

192. Toung TJK, McPherson RW, Ahn H et al: Pneumocephalus: effects of patient position on the incidence and location of aerocele after posterior fossa and upper cervical cord surgery, *Anesth Analg* 65:65-70, 1986.

193. Toung TJK, Miyabe M, McShane AJ et al: Effect of PEEP and jugular venous compression on canine cerebral blood flow and oxygen consumption in the head elevated position, *Anesthesiology* 68:53-58, 1988.

194. Toung TJK, Ngeow YK, Long DL et al: Comparison of the effects of positive end-expiratory pressure and jugular venous compression on canine cerebral venous pressure, *Anesthesiology* 61:169-172, 1984.

195. Troianos CA, Jobes DR, Ellison N: Ultrasound-guided cannulation of the internal jugular vein. A prospective, randomized study, *Anesth Analg* 72:823-826, 1991.

196. Turpie AG, Hirsh J, Gent M et al: Prevention of deep vein thrombosis in potential neurosurgical patients, *Arch Intern Med* 149:679-681, 1989.

197. Urasaki E, Wada S, Matsukado Y et al: Monitoring of short-latency somatosensory evoked potentials during surgery for cervical cord and posterior fossa lesions—changes in subcortical components, *Neurol Med Chir* 28:546-552, 1988.

198. Verstappen FTJ, Bernards JA, Kreuzer F: Effects of pulmonary gas embolism on circulation and respiration in the dog. III. Excretion of venous gas bubbles by the lung, *Pflurgers Arch* 370:67-70, 1977.

199. Vik A, Brubakk AO, Hennessy TR: Venous air embolism in swine: transport of gas bubbles through the pulmonary circulation, *J Appl Physiol* 69:237-244, 1990.

200. Von Gossein H, Samii M, Suhr D et al: The lounging position for posterior fossa surgery: anesthesiological considerations regarding air embo-

lism, *Childs Nerv Syst* 7:568-574, 1991.

201. Voorhies RM, Fraser AR: Cerebral air embolism occurring at angiography and diagnosed by computerized tomography, *J Neurosurg* 60:177-178, 1984.

202. Voorhies RM, Fraser RAR, van Poznak A: Prevention of air embolism with positive end-expiratory pressure, *Neurosurgery* 12:503-506, 1983.

203. Wade JG, Larson PC, Hickey RF et al: Effect of carotid endarterectomy on carotid chemoreceptor and baroreceptor function in man, *N Engl J Med* 282:823-829, 1970.

204. Warner DO, Cucchiara RF: Position of proximal orifice determines electrocardiogram recorded from multiorificed catheter, *Anesthesiology* 65:235-236, 1986.

205. Warren JE, Tsueda K, Young B: Respiratory pattern changes during repair of posterior-fossa arteriovenous malformation, *Anesthesiology* 45:690-693, 1976.

206. Warren LP Jr, Djang WT, Moon RE et al: Neuroimaging of scuba diving injuries to the CNS, *Am J Roentgenol* 151:1003-1008, 1988.

207. Watanabe E, Schramm J, Schneider W: Effect of a subdural air collection on the sensory evoked potential during surgery in the sitting position, *Electrocencephalogr Clin Neurophysiol* 74:194-201, 1989.

208. Watanabe E, Schramm J, Strauss C et al: Neurophysiologic monitoring in posterior fossa surgery. II. BAEP-waves I and V and preservation of hearing, *Acta Neurochir (Wien)* 98:118-128, 1989.

209. Whitby JD: Electrocardiography during posterior fossa operations, *Br J Anaesth* 35:624, 1963.

210. Whitby JD: Early cases of air embolism, *Anaesthesia* 19:579-584, 1964.

211. Wilder BL: Hypothesis: the etiology of midcervical quadriplegia after operation with the patient in the sitting position, *Neurosurgery* 11:530-531, 1982.

212. Wilkins RH, Albin MS: An unusual entrance site of venous air embolism during operation in the sitting position, *Surg Neurol* 7:71, 1977.

213. Wood EH, Lambert EH, Baldes EJ et al: Effects of acceleration in relation to aviation, *Fed Proc* 5:327-344, 1946.

214. Yahagi N, Furuya H: The effects of halothane and pentobarbital on the threshold of transpulmonary passage of venous air emboli in dogs, *Anesthesiology* 67:905-909, 1987.

215. Yahagi N, Furuya H, Yoshikazu S et al: Effect of halothane, fentanyl, and ketamine on the threshold for transpulmonary passage of venous air emboli in dogs, *Anesth Analg* 75:720-723, 1992.

216. Yates AP, Sumner E, Lindahl SG: Respiratory disturbance and posterior fossa surgery. A case report, *Anaesthesia* 41:1214-1218, 1986.

217. Young ML, Smith DS, Murtagh F et al: Comparison of surgical and anesthetic complications in neurosurgical patients experiencing venous air embolism in the sitting position, *Neurosurgery* 18:157-161, 1986.

218. Zasslow MA, Pearl RG, Larson CP et al: PEEP does not affect left atrial-right atrial pressure difference in neurosurgical patients, *Anesthesiology* 68:760-763, 1988.

17

Cerebral Aneurysms: Surgical Considerations

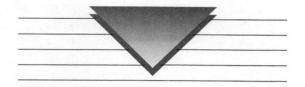

MARK J. KOTAPKA
EUGENE S. FLAMM

Intracranial aneurysms have been recognized as the cause of subarachnoid hemorrhage (SAH) at least since the late eighteenth century.[38] More than 100 years passed, however, before cerebral aneurysms were approached surgically. In 1885, Sir Victor Horsley successfully ligated the cervical carotid artery to treat a large intracranial internal carotid artery aneurysm. The first occlusion of an intracranial aneurysm with a metal clip was performed by Walter Dandy in 1937.[13] Today the surgical management of intracranial aneurysms has advanced coincident with technical developments to the extent that few aneurysms are beyond the reach of the neurosurgeon. In spite of this progress, the overall morbidity and mortality of SAH continues to be high.[33] This results from the direct effects of hemorrhage, rebleeding before definitive treatment, and delayed ischemic events. This chapter reviews the current understanding and management of ruptured and unruptured intracranial aneurysms. With an understanding of the basic princi-

ples of neurosurgical management of cerebral aneurysms, one can optimize the anesthetic management of such patients and, in turn, attain improved neurologic outcome.

EPIDEMIOLOGY

The prevalence of intracranial aneurysms in the general population of the United States has been estimated at 2% to 5%.[9,24] Rupture of an intracranial aneurysm resulting in SAH is less common, with an average incidence of 11 to 16 per 100,000 people per year.[58,71] This translates into approximately 28,000 cases of SAH per year. It is estimated that only two of every three patients who sustain an SAH survive to reach medical attention.[71] Thus diagnosis and treatment of intracranial aneurysms before hemorrhage would significantly reduce the high morbidity and mortality associated with SAH.

The age distribution of SAH reaches a peak in middle

age. At least 60% of aneurysm ruptures occur between the ages of 40 and 60.[40] There is a slight sexual preponderance, with a female-to-male ratio of approximately 3:2.

NATURAL HISTORY

The natural history of intracranial aneurysms was studied in various populations before the development of modern treatment methods. Aneurysms that have not ruptured carry a 1% to 2% per year risk of hemorrhage.[87] Aneurysms that have ruptured carry a much greater chance of future hemorrhage. Approximately 50% of ruptured aneurysms will rebleed within 6 months after the initial hemorrhage. After this period, the risk of repeat hemorrhage decreases to 3% per year.[27]

The rupture of an intracranial aneurysm carries a significant chance of death or disability. The recently published International Cooperative Study on the Timing of Aneurysm Surgery documented that, of patients who survive to be admitted to a hospital, one of three will be rendered severely disabled, vegetative, or dead after SAH.[33] Remembering that only two of three SAH victims survive to reach medical attention, we see that less than half of patients with SAH will have an acceptable outcome.

PATHOLOGY

The etiology of intracranial aneurysms has long been debated. For many years aneurysms were believed to be congenital. However, the infrequent occurrence of aneurysms in children argued against a congenital etiology.[24] In addition, recent evidence indicates that aneurysms are acquired vascular lesions secondary to degenerative changes in the muscular and elastic components of vessel walls, usually occurring at branch points of major cerebral vessels and frequently associated with hypertension.[77] Congenital influences may play a role in predisposing certain locations to aneurysm formation based on variability in vessel-wall structure.[74] A deficiency of type III collagen has been found in the arteries of patients with SAH.[51] The exact role of this biochemical abnormality has yet to be determined.

Whether there is a genetic link between cerebral aneurysms and SAH still is unknown. Certain families do suffer a greater incidence of aneurysmal SAH than would be predicted based on the known epidemiology; however, less than 100 such families have been reported.[4,22] The genetic mechanisms involved in such cases are unknown.

The pathologic anatomy of intracranial aneurysms is well documented.[62] More than 90% of cerebral aneurysms occur at the following locations: (1) the origin of the posterior communicating artery, (2) the region of the anterior communicating artery, (3) the middle cerebral artery bifurcation, (4) the apex of the basilar artery, and (5) the internal carotid artery bifurcation. Multiple intracranial aneurysms occur in a significant number of patients. Estimates

of multiplicity in cerebral aneurysms range from 5.4% to 33.3%.[60]

A considerable variation has been noted in the size of intracranial aneurysms responsible for SAH. Wiebers et al. suggested that there was little likelihood of bleeding from an asymptomatic aneurysm less than 1 cm in diameter.[85] However, the experience of most aneurysm surgeons and the data reported in the literature suggest that the majority of aneurysms that do bleed are less than 1 cm in diameter.[16] A review of 1092 aneurysms reported to the Cooperative Aneurysm Study from 1970 to 1977 revealed a mean diameter of 8.2 mm, with 71% having a diameter less than 1 cm and 13% less than 0.5 cm at the time of rupture.[30] Other studies also suggest that aneurysms greater than 0.5 cm should be considered at risk for rupture but that those less than 0.5 cm carry little risk of hemorrhage.[13,43,55] Smaller aneurysms have been documented to enlarge with time, so it is difficult to predict fully the future risk in these cases.

ASSOCIATED CONDITIONS

A variety of medical conditions are associated with the development of cerebral aneurysms and subsequent SAH. Evidence of hypertension has been found in as many as 80% of individuals with cerebral aneurysms.[9] Indeed, as previously noted, hypertension may be an etiologic factor in the development of aneurysms.[77] Many of the diseases associated with cerebral aneurysms have hypertension as an integral part of their pathophysiology. For example, coarctation of the aorta is frequently associated with cerebral aneurysms, and SAH is responsible for the death of approximately 10% of these patients.[19] Likewise, approximately 16% of patients with polycystic kidney disease are found at autopsy to have cerebral aneurysms,[11] and SAH is the cause of death in 15% of patients with this disease. In addition, fibromuscular dysplasia is associated with cerebral aneurysms. Finally, aneurysms have been found in more than 20% of those patients with disease involving the head and neck.[45]

A recent report noted a very significant association between cigarette smoking and SAH.[41] The authors report an elevenfold increase in the chance of aneurysmal hemorrhage in smokers. The chance of developing delayed ischemic events after SAH also appears to be increased in smokers.

DIAGNOSIS
Clinical Features

Aneurysms that have not ruptured may be either clinically silent or symptomatic. Asymptomatic unruptured aneurysms are either found during angiography in a patient with multiple aneurysms and SAH or are found during radiologic investigation of other processes such as carotid occlusive disease or sinusitis.

Symptomatic, but unruptured, intracranial aneurysms may present clinically in a variety of ways. The clinical syndrome of a progressive third-cranial-nerve palsy associated with an aneurysm of the posterior communicating artery is well recognized. Other presentations include that of ischemic events related to emboli originating from the aneurysm or of a variety of symptoms related to effects of the aneurysm as a mass lesion.[19]

The clinical presentation of aneurysmal SAH—the sudden onset of severe headache, with or without loss of consciousness, accompanied by signs of meningeal irritation—is well known. The diagnosis is usually easily confirmed by head computed tomography (CT) or lumbar puncture. Such hemorrhages occasionally are preceded by a variety of lesser symptoms, which may be attributed to minor hemorrhages from the aneurysm.[56]

A patient who has suffered aneurysmal rupture and SAH may be classified or graded according to one of several systems that have been devised by Botterell,[7] Hunt,[25] or the Cooperative Study.[71] These are presented in Table 17-1. Although such systems have obvious limitations, they are important in evaluating results of therapy, provide a common language for health care workers caring for such patients, and are a predictor of outcome.

Radiology

The diagnostic evaluation of a patient with SAH or with a suspected unruptured aneurysm continues to be based on four-vessel cerebral angiography.[36] Because of the occurrence of multiple intracranial aneurysms, a complete four-vessel study must be completed in all patients in whom the diagnosis of aneurysm is entertained. In the event multiple aneurysms are found, one usually can determine which aneurysm has bled from the angiogram combined with a CT of the head. Magnetic resonance (MR) imaging may be helpful several days after the hemorrhage has occurred, but, because of the signal characteristics of acute subarachnoid blood, such studies are not always helpful in the first 24 to 48 hours after SAH.

Angiography may not disclose the responsible aneurysm, in all cases, of SAH. A recent report noted negative angiograms in 45 of 469 patients with SAH.[26] A repeat study on 38 of these patients revealed eight aneurysms that were originally missed. Therefore a negative angiogram should be followed by a repeat angiogram.

Magnetic resonance angiography, a recently developed, noninvasive technique, has been shown to be applicable to the cerebral vasculature.[70] This methodology is still in its developmental stages, however, and has yet to be rigorously tested against standard angiography in the evaluation of intracranial aneurysms. Thus most aneurysm surgeons will not operate solely based on a positive magnetic resonance angiogram. In addition, the reliability of a negative study in the setting of SAH is unknown.

COMPLICATIONS OF SAH

The clinical management of cerebral aneurysms centers on the reduction of risk of hemorrhage in unruptured cases and of repeat hemorrhage in SAH. In patients whose aneurysms have ruptured, treatment must also address the various complications of SAH, which account for a significant proportion of the morbidity and mortality. Thus it is useful to discuss these complications before considering definitive treatment of cerebral aneurysms.

The major complications of SAH are aneurysmal rebleeding and delayed cerebral ischemia secondary to vasospasm. The International Cooperative Study delineated the relative contributions of these complications to the high morbidity and mortality of SAH.[33] Of 3521 patients admitted to the study, 7.5% died or were severely disabled as a result of aneurysmal rebleeding. Vasospasm was responsible for the death or disability of 13.5% of patients admitted to the study.

TABLE 17-1
Grades of Subarachnoid Hemorrhage

Grading System	Description
Botterell	1 Conscious patient with or without signs of SAH
	2 Drowsy patient without significant deficit
	3 Drowsy patient with deficit and an intracerebral clot
	4 Patient with a major deficit deteriorating because of a large intracerebral clot, or an older patient with a less severe deficit but with preexisting cerebrovascular disease
	5 Moribund patient with failing vital centers and extensor rigidity
Hunt	0 Unruptured aneurysm
	1 Ruptured aneurysm with minimal headache
	2 Moderate-to-severe headache; no deficit other than cranial nerve palsy
	3 Drowsiness/confusion or mild focal deficit
	4 Stupor, significant hemiparesis, early decerebration, vegetative disturbances
	5 Deep coma, decerebrate rigidity, moribund
Cooperative Study	1 Symptom free
	2 Minor symptoms (headache, meningeal irritation, diplopia)
	3 Major deficit but fully responsive
	4 Impaired state of alertness but capable of protective responses to noxious stimuli
	5 Poorly responsive but with stable vital signs
	6 No response to address or shaking, nonadaptive responses to noxious stimuli, and instability of vital signs

Aneurysmal Rebleeding

As noted previously, the natural history of intracranial aneurysms is such that 50% will rebleed within the first 6 months after SAH.[27] Details of the rebleeding risk during the acute period after SAH have been obtained. Early trials of conservative therapy (i.e. bed rest) in middle cerebral artery aneurysms revealed that 33% of patients treated in this manner rebled within 2 weeks, and anterior communicating artery aneurysms had a 2-week rebleed rate of 24%.[44] A subsequent randomized study of conservative treatment found that 20% of patients admitted within 7 days of SAH rebled in the first 2 weeks.[54] A study of antifibrinolytic therapy as a means to decrease aneurysmal rebleeding demonstrated that 4% of conservatively treated patients rebled within 24 hours of their initial SAH.[31] After this initial period, the average daily rate of rebleeding for the first 2 weeks after SAH was 1.5% per day. Because of the high risk of aneurysmal rebleeding with its coincident high mortality, a variety of treatment modalities have been employed to attempt to lessen the risk of rebleeding.

Blood pressure control is of critical importance in reduction of risk of aneurysmal rebleeding.[71] Practitioners are concerned about aggressive treatment of hypertension in the presence of increased intracranial pressure and/or ischemia secondary to vasospasm. Nevertheless, modest reductions in systolic pressures are generally tolerated and do reduce the risk of rebleeding.

In addition to reduction in blood pressure, other methods have been employed to prevent aneurysmal rebleeding in SAH. Antifibrinolytic agents have been used in an attempt to prevent lysis of the clot formed around the aneurysmal dome at the time of SAH. Most commonly, epsilon-aminocaproic acid in doses of 24 to 48 g IV per day has been used. Such therapy has been confirmed to significantly reduce the risk of aneurysmal rebleeding.[50,61] However, other studies have demonstrated that the overall outcome for patients with SAH is not altered by antifibrinolytic therapy secondary to an increase in ischemic complications from vasospasm.[28,32,49] Currently, the role of antifibrinolytics in the future management of SAH is unclear.[21] Because more aneurysms are surgically treated acutely, antifibrinolytic agents have become less important.

Vasospasm

Vasospasm is the leading cause of morbidity and mortality in patients who initially survive SAH. Because vasospasm was first described by Robertson in 1949, much has been learned about the nature of vasospasm, and effective treatments are being developed.[64] Radiologic evidence of vasospasm has been noted in up to 70% of angiograms performed within the first weeks after aneurysmal rupture.[83] However, clinical vasospasm occurs in approximately 30% of patients with SAH.[1]

The clinical syndrome of vasospasm consists of delayed neurologic deterioration after SAH in the absence of evidence of aneurysmal rebleeding. Patients often complain of worsening headache and then are noted to exhibit a gradual diminution in their level of consciousness and/or develop a new or exacerbated focal deficit. Clinical vasospasm usually occurs at about 4 to 9 days after SAH. It typically does not occur later than 2 weeks after aneurysmal rupture.[83]

The treatment of cerebral vasospasm has developed from several lines of research into its pathophysiology. This research has concentrated on identification of the changes in the arterial wall and the effector mechanisms involved in the production of these changes.

The changes in cerebral vessels in vasospasm have been attributed both to contraction of vascular smooth muscle and to thickening of the vessel wall. A combination of these two factors is thought to produce luminal narrowing.[42] The mechanisms by which these changes occur have yet to be fully elucidated. A variety of possibly interrelated effector systems, including prostaglandins, biologic amines and peptides, cyclic nucleotides, calcium, lipid peroxidation, and free radicals, have all been implicated.[10,46,84] However, the substance or substances responsible for initiating the sequence of events leading to vasospasm have not yet been fully identified.[61]

The diagnosis of vasospasm is generally made clinically but can be supported by a variety of measurements of vessel diameter or cerebral blood flow. Conventional cerebral angiography has traditionally been used to confirm the presence of vasospasm.[18,82] However, angiographic abnormalities may be present in individuals without clinical vasospasm. The opposite is not true. Other methodologies have been applied to the assessment of cerebral vasospasm. Xenon-enhanced CT has been demonstrated to be useful in assessing regional blood flow in patients symptomatic from vasospasm.[90] Transcranial Doppler ultrasound provides a noninvasive means of measuring flow velocities in major cerebral vessels and thus indirectly assessing vessel diameter. Transcranial Doppler flow velocities have been correlated both with cerebral blood flow measurements and with cerebral angiography.[53,75] This technique is currently being studied and widely used as a bedside method for monitoring these events.

The treatment of cerebral vasospasm is directed at preventing either its occurrence or its ischemic consequences. There appears to be a correlation between the amount of subarachnoid blood after aneurysmal rupture and the occurrence and severity of vasospasm.[47] Because of this correlation, attempts have been made to decrease the incidence of vasospasm by early surgery, which includes extensive removal of subarachnoid blood.[79] Using a different approach, others have used intrathecal thrombolytic therapy to lyse subarachnoid blood.[15] Whether such methods are truly effective in vasospasm remains to be seen.

Another approach used in the treatment of vasospasm is based on the role of calcium in vascular smooth muscle physiology and its role in cerebral ischemia. In the laboratory, calcium channel blockers have been shown to prevent induced vasoconstriction of cerebral arterial vessels.[3] Subsequent clinical studies demonstrated reduced morbidity and mortality in SAH patients treated with the calcium channel blocker nimodipine.[2,57] Nimodipine appeared to have no effect on the degree of angiographic vasospasm. Because of this discrepancy, the direct neuroprotective effect of calcium antagonists is now being investigated.[46] Currently, the calcium channel blocker nimodipine is approved for use in the United States in the treatment of SAH. A clinical trial with an additional calcium channel blocker, nicardipine, failed to show significant benefit over what has been called "triple H" therapy—hypervolemia, hemodilution, and hypertension.[17,20,65]

Volume expansion and induced hypertension have been used successfully in the treatment of ischemic complications of cerebral vasospasm.[29] Indeed, such therapy has been demonstrated to reverse the reduction in cerebral blood flow seen in symptomatic vasospasm.[69] Because of the potential worsening of cerebral edema and increased intracranial pressure, other researchers have proposed the use of isovolemic hemodilution in the treatment of vasospasm.[81,82] The beneficial effects of such regimens may be related to reduction in blood viscosity and increased flow through narrowed vessels. The management of patients with SAH has changed greatly in the past 10 years. Volume expansion and hemodilution, generally combined with the administration of the calcium channel blocker nimodipine, have become the focal points of any regimen for these patients.

A new method for treating symptomatic vasospasm involves the use of cerebral angioplasty to dilate constricted major cerebral vessels. A recent report has demonstrated the apparent efficacy and safety of this method.[52] Further studies are needed to determine the exact clinical role of this promising technique. This procedure often must be done under general anesthesia both to control respiration in critically ill patients and to permit accurate placement of the intraarterial balloon used to dilate the cerebral vessels.

Other Complications

Hydrocephalus is an important complication of aneurysmal rupture. Both acute and delayed hydrocephalus may occur. Acute hydrocephalus of the obstructive type, manifested by progressive obtundation leading to coma, requires prompt treatment with ventricular drainage. Delayed hydrocephalus of the communicating type is usually not emergent and may be managed conservatively, pending definitive treatment of the aneurysm. Intracranial pressure may be elevated after SAH without CT evidence of ventricular enlargement. In these cases, therapy aimed at reducing intracranial pressure and optimizing cerebral blood flow may be beneficial.[6]

Epilepsy is another complication of SAH. Researchers have estimated that approximately 10% of patients with SAH will develop a seizure disorder, usually within the first 18 months after SAH.[68] The occurrence of a seizure after SAH but before definitive treatment of the aneurysm may lead to disastrous rebleeding. For these reasons, most aneurysm surgeons start anticonvulsants as soon as the diagnosis of SAH is established.

DEFINITIVE TREATMENT

The definitive treatment of cerebral aneurysms has involved a variety of methods to reduce the risk of aneurysmal rupture. As noted previously, proximal ligation of the parent vessel was originally used by neurosurgeons to treat aneurysms of the internal carotid artery.[14,38] Subsequent studies have confirmed that, for proximal internal carotid artery aneurysms, ligation or occlusion of the internal carotid does confer some degree of protection against future hemorrhage, albeit with the risk of treatment-induced stroke.[72]

Direct attempts to surgically treat intracranial aneurysms originally used muscle, and then subsequently other materials such as gauze and plastics, to wrap or coat the aneurysm and thus retard future enlargement and rupture.[48,71,80] This technique, like proximal ligation, may offer some degree of protection against aneurysmal rupture.

Endovascular techniques using detachable balloons or platinum coils for occlusion of intracranial aneurysms represent a new form of treatment for these lesions. These approaches have been applied to both anterior and posterior circulation aneurysms, with favorable results.[23,66] Further studies are needed to determine the exact role of interventional radiologic techniques in the management of cerebral aneurysms.

The evolution of the direct surgical approach to treating intracranial aneurysms has been reviewed.[14] With the development of microsurgical techniques, the obliteration of intracranial aneurysms with small spring-loaded metal clips has become the standard treatment of these lesions.[35,89] The details of the surgical technique are reviewed in standard neurosurgical texts.[88] The basic surgical principles involve the meticulous identification, dissection, and preservation of the involved normal intracranial arteries, including small perforating vessels, and the total isolation of the aneurysm from the circulation (see later discussion). Microneurosurgeons have gained experience in the treatment of all types of intracranial aneurysms, including those of the posterior circulation and those previously considered too large for safe surgical treatment.[12,63] A variety of additional techniques have added to the safety of the surgical treatment of cerebral aneurysms, including the use of intraoperative electrophysiologic monitoring, cerebral protective agents such as high-dose barbiturates, induced hypotension, temporary occlusion of the parent vessel, and, in extraordinary cases, the use of hypothermia and circulatory arrest.[5,73,76]

Although the surgical clipping of intracranial aneurysms is the accepted form of treatment, there has been considerable debate concerning the timing of such surgery. The prevalent view among vascular neurosurgeons originally was that delayed surgery led to improved outcome for patients with SAH.[13] This view was popularized because of the technical advantages of operating 10 to 14 days after SAH and because early surgery demonstrated no benefit. Later studies, however, demonstrated an apparent benefit of surgery within the first days after SAH.[37] Because of these conflicting views, the International Cooperative Study on the Timing of Aneurysm Surgery was undertaken to determine the optimal time for treatment.[34] The results of this study indicate that early surgery (0 to 3 days after SAH) and late surgery (11 to 14 days after SAH) were equivalent in patient outcome. The risks of rebleeding and of vasospasm in patients receiving delayed operations were essentially equivalent to the increased operative risk with early surgery. Of interest, study patients surgically treated during an intermediate period of 7 to 10 days after SAH fared the worst, apparently being subjected to the risks of rebleeding and vasospasm, along with the increased risk of earlier surgery. Although not universally followed, a trend has arisen of early surgery within 48 hours of SAH at centers treating large numbers of patients with cerebral aneurysms.

PREOPERATIVE AND POSTOPERATIVE CARE

The preoperative treatment of patients with SAH has largely been described in preceding sections and will be summarized here.

SAH patients should be placed in a quiet environment at bed rest. If necessary, patients should be sedated. Phenobarbital, 30 to 60 mg every 6 to 8 hours, is useful in this setting. The headache of SAH may require the administration of only acetaminophen, but in some cases narcotic analgesics are required. As noted previously, strict attention is paid to blood pressure control. Realizing that a balance exists between risk of aneurysmal rupture and maintenance of adequate cerebral perfusion pressure, one should attempt mild reduction of the systolic blood pressure (i.e. 30%), with close observation for signs of neurologic deterioration. This reduction in blood pressure often is accomplished by the calcium channel blockers used as treatment or prophylaxis of vasospasm. If needed, supplemental beta-adrenergic blockers or other antihypertensives may be employed.

In addition to these measures, patients should receive anticonvulsants, stool softeners, and antacids or histamine receptor (H-2) antagonist. Steroids may be indicated in patients with evidence of cerebral swelling on head CT or in patients for whom early surgery is contemplated. Other general measures include the maintenance of adequate nutrition, elastic or compression stockings for the lower extremities, and any other items for patient comfort deemed appropriate. In the event that delayed surgery is planned, antifibrinolytic agents may be employed as outlined previously.

The postoperative management of a patient with SAH concentrates on the prevention and treatment of ischemic events related to vasospasm, along with hydrocephalus, epilepsy, and other routine postoperative concerns, as noted

previously. This is usually accomplished by the continued use of volume expansion through the use of colloid and crystalloid, along with a calcium channel blocker such as nimodipine.

Many surgeons routinely puncture the aneurysm after clip application to ensure adequate isolation from the circulation. If this is not done, a postoperative angiogram is obtained to document aneurysm obliteration. In assessing for vasospasm postoperatively, one uses transcranial Doppler ultrasonography, with repeat angiography performed as necessary, particularly if balloon angioplasty is available.

SURGICAL TECHNIQUE

The surgical technique employed in an individual case varies according to the anatomic location and configuration of the aneurysm, as well as the preferences of the surgeon. In general, however, most intracranial aneurysms are approached by the frontotemporal approach popularized by Yasargil.[88] This approach is summarized as follows.

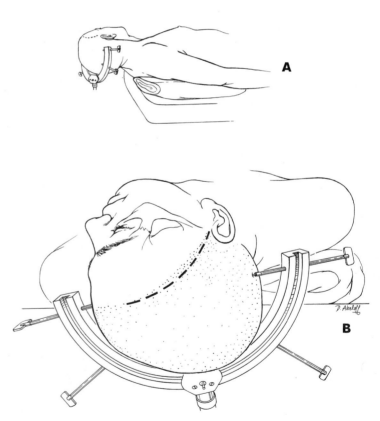

FIG. 17-1 **A,** Overall view of the patient positioned for a right pterional craniotomy. The head is turned fully to the left, and the right shoulder is elevated. **B,** Detail of the incision line, which is behind the hairline and slightly curved. *(From Flamm ES: Cerebral aneurysms at the bifurcation of the internal carotid artery. In Rengachary SS, Wilkins RH, editors: Neurosurgical operative atlas, vol 1, American Association of Neurological Surgeons, Baltimore, 1991, Williams & Wilkins, p 89.)*

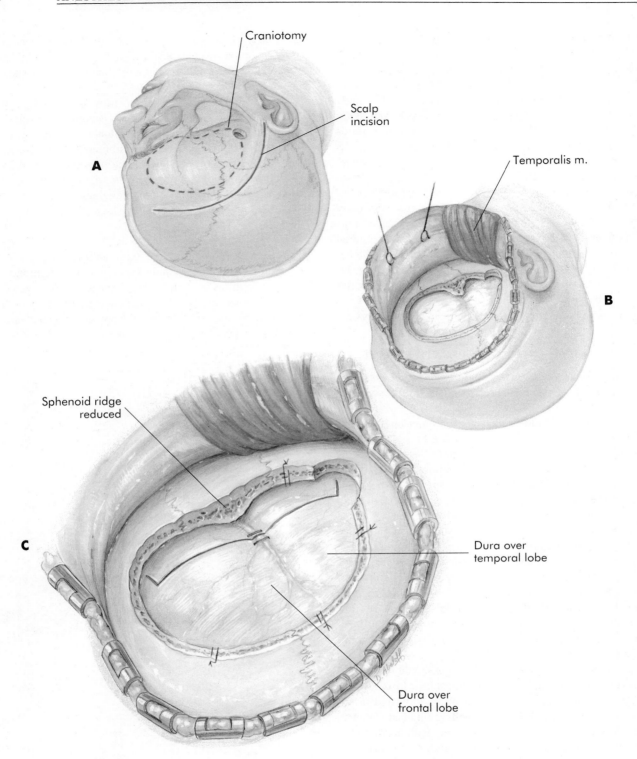

FIG. 17-2   **A,** Burr hole and bone flap superimposed within the scalp flap. **B,** Bone flap removed. **C,** Bony opening after reduction of the sphenoid wing. Dural incision is indicated. *(From Flamm ES: Cerebral aneurysms at the bifurcation of the internal carotid artery. In Rengachary SS, Wilkins RH, editors: Neurosurgical operative atlas, vol 1, American Association of Neurological Surgeons, Baltimore, 1991, Williams & Wilkins, p 90.)*

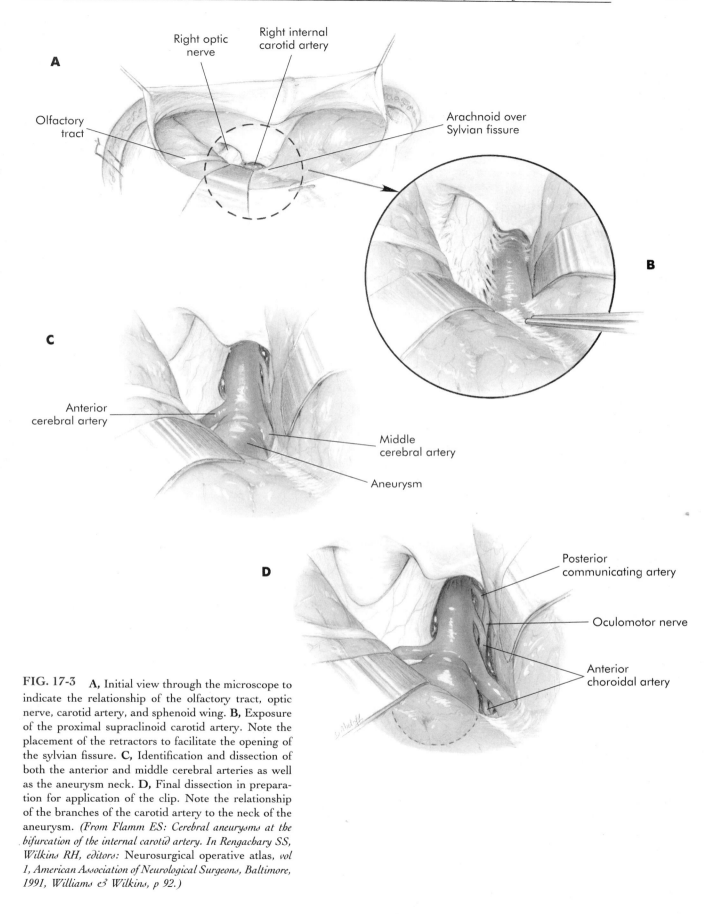

FIG. 17-3   **A,** Initial view through the microscope to indicate the relationship of the olfactory tract, optic nerve, carotid artery, and sphenoid wing. **B,** Exposure of the proximal supraclinoid carotid artery. Note the placement of the retractors to facilitate the opening of the sylvian fissure. **C,** Identification and dissection of both the anterior and middle cerebral arteries as well as the aneurysm neck. **D,** Final dissection in preparation for application of the clip. Note the relationship of the branches of the carotid artery to the neck of the aneurysm. *(From Flamm ES: Cerebral aneurysms at the bifurcation of the internal carotid artery. In Rengachary SS, Wilkins RH, editors:* Neurosurgical operative atlas, *vol 1, American Association of Neurological Surgeons, Baltimore, 1991, Williams & Wilkins, p 92.)*

The patient is positioned supine with the head laterally rotated and extended toward the floor to maximize exposure of the undersurface of the frontotemporal region (Fig. 17-1, A). In doing this, one should take care to keep the head above heart level to minimize venous hypertension. The standard scalp incision runs behind the hairline from the zygomatic arch to the midline (Fig. 17-1, B).

A frontotemporal craniotomy is performed, which exposes the base of the frontal lobe, the sylvian fissure, and the anterior temporal lobe (Fig. 17-2, A and B). The dura is opened in a fashion to allow access to the undersurface of the frontal lobe (Fig. 17-2, C).

The frontal lobe is gently retracted superiorly, and the temporal lobe retracted posteriorly (Fig. 17-3, A). The most important intracranial landmarks for the neurosurgeon are the optic nerve and proximal internal carotid artery (Fig. 17-3, A and B). The arachnoid is opened widely, and the dissection is carried out along the internal carotid artery and its branches, based on the location of the aneurysm. In this example, the dissection is carried out along the internal carotid artery to the aneurysm at the carotid bifurcation (Fig. 17-3, C). The important carotid branches, such as the posterior communicating, anterior choroidal, and anterior and middle cerebral arteries, must be fully dissected (Fig. 17-3, D). In this fashion, the aneurysm may be safely clipped with preservation of the parent arterial vessel and involved branches.

By employing the approach outlined here, the vast majority of intracranial aneurysms may be effectively treated. Aneurysms in rarer locations or those with special anatomic characteristics may require modifications of this technique or different approaches entirely.

NEUROANESTHETIC MANAGEMENT: SURGICAL PERSPECTIVES

As with any craniotomy in which the intracranial pressure (ICP) is known or suspected to be elevated, the intraoperative anesthetic management of cerebral aneurysms is concerned with the reduction of ICP and with providing adequate relaxation of the brain to obtain optimal surgical exposure and to facilitate safe and effective obliteration of the aneurysm. The techniques of hyperventilation ($Paco_2$ 25 to 30 mm Hg), osmotic diuresis (mannitol 0.5 to 1.0 g/kg), and use of anesthetic agents that do not adversely affect ICP are generally accepted and will be addressed in detail in other chapters of this text. Because of the propensity of patients with SAH to develop communicating hydrocephalus, an additional technique, often of value in aneurysm surgery, is intraoperative cerebrospinal fluid (CSF) drainage via a lumbar catheter placed before the start of surgery. In general, the catheter is opened after the dura is opened, closed after brain relaxation is adequate, and removed at the end of the procedure.

However, in addition to raised ICP, intracranial aneurysms pose special problems to the neuroanesthesiologist.

As previously discussed, the major causes of mortality and morbidity in patients who reach medical attention after SAH are aneurysmal rebleeding and delayed cerebral ischemia secondary to vasospasm. Likewise, the anesthetic management of a craniotomy for a ruptured aneurysm aims to optimize the surgical exposure and attempts to minimize the risk of intraoperative aneurysmal rupture and the likelihood of postoperative neurologic deficits secondary to intraoperative ischemic insults.

A variety of techniques are potentially useful in decreasing the likelihood of intraoperative aneurysmal rupture or in facilitating clip application after rupture of an aneurysm. Maintenance of the patient's blood pressure at or slightly below normal physiologic limits for the individual during the operative procedure is of great importance. This is especially true during induction of anesthesia and during particularly stimulating portions of the procedure (i.e., the application of a pin-fixation head holder). The use of a local anesthetic at the pin sites is recommended. However, special circumstances may require raising or lowering of the patient's blood pressure during the operation. Induced hypotension has long been used to facilitate dissection of the aneurysm and related vessels.[86] Likewise, in the event of aneurysmal rupture, induced hypotension may decrease the rate of blood loss and aid the surgeon in clip application. The drug most frequently used to induce hypotension is sodium nitroprusside. The degree and duration of hypotension recommended vary, depending on many factors, including the experience of the surgical team.

A surgical technique that essentially accomplishes goals similar to induced hypotension is that of temporary parent-vessel occlusion.[89] In this technique, a temporary aneurysm clip is applied to the parent vessel proximal to the aneurysm. This decreases the tension in the aneurysm and makes a difficult dissection less dangerous. In the event of intraoperative aneurysmal rupture, temporary clip application is also helpful in controlling the hemorrhage and enabling the surgeon to proceed safely with definitive clip application. The duration of temporary clip application that is considered safe varies and may be guided by electrophysiologic monitoring. Some surgeons have used up to 30 to 60 minutes of parent-vessel occlusion with good results.[78] More limited periods of temporary occlusion are now recommended. The advisability of continuous or intermittent occlusion remains unclear. Systemic arterial blood pressure is usually maintained at or above its usual level to help assure adequate perfusion of the remainder of the brain during parent-vessel occlusion.

A technique that has been used in treating very difficult cases is profound hypothermia and cardiac arrest.[76] This technique is reserved for the most difficult cases and is not part of the routine management of intracerebral aneurysms.

As noted previously, techniques employing hypotension or temporary vessel occlusion are limited by their potential to produce ischemic deficits. Therefore one must exercise caution with either technique, especially if vasospasm is known or suspected to exist. A variety of pharmacologic agents have been investigated for their ability to protect the nervous system from ischemic insults. The most widely used drug is pentobarbital; however, calcium channel blockers and glutamate receptor antagonists are also being investigated.

RESULTS OF TREATMENT

The International Cooperative Study on the Timing of Aneurysm Surgery recently documented the results of treatment in 3521 patients admitted to participating centers within 3 days of SAH.[33] Of the patients admitted to this study, 83% were surgically treated. Follow-up evaluations at 6 months revealed that 69% of patients surgically treated (58% of the total) had recovered to their premorbid neurologic status. One third of the patients in this study were severely disabled, vegetative, or dead at 6 months.

In addition to the morbidity and mortality documented previously, of the 28,000 estimated cases of SAH in the United States each year, only about 18,000 survive to reach medical attention.[71]

The outcome after SAH has also been assessed with regards to cognition and functional status. It has been estimated that up to half of survivors of SAH manifest evidence of late psychosocial or cognitive impairment.[39,67] Additional studies are needed to further define the extent and delineate the neurophysiology involved in these important observations.

In assessing the results of surgery for unruptured aneurysms, the outlook is much brighter. The results of elective surgery for aneurysms reveal a combined morbidity and mortality rate of under 5% for the majority of aneurysms encountered.[8,59] A recently published report of 179 unruptured aneurysms of the posterior circulation subjected to surgical treatment revealed a morbidity and mortality rate of 4.2%.[63] These results are from neurosurgical centers with extensive aneurysm experience.

Based on (1) the results of elective surgery in unruptured aneurysms, (2) the known natural history of cerebral aneurysms, and (3) the significant morbidity and mortality associated with aneurysmal rupture, it is recommended that surgical clipping be performed in the vast majority of unruptured cerebral aneurysms greater than 5 mm in diameter in patients whose life expectancies justify the expected surgical risk. This decision must be individualized for each patient and each aneurysm.

▼

SUMMARY

Cerebral aneurysms that have ruptured carry a significant overall morbidity and mortality that is in large part due to potentially treatable causes, such as vasospasm. Cerebral aneurysms that are unruptured carry a definite risk of rupture that in the average patient represents a significant health risk. In both ruptured and unruptured aneurysms, modern neurosurgical techniques may be employed in nearly all cases to safely obliterate the aneurysm and eliminate the risk of future hemorrhage.

Modern neuroanesthetic techniques facilitate safe operative treatment of aneurysms by aiding in surgical exposure and by minimizing the risk of catastrophic intraoperative hemorrhage and postoperative ischemic neurologic deficit. Improvement in the overall outcome of patients with SAH depends on advances in the treatment of the sequelae of aneurysmal rupture and on the identification and treatment of cerebral aneurysms before hemorrhage.

References

1. Adams HP, Kassell NF, Torner JC et al: Predicting cerebral ischemia after aneurysmal subarachnoid hemorrhage: influences of clinical condition, CT results, and antifibrinolytic therapy. A report of the cooperative aneurysm study, *Neurology* 37:1586-1591, 1987.
2. Allen GS, Ahn HS, Preziosi TJ et al: Cerebral arterial spasm—a controlled trial of nimodipine in patients with subarachnoid hemorrhage, *N Eng J Med* 308:619-624, 1983.
3. Allen GS, Bahr AL. Cerebral arterial spasm 10. Reversal of chronic spasm in dogs with orally administered nifedipine, *Neurosurgery* 4:43-47, 1979.
4. Andrews RJ. Familial intracranial aneurysms, *Arch Neurol* 36:524, 1979.
5. Ausman JI, Diaz FG, Malik G et al: Management of cerebral aneurysms: further facts and additional myths, *Surg Neurol* 32:21-35, 1989.
6. Bailes JE, Spetzler RF, Hadley MN et al: Management morbidity and mortality of poor grade aneurysm patients, *J Neurosurg* 72:559-566, 1990.
7. Botterell EH, Lougheed WM, Scott JW et al: Hypothermia and interruption of carotid, or carotid and vertebral circulation, in the surgical management of intracranial aneurysms, *J Neurosurg* 13:1-42, 1956.
8. Brisman R: Management of multiple and asymptomatic aneurysms. In Fein JM, Flamm ES, editors: *Cerebrovascular surgery,* New York, 1985, Springer-Verlag.
9. Chason JL, Hindman WM. Berry aneurysms of the circle of Willis: results of a planned autopsy study, *Neurology* 8:41-44, 1958.
10. Chyatte D, Sundt TM: Cerebral vasospasm: evidence supporting an inflammatory etiology. In Wilkins RH, editor: *Cerebral vasospasm,* New York, 1988, Raven Press.
11. Chester AC, Harris JP, Schreiner GE: Polycystic kidney disease, *Am Fam Physician* 16:94-101, 1977.
12. Drake CG: The treatment of aneu-

rysms of the posterior circulation, *Clin Neurosurg* 26:96-144, 1979.

13. Drake CG: Management of cerebral aneurysm, *Stroke* 12:274-282, 1981.

14. Drake C. Earlier times in aneurysm surgery, *Clin Neurosurg* 32:11-50, 1985.

15. Findlay JM, Weir BA, Gordon P et al: Safety and efficacy of intrathecal thrombolytic therapy in a primate model of cerebral vasospasm, *Neurosurgery* 24:491-498, 1989.

16. Flamm ES: The management of aneurysmal subarachnoid hemorrhage. In Fein JM, Flamm ES, editors: *Cerebrovascular surgery*, New York, 1985, Springer-Verlag.

17. Flamm ES, Adams HP, Beck DW et al: Dose escalation study of intravenous nicardipine in patients with aneurysmal subarachnoid hemorrhage, *J Neurosurg* 68:393-400, 1988.

18. Fletcher TM, Taveras JM, Pool JL: Cerebral vasospasm in angiography for intracranial aneurysms, *Arch Neurol* 1:38-47, 1959.

19. Fox JL: *Intracranial aneurysms*, New York, 1983, Springer-Verlag.

20. Haley EC, Kassell NS, Torner JC: A randomized controlled trial of high-dose intravenous nicardipine in aneurysmal subarachnoid hemorrhage. A report of the Cooperative Aneurysm Study, *J Neurosurg* 78:537-547, 1993.

21. Haley EC, Torner JC, Kassell NF: Antifibrinolytic therapy and cerebral vasospasm, *Neurosurg Clin* 1:349-356, 1990.

22. Hashimoto I: Familial intracranial aneurysms and cerebral vascular anomalies, *J Neurosurg* 46:419-427, 1977.

23. Higashida RT, Halbach VV, Cahan LD et al: Detachable balloon embolization therapy of posterior circulation intracranial aneurysms, *J Neurosurg* 71:512-519, 1989.

24. Housepian EM, Pool JL: A systematic analysis of intracranial aneurysms from the autopsy file of the Presbyterian Hospital, 1914-1956, *J Neuropathol Exp Neurol* 17:409-423, 1958.

25. Hunt WE, Kosnick EJ: Timing and preoperative care in intracranial aneurysm surgery, *Clin Neurosurg* 21:79-89, 1974.

26. Iwanaga H, Wakai S, Ochiai C et al: Ruptured cerebral aneurysms missed by initial angiographic study, *Neurosurgery* 27:45-51, 1990.

27. Jane JA, Kassell NF, Torner JC et al: The natural history of aneurysms and arteriovenous malformations, *J Neurosurg* 62:321-323, 1985.

28. Kassell NF, Haley EC, Torner JC: Antifibrinolytic therapy in the treatment of subarachnoid hemorrhage, *Clin Neurosurg* 33:137-145, 1986.

29. Kassell NF, Peerless SJ, Durward QJ et al: Treatment of ischemic deficits from vasospasm with intravascular volume expansion and induced arterial hypertension, *Neurosurgery* 11:337-343, 1982.

30. Kassell NF, Torner JC: Size of intracranial aneurysms, *Neurosurgery* 12:291-297, 1983.

31. Kassell NF, Torner JC: Aneurysmal rebleeding: a preliminary report from the cooperative aneurysm study, *Neurosurgery* 13:479-481, 1983.

32. Kassell NF, Torner JC, Adams HP: Antifibrinolytic therapy in the acute period following subarachnoid hemorrhage. Preliminary observations from the cooperative aneurysm study, *J Neurosurg* 61:225-230, 1984.

33. Kassell NF, Torner JC, Haley EC et al: The international cooperative study on the timing of aneurysm surgery. Part I: overall management results, *J Neurosurg* 73:16-36, 1990.

34. Kassell NF, Torner JC, Jane JA et al: The international cooperative study on the timing of aneurysm surgery. Part 2: surgical results, *J Neurosurg* 73:37-47, 1990.

35. Krayenbuhl H, Yasargil MG, Flamm ES et al: Microsurgical treatment of intracranial saccular aneurysms, *J Neurosurg* 37:678-686, 1972.

36. Lin JP, Kricheff IL: Neuroradiology of intracranial aneurysms. In Fein JM, Flamm ES, editors: *Cerebrovascular surgery*, New York, 1985, Springer-Verlag.

37. Ljunggren B, Brandt L, Kagstrom E et al: Results of early operations for ruptured aneurysms, *J Neurosurg* 54:473-479, 1981.

38. Ljunggren B, Brandt L, Saveland H et al: Management of ruptured aneurysm: a review, *Br J Neurosurg* 1:9-32, 1987.

39. Ljunggren B, Sonesson BS, Saveland H et al: Cognitive impairment and adjustment in patients without neurological deficits after aneurysmal SAH and early operation, *J Neurosurg* 62:673-679, 1985.

40. Locksley HB: Report of the cooperative study of intracranial aneurysms and subarachnoid hemorrhage. Section V part 1. Natural history of subarachnoid hemorrhage, intracranial aneurysms, and arteriovenous malformations, *J Neurosurg* 25:219-239, 1966.

41. Longstreth WT, Nelson LM, Koepsell TD et al: Cigarette smoking, alcohol use, and subarachnoid hemorrhage, *Stroke* 23:1242-1249, 1992.

42. Mayberg MR, Okada T, Bark DH: Morphologic changes in cerebral arteries after subarachnoid hemorrhage, *Neurosurg Clin* 1:417-432, 1990.

43. McCormick W, Acosta-Rua G: The size of intracranial saccular aneurysms: an autopsy study, *J Neurosurg* 33:422-427, 1970.

44. McKissock W, Richardson A, Walsh L: Middle cerebral aneurysms: further results in the controlled trial of conservative and surgical treatment of ruptured intracranial aneurysms, *Lancet* 2:417-421, 1962.

45. Mettinger KL: Fibromuscular dysplasia and the brain: II. Current concept of the disease, *Stroke* 13:53-58, 1982.

46. Meyer FB: Calcium, neuronal hyperexcitability, and ischemic injury, *Br Res* 14:227-243, 1989.

47. Mizukami M, Takemae T, Tazawa T et al: Value of computed tomography in the prediction of cerebral vasospasm after aneurysm rupture, *Neurosurgery* 7:583-586, 1980.

48. Mount LA, Antunes JL: Results of treatment of intracranial aneurysms by wrapping and coating, *J Neurosurg* 42:189-193, 1975.

49. Muizelaar JP: Antifibrinolytics in subarachnoid hemorrhage: a randomized double blind placebo controlled study with 479 patients, *Stroke* 15:188-189, 1984.

50. Mullan S, Dawley J: Antifibrinolytic therapy for intracranial aneurysms, *J Neurosurg* 28:21-23, 1968.

51. Neil-Dwyer G, Bartlett JR, Nicholls AC et al: Collagen deficiency and ruptured cerebral aneurysms: a clinical and biochemical study, *J Neurosurg* 59:16-20, 1983.

52. Newell DW, Eskridge JM, Mayberg MR et al: Angioplasty for the treatment of symptomatic vasospasm following subarachnoid hemorrhage, *Neurosurgery* 71:654-660, 1989.

53. Newell DW, Winn HR: Transcranial Doppler in cerebral vasospasm, *Neurosurg Clinics* 1:319-328, 1990.

54. Nibbelink DW, Torner JC, Henderson WG: Intracranial aneurysms and subarachnoid hemorrhage—report of a randomized treatment study: IV. A. Regulated bed rest, *Stroke* 8:202-218, 1977.
55. Ojemann RG, Heros RC, Crowell RM: *Surgical management of cerebrovascular disease,* Baltimore, 1985, Williams & Wilkins.
56. Okawara SH: Warning signs prior to rupture of an intracranial aneurysm, *J Neurosurg* 38:575-580, 1973.
57. Petruk KC, West M, Mohr G et al: Nimodipine treatment in poor grade aneurysm patients: results of a multicenter, double-blind, placebo-controlled trial, *J Neurosurg* 68:505-517, 1988.
58. Phillips LH, Whisnant JP, O'Fallon W et al: The unchanging pattern of subarachnoid hemorrhage in a community, *Neurology* 30:1034-1040, 1980.
59. Piepgras DG: Management of incidental intracranial aneurysms, *Clin Neurosurg* 35:511-518, 1989.
60. Poppen JL, Fager CA: Multiple intracranial aneurysms, *J Neurosurg* 16:581-589, 1959.
61. Ransohoff J, Goodgold A, Benjamin MV: Preoperative management of patients with ruptured intracranial aneurysms, *J Neurosurg* 36:525-530, 1972.
62. Rhoton AL, Fujii K, Saeki N et al: Microsurgical anatomy of intracranial aneurysms. In Fein JM, Flamm ES, editors: *Cerebrovascular surgery,* New York, 1985, Springer-Verlag.
63. Rice BJ, Peerless SJ, Drake CG: Surgical treatment of unruptured aneurysms of the posterior circulation, *J Neurosurg* 73:165-173, 1990.
64. Robertson EG: Cerebral lesions due to intracranial aneurysms, *Brain* 72:150-189, 1949.
65. Robinson M, Teasdale G: Calcium antagonists in the management of subarachnoid hemorrhage, *J Cereb Brain Metab Rev* 2:205-226, 1990.
66. Romodanov AP, Shcheglov VI: Intravascular occlusion of saccular aneurysms of cerebral arteries by means of a detachable balloon catheter, *Adv Tech Stand Neurosurg* 9:25-48, 1982.
67. Ropper AH, Zervas NT: Outcome one year after SAH from cerebral aneurysm. Management morbidity, mortality, and functional status in 112 consecutive good-risk patients, *J Neurosurg* 60:909-915, 1984.
68. Rose FC, Sarner M: Epilepsy after ruptured intracranial aneurysm, *Br Med J* 1:18-21, 1965.
69. Rosenstein J, Suzuki M, Symon L et al: Clinical use of a portable bedside cerebral blood flow machine in the management of aneurysmal subarachnoid hemorrhage, *Neurosurgery* 15:519-525, 1984.
70. Ross JS, Masaryk TJ, Modic MT et al: Magnetic resonance angiography of the extracranial arteries and the intracranial vessels: a review, *Neurology* 39:1369-1376, 1989.
71. Sahs AL, Nibbelink DW, Torner JC, editors: *Aneurysmal subarachnoid hemorrhage. Report of the cooperative study,* Baltimore, 1981, Urban and Schwarzenberg.
72. Sahs AL, Perret CE, Locksley HB et al: *Intracranial aneurysms and subarachnoid hemorrhage. A cooperative study,* Philadelphia, 1969, JB Lippincott.
73. Schramm J, Koht A, Schmidt G et al: Surgical and electrophysiological observations during clipping of 134 aneurysms with evoked potential monitoring, *Neurosurgery* 26:61-70, 1990.
74. Sekhar LN, Heros RC: Origin, growth, and rupture of saccular aneurysms: a review, *Neurosurgery* 8:248-260, 1981.
75. Sekhar LN, Weschler LR, Yonas H et al: Value of transcranial Doppler examination in the diagnosis of cerebral vasospasm after subarachnoid hemorrhage, *Neurosurgery* 22:813-821, 1988.
76. Spetzler RF, Hadley MN, Rigamonti D et al: Aneurysms of the basilar artery treated with circulatory arrest, hypothermia, and barbiturate cerebral protection, *J Neurosurg* 68:868-879, 1988.
77. Stehbens WE: Etiology of intracranial berry aneurysms, *J Neurosurg* 70:823-831, 1989.
78. Suzuki J, Kwak R, Okudaira Y: The safe time limit of temporary clamping of cerebral arteries in the direct surgical treatment of intracranial aneurysm under moderate hypothermia, *Tohoku J Exp Med* 127:1-7, 1979.
79. Taneda M: Effect of early operation for ruptured aneurysms on prevention of delayed ischemic symptoms, *J Neurosurg* 57:622-628, 1982.
80. Todd NV, Tocher JL, Jones PA et al: Outcome following aneurysm wrapping: a 10-year follow-up review of clipped and wrapped aneurysms, *J Neurosurg* 70:841-846, 1989.
81. Tu YK, Heros RC, Karacostas O et al: Isovolemic hemodilution in experimental focal cerebral ischemia. Part 1: effects on hemodynamics, hemorheology, and intracranial pressure, *J Neurosurg* 69:72-81, 1988.
82. Tu YK, Heros RC, Karacostas O et al: Isovolemic hemodilution in experimental focal cerebral ischemia. Part 2: effects on regional cerebral blood flow and size of infarction, *J Neurosurg* 69:82-91, 1988.
83. Weir B, Grace M, Hansen J et al: Time course of vasospasm in man, *J Neurosurg* 48:173-178, 1978.
84. White RP: Responses of isolated cerebral arteries to vasoactive agents, *Neurosurg Clin* 1:401-415, 1990.
85. Wiebers DO, Whisnant JP, O'Fallon WM: The natural history of unruptured intracranial aneurysms, *N Engl J Med* 304:696-698, 1981.
86. Wilson CB, Spetzler RF: Factors responsible for improved results in the surgical management of intracranial aneurysms and vascular malformations, *Am J Surg* 134:33-38, 1977.
87. Winn HR, Almaani WS, Berga SL et al: The long term outcome in patients with multiple aneurysms. Incidence of late hemorrhage and implications for treatment of incidental aneurysms, *J Neurosurg* 59:642-651, 1983.
88. Yasargil MG: *Microneurosurgery,* New York, 1984, Thieme Stratton.
89. Yasargil MG, Fox JL: The microsurgical approach to intracranial aneurysms, *Surg Neurol* 3:7-14, 1975.
90. Yonas H, Sekhar L, Johnson SW et al: Determination of irreversible ischemia by Xenon-enhanced computed tomographic monitoring of cerebral blood flow in patients with symptomatic vasospasm, *Neurosurgery* 22:368-372, 1989.

18

Cerebral Aneurysms: Anesthetic Considerations

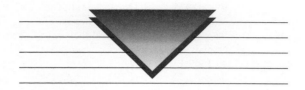

CALVIN C. ENG
ARTHUR M. LAM

Although it is simplistic, the statement by the British neurosurgeon J. Gillingham[56] that "In the early years anaesthetists spent their time pushing the brain out of the skull while in recent times they have been sucking it back in" underscores the importance and contribution of neuroanesthesia to the improved results of surgical treatment of ce-

rebral aneurysms. Other advances include the improvements in microsurgical instrumentation, such as the operating microscope, neuroradiology, and the development of specialized centers with surgeons and anesthesiologists dedicated to the treatment of patients with cerebral aneurysms. However, data published from The International Cooperative Study on the Timing of Aneurysm Surgery (Cooperative Study)[83,84] indicated that overall surgical mortality remains high, at approximately 20%. To a certain extent these results might have been biased because of the trend toward early operative intervention in high-risk patients who were previously considered unsuitable for surgery. Nonetheless, even patients admitted in good condition with a level of consciousness score equivalent to Hunt and Hess grades I and II (see later discussion) have a "good" recovery rate of only 58% and a mortality of 26%.[83] Thus much room exists for improvement in all aspects of cerebral aneurysm treatment. Considerable variations in mortality and morbidity exist between centers of the Cooperative Study, and the reasons for these variations are not apparent. The leading causes of death and disability were, in descending order, vasospasm, the direct effects of the initial bleed (massive subarachnoid, subdural, or intracerebral hematoma, permanent ischemic effects of increased intracranial pressure), rebleeding, and surgical complications.[83] Successful anesthetic management of these patients requires a thorough understanding of the natural history, pathophysiology, and surgical requirements of the procedures.

PREOPERATIVE CONSIDERATIONS

The main steps in preoperative evaluation include (1) assessment of the patient's neurologic condition and clinical grading of the subarachnoid hemorrhage (SAH); (2) a review of the patient's intracranial pathologic condition including CT scan and angiograms; (3) monitoring of intracranial pressure (ICP) and transcranial Doppler ultrasonography (TCD)[64] if available; (4) evaluation of other systemic functions, premorbid as well as the present condition, with emphasis on systems known to be affected by SAH; (5) communication with the neurosurgeon regarding positioning and special monitoring requirements; and (6) optimization of the patient's condition by correcting any existing biochemical and physiologic disturbances. The preoperative assessment allows appropriate planning of an anesthetic regimen with consideration of both the pathophysiology of all organ systems and the surgical requirements. This will ensure a smooth anesthetic for an uncomplicated aneurysm and a heightened level of preparedness for a complicated one.

THE CENTRAL NERVOUS SYSTEM

To allow better assessment of surgical risk and prognostication of outcome, Botterell et al. in 1956 first proposed the grading of subarachnoid hemorrhage[17] (Table 18-1). This was later modified by Hunt and Hess[71] (Table 18-2), and more recently a grading scale based on the Glasgow Coma Scale was introduced by the World Federation of Neurological Surgeons[45] (Table 18-3). In the World Federation classification the most important correlate with outcome is the preoperative level of consciousness.[83] These

TABLE 18-1
Botterell et al.'s Clinical Grades

Grade	Criteria
I	Conscious with or without meningeal signs
II	Drowsy without significant neurologic deficit
III	Drowsy with neurologic deficit and probable cerebral clot
IV	Major neurologic deficits present
V	Moribund with failing vital centers and extensor rigidity

TABLE 18-2
Modified Hunt and Hess's Clinical Grades*

Grade	Criteria
0	Unruptured aneurysm
I	Asymptomatic or minimal headache and slight nuchal rigidity
II	Moderate to severe headache, nuchal rigidity, but no neurologic deficit other than cranial nerve palsy
III	Drowsiness, confusion, or mild focal deficit
IV	Stupor, mild to severe hemiparesis, possible early decerebrate rigidity, vegetative disturbance
V	Deep coma, decerebrate rigidity, moribund appearance

*Serious systemic disease such as hypertension, diabetes, severe arteriosclerosis, chronic pulmonary disease, and severe vasospasm seen on arteriography result in placement of the patient in the next less favorable category.

TABLE 18-3
World Federation of Neurological Surgeons' Grading Scale

WFNS* Grade	GCS† Score	Motor Deficit
I	15	Absent
II	14-13	Absent
III	14-13	Present
IV	12-7	Present or absent
V	6-3	Present or absent

*World Federation of Neurological Surgeons.
†Glasgow Coma Scale.

clinical grading schemes allow evaluation of operative risk, communication among physicians about the patient's condition, and conduct of comparative studies of therapy on outcome. The modified Hunt and Hess grading scale remains the most commonly used grading scale, both because of familiarity and ease of application.

Although the surgical mortality and morbidity vary with different institutions, patients in good preoperative condition (grades I and II) can be expected to do well, whereas grade V patients have a high mortality and morbidity (Table 18-4). The clinical grade also indicates the severity of associated cerebral pathophysiology. The greater the clinical grade, the more likely there will be vasospasm,[7] ele-

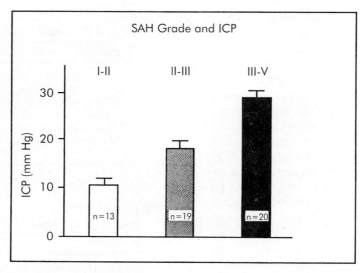

FIG. 18-1   The relationship between SAH grade (Hunt and Hess) and ICP. *(From Voldby B, Enevoldsen EM: Intracranial pressure changes following aneurysm rupture. I. Clinical and angiographic correlations,* J Neurosurg *56:186, 1982.)*

TABLE 18-4
Surgical Mortality and Major Morbidity vs. Clinical Grades*

Grade (Hunt and Hess)	Mortality (%)	Morbidity (%)
0	0-2	0-2
I	2-5	2
II	5-10	7
III	5-10	37
IV	35-60	40
V	50-70	45

*Pooled from the literature and experience in the authors' hospital.

vated ICP,[217] impaired cerebral autoregulation,[36,72,207,218] and a disordered cerebrovascular response to hypocapnia.[207,218] A worse clinical grade is also associated with a higher incidence of cardiac arrhythmia[55] and myocardial dysfunction.[35] Patients with worse clinical grades tend to be hypovolemic and hyponatremic.[40,41,138] Thus understanding the grading scale allows the anesthesiologist to communicate effectively with other physicians and facilitates assessment of the pathophysiologic derangements and planning the perioperative anesthetic management.

INTRACRANIAL PRESSURE

Intracranial pressure increases rapidly after a subarachnoid hemorrhage and may approach the levels of the systemic blood pressure. This phase lasts minutes and is thought to limit the amount of blood leakage through the ruptured aneurysm.[142,172] With recurrent rupture of the aneurysm, ICP increases further from mass effect (clot), cerebral edema, or hydrocephalus from a blocked aqueduct.[172] A communicating hydrocephalus may later develop because of arach-

noidal adhesions from the extravascular blood that interferes with reabsorption of cerebrospinal fluid (CSF).[16] In the Cooperative Study the incidence of hydrocephalus was about 15%. An increased ICP with hypovolemia may increase the likelihood of delayed cerebral ischemia and infarction.[138] The development of vasospasm can also exacerbate an increase in ICP, because the reduction in cerebral blood flow (CBF) as a result of vasoconstriction is accompanied by vasodilation in the distal vessels. This causes an increase in cerebral blood volume (CBV).[59,112] Other factors that would contribute to increases in ICP include an intracerebral (17%) or intraventricular (17%) hematoma.[83] Clinically, hydrocephalus is characterized by progressive obtundation and nonreactive small pupils. These clinical features, however, are only present in about 50% of the cases, and therefore radiologic diagnosis is essential.[213]

ICP correlates well with clinical grade. It is generally normal in grade I and II patients but is elevated in grade IV and V patients[217] (Fig. 18-1). However, a normal ICP does not necessarily imply a normal intracranial compliance. It is important not to normalize the ICP too rapidly, since it may increase the transmural pressure (TMP) gradient across the aneurysm wall and cause further hemorrhage. A cerebral perfusion pressure of 60 to 80 mm Hg is a reasonable goal.[172]

IMPAIRMENT OF AUTOREGULATION AND CO_2 REACTIVITY

Patients with SAH generally have decreased CBF and cerebral metabolic rate.[24,59,75,112] At the same time CBV increases if vasospasm develops.[59,112] These patients may also have an impaired ability to autoregulate, with the degree of impairment correlating directly with the clinical grade.[36,72,207,218] Nornes et al. observed that the lower limit of autoregulation was significantly higher in grade III patients than in grade I and II patients during intracranial surgery.[143] The development of impaired autoregulation closely correlates with the occurrence of vasospasm.[218]

If neurologic deterioration occurs, it is vital to review the hemodynamic measurements for any associated relationship. Many well-documented cases describe patients with SAH who developed a new neurologic deficit associated with a decrease in blood pressure and a subsequent reversal of the deficit with a pharmacologically induced increase in blood pressure.[78] Therefore the anesthesiologist must not allow the perfusion pressure to decrease below this lower limit perioperatively. This represents a relative contraindication to induced hypotension during surgery, as will be discussed later.

The cerebrovascular response to hyperventilation is generally preserved after SAH.[36,207,218] Although impairment of autoregulation may occur in patients assigned relatively good clinical grades, a decline in CO_2 reactivity does not occur until there is severe damage.[207] Thus hyperventilation remains effective in reducing CBF and CBV during perioperative management for most patients.

INTRAVASCULAR VOLUME STATUS AND HYPONATREMIA

The intravascular volume status has been found to be abnormally low in 36% to 100% of patients with SAH, and the degree of hypovolemia correlates with the clinical grade.[111,138,182,224,225] Moreover, patients with signs of increased ICP on CT scan have a greater likelihood of systemic hypovolemia.[138] The reasons are multifactorial and probably include bed rest, supine diuresis, negative nitrogen balance, decreased erythropoiesis, and iatrogenic blood loss.[111] Hypovolemia may exacerbate vasospasm and is associated with cerebral ischemia and infarction.[67,138,224]

Paradoxically, hypovolemia has often been observed to be associated with hyponatremia. This condition was once attributed to the development of the syndrome of inappropriate antidiuretic hormone and was treated with fluid restriction. Recent investigations, however, suggest that the hyponatremia is related to hydrocephalus that causes distention of the cerebral ventricles, which may lead to release of atrial natriuretic factors from the hypothalamus.[39-42,161] Patients in vasospasm have also been reported to have a 30% incidence of hyponatremia.[66] These observations suggest that hyponatremia associated with SAH should not be treated with fluid restriction.[224,225] Instead, these patients should be treated with normal saline and, in refractory cases, hypertonic saline (3%). Patients at risk of vasospasm should be treated with volume expansion and induced hypertension. It appears that in an ischemic brain with dysautoregulation, either volume expansion with consequent increase in cardiac output or an increase in blood pressure can independently improve cerebral perfusion.[101] However,

it is not clear whether it is the hypervolemia or the hypertension that is the most crucial factor in ameliorating the vasospasm. The prophylactic value of aggressive hypervolemic therapy to reduce the incidence of vasospasm, in any event, must be balanced against the risk of pulmonary edema (see also the later section on vasospasm).[119]

Other significant electrolyte abnormalities include hypokalemia and hypocalcemia. In a series of 406 patients with SAH, both hypokalemia (K^+ <3.4 mmol/L) and hypocalcemia (Ca^{++} <2.2 mmol/L) were noted (41% and 74%, respectively).[163]

CARDIAC EFFECTS
Electrocardiographic Changes

Abnormalities in rhythm and morphology of the electrocardiogram (ECG) are observed in 50% to 100% of patients with SAH.* The types of arrhythmias vary from benign rhythms such as sinus bradycardia, sinus tachycardia, atrioventricular dissociation, and bradycardia-tachycardia to more serious and potentially life-threatening rhythms such as ventricular tachycardia and fibrillation. Morphologic changes in the ECG include T-wave inversion, depression of the ST segment, the appearance of U waves, prolonged QT interval, and rarely Q waves.† A prolonged QT interval, which may occur in 20% to 41% of the patients, has been observed to be associated with dangerous ventricular arrhythmias.[5] These ECG changes usually occur during the first 48 hours after SAH. The duration is variable; the ECG may return to normal in 10 days[216] or may take up to 6 weeks to return to normal.[65] These abnormalities may fluctuate from day to day[55] and have been shown to also occur intraoperatively and postoperatively.[105,106]

Electrolyte disturbances may contribute to the etiology of the ECG changes. Hypokalemia may cause a depression of the ST segment, a decrease in the amplitude of the T wave, an increase in the amplitude of the U wave, as well as arrhythmias.[163] Hypocalcemia may cause prolongation of the QT interval and promote cardiac arrhythmias or myocardial depression.[163] Other factors contributing to ECG changes occur at the time of the acute bleed when the sudden increase in ICP induces a hypothalamic-mediated overwhelming sympathetic discharge and consequent cardiac changes.[31,177] Cruickshank et al.[31] have shown a strong correlation between high urinary levels of catecholamines and T-wave inversion, the presence of Q waves, and prolonged QT intervals in patients with an acute SAH. One clinicopathologic study demonstrated the coexistence of hypothalamic and myocardial lesions to further support the hypothesis that it is secondary to hypothalamic injury.[43] The catecholamines released, especially norepinephrine, may cause damage through systemic hypertension, which leads to left ventricular strain or direct tissue toxicity.[31,110] In ad-

---

*References 5, 18, 37, 55, 110, 165, 216.
†References 5, 18, 55, 110, 165, 216, 222, 223.

dition, corticosteroid levels are also increased and may render the myocardium more sensitive to the catecholamines and enhance the ability of catecholamines to cause hypokalemia.[31] However, Grad et al.[58] recently found no correlation between ECG changes and plasma norepinephrine concentrations.

Myocardial Function

Echocardiographic studies have failed to establish a relationship between ECG changes and myocardial dysfunction; however, myocardial dysfunction is correlated to the severity of the neurologic injury.[35,156]

Anesthetic Implications

Patients with prolonged QT interval, T-wave abnormalities, and Q waves should have prompt correction of electrolyte disturbances and timely treatment with antiarrhythmic drugs.[5,216] Experimentally, pharmacologic or surgical blockade of the sympathetic nervous system prevents or abolishes these ECG changes.[216,222] However, no evidence exists that the prophylactic administration of a beta-adrenergic or other autonomic antagonist significantly alters the outcome in these patients, and their use for this purpose is probably not warranted.[58,110]

Q waves and other ECG evidence of ischemia are always worrisome and, when observed in a patient with subarachnoid hemorrhage (SAH), pose a diagnostic dilemma.[168,223] Although most ECG abnormalities following SAH appear to be neurogenic rather than cardiogenic in nature,[163] diagnostic difficulty has on occasion led to a delay in surgery.[168] Moreover, microscopic hemorrhages and myocytolysis have been observed in a postmortem study,[222] although other studies have reported no signs of myocardial damage.[55]

Three possibilities exist for ECG abnormalities suggesting ischemia: coincidental acute myocardial infarction, SAH-induced myocardial infarction, and ECG changes without infarction. Cardiac enzymes and echocardiography should be obtained in suspicious cases. As with any surgical procedure, the decision to proceed with surgery depends on the urgency of the situation. Because of the risk of rebleeding, surgical therapy of a ruptured aneurysm is almost always considered urgent.

In summary, ECG changes are prevalent following SAH and likely represent hyperactivity of the sympathetic system with increased levels of norepinephrine. Although in some patients there is no myocardial pathologic condition, in others there may be necrosis and other myopathology. In suspicious cases serial myocardial enzymes should be obtained. Since the cardiac changes reflect the severity of neurologic damage and have not been shown to materially contribute to perioperative mortality or morbidity the decision to operate should not be influenced by these ECG changes. These considerations, however, may influence the decision regarding the choice of invasive monitoring.

RESPIRATORY SYSTEM

Pulmonary edema has been observed to accompany SAH, and a sympathetic mechanism is again implicated.[222] Aspiration and hydrostatic pneumonia are other potential complications.

OTHER MAJOR MEDICAL PROBLEMS

Based on the Cooperative Study, other major medical problems include systemic hypertension (21%), heart disease (3%), and diabetes mellitus (2%).[83]

CONCURRENT MEDICAL TREATMENTS

Patients receiving diuretic therapy for chronic hypertension may have preexisting fluid and electrolyte problems before SAH.

Anticonvulsant therapy such as phenytoin and carbamazepine antagonizes the actions of nondepolarizing agents such as pancuronium and vecuronium, leading to increased muscle relaxant dose requirements and a shortened duration of action.[146,147,162] Acute anticonvulsant therapy of less than 7 days' duration probably has little effect. The mechanism is unclear but is probably pharmacodynamic rather than pharmacokinetic in origin.[146] Although the results are not consistent, atracurium appears to be less affected when compared to other nondepolarizing agents.[146,204] One report suggests that anticonvulsant therapy also increases fentanyl requirements.[206]

Some hospitals continue to use antifibrinolytic agents such as epsilon aminocaproic acid or tranexamic acid to prevent rebleeding while the patient is waiting for surgery. The anesthesiologist should be aware that these patients have a greater incidence of vasospasm and hydrocephalus.[82] They also have a higher incidence of venous thrombosis and pulmonary embolism.

Calcium channel antagonists are now routinely administered for vasospasm prophylaxis. This therapy has specific anesthetic implications that will be discussed later.

TIMING OF SURGERY

The two major complications contributing to significant morbidity and mortality following SAH are rebleeding and vasospasm, with each accounting for about 7% of mortality.[83] Since the brain is acutely swollen with fresh clots following SAH, it was generally believed that early operation increases the incidence of postoperative vasospasm. Therefore until recently most surgeons waited 7 to 10 days for the acute inflammatory process to subside before any operative intervention. Indeed, results from the Cooperative Study indicate that the brain was considered "tight" in 50% of cases with early surgery (day 0 after SAH), but only 20% were rated as "tight" after 10 days[84] (Fig. 18-2). Although delaying surgery will allow brain swelling to decrease, both

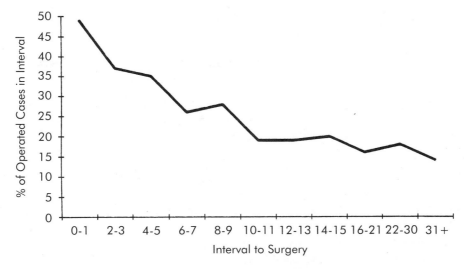

FIG. 18-2   The percent of patients with a "tight" brain during surgical exposure correlated with the day of operation after subarachnoid hemorrhage. *(From Kassell NF, Torner JC, Haley EC et al: The international cooperative study on the timing of aneurysm surgery. I. Overall management results,* J Neurosurg 73:18, 1990.)

rebleeding and vasospasm can occur during this waiting period. When surgery was delayed, antifibrinolytic agents were usually given to prevent lysis of the clot and rebleeding from the rent of the aneurysm. However, randomized clinical trials showed that, although these agents are effective in reducing the incidence of rebleeding, the incidence of vasospasm increases, leaving the overall morbidity and mortality unchanged.[80,215] In an attempt to improve the overall outcome there is a growing trend toward early operation, so that the risk of rebleeding can be eliminated and any vasospasm more aggressively treated. Results from the Cooperative Study, however, showed that the overall management results were not significantly different between early (0 to 3 days) and late (after 10 days) surgery, but the results were the worst with surgery performed between 7 and 10 days.[83] A subsequent analysis of data derived from only North American centers varied from the overall findings and indicated that the best results were achieved when surgery was planned between days 0 and 3 after SAH, therefore arguing strongly in favor of early surgery.[61] Although they should never be the primary consideration, substantial economic savings also are realized with early surgery. The trend toward early operation will probably continue, and patients in a less than ideal condition for surgery will be coming to the operating room.

REBLEEDING

Previous studies suggest that rebleeding following the initial SAH peaks at the end of the first week. The Cooperative Study indicates that rebleeding peaks at 4% during the first 24 hours and then levels off at 1.5% per day on subsequent days.[81] The overall incidence is 11%,[61] which ac-

counts for 8% of the mortality and disability.[83] The incidence is lower in patients receiving antifibrinolytic agents.[83] Rebleeding remains a major threat in hospitals where delayed surgery is the standard practice. With the trend toward early operation, the risk of rebleeding is reduced but not eliminated. A combination of antifibrinolytic therapy for rebleeding and a calcium channel blocker for vasospasm has been suggested as a possible remedy.[13]

VASOSPASM
Incidence

In patients who initially survive an SAH, cerebral vasospasm causing ischemia or infarction remains an important cause of morbidity and mortality.* In the Cooperative Study, vasospasm accounted for 13.5% of the overall mortality and major morbidity.[83] Not all patients with SAH will develop vasospasm; and its severity, time course, and prognosis are largely unpredictable.[29] The incidence and severity of delayed cerebral vasospasm have been shown to correlate with the amount and location of blood in the basal cisterns.[3,145] The frequency of occurrence as determined by angiography is estimated to be 40% to 60%.[50,80] However, clinically significant and symptomatic vasospasm occurs at a lower frequency (20% to 30%).[66,69,80] The difference may be explained by the varying degree of vasospasm. It has been established that the lower limit of CBF compatible with normal brain function is approximately 15 to 20 ml/100 g/min.[196] Thus considerable reduction in CBF can occur from vasospasm without clinical symptoms. When symptomatic vasospasm develops, approximately 50% of

*References 3, 4, 25, 50, 66, 78, 80, 83.

the patients will die or be left with a serious residual neurologic deficit.[3,25,69] Typically, angiographically detectable vasospasm is not seen until 72 hours after SAH,[194] the incidence peaks 7 days after SAH,[50,80] and it is seldom seen after 2 weeks.[4,29,128]

Pathogenesis

The vasospastic artery has structural and pathologic changes within the vessel wall, such as swelling and necrosis of the smooth muscle cells.[3] Although the exact mechanism and cause of spasm have not been completely elucidated, a reasonable hypothesis is that one or more vasoactive substances contained in the blood in the basal cisterns induce changes in the cerebral arteries to cause severe constriction.[29] The component in the blood implicated in the pathogenesis of vasospasm is currently thought to be oxyhemoglobin. Interaction with endothelium-derived relaxing factor and the endothelium may also play a part.[104] In support of this hypothesis, early intracranial operation (within 48 hours) to remove extravasated subarachnoid blood has been shown to be effective in reducing the occurrence of vasospasm and associated neurologic deterioration.[49,128,203] Delayed cerebral ischemia occurred only in patients in whom the subarachnoid blood clot remained in the cisterns.[128] Because subarachnoid blood may be widely dispersed from a ruptured aneurysm, the removal of blood must be aggressive and extensive, including tissue beyond the vicinity of the aneurysm and the adjacent cisterns.[203] Instillation of human recombinant tissue plasminogen activator (rt-PA) into the subarachnoid space is effective in lysing the clot and also reduces the severity of vasospasm.[49,145,233]

Clinical Manifestations

Delayed cerebral ischemia from vasospasm after SAH is a multivascular or diffuse process in most patients.[69] The clinical manifestations of vasospasm include a decrease in the level of consciousness, new onset of focal signs, and mutism. In a prospective study, Hijdra et al.[69] found that the majority of the patients with delayed cerebral ischemia from vasospasm had a decrease in the level of consciousness that may be accompanied by but was never preceded by focal signs. The time course for the appearance of the clinical manifestations may occur abruptly, but more commonly it appears gradually.[66,69]

Diagnosis

Following the appearance of new focal signs or a decreased level of consciousness, the diagnosis of cerebral vasospasm is confirmed by angiography. A CT scan may show hypodense lesions in brain areas that are consistent with the clinical signs. The diagnosis of vasospasm may also be predicted or anticipated before the onset of clinical vasospasm with the use of the transcranial Doppler (TCD). With vasospasm, cerebral artery flow velocities increase,[171] although confirmation with angiography is necessary. This new noninvasive technology also allows continual evalua-

tion of the patient in vasospasm without resorting to frequent angiographic investigations.

Treatment
Pharmacologic

Numerous drugs have been investigated for prevention or treatment of vasospasm, but most are ineffective.[29,226] Calcium channel blockers, of which nimodipine has been most extensively studied, are the only class of drugs that have been shown to consistently reduce the morbidity and mortality from vasospasm. Depending on the study, the incidence of poor outcome is reduced by 40% to 70%.* Interestingly, none of these favorable studies with calcium channel blocker prophylaxis was able to demonstrate any significant change in the incidence or severity of vasospasm, suggesting that the beneficial effects of nimodipine may be occurring at either a distal vessel site or a cellular level. The only study that demonstrated a significant improvement in angiographic vasospasm with a calcium channel blocker was reported recently using the experimental agent fasudil hydrochloride.[174]

Nonpharmacologic

Surgical. The presence of subarachnoid blood is related to the occurrence of vasospasm both qualitatively and quantitatively. By operating on patients with SAH within 48 hours of hemorrhage, Taneda[203] reduced the incidence of delayed ischemic deficits from 25% (11 of 44 patients who underwent surgery 10 days or more after the hemorrhage) to 11% (11 of 101 patients). Thus early operation with extensive irrigation of the cisterns may have reduced the incidence or severity of vasospasm.

Reduction of ICP. If the patient has elevated ICP, cerebral perfusion may be improved by lowering the ICP. Improvement in neurologic status with this treatment alone has been reported.[79]

Hypervolemic, Hypertensive, Hemodilution Therapy. The most consistently effective regimen now available to prevent and treat ischemic neurologic deficits caused by cerebral vasospasm uses hypervolemia, hypertension, and hemodilution (triple H therapy).† The rationale behind induced hypervolemia and hypertension is that in SAH the ischemic areas of the brain have impaired autoregulation and thus CBF depends on perfusion pressure, which partly depends on the intravascular volume and mean arterial blood pressure.[72,100,101,111]

This therapy is most successful if instituted early when the neurologic deficits are mild and before the onset of infarction.[78] However, prophylactic treatment initiated before aneurysm clipping is associated with a significant risk of rebleeding (19% in one series).[77] Other concerns include worsening of cerebral edema, increasing ICP, and causing

*References 4, 120, 137, 153, 154, 208.
†References 7, 20, 66, 78, 111, 179, 180.

hemorrhage into an infarcted area. With early surgery there is less likelihood of rebleeding from the hypervolemic, hypertensive therapy.[20,179,180] Other systemic complications include pulmonary edema (7% to 17%), myocardial infarction (2%), dilutional hyponatremia (3% to 35%), and coagulopathy (3%).[7,20,66,78]

To optimize therapy and minimize the potential cardiovascular and pulmonary complications, invasive monitors, including arterial blood pressure, central venous pressure (CVP), or, preferably, a pulmonary artery catheter, are essential. Sufficient intravenous fluids are infused to increase the CVP to 10 mm Hg or the pulmonary artery wedge pressure (PAWP) to 12 to 20 mm Hg.[20,78,100,179,180] In a recent study where a Starling curve was constructed in nine patients with a ruptured intracranial aneurysm, Levy and Giannotta[100] observed that increasing the PAWP from 8 to 14 mm Hg correlated with significant increases in left ventricular stroke work index, stroke volume index, and cardiac index. However, further volume expansion to increase PAWP to above 14 mm Hg resulted in a decline in the cardiac index. No correlation existed between changes in CVP and changes in PAWP during volume expansion. They recommend that PAWP should be the variable to observe during hypervolemic therapy.[100] This appears to be a reasonable recommendation.

Hypervolemia is generally achieved with infusions of colloids (e.g., 5% albumin) as well as crystalloids. Hetastarch and dextran solutions should be used sparingly or not at all because of the potential complication of coagulopathy.[33,34] Although intravenous fluid loading alone is often effective,[78] it is at times insufficient to raise the blood pressure or reverse ischemic symptoms; vasopressors are then initiated to induce hypertension. The most widely used vasopressors are dopamine, dobutamine, or phenylephrine. The hypertensive, hypervolemic therapy may induce a vagal response as well as a profound diuresis requiring administration of large amounts of intravenous fluids. Atropine (1 mg IM every 3 to 4 hours) may be given to maintain the heart rate between 80 and 120, and aqueous vasopressin (Pitressin) (5 units IM) may be administered to maintain the urine output at less than 200 ml/hr. With this regimen, often only small amounts of vasopressor drugs are required.[78] The blood pressure is titrated to a level necessary to reverse the signs and symptoms of vasospasm or to a maximum of 160 to 200 mm Hg systolic in patients whose aneurysm has been clipped.[7,78] If the aneurysm has not been clipped, then the systolic blood pressure is increased to only 120 to 150 mm Hg. The elevated blood pressure must be maintained until the vasospasm resolves, usually in 3 to 7 days. Response to therapy can now be monitored noninvasively using the TCD; improvement in vasospasm is associated with a decrease in flow velocity.

Hemodilution, the last component of the triple H therapy, is based on the correlation of hematocrit and whole blood viscosity.[229] As the hematocrit and the viscosity decrease, the cerebrovascular resistance correspondingly decreases and CBF increases. One argument against hemodilution is that the oxygen-carrying capacity is also decreased. Experimental studies have suggested that a hematocrit of 33% provides an optimal balance between viscosity and oxygen-carrying capacity[229] and this has been applied clinically.[7]

Transluminal Angioplasty. In all major vessels that are accessible, transluminal angioplasty has been used in patients refractory to conventional treatment and preliminary results are promising, with reversal of deficits within 12 to 48 hours in 75% of the patients treated.[139] In distal vessels that are not accessible for angioplasty, the administration of papaverine (2 mg over 10 seconds) via superselective intraarterial infusion has been shown to be effective.[77]

ANESTHETIC CONSIDERATIONS
Hypertensive Therapy

The anesthetic management of patients with vasospasm or at risk for vasospasm requires an understanding of the natural course of vasospasm, concurrent therapy, the importance of intravascular volume status, the changes in electrolyte concentration that occur with the treatment of vasospasm, and which hemodynamic variables are associated with vasospasm. Although it is generally believed that early surgery increases the risk of vasospasm, there are no substantiating data, and recent data suggest otherwise.[83,179-181]

Asymptomatic patients at risk of vasospasm include all patients who undergo surgery before the onset of vasospasm. Although it is not possible to predict the occurrence of postoperative vasospasm, patients with good SAH grades tend to have a lower incidence. These patients should be maintained in a normovolemic state with volume loading initiated toward the end of the operation, after the aneurysm has been clipped. Intraoperatively, controlled hypotension can be provided safely, if so requested by the surgeon. Treatment of postoperative hypertension should not be too aggressive.

Some physicians consider patients symptomatic from vasospasm as high risk and not eligible for surgery. Many other surgeons, however, believe the most effective treatment of vasospasm is immediate clipping of the aneurysm so that aggressive hypertensive, hypervolemic therapy can be implemented. Symptomatic patients presenting for emergency clipping of aneurysms should be treated aggressively, and hypervolemia should be maintained and guided with invasive monitoring.[20] For patients already treated with hypertensive therapy, the threshold blood pressure below which the patient becomes symptomatic must be noted and the blood pressure should not be allowed to fall below this value. Buckland et al.[20] have advocated intraoperative induced hypertension as a prophylactic measure. This, however, must be balanced against the risk of increased brain swelling and difficulty with intraoperative brain retraction.

Because the main aim must be to maintain an adequate cerebral perfusion pressure (CPP), induced hypotension is contraindicated in these patients.

With respect to asymptomatic patients operated on a delayed basis, vasospasm seldom occurs past 12 days after SAH. Therefore patients who are operated on later than 10 to 12 days after SAH have a low risk of vasospasm and can be managed in a normal fashion.

Calcium Channel Antagonists

Calcium channel antagonists have a proven efficacy in reducing the neurologic complications of vasospasm. In most institutions all patients with SAH are prophylactically treated with nimodipine or nicardipine. Clinical experience suggests that these drugs do not present any difficulty for anesthetic management, although 5% of the patients who receive nimodipine and 23% of the patients who receive intravenous nicardipine[51] develop mild hypotension as a result of systemic vasodilation.[208] A similar tendency toward lower systemic blood pressure was also observed intraoperatively,[191,192,219] and there was a reduced demand for hypotensive agents when controlled hypotension was used.[219]

PREMEDICATION

To allow accurate assessment of the patient's immediate preoperative neurologic condition and clinical grade, preoperative medications are best omitted. A proper preoperative visit by the anesthesiologist with a thorough explanation usually obviates any need for preoperative medication. However, an anxious patient may become hypertensive, with increased risk of rebleeding. On the other hand, premedications such as barbiturates and narcotics may cause respiratory depression, resulting in an increase in CBF and CBV; therefore such medication must be used judiciously in patients with elevated ICP. Premedication should be individualized. Patients with a good clinical grade may receive morphine, 1 to 5 mg, and/or midazolam, 1 to 5 mg, intravenously for sedation. Best results are achieved when administration is titrated in 1 mg increments. Patients already treated with mechanical ventilation may receive higher doses (morphine, 10 to 20 mg; midazolam, 5 to 10 mg) if hemodynamic stability is maintained. Muscle relaxants may also be required for transport of intubated patients. Patients should continue to receive their regular dose of nimodipine and dexamethasone.

INTRAOPERATIVE CONSIDERATIONS AND INDUCTION OF ANESTHESIA

The incidence of aneurysm rupture during induction of anesthesia, although rare (reported to be 2% in one series[211] but probably less than 1% with modern anesthetic techniques), is usually precipitated by a sudden rise in blood pressure during tracheal intubation and is associated with a high mortality.[211] Therefore the goal during induction of

anesthesia for aneurysm surgery is to reduce the risk of aneurysm rupture by minimizing the transmural pressure (TMP) while simultaneously maintaining an adequate cerebral perfusion pressure (CPP). As illustrated in Fig. 18-3, both TMP and CPP are determined by the same equation: MAP − ICP. Therefore these represent opposite objectives. Ideally the TMP or CPP should be maintained at the preoperative level throughout the induction period, particularly in patients with good SAH grades. This, however, is not always possible. As a general principle, the patient's blood pressure should be reduced by 20% to 25% below the baseline value, and prophylaxis for the normal hypertensive response to intubation should be instituted before attempting tracheal intubation. Another useful approach is to balance the risk of ischemia from a decrease in CPP against the benefit of a reduced chance of aneurysmal rupture from a decrease in TMP, taking into consideration the patient's clinical grade. Patients with SAH grades 0, I, and II generally have normal ICP and are not experiencing acute ischemia.[217] Therefore these patients will tolerate a bigger transient decrease in blood pressure (30% to 35%, or systolic blood pressure at about 100 mm Hg). In contrast, patients with poor clinical grades frequently have increased ICP,[217] low CPP, and often ischemia. The elevated ICP decreases the TMP and partially protects the aneurysm from rerupture. These patients may not tolerate transient hypotension as well, and the duration and magnitude of blood pressure decrease should be moderated. The same consideration applies to the use of hyperventilation. Patients with a good clinical grade should not be hyperventilated, since the reduction in CBF will lead to a reduction in ICP and consequently an increase in TMP. Conversely, patients with poor

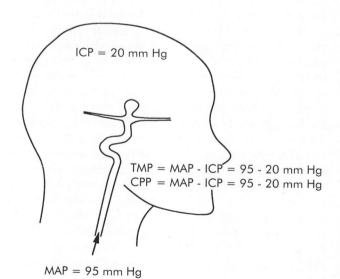

FIG. 18-3 Determinants of transmural pressure (TMP) and cerebral perfusion pressure (CPP). Both are determined by the difference between mean arterial pressure (MAP) and intracranial pressure (ICP) and are therefore numerically identical.

clinical grades should be managed with moderate hyperventilation to improve cerebral perfusion. To reduce the risk of aneurysm rupture or ischemia, the change in TMP or CPP should always be gradual and not abrupt.

If these principles and objectives are adhered to, a variety of anesthetic agents and techniques can be used successfully. Irrespective of the technique used, direct intraarterial blood pressure monitoring should be established before induction of anesthesia so that the patient's response to therapy can be continuously assessed.

Conceptually, it is convenient to think of the induction phase as consisting of two parts: (1) induction to achieve loss of consciousness and (2) prophylaxis to prevent a rise in blood pressure in response to laryngoscopy and intubation.

Induction to Achieve Loss of Consciousness

Thiopental (3 to 5 mg/kg) in combination with fentanyl (3 to 7 μg/kg) or sufentanil (0.3 to 0.7 μg/kg) is suitable. Other alternatives include etomidate (0.3 to 0.4 mg/kg) and midazolam (0.1 to 0.2 mg/kg). Propofol has a similar action to thiopental. It reduces CBF and metabolic rate,[214] and with careful titration (1.5 to 2.5 mg/kg) it can be used without compromising cerebral perfusion.

Regarding the use of narcotics, Marx et al.[113] had observed that sufentanil may cause an increase in ICP in patients with supratentorial tumors and suggested that this may be secondary to cerebral vasodilation. More recently, both fentanyl and sufentanil have been shown to increase ICP in patients with head trauma,[1,184] and Trindle et al.[210] reported that both agents increase CBF velocity. Other investigators, however, were unable to document either an increase in flow or a change in ICP with sufentanil.[114,220,221] In view of these studies, the mechanism of the increase in ICP remains unclear and may be related to the simultaneous decrease in systemic blood pressure. When used in combination with a vasoconstrictive agent such as thiopental or etomidate, these narcotics should be safe for use in patients with SAH, although hyperventilation should be instituted in patients with elevated ICP.

Prophylaxis Against Rise in Blood Pressure During Laryngoscopy

The above regimen only dealt with induction of unconsciousness, and other agents are required before tracheal intubation is attempted. Many anesthetic adjuncts have been used successfully to prevent the rise in blood pressure with laryngoscopy and tracheal intubation. These include the use of high-dose narcotics (e.g., fentanyl, 5 to 10 μg/kg, or sufentanil, 0.5 to 1.0 μg/kg),[85] beta-adrenergic antagonists (e.g., esmolol, 0.5 mg/kg),[32,166] labetalol (10 to 20 mg), intravenous or topical lidocaine (1.5 to 2.0 mg/kg),[62] a second dose of thiopental (1 to 2 mg/kg),[212] or a deep level of an inhalation anesthetic such as isoflurane.[91] Intravenous adjuncts are preferred in patients with poor SAH grades, whereas deep inhalation anesthetics are appropriate for patients with good SAH grades but should be avoided in patients with increased ICP. We routinely administer intravenous lidocaine, 1.5 mg/kg 2 to 3 minutes before intubation.

Choice of Muscle Relaxant

Although succinylcholine has been reported to increase ICP,[95] it has been used successfully in many aneurysm patients with no known sequelae. Moreover, this increase in ICP is not seen when the patients are deeply anesthetized[91] or when succinylcholine is preceded by a defasciculating dose of a nondepolarizing agent.[127,189] Another potential concern with succinylcholine is the possibility of potassium release. An early study reported this to be a significant complication,[73] but this observation was not confirmed by a recent investigation.[109] In all likelihood, succinylcholine is probably safe to use in the patient with acute SAH but should be avoided in patients with motor deficits in the subacute stages. In view of these potential complications, many anesthesiologists prefer to use a nondepolarizing agent such as vecuronium or atracurium. Vecuronium is associated with hemodynamic stability, whereas atracurium may cause systemic hypotension. Pancuronium, on the other hand, may cause tachycardia and hypertension, although this effect is attenuated by the simultaneous administration of synthetic narcotics such as fentanyl or sufentanil. The choice of muscle relaxant thus depends on the anesthesiologist's preference as well as the nature of other drugs being administered at the time of induction. For subsequent neuromuscular blockade, any of the nondepolarizing agents can be used.

To avoid coughing, the neuromuscular junction should be monitored and tracheal intubation only attempted when muscle paralysis is complete. The blood pressure should also be watched closely during laryngoscopy. Should the blood pressure begin to rise unexpectedly (above the preinduction value), the intubation attempt must cease and additional anesthetic agents or adjuncts must be given.

Although not universally accepted, the reinforced endotracheal tube is our preference to avoid intraoperative kinking.

The Patient with a Full Stomach

If the patient has a full stomach, the anesthesiologist must balance the risk of aneurysm rupture against the risk of aspiration. One approach is to treat the patient as any patient at risk of regurgitation and aspiration, using a rapid sequence induction with cricoid pressure. To obtund the hypertensive response to tracheal intubation, fentanyl, 10 μg/kg, or sufentanil, 0.1 μg/kg, should be used in combination with thiopental. Either succinylcholine (1.5 to 2.0 mg/kg) preceded by defasciculation or vecuronium (0.15 to 0.20 mg/kg) can be used for muscle relaxation. Without the ability to titrate the drugs to response, this technique is associated with a risk of systemic hypotension. An alternative approach is to accept the small risk of regurgitation and titrate in the appropriate amount of narcotics and hypnotics as indicated by the blood pressure response while maintaining oxygenation and ventilation by mask with cricoid pressure. With either approach, should the blood pressure start to rise with laryngeal stimulation, the anesthesiologist should abort the laryngoscopy, maintain ventilation with cricoid pressure, and increase the depth of anesthesia before another attempt at tracheal intubation. Esmolol (0.5 mg/kg) given intravenously may be a useful adjunct in this situation. Labetalol, 10 to 30 mg in 5 mg increments, is also effective.

The Patient with a Potentially Difficult Airway

The potential risk of aneurysm rupture is increased in patients with a difficult airway.[211]

1. *When a difficult airway is anticipated,* fiberoptic intubation is the method of choice. Because translaryngeal injection may cause coughing and hypertension, it is preferable in these cases to provide topical anesthesia by inhalation of nebulized lidocaine (4%). Sufficient time (20 to 30 minutes), however, must be allowed for this method to be effective. Intravenous fentanyl and midazolam in 50 μg and 1 mg increments, respectively, may be administered judiciously provided that the patient does not have an elevated ICP. Alternatively, after appropriate sedation as outlined above, translaryngeal injection through the cricothyroid membrane of lidocaine (2.5 to 3.0 ml of 4% lidocaine) can be performed. After obtundation of the cough reflex with intravenous narcotics, the cough response to the translaryngeal injection should be brief and attenuated. To anesthetize the upper pharynx and laryngopharynx, topical benzocaine spray can be used. Other authors advocate supplementation with bilateral superior laryngeal nerve block by injecting 0.75 ml lidocaine (2%) subcutaneously on either side of the hyoid arch. We have found the combination of topical spray and translaryngeal injection satisfactory.

2. *If there is an unexpectedly difficult airway* but ventilation is adequate while tracheal intubation is impossible, the patient should be maintained anesthetized with either intravenous or inhalation anesthetic drugs. Using an intubating mask with a portal for the fiberscope, fiberoptic intubation can then be accomplished while systemic blood pressure is continuously monitored. Alternatively, retrograde intubation over a translaryngeal guide wire can be attempted. If neither ventilation nor intubation is possible, transtracheal jet ventilation should be implemented and oxygenation maintained while fiberoptic intubation is attempted. Cricothyroidotomy or tracheostomy may be necessary.

AFTER INTUBATION
Monitoring Requirements

Following induction of anesthesia and tracheal intubation, additional monitors and catheters are placed. In addition to

ECG, a neuromuscular blocked monitor, noninvasive blood pressure, pulse oximetry, end-tidal capnography, urinary catheter, esophageal stethoscope, and temperature should be used. Monitoring for aneurysm surgery should also include direct intraarterial blood pressure measurement, preferably instituted before induction of anesthesia. Adequate intravenous access is important, and at least one 16-gauge or 14-gauge peripheral catheter should be inserted in addition to the central venous catheter or pulmonary artery catheter. To accurately reflect the CPP, the arterial transducer should be placed at the level of the base of the skull and adjusted with any change in the patient's position. Intermittent blood sampling for determinations of hematocrit, blood gases, glucose, osmolarity, and electrolytes are also important. Blood glucose exceeding 200 mg/dl should be judiciously treated with insulin. Osmolarity measurement helps to determine the efficacy of additional mannitol when the brain is judged "tight"; if serum osmolarity exceeds 320 mOsm, additional mannitol is unlikely to help. Patients placed in the seated position have other requirements, which are discussed in other chapters.

The patient is then positioned for surgery. Insertion of the pins for the Mayfield or other pin fixation device represents a very noxious stimulus and can increase the blood pressure dramatically if the patient is not pretreated. Infiltration with local anesthesia[27,70,98] and administration of additional thiopental or narcotics are an effective regimen. Alternatively, esmolol (0.5 mg/kg) or labetalol (10 to 20 mg) can be used.

Central Venous Pressure Catheter vs. Pulmonary Artery Catheter

All patients undergoing craniotomy for aneurysm surgery should have a CVP catheter placed for the following reasons: (1) the prevalence of preexisting hypovolemia, (2) large intraoperative fluid shift with the use of osmotic and loop diuretics, (3) the potential risk of aneurysm rupture necessitating blood and fluid resuscitation, and (4) the possible presence of myocardial dysfunction. Many anesthesiologists will insert a pulmonary artery catheter when one of the following conditions is present: (1) patient has known coronary artery disease or ventricular dysfunction, (2) patient has symptomatic vasospasm necessitating preoperative hypertensive therapy, or (3) patient is in poor clinical grade and at high risk of developing postoperative vasospasm, and intravascular volume expansion is planned. When the decision is made to insert a central venous catheter instead of a pulmonary artery catheter, a large-bore conduit should be placed so that a pulmonary artery catheter can be inserted later on if so indicated.

Site of Central Venous Catheter and Pulmonary Artery Catheter Placement

Central venous access can be established via the internal jugular vein, the subclavian vein, or the antecubital vein. Each route has advantages and disadvantages.

The internal jugular vein is readily accessible and easy to locate, but some neurosurgeons are concerned with potential venous obstruction. We have not found this to be a problem, and it is our method of choice. For subtemporal incisions, as well as in procedures where the extracranial internal carotid artery may be temporarily occluded, we place the catheter on the contralateral side to avoid interference with the surgical field.

The subclavian route will not interfere with cerebral venous drainage but is associated with a significant risk of pneumothorax. The antecubital approach is least invasive but has a lower success rate, which, however, can be improved with ECG guidance.[6]

Although it is customary to place the patient in Trendelenburg position to facilitate placement of the central venous catheter, this is potentially dangerous in patients with elevated ICP. We generally do not use more than 5% to 10% tilt, and in patients with known elevated ICP we prefer to attempt placement in the neutral supine position.

Because of the potential risk of intraoperative aneurysm rupture, all patients should have at least 4 to 6 units of blood typed, crossed, and available at the time of surgical incision.

Other Monitoring

Other monitoring includes jugular bulb oxygen saturation, noninvasive cerebral oximetry, and transcranial Doppler ultrasonography (TCD).

Intermittent or continuous jugular bulb oxygen saturation determination may be useful in determining the optimal level of hyperventilation because it provides an indicator of early cerebral ischemia through detecting an increase in oxygen extraction. Regional cerebral oximetry uses optical spectroscopy to measure brain vascular hemoglobin saturation in a noninvasive manner to provide similar information.[116] Continuous TCD monitoring may improve the safety of induced hypotension by correlating the blood velocity change to the decline in blood pressure. None of these modalities, however, can be considered routine clinical tools at present.

Positioning of the Patient

The location and the size of the aneurysm generally determine the position of the patient for the surgical procedure. Preoperative review of the angiogram and CT scan will facilitate proper positioning of the patient. Anterior circulation aneurysms are usually approached using a frontal temporal incision with the patient in the supine position. Basilar tip aneurysms are approached using a subtemporal incision with the patient in the lateral position or an incision allowing the patient to remain supine. Vertebral and basilar trunk aneurysms are often approached using a suboccipital incision, with the patient either in the seated position or the "park-bench" position (semiprone lateral).[88] The risk of air embolism is always present, although it is sig-

nificantly higher in the seated position compared to the supine position.[14] As a general principle, because of the duration of these surgical procedures, all bony prominences must be well padded and all extremities well supported before the surgical procedure begins. Equally important before draping is a final inspection of the head and neck position in relationship to the body and palpation of the neck to ensure that jugular venous obstruction does not occur. This is a frequent cause of unexplained intraoperative cerebral swelling. Therefore it is generally advisable to secure the tracheal tube with tapes rather than a tie around the neck since a tie may slip and tighten around the neck. Although not proven, partial venous obstruction may contribute to reported postoperative tongue swelling and airway obstruction in posterior fossa procedures.[115,131] For this reason a soft bite block is preferable to an oropharyngeal airway.

After final positioning the lung fields should be auscultated to rule out bronchial intubation. Flexion of the head will tend to advance the endotracheal tube, whereas extension of the head will have the opposite effect. Careful placement of the endotracheal tube initially and ensuring that it is between 20 and 24 cm at the teeth (in the average-sized adult) will diminish but not eliminate the possibility of bronchial intubation with flexing of the patient's head.

MAINTENANCE OF ANESTHESIA

The goals during maintenance of anesthesia are to (1) provide a relaxed or "slack" brain that will allow minimal retraction pressure, (2) maintain perfusion to the brain, (3) reduce transmural pressure if necessary during dissection of the aneurysm and final clipping, and (4) allow prompt awakening and assessment of patients with good SAH grades.

With the trend toward early surgery the anesthesiologist can expect to see more difficult conditions where maximal brain "relaxation" therapy is required. Since no data exist on the influence of anesthetic drugs on the outcome of aneurysm surgery, the choice should be based on both the brain condition and the overall management plan, taking into consideration the patient's preoperative clinical grade. In general, a patient with SAH grades I, II, or III undergoing an uneventful aneurysm clipping should be allowed to awaken and be extubated in the operating room. Either an intravenous or inhalation anesthetic or a combination of both can be used to provide such conditions.

Nitrous oxide is a cerebral vasodilator when used in combination with a potent inhaled anesthetic.[2,63,91,160] It has also been reported to cause cerebral stimulation with an increase in cerebral metabolic rate.[160] Although no outcome studies suggest that nitrous oxide may have a detrimental effect, there is little or no advantage in using it with a potent inhaled anesthetic. On the other hand, the vasodilatory properties of nitrous oxide are attenuated when used in combination with an intravenous anesthetic agent.[214] We generally omit nitrous oxide when isoflurane is used but may use it in combination with propofol and fentanyl infusion.

With regard to narcotic agents, fentanyl and sufentanil, given either in bolus (50 to 100 μg and 5 to 10 μg, respectively) in response to hemodynamic changes or in continuous infusion (1 to 2 μg/kg/hr or 0.1 to 0.2 μg/kg/hr, respectively), when combined with isoflurane (0.5% to 1.0%) provide satisfactory conditions for most patients in good condition. Desflurane (4% to 6%) appears to have similar cerebrovascular effects to isoflurane[148] and can be used as an alternative. Its low blood gas solubility is a theoretic advantage. The narcotic infusions should be discontinued approximately 1 hour before the surgical dressing is applied. The total dosage should not exceed 10 μg/kg for fentanyl and 2 μg/kg for sufentanil to allow awakening and immediate neurologic assessment. No differences among the narcotic drugs have been found with respect to observed brain "tightness"[54] or the amount of retractor pressure required for intraoperative brain retraction.[68] Fentanyl and alfentanil exhibit no significant clinical differences with respect to emergence from anesthesia.[134] Total intravenous anesthesia with propofol and alfentanil infusion has also been used successfully. High-dose narcotics (fentanyl, 50 to 100 μg/kg; sufentanil, 5 to 10 μg/kg), however, will prolong recovery and are unsuitable if rapid awakening and assessment are desired.[175] For patients with poor preoperative SAH grades, extubation of the trachea at the end of the surgical procedure is not planned, and an intravenous anesthetic-based technique is more appropriate (fentanyl– or sufentanil–nitrous oxide ± propofol). In difficult cases where the brain remains tight, continuous thiopental infusion at 5 to 6 mg/kg/hr should be considered.[178] Alternatively, etomidate (0.2 to 0.3 mg/kg/hr) or propofol (150 to 200 μg/kg/hr) infusion can be used. These two latter agents may have the added advantage of a shorter recovery time should extubation of the trachea be contemplated at the end of the procedure.

Irrespective of the anesthetic technique used, it is important to recognize that the surgical stimulus during cerebral aneurysm surgery varies at different times. Noxious stimuli begin with insertion of the pinhead holder and intensify with the raising of the bone flap; once the dura is open there is little or no surgical stimulation. The anesthetic plan must therefore take this into consideration to avoid wide fluctuations in cerebral perfusion pressure or dangerous increases in blood pressure. Of note is the fact that retraction of cranial nerves and the brain stem (posterior fossa aneurysms) may be associated with sudden increases in blood pressure or heart rate. Thus a deeper level of anesthesia needs to be maintained with these circumstances.

Brain Relaxation

Various adjuncts are used to relax the brain. Although the details of practice vary, they are all directed at the components of the intracranial vault: brain tissue volume, CSF volume, and blood volume.

To reduce brain tissue volume, 20% mannitol (0.5 to 2 g/kg) is usually given over 30 minutes to effect osmotic diuresis. The usual dose is 1 g/kg; an additional dose is given when indicated by the brain conditions. A total dose of 2 g/kg is frequently given when temporary artery occlusion is planned (also see the section on temporary occlusion). Mannitol's action begins within 4 to 5 minutes and peaks in about 30 to 45 minutes. Although the classic mechanism is believed to be movement of intracellular water into the intravascular volume along the osmotic gradient (the osmolarity of 20% mannitol is 1098 mOsm/L), some evidence exists that the rapid action of mannitol can be mediated by decreased production of CSF.[167] The cardiovascular and cerebrovascular actions of mannitol can be considered to be triphasic: transient, delayed, and late. Because of mannitol's high osmolarity, it transiently increases CBF, CBV, and ICP, which are followed by a subsequent decrease in CBV and ICP.[157,158] Systemically, an acute decrease in peripheral vascular resistance occurs, particularly when mannitol is given quickly (in less than 10 minutes). This may result in transient hypotension,[30] followed by a marked rise in CVP, PAWP, and cardiac output.[164] Therefore the full dose of mannitol should be given over 30 minutes. It also transiently reduces hematocrit, increases serum osmolarity, and causes hyponatremia, hypochloremia, and hyperkalemia.[107] Potential complications from the delayed effects therefore include fluid overload and pulmonary edema in patients with poor cardiac function. Within 45 minutes the cardiovascular effects have dissipated, and with the onset of full diuresis the intravascular volume may start to contract. Theoretically mannitol should not be given before the dura is open to minimize fluctuation in ICP. Shrinkage of the brain may also cause tearing of the bridging veins. In clinical practice, slow mannitol infusion (100 to 200 ml/hr) is frequently begun after final positioning of the patient and the infusion rate increased after the bone flap has been raised (400 to 500 ml/hr). Some practitioners routinely use furosemide (0.1 to 0.5 mg/kg) to augment the action of mannitol.[155] Additional mannitol, to a total of 2 g/kg, because of its potential brain protective effect, is often administered before temporary occlusion of major feeding arteries.[107,152,197,200]

Reducing the volume of the CSF compartment by drainage of CSF with a lumbar subarachnoid drain facilitates surgical exposure since the average adult has approximately 150 ml of CSF. Extreme care should be exercised during insertion of the drain to minimize CSF loss and a sudden decrease of ICP, or TMP may increase abruptly and result in a rebleed. Because of the risk of brain stem herniation, lumbar drainage of CSF is contraindicated in patients with intracerebral hematoma. Although in theory free drainage should only be allowed after the dura is open to minimize the risk of rebleeding, in practice 20 to 30 ml of CSF is usually drained just before dural opening to facilitate dural incision. Rapid drainage can cause sudden reflex hypertension, presumably from stimulation of the brainstem. Barker has suggested that the drainage rate should not exceed 5 ml/min.[8] The drain is usually left open during the procedure until the aneurysm is clipped or until the beginning of dural closure.

The equipment used for subarachnoid lumbar drain varies among different hospitals, and some neurosurgeons prefer not to use CSF drainage, relying on mannitol and hyperventilation instead. We use a standard commercially available kit (Lumbar Catheter Accessory Kit by Cordis, Miami), which essentially consists of a 14-gauge Touhy needle and a soft flexible catheter having multiple orifices at the end. In essence the subarachnoid drain differs from a subarachnoid catheter inserted for continuous spinal analgesia only in size. Regular lumbar epidural kits designed for epidural anesthesia are generally not satisfactory because the size of the catheter is too small, and in patients with acute SAH, blood clots frequently block the drainage. Pediatric feeding catheters have also been used with success, but the stiffness of these catheters increases the risk of potential spinal cord damage. On the other hand, caution must be exercised with the removal of the soft, flexible catheter at the end of the procedure. Because the catheter is placed with the patient in the flexed position but often is removed in the extended or neutral position, the catheter has been known to break off at the site of compression between the vertebral bodies. The patient should therefore be placed in the flexed position whenever difficulty with removal is encountered. To avoid the difficulty with insertion and removal of these catheters, some hospitals use malleable spinal needles and simply bend the needle to the patient's contour after placement. This approach is most suited to patients who have been placed in the lateral position.

CBV can be reduced. Within the physiologic range of $Paco_2$ (20 to 70 mm Hg), CBF bears an almost linear relationship to arterial $Paco_2$, changing 2% to 3% per mm Hg change in $Paco_2$. Controlled hyperventilation therefore can be used to decrease the CBV, which probably changes by about 1% per mm Hg change in $Paco_2$. Although anesthetic agents may influence the response to CO_2, the changes are small and CO_2 reactivity is generally well preserved. CO_2 reactivity is normal in patients with good SAH grades but may be impaired in those with poor SAH grades. Although it is generally safe to maintain $Paco_2$ in the range of 25 to 35 mm Hg, it should be individualized according to the operating conditions. A reasonable approach is to institute mild hypocapnia (30 to 35 mm Hg) before the dura is open, moderate hypocapnia (25 to 30 mm Hg) after the dura is open, and relative normocapnia during induced hypotension[193] and after the aneurysm is clipped. The advantages of extreme hypocapnia in reducing CBV should always be balanced against the risk of potential cerebral ischemia. Since the objective is to relax the brain without causing ischemia, the efficacy of hyperventilation should be continuously assessed by observing the intraoperative brain relaxation in order to achieve the optimal $Paco_2$.

In difficult situations, brain relaxation may remain unsatisfactory and refractory to the above regimen. If this oc-

curs make sure there is no hypoxemia or systemic hypertension. Check the patient's neck to rule out venous obstruction. Inspect the subarachnoid drain to ensure patency and proper drainage of CSF. Since nitrous oxide is a cerebral vasodilator when used in conjunction with an inhaled anesthetic,[2,63,91,160] discontinue nitrous oxide. After communication with the surgeon, a head-up tilt can be implemented to facilitate venous blood and CSF drainage. Finally, a test dose of thiopental (150 to 200 mg) is given and if brain relaxation improves, a continuous infusion is started (4 to 5 mg/kg/hr). This will usually, but not always, produce a prolonged recovery from anesthesia. Occasionally uncontrolled intraoperative swelling may be due to an intracerebral hematoma.

Fluid and Electrolyte Balance

Fluid should be administered according to the patient's need and guided by intraoperative blood loss, urine output, and CVP or PAWP. Intravenous fluid should not be withheld if induced hypotension is planned, since hypovolemic hypotension is detrimental to organ perfusion. The aim is to maintain normovolemia before aneurysm clipping and slight hypervolemia after clipping. Electrolytes should be replaced as needed. Glucose-containing solutions should not be given, because evidence exists that hyperglycemia may aggravate both focal and global transient cerebral ischemia.[93,96] Because lactated Ringer's solution is relatively hypoosmolar, a more physiologic solution such as Plasmalyte, Normo-sol, or normal saline is preferred. Some practitioners use 5% albumin after clipping of the aneurysm, but the advantages of this protocol have not been documented. On the other hand, hetastarch should probably not be used or used in small amounts (less than 500 ml) because of the risk of intracranial bleeding.[33,34]

OTHER CONSIDERATIONS
Controlled Hypotension vs. Temporary Occlusion

Because of the enlargement of the aneurysmal sac, the wall stress increases disproportionately to increases in blood pressure[48] (Fig. 18-4); hence large aneurysms are more likely to rupture than small ones. Therefore traditionally the blood pressure is lowered during microscopic dissection of the aneurysm, particularly during clip placement, to reduce the risk of rupture. Hypotension also decreases bleeding, which allows better visualization of the anatomy of the aneurysm and the perforating vessels. Although the risk of hypotension-induced global cerebral ischemia always exists, deliberate hypotension has been used successfully for many years without apparent ill effects. However, the demonstration of impairment of autoregulatory capacity following SAH[36,72,207,218] and the unpredictable cerebrovascular response to induced hypotension[47] have led to reassessment of routine deliberate hypotension. For example, patients in vasospasm as evidenced by angiography or symptoms are particularly at risk of ischemia during hypotension. To re-

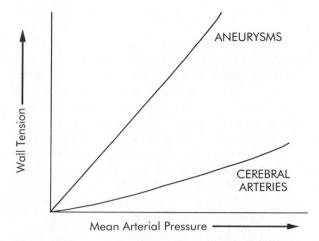

FIG. 18-4   The relationship between wall tension and mean arterial pressure (ICP = 0 when dura is open). For any given pressure, wall stress and therefore the tendency to rupture are higher in an aneurysmal sac than in a normal cerebral artery. *(From Ferguson GG: The rationale for controlled hypotension. In Varkey GP, editor:* Anesthetic considerations in the surgical repair of intracranial aneurysms, *Boston, 1982, Little, Brown.)*

duce the risk of aneurysm rupture without using hypotension, many surgeons are now using temporary occlusion of the major feeding artery.[74,117,129,130] The potential risks of temporary occlusion include focal cerebral ischemia and subsequent infarction as well as damage to the feeding artery from the occlusion. With improved design of temporary clips the latter complication is now of less concern.[198] The risk of cerebral infarction remains and depends on the duration of the temporary occlusion as well as the state of the collateral circulation. The anesthetic management of patients during induced hypotension clearly differs from management during temporary occlusion.

Controlled Hypotension

The major concerns with controlled hypotension are avoidance of cerebral ischemia and maintenance of organ perfusion. No ideal hypotensive agents exist, but many hypotensive drugs and techniques have been used successfully and are discussed in detail elsewhere in this book.

Temporary Occlusion

Because the tolerable duration of temporary occlusion varies with different arteries as well as with different individuals, it is difficult to predict the upper time limit in any given situation. Five to seven minutes of occlusion with prompt reperfusion are usually well tolerated, but this time period is generally insufficient for clipping difficult or giant aneurysms. Although no randomized clinical trials have been conducted, a number of regimens have been used to extend the occlusion duration. Suzuki introduced the technique of high-dose mannitol (2 g/kg) for temporary arterial occlusion,[197,199,200,232] and experimental studies have supported a brain-protective role for mannitol.[102,231,232] Be-

cause neuronal damage may be mediated by the production of free radicals, Suzuki advocates a combination of mannitol (500 ml of a 20% solution, or 100 g), vitamin E (500 mg), and dexamethasone (50 mg), often referred to as the Sendai cocktail,[197] for temporary arterial occlusion. Up to 60 or more minutes of temporary arterial occlusion have been obtained using this regimen without apparent postoperative neurologic deficits. Other surgeons use pharmacologic metabolic suppression, theorizing that, by decreasing cerebral metabolic rate, the tissues distal to the occlusion can tolerate a longer period of ischemia. Both thiopental[117,133] and etomidate[9] have been used for this purpose. The end point with either agent should be burst suppression, as indicated by electroencephalogram (EEG) monitoring. Thiopental, 5 to 6 mg/kg, or etomidate, 0.4 to 0.5 mg/kg, administered intravenously before temporary occlusion would achieve this aim in 2 to 3 minutes. Additional doses may be given as indicated by EEG. However, the additional doses may not be effective if collateral circulation is inadequate for delivery of the agent. On the other hand, in this situation the thiopental or etomidate that has been given would also stay in the ischemic area longer because of the diminished blood flow for washout. Although there have been no controlled clinical studies, good results have been reported whether thiopental,[117,133] etomidate,[9] or mannitol[197,199] is used for cerebral protection. Because there is less associated systemic hypotension, etomidate may be preferable to thiopental. To use pharmacologic protection efficiently, it is necessary to monitor the EEG to define the end point, since no further metabolic benefits can be derived with doses greater than those needed to produce burst suppression or electrical silence.[121] Electrophysiologic monitoring also can be used to determine the upper limit of occlusion duration, thus allowing the surgeon to proceed without haste as long as the monitoring suggests normal function. This approach allows one to recognize the need for brief periods of reperfusion when the monitoring indicates deterioration. Either EEG or evoked potentials (EPs) can be used for such purposes when mannitol is used for cerebral protection. Obviously only the latter can be used when anesthetic pharmacologic protection is utilized. Some surgeons use mild hypotension during dissection and then apply temporary arterial occlusion during actual placement of the clip. It is important to restore the blood pressure to normal before the placement of the temporary clips to maximize collateral blood flow.

Moderate hypothermia (28° to 32° C) has also been used to extend the duration of tolerable occlusion.[197] Although it is clear that metabolic suppression is achieved, potential complications include ventricular arrhythmia, myocardial depression, coagulopathy, and postoperative shivering. Pharmacologic metabolic suppression or mannitol appears to provide the same degree of brain protection without the complications, and moderate hypothermia is now seldom utilized. In our hospital we prefer to use additional mannitol to a total of 2 g/kg just before the proximal vessel occlusion. In patients where the collateral circulation has been demonstrated to be poor or nonexistent angiographically and yet temporary occlusion is deemed necessary, we would induce burst suppression with thiopental in addition to the use of mannitol. Prior communication between the neurosurgeon and the anesthesiologist is clearly needed for the successful management of these patients. The placement of EEG electrodes must not interfere with the surgical field and must be well shielded and protected from the prep solution and blood to allow proper monitoring of EEG intraoperatively. Fortunately, a simple bihemispheric frontooccipital montage will suffice. This can be accomplished by placing surface gel electrodes over the forehead just above the eyes referenced to the respective electrodes placed over the ipsilateral mastoid process and then shielded with occlusive dressings.

With improvement in cardiopulmonary bypass technology and coagulation management, interest in the use of profound hypothermia and circulatory arrest for complex or giant aneurysms has been revived. Recent experimental studies in cerebral ischemia have demonstrated that even mild hypothermia can exert significant cerebroprotective effects by suppressing release of excitotoxic amino acids.[21,22,124,125] Thus not only is it reasonable to maintain the body temperature between 33° and 35° C during the periods when the patient is considered to be at risk of cerebral ischemia, but also any increase in body temperature above normal must be vigorously treated.

Electrophysiologic Monitoring

Electrophysiologic monitoring such as EEG and evoked potentials (EPs) may allow intraoperative detection of cerebral ischemia, leading to a change in surgical technique that improves perfusion. However, they are not routinely used because their changes are not always specific and the recording sites not always accessible.

EEG has been used to determine the lowest blood pressure tolerable during induced hypotension, but the results are not consistent.[15,76] This is not surprising since a significant decrease in EEG activity can be compatible with normal neurologic recovery. A recent report described the use of intraoperative bihemispheric computer-processed EEG and found that changes correspond to postoperative outcome.[205] However, the series is too small for any conclusions. In contrast, EEG monitoring may be indicated when temporary occlusion is planned, either to determine the duration of tolerance or for titration of anesthetic agents when pharmacologic metabolic suppression is desired.

Somatosensory evoked potential (SSEP) monitoring has been investigated for use during procedures on both anterior and posterior circulation aneurysms, whereas brain stem auditory evoked potential (BAEP) has been primarily investigated for use during procedures on vertebral-basilar aneurysms.* Both monitors are probably most useful when temporary or permanent vessel occlusion is planned. EPs can be recorded even when the EEG is suppressed with high-dose barbiturates and are therefore the only electrophysiologic monitor available when maximal pharmacologic metabolic suppression is used. Common to all electrophysiologic monitoring, even during temporary occlusion, SSEP monitoring lacks specificity and a high false-alarm rate can be expected. The false-negative rate (SSEP unchanged but neurologic deficit occurs) is lower but remains significant in most series. Table 18-5 summarizes the reported series on use of SSEP during temporary arterial occlusion. Most series report a high false-positive rate as well as a considerable false-negative rate. In view of these results, routine use of EP monitoring cannot be advocated. In selected cases where permanent occlusion of a major vessel is anticipated, SSEP or BAEP monitoring may be useful.

Spontaneous breathing has been used in the past as an indicator of brain stem function, particularly when extreme hypotension is used. It is seldom used today, because optimal brain relaxation is difficult to achieve and extreme hypotension is no longer used. However, with aneurysms involving the low basilar artery and the vertebral arteries where temporary or permanent occlusion of the feeding vessel is contemplated, spontaneous breathing may provide additional and more specific information than cardiovascular monitoring. Disturbances ranging from tachypnea to apnea have been observed.[90] Fortunately these situations are extremely rare.

*References 53, 86, 90, 94, 108, 129, 130, 169, 202.

TABLE 18-5
SSEP Monitoring in Temporary Arterial Occlusion for Cerebral Aneurysm Surgery

Authors	No. of Patients	No. of Patients with Temporary Occlusion	False-Positive Results	False-Negative Results
Schramm et al. (1990)[169]	113	34	40%	34%
Manninen et al. (1990)[108]	157	97	43%	14%
Mooij et al. (1987)[130]	5	5	?	0%
Momma et al. (1987)[129]	40	40	60%	5%
Kikooka et al. (1987)[86]	31	15	38%	22%
Symon and Vajda (1984)[201]	34	15	40%	7%

Intraoperative Aneurysm Rupture

The incidence of aneurysm rupture varies with the size and the anatomic location of the aneurysm. There also appear to be differences between institutions. In the Cooperative Study an intraoperative aneurysm leak occurred about 6% of the time, whereas frank rupture occurred in 13%,[84] for a combined incidence of 19%. These findings are similar to the series reported by Batjer.[9,84] In approximately 8% of these cases the rupture resulted in frank hemorrhagic shock.[84] In Batjer and Samson's series, 7% of the ruptures occurred before dissection of the aneurysm, 48% during dissection, and 45% during clip application.[10] Mortality and morbidity are increased with intraoperative rupture. Management will partially depend on the ability to maintain the blood volume during rupture. If the leak is small and dissection is complete, the surgeon can gain control with suction and then apply the permanent clip to the neck of the aneurysm. Alternatively, temporary clips can be applied proximally and distally to the aneurysm to gain control. The key to anesthetic management is good communication with the surgeon and close monitoring of the patient's vital signs as well as the surgical conditions. Video monitors allowing the anesthesiologist to view the surgical field greatly facilitate patient care during this acute, rapidly changing situation. If temporary occlusion is not planned or not possible and blood loss is not significant, the mean arterial pressure should be decreased transiently to 50 mm Hg or even lower to facilitate surgical control. Proximal and distal temporary occlusion, however, is the preferred method. Thiopental or etomidate may be given to provide some protection before placement of the temporary clip. The latter agent is preferable if the status of blood volume is uncertain. If frank hemorrhage occurs, aggressive fluid resuscitation and blood transfusion must begin immediately. Administration of a cerebroprotective agent may not be possible because of the associated hemodynamic effects. Induced hypotension under these circumstances may not be possible, because the intravascular volume must be restored first. During temporary occlusion, normotension must be maintained to maximize collateral perfusion. Excellent results have been achieved by Batjer using temporary occlusion for intraoperative rupture.[10]

EMERGENCE AND RECOVERY

Communication between the surgeon and the anesthesiologist is again essential for optimal management of emergence from anesthesia. If the surgical procedure is uneventful, SAH grade I and II patients should be allowed to awaken and their tracheas may be extubated in the operating room. To minimize coughing, particularly during movement of the head when the surgical dressing is applied, intravenous lidocaine, 1.5 mg/kg, is effective, but its duration of action is only about 3 to 5 minutes. It can be safely repeated if necessary. Because hypertensive therapy is effective in reversing delayed cerebral ischemia from vasospasm, mod-

est levels of postoperative hypertension (<180 mm Hg systolic) are not aggressively treated. Nonetheless, severe hypertension (>200 mm Hg systolic) may cause increased swelling or cerebral hemorrhage. Labetalol and esmolol are both effective in controlling emergence hypertension.[135] Labetalol is usually given in 5 to 10 mg increments and esmolol in 0.1 to 0.5 mg/kg increments until blood pressure is controlled. Other hypotensive drugs, including sodium nitroprusside, nitroglycerin, hydralazine, and nicardipine, can also be used. However, these drugs may cause cerebral vasodilation and increase ICP. In institutions where ICP monitors are placed routinely at the end of the surgical procedure and ICP is monitored postoperatively, it is safe to use these vasodilators for control of blood pressure. They are equally safe in patients who are awake and whose neurologic signs are being continually monitored.

Depending on their preoperative ventilatory status and the duration and difficulty of the surgical procedure, SAH grade III patients may or may not have their tracheal tube removed in the operating room. In general, one should err on the side of conservatism. Only when the surgical procedure is uneventful, brain relaxation has not been a problem, and the patient can maintain adequate ventilation with intact laryngeal reflexes should extubation of the trachea be considered. Patients with preoperative SAH grades of IV and V usually require postoperative ventilatory support and continuous neurointensive care. Patients with multiple aneurysms must continue to have their systemic blood pressure under strict control (within 20% of their normal blood pressure) to prevent rupture of unclipped aneurysms during emergence and recovery from anesthesia.

Patients who have experienced intraoperative aneurysm rupture and patients with vertebral-basilar aneurysms must be considered individually irrespective of their preoperative clinical SAH grade. In both instances their recovery may be slow, and immediate tracheal extubation may not be possible. In the former situation intraoperative cerebral ischemia may have occurred, and in the latter instance, transient or permanent cranial nerve dysfunction may result from perforator vessel occlusion or brain stem retraction.

POSTOPERATIVE CONSIDERATIONS

In the immediate postoperative period the anesthesiologist should assess the patient to ensure that the recovery is satisfactory and consistent with the anesthetic given. The time of recovery clearly depends on the type of anesthetic and the dose of anesthetic given as well as the patient's sensitivity to drugs given. There is no hard and fast rule to discriminate between anesthetic effects and surgical complications. It is nevertheless important to distinguish residual anesthesia from surgical complications such as development of subdural or epidural hematomas. Some general guidelines are useful: (1) anesthesia causes global depression, and any new focal neurologic deficit should alert to a surgical cause; (2) the effect of potent inhaled anesthetics should have largely dissipated after 30 to 60 minutes; (3) patients whose pupils are mid-sized and reactive to light and whose respirations are not depressed are unlikely to be experiencing narcotic overdose; and (4) unequal pupils not present before operation always suggests a surgical event. The neurologic status should be assessed every 15 minutes in the recovery room or intensive care unit, and in some patients an immediate CT scan or angiogram may be necessary.

SUBARACHNOID HEMORRHAGE AND PREGNANCY

Intracranial hemorrhage from either a cerebral aneurysm or arteriovenous malformation (AVM) is seen in 0.01% to 0.05% of all pregnancies,[38,126,170] which is not different from their occurrence in the general population. Thus pregnancy does not predispose the patient to the development of SAH,[52] and the occurrence of SAH is not related to parity.[126] Most intracranial hemorrhages are caused by aneurysmal rupture (77%) rather than by AVM (23%) leakage.[38] The mean age for patients with aneurysmal hemorrhage was 28 to 30 years.[38,52,126]

Time Course of Bleeding

Most studies have found that aneurysms bleed more frequently during the third trimester, although bleeding has occurred as early as 6 weeks of gestation.[28,38,52,126] The tendency to bleed as pregnancy progresses may be due to cardiovascular changes. Cardiac output increases with pregnancy, with peak periods at 28 to 32 weeks, labor and delivery, and the initial postpartum period. Maternal blood volume, systolic blood pressure, stroke volume, and heart rate increases continually throughout pregnancy and reach maximum at term. During labor and delivery the cardiac output and blood pressure both increase in short bursts with uterine contractions secondary to pain and autotransfusion. The importance of these short bursts in facilitating aneurysmal rupture is uncertain; one author is of the opinion that labor is not a precipitating factor and that aneurysmal rupture during labor is a rare event.[52] Of note, these cardiovascular changes associated with contractions can be blunted with epidural anesthesia.

Maternal and Fetal Outcome

The reported maternal mortality from aneurysmal SAH was 35%, which is similar to the nongravid population, and the fetal mortality was 17%.[38] The maternal mortality varied directly with the Hunt and Hess clinical grade.[38] Both maternal mortality (11% vs. 63%) and fetal mortality (5% vs. 27%) are significantly better with surgical treatment compared to conservative management.[38]

Diagnosis

The clinical features of SAH in pregnant patients are similar to those of the general population. However, other dis-

orders associated with pregnancy may mimic SAH and must be ruled out; these include pituitary apoplexy, cerebral sinus thrombosis, intracranial arterial occlusion, migraine headaches, postdural puncture headaches, and preeclampsia. Other disorders causing neurologic symptoms suggestive of elevated ICP that may be confused with SAH include intracranial tumors or other mass lesions, meningitis, encephalitis, or demyelinating disease. A high index of suspicion is necessary to make the diagnosis of SAH in a pregnant patient. Preeclampsia, which is defined as hypertension, proteinuria, and peripheral edema, is another common cause of intracranial hemorrhage during the third trimester of pregnancy.[52,170] The diagnosis is confirmed by CT scan or lumbar dural puncture followed by angiography.[52] With proper shielding of the uterus, radiation exposure to the fetus is minimal. Iodinated contrast agents do not cross the placental barrier and pose little risk to the fetus. However, because of their osmotic effect, fetal dehydration may occur. Consequently, the mother should have adequate intravenous hydration during and after receiving contrast and the serum osmolarity and urine output should be monitored to avoid fetal dehydration.

Obstetric Management of SAH in Pregnancy

Although the treatment of choice for SAH during pregnancy is clearly surgical,[126] management depends on the gestational age of the fetus as well as the clinical status of the mother. Before fetal viability (<32 weeks) and in patients with good SAH grades, surgical clipping should be performed as soon as possible to prevent rebleeding.[52,126] Approximately 80% of aneurysm ruptures occur before 36 weeks of pregnancy. In these patients, aneurysm clipping followed by delivery at full term generally results in a satisfactory outcome for both the mother and infant.[28] During craniotomy, continuous fetal heart rate monitoring should be used with an obstetric team available. If fetal distress develops, cesarean delivery may be considered. If labor begins and delivery appears imminent, the craniotomy should be temporarily halted and the fetus delivered by cesarean section.[38] If the fetus is near term or signs of fetal distress are apparent, the fetus should be delivered by cesarean section first and then the aneurysm should be clipped.[38] Oxytocic drugs have been used to decrease uterine atony and bleeding after delivery without causing deleterious neurologic effects, although they have not been studied extensively in this setting.[87] The most common hemodynamic alteration with oxytocin is hypotension, whereas hypertension is associated with methylergonovine maleate (Methergine) and prostaglandins.

In gravid patients with a surgically inaccessible or undetermined aneurysm and in whom delivery is scheduled, obstetric management is controversial. The risk of bleeding during vaginal delivery is not significantly different from that during cesarean delivery. Although some authors contend that these patients should all have cesarean deliveries to avoid the strain induced by labor, no significant differences exist in maternal and fetal mortality between vaginal and cesarean delivery in untreated aneurysms.[38]

One unusual circumstance where emergency cesarean delivery is indicated is a patient in her third trimester who has bled, is now moribund, and is undergoing neuroresuscitation.[52,87]

Physiologic Changes in Pregnancy

Pregnancy is accompanied by a progressive increase in minute ventilation and a decrease in functional residual capacity. These changes make pregnant women prone to develop hypoxemia. The minimum alveolar concentration for inhaled anesthetics decreases.[150] The increased minute ventilation that occurs with pregnancy lowers the $Paco_2$ to approximately 32 mm Hg and changes the set point for the cerebrovascular response to hyperventilation. Attempts to lower ICP therefore necessitate lowering $Paco_2$ to 25 mm Hg or less. Further decreases in $Paco_2$, however, may cause fetal hypoxia and acidosis by decreasing uterine blood flow and reduced release of oxygen secondary to a shift of the hemoglobin-oxygen dissociation curve to the left. For these reasons, maternal $Paco_2$ should be maintained at approximately 30 mm Hg.

Uterine Blood Flow

Uterine blood flow is not autoregulated. It varies directly with systemic maternal blood pressure and is inversely proportional to uterine vascular resistance.[97] A maternal systolic blood pressure of less than 100 mm Hg may produce uterine hypoperfusion and fetal bradycardia. Hypotension during aneurysm clipping may occur as a result of hypovolemia, administration of anesthetic agents, excessive positive pressure ventilation, hemorrhage, or the use of nimodipine. Whatever the cause, maternal hypotension must be treated vigorously. Although induced hypotension may have adverse effects on the fetus, it has been used successfully to facilitate aneurysm clipping.[141,228] Positioning of the patient in the third trimester also affects uterine blood flow; a supine or right lateral position may cause the aorto-vena caval syndrome resulting in maternal hypotension.[97] Therefore left uterine displacement must be maintained with a roll or wedge under the right hip. Uterine blood flow may decrease during controlled ventilation secondary to the effect of hypocapnia on the uterine blood vessels[97,99,132] or the mechanical effect of positive pressure ventilation on cardiac output.[97,99]

Anesthetic Management

Because these aneurysms present primarily in the third trimester of pregnancy, the anesthesiologist must face the possible complications associated with pregnancy as well as the special considerations for aneurysm clipping. The anesthetic management also depends on the gestational age and obstetric plan, that is, whether delivery of the fetus will precede the neurosurgical procedure or whether the aneurysmal clipping will be done followed by normal maturation of the fetus with subsequent delivery at term. Benefits of anesthetic drugs and technique used for the mother must always be balanced against potential risks to the fetus.

General Principles

The goals of anesthesia during pregnancy are to ensure the recovery of the mother and the normal continuation of pregnancy without damage to the fetus. The anesthetic management should be the same as for the nonpregnant aneurysm patient except that one is taking care of two patients. Pregnant patients have special needs because of the physiologic changes that occur during pregnancy, including (1) consideration for the decrease in mean alveolar concentration (MAC),[150] (2) an increased potential for aspiration and having a difficult airway, (3) special positioning, (4) the influence of anesthetic-induced depression on maternal blood pressure, and (5) the risk of inducing premature labor. Special needs with respect to the fetus are (1) adequate fetal-maternal oxygen exchange, which depends on adequate maternal blood pressure, (2) potential for teratogenic effects secondary to drugs, and (3) perioperative monitoring of the fetus.[38]

Measures should be taken to prevent aspiration of gastric contents, since all pregnant patients are considered to have full stomachs, and to prevent the hypertensive response to intubation that may increase the potential of cerebral aneurysm rupture.[141] Pregnant patients should fast overnight, receive an H_2 receptor antagonist such as ranitidine, and be given metoclopramide preoperatively to reduce the volume of gastric contents. The induction technique is essentially the same as for a nonpregnant patient with a full stomach, and the reader is referred to the previous section on this topic.

When positioning the patient in the third trimester of pregnancy, it is important to prevent aortocaval compression by using left uterine displacement. Immediately after positioning, the fetal heart rate should be monitored, because this is the only practical way of monitoring fetal well-being during anesthesia.

Loss of beat-to-beat variation in heart rate may be an early sign of fetal hypoxia during awake conditions but is normal for the anesthetized fetus.[103] Interpretation of the intraoperative fetal heart rate should be made with comparison of a preinduction recording to the various changes during the course of anesthesia and surgery.[103] If the fetus develops tachycardia or bradycardia during maternal hypotension, the surgeon should be immediately informed, the blood pressure increased, and an obstetrician consulted.

Use of Induced Hypotension

Induced hypotension has been employed with success to facilitate aneurysm clipping during pregnancy.[126,141] Hypotensive agents that have been used include sodium nitroprusside,[159,170,228] trimethaphan, and high concentrations of isoflurane.[141] Sodium nitroprusside acts directly on the smooth muscle of the blood vessel and is freely permeable to the placenta, although this property is probably species dependent.[136,228] It may decrease uterine blood flow[228] as well as cause fetal cyanide toxicity.[136] Although trimethaphan has been used for hypotension during pregnancy, it causes reductions in both cardiac output and CBF[190] and therefore may be unsuitable for this purpose. Isoflurane is an alternative, because it has little effect on cardiac output[89] and CBF.[140] In the pregnant ewe at 1.5 MAC, uteroplacental blood flow was maintained and did not cause fetal hypoxemia or metabolic acidosis.[149] The use of hypotension, however, remains controversial, and several authors have suggested that this technique be avoided in pregnant patients.[23,52] With the trend toward temporary occlusion, there should be no need for induced hypotension during pregnancy. If hypotension is to be used, the fetal heart rate must be monitored closely and the BP raised should fetal bradycardia or tachycardia occur.

Other Considerations

Mannitol has been shown to cross the placenta and may accumulate in the fetus and lead to changes in fetal osmolality, volume, and the concentrations of various electrolytes. Mannitol infusions of 12.5 g/kg in pregnant rabbits shift free water from the fetus to the mother, which increases fetal osmolality by 22%, increasing plasma sodium to 162 mEq/L and decreasing plasma volume by 50%.[19] In a human study the administration of 200 g of mannitol to the mother before delivery altered the volume, osmolality, and concentration of solutes in the fetus.[11] However, in dosages used clinically in aneurysm clipping (0.5 to 1.0 g/kg), mannitol is unlikely to cause severe fluid or electrolyte ab-

TABLE 18-6
Adverse Uteroplacental Drug Effects

Drugs	Adverse Effects
Phenytoin	Minimal
Thiopental	Neonatal depression (>8 mg/kg in humans); worsening of preexisting fetal distress caused by maternal hemodynamic effects
Lidocaine	Uterine hypertonus and vasoconstriction with fetal distress (toxic doses in sheep); worsening of preexisting fetal distress
Mannitol	Oligohydramnios with fetal hyperosmolarity, hypernatremia, dehydration, cyanosis, bradycardia (12.5 g/kg in rabbits); fetal hyperosmolarity in humans 1 hr after 200 g IV
Furosemide	Possible dilation of ductus arteriosus; electrolyte abnormalities
Nitroprusside	Decreased uterine vascular resistance; lethal fetal cyanide levels with onset of maternal tachyphylaxis in sheep
Nitroglycerin	Decreased uterine vascular resistance
Hydralazine	Decreased uterine vascular resistance
Propranolol	Decreased umbilical blood flow in sheep; premature labor, worsening of preexisting fetal distress; neonatal acidosis, bradycardia, hypoglycemia, apnea, diminished response to hypoxia and acidosis

normalities in the fetus. Mannitol is also not always essential for brain relaxation; however, if it is required, moderate doses should be used.[141]

Beta-adrenergic antagonists have been reported to cause intrauterine growth retardation, premature labor, worsening of preexisting fetal distress, neonatal acidosis, bradycardia, hypoglycemia, apnea, and diminished response to hypoxia and acidosis.[60,87,228] To what extent these theoretic considerations should influence clinical decisions regarding the use of beta blockers is not clear. A rational approach would be to limit the use of these agents to clear indications and always be aware of these potential adverse effects. Table 18-6 contains a summary of the effects of some drugs on the uterus/placenta.

Preterm Clipping of Aneurysm with Normal Delivery at Term

The emphasis here is to treat the patient as any patient with SAH while being cognizant of the effects of anesthetic drugs and techniques on fetal well-being. Since delivery is not immediate, neonatal depression is not a significant concern. Perioperative and postoperative fetal heart rate monitoring is mandatory. Patients who have had successful clipping of their aneurysm do not require specialized management of labor or delivery and may receive an oxytocic agent for induction of labor for vaginal delivery unless there are obstetric indications for abdominal delivery.[52,126]

Cesarean Delivery Followed by Aneurysm Clipping

The aim here is to prevent rupture of the aneurysm while the cesarean delivery is being performed. A light anesthetic, although normally appropriate to minimize neonatal depression, may allow for maternal hypertension and rupture of the aneurysm. Both intravenous and inhaled anesthetic agents, however, will cross the placental barrier, resulting in neonatal depression. On balance, one should anesthetize the patient to an adequate depth of anesthesia with the aim of preventing aneurysmal rupture during induction as well as during maintenance and accept the price of neonatal depression. Equipment and personnel for neonatal resuscitation should be at hand when delivery occurs.

GIANT ANEURYSMS

Giant cerebral aneurysms are defined as those greater than 2.5 cm in diameter, representing a subset of cerebral aneurysms that may present technical difficulty because of their size or lack of an anatomic neck. They often have perforating vessels originating in the wall of the neck, as well as a high likelihood of atheromatous changes. The incidence of giant aneurysm is 2% of all patients in the Cooperative Study.[83] Most giant aneurysms present with symptoms of a mass lesion, such as headache, visual disturbance, or cranial nerve palsies. The surgical treatment of these aneurysms is associated with significant perioperative morbidity and mortality. In a series of 174 patients with giant aneurysms who underwent standard surgical treatment, Drake[44] reported that 71.5% of the patients had good outcomes, 13% were severely disabled, and 15.5% died. The series of 174 included 73 patients with giant basilar aneurysms that were associated with a complication rate of near 50% (23% had poor outcome and 25% died). Surgery for giant aneurysm remains a formidable challenge, and some neurosurgeons advise their patients against operative intervention unless immediate life-threatening risks are present.[183] Two surgical techniques are used for the management of giant aneurysms considered otherwise inoperable: (1) the use of proximal and distal temporary occlusion to collapse the aneurysm and (2) the use of circulatory arrest under profound hypothermia.[46] Although the former approach has been advocated by some surgeons,[10,201] it is not considered uniformly applicable. The latter approach had been used as a general approach for all cerebral aneurysms but fell into disfavor as improvements in microsurgical technique and neuroanesthesia allowed conventional approaches to achieve better results. Recently, however, interest has been revived in using hypothermic circulatory arrest for giant aneurysms, with several groups reporting good results and a mortality ranging from 0% to 25%.* The main advantages of hypothermic circulatory arrest for giant aneurysm include (1) decompression of the aneurysmal sac, (2) better visualization of the anatomy, (3) a totally bloodless field, and (4) easy manipulation and placement of the clip. Circulatory arrest can be performed using closed chest femoral vein–femoral artery bypass or open chest with median sternotomy and ventricular venting. The closed chest method is associated with lower morbidity and is preferred.

The anesthetic management of temporary occlusion has been discussed elsewhere in this chapter; therefore only circulatory arrest under profound hypothermia will be discussed here. The major issues concern brain protection and complications of cardiopulmonary bypass. For details on physiology and management of cardiopulmonary bypass, the reader should consult a standard textbook on cardiovascular anesthesia.

Brain Protection in Circulatory Arrest

Cerebral hypoxia and ischemia are the factors that limit the duration of the circulatory arrest. The metabolic oxygen consumption of the brain may be divided into an active component, which can be regarded as any neuronal activity, and a basal component, which is related to maintenance of cellular integrity. Pharmacologic and nonpharmacologic methods that decrease metabolic oxygen consumption will increase the duration of arrest tolerated. At the present time, these include the use of barbiturates and profound hypothermia. A number of investigators have reported good results with giant aneurysms utilizing the combination of barbiturate therapy and profound hypothermia during circulatory arrest.[12,183,185,209] However,

*References 12, 57, 118, 176, 183, 185, 227.

similar results have also been obtained with profound hypothermia alone.[227]

Barbiturates

Barbiturates can reduce the cerebral metabolic rate (CMR_{O_2}), attributed to the active component to zero and, therefore, reduce the overall CMR_{O_2} to a maximum of 50%. Additional barbiturate administration beyond what is required to cause electrical silence in the EEG will not decrease the metabolic rate further.[121] However, barbiturates may have other actions, including free radical scavenging and membrane stabilization.[185] Therefore barbiturates may provide additional cerebral protection even during profound hypothermia, but this remains controversial. Barbiturate therapy is most effective in preventing cerebral injury secondary to temporary focal ischemia.[173] It is less well established in the situation of temporary global ischemia.[187] Two modes of administering barbiturates (primarily sodium thiopental) before cooling and arrest are used: a single bolus or a con tinuous infusion. Where a single dose of thiopental was given, the amount ranged from 30 to 40 mg/kg administered over 30 minutes.[12,176,209] In most of the reported series, however, EEG monitoring was not used to determine the end point. Monitoring the EEG allows the anesthesiologist to titrate the loading dose and the maintenance infusion to achieve EEG burst suppression throughout the procedure.[144,185] A simple bihemispheric two-channel EEG device will suffice. Burst suppression may be accomplished with an initial loading dose of thiopental, 3 to 5 mg/kg, followed by a continuous infusion varying from 0.1 to 0.5 mg/kg/min for the entire period of cardiopulmonary bypass. With profound hypothermia at temperatures below 18° C, the EEG is rendered isoelectric even without pharmacologic suppression (in contrast, evoked responses are abolished between 15° and 18° C). It is recommended that the thiopental infusion rate established during normothermia be maintained during circulatory arrest.[183]

Hypothermia

Hypothermia (Table 18-7) is a nonpharmacologic method of reducing the CMR_{O_2} and is different from barbiturates in that it reduces not only the active component but also the basal component of the CMR_{O_2}.[188] Hypothermia causes a significant reduction in cerebral oxygen consumption and has been demonstrated to protect the brain during anoxic conditions.[186] The period of circulatory arrest tolerated at

TABLE 18-7
Hypothermia

Body Temperature (°C)	Normal Cerebral Metabolic Rate (%)	Period of Tolerated Circulatory Arrest (min)
38	100	4-5
30	50	8-10
25	25	16-20
20	15	32-40
10	10	64-80

normothermia is only 4 to 5 minutes, but it doubles for every 8° C temperature reduction.[123] Thus the $CMRo_2$ decreases to 50% of normal with hypothermia to 30° C, 25% of normal at 25° C, 15% of normal at 20° C, and 10% of normal at 15° C. At 15° C continuous circulatory arrest can be tolerated for 32 to 40 minutes. The maximum time of deep hypothermic arrest has not been definitively established, but in clinical practice it has been safely used for up to 60 minutes.[227]

Because substantial gradients in temperature can develop between the brain and the periphery during cooling and rewarming, it is important to monitor the brain temperature accurately before circulatory arrest. Williams et al.[227] reported close correlation of brain temperature measured with esophageal, tympanic membrane, and nasopharyngeal sensors. In contrast, rectal and bladder temperatures are unreliable. Direct brain temperature monitoring has also been advocated.[183] To improve safety, at least two temperature monitoring sites should be used.

The depth of hypothermia and duration of circulatory arrest reported in various series for treatment of giant aneurysms are summarized in Table 18-8. Note that the amount of time necessary for the clipping is usually less than the tolerable safe limit at the temperature used. Compared to early experience, the mortality and morbidity have declined substantially. The more recent series suggest that temperature should be decreased to 15° to 18° C, since the series with the highest mortality (25%) was associated with circulatory arrest at 25° C.[151]

Cardiovascular Effects of Hypothermia. Hypothermia induces characteristic cardiovascular changes.[123,185] As temperature decreases, systemic vascular resistance increases while cardiac output decreases. To allow high pump flow to facilitate rapid cooling and subsequent rewarming, use of vasodilators such as sodium nitroprusside may be necessary. Progressive bradycardia occurs as the temperature approaches 30° C, and the atrium frequently begins to develop flutter or fibrillation below 30° C. The ventricles usually fibrillate below 28° C. Because continuous ventricular fibrillation may cause ischemic injury to the heart, electrical activity should be terminated with administration of 40 to 80 mEq of potassium chloride to the pump or with cardioversion (100 to 250 watts/sec).

Hematologic Effects of Hypothermia. The coagulation system is severely perturbed by hypothermia, and the problem is compounded by inadequate surgical hemostasis or incomplete reversal of heparin with protamine.[12,26,185,227] Hypothermia-induced coagulopathy is caused by a multitude of factors: (1) hypothermia reduces the platelet count, probably from splenic sequestration; (2) it causes a reversible platelet dysfunction by decreasing adhesiveness; (3) it slows down the enzyme-mediated steps in the coagulation cascade; and (4) it decreases the metabolism of heparin. The dilutional effect of priming solutions with cardiopulmonary bypass on factors I, II, V, VII, and XIII also contributes to difficulty with hemostasis.

Hypothermia also causes an increase in viscosity, leading to sludging of the red blood cells. However, this can be effectively treated by deliberately lowering the hematocrit with phlebotomy and simultaneously replacing the blood volume with a crystalloid solution. The phlebotomy not only decreases the hematocrit, but also preserves platelet-rich autologous blood for subsequent transfusion during the rewarming phase. The decreased hematocrit re-

TABLE 18-8
Circulatory Arrest for Treatment of Giant Aneurysms

Authors	No. of Cases	Body Temperature (° C)	Duration of Arrest		Major Morbidity (%)	Mortality (%)
			Median (min)	Range (min)		
Woodhall et al. (1960)[230]	1*	12	30	—	100	0
Patterson and Ray (1962)[151]	7	14-17	25	9-43	0	30
Michenfelder et al. (1964)[122]	15	13-16	17	0-39	40	20
Drake et al. (1964)[46]	10	13-17	14	2-18	40	30
Sundt et al. (1972)[195]	1	13	30	—	100	0
McMurtry et al. (1974)[118]	12†	28-29	9	1-28	50	8
Baumgartner et al. (1983)[12]	15‡,§	16-21.5	19	0-51	20	0
Gonski et al. (1986)[57]	40	25	10	0-35	23	25
Spetzler et al. (1988)[185]	7	17.5-21	11	7-53	29	14
Thomas et al. (1990)[209]	1‡	15.4	35	—	0	0
Solomon et al. (1991)[183]	14‡	15-22.5	22	8-51	50	0
Williams et al. (1991)[227]	10‖	8.4-13.7	25	1.25-60	20	10

*Patient with metastatic bronchogenic carcinoma.
†One of the twelve patients had an AVM.
‡Barbiturate therapy also used.
§Two of the fifteen were patients with medullary hemangioblastoma.
‖Only 4 out of the 10 patients had giant aneurysms. The patient who died had an arteriovenous malformation (AVM); the patients with morbidity included one with an AVM and one with an aneurysm.

duces oxygen-carrying capacity, but this is partially compensated for by the increased amount of dissolved oxygen caused by the increased oxygen solubility that occurs with hypothermia. The hemoglobin-oxygen dissociation curve, however, is also shifted to the left and may reduce unloading of oxygen in ischemic tissue.

Hyperglycemia

Hypothermia prevents proper utilization and metabolism of glucose and may cause hyperglycemia. As mentioned above, hyperglycemia may exacerbate neuronal damage during ischemia[93,95] and therefore should be treated with insulin. Frequent monitoring of serum glucose and electrolytes in addition to acid-base balance is therefore essential.

Anesthetic Considerations

In addition to the normal evaluation of the patient with SAH, preoperative consideration of patients scheduled for hypothermic circulatory arrest must include special emphasis on coexisting cardiac, pulmonary, hematologic, or neurologic disorders that may modify or exclude the patient from this form of therapy. For example, patients with aortic valve insufficiency may require the open-chest method of cardiopulmonary bypass to prevent ventricular distention. On the other hand, patients with poor ventricular function, existing coagulopathy, or significant carotid artery disease may be considered unsuitable for this procedure.

Although induction of anesthesia is similar to what has been covered previously regarding monitors, blood pressure control, and intubation, several additional monitors should be considered. These include electroencephalography (EEG), somatosensory evoked potentials (SSEP), brain stem auditory evoked potentials (BAEP), transesophageal echocardiography, and transcranial Doppler (TCD). The EEG monitors cortical activity and is necessary as an end point for barbiturate-induced burst suppression when barbiturates are used for added protection. SSEP, on the other hand, is a measure of the sensory conduction to the cortex and can be recorded even during a barbiturate-induced silent EEG. BAEP reflects the function of the auditory pathway through the brain stem and may be useful during procedures on vertebral-basilar aneurysms.[185] However, during profound hypothermia at 15° to 18° C, all electrophysiologic activity is abolished. Nevertheless, SSEP monitoring may allow assessment of neurologic function during cooling as well as rewarming and may have prognostic value. Transesophageal echocardiography allows visualization of the cardiac chambers and assessment of ventricular function and is useful in management of patients with cardiac disease.[183] In addition, TCD has been used during these procedures,[183] presumably to monitor cerebral blood flow velocity and emboli, although its value has not been established.

The overall management necessitates a team effort requiring effective communication from all participants. To administer anesthesia safely for hypothermic circulatory arrest, a thorough understanding of the cardiovascular and hematologic perturbations in response to hypothermia must be appreciated. The technique also demands a knowledge of the use of the various electrophysiologic monitors that guide efforts to provide cerebral protection. Although the actual practice varies among different institutions, a suggested protocol is appended.

The major and most feared postoperative complication associated with hypothermic cardiac arrest for aneurysm surgery is coagulopathy leading to cerebral hemorrhage. A small leak at the operative site can be disastrous. To reduce this risk the surgeon should complete the dissection of the aneurysm and verify absolute hemostasis before initiating hypothermic circulatory arrest. Heparinization should be evaluated and followed with the activated clotting time (ACT) and maintained within 400 to 450 seconds. Once rewarming has occurred and the patient no longer requires bypass, protamine sulfate is titrated to reverse the effect of heparin until the ACT is between 100 and 150 seconds. The phlebotomized blood removed earlier is retransfused, and additional blood products such as fresh frozen plasma, cryoprecipitate, and platelets are often required. Meticulous surgical hemostasis is again necessary before dural closure begins.

The anesthesiologist must also watch for any cardiovascular complications associated with cardiopulmonary bypass, including hypotension, low cardiac output, and hypertension, and correct any rhythm abnormalities during the cooling or rewarming phase. The patient may also require inotropic support during the warming and immediate postoperative course. With or without additional barbiturate protection, the patient is generally transferred directly to the intensive care unit for continued care. Extubation of the trachea and assessment of neurologic function can usually be accomplished within 12 to 24 hours postoperatively.

SUMMARY

Because of the associated systemic effects and the surgical requirements, patients with cerebral aneurysms present a unique challenge to the anesthesiologist. This chapter has a highlighted the major considerations and suggested rational approaches. The important steps are (1) thorough understanding of the patient's pathophysiology in relation to the subarachnoid hemorrhage as well as other related systemic effects; (2) communication with the neurosurgeon to clarify the surgical approach and the need for any specific monitoring; (3) outline of the an-

Continued.

esthetic objectives; (4) formulation of anesthetic plan to meet the objectives, taking into consideration one's knowledge of anesthetic drugs and clinical experience (this should also include planning for untoward events intraoperatively such as rupture of the aneurysm); and (5) implementation of the plan. There will always be patients who, despite our best efforts, fail to benefit from the surgical procedure. It is hoped, however, that with proper planning, optimal results can be achieved.

References

1. Albanese J, Durbec O, Viviand X et al: Sufentanil increases intracranial pressure in patients with head trauma, *Anesthesiology* 79:493, 1993.

2. Algotsson L, Messeter K, Rosen I et al: Effects of nitrous oxide on cerebral haemodynamics and metabolism during isoflurane anaesthesia in man, *Acta Anaesthesiol Scand* 36:46, 1992.

3. Allen GS: Role of calcium antagonists in cerebral arterial spasm, *Am J Cardiol* 55:149B, 1985.

4. Allen GS, Ahn HS, Preziosi TJ et al: Cerebral arterial spasm: a controlled trial of nimodipine in patients with subarachnoid hemorrhage, *N Engl J Med* 308:619, 1983.

5. Andreoli A, di Pasquale G, Pinelli G et al: Subarachnoid hemorrhage: frequency and severity of cardiac arrhythmias. A survey of 70 cases studied in the acute phase, *Stroke* 18:558, 1987.

6. Artru AA, Colley PS: Placement of multiorificed CVP catheters via antecubital veins using intravascular electrocardiography, *Anesthesiology* 69:132, 1988.

7. Awad IA, Carter LP, Spetzler RF et al: Clinical vasospasm after subarachnoid hemorrhage: response to hypervolemic hemodilution and arterial hypertension, *Stroke* 18:365, 1987.

8. Barker J: An anaesthetic technique for intracranial aneurysms, *Anaesthesia* 30:557, 1975 (letter).

9. Batjer HH, Frankfurt AI, Purdy PD et al: Use of etomidate, temporary arterial occlusion, and intraoperative angiography in surgical treatment of large and giant cerebral aneurysms, *J Neurosurg* 68:234, 1988.

10. Batjer H, Samson D: Intraoperative aneurysmal rupture: incidence, outcome, and suggestions for surgical management, *Neurosurgery* 18:701, 1986.

11. Battaglia F, Prystowski H, Smisson C et al: Fetal blood studies. XIII. The effect of the administration of fluids intravenously to mothers upon the concentrations of water and electrolytes in plasma of human fetuses, *Pediatrics* 25:2, 1960.

12. Baumgartner WA, Silverberg GD, Ream AK et al: Reappraisal of cardiopulmonary bypass with deep hypothermia and circulatory arrest for complex neurosurgical operations, *Surgery* 94:242, 1983.

13. Beck DW, Adams HP, Flamm ES et al: Combination of aminocaproic acid and nicardipine in treatment of aneurysmal subarachnoid hemorrhage, *Stroke* 19:63, 1988.

14. Black S, Ockert DB, Oliver WC et al: Outcome following posterior fossa craniectomy in patients in the sitting or horizontal positions, *Anesthesiology* 69:49, 1988.

15. Blume WT: Monitoring the safe levels of hypotension. III. The role of electroencephalography, *Int Anesthesiol Clin* 20:125, 1982.

16. Borgmann R: Natural course of intracranial pressure and drainage of CSF after recovery from subarachnoid hemorrhage, *Acta Neurol Scand* 81:300, 1990.

17. Botterell EH, Lougheed WM, Scott JW et al: Hypothermia and interruption of the carotid or carotid and vertebral circulation in the surgical management in intracranial aneurysms, *J Neurosurg* 13:1, 1956.

18. Brouwers PJAM, Wijdicks EFM, Hasan D et al: Serial electrocardiographic recording in aneurysmal subarachnoid hemorrhage, *Stroke* 20:1162, 1989.

19. Bruns PD, Londer RO, Drose VE et al: The placental transfer of water from fetus to mother following the intravenous infusion of hypertonic mannitol to the maternal rabbit, *Am J Obstet Gynecol* 86:160, 1963.

20. Buckland MR, Batjer HH, Giesecke AH: Anesthesia for cerebral aneurysm surgery: use of induced hypertension in patients with symptomatic vasospasm, *Anesthesiology* 69:116, 1988.

21. Busto R, Dietrich WD, Globus MY-T et al: The importance of brain temperature in cerebral ischemic injury, *Stroke* 20:1113, 1989.

22. Busto R, Globus MT-T, Dietrich WD et al: Effect of mild hypothermia on ischemia-induced release of neurotransmitters and free fatty acids in rat brain, *Stroke* 20:904, 1989.

23. Cannell DE, Botterell EH: Subarachnoid hemorrhage and pregnancy, *Am J Obstet Gynecol* 12:844, 1956.

24. Carpenter DA, Grubb RL, Temperl LW et al: Cerebral oxygen metabolism after aneurysmal subarachnoid hemorrhage, *J Cereb Blood Flow Metab* 11:837, 1991.

25. Chyatte D, Sundt TM: Cerebral vasospasm after subarachnoid hemorrhage, *Mayo Clin Proc* 59:498, 1984.

26. Cohen JA, Frederickson EL, Kaplan J: Plasma heparin activity and antagonism during cardiopulmonary bypass with hypothermia, *Anesth Analg* 56:564, 1977.

27. Colley PS, Dunn R: Prevention of blood pressure response to skull-pin head holder by local anesthesia, *Anesth Analg* 58:241, 1979.

28. Conklin KA, Herr G, Fung D: Anesthesia for cesarean section and cerebral aneurysm clipping, *Can Anaesth Soc J* 34:451, 1984.

29. Cook DA: The pharmacology of cerebral vasospasm, *Pharmacology* 29:1, 1984.

30. Cote CJ, Greenhow E, Marshall BE: The hypotensive response to rapid intravenous administration of hypertonic solutions in man and rabbit, *Anesthesiology* 50:30, 1979.

31. Cruickshank JM, Neil-Dwyer G, Stott AW: Possible role of catecholamines, corticosteroids, and potas-

sium in production of electrocardiographic abnormalities associated with subarachnoid haemorrhage, *Br Heart J* 36:697, 1974.

32. Cucchiara RF, Benefiel DJ, Matteo RS et al: Evaluation of esmolol in controlling increases in heart rate and blood pressure during endotracheal intubation in patients undergoing carotid endarterectomy, *Anesthesiology* 65:528, 1986.

33. Cully MD, Larson CP Jr, Silverberg GD: Hetastarch coagulopathy in a neurosurgical patient, *Anesthesiology* 66:706, 1987.

34. Damon L, Adams M, Stricker RB et al: Intracranial bleeding during treatment with hydroxyethyl starch, *N Engl J Med* 317:964, 1987.

35. Davies KR, Gelb AW, Manninen PH et al: Cardiac function in aneurysmal subarachnoid haemorrhage: a study of electrocardiographic and echocardiographic abnormalities, *Br J Anaesth* 67:58, 1991.

36. Dernbach PD, Little JR, Jones SC et al: Altered cerebral autoregulation and CO_2 reactivity after aneurysmal subarachnoid hemorrhage, *Neurosurgery* 22:822, 1988.

37. Di Pasquale G, Pinelli G, Andreoli A et al: Holter detection of cardiac arrhythmias in intracranial subarachnoid hemorrhage, *Am J Cardiol* 59:596, 1987.

38. Dias MS, Sekhar LN: Intracranial hemorrhage from aneurysms and arteriovenous malformations during pregnancy and the puerperium, *Neurosurgery* 27:855, 1990.

39. Diringer MN, Kirsch JR, Ladenson PW et al: Cerebrospinal fluid atrial natriuretic factor in intracranial disease, *Stroke* 21:1550, 1990.

40. Diringer MN, Ladenson PW, Stern BJ et al: Plasma atrial natriuretic factor and subarachnoid hemorrhage, *Stroke* 19:1119, 1988.

41. Diringer MN, Lim JS, Kirsch JR et al: Suprasellar and intraventricular blood predict elevated plasma atrial natriuretic factor in subarachnoid hemorrhage, *Stroke* 22:577, 1991.

42. Doczi T, Joo F, Vecsernyes M et al: Increased concentration of atrial natriuretic factor in the cerebrospinal fluid of patients with aneurysmal subarachnoid hemorrhage and raised intracranial pressure, *Neurosurgery* 23:16, 1988.

43. Doshi R, Neil-Dwyer G: Hypothalamic and myocardial lesions after subarachnoid haemorrhage, *J Neurol Neurosurg Psychiatry* 40:821, 1977.

44. Drake CG: Giant intracranial aneurysms: experience with surgical treatment in 174 patients, *Clin Neurosurg* 26:12, 1979.

45. Drake CG: Report of World Federation of Neurological Surgeons Committee on a universal subarachnoid hemorrhage grading scale, *J Neurosurg* 68:985, 1988.

46. Drake CG, Barr HWK, Coles JC et al: The use of extracorporeal circulation and profound hypothermia in the treatment of ruptured intracranial aneurysm, *J Neurosurg* 21:575, 1964.

47. Farrar JK, Gamache FW, Ferguson GG et al: Effects of profound hypotension on cerebral blood flow during surgery for intracranial aneurysms, *J Neurosurg* 55:857, 1981.

48. Ferguson GG: The rationale for controlled hypotension. In Varkey GP, editor: *Anesthetic considerations in the surgical repair of intracranial aneurysms,* vol 20, Boston, 1982, Little, Brown.

49. Findlay JM, Weir BKA, Gordon P et al: Safety and efficacy of intrathecal thrombolytic therapy in a primate model of cerebral vasospasm, *Neurosurgery* 24:491, 1989.

50. Fisher CM, Roberson GH, Ojemann RG: Cerebral vasospasm with ruptured saccular aneurysm: the clinical manifestations, *Neurosurgery* 1:245, 1977.

51. Flamm ES, Adams HP, Beck DW et al: Dose-escalation study of intravenous nicardipine in patients with aneurysmal subarachnoid hemorrhage, *J Neurosurg* 68:393, 1988.

52. Fliegner JFH, Hooper RS, Kloss M: Subarachnoid haemorrhage in pregnancy, *J Obstet Gynaecol Br Commonwealth* 76:912, 1969.

53. Friedman WA, Chadwick GM, Verhoeven FJS et al: Monitoring of somatosensory evoked potentials during surgery for middle cerebral artery aneurysms, *Neurosurgery* 29:83, 1991.

54. From RP, Warner DS, Todd MM et al: Anesthesia for craniotomy: a double-blind comparison of alfentanil, fentanyl, and sufentanil, *Anesthesiology* 73:896, 1990.

55. Galloon S, Rees GAD, Briscoe CE et al: Prospective study of electrocardiographic changes associated with subarachnoid haemorrhage, *Br J Anaesth* 44:511, 1972.

56. Gillingham J: Historical perspectives presented to the society of neurological surgeons, Chicago, May 1981.

57. Gonski A, Acedillo AT, Stacey RB: Profound hypothermia in the treatment of intracranial aneurysms, *Aust NZ J Surg* 56:639, 1986.

58. Grad A, Kiauta T, Osredkar J: Effect of elevated plasma norepinephrine on electrocardiographic changes in subarachnoid hemorrhage, *Stroke* 22:746, 1991.

59. Grubb RL, Raichle ME, Eichling JO et al: Effects of subarachnoid hemorrhage on cerebral blood volume, blood flow, and oxygen utilization in humans, *J Neurosurg* 46:446, 1977.

60. Habib A, McCarthy JS: Effects on the neonate of propranolol administered during pregnancy, *J Pediatr* 91:808, 1977.

61. Haley Jr EC, Kassell NF, Torner JC: The International Cooperative Study on Timing of Aneurysm Surgery: the North American experience, *Stroke* 23:205, 1992.

62. Hamill JF, Bedford RF, Weaver DC et al: Lidocaine before endotracheal intubation: intravenous or laryngotracheal? *Anesthesiology* 55:578, 1981.

63. Hansen T, Warner D, Todd M et al: Effects of nitrous oxide and volatile anaesthetics on cerebral blood flow, *Br J Anaesth* 63:290, 1989.

64. Harders AG, Gilsbach JM: Time course of blood velocity changes related to vasospasm in the circle of Willis measured by transcranial Doppler ultrasound, *J Neurosurg* 66:718, 1987.

65. Harries AD: Subarachnoid haemorrhage and the electrocardiogram: a review, *Postgrad Med J* 57:294, 1981.

66. Hasan D, Vermeulen M, Wijdicks EFM et al: Effect of fluid intake and antihypertensive treatment on cerebral ischemia after subarachnoid hemorrhage, *Stroke* 20:1511, 1989.

67. Hasan D, Wijdicks EFM, Vermeulen M: Hyponatremia is associated with cerebral ischemia in patients with aneurysmal subarachnoid hemorrhage, *Ann Neurol* 27:106, 1990.

68. Herrick IA, Gelb AW, Manninen PH et al: Effects of fentanyl, sufentanil, and alfentanil on brain retractor pressure, *Anesth Analg* 72:359, 1991.

69. Hijdra A, van Gijn J, Stefanko S et al: Delayed cerebral ischemia after

aneurysmal subarachnoid hemorrhage: clinicoanatomic correlations, *Neurology* 36:329, 1986.

70. Hillman DR, Rung GW, Thompson WR et al: The effect of bupivacaine scalp infiltration on the hemodynamic response to craniotomy under general anesthesia, *Anesthesiology* 67:1001, 1987.

71. Hunt WE, Hess RM: Surgical risk as related to time of intervention in the repair of intracranial aneurysms, *J Neurosurg* 28:14, 1968.

72. Ishii R: Regional cerebral blood flow in patients with ruptured intracranial aneurysms, *J Neurosurg* 50:587, 1979.

73. Iwatsuki N, Kuroda N, Amaha K et al: Succinylcholine-induced hyperkalemia in patients with ruptured cerebral aneurysms, *Anesthesiology* 53:64, 1980.

74. Jabre A, Symon L: Temporary vascular occlusion during aneurysm surgery, *Surg Neurol* 27:47, 1987.

75. Jakobsen M, Enevoldsen E, Bjerre P: Cerebral blood flow and metabolism following subarachnoid hemorrhage: cerebral oxygen uptake and global blood flow during the acute period in patients with SAH, *Acta Neurol Scand* 82:174, 1990.

76. Jones TH, Chiappa KH, Young RR et al: EEG monitoring for induced hypotension for surgery of intracranial aneurysms, *Stroke* 10:292, 1979.

77. Kaku Y, Yonekawa Y, Tsukahara T et al: Superselective intra-arterial infusion of papaverine for the treatment of cerebral vasospasm after subarachnoid hemorrhage, *J Neurosurg* 77:842, 1992.

78. Kassell NF, Peerless SJ, Durward QJ et al: Treatment of ischemic deficits from vasospasm with intravascular volume expansion and induced arterial hypertension, *Neurosurgery* 11:337, 1982.

79. Kassell NF, Peerless SJ, Reilly PL: Intracranial pressure, aneurysms and subarachnoid hemorrhage. In Deks JWF, Bosch DA, Brock M, editors: *Intracranial pressure III*, Berlin, 1976, Springer-Verlag.

80. Kassell NF, Sasaki T, Colohan ART et al: Cerebral vasospasm following aneurysmal subarachnoid hemorrhage, *Stroke* 16:562, 1985.

81. Kassell NF, Torner JC: Aneurysmal rebleeding: a preliminary report from the cooperative aneurysm study, *Neurosurgery* 13:479, 1983.

82. Kassell NF, Torner JC, Adams HP: Antifibrinolytic therapy in the acute period following aneurysmal subarachnoid hemorrhage, *J Neurosurg* 61:225, 1984.

83. Kassell NF, Torner JC, Haley EC et al: The International Cooperative Study on the Timing of Aneurysm Surgery. I. Overall management results, *J Neurosurg* 73:18, 1990.

84. Kassell NF, Torner JC, Haley C et al: The International Cooperative Study on the Timing of Aneurysm Surgery. II. Surgical results, *J Neurosurg* 73:37, 1990.

85. Kautto UM: Attenuation of the circulatory response to laryngoscopy and intubation by fentanyl, *Acta Anaesth Scand* 26:217, 1982.

86. Kidooka M, Nakasu Y, Watanabe K et al: Monitoring of somatosensory-evoked potentials during aneurysm surgery, *Surg Neurol* 27:69, 1987.

87. Kofke WA, Wuest HP, McGinnis LA: Cesarean section following ruptured cerebral aneurysm and neuroresuscitation, *Anesthesiology* 60:242, 1984.

88. Lam A: Proper positioning of the patient. In Varkey GP, editor: *Anesthetic considerations in the surgical repair of intracranial aneurysms. International anesthesiology clinics*, vol 20, Boston, 1982, Little, Brown.

89. Lam AM, Gelb AW: Cardiovascular effects of isoflurane-induced hypotension for cerebral aneurysm surgery, *Anesth Analg* 62:742, 1983.

90. Lam AM, Keane JF, Manninen PH: Monitoring of brainstem auditory evoked potentials during basilar artery occlusion in man, *Br J Anaesth* 57:924, 1985.

91. Lam AM, Mayberg TS, Cooper JO et al: Nitrous oxide–isoflurane anesthesia causes more cerebral vasodilation than an equipotent dose of isoflurane in humans, *Anesth Analg* (1994, in press).

92. Lam AM, Nicholas JF, Manninen PH: Influence of succinylcholine on lumbar cerebral spinal pressure in man, *Anesth Analg* 63:240, 1984.

93. Lam AM, Winn HR, Cullen BF et al: Hyperglycemia and neurologic outcome in patients with head injury, *J Neurosurg* 75:545, 1991.

94. Landi A, Demo P, Carraro JR et al: Intraoperative monitoring by means of somatosensory evoked potentials during cerebral aneurysm surgery, *Agressologie* 31:363, 1990.

95. Lanier WL, Milde JH, Michenfelder JD: Cerebral stimulation following succinylcholine in dogs, *Anesthesiology* 64:551, 1986.

96. Lanier W, Stangland K, Scheithauer B et al: The effects of dextrose infusion and head position on neurologic outcome after complete cerebral ischemia in primates: examination of a model, *Anesthesiology* 66:39, 1987.

97. Lennon RL, Sundt Jr TM, Gronert GA: Combined cesarean section and clipping of intracerebral aneurysm, *Anesthesiology* 60:240, 1984.

98. Levin R, Hesselvik JF, Kourtopoulos H et al: Local anesthesia prevents hypertension following application of the Mayfield skull-pin head holder, *Acta Anaesthesiol Scand* 33:277, 1989.

99. Levinson G, Shnider SM, DeLorimier AA et al: Effects of maternal hyperventilation on uterine blood flow and fetal oxygenation and acid-base balance, *Anesthesiology* 40:340, 1974.

100. Levy ML, Giannotta SL: Cardiac performance indices during hypervolemic therapy for cerebral vasospasm, *J Neurosurg* 75:27, 1991.

101. Levy ML, Rabb CH, Zelman V et al: Cardiac performance enhancement from dobutamine in patients refractory to hypervolemic therapy for cerebral vasospasm, *J Neurosurg* 19:494, 1993.

102. Little JR: Modification of acute focal ischemia by treatment with mannitol, *Stroke* 9:4, 1978.

103. Liu PL, Warren TM, Ostheimer GW et al: Foetal monitoring in parturients undergoing surgery unrelated to pregnancy, *Can Anaesth Soc J* 32:525, 1985.

104. Macdonald RL, Weir BK: A review of hemoglobin and the pathogenesis of cerebral vasospasm, *Stroke* 22:971, 1991.

105. Manninen PH, Gelb AW, Lam AM et al: Perioperative monitoring of the electrocardiogram during cerebral aneurysm surgery, *J Neurosurg Anesth* 2:16, 1990.

106. Manninen PH, Lam AM, Gelb AW: Electrocardiographic changes during and after isoflurane-induced hypotension for neurovascular surgery, *Can J Anaesth* 34:549, 1987.

107. Manninen PH, Lam AM, Gelb AW et al: The effect of high-dose mannitol on serum and urine electrolytes

and osmolality in neurological patients, *Can J Anaesth* 34:442, 1987.

108. Manninen PH, Lam AM, Nantau W: Monitoring of somatosensory evoked potentials during temporary arterial occlusion in aneurysm surgery, *J Neurosurg Anesth* 2:97, 1990.

109. Manninen PH, Mahendran B, Gelb AW et al: Succinylcholine does not increase serum potassium levels in patients with acutely ruptured cerebral aneurysm, *Anesth Analg* 70:172, 1990.

110. Marion DW, Segal R, Thompson ME: Subarachnoid hemorrhage and the heart, *Neurosurgery* 18:101, 1986.

111. Maroon JC, Nelson PB: Hypovolemia in patients with subarachnoid hemorrhage: therapeutic implications, *Neurosurgery* 4:223, 1979.

112. Martin WRW, Baker RP, Grubb RL et al: Cerebral blood volume, blood flow, and oxygen metabolism in cerebral ischaemia and subarachnoid haemorrhage: an in-vivo study using positron emission tomography, *Acta Neurochirurgica* 70:3, 1984.

113. Marx W, Shah N, Long C et al: Sufentanil, alfentanil, and fentanyl: impact on cerebrospinal fluid pressure in patients with brain tumors, *J Neurosurg Anesth* 1:3, 1989.

114. Mayer N, Weinstabl C, Podreka I et al: Sufentanil does not increase cerebral blood flow in healthy human volunteers, *Anesthesiology* 73:240, 1990.

115. McAllister RG: Macroglossia: a positional complication, *Anesthesiology* 40:199, 1974.

116. McCormick PW, Stewart M, Goetting MG et al: Regional cerebrovascular oxygen saturation measured by optical spectroscopy in humans, *Stroke* 22:596, 1991.

117. McDermott MW, Durity FA, Borozny M et al: Temporary vessel occlusion and barbiturate protection in cerebral aneurysm surgery, *Neurosurgery* 25:54, 1989.

118. McMurtry JG, Housepian EM, Bowman FO et al: Surgical treatment of basilar artery aneurysms, elective circulatory arrest with thoracotomy in 12 cases, *J Neurosurg* 40:486, 1974.

119. Medlock MD, Dulebohn SC, Elwood PW: Prophylactic hypervolemia without calcium channel blockers in early aneurysm surgery. *Neurosurgery* 30:12, 1992.

120. Mee E, Dorrance D, Lower D et al: Controlled study of nimodipine in aneurysm patients treated early after subarachnoid hemorrhage. *Neurosurgery* 22:484, 1988.

121. Michenfelder JD: The interdependency of cerebral functional and metabolic effects following massive doses of thiopental in the dog, *Anesthesiology* 41:231, 1974.

122. Michenfelder JD, Kirklin JW, Uihlein A et al: Clinical experience with a closed-chest method of producing profound hypothermia and total circulatory arrest in neurosurgery, *Ann Surg* 159:125, 1964.

123. Michenfelder JD, Terry HR, Daw EF et al: Induced hypothermia: physiologic effects, indications and techniques, *Surg Clin North Am* 45:889, 1965.

124. Minamisawa H, Nordstrom C-H, Smith M-L et al: The influence of mild body and brain hypothermia on ischemic brain damage, *J Cereb Blood Flow Metab* 10:365, 1990.

125. Minamisawa H, Smith M-L, Siesjo BK: The effect of mild hyperthermia and hypothermia on brain damage following 5, 10, and 15 minutes of forebrain ischemia, *Ann Neurol* 28:26, 1990.

126. Minielly R, Yuzpe AA, Drake CG: Subarachnoid hemorrhage secondary to ruptured cerebral aneurysm in pregnancy, *Obstet Gynecol* 53:64, 1979.

127. Minton MD, Grosslight K, Stirt JA et al: Increases in intracranial pressure from succinylcholine: prevention by prior nondepolarizing blockade, *Anesthesiology* 65:165, 1986.

128. Mizukami M, Kawase T, Usami T et al: Prevention of vasospasm by early operation with removal of subarachnoid blood, *Neurosurgery* 10:301, 1982.

129. Momma F, Wang AD, Symon L: Effects of temporary arterial occlusion on somatosensory evoked responses in aneurysm surgery, *Surg Neurol* 27:343, 1987.

130. Mooij JJ, Buchthal A, Belopavlovic M: Somatosensory evoked potential monitoring of temporary middle cerebral artery occlusion during aneurysm operation, *Neurosurgery* 21:492, 1987.

131. Moore JK, Chaudhri S, Moore AP et al: Macroglossia and posterior fossa disease, *Anaesthesia* 43:382, 1988.

132. Motoyama EK, Rivard G, Acheson F: The effect of changes in maternal pH and CO_2 on the Po_2 of fetal lambs, *Anesthesiology* 28:891, 1967.

133. Muizelaar JP: The use of electroencephalography and brain protection during operation for basilar aneurysms, *Neurosurgery* 25:899, 1989.

134. Mutch WA, Ringaert KR, Ewert FJ et al: Continuous opioid infusions for neurosurgical procedures: a double-blind comparison of alfentanil and fentanyl, *Can J Anaesth* 38:710, 1991.

135. Muzzi DA, Black S, Losasso TJ et al: Labetalol and esmolol in the control of hypertension after intracranial surgery, *Anesth Analg* 70:68, 1990.

136. Naulty J, Cefalo RC, Lewis PE: Fetal toxicity of nitroprusside in the pregnant ewe, *Am J Obstet Gynecol* 139:708, 1981.

137. Neil-Dwyer G, Mee E, Dorrance D et al: Early intervention with nimodipine in subarachnoid hemorrhage, *Eur Heart J* 8:41, 1988.

138. Nelson RJ, Roberts J, Rubin C et al: Association of hypovolemia after subarachnoid hemorrhage with computed tomographic scan evidence of raised intracranial pressure, *Neurosurgery* 29:178, 1991.

139. Newell DW, Eskridge JM, Mayberg MR et al: Angioplasty for the treatment of symptomatic vasospasm following subarachnoid hemorrhage, *Neurosurgery* 71:654, 1989.

140. Newman B, Gelb AW, Lam AM: The effect of isoflurane-induced hypotension on cerebral blood flow and cerebral metabolic rate for oxygen in humans, *Anesthesiology* 64:307, 1986.

141. Newman B, Lam AM: Induced hypotension for clipping of a cerebral aneurysm during pregnancy: a case report and brief review, *Anesth Analg* 65:675, 1986.

142. Nornes H: The role of intracranial pressure in the arrest of hemorrhage in patients with ruptured intracranial aneurysm, *J Neurosurg* 39:226, 1973.

143. Nornes H, Knutzen B, Wikeby P: Cerebral arterial blood flow and aneurysm surgery. II. Induced hypotension and autoregulatory capacity, *J Neurosurg* 47:819, 1977.

144. Nussmeier NA, Arlund C, Slogoff S: Neuropsychiatric complications after cardiopulmonary bypass: cerebral

protection by a barbiturate, *Anesthesiology* 64:165, 1986.

145. Ohman J, Servo A, Heiskanen O: Effect of intrathecal fibrinolytic therapy on clot lysis and vasospasm in patients with aneurysmal subarachnoid hemorrhage, *J Neurosurg* 75:197, 1991.

146. Ornstein E, Matteo RS, Schwartz AE et al: The effect of phenytoin on the magnitude and duration of neuromuscular block following atracurium or vecuronium, *Anesthesiology* 67:191, 1987.

147. Ornstein E, Matteo RS, Young WL et al: Resistance to metocurine-induced neuromuscular blockade in patients receiving phenytoin, *Anesthesiology* 63:294, 1985.

148. Ornstein E, Young WL, Fleisher et al: Desflurane and isoflurane have similar effect on cerebral blood flow in patients with intracranial mass lesions, *Anesthesiology* 79:498, 1993.

149. Palahniuk FJ, Shnider SM: Maternal and fetal cardiovascular acid-base changes during halothane and isoflurane anesthesia in the pregnant ewe, *Anesthesiology* 41:462, 1974.

150. Palahniuk FJ, Shnider SM, Eger EI: Pregnancy decreases the requirements for inhaled anesthetic agents, *Anesthesiology* 41:82, 1974.

151. Patterson RH, Ray BS: Profound hypothermia for intracranial surgery: laboratory and clinical experience with extracorporeal circulation by peripheral cannulation, *Ann Surg* 156:377, 1962.

152. Peerless SJ, Drake CG: Posterior circulation aneurysms. In Wilkins RH, Rengachary SG, editors: *Neurosurgery,* New York, 1987, McGraw-Hill.

153. Petruk KC, West M, Mohr G et al: Nimodipine treatment in poor-grade aneurysm patients: results of a multicenter double-blind placebo-controlled trial, *J Neurosurg* 68:505, 1988.

154. Pickard JD, Murray GD, Illingworth R et al: Effect of oral nimodipine on cerebral infarction and outcome after subarachnoid haemorrhage: British Aneurysm Nimodipine Trial, *Br Med J* 298:636, 1989.

155. Pollay M, Fullenwider C, Roberts PA et al: Effect of mannitol and furosemide on blood-brain osmotic gradient and intracranial pressure, *J Neurosurg* 59:945, 1983.

156. Pollick C, Cujec B, Parker S et al: Left ventricular wall motion abnormalities in subarachnoid hemorrhage: an echocardiographic study, *J Anesth Crit Care* 12:600, 1988.

157. Ravussin P, Archer DP, Meyer E et al: The effect of rapid infusion of saline and mannitol on cerebral blood volume and intracranial pressure in dogs, *Can Anaesth Soc J* 32:506, 1985.

158. Ravussin P, Archer DP, Tyler JL et al: Effects of rapid mannitol on cerebral blood volume, *J Neurosurg* 64:104, 1986.

159. Rigg D, McDonogh A: Use of sodium nitroprusside for deliberate hypotension during pregnancy, *Br J Anaesth* 53:985, 1981.

160. Roald OK, Forsman M, Heier MS et al: Cerebral effects of nitrous oxide when added to low and high concentrations of isoflurane in the dog, *Anesth Analg* 72:75, 1991.

161. Rosenfeld JV, Barnett GH, Sila CA et al: The effect of subarachnoid hemorrhage on blood and CSF atrial natriuretic factor, *J Neurosurg* 71:32, 1989.

162. Roths S, Ebrahim ZY: Resistance to pancuronium in patients receiving carbamazepine, *Anesthesiology* 66:691, 1987.

163. Rudehill A, Gordon E, Sundqvist K et al: A study of ECG abnormalities and myocardial specific enzymes in patients with subarachnoid haemorrhage, *Acta Anaesth Scand* 26:344, 1982.

164. Rudehill A, Lagerkranser M, Lindquist C et al: Effects of mannitol on blood volume and central hemodynamics in patients undergoing cerebral aneurysm surgery, *Anesth Analg* 62:875, 1983.

165. Rudehill A, Olsson GL, Sundquist K et al: ECG abnormalities in patients with subarachnoid haemorrhage and intracranial tumors, *J Neurol Neurosurg Psychiatry* 50:1375, 1987.

166. Safwat AM, Reitan JA, Misle GR et al: Use of propranolol to control rate-pressure product during cardiac anesthesia, *Anesth Analg* 60:732, 1981.

167. Sahar A, Tsipstein E: Effects of mannitol and furosemide on the rate of formation of cerebrospinal fluid, *Experimental Neurology* 60:584, 1978.

168. Samra SK, Kroll DA: Subarachnoid hemorrhage and intraoperative electrocardiographic changes simulating myocardial ischemia: anesthesiologist's dilemma, *Anesth Analg* 64:86, 1985.

169. Schramm J, Koht A, Schmidt G et al: Surgical and electrophysiological observations during clipping of 134 aneurysms with evoked potential monitoring, *Neurosurgery* 26:61, 1990.

170. Scudmore JH, Moir JC: Rupture of an intracranial aneurysm during pregnancy, *J Obstet Gynaecol Br Commonwealth* 73:1019, 1966.

171. Seiler RW, Grolimund P, Aaslid R et al: Cerebral vasospasm evaluated by transcranial ultrasound correlated with clinical grade and CT-visualized subarachnoid hemorrhage, *J Neurosurg* 64:594, 1986.

172. Shapiro MH: Intracranial hypertension: therapeutic and anesthetic considerations, *Anesthesiology* 43:445, 1975.

173. Shapiro MH: Barbiturates in brain ischaemia, *Br J Anaesth* 57:82, 1985.

174. Shibuya M, Suzuki Y, Sugita K et al: Effect of AT877 on cerebral vasospasm after aneurysmal subarachnoid hemorrhage: results of a prospective placebo-controlled double-blind trial, *J Neurosurg* 76:571, 1992.

175. Shupak RC, Harp JR: Comparison between high-dose sufentanil-oxygen and high-dose fentanyl-oxygen for neuroanesthesia, *Br J Anaesth* 57:375, 1985.

176. Silverberg G, Reitz B, Ream A: Hypothermia and cardiac arrest in the treatment of giant aneurysms of the cerebral circulation and hemangioblastoma of the medulla, *J Neurosurg* 55:337, 1981.

177. Smith M, Ray CT: Cardiac-arrhythmias, increased intracranial pressure, and the autonomic nervous system, *Chest* 61:125, 1972.

178. Sokoll MD, Kassell NF, Davies LR: Large dose thiopental anesthesia for intracranial aneurysm surgery, *Neurosurgery* 10:555, 1982.

179. Solomon RA, Fink ME, Lennihan L: Early aneurysm surgery and prophylactic hypervolemic hypertensive therapy for the treatment of aneurysmal subarachnoid hemorrhage, *Neurosurgery* 23:699, 1988.

180. Solomon RA, Fink ME, Lennihan L: Prophylactic volume expansion therapy for the prevention of delayed cerebral ischemia after early aneurysm surgery: results of a preliminary trial, *Arch Neurol* 45:325, 1988.

181. Solomon RA, Onesti ST, Klebanoff L: Relationship between the timing of aneurysm surgery and the development of delayed cerebral ischemia, *J Neurosurg* 75:56, 1991.

182. Solomon RA, Post KD, McMurtry III JG: Depression of circulating blood volume in patients after subarachnoid hemorrhage: implications for the management of symptomatic vasospasm, *Neurosurgery* 15:354, 1984.

183. Solomon RA, Smith CR, Raps EC et al: Deep hypothermic circulatory arrest for the management of complex anterior and posterior circulation aneurysms, *Neurosurgery* 29:732, 1991.

184. Sperry RJ, Bailey PL, Reichman MV et al: Fentanyl and sufentanil increase intracranial pressure in head trauma patients, *Anesthesiology* 77:416, 1992.

185. Spetzler RF, Hadley MN, Rigamonti D et al: Aneurysms of the basilar artery treated with circulatory arrest, hypothermia, and barbiturate cerebral protection, *J Neurosurg* 68:868, 1988.

186. Steen PA, Michenfelder JD: Barbiturate protection in tolerant and nontolerant hypoxic mice: comparison with hypothermic protection, *Anesthesiology* 50:404, 1979.

187. Steen PA, Milde JH, Michenfelder JD: No barbiturate protection in a dog model of complete cerebral ischemia, *Ann Neurol* 5:343, 1979.

188. Steen PA, Newberg L, Milde JH et al: Hypothermia and barbiturates: individual and combined effects on canine cerebral oxygen consumption, *Anesthesiology* 58:527, 1983.

189. Stirt JA, Grosslight KR, Bedford RF et al: Defasciculation with metocurine prevents succinylcholine-induced increases in intracranial pressure, *Anesthesiology* 67:50, 1987.

190. Stoyka WW, Schutz H: The cerebral response to sodium nitroprusside and trimethaphan controlled hypotension, *Can Anaesth Soc J* 22:275, 1975.

191. Stullken EH, Balestrieri FJ, Prough DS et al: The hemodynamic effects of nimodipine in patients anesthetized for cerebral aneurysm clipping, *Anesthesiology* 62:346, 1985.

192. Stullken EH, Johnston WE, Prough DS et al: Implications of nimodipine prophylaxis of cerebral vasospasm on anesthetic management during intracranial aneurysm clipping, *J Neurosurg* 62:200, 1985.

193. Sullivan HG, Keenan RL, Isrow L et al: The critical importance of P_{aCO_2} during intracranial aneurysm surgery, *J Neurosurg* 52:426, 1980.

194. Sundt TM, Kobayashi S, Fode NC et al: Results and complications of surgical management of 809 intracranial aneurysms in 722 cases related and unrelated to grade of patient, type of aneurysm, and timing of surgery, *J Neurosurg* 56:753, 1982.

195. Sundt TM, Pluth JR, Gronert GA: Excision of giant basilar aneurysm under profound hypothermia: report of a case, *Mayo Clin Proc* 47:631, 1972.

196. Sundt TM, Sharbrough FW, Piepgras DG et al: Correlation of cerebral blood flow and electroencephalographic changes during carotid endarterectomy with results of surgery and hemodynamics of cerebral ischemia, *Mayo Clin Proc* 56:533, 1981.

197. Suzuki J: Temporary occlusion of trunk arteries of the brain during surgery. In Suzuki J, editor: *Treatment of cerebral infarction: experimental and clinical study*, New York, 1987, Springer-Verlag.

198. Suzuki J, Komada N, Homma M: New clips and flexible clip forceps for neurosurgery. In Suzuki J, editor: *Cerebral aneurysms*, Tokyo, 1979, Neuron.

199. Suzuki J, Onuma T, Yoshimoto T: Results of early operation on cerebral aneurysms, *Surg Neurol* 11:407, 1979.

200. Suzuki J, Yoshimoto T: The effect of mannitol in prolongation of permissible occlusion time of cerebral arteries: clinical data of aneurysm surgery. In Suzuki J, editor: *Cerebral aneurysms*, Tokyo, 1979, Neuron.

201. Symon L, Vajda J: Surgical experiences with giant intracranial aneurysms, *J Neurosurg* 61:1009, 1984.

202. Symon L, Wang AD, Costa E et al: Perioperative use of somatosensory evoked responses in aneurysm surgery, *J Neurosurg* 60:269, 1984.

203. Taneda M: Effect of early operation for ruptured aneurysms on prevention of delayed ischemic symptoms, *J Neurosurg* 57:622, 1982.

204. Templehoff R, Modica PA, Jellish WS et al: Resistance to atracurium-induced neuromuscular blockade in patients with intractable seizure disorders on chronic anticonvultant therapy, *Anesth Analg* 71:665, 1990.

205. Tempelhoff R, Modica PA, Rich KM et al: Use of computerized electroencephalographic monitoring during aneurysm surgery, *J Surgery* 71:24, 1989.

206. Tempelhoff R, Modica PA, Spitnagel EL: Anticonvulsant therapy increases fentanyl requirements during anesthesia for craniotomy, *Can J Anaesth* 37:327, 1990.

207. Tenjin H, Hirakawa K, Mizukawa N et al: Dysautoregulation in patients with ruptured aneurysms: cerebral blood flow measurements obtained during surgery by a temperature-controlled thermoelectrical method, *Neurosurgery* 23:705, 1988.

208. Tettenborn D, Dycka J: Prevention and treatment of delayed ischemic dysfunction in patients with aneurysmal subarachnoid hemorrhage, *Stroke* 21(suppl IV):85, 1990.

209. Thomas AN, Anderton JM, Harper NJN: Anaesthesia for the treatment of a giant cerebral aneurysm under hypothermic circulatory arrest: case report, *Anaesthesia* 45:383, 1990.

210. Trindle MR, Dodson BA, Rampil IJ: Effects of fentanyl versus sufentanil in equianesthetic doses on middle cerebral artery blood flow velocity, *Anesthesiology* 78:454, 1993.

211. Tsementzis SA, Hitchcock ER: Outcome from "rescue clipping" of ruptured intracranial aneurysms during induction anaesthesia and endotracheal intubation, *J Neurol Neurosurg Psychiatry* 48:160, 1985.

212. Unni VKN, Johnston RA, Young HSA et al: Prevention of intracranial hypertension during laryngoscopy and endotracheal intubation: use of a second dose of thiopentone, *Br J Anaesth* 56:1219, 1984.

213. Van Gijn J, Hijdra A, Wijdicks EF et al: Acute hydrocephalus after aneurysmal hemorrhage, *J Neurosurg* 63:355, 1985.

214. Van Hemelrijck J, Fitch W, Mattheussen M et al: Effect of propofol on cerebral circulation and autoregulation in the baboon, *Anesth Analg* 71:49, 1990.

215. Vermulen M, Lindsay KW, Murray GD et al: Antifibrinolytic treatment in subarachnoid hemorrhage, *N Engl J Med* 311:432, 1984.

216. Vidal B, Dergal E, Cesarman E et al:

Cardiac arrhythmias associated with subarachnoid hemorrhage: prospective study, *Neurosurgery* 5:675, 1979.

217. Voldby B, Enevoldsen EM: Intracranial pressure changes following aneurysm rupture. I. Clinical and angiographic correlations, *J Neurosurg* 56:186, 1982.

218. Voldby B, Enevoldsen EM, Jensen FT: Cerebrovascular reactivity in patients with ruptured intracranial aneurysms, *J Neurosurg* 62:59, 1985.

219. Warner DS, Sokoll MD, Maktabi M et al: Nicardipine HCL: clinical experience in patients undergoing anaesthesia for intracranial aneurysm clipping, *Can J Anaesth* 36:219, 1989.

220. Weinstabl C, Mayer N, Richling B et al: Effect of sufentanil on intracranial pressure in neurosurgical patients, *Anaesthesia* 46:837, 1991.

221. Weinstabl C, Mayer N, Spiss CK: Sufentanil decreases cerebral blood flow velocity in patients with elevated intracranial pressure, *Ger J Anaesthesiol* 9:481, 1992.

222. Weintraub BM, McHenry LC: Cardiac abnormalities in subarachnoid hemorrhage: a resume, *Stroke* 5:384, 1974.

223. White JC, Parker SD, Rogers M: Preanesthetic evaluation of a patient with pathologic Q waves following subarachnoid hemorrhage, *Anesthesiology* 62:351, 1985.

224. Wijdicks EFM, Vermeulen M, Hijdra A et al: Hyponatremia and cerebral infarction in patients with ruptured intracranial aneurysms: is fluid restriction harmful? *Ann Neurol* 17:137, 1985.

225. Wijdicks EFM, Vermeulen M, ten Haaf JA et al: Volume depletion and natriuresis in patients with a ruptured intracranial aneurysm, *Ann Neurol* 18:211, 1985.

226. Wilkins RH: Attempted prevention or treatment of intracranial arterial spasm: an update, *Neurosurgery* 18:808, 1986.

227. Williams MD, Rainer WG, Fieger HG et al: Cardiopulmonary bypass, profound hypothermia, and circulatory arrest for neurosurgery, *Ann Thorac Surg* 52:1063, 1991.

228. Willoughby JS: Sodium nitroprusside, pregnancy and multiple intracranial aneurysms, *Anaesth Intensive Care* 12:358, 1984.

229. Wood JM, Kee DB: Hemorrheology of the cerebral circulation in stroke, *Stroke* 16:765, 1985.

230. Woodhall B, Sealy WC, Hall KD et al: Craniotomy under conditions of quinidine-protected cardioplegia and profound hypothermia, *Ann Surg* 152:37, 1960.

231. Yoshimoto T, Sakamoto T, Watanabe T et al: Experimental cerebral infarction. III. Protective effect of mannitol in thalamic infarction in dogs, *Stroke* 9:217, 1978.

232. Yoshimoto T, Suzuki J: Intracranial definitive aneurysm surgery under normothermia and normotension-utilizing temporary occlusion of major cerebral arteries and pre-operative mannitol administration, *Neurol Surg (Tokyo)* 4:775, 1976.

233. Zabramski JM, Spetzler RF, Lee KS et al: Phase I trial of tissue plasminogen activator for the prevention of vasospasm in patients with aneurysmal subarachnoid hemorrhage, *J Neurosurg* 75:189, 1991.

APPENDIX 1

Protocol For Circulatory Arrest

1. Place intraarterial and large-bore intravenous catheters before induction of anesthesia. The usual precautions for induction of anesthesia in patients with a cerebral aneurysm apply.
2. Once anesthesia is induced and the trachea intubated, place the following: either a central venous line or pulmonary artery catheter, a second intraarterial catheter to allow phlebotomy, a lumbar subarachnoid drain, electrophysiologic monitors (EEG and/or SSEP), and both nasopharyngeal and esophageal temperature probes. Anticipate periods of stimulation such as tracheal intubation, head pinning, and periosteal retraction, which can cause hypertension.
3. Begin surface cooling by using a cooling blanket and lowering the room temperature. The rate of decrease should proceed at approximately 0.2° C/min.
4. If barbiturates are to be used, administer a 3 to 5 mg/kg bolus of thiopental to induce either a burst suppression pattern at a 1:5 ratio (i.e., time period in burst relative to electrical silence) or an isoelectric EEG. This can be followed by a continuous infusion of thiopental at 0.1 to 0.5 mg/kg/min. Once cooling begins, the infusion is continued at this rate for the entire period on cardiopulmonary bypass.
5. Hemodilute to a hematocrit of 28% to 30% by collecting blood into an anticoagulant solution kept at room temperature. Maintain intravascular volume with up to 4 L of cold intravenous saline containing potassium chloride (4 to 6 mEq/L).
6. After the aneurysm is dissected and hemostasis obtained, extracorporeal circulation via femoral artery–femoral vein bypass is begun when the patient's temperature reaches 34° C. Just before initiating bypass, ensure surgical hemostasis and then give heparin, 300

to 400 IU/kg, to maintain the ACT between 450 and 480 seconds.
7. Cool the patient to between 18° and 22° C. Be aware of ECG changes; at 28° C the myocardium is extremely irritable and may fibrillate continuously. Fibrillation should be stopped with 40 to 80 mEq of potassium chloride, but if fibrillation is persistent, cardiovert with 100 to 250 watts/sec.
8. Circulatory arrest occurs between 15° and 18° C and should be limited to the period of clip application. The EEG should be isoelectric before arrest. If barbiturates were not used earlier, they may be added at this point to achieve a silent EEG. Elevate the patient's head slightly to facilitate venous drainage, keeping in mind that this position increases the potential risk of air embolism and no-reflow phenomenon in small vessels.
9. Once the aneurysm is clipped, bypass is reestablished and the patient is rewarmed at a rate of 0.2° to 0.5° C/min. Too rapid rewarming can cause tissue acidosis and hypoxia. Sodium nitroprusside may be used to allow a more homogeneous rewarming.
10. With rewarming, the heart will fibrillate. Cardiovert with 200 to 400 joules through external defibrillating pads. Antiarrhythmic drugs may be required to restore a normal sinus rhythm. In addition, the patient may require inotropic support.
11. Extracorporeal circulation is discontinued when the patient's temperature is 34° C and the heart can maintain a normal cardiac output and sinus rhythm.
12. The ACT is corrected to 100 and 150 seconds with protamine sulfate. The autologous blood containing platelet-rich plasma is transfused. Other blood products may be necessary to restore hemostasis.

19

Interventional Neuroradiology and the Anesthetic Management of Patients with Arteriovenous Malformations

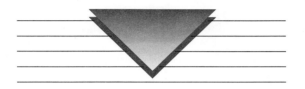

BARBARA A. DODSON

CEREBRAL ARTERIOVENOUS MALFORMATIONS

Patients with cerebral arteriovenous malformations (AVMs) have, in the past, been treated with minimal surgical intervention because many thought that these lesions carried unacceptable surgical risks.[21,22] However, with the development of microsurgical techniques in the 1960s and the explosive use of adjunct endovascular embolization procedures in the 1980s, many patients can now have surgical resection of lesions previously considered inoperable.*

Cerebral arteriovascular malformations belong to a group of vascular abnormalities that involve the central nervous system. This group includes capillary telangiectasias, venous malformations, cavernous angiomas, and classic arteriovenous malformations.[60,91]

Capillary telangiectasias occur deep in the brain parenchyma, often in the brainstem. They are usually associated with the Weber-Osler disorder and are thought to have little clinical significance.[76] Venous malformations are composed of anomalous medullary veins that converge in a centrally located dilated trunk, giving them a characteristic "caput medusae" angiographic appearance.[101] The surrounding brain parenchyma is normal. Their clinical significance remains controversial, and catastrophic infarction of normal brain can occur with resection of the malformation. Therefore surgical removal is generally not recommended.[78] Cavernous angiomas may compose a subtype of AVMs. They are distinguished from classic AVMs by the presence of dilated sinusoidal channels, which form the majority of these lesions. They are rare, reportedly less than 1% of all intracranial vascular lesions and 15% of all cerebral vascular

---

*References 3, 39, 70, 87, 95, 103, 110.

malformations.[60,77,105,107] The most common presentation is seizure. Unlike the classic AVM, approximately 25% of patients with cavernous angiomas become symptomatic during the first 2 decades of life. There are two forms, sporadic and familial. The familial form is transmitted in an autosomal dominant fashion, with an increased frequency in a Hispanic population.[77]

Classic AVMs are generally congenital in origin, arising early in fetal life during the development of primitive vasculature into arteries, veins, and capillaries (this occurs at approximately 3 weeks gestation). During this period direct arterial-to-venous communications develop without an intervening capillary bed. Initially, only arteries within the zone of abnormal shunting are involved in the AVM. However, as blood flow through the lesion gradually increases because of the decreased resistance of the shunt, the feeding arteries and draining vein also increase. The high-flow, low-resistance shunt may be sufficient to divert flow from other hemispheric or counterhemispheric areas through enlarging collaterals. This process increases the size of the AVM and produces clinical symptoms. The degree and rate with which these vascular changes occur depend on the original characteristics of the embryonic AVM.[51]

Anatomic Features

There are four anatomic components to an AVM: the nidus, the arterial feeders, the arterial collaterals, and the venous outflow.[59] The nidus is that portion of an AVM containing the plexus of abnormal arterial-to-venous connections. These are thin-walled vessels, lacking in normal smooth muscle and elastic laminae,[60] and it may be histologically impossible to differentiate arteries from veins. Normal brain parenchyma is largely replaced by this tight cluster of abnormal vessels, and the actual margins of the nidus may be difficult to define. Although these vessels are usually small, in some AVMs there may be one to several large fistulae. As will be discussed, these fistulae can constitute a large arterial-to-venous shunt, sufficient to produce cerebral and/or systemic effects. The major vascular supply to the AVM is the arterial feeders. They are usually pial in origin, arising most commonly from the middle cerebral artery. However, some AVMs have feeding arteries of dural origin. The high-flow low-resistance shunt in the nidus is also capable of recruiting additional arterial vessels, which serve as collaterals and increase flow. Venous outflow channels then drain into superficial and/or deep draining veins.

The vast majority (70% to 90%) of AVMs are supertentorial[61,72] (Fig. 19-1). Approximately 10% occur in the posterior fossa. AVMs can also occur intracerebrally, with approximately 18% occurring within the basal ganglia or internal capsule. Dural AVMs or fistulae are relatively rare, making up 10% to 15% of all intracranial AVMs. These most frequently involve the cavernous, transverse, or sigmoid sinus.[2] Dural AV fistulae can present with a wide range of clinical symptoms, depending on their location and

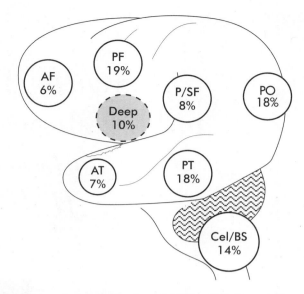

FIG. 19-1 Anatomic location of AVMs: This figure indicates the location of AVMs as a percentage of angiographically demonstrable intraparenchymal AVMs (n = 280 patients). *AF*, anterofrontal; *PF*, posterofrontal; *AT*, anterotemporal; *PT*, posterotemporal; *P/SF*, parietal/Sylvian fissure; *PO*, parietooccipital; *Cel/BS*, cellebellum/brainstem. Percentages in deep structures include 3% in basal ganglia, 4% in corpus collosum, and 3% intraventricular. (*Modified from Piepgras DG, Sundt TJ, Ragoowansi AT et al:* J Neurosurg 78:5-11, 1993.)

venous drainage. Many are asymptomatic or present with a bruit or headache. Others, however, particularly those involving the transverse or sigmoid sinuses, are particularly prone to hemorrhage. AVMs can also occur within the neural elements of the spine. They can occur as either intramedullary or perimedullary AVMs or dural fistulae.

Sometimes an AVM is referred to as *cryptic*. Cryptic AVMs or cryptic vascular malformations constitute a group of angiographically invisible cerebrovascular and spinovascular lesions that are capable of both bleeding and inducing seizure. Features common to cryptic vascular malformations include a collection of abnormal vessels that are invisible angiographically but that have typical or highly suggestive characteristics on T_1-weighted and T_2-weighted magnetic resonance images (MR).[107]

There is a 4% to 10% incidence of aneurysms associated with AVMs.[16,72,92] The majority of these aneurysms are located on AVM arterial feeding vessels. The aneurysms associated with AVMs can occur within the nidus (sometimes called pseudoaneurysms) and in the feeding arteries either at typical bifurcation sites or at atypical sites. Three theories have been proposed to explain the coexistence of these two different neurovascular lesions. The first is coincidence. The second invokes a generalized vascular maldevelopment leading to two congenital abnormalities. The third and most popular theory is that increased flow through the AVM leads to aneurysm formation.[16] Feeding artery aneurysms are a frequent source of AVM hemorrhage. They may require surgical clipping before embolization and removal of the AVM, particularly if they are a source of hemorrhage.[109] It has been noted that, unlike the usual natural history of intracranial aneurysm, many of these aneurysms resolve after AVM resection. Nevertheless, the coexistence of an aneurysm and an AVM should be a consideration when formulating an anesthetic plan.

Most AVMs produce high-flow, low-resistance shunts with mean transmural pressures that are 45% to 60% of the systemic mean arterial blood pressure (MAP). Measurements have shown pressures in arterial feeding vessels to be uniformly less than systemic pressure, ranging from 40 to 80 mm Hg.[66,87] The shunts through the AVM can be large enough to induce secondary systemic effects, such as congestive heart failure (CHF) or cerebral ischemia. Although CHF is a relatively rare presentation in adults, it is a frequent initial presentation in infants with AVMs of the vein of Galen and a common cause of mortality in these cases.[40,58,63] The more common clinical effect of large shunts in adults is the development of cerebral ischemia with secondary neurologic deficits. This will be discussed in more detail following.

Clinical Presentation

Most patients with an AVM develop symptoms some time between their third and fifth decades of life (i.e., 20 to 40 years old). Less than 10% of patients with symptomatic lesions are under 10 years old.[51] Approximately 80% of all patients with an AVM develop symptoms by the time they are 40 years old. The incidence of initial symptoms declines after the age of 50, and approximately 20% of all AVMs are clinically asymptomatic.[53] This number will probably decrease in the future with the increasing use of computed tomography (CT) and MR scans.

The most common initial presentation is spontaneous hemorrhage. It occurs in approximately 50% of lesions and is the initial presentation in 80% of patients.[16,26,51,65] The ongoing risk of hemorrhage is approximately 1% to 3% per year, and the risk of recurrent hemorrhage is 6% in the first year and 2% to 4% thereafter.[16,26,51,65] Hemorrhage usually appears in patients between 10 and 35 years old and decreases with increasing age. AVM features that have been associated, in some studies, with a higher risk of hemorrhage include small size, location, and high hemodynamic resistance or shunt resistance.[16,31]

The second-most-common clinical presentation is seizures. The incidence of patients with AVMs presenting with seizures without clinical evidence of hemorrhage ranges from 17% to 40% in most published series.[19,72] In general, the seizure pattern appears to be correlated with the location of the AVM. Frontal lobe AVMs generally present with generalized seizures without aura, temporal lobe AVMs with complex partial seizures progressing to generalized seizures, and parietal or occipital AVMs with simple par-

tial seizures.[49] AVMs involving the posterofrontal and temporal lobes are more likely to present with seizures as compared with AVMs overall.[19,20,73] However, the epileptic foci may be distal to the AVM location. Surgical intervention for AVMs associated with seizures has been controversial. Several studies suggest an increase rather than a decrease in seizure frequency after AVM surgery.[19,20,29] Indeed, Foy et al.[29] reported a 50% incidence of seizures after AVM surgery, as compared with a 17% incidence for patients undergoing a supratentorial craniotomy. However, recent studies suggest that the vast majority of patients with multiple preoperative seizures had significant improvement in their seizure frequency postoperatively[37,73,111,112] (Fig. 19-2). In an analysis of 280 patients, Piepgras et al.[73] found a significant reduction in seizure frequency and improvement in neurologic recovery in patients who underwent resection of their AVMs. Although some patients without a prior history of seizures can develop seizures postoperatively, the incidence of late postoperative seizures appears to be low, approximately 7%, and these seizures can be well controlled with medication.[37,73,111,112]

Severe headaches, often described as migrainelike, are another common clinical presentation.[32] Although the origin of the headaches is unknown, increased intracranial pressure secondary to the increased blood flow shunting through the lesion is thought to play a substantial role.[9,17]

Increasing neurologic deficits are also a presenting feature of AVMs. Indeed, some patients' initial presentation may be increased intracranial pressure.[9,17] Others may present with symptoms suggestive of transient or progressive ischemic deficits.[28,47,53] The high-flow, low-resistance nature of the AVM can shunt a large volume of CBF away from the higher-resistance capillary bed of the surrounding normal brain. In time, CBF in the surrounding area can decrease, resulting in hypoperfusion and cerebral ischemia in surrounding brain regions.[83] Feidel and Perot coined the term "steal" to describe the absent or delayed angiographic perfusion of tissue surrounding an AVM.[28] Angiographic steal may be present in patients with no evidence of clinical steal. There is a significant correlation between AVM size, peripheral venous drainage, development of arterial collaterals, and the clinical symptoms of steal.[56]

Unlike aneurysms, there appears to be little correlation between chronic or acute hypertension and spontaneous hemorrhage for AVMs. In an analysis of 545 patients, hemorrhage occurred during sleep in 36% of the patients, compared with an incidence of less than 25% during traditional high-systemic-pressure activities such as heavy lifting, straining while defecating, coitus, or "emotional distress."[72] Szabo et al.[97] in a combined prospective/retrospective study found no incidence of hemorrhage in awake patients undergoing radiosurgery for AVM obliteration despite a documented 30% increase in systemic arterial pressure during application of the stereotactic head frame.

Some investigators have suggested an increase in hemorrhage from AVM during pregnancy. Intracranial hemor-

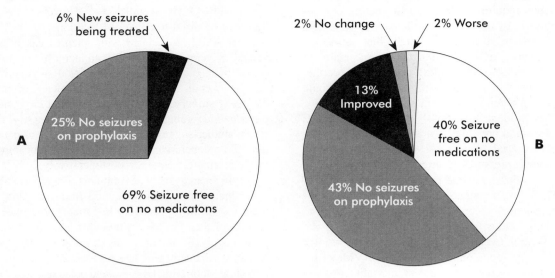

FIG. 19-2   Incidence of postoperative seizures in patients undergoing total resection of AVM. **A,** Patients (n = 136) who had no preoperative seizure history. **B,** Patients (n = 102) with history of preoperative seizures. *(Modified from Piepras DG, Sundt TJ, Ragoowansi AT et al:* J Neurosurg *78:5-11, 1993.)*

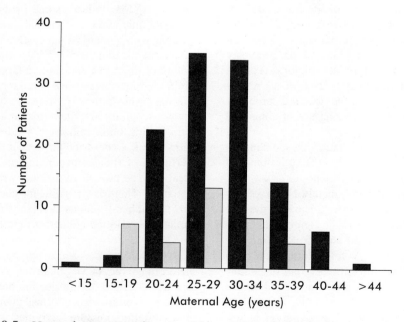

FIG. 19-3   Maternal age at time of intracranial hemorrhage during pregnancy: this figure demonstrates the age distribution for patients presenting with an intracranial hemorrhage during pregnancy from either an aneurysmal rupture *(closed bars;* n = 118) or an AVM bleeding *(stippled bars;* n = 36). This distribution is similar to that for the general population with respect to age at time of initial hemorrhage. *(Modified from Dias MS, Sekhar LN:* Neurosurgery *27:855-866, 1990.)*

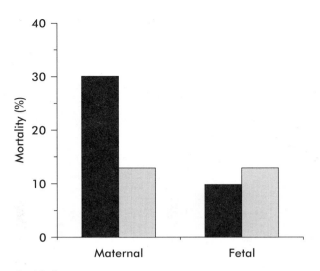

FIG. 19-4 Effect of obstetric management on outcome after AVM hemorrhage: this figure shows the maternal and fetal mortality (in percent) associated with vaginal delivery *(closed bars)* or cesarean section *(stippled bars)* in patients with hemorrhage from an AVM. There are no statistically significant differences in either fetal or maternal outcomes between the two obstetric techniques. *(Modified from Dias MS, Sekhar LN:* Neurosurgery *27:855-866, 1990.)*

BOX 19-1

CLINICAL AND ANGIOGRAPHIC RISK FACTORS PREDICTING AN AGGRESSIVE CLINICAL COURSE

History of progressive neurologic deficits, not caused by seizure and/or hemorrhage, suggesting cerebral ischemia secondary to cerebral steal from the AVM
Size greater than 4 to 5 cm
Age greater than 40 years
AVM within 2 to 3 cm of internal carotid artery
Angiographic indications of diversion of blood flow to AVM from areas in contralateral hemisphere distal from AVM (e.g., angiographic steal)
Blood supply to the AVM by leptomeningeal collaterals via the external carotid system
Poor angiographic filling of the arterial bed within 2 cm of the AVM margin
AVM filling from two or three major arterial feeders rather than multiple small arterial feeders

Modified from Young WL, Prohovnik L, Ornstein E et al: *Neurosurgery* 27:257-266, 1990.

---

rhage (ICH) can be a grave complication of pregnancy, occurring in 0.01% to 0.05% of all pregnancies. Although rare, ICH accounts for 5% to 12% of all maternal deaths.[7,25,41,79,80] Between 23% and 50% of intracranial hemorrhages occurring during pregnancy were the result of a ruptured AVM. In a widely quoted study by Robinson et al.,[79] risk for AVM hemorrhage during pregnancy was placed at 87%. However, other investigators found no increased risk for initial hemorrhage or rebleeding in pregnant women without a previous hemorrhage compared with the general population of patients with unruptured AVMs.[41,80] Distribution of these lesion follows that for the general population, with a peak incidence in the 20-to-40 age group (Fig. 19-3). Some investigators believe there is an increase in the frequency of AVM rupture during the second and third trimester, coinciding with the rise in cardiac output,[80] although others have found no relationship between period of gestation and hemorrhage.[41] In most neurosurgical practices, patients with unruptured AVMs and stable posthemorrhage patients are allowed to reach term with excision of the AVM performed electively after delivery.[7,25,41,79,80] The method of delivery, vaginal vs. cesarean section, appears to have no influence on either fetal or maternal outcome[25] (Fig. 19-4). Therefore the method of delivery should be based on obstetric rather than neurosurgical considerations.

Outcome

Because AVM transmural pressure is less than the transmural pressure in aneurysms, rupture is usually less devas-

tating. However, spontaneous hemorrhage still has a high morbidity and mortality. Reports on the mortality associated with initial hemorrhage range from 10% to 29% and increase with each bleeding episode.[16,31,72] The rate of serious morbidity (i.e., neurologic deficits) varies from 23% to 80% for each hemorrhagic episode.[38,106] Indications for surgical resection of AVMs have traditionally been hemorrhage, intractable epilepsy, and progressive neurologic deficits. Unruptured AVMs were originally thought to be relatively benign lesions, and most believed that surgical risks outweighed the natural history of the lesions. However, more recent studies have shown that unruptured AVMs represent a major threat for patients less than 50 years old, with a combined mortality and serious morbidity rate of 35% to 50% over 15 to 20 years.[16,38] Therefore, together with improved surgical outcomes from the use of microsurgical and endovascular techniques, a more aggressive neurosurgical stance has developed toward the excision of unruptured AVMs.

Certain clinical and angiographic features appear to be risk factors in the development of an aggressive neurologic course, where the term *aggressive neurologic course* is defined as hemorrhage or progressive focal neurologic deficits other than ophthalmoplegia (Box 19-1). In particular, AVMs with meningeal venous drainage, variceal or aneurysmal venous dilations, and/or galenic drainage appear to pose significant risks for an aggressive clinical course.[5] Dural AVMs of the anterior cranial fossa appear particularly prone to present as massive ICH.[57] Smaller AVMs appear to be at greater risk for hemorrhage than larger lesions.[19,31,85] In general, smaller AVMs have higher perfusion pressure in their feeding vessels than larger AVMs, and perfusion pressure within the AVM rather than blood volume within the AVM nidus is thought to be the primary factor in the development of bleeding.[85]

Great Vein of Galen Malformations

Vein of Galen malformations are congenital neurovascular lesions consisting of connections between intracerebral vessels and the great vein of Galen or the adjacent midline middle cerebral vein. The arterial feeders usually arise from the anterior and posterior choroidal vessels, thalamoperforators, and pericallosal branches of the anterior cerebral arteries.[48] There can be multiple, small connections or large fistulae between the arterial feeders and the vein of Galen or middle cerebral vein. Patients with vein of Galen malformations fall into three groups according to their clinical presentation: neonates with intractable congestive heart failure at birth, infants who present with hydrocephalus and seizures, and older children with hemorrhage as their presenting symptom.[30] The vast majority of patients with vein of Galen malformations present while neonates. These lesions have the largest shunt, the poorest prognosis, and are nearly always fatal without treatment.[40,63] Surgical treatment with ligation of the fistulae has been disappointing and has an extremely high mortality rate.[43,58] However, embolization can produce a marked reduction of the shunt and has emerged as a promising palliative treatment that allows the neonate to grow to a size and age where more definitive treatment can be safely undertaken.[18,27]

Anatomic Grading Systems

Several grading systems have been advanced for estimating the surgical risk for AVM resection.[86,89,98] Features that influence outcome include:

- Size: A number of studies have shown that the smaller the AVM, particularly less than 3 cm, the better the outcome (Fig. 19-5). Technically, the ability to perform a total resection is higher with smaller AVMs.
- Location: Resection of AVMs located in deep structures such as the basal ganglia, corpus callosum, and walls of lateral ventricles have a poorer outcome than resection of AVMs in more superficial locations.
- The number and origin of feeding arteries: A poorer outcome is associated with both an increased number of feeding arteries and the number of different systems feeding the AVM (i.e., feeders from anterior, middle, or posterior cerebral arteries; anterior or posterior choroidal arteries; lenticulostriate or thalamoperforating arteries; and superior, anterior inferior, or posterior inferior cerebellar arteries).
- The pattern of venous drainage draining vessels—superficial vs. deep: Venous drainage is considered superficial if the AVM drains through the cortical venous system. A deep venous drainage is one where any of the drainage is through deep veins such as the internal cerebral veins, basal vein, or precentral cerebellar vein and is associated with a poorer outcome.

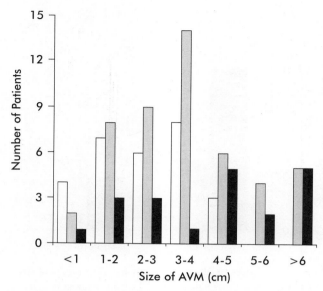

FIG. 19-5 Surgical outcome as a function of AVM size. There is a good correlation between the size of an AVM (in cm) and the surgical outcome. The *open bars* represent excellent outcomes, the *stippled bars* good-to-fair outcomes, and the *closed bars* poor outcomes at time of discharge from the hospital. Outcomes clearly are better for AVMs of less than 4 cm. *(Modified from Tamaki N, Ebara K, Lin T et al:* Neurosurgery 29:856-861, 1991.)

TABLE 19-1

Grading System of Spetzler and Martin for Arteriovenous Malformations

Graded Feature	Points Assigned
AVM Size	
Small (<3 cm)	1
Medium (3-6 cm)	2
Large (>6 cm)	3
Eloquence* of Adjacent Brain	
Noneloquent	0
Eloquent	1
Pattern of Venous Drainage	
Superficial only	0
Deep	1

Grade = Size + Eloquence + Venous Drainage

Examples:
Grade 1: small, noneloquent, superficial drainage
1 + 0 + 0 = 1

Grade 5: large, eloquent areas involved, deep venous drainage
3 + 1 + 1 = 5

*See text for definition.
From Spetzler RF, Martin NA: *J Neurosurg* 65:476-483, 1986.

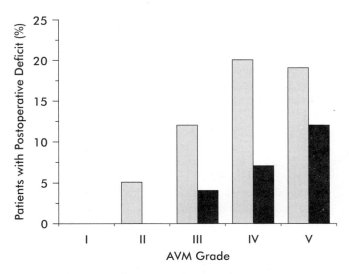

FIG. 19-6 Surgical outcome after AVM resection as function of grade of AVM. This figure demonstrates the surgical outcome of 100 patients as a function of the severity of their AVM using the grading system of Spetzler and Martin (see Table 19-1). There is a good correlation between degree of major *(closed bars)* and minor *(stippled bars)* deficits and the preoperative grade of the AVM. *(Modified from Spetzler RF, Martin NA:* J Neurosurg *65:476-483, 1986.)*

- Eloquent vs. noneloquent location of AVM: An eloquent brain area is defined as a region with a readily identifiable neurologic function whose injury would result in a disabling neurologic deficit. Eloquent areas include cerebral cortex (motor, sensory, language, and visual areas), thalamus, hypothalamus, internal capsule, brainstem, deep cerebellar nuclei, and cerebellar peduncles. Clearly, removal of an AVM adjacent to eloquent areas has a much higher risk of postoperative neurologic morbidity than resection from noneloquent areas. Damage to these structures may occur intraoperatively during retraction and resection or postoperatively from edema or hemorrhage.
- Degree of steal from adjacent brain.
- The rate of flow through the lesion.

Of these six factors, the most important appear to be size, pattern of venous drainage, and eloquence of the surrounding area. Most neurosurgeons use the grading system of Spetzler and Martin in assessing surgical risk for resection (Table 19-1).[86] There appears to be a good correlation between AVM grading with this system and postoperative neurologic complications[89] (Fig. 19-6).

TREATMENT
Conservative

Surgical treatment of an AVM is generally indicated if the risk of operation is less than the risk from nonoperative treatment. Certain extremely large, diffuse AVMs that are dispersed through eloquent brain areas or AVMs whose ni-

dus encompasses vital brain areas such as the brainstem or hypothalamus are often considered inoperable (grade 6). Because surgical resection of these lesions carries a very high risk of death or totally disabling deficits, conservative treatment is often advocated.[37] However, the use of radiosurgery and/or endovascular embolization also has been advocated as palliative and possibly definitive treatment for these lesions.[23]

Radiation Therapy

Radiosurgery has been used in the treatment of AVMs not amenable to surgical resection. Small AVMs in critical locations, such as the basal ganglia or posterior fossa, considered unsuitable for surgical excision because of unacceptable risks for developing profound neurologic deficits, are the lesions most frequently referred for radiosurgery. Radiation can induce fibrosis in the irradiated vessels, resulting in a gradual obliteration of the vessel lumen.[94]

Conventional radiation was used in the past for the treatment of symptomatic AVMs. However, it is ineffective and is no longer in current use.[68] At present, stereotactic radiosurgery of AVMs is performed using the Cobalt-60 gamma knife,[23,55] megavoltage linear accelerator-based radiosurgery,[14] or Bragg peak proton beams.[46,93] The role of radiosurgery in the treatment of AVMs remains controversial. Some neurosurgeons believe radiosurgery alone is totally ineffective for treating AVMs. The best results occur in small inoperative lesions. Lunsford et al.[55] reported a 2-year obliteration rate of greater than 85% for lesions less than 4 cm in size. Radiation may be useful as an adjunct for larger AVMs. However, the rebleed rate for AVMs treated but not obliterated is the same as if no treatment had been given.[26,55]

Complications from radiosurgery immediately after treatment include new onset seizures, an increase in previous seizure frequency, and new neurologic deficits. Over the long term, hemorrhage remains the most significant reason for posttreatment morbidity and mortality. Radiation-induced fibrosis requires more than 24 months to develop, with the patient at risk for hemorrhage during this period.[94] Stereotactic radiosurgery can also induce radiation necrosis of normal brain matter. Radiation-induced complications are related to the dose and volume of the tissue irradiated.[68] There is limited availability of radiosurgery because the machines are very expensive and available in only a few centers.

ENDOVASCULAR EMBOLIZATION

One of the major changes in the treatment of AVMs has been the use of endovascular embolization. Although embolization of an AVM was first reported in 1960,[54] not until the 1980s with the development of microcatheters and embolic materials did embolization become an increasingly popular therapeutic modality.[3,87] The use of endovascular techniques to reduce the size of an AVM has greatly reduced the morbidity and mortality for surgical excision. Many patients who have previously been thought to have inoperable AVMs are now treated with endovascular embolization either before surgery or combined with either one-stage or multistaged surgical removal.[3,70,87,103]

The therapeutic goal is complete obliteration of the AVM nidus.[26,42,53,104] However, this is rarely accomplished, and there is a very low cure rate for AVMs treated only by embolization.[26,104] One reason for this lack of success is that not all feeders are amenable to embolization. This can be because a vessel may also involve associated branches to adjacent normal brain, a vessel may be too small for passage of the catheter, or the AVM nidus may be distal from the feeding artery. Particularly difficult to embolize are the deep-penetration arteries.

One problem with preoperative embolization is the recruitment of deep, collateral feeding arteries after the occlusion of more superficial vessels.[26,42,53] This can significantly complicate surgical resection of an AVM and is considered by some to be a major disadvantage of preoperative embolization.

Permanent obliteration of an AVM by embolization does not usually occur because of vessel recanalization and/or collateral development after embolization. Cure rates are low, ranging from 8% to 16%, with a serious morbidity rate of 13.5% to 22%.[34] The exceptions are dural arteriovenous fistulae, particularly those involving the cavernous sinus, which often are curable by embolization alone.[34,35,81,109] The use of embolization as a palliative procedure is controversial. There appears to be no difference in outcomes in AVMs between partially occluded and untreated lesions.

Embolization usually is part of a staged procedure that includes the surgical resection of the AVM.[3,87,103] However, the timing of surgery after embolization remains a subject of debate. Preoperative embolization decreases blood flow to the AVM, making it more amenable to surgical resection. However, embolization also can direct large volumes of blood from the high-flow, low-resistance shunt of the AVM into the previously hypoperfused surrounding brain area, raising the possibility of hyperemic complications (see later discussion). The time necessary for resolution of the postocclusion hyperemia must be weighed against recanalization of the AVM or development of new, possibly deep collaterals.

The embolizing material is introduced through catheters placed via percutaneous puncture of either the femoral or carotid artery. Superselective angiography using soft microcatheters is necessary to define the angiographic architecture of the AVM. The hemodynamics of the vessels are also monitored during the procedures because the cerebrohemodynamics of an AVM can change very dramatically and abruptly with small amounts of embolic material.[87]

Two endovascular techniques are currently in use; these differ in the material used for embolization. The first method uses liquid polymerization agents, which are injected into the nidus of the AVM. In North America, normobutyl cyanoacrylate (NBCA) is the most commonly used liquid polymer[32,39,42] and appears to be the most resistant to recanalization. However, cyanoacrylate also carries a higher risk of complications because of the changes in flow patterns induced during injection of the polymerizing material.[109] Many surgeons also complain that embolization of an AVM with cyanoacrylate makes surgical resection more difficult, in that the embolized AVM is a solid, brittle mass that is difficult to manipulate and resect.[42,87] This is particularly true for AVMs embolized with isobutyl 2-cyanoacrylate. However, lesions embolized with NBCA appear to be much softer and easier to manipulate.[42]

The second endovascular technique uses vessel embolization by particulate materials. Polyvinyl alcohol (PVA) is the most commonly used particulate material. It is available in particle sizes ranging from 150 μm to more than 2 mm in diameter. Other agents include steel and platinum microcoils, silicon beads, gelfoam, and collagen. Complications include the passage of the particulate material into the systemic circulation and the inadvertent embolization of a vessel feeding normal brain. Recanalization is also reported to be a problem after embolization with PVA. However, recanalization was not found to complicate the surgical resection of 54 patients embolized with PVA 1 to 4 weeks before surgery.[75] Most neuroradiologists use a combination of the two techniques, depending on the size and angiographic architecture of the AVM.

▼

BOX 19-2

ANESTHETIC CONSIDERATIONS FOR EMBOLIZATION PROCEDURES

A. General anesthesia vs. sedation
  1. Need for intraoperative neurologic testing (e.g., speech, vision)
  2. Need for controlled ventilation
  3. Ability of patient to lie still for long periods
    a. Preexisting medical conditions (i.e., arthritis or cough)
    b. History of claustrophobia
    c. Patient cooperation
    d. Neurologic status
  4. Contrast dye load with possibly rapid volume overload or induced hypovolemia
B. Radiation precautions
C. Possible complications
  1. New neurologic deficits
  2. Seizures
  3. Pulmonary embolism
  4. Inability to handle the contrast dye load
  5. Severe acute bleeding
  6. Hyperemic complications (normal perfusion pressure breakthrough syndrome and/or venous outflow obstruction)

In general, the overall goal of preoperative embolization is to reduce the arteriovenous shunt, decreasing the risks of intraoperative bleeding and postoperative hyperemic complications, and to increase the ease of surgical resection by embolizing those feeding vessels most difficult to access.

Anesthetic Management for Embolization Procedures

Box 19-2 presents anesthetic considerations for embolization procedures.

Preoperative Evaluation

The patient's neurologic status as well as general physical condition must be evaluated before embolization. Preexisting neurologic deficits, particularly those suggesting the presence of intracerebral steal, should alert the anesthesiologist to the risk of cerebral ischemia if systemic blood pressure should fall. The patient should also be evaluated for signs of increased ICP secondary to the mass effect from a recent ICH. It is important to evaluate the ability of a patient to lie still for periods of up to 6 to 8 hours. Medical conditions such as severe arthritis, cough, or a history of claustrophobia may prevent a patient from remaining still for these long periods of time.

Anesthetic Technique

Embolization procedures may be performed under local anesthesia with sedation or under general anesthesia; there are strong advocates for both techniques. Although the procedures are often long and can be uncomfortable, they generally are not painful enough to require a general anesthetic. In addition, the ability to communicate with the patient permits ongoing neurologic evaluation. This can be exceedingly important during embolization procedures involving eloquent areas, such as speech. However, certain patients are not good candidates for a sedation technique. They include young children (generally less than 12 to 13 years), patients with severe arthritis or claustrophobia, or those who are unable to cooperate. General anesthesia with controlled ventilation should be used in patients in whom hypercapnia from sedation may exacerbate ICP.

Many agents have been used for sedation. Modest doses of droperidol, midazolam, fentanyl, or propofol have all been used with good effect. However, patients must be closely watched for signs of oversedation. Monitors should include those for BP, ECG, and pulse oximetry. Oxygen via nasal prongs should be administered to all patients. Nasal prongs also provide a useful port for monitoring end-tidal CO_2 via capnography.

The choice of agents for the induction and maintenance of general anesthesia should reflect both the need for rapid emergence at the end of the procedure and the medical and neurologic requirements of the patient. Thiopental is most commonly used for induction. Nitrous oxide/narcotics (particularly fentanyl), inhalational agents (usually isoflurane),

and propofol have been used alone and in combination for maintenance of anesthesia. Deep levels of anesthesia are generally not required. Close attention must be given to blood pressure control. Hypotension may worsen ischemia from intracerebral steal, whereas hypertension may dangerously elevate ICP, in addition to exacerbating other preexisting systemic diseases, such as coronary artery disease. Intraarterial monitoring should be used in patients at risk from systemic blood pressure changes or in whom the use of deliberate hypotension is contemplated. (The use of deliberate hypotension in patients with AVMs will be discussed later.) Because patient immobility is necessary during the endovascular procedures, many patients are best managed with muscle relaxants and controlled ventilation.

The neuroradiology suite itself can be a difficult environment in which to perform a safe anesthetic. Equipment placement and patient positioning can prevent rapid access to a patient's airway. Lighting levels are often low to facilitate imaging and can interfere with visual assessment of a patient's coloring and respiratory efforts. These features must be considered in the formulation of any anesthetic plan. In addition, the extensive use of fluoroscopy in endovascular procedures necessitates comprehensive radiation precautions for both the patient and the anesthesiologist.

Possible Complications

Endovascular embolization procedures have been reported to have morbidity and mortality rates ranging from 10% to 12% and 2.7% to 4%, respectively.[32,39,42,102] The most common complication related to embolization is neurologic deficits secondary to inadvertent occlusion of normal vessels. Many neuroradiologists and neurosurgeons prefer to perform endovascular embolization under local anesthesia so that they may continuously monitor the neurologic status of their patients. The deficits may manifest as either progressive ischemic deficits, such as aphasia, hemianopsia, or hemiplegia, or as seizures. In some institutions, amobarbital 30 mg (sometimes referred to as the superselective Amytal test[75]) is injected into an artery potentially feeding eloquent areas to determine the neurologic function of the vascular area before arterial occlusion.[75,103] This can be particularly important when the area may involve language or sensorimotor cortices.

Seizures, either of new onset or a continuation of a preexisting epileptic state, may occur during the embolization procedure. Close attention should be paid to a preoperative history of seizures. Medical treatment of intraoperative seizures includes the use of short-acting benzodiazepines or barbiturates. A short-acting barbiturate, such as methohexital (30 mg), can be particularly useful in treating seizures in a previously alert patient. Attention must be given to the maintenance of a patent airway. Normal respiration, if interrupted, generally returns within 2 minutes after administration of this dose of methohexital.

Pulmonary embolism may also result from the shunting into the system circulation of particulate material used in the embolization procedure. This most frequently occurs during embolization of AVMs of the great vein of Galen or lesions containing large fistulae.

The contrast medium can result in a variety of complications, including adverse reactions to the contrast medium itself. The osmotic load from the contrast dye may be sufficient to induce congestive heart failure in some patients. The contrast medium also induces an osmotic diuresis that can result in hypovolemia and electrolyte abnormalities. Close attention should be given to the fluid status, urine output, and electrolyte status of these patients.

Acute, severe bleeding can occur during embolization procedures.[33,74] This may be the result of perforation of a feeding artery by a guidewire or catheter or rupture of an aneurysm associated with the AVM, or secondary to hyperemic complications (see later discussion). Perforation of a feeding artery by a guidewire or catheter appears to have a better prognosis than rupture of a dysplastic vessel or aneurysm because the muscular wall of a normal artery contracts to seal a small perforation.[33] Treatment depends on the etiology of the bleeding. Small perforations may be treated conservatively without immediate neuroradiologic or neurosurgical intervention. In many cases, the catheter itself may be used to occlude the perforation. Radiologic intervention may include embolization of the vessel proximal to the site of bleeding. In some cases, the perforating catheter may be left in place, occluding the bleeding site, while the patient undergoes an emergency craniotomy for aneurysm clipping. The outcome of emergency surgical intervention to control severe hemorrhage is grim.[33] There is continued intracerebral hemorrhage during the considerable time that it takes to perform the most expeditious craniotomy. In addition, vessels most frequently embolized are surgically inaccessible, deep to the AVM. Most of these patients die intraoperatively from exsanguination or uncontrollable cerebral hypertension.

The anesthetic management of patients with vessel perforations depends on their neurologic status. After the anesthesiologist discusses the situation with the neuroradiologist, systemic anticoagulants should be reversed immediately. Awake patients complain almost immediately of a severe headache. Many also have nausea; therefore it is important to make a cardiovascularly stable patient comfortable with antiemetics and analgesics. Extravasation of contrast material into brain parenchyma can induce seizures, so anticonvulsant therapy should be initiated. If an emergency craniotomy is deemed necessary, multiple large-bore intravenous catheters should be placed and a rapid transfusion device prepared.

Embolization can cause sudden changes in vessel pressures, which can result in hyperemic complications (to be discussed in detail). Embolization can result in edema and hemorrhage from venous thrombosis. The thrombosis can arise either from inadvertent embolization of a draining vessel or by decreased blood flow through the occluded AVM bed. Perioperative edema and hemorrhage may also result

---

> **BOX 19-3**
> **INCREASED RISK FOR UNFAVORABLE SURGICAL OUTCOMES**
>
> 1. Age > 50 years
> 2. Involvement of perforating vessels
> 3. Right hemispheric AVM
> 4. Large size AVM (>4 to 5 cm)
> 5. Depressed total cerebral blood flow
> 6. Progressive neurologic deficit
> 7. Angiographic evidence of steal
> 8. Hyperemic complications (perioperative edema or hemorrhage)
>
> Modified from Batjer HH, Devous MS, Seibert GB et al: *Neurosurgery* 24:75-79, 1989.

from increased blood flow through areas previously hypoperfused with possibly altered cerebral autoregulation. This syndrome has been termed *normal perfusion pressure breakthrough* and will be discussed in detail. The staged removal of an AVM from cerebral circulation has been advocated as a way to prevent these complications.

SURGICAL RESECTION

Surgical resection either alone or in combination with preoperative and/or intraoperative embolization remains the treatment of choice for AVMs.* Microsurgical techniques, combined with embolization and improvements in neuroanesthesia, have enabled the total resection of lesions previously considered inoperative. Surgical mortality ranges from 0.6% to 14% and correlates with the preoperative grade of the AVM; that is, the larger and more involved the AVM, the greater the incidence of postoperative morbidity and mortality. Early postoperative morbidity ranges from 17% to 28%.† Of interest is the long-term outcome from surgical resection. Not only is the risk of hemorrhage virtually eliminated with surgical resection of the lesion, but there is an overall improvement in neurologic outcome with time. Heros et al.,[37] in a retrospective survey of 153 consecutive patients, reported an improvement in serious morbidity of 24.2% to 7.8%, with more than 90% of patients subjectively feeling capable of working full-time. Similar improvements in neurologic outcomes over time have been reported by Wilson et al.[110] and Stein and Wolpert.[92] In addition to the preoperative grade of the AVM, several other factors have been identified as predictors of increased surgical risks. These include age greater than 50 years, preoperative hemorrhage, presence of right vs. hemispheric AVM, and recruitment of perforating vessels[12] (Box 19-3).

---

*References 3, 26, 37, 38, 87, 90-92, 95, 110.
†References 3, 26, 37, 38, 87, 90-92, 95, 110.

<hr>

<table>
<tr><td>

BOX 19-4

ANESTHETIC CONSIDERATIONS FOR SURGICAL
RESECTION OF AN AVM

A. Preoperative
  1. Preexisting medical condition
  2. Neurologic status (e.g., history of seizures, symptoms of intracerebral steal or mass effect)
  3. Fluid and electrolyte status
  4. Preoperative diagnostic studies (e.g., location and size of AVM, cranial nerve involvement, presence of aneurysm)
  5. Planned surgical approach
B. Induction
  1. Monitors
  2. Blood pressure control
C. Maintenance of anesthesia
  1. Choice of agent
    a. Need for neurologic testing
      (i) General anesthesia vs. sedation
      (ii) Use of EEG and/or evoked potentials
    b. Use of high-dose barbiturates
  2. Use of deliberate hypotension
  3. Ability to evaluate neurologic status in early postoperative period
D. Possible complications
  1. New neurologic deficits
  2. Severe intraoperative blood loss
  3. Hyperemic complications
    a. Normal perfusion pressure breakthrough syndrome
    b. Venous obstruction

</td></tr>
</table>

Anesthetic Management

Box 19-4 presents the anesthetic considerations for surgical resection of an AVM.

Preoperative Evaluation

As previously discussed for patients undergoing endovascular procedures, patients scheduled for AVM surgery should have a thorough preoperative anesthetic examination. Special attention should be given to both preexisting medical conditions and the preoperative neurologic status. Preoperative neurologic deficits should be noted. Of particular concern are preexisting symptoms of intracerebral steal and mass effect with increased ICP secondary to ICH. Patients should be evaluated for a history of seizures. Attention should be given to preoperative medications, such as antiseizure medications and steroids. The fluid and electrolyte status of a patient should be reviewed preoperatively. Patients who have undergone preoperative embolization are particularly prone to fluid and electrolyte abnormalities secondary to contrast media–induced diuresis.

Preoperative diagnostic studies should be examined for other abnormalities, such as the presence of an aneurysm within the AVM or a midline shift suggestive of a mass effect. The location of the AVM should also be evaluated for possible intraoperative and/or postoperative complications. For example, surgical excision of an AVM near the brain-stem can result in brainstem and/or cranial nerve dysfunction. In these cases, surgical stimulation of cranial nerves V and/or X can result in intraoperative hemodynamic changes, and involvement of cranial nerves IX and/or X can produce postoperative respiratory problems.

Patient positioning during surgery should also be considered before surgery. The patient should be questioned about any preexisting conditions, such as arthritis, that might complicate positioning. Premedication should be tailored to reflect the patient's medical and neurologic status. Care must be taken to avoid oversedation leading to hypercarbia in patients at risk for increased ICP.

Induction of Anesthesia

Appropriate monitoring devices should be placed before the induction of anesthesia. These monitors include ECG, pulse oximetry, capnography, and intraarterial blood pressure monitoring. Patients can undergo extensive and rapid blood loss during surgical resection of an AVM. Therefore venous access must be sufficient to permit the rapid transfusion of several units of blood. A central venous catheter or a pulmonary artery catheter may be useful in monitoring fluid replacement in patients with underlying cardiovascular disease.

Induction must be smooth with impeccable blood pressure control. Decreased blood pressure may produce ischemic changes in hypoperfused areas. Hypertension may rupture an aneurysm or worsen cerebral hypertension by increasing the mass effect of a hemotoma. The ability to control hemodynamics and ICP during induction is the most important consideration in choosing an induction agent. Thiopental is frequently used, and propofol may also prove helpful as an induction drug in these patients. Hemodynamic responses to laryngoscopy, intubation, and placement of pin head fixation must be anticipated. Several agents have been used successfully to blunt these responses. These agents include lidocaine (1.5 mg/kg), esmolol (0.5 to 1 mg/kg), and further doses of the induction agent.

Maintenance of Anesthesia

Several different techniques have been advocated for maintenance of anesthesia. As with induction, one must consider surgical requirements and the patient's medical and neurologic status in choosing a technique. For example, in some cases where the AVM is small and in an eloquent area, the craniotomy may be best performed under local anesthesia with sedation. The need for neurologic testing using EEG or evoked potentials may also influence the choice of agent. In general, both nitrous oxide/narcotic (particularly fentanyl) and volatile anesthetic (usually isoflurane) techniques have been used successfully in these patients.

Surgical exposure is usually facilitated by mild hyperventilation (Paco$_2$ of 30 to 35 mm Hg). However, further decreases in Paco$_2$, the use of diuretics (usually mannitol and/or furosemide), and CSF drains may be necessary for surgical access to AVMs located deep in the brain or large AVMs, or in patients with brain swelling secondary to ICH. The use of crystalloids for fluid replacement should be limited. Replacement with colloid rather than crystalloid is preferred to maintain intravascular volume and to decrease the risk of intracerebral swelling from increased brain intracellular water.

Severe intraoperative bleeding always remains a possibility in patients undergoing surgical resection of AVMs. Indeed, the morbidity and mortality associated with massive intraoperative bleeding have been the underlying reasons for the traditionally conservative treatment of AVMs.[21,22] Although preoperative endovascular embolization has been shown to reduce intraoperative blood loss,[3,42,87,89,103] bleeding can be difficult to control, and it can be massive and rapid. At particular risk for massive bleeding are patients with dural AV fistulae involving the major sinuses, especially the transverse or sigmoid sinuses or those involving the great vein of Galen.[8,96] Bleeding may also result in malignant cerebral edema.

Deliberate Hypotension

Some neurosurgeons have advocated the use of deliberate hypotension on a routine basis during AVM resection as a way both to decrease blood loss during resection and to decrease the risk of hyperemic complications.[69,87,89] Deliberate hypotension may be of greatest usefulness during resection of deep feeder arteries because they are difficult to visualize and ligate. However, the use of deliberate hypotension must be balanced against the overall low transmural pressure of AVMs. Indeed, any hypotension may induce ischemic changes in areas already at risk from hypoperfusion with normal blood pressure. In addition, there is concern that hypotension may predispose the venous system to venous outflow thrombosis and obstruction.[1] Moderate hypotension may have a role in the treatment of brain edema secondary to normal perfusion pressure breakthrough (NPPB) syndrome. In any case, its use must be determined on a case-by-case basis.

Use of High-Dose Barbiturates

High-dose barbiturates (up to 2 to 5 g of thiopental) have been advocated for prophylactic use in all AVM surgery.[84,87] The argument for using high-dose barbiturates is based primarily on brain protection although their ability to prevent or decrease the occurrence of hyperemic complications remains largely anecdotal.[24,84,87] However, a recent prospective study by U, Kerber, and Todd[100] suggests that high-dose barbiturate anesthesia (which they defined as 10 to 15 mg/kg of pentobarbital given over 30 to 60 minutes, with the dosage thereafter titrated to maintain deepburst suppression on the EEG) may decrease surgical morbidity and mortality from hyperemic complications as compared with a nitrous oxide/fentanyl technique in patients undergoing resection of deep-seated AVMs, such as those in the basal ganglia. Although there was a significant difference in outcomes in the two groups, the study population was small,[20] and larger studies will be necessary to determine the effectiveness of this technique. The use of high-dose barbiturates must be decided patient-by-patient, with the possible advantages weighed against the possible complications. For example, in patients with symptoms of a clinically significant steal phenomenon, high-dose barbiturates may induce hypotension that would place the already hypoperfused brain at an even higher risk for ischemic injury. In addition, the use of high-dose barbiturates frequently prolongs patients' emergence from anesthesia, thus delaying neurologic evaluation upon completion of surgery. Indeed, proponents of the use of high-dose barbiturates electively maintain mechanical ventilation and sedation in their patients for the first postoperative day.[100] Because of these problems, the use of mild hypothermia (32 to 34° C), instead of barbiturate coma, has grown in popularity as a technique for brain protection.

Emergence

In general, the anesthetic technique should be tailored to permit a prompt awakening on completion of the surgical procedure whenever possible. The ability to neurologically evaluate a patient in the immediate postoperative period can allow for the early diagnosis and treatment of operative complications, such as hematoma formation. Care should be taken to prevent hypertension during and after surgical closure, which can lead to bleeding in the AVM bed, rupture of associated aneurysms, or hyperemic complications (to be discussed following). Sympathetic blockers such as esmolol, labetalol, and propranolol, and vasodilators such as hydralazine and sodium nitroprusside have all been used successfully for blood pressure control. Systemic blood pressure should be maintained within the patient's normal range. In patients with incomplete AVM resection or at risk for the NBBP syndrome (to be discussed following), a mild degree of deliberate hypotension may be necessary during the postoperative period.

POSTOPERATIVE COMPLICATIONS
Hyperemic Complications

Hyperemic complications, defined as perioperative edema or hemorrhage, constitutes the major source of postoperative morbidity and mortality after AVM surgery.[82,91,92] Batjer et al.[12] reported that less than half of patients who had hyperemic complications had a good outcome (46%) as compared with patients without hyperemic complications.[92] The mechanism(s) behind the high occurrence of hyperemic complications remains unclear. Several theories have been advanced to explain this phenomenon. The best known is the normal perfusion pressure breakthrough theory of Spetzler et al.[88] Another, recently proposed by Al-Rodhan et al.,[1] is the occlusive hyperemia theory. These both will be discussed. Postoperative bleeding may also arise from either an incomplete resection of the AVM or from incomplete hemostasis. Hemostasis can be extremely difficult after AVM resection.

Normal Perfusion Pressure Breakthrough Syndrome

Pathogenesis

The high-flow, low-resistance shunt that is associated with AVMs can be large enough to lead to chronic hypoperfusion in the surrounding brain tissue. The abrupt removal of the shunt from circulation, either by embolization or surgery, has been reported to induce cerebral edema, hyperemia, and subsequent hemorrhage into these surrounding areas.[11,36,82,88] It has been suggested that infants with vein of Galen malformations may be at particularly high risk for these complications and that malignant brain swelling with hemorrhage may be an important factor in the poor surgical outcomes of these patients.[43,63] The clinical syndrome of cerebral hyperperfusion with normal cerebral perfusion pressures has been called *normal perfusion pressure breakthrough (NPPB)*. The mechanism underlying this phenomenon was first hypothesized by Spetzler et al. in 1978.[88] They suggested that the chronic hypoperfusion and/or ischemia in the brain area surrounding a large shunt leads to vasomotor paralysis with a loss of cerebral autoregulation. With the abrupt removal of the shunt from the circulation, either by embolization or surgery, the previously hypoperfused areas receive a normal CBF. This sudden increase in CBF into areas without autoregulation can lead to cerebral edema and hemorrhage.

There is still considerable controversy surrounding the existence and clinical significance of NPPB.[1,108] There are substantial theoretic grounds supporting the existence of this phenomenon.[66] However, much of the clinical evidence is based on anecdotal experiences in which other explanations, such as bleeding from an unidentified, unresected AVM or insufficient hemostasis in areas with postoperatively increased blood flow, cannot be rigorously excluded.* The carotid-jugular fistula animal models of Spetzler et al.[88] and Morgan et al.[62] have provided most of the experimental evidence for the syndrome.

Recent reports have documented changes in cerebral blood flow and perfusion pressure during occlusion of AVMs and, in some cases, development of cerebral hyperemia and edema. Batjer et al.[13] described serial hemodynamic measurements of both cerebral blood flow and flow velocity using xenon wash-out and transcranial Doppler ultrasonography in three patients during treatment for AVMs. They found substantial hyperemia developing after both resection and embolization. Restoration of normal regional

---

*References 3, 26, 52, 65, 66, 82, 87, 110.

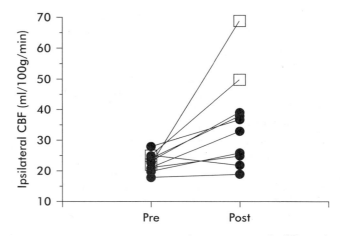

FIG. 19-7 Changes in CBF with AVM removal: the graph demonstrates CBF as measured by the ^{133}Xe technique in individual patients before *(pre)* and after *(post)* AVM resection. The changes in CBF in two patients who displayed clinical evidence of the NPPB syndrome are shown with the open squares. *(Modified from Young WL, Prohovnik I, Ornstein E et al: Anesth Analg 67:1011-4, 1988.)*

cerebral blood flow was noted after embolization in one patient who had cerebral hypoperfusion before treatment. In another patient, postoperative hyperemia was associated with both persistently elevated blood-flow velocities and hemispheric neurologic deficits. Using the ^{133}Xe wash-out technique to measure CBF, Young et al.[114,115] found bilateral increases in cortical blood flow after surgical obliteration of the shunt (Fig. 19-7). Of particular interest, the two patients with the highest increases in blood flow developed clinical symptoms postoperatively consistent with the NPPB syndrome. Jungreis et al.[44,45] found abrupt changes in the MAP of arterial feeders immediately after embolization.

Reports of the overall incidence of clinically significant NPPB have been variable. Frequency estimates range from 1.4% to 18%.[12,53,63,110] For larger AVMs (>4 to 5 cm) the reported incidence is significantly higher, ranging from 19% to 37%.[53,98] This is most likely a factor secondary to the correlation of AVM size and extent of loss of autoregulation and/or decrease in CBF in the area surrounding an AVM.[6,98] The phenomenon of NPPB has been reported in other situations, such as carotid endarterectomy, where there is a restoration of CBF to previously ischemic areas.

Mechanism

Smooth muscle derangements in the cerebral vasculature have been advanced as a possible mechanism for the NPPB syndrome.[10] Batjer and Devous examined the effect of acetazolamide (a cerebral vasodilator) on regional CBF in patients scheduled for AVM resection. They found an abnormally enhanced vasoreactivity (vasodilation) to acetazolamide stimulation in the hypoperfused brain areas of patients with preoperative angiographic steal phenomena as well as in patients who developed hyperemic complications postoperatively.[10] Impaired CO_2 reactivity has also been reported to exist before resection in brain areas surrounding an AVM.[6,88] However, in the majority of studies, CO_2 reactivity appeared to return to normal after resection. Furthermore, Young et al.[114,116] reported CO_2 reactivity to be intact both before and after resection despite acute increases in cerebral perfusion pressure with shunt obliteration. These findings suggest a possible uncoupling of vasoconstrictive and vasodilatory responses. This "dissociative vasoparalysis" has been described in tumor patients and in patients after head trauma.[67,71] The fact that chronically hypoperfused areas surrounding AVMs can be capable of vasodilatory reactivity in response to pharmacologic or metabolic stimuli such as acetazolamide and CO_2 but incapable of vasoconstrictive reactivity in response to increased perfusion pressure supports the existence of a dissociative vasoparalysis as a possible mechanism for the NBBP syndrome.[11]

Not all patients who undergo AVM resection either as a single or staged procedure develop symptoms consistent with the NPPB syndrome. Indeed, there are four possible hemodynamic responses that patients may display in response to AVM resection: (1) no change in arteriovenous pressure gradient with shunt occlusion, (2) an increased pressure gradient with appropriate autoregulatory response, (3) an increased pressure gradient with impaired autoregulatory response and a resultant increase in CBF, and (4) an increased pressure gradient with impaired autoregulatory responses and a resultant increase in CBF sufficient to induce NPPB complications.[114] At particular risk of developing NPPB are patients who present with neurologic findings of cerebral ischemia secondary to the high-flow, low-resistance shunt of the AVM. These patients are at a higher risk than patients whose presenting symptoms are intracerebral hemorrhage from a ruptured AVM. Angiographic features associated with high risk of NPPB include: (1) large high-flow AVM, (2) multiple, large-diameter feeding arteries, (3) an AVM location in a border zone (e.g., superior parietal lobe), and (4) a shift in CBF toward the AVM (e.g., inverse steal).[50]

Prevention

A key element in the surgical treatment of AVMs has been the removal of the AVM by staged excision, occlusion, and/or embolization of the feeding vessels combined with later surgery.[3,87] The technique underlying staged removal is to decrease the size of the AVM, permitting a staged removal of the shunt from circulation, thus allowing the surrounding brain tissue to regain its autoregulation.

Other modalities suggested to prevent NPPB include clamping of the cervical carotid artery,[15,99] induced hypotension, and barbiturate treatment (see later discussion).[84,87] Some surgeons do not believe these treatments change the incidence of NPPB, particularly with respect to postoperative complications. Rather, they allege that one-

stage operations are safer.[15,64,99] They argue that staged procedures increase the risk of hemorrhage by repeatedly inducing acute hypoperfusion on the chronic hypoperfusion during a staged resection. There is, in addition, the problem of a rebleed occurring between the initial and final resection. Staging also may increase the difficulty of resection by diverting flow from large, readily accessible feeding arteries to deep penetrating vessels. Finally, quantification of the degree of flow reduction after subtotal resection is difficult, the time necessary for correction of a disordered autoregulation is unclear, and the remaining AVM can rapidly collateralize.[64] This is, in general, a minority opinion, and the current trend is toward staged removal.

Treatment

Because the mechanisms that lead from hyperperfusion to frank hemorrhage remain unclear, treatment of symptoms consistent with the NPPB syndrome (i.e., cerebral edema, increased ICP, hemorrhage), remains controversial. There are few, if any, prospective studies comparing clinical therapies. Most treatment is based on anecdotal case reports and consists of commonly used modalities for treating increased ICP and providing brain protection.[4,24,36,64,113] In general, one should initiate the usual steps for reducing increased ICP, such as osmotic diuretics (usually mannitol), head-up position, and hyperventilation although their usefulness has not been determined. Several centers suggest the use of deep barbiturate anesthesia both prophylactically during all surgical and endovascular procedures involving AVM removal and as treatment for the NPPB syndrome.[24,84,87] The judicious use of deliberate hypotension may be helpful. The optimal degree of hypotension is a function of both the severity of the cerebral hyperperfusion and systemic and/or cerebrovascular ischemic concerns. The use of moderate hypothermia has also been suggested. In general, prevention and treatment await a better understanding of the pathophysiology underlying the phenomenon and better devices for monitoring cerebral hemodynamics in the perioperative period.

Venous Outflow Obstruction

Perioperative edema and hemorrhage may be secondary to venous outflow obstruction. The venous outflow of an AVM may also function as the draining vessels for the normal brain parenchyma surrounding the AVM. As the AVM is removed from the circulation, blood is shunted back into the surrounding area. However, Nornes and Grips[66] found the perfusion pressure in AVM draining veins to decrease from approximately 15 mm Hg before resection to virtually zero after resection. This decreased flow predisposes the draining veins to thombosis, which may induce hyperemia and possibly hemorrhage within the surrounding brain regions also drained by these vessels. Venous outflow obstruction also may be induced by surgical ligation or embolization of the draining veins. Venous outflow obstruction in the face of incomplete occlusion of an arterial feeder can lead to massive hemorrhage. Al-Rodhan et al.[1] have proposed that venous outflow obstruction, which they have termed "occlusive hyperemia," may be the major cause of hyperemic complications after AVM excision. Furthermore, they suggest that, in addition to venous obstruction, there is stagnant CBF in the former arterial feeders and their parenchymal branches, leading to a worsening of preexisting hypoperfusion and cerebral ischemia in the area surrounding the AVM. Measures suggested to prevent the occurrence of venous outflow occlusion include the avoidance of excessive hypotension (MAP <70 to 80 mm Hg) during AVM resection. Whereas moderate hypotension may aid during some resections, its use must be weighed against both low arterial perfusion pressures resulting in ischemic injury in areas already hypoperfused and low venous perfusion pressures resulting in venous thombosis.[1]

Monitoring Changes in CBF

Altered cerebral hemodynamics contribute significantly to postoperative complications.[6,98] Therefore improved outcomes depend on the prevention and/or treatment of hyperemic complications. Intraoperative monitoring may help predict and/or diagnose patients at high risk for developing hyperemic complications. Important factors in the development of hyperemic complications that might be amenable for monitoring include: (1) CBF in the brain area surrounding the AVM nidus, (2) pressure in the feeding vessels before AVM removal, (3) pressure in the venous outflow vessels, (4) rapid return to normal of arterial and venous pressures after AVM removal, and (5) significant increases in CBF after embolization and/or after AVM removal.[44,45] Sequential hemodynamic measurements may predict patients at risk for perioperative complications as well as provide some clinical guidelines for the extent and timing of embo-

lization and surgery.[13] Jungreis et al.[44,45] have suggested monitoring blood pressure changes in arterial feeders during therapeutic embolization. The ability to measure rCBF during surgery currently is restricted to a few academic centers. Other promising techniques for monitoring CBF during shunt obliteration by either AVM removal or embolization are transcranial Doppler ultrasonography and thermal diffusion flow probes. ICP monitors may be of use in the postoperative period. Improved monitoring during AVM surgery requires the development of better monitoring devices.

▼

SUMMARY

The anesthetic management of patients undergoing procedures for the embolization and/or surgical resection of AVMs requires a clear understanding of the high-flow, low-resistance nature of these lesions. That is, before surgery, AVMs may produce shunts sufficiently large to induce intracerebral steal, resulting in ischemia in the surrounding brain parenchyma. During surgical resection, their diffuse vascularity can lead to rapid and massive blood loss that can be difficult to control. Finally, the removal of these shunts from the cerebral circulation, by either embolization or surgical resection, can result in brain swelling and possible hemorrhage, either from the rapid return of blood flow to areas with dysfunctional cerebral autoregulation or from venous thrombosis and obstruction. Knowledge of the pathophysiology that underlies these potential complications is necessary for the formulation of a rational anesthetic plan.

References

1. Al-Rodhan NRF, Sundt TM, Piepgras DG et al: Occlusive hyperemia: a theory for the hemodynamic complications following resection of intracerebral arteriovenous malformations, *J Neurosurg* 78:167-175, 1993.

2. Aminoff MJ: Vascular anomalies in the intracranial dural mater, *Brain* 96:601-612, 1973.

3. Andrews BT, Wilson CB: Staged treatment of arteriovenous malformations of the brain, *Neurosurgery* 21:314-323, 1987.

4. Aoki N, Mizutani H: Arteriovenous malformation in the territory of the occluded middle cerebral artery with massive intraoperative brain swelling: case report, *Neurosurgery* 16:660-662, 1985.

5. Awad IA, Little JR, Akarawi WP et al: Intracranial dural arteriovenous malformations: factors predisposing to an aggressive neurological course, *J Neurosurg* 72:839-50, 1990.

6. Barnett GH, Little JR, Ebrahim ZY et al: Cerebral circulation during arteriovenous malformation operation, *Neurosurgery* 20:836-842, 1987.

7. Barno A, Freeman DW: Maternal deaths due to spontaneous subarachnoid hemorrhage, *Am J Obstet Gynecol* 125:384-392, 1976.

8. Barnwell SL, Halbach VV, Higashida RT et al: Complex dural arteriovenous fistulas. Results of combined endovascular and neurosurgical treatment in 16 patients, *J Neurosurg* 71:352-8, 1989.

9. Barrow DL: Unruptured cerebral arteriovenous malformations presenting with intracranial hypertension, *Neurosurgery* 23:484-90, 1988.

10. Batjer HH, Devous MS: The use of acetazolamide-enhanced regional cerebral blood flow measurement to predict risk to arteriovenous malformation patients, *Neurosurgery* 31:213-7, 1992.

11. Batjer HH, Devous MS, Meyer YJ et al: Cerebrovascular hemodynamics in arteriovenous malformation complicated by normal perfusion pressure breakthrough, *Neurosurgery* 22:503-9, 1988.

12. Batjer HH, Devous MS, Seibert GB, et al: Intracranial arteriovenous malformation: relationship between clin-

ical factors and surgical complications, *Neurosurgery* 24:75-79, 1989.

13. Batjer HH, Purdy PD, Giller CA et al: Evidence of redistribution of cerebral blood flow during treatment for an intracranial arteriovenous malformation, *Neurosurgery* 25:599-604, 1989.

14. Betti DO, Munari C, Rosler R: Stereotactic radiosurgery with the linear accelerator. Treatment of arteriovenous malformations, *Neurosurgery* 24:311-321, 1989.

15. Bonnal J, Born JD, Hans P: One-stage excision of high-flow arteriovenous malformation, *Neurosurgery* 62:75-79, 1985.

16. Brown RJ, Wiebers DO, Forbes G et al: The natural history of unruptured intracranial arteriovenous malformations, *J Neurosurg* 68:352-7, 1988.

17. Chimowitz MI, Little JR, Awad IA et al: Intracranial hypertension associated with unruptured cerebral arteriovenous malformations, *Ann Neurol* 27:474-9, 1990.

18. Ciricillo SF, Edwards MS, Schmidt KG et al: Interventional neuroradiological management of vein of Galen malformations in the neonate, *Neurosurgery* 27:22-7, 1990.

19. Crawford PM, West CR, Chadwick DW et al: Arteriovenous malformations of the brain: natural history in unoperative patients, *J Neurol Neurosurg Psychiatry* 49:1-10, 1986.

20. Crawford PM, West CR, Shaw MDM et al: Cerebral arteriovenous malformations and epilepsy: factors in the development of epilepsy, *Epilepsia* 27:270-275, 1986.

21. Cushing H, Bailey P: *Tumors arising from the blood vessels of the brain: angiomatous malformations and hemangioblastomas,* Springfield, Ill, 1928, Charles C. Thomas.

22. Dandy WE: Venous abnormalities and angiomas of the brain, *Arch Surg* 17:715-793, 1928.

23. Dawson R III, Tarr RW, Hecht ST et al: Treatment of arteriovenous malformations of the brain with combined embolization and stereotactic radiosurgery: results after 1 and 2 years, *Am J Neuroradiol* 11:857-64, 1990.

24. Day A, Friedman W, Sypert G et al: Successful treatment of the normal perfusion breakthrough syndrome, *Neurosurgery* 11:625-630, 1982.

25. Dias MS, Sekhar LN: Intracranial hemorrhage from aneurysms and arteriovenous malformations during pregnancy and the puerperium, *Neurosurgery* 27:855-866, 1990.

26. Drake CG: Cerebral arteriovenous malformations: considerations for and experience with surgical treatment in 166 cases, *Neurosurgery* 26:145-206, 1979.

27. Edwards MSB, Hieshima GB, Higashida RT et al: Management of vein of Galen malformations in the neonate, *Intervent Pediatr* 3:184-188, 1988.

28. Feindel W, Perot P: Red cerebral veins. A report on arteriovenous shunts in tumors and cerebral scars, *J Neurosurg* 22:315-325, 1965.

29. Foy PM, Copeland GP, Shaw MDM: The incidence of postoperative seizures, *Acta Neurochir* 55:253-264, 1981.

30. Gold AP, Ranssohoff JR, Carter S: Vein of Galen malformation, *Acta Neurol Scand Suppl* 40:5-31, 1964.

31. Graf CJ, Perret GE, Torner JC: Bleeding from cerebral arteriovenous malformations as part of their natural history, *J Neurosurg* 58:331-338, 1984.

32. Graves VB, Duff TA: Intracranial arteriovenous malformations. Current imaging and treatment, *Invest Radiol* 25:952-960, 1990.

33. Halbach VV, Higashida RT, Dowd CF, et al: Management of vascular perforations that occur during neurointerventional procedures, *Am J Neuroradiol* 12:319-27, 1991.

34. Halbach VV, Higashida RT, Hieshima GB: Interventional neuroradiology, *Am J Roentgenol* 153:467-76, 1989.

35. Halbach VV, Higashida RT, Hieshima GB et al: Dural fistulae involving the cavernous sinus: results in 30 patients, *Radiology* 163:437-442, 1987.

36. Halbach VV, Higashida RT, Hieshima GB et al: Normal perfusion pressure breakthrough occuring during treatment of carotid and vertebral fistulas, *Am J Neuroradiol* 8:751-756, 1987.

37. Heros RC, Korosue K, Diebold PM: Surgical excision of cerebral arteriovenous malformations: late results, *Neurosurgery* 26:570-7, 1990.

38. Heros RC, Tu YK: Is surgical therapy needed for unruptured arteriovenous malformations? *Neurology* 37:279-286, 1987.

39. Higashida RT, Hieshima GB, Halbach VV: Advances in the treatment of complex cerebrovascular disorders by interventional neurovascular techniques, *Circulation* 83:196-206, 1991.

40. Holden AM, Fyler DC, Shillito J et al: Congestive heart failure from intracranial arteriovenous fistula in infancy, *Pediatrics* 49:30-39, 1972.

41. Horton JC, Chambers WA, Lyons SL, et al: Pregnancy and the risk of hemorrhage from cerebral arteriovenous malformations, *Neurosurgery* 27:867-871, 1990.

42. Jafar JJ, Davis AJ, Berenstein A et al: The effect of embolization with N-butyl cyanoacrylate prior to surgical resection of cerebral arteriovenous malformations, *J Neurosurg* 78:60-9, 1993.

43. Johnston IH, Whittle IR, Besser M et al: Vein of Galen malformation: diagnosis and management, *Neurosurgery* 20:747-758, 1987.

44. Jungreis CA, Horton JA: Pressure changes in the arterial feeder to a cerebral AVM as a guide to monitoring therapeutic embolization, *Am J Neuroradiol* 10:1057-60, 1989.

45. Jungreis CA, Horton JA, Hecht ST: Blood pressure changes in feeders to cerebral arteriovenous malformations during therapeutic embolization, *Am J Neuroradiol* 10:575-7, 1989.

46. Kjellberg RK, Hanamura T, Davis KR et al: Bragg-peak proton-beam therapy for arteriovenous malformations of the brain, *N Engl J Med* 309:269-274, 1983.

47. Kusske JA, Kelly WA: Embolization and reduction of the "steal" syndrome in cerebral arteriovenous malformations, *J Neurosurg* 40:313-321, 1974.

48. Lasjaunias P, Ter Brugge K, Lopez-Ibor L et al: The role of dural anomalies in vein of Galen aneurysms: report of six cases and review of literature, *AJNR* 8:185-192, 1987.

49. Leblanc R, Feindel W, Ethier R: Epilepsy from cerebral arteriovenous malformations, *Can J Neurol Sci* 10:91-95, 1983.

50. Leblanc R, Little JR: Hemodynamics of arteriovenous malformations, *Clin Neurosurg* 36:299-317, 1990.

51. Luessenhop AJ: Natural history of cerebral arteriovenous malforma-

tions. In Wilson CB, Stein BM, editors: *Intracranial arteriovenous malformations,* Baltimore, 1984, William & Wilkins, pp 12-23.

52. Luessenhop AJ, Ferraz FM, Rosa L: Estimate of the incidence and importance of circulatory breakthrough in the surgery of cerebral arteriovenous malformations, *Neurol Res* 4:177-190, 1982.

53. Luessenhop AJ, Rosa L: Cerebral arteriovenous malformations. Indications for and results of surgery, and the role of intravascular techniques, *Neurosurgery* 60:14-22, 1984.

54. Luessenhop AJ, Spence WT: Artificial embolization of cerebral arteries. Report of use in a case of arteriovenous malformation, *JAMA* 172:1153-115, 1960.

55. Lunsford LD, Kondziolka D, Flickinger JC et al: Stereotactic radiosurgery for arteriovenous malformations of the brain, *J Neurosurg* 75:512-24, 1991.

56. Marks MP, Lane B, Steinberg G et al: Vascular characteristics of intracerebral arteriovenous malformations in patients with clinical steal, *AJNR* 12:489-496, 1991.

57. Martin NA, King WA, Wilson CB et al: Management of dural arteriovenous malformations of the anterior cranial fossa, *J Neurosurg* 72:692-7, 1990.

58. Matjasko J, Robinson W, Eudaily D: Successful surgical and anesthetic management of vein of Galen aneurysm in a neonate in congestive heart failure, *Neurosurgery* 22:908-910, 1988.

59. McCormick WF: The pathology of vascular ("arteriovenous") malformations, *J Neurosurg* 24:807-816, 1966.

60. McCormick WF: Pathology of vascular malformations of the brain. In Wilson CB, Stein BM, editors: *Intracranial arteriovenous malformations,* Baltimore, 1984, Williams & Wilkins, pp 44-63.

61. Michelson WJ: Natural history and pathology of arteriovenous malformations, *Clin Neurosurg* 26:145-208, 1979.

62. Morgan MK, Johnston I, Besser M et al: Cerebral arteriovenous malformations, steal, and the hypertensive breakthrough threshhold. An experi-

mental study in rats, *J Neurosurg* 66:563-567, 1987.

63. Morgan MK, Johnston IH, Sundt TJ: Normal perfusion pressure breakthrough complicating surgery for the vein of Galen malformation: report of three cases [see comments], *Neurosurgery* 24:406-10, 1989.

64. Morgan MK, Sundt TJ: The case against staged operative resection of cerebral arteriovenous malformations, *Neurosurgery* 25:429-35, 1989.

65. Mullan S, Brown FD, Patronas NJ: Hyperemic and ischemic problems of surgical treatment of arteriovenous malformations, *J Neurosurg* 51:757-764, 1979.

66. Nornes H, Grip A: Hemodynamic aspects of cerebral arteriovenous malformations, *J Neurosurg* 53:456-464, 1980.

67. Obrist WD, Langfitt TW, Jaggi JL et al: Cerebral blood flow and metabolism in comatose patients with acute head injury, *J Neurosurg* 61:241-253, 1984.

68. Ogilvy CS: Radiation therapy for arteriovenous malformations: a review [see comments], *Neurosurgery* 26:725-35, 1990.

69. Ornstein E, Young WL, Ostapkovich N et al: Deliberate hypotension in patients with intracranial arteriovenous malformations: esmolol compared with isoflurane and sodium nitroprusside, *Anesth Analg* 72:639-644, 1991.

70. Pasqualin A, Scienza R, Cioffi F et al: Treatment of cerebral arteriovenous malformations with a combination of preoperative embolization and surgery, *Neurosurgery* 29:358-68, 1991.

71. Paulson OB, Olesen J, Christensen MS: Restoration of autoregulation of cerebral blood flow by hypocapnia, *Neurology* 22:286-293, 1972.

72. Perret G, Grip A: Report on the cooperative study of intracranial aneurysms and subarachnoid hemorrhage. Section VI. Arteriovenous malformations. An analysis of 545 cases of craino-cerebral arteriovenous malformations and fistulae reported to the Cooperative Study, *J Neurosurg* 25:467-490, 1966.

73. Piepgras DG, Sundt TJ, Ragoowansi AT et al: Seizure outcome in patients with surgically treated cerebral arte-

riovenous malformations, *J Neurosurg* 78:5-11, 1993.

74. Purdy PD, Batjer HH, Samson D: Management of hemorrhagic complications from preoperative embolization of arteriovenous malformations, *J Neurosurg* 74:205-11, 1991.

75. Purdy PD, Samson D, Batjer HH et al: Preoperative embolization of cerebral arteriovenous malformations with polyvinyl alcohol particles: experience in 51 adults, *Am J Neuroradiol* 11:501-10, 1990.

76. Reagan TJ, Bloom WH: The brain in hereditary hemorrhagic telangiectasia, *Stroke* 2:361-368, 1971.

77. Rigamonti D, Hadley MN, Drayer BP et al: Cerebral cavernous malformations. Incidence and familial occurrence, *N Engl J Med* 319:343-7, 1988.

78. Rigamonti D, Spetzler RF, Medina M et al: Cerebral venous malformations, *J Neurosurg* 73:560-564, 1990.

79. Robinson JL, Hall CS, Sedzimir CB: Arteriovenous malformations, aneurysms and pregnancy, *J Neurosurg* 41:63-70, 1974.

80. Sadasivan B, Ghaus MM, Lee C et al: Vascular malformations and pregnancy, *Surg Neurol* 33:1990.

81. Seeger JF, Gabrielson TO, Giannotta SL et al: Carotid cavernous sinus fistulae and venous thombosis, *Am J Neuroradiol* 1:141-148, 1980.

82. Solomon RA, Michelsen WJ: Defective cerebrovascular autoregulation in regions proximal to arteriovenous malformation of the brain: a case report and topic review, *Neurosurgery* 14:78-82, 1984.

83. Spetzler R, Martin N: Pathophysiology of cerebral ischemia accompanying arteriovenous malformations. In Wilson CB, Stein BM, editors: *Intracranial arteriovenous malformations,* Baltimore, 1984, Williams & Wilkins, pp 24-31.

84. Spetzler RF, Hadley MN: Protection against cerebral ischemia: the role of barbiturates, *Cerebrovasc Brain Metab Rev* 1:212-29, 1989.

85. Spetzler RF, Hargraves RW, McCormick PW et al: Relationship of perfusion pressure and size to risk of hemorrhage from arteriovenous malformations, *J Neurosurg* 76:918-23, 1992.

86. Spetzler RF, Martin NA: A proposed

grading system for arteriovenous malformations, *J Neurosurg* 65:476-483, 1986.

87. Spetzler RF, Martin NA, Carter LP et al: Surgical management of large AVMs by staged embolization and operative excision, *J Neurosurg* 67:17-28, 1987.

88. Spetzler RF, Wilson CB, Weinstewin P et al: Normal perfusion pressure breakthrough, *Clin Neurosurg* 25:651-672, 1978.

89. Spetzler RF, Zabramski JM: Grading and staged resection of cerebral arteriovenous malformations, *Clin Neurosurg* 36:318-37, 1990.

90. Stein BM, Kader A: Intracranial arteriovenous malformations (honored guest lecture), *Clin Neurosurg* 39:76-113, 1992.

91. Stein BM, Wolpert SM: Arteriovenous malformations of the brain: I. current concepts and treatment, *Arch Neurol* 37:1-5, 1980.

92. Stein BM, Wolpert SM: Arteriovenous malformations of the brain: II. current concepts and treatment, *Arch Neurol* 37:69-75, 1980.

93. Steinberg GK, Fabrikant JI, Marks MP et al: Sterotactic heavy-charged-particle Bragg-peak radiation for intracranial arteriovenous malformations, *N Engl J Med* 323:96-101, 1990.

94. Steiner L: Treatment of arteriovenous malformations by radiosurgery. In Wilson CB, Stein BM, editors: *Intracranial arteriovenous malformations,* Baltimore, 1984, Williams & Wilkins, pp 295-313.

95. Sundt TJ, Piepgras DG, Stevens LN: Surgery for supratentorial arteriovenous malformations, *Clin Neurosurg* 37:49-115, 1991.

96. Sundt TM, Piepgras DG: The surgical approach to arteriovenous malformations of the lateral and sigmoid dural sinuses, *J Neurosurg* 59:32-39, 1983.

97. Szabo MD, Crosby G, Sundaram P et al: Hypertension does not cause spontaneous hemorrhage of intracranial arteriovenous malformations, *Anesthesiology* 70:761-763, 1989.

98. Tamaki N, Ehara K, Lin TK et al: Cerebral arteriovenous malformations: factors influencing the surgical difficulty and outcome, *Neurosurgery* 29:856-61, 1991.

99. Tamaki N, Lin T, Asada M et al: Modulation of the blood flow following excision of a high flow cerebral venous arteriovenous malformation, *J Neurosurg* 72:509-512, 1990.

100. U HS, Kerber CW, Todd MM: Multimodality treatment of deep periventricular cerebral arteriovenous malformations, *Surg Neurol* 38:192-203, 1992.

101. Valavanis A, Wellauer J, Yasargil MG: The radiological diagnosis of cerebral venous angioma: cerebral angiography and computed tomography, *Neuroradiology* 24:193-199, 1983.

102. Vineula F, Dion J, Lylyk P et al: Update on interventional neuroradiology, *AJR* 153:23-33, 1989.

103. Vinuela F, Dion JE, Duckwiler G et al: Combined endovascular embolization and surgery in the management of cerebral arteriovenous malformations: experience with 101 cases, *J Neurosurg* 75:856-64, 1991.

104. Vinuela FV, Debrun GM, Fox AJ et al: Dominant hemisphere arteriovenous malformations: therapeutic embolization with isobutyl-2-cyanoarcrylate, *AJNR* 4:959-966, 1983.

105. Voight K, Yasagil MG: Cerebral cavernous hemangiomas or cavernomas, *Neurochir* 19:59-68, 1976.

106. Wilkens RH: Natural history of intracranial vascular malformations: a review, *Neurosurgery* 16:421-430, 1985.

107. Wilson CB: Cryptic vascular malformations, *Clin Neurosurg* 38:49-84, 1992.

108. Wilson CB, Hieshima G: Occlusive hyperemia: a new way to think about an old problem, *J Neurosurg* 78:1993.

109. Wilson CB, Hieshima GB, Higashida RT et al: Interventional radiologic adjuncts in cerebrovascular surgery, *Clin Neurosurg* 37:332-52, 1991.

110. Wilson CB, UHS, Domingue J: Microsurgical treatment of intracranial vascular malformations, *J Neurosurg* 51:446-454, 1979.

111. Yeh HS, Kashiwagi S, Tew JMJ et al: Surgical management of epilepsy associated with cerebral arteriovenous malformations, *J Neurosurg* 72:1990.

112. Yeh HS, Tew JM, Gartner M: Seizure control after surgery on cerebral arteriovenous malformations, *J Neurosurg* 78:12-18, 1993.

113. Young WL, McCormick PC: Perioperative management of intracranial catastrophes, *Crit Care Clin* 5:821-44, 1989.

114. Young WL, Prohovnik I, Ornstein E et al: The effect of arteriovenous malformation resection on cerebrovascular reactivity to carbon dioxide, *Neurosurgery* 27:257-66, 1990.

115. Young WL, Prohovnik I, Ornstein E et al: Monitoring of intraoperative cerebral hemodynamics before and after arteriovenous malformation resection, *Anesth Analg* 67:1011-1014, 1988.

116. Young WL, Solomon RA, Prohovnik I et al: 133Xe blood flow monitoring during arteriovenous malformation resection: a case of intraoperative hyperperfusion with subsequent brain swelling, *Neurosurgery* 22:765-9, 1988.

20

Induced Hypotension

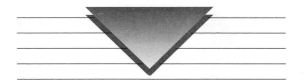

JAMES E. COTTRELL
JOHN HARTUNG

CLINICAL CONSIDERATIONS
    Laplace's law and aneurysm rupture
    How low can MAP be reduced?
COMMONLY USED DRUGS
    Sodium nitroprusside
    Nitroglycerin

Effects of nitroprusside and nitroglycerin
    on microcirculation
    Trimethaphan
POTENT INHALATIONAL
    ANESTHETICS
    Isoflurane

LESS COMMONLY USED, NEW, AND
    EXPERIMENTAL DRUGS
    Adenosine triphosphate
    Esmolol and labetalol
SUMMARY

Having observed in 1946 that neurosurgeons "make extremely slow progress with the removal of tumors until the patient's blood pressure falls as a result of loss of blood," Gardner reported the first case of intentionally "lowering a patient's blood pressure by venipuncture in order that bleeding from the tumor might be more readily controlled (and) the patient's own blood could be returned instead of transfusing blood from a donor."[25]

The idea caught on. Just 9 years later, Little was able to collect information on 27,930 cases of induced hypotension across the United States and Great Britain. Techniques ranged from arteriotomy to administration of trimethaphan. The U.S. complication rate was 1 in 27, with a mortality rate of 1 in 136. Tempering his conclusion that we might want to "dismiss 'controlled hypotension' as a menace to humanity," Little conceded that it should be considered "for an urgent and rational indication . . . in the carefully selected case."[46,47]

Enthusiasm for inducing hypotension has waxed[44] and waned[82] several times since the mid-1950s. In 1982 Michenfelder called the technique anesthesiology's preeminent contribution to reduction of mortality from aneurysm surgery during the preceding decade.[58] However, the succeeding decade has seen improvements in surgical technique that enable increased employment of temporary vascular clips to achieve hypotension that is limited to the aneurysm and its immediately distal area of cerebral blood flow (CBF).[3,36] When combined with recent evidence that compromised neural tissue is jeopardized by any substantive diminution in CBF,[9,11,34,53,94] advances in surgical technique have swung the pendulum of induced hypotension's popularity back toward Little's "public menace" position. Drummond recently recommended that "it is preferable to minimize blood pressure reduction and to reserve hypotension for the control of intraoperative rupture or perhaps for brief periods preceding clip application."[19]

Nevertheless, clipping is not always possible after aneurysm rupture, more than a few neurosurgeons are wary of placing temporary clips routinely,[14] and induced hypotension is still a preferred technique for arteriovenous malformations (AVM) and may come to be preferred for closed-cranium embolization of AVMs and saccular aneurysms.[15] Accordingly, we need to know how to do it.

425

CLINICAL CONSIDERATIONS
Laplace's Law and Aneurysm Rupture

Unfortunately, as recognized by Laplace, when an aneurysm grows larger and its wall becomes thinner, less pressure is required to expand it to the breaking point (Fig. 20-1).[23] Accordingly, either an increase in mean arterial pressure (MAP) or a fall in cerebrospinal fluid (CSF) pressure or brain tissue pressure will increase transmural pressure, the wall stress, and the risk of rupture (Fig. 20-2).[8] Nevertheless, it is difficult to confirm the usefulness of deliberate hypotension in prevention of aneurysm rupture. The only published study directly comparing hypotension with normotension found no difference in the frequency of aneurysm rupture during surgery.[17] In addition, Giannota et al. recently reviewed 41 cases of perioperative or intraoperative aneurysm rupture and found that patients treated by ipsilateral carotid artery tamponade or temporary clips had better outcomes than those in whom hypotension was induced.[27]

How Low Can MAP Be Reduced?

Most practitioners agree that reduction of MAP to 50 mm Hg can be tolerated well by the normal, healthy brain.[86] However, patients with chronic hypertension usually lose cerebral blood flow autoregulation at 50 mm Hg, so their blood pressure should be reduced only to 50 mm Hg below

their normal pressure.[64] Other contraindications to all but the most moderate reductions in blood pressure (20 to 30 mm Hg) include fever, anemia, occlusive cerebrovascular disease, prolonged retractor pressure,[49] and intracerebral hematoma. Although hyperventilation is a useful technique for reducing intramural pressure through cerebral vasoconstriction, its use in conjunction with hypotension may aggravate the risk of partial ischemia,[30] so ventilation during hypotension should be adjusted to maintain normocarbia.

COMMONLY USED DRUGS
Sodium Nitroprusside

Sodium nitroprusside (SNP) ($Na_2Fe[CN]_5NO.2H_2O$) continues to be the most widely used drug for intravenous induction of hypotension. Like all nitrovasodilators, SNP decreases peripheral vascular resistance by metabolic or spontaneous reduction to nitric oxide (NO).[39] Adequate blood flow to vital organs is maintained at perfusion pressures above 50 mm Hg. Sodium nitroprusside has rapid onset and a short half-life and primarily dilates resistance vessels without affecting cardiac output (CO).

Adverse effects may result from SNP infusion. These include cyanide (CN) and thiocyanate toxicity, rebound hypertension, intracranial hypertension, blood coagulation abnormalities, increased pulmonary shunting, and hypothyroidism.* In addition, myocardial, liver, and skeletal muscle oxygen reserves are decreased by SNP, and mitochondria may be damaged.[21] Death from SNP-induced

---

*References 10, 15, 18, 33, 56, 61, 62.

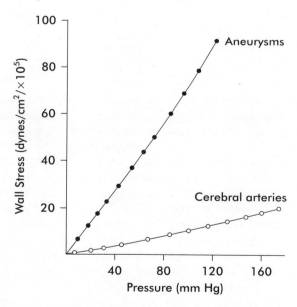

FIG. 20-1 Wall stress for aneurysms and cerebral arteries as a function of intraluminal pressure, calculated from the elastic diagrams for each. Wall stress (dynes/cm²) equals wall tension (dynes/cm) divided by wall thickness (cm). The value for minimum wall thickness of cerebral arteries was designated as 175 μm, and a figure of 25 μm was chosen for aneurysms. *(From Ferguson GG: The rationale for controlled hypotension. In Varley GP, editor: Anesthetic considerations in the surgical repair of intracranial aneurysms, Int Anesth Clin, vol 20, Boston, 1982, Little Brown.)*

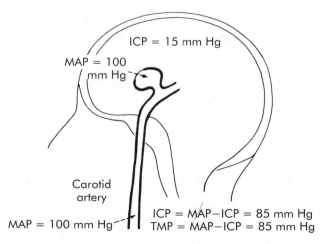

FIG. 20-2 Transmural pressure of aneurysm (TMP) is the same as the cerebral perfusion pressure (CPP) and is equal to the difference between mean arterial pressure (MAP) and intracranial pressure (ICP). Rupture of a surgically exposed aneurysm occurs when TMP exceeds the tensile strength of the aneurysm wall. *(From Boarini DJ, Kassell NF: Cerebral management. In Cottrell JC, Turndorf H, editors: Anesthesia and neurosurgery, ed 2, St Louis, 1986, CV Mosby.)*

severe acidosis has occurred after infusion of 750 mg over a 5-hour period.[57]

Cyanide is produced when SNP is metabolized (Fig. 20-3). SNP contains CN at a level of .44 mg CN/mg SNP. Toxic blood levels (greater than 100 $\mu g/dl^{-1}$) occur when more than 1 mg/kg SNP is administered within 2 1/2 hours or when more than 0.5 mg/kg/hr is administered within 24 hours. Death from SNP secondary to CN has been reported in a pediatric patient when blood CN level was 400 $\mu g/dl^{-1}$.[18] Greater risk of CN toxicity exists in patients who are nutritionally deficient in cobalamine (vitamin B_{12} compounds) or in dietary substances containing sulfur. Measurement of blood CN and pH enables detection of abnormalities in high-risk patients for whom larger-than-recommended amounts of SNP have been used. Treatment should consist of intravenous thiosulfate, except in those patients with abnormal renal function, for whom hydroxocobalamin is recommended (Fig. 20-4).[4] Circulating levels of thiocyanate increase when renal function is compromised, and central nervous system abnormalities result when thiocyanate levels reach 5 to 10 mg/dl^{-1}. Fortunately, captopril can be used to lower the dose requirement of SNP and thereby reduce the consequent build-up of cyanide (Fig. 20-5).[93,102] Another recently advocated strategy for reducing the potential for cyanide toxicity is to maintain SNP-like pharmacodynamics while greatly reducing SNP dosage in a 1:10 mixture with trimethaphan.[65,66] Diltiazem,[7] metoprolol,[6] and esmolol have also been shown to effectively reduce SNP requirements, but esmolol does so at the cost

of dose-dependent reductions in left ventricular contractility.[84]

Systemic and pulmonary hypertension occur after abrupt discontinuance of SNP.[15] This results from increased plasma renin activity (PRA) caused by either ischemic or dilated renal vessels. Gradual SNP discontinuance, preoperative propranolol, and converting enzyme inhibitors (captopril) attenuate this response until increased PRA returns to normal (plasma half-life = 30 minutes).

Based on results obtained in dogs, Michenfelder and Milde have argued that SNP dilates cerebral capacitance vessels regardless of anesthetic background and also dilates cerebral resistance vessels when autoregulation is blunted by a volatile agent.[59,80] More recently, Stånge, et al. have found evidence in pigs that SNP directly impairs cerebral autoregulation.[89] Under either circumstance, if venous return is impeded by a mass lesion, SNP causes an increase in cerebral blood volume (CBV). Accordingly, SNP causes increased intracranial pressure (ICP) in patients with low intracranial elastance (Table 20-1).[16] In the closed cranium an increase in ICP can cause hemispheric reductions in CBF because of regional reductions in cerebral perfusion pressure (CPP = MAP − ICP). In the open cranium with open dura, SNP-induced cerebral vasodilation is not likely to affect regional CBF[76] but may cause brain swelling and disturb local perfusion, especially in areas under retraction and areas that are distant from the site of small-to-moderate sized craniotomies.

Sodium nitroprusside can cause platelet disintegration

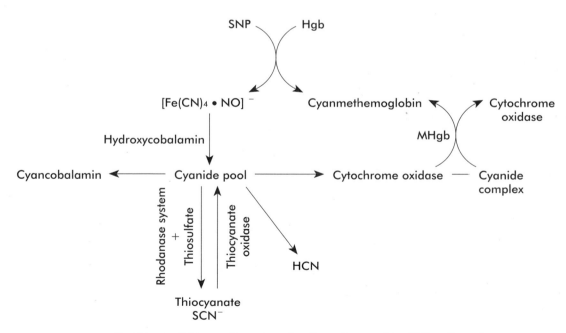

FIG. 20-3 Red blood cell biotransformation of sodium nitroprusside. *SNP*, sodium nitroprusside; *Hgb*, hemoglobin; *mHgb*, methemoglobin; *SCN*, thiocyanate; *HCN*, hydrogen cyanide. *(From Bendo AA, Kass IS, Hartung JH et al: Neurophysiology and neuroanesthesia. In Barash PG, Cullen BF, Stoelting RH, editors: Clinical anesthesia, ed 2, Philadelphia, 1992, JB Lippincott.)*

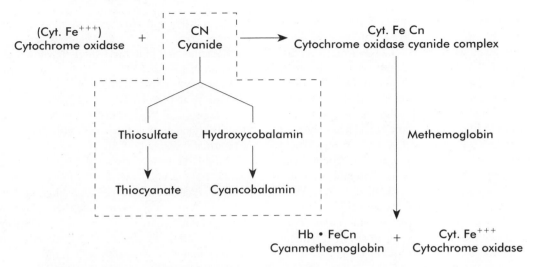

FIG. 20-4   Tissue cytochrome oxidase combines with cyanide to form cytochrome oxidase–cyanide complex. Methemoglobin frees cyanide from the complex, forming cyanmethemoglobin. Other potential pathways to prevent toxicity include the additon of thiosulfate or hydroxocobalamin. The *dashed line* indicates treatment of cyanide toxicity. *(From Bendo AA, Kass IS, Hartung JH et al: Neurophysiology and neuroanesthesia. In Barash PG, Collen BF, Stoelting RH, editors: Clinical anesthesia, ed 2, Philadelphia, 1992, JB Lippincott.)*

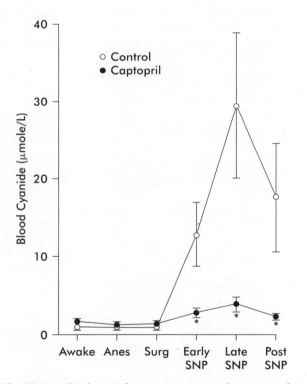

FIG. 20-5   Blood cyanide in two groups of patients whose blood pressure was decreased by sodium nitroprusside. Patients pretreated with captopril (3 mg/kg) had significantly less cyanide than those not treated even though a similar degree of hypotension was obtained. Total sodium nitroprusside infused was significantly less in patients treated with captopril. *(From Woodside J Jr, Garner L, Bedford RJ: Anesthesiology 60:413, 1984.)*

and inhibition of platelet aggregation;[33,56] however, recent evidence indicates that this complication is reversible and transitory.[31] Nevertheless, SNP-induced abnormalities in blood coagulation can exacerbate increased intraoperative bleeding caused by vasodilation.[33]

Increased pulmonary shunting occurs in patients with normal pulmonary function after SNP-induced hypotension, but fibrosed pulmonary vessels of patients with chronic obstructive lung disease show little response to SNP, and shunting increases are not significant.[10] Subsequent work has demonstrated a significant relationship between age and SNP sensitivity, with lower doses capable of inducing equally profound hypotension in older patients.[101] It is possible that further elucidation of this age/dose relationship will allow more appropriate age-specific administration of SNP with a consequent amelioration of SNP-related complications.

Nitroprusside is obtained in a 5 ml amber rubber-stopper vial containing 50 mg of sodium nitroprusside dihydrate. It can be dissolved in 5% dextrose in water (D_{5W}) to the concentration desired; 50 mg of sodium nitroprusside in 250, 500, or 1000 ml of D_5W makes a concentration of 200 μg, 100 μg, or 50 μg/ml respectively. After it is dissolved, sodium nitroprusside deteriorates in the presence of light. Therefore the container should be wrapped in aluminum foil. An unstable sodium nitroprusside ion in aqueous solution reacts with a variety of substances within 3 to 4 hours, forming colored salts. Other drugs should not be infused in the same solution as sodium nitroprusside.

Because vascular response to sodium nitroprusside can be dramatic, sodium nitroprusside should be administered

TABLE 20-1
Cerebral Perfusion Pressure After Hypotension Induced
by Sodium Nitroprusside

Measurement (mm Hg)	Before Sodium Nitroprusside	After Sodium Nitroprusside
MAP	104 ± 2.55	70.9 ± 3.61*
ICP	14.58 ± 1.76	27.61 ± 3.16
CPP	89.32 ± 3.57	43.23 ± 4.60

*Mean arterial pressure *(MAP)* reduced by 33%; *ICP*, intracranial pressure; *CPP*, cerebral perfusion pressure.
From Cottrell JE, Patel KD, Ransohoff JR: *J Neurosurg* 48:329, 1978.

with an infusion pump or a Volutrol IV set. When microdrip techniques are used, a continuous increase in flow rate or increased height of the infusion may be required.

The usual dose of sodium nitroprusside is 0.5 to 10 µg/kg/min. Infusion is begun at 1 µg/kg/min and is increased to achieve the desired MAP. If adequate reduction of blood pressure is not obtained with 10 µg/kg/min within 10 to 15 minutes, the infusion should be stopped to avoid cyanide toxicity. Direct arterial manometry should be used during sodium nitroprusside infusion.

Nitroglycerin

Nitroglycerin (NTG) directly dilates capacitance vessels[54] and has a short half-life and no clinically significant toxic metabolites. Resistance to NTG has been reported in some patients receiving volatile anesthetics.[14,77] As with SNP, high intracranial elastance contraindicates NTG use before dural opening unless steroids, diuretics, or sedatives have improved elastance. Even with the dura open, both nitrates entail some risk of increased CBV and significant brain swelling.[14,15] Also similar to SNP, after NTG-induced hypotension, pulmonary shunting increases in patients with normal pulmonary function in contrast to those with chronic obstructive pulmonary disease (COPD). One research report indicates that NTG reduces cardiac index compared with SNP at a mean arterial blood pressure of 40 mm Hg.[52]

Nitroglycerin is supplied in a variety of formulations from various manufacturers, some of which require dilution. As obtained from the manufacturer, NTG is relatively stable when exposed to light and can be kept up to 2 years without refrigeration. The drug is administered continuously for deliberate hypotension or to control increased blood pressure, using a direct intravenous infusion without dilution. Nitroglycerin is absorbed by plastic bags and should be infused from glass bottles or from high-density polyethylene syringes and tubings.[13] An infusion pump is best for infusion at a beginning rate of 1 to 2 µg/kg/min with increases to achieve the desired blood pressure level. Good hypotensive response is usually seen at 2 µg/kg/min. Upper limits of infusion have not been set because toxic effects have not been described, but the concentration of the infused solution should not exceed 400 µg/ml.

Effects of Nitroprusside and Nitroglycerin on Microcirculation

In animal experiments that have continuously monitored local tissue Po_2 in skeletal muscle, liver, and myocardium, tissue Po_2 is dramatically reduced while arterial Po_2 remains within normal range during sodium nitroprusside infusion.[32] This clinically relevant finding has been confirmed by measurement in patients. In support of these findings, Franke et al. have shown by capillaroscopy that sodium nitroprusside predominantly dilates precapillaries, but nitroglycerin acts on all microvascular segments.[24] During hypotension, with the use of either drug, pressure is decreased to the same extent on the arteriolar side, but on the venous side there is a decrease only with nitroglycerin. Accordingly, the pressure difference between the arteriolar side and the venule side, which is of great importance for capillary perfusion, remains unchanged with nitroglycerin but decreases significantly with sodium nitroprusside. Furthermore, Franke et al. found that a significant volume of blood is diverted through arteriovenous shunts during sodium nitroprusside hypotension.[24] These results imply that NTG has a higher therapeutic index than SNP, at least in patients who are not NTG-refractory and/or do not respond with tachyphylaxis.

Trimethaphan

Trimethaphan (TMP) blocks sympathetic ganglia, resulting in resistance and capacitance vessel relaxation, which usually decreases arterial pressure. Trimethaphan's short plasma half-life makes for easy control, but histamine release has been reported to cause bronchospasms[35] and potential ICP increases.[90] The speed of infusion and altered autoregulation may also influence trimethaphan's effect on ICP.[40] Myoneural blockade has been reported after administration of trimethaphan, probably because of its chemical resemblance to neuromuscular blocking agents.

Trimethaphan is not recommended for hypotension below 55 mm Hg MAP because electroencephalographic (EEG) suppression occurs below this level[92] although that effect may be less frequent when isoflurane is used as a background anesthetic.[48] Laboratory results show that cortical CBF and tissue oxygenation are reduced during profound TMP-induced hypotension (MAP 30 to 35 mm Hg) relative to SNP-induced hypotension[51] and that TMP hypotension below MAP 50 mm Hg causes increased brain lactate concentrations.[60] These findings accord well with recent evidence that TMP reduces local CBF during neuroleptanalgesia in humans, even when MAP is maintained at 70 mm Hg.[1] When these cerebral effects are considered in light of experimental evidence that TMP-induced hypotension reduces arterial basoreflex response to rapid blood loss from exsanguination,[91] it seems reasonable to conclude that TMP should not be used as a sole agent for producing hypotension during neurosurgical procedures.

Potent Inhalational Anesthetics

Halothane, enflurane, isoflurane, desflurane, and sevoflurane hypotension are produced by increasing their respective inspired concentrations. Decreased blood pressure results from varying degrees of myocardial depression and peripheral vascular dilation. Potential adverse effects include autoregulatory loss of vital organ blood flow, reduction in cerebral perfusion pressure (CPP) as MAP decreases, ICP increase in patients with intracranial masses, increased cerebral edema, and accumulation of anaerobic metabolites.

Halothane-induced hypotension entails the risk of adverse myocardial depression,[78] loss of autoregulation,[41] and increases in ICP that cannot be resolved through hyperventilation.[37,38] In addition to reducing cardiac output, high-dose or prolonged enflurane anesthesia has been shown to increase CSF production in the laboratory[2] and induce seizures in some patients, especially during hypocapnia.

Laboratory evidence suggests that desflurane hypotension causes substantial reduction in CPP and CBF with a concomitant decrease in oxygen metabolism (CMR_{O_2}).[63] Recent results derived from humans indicated that the blood pressure response to changes in inspired concentration of sevoflurane is more rapid than the response to changes in concentration of isoflurane.[75]

Isoflurane

The only inhalation agent currently recommended for deliberate hypotension is isoflurane.[44] Macnab et al. have determined that, relative to SNP, isoflurane blunts the stress response to induced hypotension.[55] The hypotension that results from isoflurane is primarily a consequence of peripheral vascular dilation, with maintenance of CO except at higher inspired concentrations. Reports of worsening of ST-segment changes and shunting of blood from collateral-dependent regions in the myocardium have caused concern about using isoflurane in patients with myocardial disease.[79] Pulmonary shunting and dead space are not increased during isoflurane-induced hypotension.

Because of isoflurane's ability to reduce CMR_{O_2} while maintaining cerebral blood flow,[29,50,81] cerebral protection seems likely. However, Bendo et al.[5] have found that clinical doses of isoflurane are not as protective as thiopental in the in vitro hippocampal slice model, and Nehls et al.[67] have demonstrated that isoflurane does not provide protection after focal ischemia. Gelb et al. have tested the hypothesis that isoflurane-induced hypotension provides a measure of protection relative to SNP-induced hypotension during middle cerebral artery occlusion in monkeys.[26] Unfortunately, they found no difference in neurologic scores or lesion size between the isoflurane and SNP groups. These results are consonant with Sano et al.'s recent laboratory finding that isoflurane does not provide more cerebral protection than halothane.[83]

In a nonhuman primate, Van Aken et al.[97] have demonstrated loss of autoregulation for 60 minutes after discontinuance of isoflurane and increases in CBF, which could worsen edema and ischemia and increase neurologic deficits. Endlund et al. have found that adenylate kinase, a marker of brain cell injury, increased 400% in the CSF of patients in whom hypotension was induced by isoflurane to MAP 50 to 65 mm Hg for 20 to 170 minutes.[22] Although high-dose isoflurane per se is not implicated by this result because of lack of a control or alternate hypotensive regimen, recent evidence indicates that equivalent degrees of hypotension can be obtained with less than 1% isoflurane if either labetalol[96] or the angiotension-converting enzyme enalaprilat[98] are used in conjunction with the isoflurane.

Less Commonly Used, New, and Experimental Drugs

Adenosine Triphosphate

Adenosine and adenosine triphosphate (ATP) have been used to induce hypotension in humans.[42,68,73,74,88] Advantages include prompt onset and short duration. Adenosine triphosphate is metabolized to adenosine and PO_4, with adenosine being responsible for vasodilation. Adenosine is metabolized to uric acid, and there are conflicting reports about the amount that accumulates. Unfortunately, ATP and adenosine dilate cerebral vessels.[85]

Thus adenosine-induced hypotension has been shown to increase ICP in dogs with or without preexisting intracranial hypertension.[99] Conversely, adenosine hypotension appears to have little effect on canine formation or reabsorption of cerebrospinal fluid,[94] does not appreciably reduce CBF if CPP is maintained above the lower limits of autoregulation,[43] and improves cardiac flow/metabolism ratios compared with controls during coronary ischemia.[87] Concern remains regarding adenosine's effect on CBF autoregulation in humans. Lagerkranser et al. reported a 15% increase in posthypotension CBF in a sample of six hyperventilated patients[42]; in an earlier study, they found 23% to 85% increases during adenosine-induced hypotension in normoventilated patients.[88]

Esmolol and Labetalol

Esmolol, an ultra-short-acting cardioselective beta-adrenergic blocker with an estimated half-life of approximately 9 minutes has been used to decrease blood pressure by itself[71,72] or in combination with other drugs.[20] Esmolol's cardiac depressant properties indicate caution in attempting to use it as a primary hypotensive agent.

Labetalol, a combined alpha- and beta-blocker, has also been used as a sole hypotensive agent in humans.[12,28,69] Like esmolol, labetalol is probably better used in combination therapies[95] when inducing hypotension, not only because of bradycardia, but also because of its lack of potency.[20] Both esmolol and labetalol have properties advantageous to neurosurgical hypotension because they do not dilate cerebral vessels, increase heart rate, cause rebound hypotension, or produce toxic metabolites under laboratory conditions.[100]

SUMMARY

More effort currently is being directed toward avoiding the need to induce hypotension during neurosurgery than toward developing new hypotensive drugs and pharmacologic combinations. That trend is likely to continue until substantial intraoperative brain protection becomes practicable, at which time the popularity of induced hypotension may swing back to its former status as a routine procedure during neurosurgery. Meanwhile, "for urgent and rational indication in the carefully selected case,"[2] a clinician's best choice among the better known agents is probably the drug or drug combination with which he/she has the most experience.

References

1. Abe K, Demizu A, Kamada K et al: Local cerebral blood flow with prostaglandin E₁ or trimethaphan during cerebral aneurysm clip ligation, *Can J Anaesth* 38:831-36, 1991.

2. Artru AA: Enflurance causes a prolonged and reversible increase in the rate of CSF fluid in the dog, *Anesthesiology* 57:255, 1982.

3. Ausman JI, Diaz FG, Malik GM et al: Management of cerebral aneurysms: further facts and additional myths, *Surg Neurol* 32:21-35, 1989.

4. Bendo AA, Kass IS, Hartung JH et al: Neurophysiology and neuroanesthesia. In Barash PG, Collen BF, Stoelting RH, editors: *Clinical anesthesia,* ed 2, Philadelphia, 1992, JB Lippincott, p 903.

5. Bendo AA, Kass IS, Cottrell JE: Comparison of the protective effect of thiopental and isoflurance against damage in the rat hippocampal slice, *Brain Res* 403:136, 1987.

6. Bemann, Jensen KA, Riisager S et al: Cerebral blood flow and metabolism during hypotension induced with sodium nitroprusside and metoprolol, *Eur J Anaesthesiology* 8:197-201, 1991.

7. Bernard J-M, Moren J, Demeure D et al: Diltiasem reduces the nitroprusside doses for deliberate hypotension, *Anesthesiology* 77;3A:427, Abstracts, 1992.

8. Boarini DJ, Kassell NF: Cerebral management. In Cottrell JC, Turndorf H, editors: *Anesthesia and neurosurgery,* ed 2, St Louis, 1986, CV Mosby, p 413.

9. Bouma GJ, Muizelaar JP, Choi SC et al: Cerebral circulation and metabolism after severe traumatic brain injury: the elusive role of ischemia, *J Neurosurg* 75:685-93, 1991.

10. Casthely PA, Learn S, Cottrell JE et al: Intrapulmonary shunting during induced hypotension, *Anesth Analg* 61:231, 1982.

11. Cole DJ, Drummond JC, Shapiro HM et al: Influence of hypotension and hypotensive technique on the area of profound reduction in cerebral blood flow during focal cerebral ischaemia in the rat, *Br J Anaesth* 64:498-502, 1990.

12. Cope DHP, Crawford MC: Labetalol in controlled hypotension, *Br J Anaesth* 51:1, 1979.

13. Cossum, PA, Roberts MS, Galbraith AJ et al: Loss of nitroglycerin from intravenous infusion sets, *Lancet* 2:345-350, 1978.

14. Cottrell JE, Gupta B, Rappaport H et al: Intracranial pressure during nitroglycerin-induced hypotension, *J Neurosurg* 53:309, 1980.

15. Cottrell JE, Illner P, Kittary MJ et al: Rebound hypertension after sodium nitroprusside-induced hypotension, *Clin Pharmacol Ther* 27:32, 1980.

16. Cottrell JE, Patel KP, Ransohoff JR: Intracranial pressure changes induced by sodium nitroprusside in patients with intracranial mass lesions, *J Neurosurg* 48:329, 1978.

17. Dahlgren BE, Gordon E, Steiner L: Evaluation of controlled hypotension during surgery for intracranial arterial aneurysms, *Excerpta Med Congr Series* 200:1232, 1968.

18. Davies DW, Kadar D, Steward DJ et al: A sudden death associated with the use of sodium nitroprusside for induction of hypotension during anesthesia, *Can Anaesth Soc J* 22:547, 1975.

19. Drummond JC: Deliberate hypotension for intracranial aneurysm sur-gery: changing practices (letter), *Can J Anaesth* 38:935-946, 1991.

20. Edmonson R, Del Valle O, Shah N et al: Esmolol for potentiation of nitroprusside-induced hypotension: impact on the cardiovascular, adrenergic, and reninangiotensin systems in man, *Anesth Analg* 69:202, 1989.

21. Endrich B, Franke N, Peter K et al: Induced hypotension: action of sodium nitroprusside and nitroglycerin on the micro-circulation. A micropuncture investigation, *Anesthesiology* 66:605, 1987.

22. Enlund M, Ahlstedt B, Revenas B et al: Adverse effects of the brain in connection with isoflurane-induced hypotensive anaesthesia, *Acta Anaesth Scand* 33:413-415, 1989.

23. Ferguson GG: The rationale for controlled hypotension. In Varley GP, editor: *Anesthetic considerations in the surgical repair of intracranial aneurysms, International Anesthesiology Clinics 20,* Boston, 1982, Little, Brown, p 91.

24. Franke N, Endrich B, Messmer K: Verdangerungen der Mikrozirkulation bei gabe von natriumnitroprusside [unten] nitroglycerin, *Schweiz Med Wochenschr* 111:1017, 1981.

25. Gardner WJ: The control of bleeding during operation by induced hypotension, *JAMA* 132:572-574, 1946.

26. Gelb AW, Boisvert DP, Tang C et al: Primate brain tolerance to temporary focal cerebral ischemia during isoflurane or sodium nitroprusside-induced hypotension, *Anesthesiology* 70:678, 1989.

27. Giannotta SL, Oppenheimer JH, Levy ML et al: Management of intraoperative rupture of aneurysm without hypotension, *Neurosurgery* 28:531-36, 1991.

28. Goldberg ME, McNulty SE, Azad SS et al: A comparison of labetalol and nitroprusside for inducing hypotension during major surgery, *Anesth Analg* 70:537-542, 1990.

29. Haraldsted VY, Asmussen J, Herlevsen P et al: Cerebral arteriovenous difference of oxygen during gradual and sudden increase of the concentration of isoflurane for induction of deliberate hypotension, *Acta Anaesth Scand* 36:142-144, 1992.

30. Harp JR, Wollman H: Cerebral metabolic effects of hyperventilation and deliberate hypotension, *Br J Anaesth* 45:256, 1973.

31. Harris SN, Escobar A, Rinder C et al: Nitroprusside induced platelet dysfunction: a reversible phenomenon? *Anesthesiology* 77;3A:145, abstract, 1992.

32. Hauss J, Schonleven K, Spiegel H et al: Nitroprusside- and nitroglycerin-induced hypotension: effects on hemodynamics and on the microcirculation, *World J Surg* 6:241, 1962.

33. Hines R, Barash PG: Infusion of sodium nitroprusside induces platelet dysfunction in vitro, *Anesthesiology* 70:611, 1989.

34. Ishige N, Pitts LH, Berry I et al: The effect of hypoxia on traumatic head injury in rats. Alterations in neurologic function, brain edema, and cerebral blood flow, *J Neurosurg* 68:129-136, 1988.

35. Ivankovitch AD, Miletich DJ, Tinker JH: Nitroprusside and other short acting hypotensive agents, *Int Anesthesth Clin* 16:132, 1978.

36. Jabre A, Symon L: Temporary vascular occlusion during aneurysm surgery, *Surg Neurol* 27:47-63, 1987.

37. Jennett WB, Barker J, Fitch W et al: Effects of anesthesia on intracranial pressure in patients with space occupying lesions, *Lancet* 1:61, 1969.

38. Jennett WB, McDowall DG, Barker J: The effect of halothane on intracranial pressure in cerebral tumors: report of two cases, *J Neurosurg* 26:270, 1967.

39. Johns RA: Endothelium-derived relaxing factor. Basic review and clinical implications, *J Cardiothorac Vasc Anesth* 5:69-79, 1991.

40. Karlin AD, Hartung J, Cottrell JE: Rate of induction of hypotension with trimethaphan modifies the intracranial pressure response in cats, *Br J Anaesth* 61:161, 1988.

41. Keaney NP, Pickerodt VWA, McDowall DG: CBF, autoregulation, CSF acid base parameters and deep halothane hypotension, *Stroke* 4:324, 1973.

42. Lagerkranser M, Bergstrand G, Gordon E et al: Cerebral blood flow and metabolism during adenosine-induced hypotension in patients undergoing cerebral aneurysm surgery, *Acta Anaesth Scand* 33:15, 1989.

43. Lam AM, Artru AA: Autoregulation of cerebral blood flow in response to adenosine-induced hypotension in dogs, *J Neurosurg Anesth* 4:120-127, 1992.

44. Lam AM, Gelb AW: Cardiovascular effects of isoflurane-induced hypotension for cerebral aneurysm surgery, *Anesth Analg* 62:742, 1983.

45. Langerkranser M: Controlled hypotension in neurosurgery '92: pro, *J Neurosurg Anesthesth* 3:150-152, 1992.

46. Lindop MJ: Complications and morbidity of controlled hypotension, *Br J Anaesth* 47:799-803, 1975.

47. Little DM Jr: Induced hypotension during anesthesia and surgery, *Anesthesia* 16:320-332, 1955.

48. Lloyd-Thomas AR, Cole PV, Prior PF: Isoflurane prevents EEG depression during trimethaphan-induced hypotension in man, *Br J Anaesth* 65:313-318, 1990.

49. Lownie S, Wu X, Karlik S et al: Brain retractor edema during induced hypotension: the effect of the rate of return of blood pressure, *Neurosurgery* 27:901-906, 1990.

50. Madsen JB, Cold GE, Hansen ES: Cerebral blood flow and metabolism during isoflurane-induced hypotension in patients subjected to surgery for cerebral aneurysms, *Br J Anaesth* 59:1204, 1987.

51. Maekawa T, McDowall DG, Okuda Y: Brain-surface oxygen tension and cerebral cortical blood flow during hemorrhagic and drug-induced hypotension in the cat, *Anesthesiology* 51:313-320, 1979.

52. Maktabi M, Warner D, Sokoll M: Comparison of nitroprusside, nitroglycerin, and deep isoflurane for induced hypotension, *J Neurosurg* 19:350, 1986.

53. Marmarou A, Anderson RL, Ward JD et al: Impact of ICP instability and hypotension on outcome in patients with severe head trauma, *J Neurosurg* 75:S59-S66, 1991.

54. Mason DT, Zelis R, Amsterdam EA: Actions of the nitrates on the peripheral circulation and myocardial oxygen consumption: significance in the relief of angina pectoris, *Chest* 59:296, 1971.

55. Mcnab MSP, Manninen PH, Lam AM et al: The stress response to induced hypotension for cerebral aneurysm surgery: a comparison of two hypotensive techniques, *Can Anaesth Soc J* 35:111, 1988.

56. Mehta P, Mehta J, Miale TD: Nitroprusside lowers platelet count, *N Engl J Med* 299:1134, 1978.

57. Merrifield AJ, Blundell MD: Toxicity of sodium nitroprusside (letter), *Br J Anaesth* 46:324, 1974.

58. Michenfelder JD, Foreword: In Varkey GP, editor: *Anesthetic considerations in the surgical repair of intracranial aneurysms*, Boston, 1982, Little Brown & Co, pp xii-xiv.

59. Michenfelder JD, Milde JH: The interaction of sodium nitroprusside, hypotension, and isoflurane in determining cerebral vasculature effects, *Anesthesiology* 69:870, 1988.

60. Michenfelder JD, Theye RA: Canine systemic and cerebral effects of hypotension induced by hemorrhage, trimethaphan, halothane or nitroprusside, *Anesthesiology* 46:188, 1977.

61. Michenfelder JD, Theye RA: Canine systemic and cerebral effects of hypotension induced by hemorrhage, trimethaphan, halothane, or nitroprusside, *Anesthesiology* 46:188, 1977.

62. Michenfelder JD, Tinker JH: Cyanide toxicity and thisulfate protection during chronic administration of sodium nitroprusside in the dog, *Anesthesiology* 47:441, 1977.

63. Milde LN, Milde JH: Cerebral and systemic hemodynamic and metabolic effects of desflurane-induced hypotension in dogs, *Anesthesiology* 74:513, 1991.

64. Miller ED Jr: Deliberate hypotension. In Miller RD, editor: *Anesthesia*, ed 3, New York, 1990, Churchill-Livingstone, pp 1347-1367.

65. Miller R, Toth C, Silva DA: Nitroprusside vs. a nitroprussed-trimethaphan mixture: a comparison of dosage requirements and hemodynamic effects during induced hypo-

tension for neurosurgery, *Mt Sinai J Med (NY)* 54:308, 1987.

66. Nakazawa K, Taneyama C, Benson KT et al: Mixtures of sodium nitroprusside and timethaphan for induction of hypotension, *Anesth Analg* 73:59-63, 1991.

67. Nehls DG, Todd MM, Spetzler RF et al: A comparison of the cerebral protective effects of isoflurane and barbiturates during temporary focal ischemia in primates, *Anesthesiology* 66:453, 1987.

68. Numajiri Y, Mokuhi T, Kagami K: ATP induced hypotensive anesthesia during prosthetic hip surgery (in Japanese), *J Clin Anesth* 3:279, 1979.

69. Okasha AS, Et-Attar AM, El-Gamal NA: Hemodynamic changes and glucose utilization during controlled hypotensive anesthesia with labetalol and sodium nitroprusside, *MEJ Anesth* 9:395-402, 1988.

70. O'Mahony J, Bolsin SNC: Anaesthesia for closed embolisation of cerebral arteriovenous malformations, *Anaesth Intens Care* 16:318-323, 1988.

71. Ornstein E, Matteo RS, Weinstein JA et al: A controlled trial of esmolol for the induction of deliberate hypotension, *J Clin Anesth* 1:31, 1988.

72. Ornstein E, Young WL, Ostapkovich N et al: Deliberate hypotension in patients with intracranial arteriovenous malformations: esmolol compared with isoflurane and sodium nitroprusside, *Anesth Analg* 72:639, 1991.

73. Owall A, Jarnberg PO, Brodin LA et al: Effects of adenosine-induced hypotension on myocardial hemodynamics and metabolism in fentanyl anesthetized patients with peripheral vascular disease, *Anesthesiology* 68:416, 1988.

74. Owall A, Lagerkranser M, Sollevi A: Effects of adenosine-induced hypotension on myocardial hemodynamics and metabolism during cerebral aneurysm surgery, *Anesth Analg* 67:228, 1988.

75. Philip JH, Ji XB, Calalang BS et al: Sevoflurane controls blood pressure faster than isoflurane, *Anaesthesiology* 77:A384, 1992.

76. Pinaud M, Souron R, Lelausque JN et al: Cerebral blood flow and cerebral oxygen consumption during nitroprusside-induced hypotension to less than 50 mm Hg, *Anesthesiology* 70:255, 1989.

77. Porter SS, Asher M, Fox DK: Comparison of intravenous nitroprusside, nitroprusside-captopril, and nitroglycerin for deliberate hypotension during posterior spine fusion in adults, *J Clin Anesth* 1:87-95, 1988.

78. Prys-Roberts C, Lloyd JW, Fisher A et al: Deliberate profound hypotension induced with halothane: studies of hemodynamics and pulmonary gas exchange, *Br J Anaesth* 46:105, 1974.

79. Reiz S, Balfors E, Bredgaard M: Coronary hemodynamic effects of general anesthesia and surgery, *Regional Anesth* 7(Suppl):S8-S18, 1982.

80. Rogers AT, Prough DS, Gravlee GP et al: Sodium nitroprusside does not dilate cerebral resistance vessels during hypothermic cardiopulmonary bypass, *Anesthesiology* 74:820-826, 1991.

81. Roth S, Jones SC, Ebrahim ZY et al: Local cortical blood flow and oxygen consumption during isoflurane-induced hypotension, *Cleve Clin J Med* 56:766-770, 1989.

82. Ruta TS, Mutch WAC: Controlled hypotension for cerebral aneurysm surgery: are the risks worth the benefits? *J Neurosurg Anesthesth* 3:153-156, 1992.

83. Sano T, Drummond JC, Patel PM et al: A comparison of the cerebral protective effects of isoflurane and mild hypothermia in a model of incomplete forebrain ischemia in the rat, *Anesthesiology* 76:221-228, 1992.

84. Shah N, Del Valle O, Edmondson R et al: Esmolol infusion nitroprusside-induced hypotension: impact on hemodynamics, ventricular performance, and venous admixture, *J Cardiothorac Vasc Anesthesia* 6:196-200, 1992.

85. Shapira Y, Artru AA, Lam AM: Changes in the rate of formation and resistance to reabsorption of cerebrospinal fluid during deliberate hypotension induced with adenosine or hemorrhage, *Anaesthesiology* 76:432-439, 1992.

86. Shapiro HM: Neurosurgical anesthesia and intracranial hypertension. In Miller RD, editor: *Anesthesia,* ed 2, New York, 1986, Churchill Livingstone, pp 1563-1620.

87. Sidi A, Rush W: Adenosine for controlled hypotension: systemic compared with intracoronary infusion in

dogs, *Anesth Analg* 75:319-328, 1992.

88. Sollevi A, Ericson K, Eriksson L et al: Effect of adenosine in human cerebral blood flow as determined by positron emission tomography, *J Cereb Blood Flow Metab* 7:673-678, 1987.

89. Stånge K, Lagerkranswer M, Solevi A: Nitroprusside-induced hypotension and cerebrovascular autoregulation in the anesthetized pig, *Anesth Analg* 73:745-752, 1991.

90. Stoyka WW, Schutz H: The cerebral response to sodium nitroprusside and trimethaphan controlled hypotension, *Can Anaesth Soc* 22:275, 1975.

91. Taneyama C, Goto H, Goto K et al: Attenuation of arterial baroreceptor reflex response to acute hypovolemia during induced hypotension, *Anesthesiology* 73:433-440, 1990.

92. Thomas WA, Cole PV, Etherington NJ et al: Electrical activity of the cerebral cortex during induced hypotension in man, *Br J Anesth* 57:134-141, 1985.

93. Thomsen LJ, Riisager S, Jensen KA et al: Cerebral flood flow and metabolism during hypotension induced with sodium nitroprusside and captopril, *Can J Anaesth* 36:392-96, 1989.

94. Tinjen H, Kimiyoshi H, Mizykawa N et al: Dysautoregulations in patients with ruptured aneurysms: cerebral blood flow measurements obtained during surgery by a temperature-controlled thermoelectrical method, *Neurosurgery* 23:705-709, 1988.

95. Toivonen J: Plasma renin, catecholamines, vasopressin and aldosterone during hypotension induced by labetalol with isoflurane, *Acta Anaesth Scand* 35:496-501, 1991.

96. Toivonen J, Virtanen H, Kaukinen S: Labetalol attenuates the negative effects of deliberate hypotension induced by isoflurane, *Acta Anaesth Scand* 36:84-88, 1992.

97. Van Aken H, Fitch W, Graham DI: Cardiovascular and cerebrovascular effects of isoflurane-induced hypotension in the baboon, *Anesth Analg* 65:565, 1986.

98. Van Aken J, Leusen I, Lacroix E et al: Influence of converting enzyme inhibition on isoflurane-induced hypotension for cerebral aneurysm surgery, *Anesthesia* 47:261-264, 1992.

99. Van Aken H, Puchstein C, Anger C et al: Changes in intracranial pressure

and compliance during adenosine triphosphate-induced hypotension in dogs, *Anesth Analg* 63:381, 1984.

100. Van Aken H, Puchstein C, Schweppe ML et al: Effect of labetalol on intracranial pressure in dogs with and without intracranial hypertension, *Acta Anaesth Scand* 26:615, 1982.

101. Wood M, Hyman S, Wood AJJ: A clinical study of sensitivity to sodium nitroprusside during controlled hypotensive anesthesia in young and elderly patients, *Anesth Analg* 66:132, 1987.

102. Woodside J Jr, Garner L, Bedford RJ: Captopril reduces the dose requirement for sodium nitroprusside induced hypotension, *Anesthesiology* 60:413, 1984.

21

Anesthesia for Diagnostic Neuroradiology

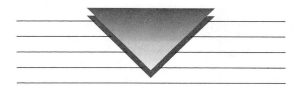

MITCHELL TOBIAS
DAVID S. SMITH

HISTORY

Diagnostic radiology has had a tremendous effect on the practice of neurosurgery. The serendipitous demonstration of air within the cerebral ventricles of one unfortunate patient after a motor vehicle accident was recognized as having diagnostic potential by Dandy, who initially used the technique for visualization of the ventricles.[26] Pneumoencephalography is now only of historic interest. With respect to dye contrast radiography, the first injectable contrast medium used in the subarachnoid space was Lipiodal, a high-density iodinated substance that had to be aspirated out of the subarachnoid space after the study.[92] Myelography continues to be a valuable radiologic investigation, particularly as an adjunct to computed tomographic (CT) studies; how-

ever, water-soluble contrast dyes are now used. Angiography was first demonstrated through tenacious experimentation using direct carotid puncture in animals and humans.[62] This contribution allowed the growth of interventional neuroradiology, which is discussed in another chapter. The explosion of computer technology through the 1970s and 1980s provided a basis for the development of other imaging techniques, including digital subtraction angiography (DSA), CT, and magnetic resonance imaging (MR).

GENERAL CONSIDERATIONS

A unifying factor in all radiologic examinations is the need for the patient to remain relatively motionless for the duration of image acquisition. Longer acquisition times, such as are required for MR, render the study more sensitive to movement artifact. Obtunded or neurologically affected patients frequently cannot cooperate. Infants, children, and patients with seizures or tremors may also be unable to provide good examinations if unassisted. These groups of patients may require an anesthesiologist's intervention to obtain successful studies. However, many radiologic suites are not easily adaptable to the requirements of safe administration of anesthesia. Older facilities are often crowded, unfamiliar, and dark. The patient may be situated at a distance from the anesthesiologist or on a mobile table (myelography). Bulky radiologic equipment may limit patient access, visibility, or both. Nonetheless, the equipment for operating room standards of monitoring and the administration of general anesthesia must be available before agreeing to assume care for one who is, or may rapidly, become a critically ill patient.

Neurodiagnostic procedures are often noninvasive or without stimulation. Although some are painful, they may be safely executed without resorting to general anesthesia. Little is gained from a technique that yields an inadequate study. Many of the studies are long and tedious. The anesthesiologist must treat each patient as unique and not abide by routine.

Magnetic Resonance Imaging

MR represents a major development in diagnosis through its enhanced resolution of anatomic structures. In many instances the resolution is superior to that obtained by CT scan.[17,49] As noted earlier, the excellent resolution of MR can be severely degraded by any patient movement. In addition, the required intense magnetic fields create unique problems with the use of physiologic monitors, standard anesthesia machines, and ventilators. Thus the restrictive environment of this technology presents unique challenges to the anesthesiologist.

Physical Basis of Magnetic Resonance

In 1946 both Purcell[74] and Bloch et al.[8] independently published work, for which they shared the 1952 Nobel Prize in physics, describing the phenomenon of nuclear induction. Use of nuclear magnetic resonance phenomena to create images was suggested by Damidian[25] and Lauterbur.[59] A subsequent decade of intense scientific effort produced the current high-resolution MR techniques, which, by their nature, avoid ionizing radiation or dependence on iodinated contrast media.

The physical and technical fundamentals are covered more fully elsewhere.[17,34,107] Briefly, atomic nuclei with an odd number of protons or neutrons have the potential to act as magnetic dipoles. Although this property is held by all paramagnetic elements (^{13}C, ^{31}P, ^{19}F, ^{23}Na, ^{1}H, and ^{2}H), clinical MR uses the most abundant element, hydrogen, whose nucleus comprises a single proton. Normally the large numbers of hydrogen protons in a given specimen are oriented randomly, and there is no net magnetic field. If, however, a biologic specimen is placed within a powerful homogeneous magnetic field, the hydrogen nuclei align their axes so that there is a slight net magnetization. To produce this alignment, MR units typically operate with static magnetic fields of 0.5 to 1.5 Tesla; as a point of reference, the earth's magnetic field measures 0.00006 Tesla. Pulsed radiofrequency (RF) energy of an appropriate frequency and duration forces these protons out of alignment with the static magnetic field and into a higher energy state. When the RF pulse is discontinued, the protons return to the "aligned" (lower energy state) and, in doing so, emit RF energy related to their quantity, chemical identity, and relationship with surrounding nuclei. Location within a tissue can be obtained by superimposing another magnetic field with a specific and changing field strength on the static magnetic field. The emitted RF signals are received by a receiver antenna within the bore of the MR unit or by a surface coil placed directly on the patient's body. These surface coils enhance the signal-to-noise ratio if more detailed imaging is desired.

Thus diagnostic imaging using magnetic resonance requires large, powerful superconducting magnets with very homogeneous static magnetic fields, controllable electromagnetic coils to create magnetic gradients, and a source of pulsed energy at a specific RF to change the energy state of the protons. Sophisticated computers control the timing, strength, and sequencing of the RF pulses; change the gradient magnetic fields; and collect and process the magnetic resonance information to construct the resulting images. The signals of interest have relatively low intensity and may be hard to differentiate from the surrounding "noise." MR signals from brains of anesthetized and unanesthetized patients differ, indirectly giving some insight into the chemical activity of anesthetic action.[104]

Hazards

The anesthetic considerations for patients having MR studies reflect some unique hazards as well as the problems associated with physiologic monitors in proximity to this unique equipment. Hazards may result from the intense static magnetic field, the magnetic gradient, RF energy, released cryogens, or injected contrast material.[102] MR currently is thought to carry no major biologic effects despite long-term exposure.[69,89]

Static and Time-Varied Magnetic Field Effects

The potential effects of static magnetic fields on biologic tissue may be divided into effects on (1) normal cellular and physiologic function and (2) implanted prostheses. In addition, these strong magnetic fields attract any ferromagnetic material that is on the patient and attending medical personnel, or material introduced into the environment as part of the monitoring or anesthesia equipment.

Physiologic effects of strong, localized magnetic field exposure in humans have included skeletogenesis,[70] improved bone fracture repair,[7] and changes in erythrocyte rheology.[12] Nonsickled homozygous erythrocytes have normal flow patterns during MR.[11] However, irreversibly sickled erythrocytes align themselves perpendicularly to a magnetic field in vitro.[12,64] The potential for worsening an acute sickle cell occlusive crisis by this magnetic effect in vivo is the subject of investigation. The addition of hypertonic intravenous MR contrast media may contribute to this potential (see later discussion on reactions to contrast media).

Other magnetically induced effects include (1) changes in electrocardiogram (ECG) signals related to induced voltages from blood flowing perpendicular to the magnetic field, (2) visual phosphenes secondary to current-induced retinal stimulation,[16] (3) evoked potentials and nerve conduction,[99] and (4) induced alterations in the sensitivity of rat pineal gland,[15,78,103] *E. coli* enzyme synthesis,[1] and avian navigation sense.[106]

Of greater concern, however, are the potentially dangerous effects of the powerful magnetic field on in vivo metals such as are contained in (1) pacemakers, (2) automatic implanted cardiac defibrillators (AICD), (3) synthetic cardiac valves, (4) spiral wire tracheal tubes, or (5) metallic objects such as shrapnel or vascular clips. Certain metal alloys have been shown to manifest sufficient attraction and movement within clinically relevant magnetic fields to present a risk of dislodgment, hemorrhage, or motile injury to adjacent sensitive structures (e.g., brain).[28] Steel alloys with adequate nickel content (approximately 10% to 40%) have low ferromagnetic properties and tend not to be hazardous at the magnetic field strengths used for MR.[66] Suitable alloys are designated austentitic by the American Iron and Steel Institute. Clips made of austentitic alloys are currently used during vascular surgery and neurosurgery.

Cardiac pacemakers have ferromagnetic parts or casings that may move in magnetic fields. Newly implanted pacemakers may shift position and cause pain or may be dislodged. A more likely occurrence is closure of the reed switch, changing the pacemaker function from synchronous to asynchronous modes. Inducted pulses as high as 20 mV can lead to inhibition of pacemaker discharge.[72] This occurs in both synchronous and asynchronous modes. Magnetic fields may also deactivate AICDs. However, direct cardiac stimulation by electrical currents induced by the gradient magnetic fields does not occur. These induced currents are orders of magnitude below the required threshold.[67] Although measurable current can be induced in pacemaker wires by the changing magnetic fields, it is well below that needed for depolarization or microshock. However, burns under ECG electrodes have been reported, and high-resistance ECG cables should be used to minimize current generation. Implanted microcircuitry (e.g., insulin, chemotherapeutic or intrathecal pumps) may malfunction within the magnetic field. Thus patients with pacemakers, AICDs,

implanted pumps, or vascular clips of a magnetic or an unknown alloy are generally barred from MR examinations.

Ferromagnetic objects, if brought sufficiently close to the magnet, may launch toward the magnet with considerable force. The force exerted on an object is inversely proportional to the fourth power of its distance from the magnet's center and is directly related to the mass of the object. An object brought too near the magnet may literally fly into the magnet or an interposed obstruction such as a patient. Many anecdotes have been published describing the ballistic consequence of ferrous objects ranging from scissors to forklift truck prongs.[33]

RF Generation

RF energy can be absorbed by tissue or other objects and converted to heat. Body surfaces absorb markedly more energy than deep tissues. Superficial tissues with decreased vascularity (and therefore less ability to dissipate heat) may be more subject to heating.[15] Current MR machines are unlikely to increase tissue temperature more than 1° C; however, febrile patients or those who are unable to perspire may be at increased risk. With implants, the amount of heating is directly related to the size and conductive properties of the implant.[27] Relatively avascular tissue (e.g., the cornea or a hip joint adjacent to a large ferrous implant) may sustain a greater effect of RF absorption than highly vascular or deeper tissues. Currents induced by a surface coil near the body are capable of producing local cutaneous burns. Reorientation of the surface coil or permitting air circulation between the coil and the patient's skin should decrease this potential problem.[9,15] Core and peripheral temperature monitoring in humans during MR examinations confirms the clinical impression that thermal effects are minimal and well tolerated.[83,88,90,91,98]

Magnetic Gradients

The switching on and off of the magnetic gradient coils creates loud noises, which frighten some patients. In one study, the incidence of emotional distress during MR was 4.3%. The distress was related, in part, to gradient noise, but claustrophobia and fear of the diagnosis also played a role.[32] This pulsing sound also creates difficulties in communication between the anesthesiologist and patient. Visualization of the patient who lies within the magnet bore is poor; therefore verbal communication is essential.

Cryogen Release

The magnet uses superconductivity to maintain its strong homogenous field. Despite recent advances, superconductors require temperatures approaching 0° Kelvin (−273° C). These austere cryostatic conditions are maintained by encasing the MR magnetic coil with liquid helium and liquid nitrogen. In the very rare event of a cryogen leak or emergency shutdown caused by a sudden increase in superconducting coil resistance with subsequent heating and boiling off of the cryogens (quench), an MR room may have its available oxygen displaced by sudden release of this dangerously cold helium and nitrogen.[107] Frostbite will occur with only momentary tissue contact with liquid helium or nitrogen. Hair and clothes entrap the liquids and facilitate skin burning. Eyes are also extremely susceptible to injury. MR rooms are designed with special venting to help prevent these consequences of cryogen release although external vents may be blocked by refuse, nests, leaves, or other material.

Clinical Considerations

Patients scheduled for MR are similar to those who come to the operating room. Critically ill adults or infants and children may require general anesthesia and neuromuscular blockade to eliminate movement. Claustrophobic or excitable patients may be adequately studied with sedation. The same careful preoperative evaluation applies to patients undergoing this procedure as applies to an operative procedure. With varying degrees of difficulty, most of the standards of care adopted by the American Society of Anesthesiologists can be met in the MR environment (Table 21-1).

A list of reportedly MR-compatible apparati has been published.[71] There are also several thoughtful reviews on issues related to monitoring during MR.[10,18,36,39,50,52,80,87,96]

Specific considerations for the anesthesiologist relate to (1) the effect of the static magnetic field, gradient magnetic fields, RF emission, and electromagnetic interference (EMI) on monitoring equipment, (2) the disruptive effects of physiologic monitors on image quality, and (3) the remote access to the patient. The compatibilities of specific brands and types of monitoring devices and the brand of MR machine employed vary.

The monitoring equipment commonly used by anesthesiologists in the operating room generates significant amounts of EMI, which may degrade the quality of the image acquired. Wires from monitors to the patient may act as antennae and attract ambient or emitted RF energy, thereby contributing to image degradation. A valuable rule obtained through clinical experience is that running data or power cables parallel to the Z axis of the static magnetic field aids in limiting artifacts. In addition, locating monitoring equipment, anesthesia apparatus, and other equip-

TABLE 21-1
Standards of Anesthetic Care and MR*

Standard	Possible Approaches and Problems with Meeting Standard During MR
Continuous presence of qualified personnel	Can be in room with patient; no known significant hazard to personnel
Evaluation of oxygenation	
Inspired oxygen	O_2 analyzers on inspiratory limb have been used; need to be fixed firmly and sufficiently far from the magnet to minimize attraction; batteries are ferromagnetic
Blood oxygenation	
Observation	Observation of lips and fingers is often impossible, especially during head or neck studies; toes may be outside the magnet and visible
Pulse oximetry	If not specially designed for MR or shielded, these devices tend to degrade the image and are unusable
Evaluation of ventilation	
Observation of clinical signs, chest excursion, reservoir bag, auscultation	Long-magnet bore makes observation difficult; noise generated during imaging makes auscultation difficult to impossible; observation of reservoir bag, if present, is possible; placement of a paper cup on the chest may aid visualization of excursion
End-tidal CO_2 analysis	Has been reported using units that sample the exhaled gas stream by aspiration; all devices have a ferromagnetic risk; Pa_{CO_2} may be underestimated; some units may generate electromagnetic interference
Volume of expired gas	Respirometers may be used if not ferromagnetic, or if placed and fixed at a safe distance
Ventilator disconnect alarm	Depends on design and distance from the magnet
Evaluation of circulation	
Continuous ECG	May be distorted and uninterpretable during image acquisition; wiring may attract RF; induced currents may burn patient
Arterial blood pressure and heart rate every 5 min	Oscillotonometry and sphygmomanometry, both manual and automated, have been used with success
Continuous monitoring	
Palpation of pulse	May be difficult to impossible
Auscultation of heart sounds	May be difficult to impossible
Intraarterial pressure trace	Ferromagnetic risk; many units generate interfering RF radiation
Ultrasound peripheral pulse monitoring	No reported experience
Pulse plethysmography	Standard on Siemens magnetom
Measurement of body temperature	Success with thermistor-based units

*Standards of Care adapted from American Society of Anesthesiologists' "Standards for Basic Intra-operative Monitoring" (approved by House of Delegates, October 21, 1986). In these standards, "continuous" means "prolonged without any interruption at any time" and "continual" means "repeated regularly and frequently in steady succession."

ment beyond the 100 gauss line will limit artifact and projectile risk.

Ventilatory Support and Inhalational Anesthetic Delivery

Some monitoring equipment may be rendered inoperative by EMI or the force of the static magnetic field. Standard anesthesia or intensive care unit ventilators employ electronic or mechanical regulation, which may malfunction within the magnetic field. A distance of 5 m from the magnet's bore is the minimum distance recommended if non-MR-modified equipment is being used.[82] The Siemens servo ventilator functions well within the MR room, and it has been used to anesthetize a patient by introducing fresh gas flow through its low-pressure inlet. However, sufficient distance between this ventilator and the magnet must be maintained. This ventilator has malfunctioned when placed in close proximity (within 4 feet) to the magnet. Fluidic ventilators[29,94] (Monaghan Medical Corp.) and manual jet ventilators, which do not depend on electronic or ferrous mechanical parts, have been employed successfully without patient or image compromise. All metal parts of such apparati need to be of aluminum or another nonferromagnetic material. Spontaneous or controlled ventilation using a reservoir bag obviates the need for any electronic equipment to deliver positive pressure ventilation. The use of oxygen delivered from a central system eliminates the need for pressurized oxygen tanks, which are strongly ferromagnetic.[77] The large amount of oxygen required to drive the bellows of fluidic ventilators makes small aluminum tanks impractical for positive pressure ventilation.[5]

There are reports of modifications to preexisting apparati to reduce ferric components, most of which are contained within the frame and castors.[46,60,76] Most anesthesia vaporizers contain little or no ferromagnetic materials and if kept several feet from the magnet and well attached to a fixed support will function and not become projectiles. Ohmeda, Inc. now produces an anesthesia machine designed for MR service (Ohmeda Excel MRI).

The long breathing circuit needed to ventilate a patient deep within the magnet necessitates elevated compression volumes.[6] Tidal volumes need to be adjusted with this in mind, particularly for pediatric patients or patients with low pulmonary compliance. Use of noncorrugated Tygon tubing can reduce the required compression volumes. For thoracic studies, image acquisition gated to one point of the respiratory cycle diminishes motion artifact during positive pressure ventilation and may be preferable to spontaneous ventilation.[45] Gating lengthens MR scan time appreciably unless high-frequency ventilation is employed.

Monitoring
Respiration

The respirometer on the expiratory limb of many ventilators can be used to monitor respiratory rate. The volume data must be interpreted with consideration for the increased compression volumes, as previously discussed. Adequacy of minute ventilation may be accurately monitored by an infrared end-tidal carbon dioxide monitor that aspirates respiratory gas. A lengthened sampling tube may be needed to place the monitor distant from the magnet if it leaks a significant amount of RF energy or shows attraction to the magnet. The extra length of tubing produces mixture distortion of the capnogram; the carbon dioxide plateau may not be well delineated, and peak measured end-tidal carbon dioxide may be less than the actual value. Placement of a paper cup on the patient's chest may facilitate visual verification of thoracic excursion. A microphonic device for detecting breath sounds has also been described.[46]

Oxygenation

Polarographic and fuel cell oxygen analyzers function well in the MR environment. Polarographic oxygen analyzers use batteries that may be ferromagnetic, and the unit should be secured against movement.

The pulse oximeter can be a serious RF source of image distortion. If the probe is placed on the toe, which is often outside the magnet, image quality may improve. Shielding of the cable[81] or substitution of a fiberoptic cable has reportedly minimized the artifactual effect upon some MR machines. Placement of a specially designed pulse oximeter (Biochem 1042A) 8 feet from the magnet has allowed continuous and accurate monitoring of oxygen saturation in a Siemens MR unit. The In Vivo Research, Inc. model 3109-1 is reported to be specifically tailored for use with General Electric MR units.

Cardiovascular Status

Blood Pressure. Both invasive and noninvasive pressure monitoring has been successfully used during MR. Oscillotonometric monitors may be sufficiently removed from the magnet by using lengthened connecting tubing. Cuff-to-tubing connectors should be nonferromagnetic.

Pressure transducers connected to intravascular catheters for central venous, arterial, or pulmonary artery pressure monitoring may function near the magnet. An increased length of tubing may be required to reach the patient, and this may give either an overshoot or a dampening of the pressure waveform. The monitor's amplifiers and screens may produce interfering RF signals. A technique for continuous measurement of arterial BP using an intraarterial catheter connected to a water manometer has been described.[31]

The cathode ray oscilloscope, which uses an electron beam incident on a phosphorous screen, is sensitive to magnetic interference. It must be placed sufficiently distant from the magnet to prevent distortion of the screen.

Electrocardiogram. The ECG is altered both by RF energy and static magnetic fields. The RF creates an artifact that may render the ECG unusable. The amount of disturbance depends on electrode and cable material, which act as antennae, and on the frequency of the RF pulsing.[101] Telemetric broadcast of ECG can reduce wiring and improve ECG quality. The quality of the image obtained by MR is highly sensitive to motion artifact. Synchronization of MR data acquisition with the ECG permits optimization of image quality, particularly of the thorax and heart, by minimizing motion artifact.[79]

The static magnetic field produces a peaked T wave secondary to the induction of electromotive force by the perpendicular flow of blood.[67] The distortion simply needs to be interpreted in the context of MR.

Pulse Rate.   The patient's pulse may be monitored by many modalities. A nonferromagnetic precordial or esophageal stethoscope may be employed, but its utility is impaired by the loud gradient coil noise during image acquisition. The pulse oximeter, oscillotonometer, Doppler, or intravascular arterial pressure monitors also provide heart rate information. Techniques for pulse rate determination using microphonics,[46] light beam displacement,[84] and a pneumatic detector[100] have been described.

Temperature

Patient temperature monitoring is a standard of care, but it can be difficult to implement. Pediatric patients are probably most in need of temperature monitoring because of the cold MR suite. Liquid crystal devices are unreadable during scanning because of the remote location of the patient. Remote readout monitoring devices are more appropriate but must be considered ferromagnetic because batteries are usually encased in ferrous metals. The wires conducting the signal from the thermistor or thermocouple may function as an antenna for stray RF signals and produce image artifact. Burns from temperature monitoring have been reported.[43] Many have ignored temperature monitoring during MR, recognizing that body exposure can be minimized.

Neuromuscular Blockade

The use of neuromuscular blocking drugs can be valuable because image quality highly depends on patient immobility. In addition, paralysis can improve pulmonary compliance in some patients. With respect to monitoring the degree of blockage, the nerve simulators currently used are limited within the MR environment because they are battery powered. Visual inspection of a lower extremity undergoing peroneal nerve stimulation remains a monitoring option. However, the wires of the nerve stimulator may allow degradation of image quality by acting as antennae for exogenous RF signals. Moreover, the pediatric patient will be so remote from the anesthesiologist that visualization of induced motor activity is prevented.

For patient safety, the array of monitors should be placed together so they can easily and simultaneously be scanned. Red light emitting diode displays make reading easier because the monitors are often located at some distance from the anesthesiologist and the patient. An MR-compatible an-

esthesia machine may be placed considerably closer to the patient. The anesthesiologist should be positioned to enable the best possible view of the patient. During a study, the anesthesiologist often remains in the MR room with the patient.

Intracranial Pressure

In patients requiring intracranial pressure monitoring, intracranial bolts of plastic are preferable to metallic bolts, which, even if not ferromagnetic, have some heating hazard and may produce local artifact during head imaging. Fiberoptic intracranial pressure monitor cables must be disconnected because the amplifier box contains ferromagnetic parts.

Resuscitation

The time required to decrease the magnetic field to a normal level is 3 to 20 minutes for most machines. Thus the magnetic field will be present during any resuscitation. Resuscitation teams are generally not prepared for high magnetic fields, in which beepers, hemostats, and laryngoscopes may become unwieldy or ballistic. Plans must be made for rapid removal of the compromised patient from the magnet room. A fully stocked resuscitation cart, defibrillator, and oxygen source should be available immediately outside the magnet room.

Anesthesia Approaches

The techniques employable include intravenous anesthesia, inhalational anesthesia, or sedation, according to the specific needs of the individual patient.

Sedation

Table 21-2 describes various approaches to sedation for patients undergoing MR. Oral chloral hydrate has been used in younger children who are being supervised by a nurse or the patient's mother.

General Anesthesia

Our experience with general anesthesia has included adults who have had head injury, involuntary muscle movement, and claustrophobia. For outpatients we have attempted light sedation as our technique of choice but have used general endotracheal tube anesthesia for outpatients as well as inpatients.

We usually induce general anesthesia in an alcove immediately adjacent to the magnet. This area has piped-in oxygen and suction. We supply an anesthesia machine and appropriate portable monitors, including ECG oscilloscope, blood pressure oscillotonometer, pulse oximeter, capnograph oxygen analyzer, and temperature detector. The patient gurney we use can be easily placed in the Trendelenburg position. Thus our induction area for MR is equipped similarly to operating room anesthesia locations.

After anesthesia induction, intubation, and stabilization,

TABLE 21-2
Examples of Sedation for MR in Children* and Adults

Age (Years)	Medication	Dosage (mg/kg)	Comments
Under 1.5	Chloral hydrate, PO	75-120, not to exceed 2 g	Give 30 min before scan
1.5 to 6	Pentobarbital, IV	2-4, not to exceed 150 mg	Give 5 min before scan
	or		
	Midazolam, IV	0.05 to 0.1	
	or		
	Pentobarbital + meperidine, PO	34	Give 1 hr before scan
Over 6	Midazolam + fentanyl, IV	0.025 to 0.1 0.75 to 3 µg/kg	Give 5 min before scan

*These approaches are currently used at the Children's Hospital of Philadelphia.

the patient is transferred to the MR gurney and transported to the MR room (these rooms are also equipped with piped-in oxygen and suction). We have used total intravenous techniques during MR, thus eliminating the need for an anesthesia machine in the MR room. We have used combinations of pentobarbital or midazolam, together with fentanyl and vecuronium. Propofol infusions in combination with a narcotic and muscle relaxant also work well. We have used the Monaghan MR ventilator during the MR study and have monitored the patients with an esophageal stethoscope, automated oscillotonomometer, capnography, respirometer, and pulse oximeter. As discussed earlier, the Monaghan MR ventilator is not ferromagnetic and can be positioned next to the magnet. In contrast, most monitoring devices are highly ferromagnetic, and, if not permanently installed, they must be moved into and removed from the MR suite with great care. The equipment should be fixed to a support while it is in the MR suite. We have found that locating the monitors against the wall near the door of the MR suite places them sufficiently far from the magnet. In our unit, the magnetic field at this location is about .01 Tesla, and the magnetic attraction, although present, tends to be weak. We typically tape the monitors to the floor to decrease the risk of movement. We have not felt a need to monitor muscle paralysis, relying on average doses and the fact the vecuronium is relatively short acting. We have not monitored temperature in adults during the MR study, but temperature monitoring is used for children.

After completion of the study, patients are returned to the anesthesia induction area, allowed to emerge from anesthesia, and are generally extubated before transport to the recovery room. Because our MR suite is located some distance from the recovery room, extubated patients receive supplemental oxygen during transport. Because the MR examination itself is not painful, the major requirements for the anesthetic are amnesia and elimination of muscle movement; thus large doses of anesthetic agent generally are not needed, and emergence has been rapid and uncomplicated.

For head-injured patients, we have studied only those whose cerebral compliance is sufficiently high to allow their assumption of the supine position for the 30 to 60 minutes required for the MR study.[42] We have used barbiturates (most often pentobarbital) together with narcotics (fentanyl) and muscle relaxants (vecuronium) and have begun both the barbiturate and narcotic, and occasionally the muscle relaxant, before patient transport to minimize hypertension and intracranial pressure increases that may occur during patient movement. We typically obtain an arterial blood gas measurement shortly after transfer into the magnet to assure adequacy of hyperventilation.

Anesthesia and sedation during MR have a unique set of constraints because of the highly magnetic fields and the sensitivity of the resulting image to EMI. However, most of the standards of modern, safe anesthetic care can be met in this environment. The growing experience at many hospitals has demonstrated that a wide range of patients can receive safe care during MR.

COMPUTED TOMOGRAPHY

Computed tomography (CT) constructs a two-dimensional cross-sectional image derived from the measured attenuation of an x-ray beam rotating around a subject. Attenuation depends on the absorbencies of tissues, which in turn depend on tissue specific gravities and chemical composition. Manipulation of the intravascular radiation absorbence is accomplished by iodinated contrast medium. Contrast is particularly valuable in studies of vascular malformations, vascularized tumors, and blood-brain barrier deficits.[35] The CT scanner uses ionizing radiation, and leakage can irradiate the anesthesiologist. Machines have been estimated to expose the anesthesiologist to only 1 to 2 mrads/hr.[3] An exposure badge should be worn, but there is little hazard to the anesthesiologist. Patients can absorb 2 to 4 rads/hr during a typical CT scan, which is about the amount of radiation involved in a traditional skull x-ray. Many anesthesia issues are similar to those of MR, (i.e., remote access, cold rooms, and movement artifact).[24,61,95] In addition, iodinated contrast medium carries specific risks (see later discussion). Most CT examinations may be performed without an anesthesiologist's involvement. Many hospitals perform pediatric examinations using oral or intravenous sedation without an anesthesiologist present. CT examinations, however, use oral contrast and sedation, violating "nothing by mouth" status.[53] Extreme caution must be taken by radiology or pediatric personnel in the airway management of children and infants who have been sedated.

A survey of radiology personnel regarding the practice of performing pediatric CT examinations provides some insight into current practice.[54] Sedation is used for many pediatric CT examinations, including those in which oral contrast material was used. In many situations, the practice deviates from the recommendations of the American Academy of Pediatrics (AAP) regarding the relationship of last oral intake and the examination. In addition, monitoring during the CT scan appears to fall short of the recommendations of the AAP because about 25% of the responding hospitals did not appear to provide the level of monitoring thought necessary for safety. If general anesthesia is planned, one must remember that oral contrast agents may have been given 5 min to 4 hours before intubation, and, depending on the volume administered, this could present a risk for aspiration.

Hospitals use various levels of sedation. Light sedation techniques are defined as producing a minimally depressed level of consciousness and a patient who can still respond appropriately to physical stimulation. In these situations, an anesthesiologist or a nurse anesthetist is rarely present.

Deep sedation is defined as a depression in the level of consciousness from which the patient is not easily aroused. However, anesthesiologists and nurse anesthetists are in attendance for only 54% of these examinations. Most typically, the patient is monitored by the regular CT technician. With respect to monitoring, only 20% of the respondents noted use of pulse oximetry, 56% noted the use of intermittent patient inspection along with blood pressure and respiration measurements, 45% noted the use of ECG, and only 15% noted the use of an automatic blood pressure device. The relative absence of oximetry in this environment is a distinct contrast to standard operating room procedures, in which all patients undergoing sedation have pulse oximetry and blood pressure and ECG monitoring. Oral chloral hydrate or barbiturates were the most frequent sedatives. Augmentation of sedation was achieved either with the same sedatives or with various combinations of meperidine, diphenhydramine, promethazine, and chlorpromazine. Rectal midazolam (0.6 mg/kg) has proved inadequate for successful studies.[23] However, 30 mg/kg of midazolam provided conditions for satisfactory scans although there was a prolonged sleep time.[41] Sedation with IV propofol (1.5 to 2.0 mg/kg IV) or thiopental (3.0 to 4.0 mg/kg IV) has been successfully used for cranial CT. Propofol provides shorter recovery times.[97]

Monitoring should be held to the same standard of care

as in the operating room. Critically ill patients should have invasive monitoring, including intracranial pressure monitoring if deemed appropriate. Unlike MR equipment, CT apparati do not interfere with monitoring. Remote access and an unfamiliar, poorly equipped environment are still issues.

ANGIOGRAPHY

Spinal or cerebral angiography is performed using a retrograde catheterization through the femoral artery or, less commonly, other arteries. Digital subtraction angiography (DSA) eliminates the risks of arterial catheterization but requires central venous cannulation and the administration of larger doses of contrast material. Many indications for angiography have been supplanted by noninvasive (CT, MR) radiologic examinations, but examinations are still performed for the evaluation of vascular lesions such as cerebral aneurysm, arteriovenous malformations, and certain tumors.[38,47,68]

Historically, the technique was performed by direct cannulation of the carotid and vertebral arteries, followed by injection of hyperosmolar medium that caused significant facial pain. General anesthesia was the preferred method of increasing patient tolerance of this pain. There was also a supposed improvement in study quality with hyperventilation.[30] A survey revealed that departmental policies in England still dictate the use of general anesthesia for angiography.[105] However, a randomized study[21] has demonstrated that local anesthesia with sedation provided superior hemodynamic stability without a significant difference in $Paco_2$ and, most important, with equivalent study quality. This may influence a shift in the United Kingdom to the current U.S. consensus that local anesthetic techniques allow a better check on neurologic status and incur less hemodynamic instability during and after angiography. Complications of cranial arteriography include arterial spasm, embolization of plaque or air, thrombosis, vessel perforation, hematoma, and intimal dissection.

MYELOGRAPHY

Myelography is a technique of obtaining X-ray films after instillation of iodinated contrast into the subarachnoid space. This is generally a benign procedure, but a severe radiculopathy may render the patient unable to lie still for a long myelographic examination, which involves positional changes and often a postmyelographic CT scan. One of the authors (MDT) had 5 mg of tetracaine placed with the hyperbaric water-soluble contrast medium and received a satisfactory saddle block, alleviating pain for the subsequent myelogram. Movement of the myelographic table can interfere with monitor cables or an anesthesia circuit. Postural hypotension may complicate position changes. The major dangers of myelography are related to reactions to the contrast medium.

REACTIONS TO CONTRAST MEDIA

Contrast media may be administered orally or, more commonly, injected intravascularly, lymphatically, or directly into the CSF. Although most injected contrast media are water soluble, radiodense, and contain iodine, paramagnetic contrast material (typically not iodinated) is available for MR studies.

Intravascular Iodinated Contrast Media (ICM)

Ever since angiography was first performed, complications of the procedure have been noted. The sixth patient studied by Moniz died of cerebral thrombosis within hours of injection. An excellent discussion of ICM has been published.[37] About 4.7% of intravascular contrast administrations result in adverse systemic reactions, of which one third require immediate treatment (Table 21-3).[85,86] Most reactions respond well to therapy, but there are an estimated 500 fatalities per year in the United States related to ICM. This rate of reaction has been supported by others.[4] The route, rate, and dosage of ICM administered influence the incidence of adverse reactions. A history of atopy, asthma, or allergy (particularly to iodine or seafood) increases the incidence of reaction to 10% to 15%. A previous reaction to ICM increases the risk during future studies to 35%.[40] Heart disease also predisposes to dangerous ICM reactions.[4]

Predictable Reactions to ICM

Radiocontrast media are iodinated organic molecules. These water-soluble molecules are filtered by the glomeruli and not reabsorbed by the renal tubules. More than 90% of ICM is normally excreted within 24 hours, with maximal renal opacification within 1 minute after IV administration.

Contrast media are hypertonic relative to most patients' plasma, and all patients experience side effects from this property that include transient hypotension, increased central venous, systemic, and pulmonary artery pressures, and increased cardiac output.[22] There is also a significant decrease in hematocrit and systemic vascular resistance. Serum osmolarity may increase 10% or more.[63] Hypertonic media can cause normal human erythrocytes to crenate and clump in a way that resembles an agglutination reaction.[20]

Erythrocytes from patients with homozygous sickle cell disease sickle irreversibly in hypertonic solution.[48] This observation suggests that hypotonic fluids such as dextrose (5%) in water be given to such patients during anesthesia to avoid red cell precipitation, thromboses, and crisis.[48]

Other osmotic side effects include cerebral edema[57] and osmotic diuresis. The osmotic diuresis can lead to hypovolemia. The relative hypovolemia renders patients with compromised renal function at greater risk for radiographic contrast-induced acute renal failure. Newer nonionic media with lower osmolalities (400 to 800 mOsm/kg) may have a lower incidence of these adverse reactions.

For the ionic species, prepared as various salts containing iodine, the cationic composition must be carefully balanced. If the sodium-to-meglumine ratio is greater than a narrow range for coronary angiography, ventricular fibrillation can occur.[37] Radiographic ICM contain iodine, which can interfere with thyroid function studies. Furthermore, hyperthyroid patients have had thyroid storm after ICM administration.

Gadopentetate dimeglumine is an MR contrast medium that is administered intravenously. It alters the T_1 relaxation time. Gadopentetate dimeglumine has been shown to alter normal red blood cell membranes in nonhuman species, resulting in increased cell hemolysis in the spleen. Patients with preexisting hemolytic anemia or sickle cell anemia have not yet been evaluated. As previously mentioned, irreversibly sickled erythrocytes have been shown to align perpendicularly to magnetic fields, and the effect of gadopentetate dimeglumine on this phenomenon is being studied. Gadopentetate dimeglumine is hyperosmolar, and hypotension has accompanied rapid intravenous administration of the agent. Headache and nausea are other common side effects. Allergic-like reactions of varying severity have also been reported.

Contrast media can alter pharmacodynamics by displacing other drugs from serum protein binding sites. Examples of such drugs studied include pentobarbital, warfarin, and isoniazid.[58]

Idiosyncratic Reactions to ICM

Idiosyncratic reactions range from mild ones such as nausea, vomiting, and facial flushing, to moderate or severe, such as an anaphylactoid-like response (IgE or immune

TABLE 21-3
Reactions to ICM After 302,082 Administrations

Grade of Reaction	Signs	Number of Reactions	Percent of Total
Mild	Nausea, vomiting, erythema	14,301	3.3
Moderate	Edema, bronchospasm, hypotension	9943	1.4
Severe	Angina, ventricular fibrillation, convulsions, prolonged hypotension	216	0.07
Fatal	Refractory hypotension, pulmonary edema, ventricular fibrillation, convulsions, anoxia	19	0.006

From Shehadi WH, Toniolo G: *Radiology* 137:299, 1980.

complexes generally are not recoverable from the affected patients' serum) (Table 21-3). Moderate symptoms of edema, hypotension, and bronchospasm may progress to severe signs such as seizures, dysrhythmia, and cardiovascular collapse. More than 50% of the reactions can be classified as mild.

Theories of Reactions to ICM

Circulating immune complexes during acute idiosyncratic reaction to ICM have not been consistently found.[93] Patients have had reactions to ICM without prior exposure, and patients with a history of reactions do not necessarily have repeat occurrences with readministration, thus calling into question hypersensitivity mechanisms although this area is very controversial.[37]

ICM appears to have direct toxic effects on the myocardium,[73] with signs of ischemia and dysrhythmia in 23% of New York Heart Association class II to IV patients. This has been hypothesized to be due to calcium chelation by DTA or citrate in the ICM, by histamine effects on the coronary arteries or artrial-ventricular node, or by the hemodynamic responses of increased pulmonary artery and right atrial pressure or plasma volume that accompany injection of ICM.

The CNS is affected by ICM, and ICMs have been found to cross the blood-brain barrier.[56] Intracisternal ICM is said to have approximately 1000 times the convulsive properties of a similar intravenous concentration,[56] with the cause of death being pulmonary edema and cardiac arrest.[37] A hypothesis suggests that ICM reactions are related to CNS toxicity in patients with increased choroid plexus permeability to ICM.[55] The CNS may manifest a range of signs or symptoms from mild to severe or fatal manifestations, depending on the susceptibilities of various brain centers. The CNS toxicity theory has received support from autopsy evidence of cerebral edema after fatal reactions.

Contrast Reactions after Intrathecal ICM Administration

Idiosyncratic reactions to subarachnoid injection of water-soluble contrast media may produce the same effects as do media given intravascularly. In addition, they may cause headache, neck and back pain, or other meningeal symptoms. Seizures are uncommon, but they are generally related to intracranial passage of the hyperbaric medium, an overdose, preexisting seizure disorder, or possibly coadministration of medications (methohexital, enflurane, phenothiazine, meperidine, tricyclic antidepressants, monoamine oxidase inhibitors, ketamine) that lower the seizure threshold.[75] This last predisposition has been contested but not disproved.[44] Metrizamide has been demonstrated to uncouple cerebral metabolism from cerebral blood flow, with the production of seizures in baboons under thiopental anesthesia.[51] The late complication of arachnoiditis is almost eliminated with intrathecal water-soluble media.

▼

BOX 21-1
TREATMENT OF ICM REACTIONS

- Discontinue ICM administration
- Monitor ECG and blood pressure
- Provide supplemental O_2 if reaction progresses
- Obtain IV access and administer fluids as required to maintain blood pressure
- Administer IV drug regimen as needed:

Anticholinergics	Atropine	0.5 mg IV
Antihistamines	Diphenhydramine	25-50 mg IV
Methylxanthines	Aminophylline	5 mg/kg IV loading dose
Steroids	Methylprednisolone	Up to 1 g IV
Catecholamine	Epinephrine	3-5 µg/kg IV bolus
		1-4 µg/kg/min IV infusion

- Be prepared for full resuscitative measures, including catecholamine administration

TREATMENT OF REACTIONS TO IODINATED CONTRAST MEDIA

All radiology areas should have resuscitation medication and equipment available. ECG and BP monitoring should be used for all administrations of ICM to high-risk patients. Reliable intravenous access should be in place for administration of fluids for hydration and drugs for resuscitation.

There are five classes of drugs, in addition to oxygen and intravenous fluids, used to treat moderate-to-severe reactions (Box 21-1). Mild reactions (nausea, flushing, itching, rash) can be observed and treated with reassurance. Some patients rapidly recover (over a few minutes), while others may proceed to moderate reactions with bronchospasm, airway edema, and/or hypotension. The rapid administration of oxygen and fluid, and the use of the full armamentarium of drugs, including epinephrine, is most often efficacious in attenuating the most severe reactions, including airway obstruction, pulmonary edema, myocardial infarction, and shock.

PROPHYLAXES AGAINST IODINATED CONTRAST MEDIA REACTIONS

Pretesting has generally been thought to be of little value. However, studies have demonstrated the tremendous value of prophylactic pretreatment of high-risk patients with prednisone before the administration of contrast media (Box 21-2).[40] In a series of 142 patients with histories of previous reaction to ICM or allergy to iodine and shellfish, none had any serious reaction after prednisone 50 mg, orally (three doses, 6 hours apart) and diphenhydramine (50 mg) IV before exposure.

▼

BOX 21-2
ICM REACTION PROPHYLAXIS REGIMEN SUGGESTED FOR HIGH-RISK PATIENTS

- Prednisone 50 mg PO (three doses given 6 hours apart)
- Diphenhydramine 50 mg IM 1 hr before the study

From Greenberger P. Patterson R, Lelly J: Administration of radiographic contrast media in high risk patients, *Invest Radiol* 15:540-543, 1980.

▼

SUMMARY

The anesthesiologist plays an important role in the case of some patients during radiologic diagnostic studies. Of importance is the recognition of the need for appropriate equipment for monitoring and providing anesthesia care despite the remote location and often cramped quarters. This applies also to a plan for resuscitation, not only for those patients under the direct care of the anesthesiologist, but also for those who may have ICM reactions. Having equipment and drugs available for appropriate resuscitation can be the difference between successful outcome and lasting disability or death.

References

1. Aarholt E, Flinn EA, Smith CW: Magnetic fields affect the lac operon system, *Phys Med Biol* 27:606-610, 1982.
2. Adair ER, Berglund LG: On the thermoregulatory consequences of MR imaging, *Magn Reson Imaging* 4:321-333, 1986.
3. Aidinis SJ, Zimmerman RA, Shapiro HM et al: Anesthesia for brain computer tomography, *Anesthesiology* 44:420-425, 1976.
4. Ansell G, Tweedie MCK, West CR et al: The current status of reactions to intravenous contrast media, *Invest Radiol* 15:S32-S39, 1980.
5. Barnett GH, Ropper AH, Johnson KA: Physiological support and monitoring of critically ill patients during magnetic resonance imaging, *J Neurosurg* 68:246-250, 1988.
6. Bartel LP, Bazik JR, Powner DJ: Compression volume during mechanical ventilation: comparison of ventilators and tubing circuits, *Crit Care Med* 13:851-854, 1985.
7. Bassett CA, Mitchell SN, Gaston SR: Treatment of ununited tibial diaphyseal fractures with pulsing electromagnetic fields, *J Bone Joint Surg* 63(Am):511-528, 1981.
8. Bloch F, Hanson WW, Packard M: The nuclear induction experiment, *Phys Rev* 70:474-485, 1946.
9. Boesiger P, Buchli R, Saner M et al: Increased radiofrequency power absorption in human tissue due to coupling between body coil and surface coil, *Ann NY Acad Sci* 649:260, 1992.
10. Boutros A, Pavlicek W: Anesthesia for magnetic resonance imaging, *Anesth Analg* 66:367-374, 1987.
11. Brody AS, Embury SH, Mentzer WC et al: Preservation of sickle cell blood-flow patterns during MR imaging: an in vivo study, *AJR* 151:139-141, 1988.
12. Brody AS, Sorette MP, Gooding CA et al: Induced alignment of flowing sickle erythrocytes in a magnetic field—a preliminary report, *Invest Radiol* 20:560-566, 1985.
13. Buchli R, Boesiger P, Meier D: Heating effects of metallic implants by MR examinations, *Magn Reson Med* 7:255-261, 1988.
14. Buchli R, Saner M, Meier D et al: Increased RF power absorption in MR imaging due to RF coupling between body coil and surface coil, *Magn Reson Med* 9:105-112, 1989.
15. Budinger TF, Cullander C: Health effects of in vivo nuclear magnetic resonance. In James TL, Margulis AR, editors: *Biomedical Magnetic Resonance,* San Francisco, 1984, Radiology Research and Education Foundation, pp 421-441.
16. Lovsund P, Oberg PA, Nilsson et al: Magnetophosphones: a quantitative analysis of thresholds, *Med Biol Eng Comput* 18:326-334, 1980.
17. Budinger TF, Lauterbur PC: Nuclear magnetic resonance technology for medical studies, *Science* 226:288-298, 1984.
18. Burk NS: Anesthesia for magnetic resonance imaging, *Anesth Clin North Am* 7:707-721, 1989.
19. Campkin TV: General anaesthesia for neuroradiology, *Br J Anaesth* 48:783-789, 1976.
20. Chaplin H, Carlsson E: Changes in human red blood cells during in vitro exposure to several roentgenologic contrast media, *Am J Roentgenol Rad Ther Nuc Med* 86:1127, 1961.
21. Clayton DG, O'Donoghue BM, Stevens JE: Cardiovascular response during cerebral angiography under general and local anesthesia, *Anaesthesia* 44:599, 1989.
22. Coté CJ, Greenhow DE, Marshall BE: The hypotensive response to rapid intravenous administration of hypertonic solutions in man and in the rabbit, *Anesthesiology* 50:30-35, 1979.
23. Coventry DM, Martin CS, Burke AM: Sedation for paediatric computerized tomography—a double-blind assessment of rectal midazolam, *Eur J Anaesth* 8:29-32, 1991.
24. Daitch JS, Lantos G: Anesthesia for neuroradiology. In Frost EAM, editor: *Clinical anesthesia in neurosurgery,* Boston, 1991, Butterworth-Heinemann, pp 147-162.
25. Damadian R: Tumor detection by nuclear magnetic resonance, *Science* 171:1151-1153, 1971.
26. Dandy WE: Ventriculography following the injection of air into the cerebral ventricles, *Ann Surg* 68:5, 1918.
27. Davis PL, Crooks L, Arakawa M et al: Potential hazards in NMR imaging heating effects of changing magnetic fields and RF fields on small metallic implants, *AJR* 137:857-860, 1981.

28. Dujovny M, Kossovsky N, Kossowsky R et al: Aneurysm clip motion during magnetic resonance imaging: in vivo experimental study with metallurgical factor analysis, *Neurosurgery* 17:543-548, 1985.

29. Dunn V, Coffman CE, McGowan JE et al: Mechanical ventilation during magnetic resonance imaging, *Magn Res Imaging* 3:169-172, 1985.

30. Edmonds-Seal J, du Boulay G, Bostick T: The effect of intermittent positive pressure ventilation upon cerebral angiography with special reference to the quality of the films—a preliminary communication, *Br J Radiol* 40:957, 1967.

31. Emmons SW, Martin HB: Continuous arterial pressure monitoring during magnetic resonance imaging—an alternative method, *Anesth Analg* 74:315-316, 1992.

32. Flaherty JA, Hoskinson K: Emotional distress during magnetic resonance imaging, *N Engl J Med* 320:467-468, 1989.

33. Fowler JR, terPenning B, Syverud SA et al: Magnetic field hazard, *N Engl J Med* 314:1517, 1986.

34. Gadian DA: *Nuclear magnetic resonance and its application to living systems,* Oxford, England, 1982, Clarendon Press.

35. Gado MH, Phelps ME, Coleman RE: An extravascular component of contrast enhancement in cranial computed tomography, *Radiology* 117:595-597, 1975.

36. Geiger RS, Cascorbi HF: Anesthesia in an NMR scanner, *Anesth Analg* 63:622-623, 1984.

37. Goldberg M: Systematic reactions to intravascular contrast media, *Anesthesiology* 60:46-56, 1984.

38. Gonzales CF, Moret J: Balloon occlusion of the carotid artery prior to surgery for neck tumors, *AJNR* 11:649-652, 1990.

39. Goudsouzian N: Current questions in patient safety, *Anesthesia Patient Safety Foundation Newsletter,* Overland Park, KS, 1987, Anesthesia Patient Safety Foundation, p 33.

40. Greenberger P, Patterson R, Lelly J et al: Administration of radiographic contrast media in high risk patients, *Invest Radiol* 15:540-543, 1980.

41. Griswold JD, Liu LMP: Rectal methohexatol in children undergoing computerized cranial tomography and MR scans, *Anesthesiology* 67:A494, 1987.

42. Hadley DM, Teadale GM, Jenkins A et al: Magnetic resonance imaging in acute head injury, *Clin Radiol* 39:131-9, 1988.

43. Hall SC, Stevenson GW, Suresh S: Burn associated with temperature monitoring during magnetic resonance imaging, *Anesthesiology* 76:152, 1992.

44. Hanus PM: Metrizamide: a review with emphasis on drug interactions, *Am J Hosp Pharm* 37:510-513, 1980.

45. Hedlund LW, Deitz J, Nassar R et al: A ventilator for magnetic resonance imaging, *Invest Radiol* 21:18-23, 1986.

46. Henneberg S, Hök B, Wiklund L et al: Remote auscultatory patient monitoring during magnetic resonance imaging, *J Clin Monit* 8:37-43, 1992.

47. Higashida RT, Halbach VV, Dowd CF et al: Intracranial aneurysms: interventional neurovascular treatment with detachable balloons—results in 215 cases, *Radiology* 178:663-670, 1991.

48. Huntsman RG, Lehman H: Treatment of sickle cell disease, *Br J Haematol* 28:437, 1974.

49. Jenkins A, Hadley DM, Teasdale GM et al: Magnetic resonance imaging of acute subarachnoid hemorrhage, *J Neurosurg* 68:731-736, 1988.

50. Kanal E, Shellock FG: Patient monitoring during clinical MR imaging, *Radiology* 185:623-629, 1992.

51. Karanjia P, Eidelman B, DeCesare S et al: The effect of metrizamide on cerebral blood flow and metabolism, *J Cereb Blood Flow Metab* 3:S534-S535, 1983.

52. Karlik S, Heatherley T, Pavan F et al: Patient anesthesia and monitoring at a 1.5-T MR installation, *Magn Res Med* 7:210-221, 1988.

53. Kaufman RA: Technical aspects of abdominal CT in infants and children, *AJR* 153:549, 1989.

54. Keeter S, Benator RM, Weinberg SM et al: Sedation in pediatric CT: national survey of current practice, *Radiology* 175:745-752, 1990.

55. Lalli AF: Contrast media reactions: data analysis and hypotheses, *Radiology* 134:1-12, 1980.

56. Lampe KF, James G, Erbesfeld M et al: Cerebrovascular permeability of a water soluble contrast material, hypaque (sodium diatrizoate). Experimental study in dogs, *Invest Radiol* 5:79, 1970.

57. Lantos G: Cortical blindness due to osmotic disruption of the blood-brain barrier by angiographic contrast agents, *Neurology* 39:567-571, 1989.

58. Lasser EC, Elizondo-Martel G, Granke RC: Potentation of pentobarbital anesthesia by competitive protein binding, *Anesthesiology* 24:665, 1963.

59. Lauterbur PC: Image formation by induced local interactions: examples employing nuclear magnetic resonance, *Nature* 242:190, 1973.

60. Liao JC, Belani KG, Mikhail S et al: Use of new anesthesia circuit for remote ventilation during magnetic resonance imaging, *Anesth Analg* 65:S88, 1986.

61. Manninen PH: Anaesthesia outside the operating room, *Can J Anaesth* 38:R126-R129, 1991.

62. Moniz E: L'Encéphaloghie artérielle, son importance dans la localisation des tumeurs cérébrales, *Rev Neurol* 3:72-90, 1927.

63. Morisette M, Gagnon RM, Lamoureux J et al: Effects of angiographic contrast media on colloid oncotic pressure, *Am Heart J* 100:319, 1980.

64. Murayama M: Orientation of sickled erythrocytes in a magnetic field, *Nature* 206:420-422, 1965.

65. National Radiological Protection Board Exposure to nuclear magnetic resonance clinical imaging, *Radiography* 258-260, 1981.

66. New PFJ, Rosen BR, Brady TJ et al: Potential hazards and artifacts of ferromagnetic and nonferromagnetic surgical and dental materials in magnetic resonance imaging, *Radiology* 147:139-148, 1983.

67. Nixon C, Hirsch NP, Ormerod IEC et al: Nuclear magnetic resonance. Its implications for the anaesthetist, *Anaesthesia* 41:131-137, 1986.

68. O'Mahony BJ, Bolsin SNC: Anaesthesia for closed embolization of cerebral arteriovenous malformations, *Anaesth Intens Care* 16:318-323, 1988.

69. Osbakken M, Griffith J, Taczanowsky P: A gross morphologic, histologic, hematologic, and blood chemistry study of adult and neonatal mice chronically exposed to high

magnetic fields, *Magn Res in Med* 3:502-517, 1986.

70. Papatheofanis FJ: A review on the interaction of biological systems with magnetic fields, *Physiol Chem Phys Med NMR* 16:251-255, 1984.

71. Patteson SK, Chesney JT: Anesthetic management for MR: problems and solutions, *Anesth Analg* 74:121-128, 1992.

72. Pavlicek W, Geisinger M, Castle L et al: The effects of nuclear magnetic resonance on patients with cardiac pacemakers, *Radiology* 147:149-153, 1983.

73. Pfister RC, Hutter AM Jr: Cardiovascular radiology. Cardiac alterations during intravenous urography, *Invest Radiol* 15(suppl 6):S239-S242, 1980.

74. Purcell EM, Torrey HC, Pound PV: Resonance absorption by nuclear magnetic moments in a solid, *Phys Rev* 69:37-38, 1946.

75. Pyles ST, Pashayan AG: Anesthesia and neuroradiology: considerations regarding metrizamide, *Anesthesiology* 58:590-591, 1983.

76. Ramsay JG, Gale L, Sykes MK: A ventilator for use in nuclear magnetic resonance studies, *Br J Anaesth* 58:1181-1184, 1986.

77. Rao CC, McNiece WL, Emhardt J: Modification of an anesthesia machine for use during magnetic resonance imaging, *Anesthesiology* 68:640-641, 1988.

78. Reuss ST, Semm P, Vollrath L: Different types of magnetically sensitive cells in the rat pineal gland, *Neurosci Lett* 40:23-26, 1983.

79. Rokey R, Wendt RE, Johnston DL: Monitoring of acutely ill patients during nuclear magnetic resonance imaging. Use of a time-varying filter electrocardiographic gating device to reduce gradient artifacts, *Magn Res Med* 6:240-245, 1988.

80. Roth JL, Nugent M, Gray JE et al: Patient monitoring during magnetic resonance imaging, *Anesthesiology* 62:80-83, 1985.

81. Salvo I, Colombo S, Capocasa T et al: Pulse oximetry in MR units, *J Clin Anesth* 2:65-66, 1990.

82. Sanders EG, Martin TW: Anesthesia for magnetic resonance imaging procedures, *Prob Anesth* 6:430-442, 1992.

83. Schaefer DJ: Dosimetry and effects of MR exposure to RF and switched magnetic fields, *Ann NY Acad Sci* 649:225-236, 1992.

84. Selldèn H, De Chateau P, Ekman G et al: Circulatory monitoring of children during anaesthesia in low-field magnetic resonance imaging, *Acta Anaesthesiol Scand* 34:41-43, 1990.

85. Shehadi WH: Adverse reactions to intravascularly administered contrast media, *Am J Roentgenol Radium Ther Nucl Med* 124:145, 1975.

86. Shehadi WH, Toniolo G: Adverse reactions to contrast media. A report from the Committee on Safety of Contrast Media of the International Society of Radiology, *Radiology* 137:299, 1980.

87. Shellock FG: Monitoring during MR: an evaluation of the effect of high field MR on various patient monitors, *Med Electron* 9:93-97, 1986.

88. Shellock FG: Thermal responses in human subjects exposed to magnetic resonance imaging, *Ann NY Acad Sci* 649:260, 1992.

89. Shellock FG, Bierman H: The safety of MRI, *JAMA* 261:3412, 1989.

90. Shellock FG, Crues JV: Temperature, heart rate, and blood pressure associated with clinical MR imaging at 1.5 T, *Radiology* 163:259-69, 1987.

91. Shellock FG, Schaefer DJ, Gordon CJ: Effect of a 1.5 tesla static magnetic field on body temperature of man, *Magn Reson Med* 3:644-647, 1986.

92. Sicard JA, Forestier J: Méthode générale d'exploration radiologique par l'huile iodée (Lipiodol), *Bull Mem Soc Med Hoos Paris* 46:463, 1922.

93. Siegle RL, Lieberman P: Measurement of histamine, complement components and immune complexes during patient reactions to iodinated contrast material, *Invest Radiol* 11:98, 1976.

94. Smith DS, Askey P, Young ML et al: Anesthetic management of acutely ill patients during magnetic resonance imaging, *Anesthesiology* 65:710-711, 1986.

95. Trankina MF, Houser WO, Cucchiara RF: Neurodiagnostic procedures. In: Cucchiara RF, Michenfelder JD, editors: *Clinical neuroanesthesia,* New York, 1990, Churchill-Livingstone, pp 421-435.

96. Vacanti FX: Addendum to current questions in patient safety, *APSF Newsletter,* Dec, 1987, pp 34-35.

97. Valtonen M: Anaesthesia for computerized tomography of the brain in children: a comparison of propofol and thiopentone, *Acta Anaesthesiol Scand* 33:170-173, 1989.

98. Vogl TJ, Krimmel K, Fuchs A et al: Influence of magnetic resonance imaging on human body core and intravascular temperature, *Med Phys* 15:562-566, 1988.

99. Vogl TJ, Paulus W, Fuchs A et al: Influence of magnetic resonance imaging on evoked potentials and nerve conduction in humans, *Invest Radiol* 26:432-437, 1991.

100. Volgyesi GA, Doyle DJ, Kucharczyk W et al: Design and evaluation of a pneumatic pulse monitor for use during magnetic resonance imaging, *J Clin Monit* 7:186-188, 1991.

101. Watkinson WP, Gordon CJ: Improved technique for monitoring electrocardiograms during exposure to radio-frequency radiation, *Am J Physiol* 250:H320-H324, 1986.

102. Weinreb JC, Maravilla KR, Peshock R et al: Magnetic resonance imaging: improving patient tolerance and safety, *AJR* 143:1285-1287, 1984.

103. Welker HA, Semm RP, Willig RP et al: Effects of an artificial magnetic field on serotonin n-acetyltransferase activity and melatonin content of rat pineal gland, *Exp Brain Res* 50:426, 1983.

104. Whitfield A, Douglas RHB: Effect of general anaesthesia on the magnetic resonance imaging signal from the brain, *Br J Anaesth* 62:694-696, 1989.

105. Wright PJ: Anaesthetic practice and neuroradiology, *Anaesthesia* 43:809, 1988.

106. Yorke E: Sensitivity of pigeons to small magnetic field variations, *J Theor Biol* 89:533, 1981.

107. Young SW: *Nuclear magnetic resonance imaging, basic principles,* New York, 1984, Raven Press.

22

Anesthetic Management of Patients Undergoing Blood-Brain Barrier Disruption

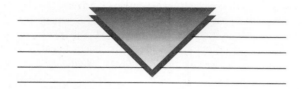

WILLIAM J. PERKINS
EDWARD A. NEUWELT

BACKGROUND
MECHANISM
PHYSIOLOGIC EFFECTS OF
  OSMOTIC BBBD

PREOPERATIVE STUDIES
ANESTHESIA CONSIDERATIONS
PROCEDURE

RESULTS
COMPLICATIONS
SUMMARY

Significant and durable responses to chemotherapy have been obtained for a number of disseminated systemic malignancies, such as non-Hodgkin's and Hodgkin's lymphoma, even when the tumor is found in multiple metastatic sites.[16,37] When these responsive tumors are identified as metastatic foci in the central nervous system (CNS), however, systemic chemotherapy fails to reduce or eliminate the tumor mass.[65,101] Indeed, patients in remission from systemic lymphoma during a course of chemotherapy have developed CNS lymphoma.[41] Neither systemic nor intrathecal chemotherapy has had a major effect on primary CNS tumors.[35] This failure in therapy may be related to either inadequate delivery[72] or the ineffectiveness of the agent. Systemic tumor regression with persistence of brain metastases after chemotherapy suggests that agents are effective when sufficiently high concentrations reach the target tissue. A technique that increases delivery of chemotherapeutic agents to the brain is therefore of clinical interest. To formulate strategies that optimize chemotherapeu-

tic drug delivery to the brain, it is necessary to consider factors constraining blood-to-brain and blood-to-tumor transfer of these agents.

A barrier to the passage of systemically administered substances into the brain was first described in the late nineteenth and early twentieth century.[18,28,29] This barrier, later termed the blood-brain barrier (BBB), consists of extensive tight junctions (zonulae occludens) between endothelial cells in the capillaries of the CNS.[4,103] These junctions are circumferential and restrict diffusion of proteins, ions, and water-soluble nonelectrolytes between endothelial cells and from the vascular lumen to brain parenchyma. The barrier to transfer of systemically administered agents imposed by the BBB takes on particular significance when considering therapy for tumors in the CNS. Although brain tumors previously were believed to have no effective BBB,[122] recent work indicates that a partially intact BBB exists in some tumors.[31,32,74,80] Even the well-vascularized, proliferative edge of a tumor, or the brain adjacent to tumor (BAT), has a complex and significant degree of BBB integrity.[59,60] The variable presence of the BBB in brain tumors has been suggested as an explanation for their poor response to systemically administered chemotherapy.[30] It is also possible that as a tumor responds to chemotherapy, its BBB permeability and blood-to-tumor drug transfer decrease.

The BBB plays a critical role in limiting the CNS access to many chemotherapeutic agents. With the exception of molecules transported by specific carrier systems, drug passage across the BBB is determined by molecular weight, lipid solubility, and ionization.[71] The BBB normally prevents passage of ionized, water-soluble drugs with a molecular weight greater than 180 daltons.[25,63] Most chemotherapeutic agents have molecular weights of 200 to 1200 daltons. Methotrexate (MTX), daunorubicin, and cyclophosphamide, for example, have molecular weights of 454, 544, and 261 daltons, respectively. The CNS access of these agents is thus impeded at the BBB on the basis of molecular weight. In addition, many of the chemotherapeutic agents are highly ionized at physiologic pH. For example, MTX is 99.8% ionized at pH 7.4, has a methanol:water partition coefficient of only 4.7, and is thus relatively lipid insoluble.

Increasing the delivery of currently used chemotherapeutic agents to the CNS requires either very high plasma drug levels for prolonged periods of time, a pathologically abnormal BBB, or enhanced blood-to-brain drug transfer despite a normally intact BBB. The latter objective has been accomplished in patients with brain tumors by reversible osmotic disruption of the BBB (BBBD).[78] This method markedly increases brain drug levels and significantly increases survival in patients with selected CNS tumors. Although osmotic BBBD is currently limited to clinical trials at only a few institutions worldwide,[34] it is anticipated that the recent success of this technique in treating primary CNS lymphoma[85] will result in more widespread use.

Background

BBB is rendered more permeable by a number of insults to the brain, such as hypertension, freezing, and trauma, but most of these produce irreversible brain damage and edema.[103] Early observations on the effect of progressively concentrated solutions of both topical and intracarotid (IC) solutes on the BBB[6,102,108,115,116] led to the suggestion that concentrated solutions could act osmotically to open the BBB. Applying hypertonic solutions to the pia-arachnoid, Rapoport observed passage of IV-administered Evans blue into brain parenchyma.[109] This effect was reversible for polar solutes, was a function of the osmolarity rather than the chemical nature of the solute, and correlated inversely with the ability of the solute to penetrate the cell membrane. IC injection of 3.4 M urea resulted in diffuse, reversible ipsilateral opening of the BBB to Evans blue–albumin in rabbits.[109] Subsequent animal studies demonstrated that there is a threshold concentration below which BBBD does not

occur. This threshold varies inversely with the lipid solubility of the solute and is relatively low, 1.6 molal, for both mannitol (25% mannitol) and arabinose,[44,107] the two most commonly used agents for osmotic BBBD. Reversibility of BBBD was demonstrated by the absence of any Evans blue–albumin extravasation when administered 30 to 60 minutes after the hypertonic IC infusion. Many other hypertonic solutions have been tried for BBBD in animals but suffer from disadvantages such as irreversibility (propylene glycol),[103] neurotoxicity (urea), and EEG changes of several hours duration (contrast agents).[92]

The goal of osmotic BBBD is to maximize drug delivery to the brain tumor, yet minimize systemic exposure and toxicity. In addition to molecular characteristics, pharmacokinetic factors such as drug metabolism and serum half-life affect drug delivery to the brain.[23] The method (i.e., bolus, slow or rapid infusion) and route of administration (intravenous vs. intracarotid) may also affect delivery.[22,23] IC drug infusion was selected because this method was predicted to result in optimal delivery of drug to the brain.[24] Corroborating this, there is a tenfold increase in brain MTX delivery with IC vs. IV administration after BBBD.[40,82,95] Brain MTX levels are increased ninetyfold when osmotic BBBD preceded IC drug administration compared with IV administration alone.[79,80,93] Enhanced MTX delivery occurs ipsilateral to the hyperosmotic infusion, and contralateral brain MTX levels are not significantly different from those of IC injection alone.[77] The highest brain MTX levels are found in regions supplied by the vessel into which the hyperosmotic solution is injected. For example, when MTX is injected into one of the vertebral arteries, the cerebellum, the medulla, the pons, and the posterior cerebrum have the highest drug levels.[83] MTX injected into an internal carotid artery distributes to the ipsilateral middle and anterior cerebral arterial circulation. Drug levels after osmotic BBBD were consistently higher in gray matter,[71] possibly because of the higher blood flow in this tissue.

Brain MTX levels after IC injection with BBBD are significantly increased as long as the drug is infused within 15 to 30 minutes after the IC hyperosmotic infusion.[82] Brain MTX concentration after IC injection alone is an order of magnitude lower than serum levels. After osmotic BBBD with IC MTX, ipsilateral brain MTX levels are greater than serum levels for more than 12 hours. At 6 to 12 hours after BBBD, brain MTX levels exceed serum levels by an order of magnitude.[82] For more than 12 hours after IC MTX administration with BBBD, brain MTX levels significantly exceed a possible minimum therapeutic level, 10^{-6} M.[48] The brain $t_{1/2}$ of MTX after BBBD is 30 to 90 minutes, significantly longer than that reported for nonpolar molecules such as sucrose and metrizamide.[86,94] Qualitatively similar results have been obtained for other chemotherapeutic agents, including adriamycin,[89] 5-fluorouracil, bleomycin, cisplatinum and cyclophosphamide.[75]

The preceding data indicate that the blood-to-brain transfer of a chemotherapeutic agent is increased by IC infusion after BBBD. The more relevant blood-to-tumor transfer is also increased by osmotic BBBD.[73,80] Most of the increased drug delivery, however, is to normal brain ipsilateral to the BBBD in subjects with a brain tumor.[3,44,127] For example, in rats having avian sarcoma virus tumor, BBBD increased MTX levels to tumor, BAT, and brain distant to tumor by 426%, 195%, and 934%, respectively.[73] This pattern of drug distribution increases possible brain-to-tumor drug transfer and minimizes the sink effect (tumor-to-brain transfer);[125] it also exposes normally protected brain to potentially neurotoxic chemotherapeutic agents.[33] The potential neurotoxic effects of IC-administered chemotherapeutic agents after BBBD have therefore been examined in animal models.[75,84,89] Of the agents tested (adriamycin, bleomycin, cisplatinum, cyclophosphamide, 5-fluorouracil, methotrexate, and mitomycin-C), IC carboplatinum, etoposide, and MTX do not have significant neurotoxic effects when administered after BBBD.

In the animal studies mentioned, drug levels were measured in brain samples, through radioimmunoassay and radionuclide counting techniques.[82] Because this is not feasible in patients, indirect methods for estimating brain drug levels were examined. Meglumine iothalamate (Conray) injected intravenously within 15 minutes of BBBD partitions into the brain parenchyma.[86] There is a linear relationship between the computed tomographic (CT) absorption value and the delivery of contrast agent.[17] Significant correlation between CT number, brain MTX levels, and Evan's blue–albumin staining was subsequently observed in normal dogs receiving MTX after osmotic BBBD.[86,87] This technique thus provides a noninvasive monitor of the degree, time course, and localization of osmotic BBBD. In addition, there were no contrast-agent–related adverse effects in normal dogs.

The ionic contrast agent initially used (meglumine iothalamate) in phase II (efficacy) clinical trials of chemotherapy with BBBD increased seizure incidence in patients with brain tumors.[98,99] Seizures related to IV contrast agent administration are rare, occurring in approximately 0.01% of the general population.[133,134] A 6% to 19% incidence of seizures, however, has been reported in patients with brain tumors receiving ionic IV contrast agents.[98] Risk factors included presence of a brain tumor, a history of seizures, and prior exposure to contrast agent and chemotherapy. Prophylactic diazepam treatment (5 mg IV) in glioma patients receiving IV meglumine iothalamate decreased the incidence of seizures from 16% to 2%.[98] The incidence of focal motor and grand mal seizures in patients receiving IV ionic contrast after osmotic BBBD is 15% to 20%.[78] Diazepam (10 mg IV) does not significantly decrease the incidence of seizures when ionic contrast agent is given after osmotic BBBD. To possibly decrease the incidence of seizures, radionuclide brain scanning using ^{99m}Tc-gluheptonate, a gamma-emitting ion normally excluded by the BBB, was studied as an alternative means of quantitating the degree

of BBBD. This method reduced the incidence of seizures to 7%, suggesting that the high incidence of seizures observed with contrast-enhanced CT was related to the contrast agent rather than the BBBD procedure. The number of gamma emissions correlated with the extent and distribution of the osmotic BBBD, but the technique had a lower sensitivity and spatial resolution than those obtained with a contrast-enhanced CT scan.[78] In addition, BBBD in the posterior cranial fossa could not be reliably quantitated with this method. More recently, an isosmotic, nonionic contrast agent, iopamidol (Isovue 300), has been evaluated for quantitative CT assessment of BBBD. The incidence of seizures in these patients is 5.7%, comparable with that observed with ^{99m}Tc-gluheptonate. Accordingly, contrast-enhanced CT is once again used to quantitate and localize BBBD. The increased seizure frequency in patients with brain tumors receiving IV contrast with or without BBBD is unexplained. The nature of the contrast agent plays a significant role because ionic agents result in a higher incidence of seizures than nonionic agents. Seizures with cerebral angiography, in which lower volumes of the same contrast agents are injected intraarterially, are very rare, suggesting that dose and route of administration also play a role.

MECHANISM

Two hypotheses have been proposed to explain reversible osmotic opening of the BBB: (1) a tight junctional or cell shrinkage model and (2) increased vesicular transport. The tight junctional hypothesis suggests that concentration-dependent, reversible opening of the BBB by water-soluble solutes is mediated by osmotically induced shrinkage of cerebrovascular endothelial cells and consequent modification of interendothelial tight junctions.[107] This hypothesis was questioned when structural alterations of interendothelial tight junctions or separation of adjacent membrane leaflets were not readily demonstrated by electron microscopy (EM).[20] Apparent stimulation of vesicular transport or possible formation of transendothelial channels by osmotic BBB provided support for the vesicular transport model.[2,39,47] EM studies with horseradish peroxidase or other tracers showed intraendothelial vesicles on abluminal endothelial surfaces filled with intravascular tracer that had passed into the abluminal basement membrane, as well as loaded vesicles within the endothelial cytoplasm. The similarity between EM images of the cerebral vascular endothelium after osmotic or other insults to the brain and EM images of fenestrated capillaries with vesicles also supported the vesicular transport model.[53,54,124]

A number of other observations, however, are not easily reconciled with the vesicular transport model. The osmotic threshold for BBBD is inversely related to solute lipid solubility, probably because lipid-soluble solutes are able to diffuse intracellularly and decrease the osmotic gradient across the cell membrane.[111] Although an osmotic gradient is a critical determinant of BBBD, it has not been shown to stimulate vesicular transport in other tissues. In addition, a phenothiazine derivative, dixyrazine, which inhibits endocytosis and exocytosis in various membranes, reduces protein extravasation associated with acute hypertension but does not influence osmotic BBBD.[49]

There is also structural evidence that osmotic BBBD results from an opening of tight junctions in cerebral endothelium. After IC injection of 3 molal urea, gaps between interendothelial tight junctions within an entire junctional complex fill with intravascular horseradish peroxidase.[5] Similar results have been reported using intravascular colloidal lanthanum.[70] The most convincing structural evidence for the interendothelial hypothesis is the opening of interendothelial junctions to both the vessel lumen and perivascular space in frog pial capillaries after treatment with hypertonic urea (Fig. 22-1).[69] The frequency of opened tight junctions was increased ninetyfold in animals treated with hyperosmotic urea compared with controls. The number of intraendothelial pits or vesicles was not, however, significantly increased by treatment with urea.

Osmotic BBBD is rapidly reversible, with the greatest increase in permeability observed within the first 30 minutes after an IC injection of a hypertonic solute.[107,136,137] After osmotic opening, the BBB also recloses more rapidly to large molecules compared with small molecules. For example, the permeability–surface area product (PA) of sucrose, inulin, and dextran molecular weight (MW) (340, 5500, and 79,000, respectively) increases markedly in the first 6 minutes after osmotic BBBD. The PA of dextran and inulin decreases to control values within 35 and 55 minutes, respectively, whereas the PA of sucrose remains significantly elevated at 55 minutes.[136,137] The size selectivity of BBB permeability at various times after osmotic opening has been mathematically modeled.[113] Experimental data are consistent with osmotically created pores or slits of about 200 Å and a density of about 1 pore per 200 μm^2 of membrane surface. The size dependence of BBB permeability is, in this model, inconsistent with enhanced vesicular transport. Although much of the literature supports the intercellular hypothesis, the structural evidence is not yet extensive enough to fully accept this as the correct model for osmotically enhanced BBB permeability.

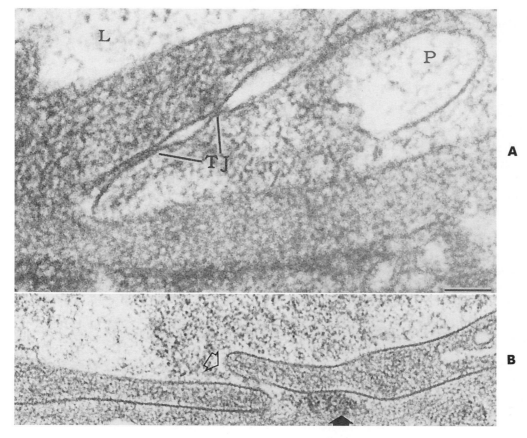

FIG. 22-1   **A,** Normal tight junction *(arrow)* in frog pial arterial endothelium. **B,** Open interendothelial tight junction *(arrow)* in the same species after exposure of the vessel to 3 M urea. Rapid cryofixation was used in both instances. *(From Nagy Z, Brightman MW: Brain Res 440:315-327, 1988).*

PHYSIOLOGIC EFFECTS OF OSMOTIC BBBD

Unilateral IC injection of a hyperosmotic solution in the anesthetized, spontaneously breathing rat resulted in apnea during the injection.[8,12] Normal ventilation resumed spontaneously within 10 to 20 seconds. Transient apnea after IC injection of a hyperosmotic solution has also been observed in the lightly anesthetized dog[82] and monkey.[106] These observations and a similar observation in early clinical trials with anesthetized, spontaneously ventilating patients led to the use of controlled or assisted ventilation during osmotic BBBD in anesthetized patients.[78] The cause of apnea in subjects undergoing BBBD has not been determined.

IC infusion with or without BBBD has no effect on blood pressure, temperature, hematocrit, and arterial blood gases in the rat.[100] In contrast with this result, mean arterial pressure decreased by 27% ± 8% (range −4 to 77%) in 10 normal monkeys during IC perfusion with 2 M urea.[103] Significant bradycardia of 10 to 150 seconds duration occurred in six of these subjects. Hypotension and bradycardia after IC infusion of hypertonic urea were associated with an increased incidence of neurologic deficit. IC perfusion with either hypertonic arabinose or lactamide also reduced systemic blood pressure by 40 mm Hg for 2 minutes in monkeys,[43] but without significant neurologic sequelae. Both hypertension and hypotension have been reported in patients after BBBD. In the first five patients with brain tumors to undergo BBBD, four experienced significant bradycardia and hypertension during the IC infusion of 25% mannitol.[81] The bradycardia and hypertension resolved 5 to 10 minutes after the IC infusion. In a clinical series of 60 BBBD procedures in 15 isoflurane-anesthetized patients, bradycardia and hypotension occurred frequently during the IC infusion of 25% mannitol.[132] Pretreatment with atropine effectively prevented the bradycardia and hypotension. The observed bradycardia and hypotension were thought to be due to carotid sinus stretching because blood that would normally enter the internal carotid artery is prevented from doing so by the high flow (6 to 12 ml/sec) IC injection of mannitol.

A rapid IC infusion could increase intracranial pressure (ICP) through both an acute increase in cerebral blood volume and an increase in brain water content. BBBD causes an increase (1.5%)[107] in brain water content in normal animals that lasts less than 48 hours.[110] This increase in brain water content has not been correlated with an increase in ICP. The effect of BBBD on brain water content in patients has not been studied. CT and magnetic resonance (MR) images give little indication of clinically significant cerebral edema after BBBD. In normal, anesthetized dogs there is a transient (< 2 hours), mild increase (5 mm Hg) in ICP with mannitol, but not with saline IC infusion.[82] Subdural intracranial pressure (ICP) increased an average of 15 mm Hg (from 4 to 19 mm Hg) in four of five patients with brain tumor undergoing phase I clinical trials of osmotic BBBD.[81] The ICP began to decrease immediately after the IC infusion, returning to normal within 30 minutes. The association of bradycardia and hypertension with the transiently elevated ICP is suggestive of a Cushing reflex. The CT scans and neurologic examination obtained after the procedure, however, did not differ from those obtained before infusion. Although ICP may increase significantly during an osmotic BBBD in patients with decreased intracranial compliance, it did not result in neurologic complications.

IC injection of hypertonic urea or lactamide in the monkey produced diffuse Evans blue–albumin staining of the aqueous and vitreous humors of the ipsilateral eye, indicating that the blood-ocular barrier is also opened by the procedure.[106,112] Intraocular pressure was decreased and the ciliary epithelium was altered in monkeys after osmotic BBBD.[96,97] In spite of these effects, visual acuity seems to be preserved in monkeys after osmotic BBBD.[71] Eleven patients treated multiple times with osmotic BBBD eventually developed retinal pigmented epithelial changes on the side of the carotid infusion. The severity of the epithelial changes varied directly with the total dosage of the chemotherapeutic agents and the number of BBB disruptions. The macular region was the most affected, with the remainder of the retina relatively unchanged. Visual loss was mild to moderate; no patient had visual acuity of less than 20/60 that could be related to the therapy, and no significant changes in visual fields have been reported.[66]

IC injection of a solution results in cortical blanching when the flow of the injectate exceeds that of blood through the internal carotid artery.[106] At sufficiently high flows there is replacement of blood in pial vessels with the injectate.[106] This results in ischemia in brain regions supplied by the perfused artery for the duration of the infusion. Intraarterial infusion of hypertonic solution at the lowest flow rate that causes complete cortical blanching results in BBBD within 25 to 30 seconds. Focal cerebral ischemia of such short duration probably has no significant effect on either neurologic or histopathologic outcome. Facial blanching in the medial forehead area also occurs during intracarotid injection of 25% mannitol, because the internal carotid artery supplies the supraorbital and supratrochlear arteries. The facial blanching lasts only as long as the IC infusion and is not associated with adverse sequelae.

After osmotic BBBD in the awake, restrained rat, local cerebral glucose utilization (LCGU) nearly doubled in the perfused hemisphere and decreased 25% in the contralateral hemisphere.[100] The increased LCGU after BBBD was prevented by diazepam, suggesting that the focal areas of intense metabolic activity reflect seizure activity. LCGU returned to normal values within 2 to 3 hours of the osmotic BBBD. In the same study, regional cerebral blood flow significantly decreased in the mannitol-perfused hemisphere. The effects of BBBD on cerebral blood flow and metabolism in humans have not been studied.

Electroencephalograms (EEGs) taken 1 day after IC urea perfusion in monkeys showed decreased amplitude in areas ipsilateral to the perfusion.[112] This EEG effect was transient and was not present 5 to 10 days after BBBD. Although EEG changes after osmotic BBBD have been reported in very few patients,[81] the 5% to 7% incidence of seizures during and after the procedure indicates that they are present in a significant number of cases.[85]

Behavioral disturbances occur during IC perfusion of hypertonic mannitol in the conscious rat.[100] Animals perfused with normal saline, which did not result in osmotic BBBD, did not exhibit any specific reaction and remained alert and normally inquisitive throughout the period of infusion. Animals perfused with IC mannitol, in which BBBD was verified with Evan's blue–albumin, reacted with head shaking and jumping and lost consciousness 20 seconds after the infusion was started. At 5 minutes after the infusion, animals with mild BBBD were again alert and responsive. Subjects with more pronounced BBBD were unresponsive for a longer period of time, suggesting that the behavioral effects of BBBD are related to the extent of barrier modification. No long-term behavioral or neurologic sequelae were observed in the rat, dog, or rhesus monkey[112] after moderate BBBD. Right-sided weakness and decreased activity were observed, however, in one of eight rhesus monkeys after extensive BBBD using 2.5 M D,L-lactamide.[106,110] Other than an anecdotal report of a severe burning sensation in the face of a lightly anesthetized patient, there is no published information about behavioral effects associated with BBBD in humans.

PREOPERATIVE STUDIES

All new patients are evaluated with a complete neurologic history and physical examination, including assessment of functional status using the Karnofsky Performance Scale,[52,78] an extensive battery of neuropsychologic assessment tests,[85,131] and a detailed audiologic and ophthalmologic examination. Focal neurologic deficits are documented for comparison with the posttreatment neurologic examination. Clinical symptoms consistent with elevated ICP are noted and used in conjunction with radiologic images in the decision to proceed with osmotic BBBD. Prior history of radiation and chemotherapy is documented. The same evaluations are performed after BBBD chemotherapy.

CT scans of the head are obtained with IV contrast to determine the initial size and location of the neoplasm. The presence of significant midline shift or of incipient herniation of intracranial contents on the CT or magnetic resonance (MR) scan is a contraindication for osmotic BBBD, because rapid introduction of 25% mannitol into the internal carotid or vertebrobasilar circulations acutely increases ICP.[78,81]

Indications for chemotherapy with BBBD are not established but currently include the presence of a brain tumor that is thought to be responsive to chemotherapy, a Karnofsky Performance Scale score greater than 60, and an estimated survival of greater than 60 days.

Patients are excluded if they have a creatinine clearance less than 60 ml/min or severe general medical illnesses, such as cardiovascular, pulmonary, or ischemic cerebrovascular disease. This is to avoid possible risks associated with multiple general anesthetics (patients with CNS lymphoma undergo 24 BBBD treatments), cerebral angiography, and the significant fluid shifts that occur after BBBD. Patients with intracranial tumors that do not have a significant blood-brain barrier, such as meningiomas, or who have tumors unresponsive to chemotherapy are also excluded. For patients who have been receiving chemotherapy with BBBD and are either febrile or leukopenic (white blood cell count less than 2700), the treatment is postponed until their condition improves.

New patients are admitted to the hospital the night before the procedure for IV administration of a loading dose of dilantin and/or phenobarbital. For patients receiving corticosteroid treatment, this treatment is tapered over a 2-week period before BBBD. Steroid administration greatly interferes with the increase in drug delivery to tumors with osmotic BBBD[73] possibly because of a steroid-related membrane-stabilizing effect. Premedications are kept to a minimum because CNS pharmacokinetics of most agents after BBBD are unknown. Diazepam, midazolam, and phenobarbital, however, have been administered as premedication and seizure prophylaxis without clinically apparent changes in either potency or duration of action.

ANESTHESIA CONSIDERATIONS

Osmotic BBBD may cause severe facial discomfort during the IC infusion of hyperosmotic fluid. Patients also may become apneic or experience hemodynamic changes and seizures of varying duration after BBBD. General anesthesia with controlled ventilation is, therefore, administered to all patients undergoing chemotherapy with BBBD. The major anesthetic issues in these patients are decreased intracranial compliance, altered cerebral drug pharmacokinetics, the possibility of seizures, possible adverse drug interactions, and the effects of anesthetic management on blood-to-brain transfer of chemotherapeutic substances.

Anesthetic considerations for patients with decreased intracranial compliance are discussed in detail in another chapter. Measures to decrease the likelihood of an anesthesia-related increase in ICP include a sodium thiopental induction and moderate hyperventilation with coadministration of isoflurane in oxygen. Muscle paralysis for tracheal intubation is obtained using succinylcholine, despite possible concerns about its effects on CBF[55,56] and ICP.[13,38,67] Succinylcholine, which has been used in neurosurgical patients with brain tumors without adverse outcome,[61] is selected to avoid significant muscle relaxant brain levels during osmotic BBBD. The ICP effect of succinylcholine in patients undergoing BBBD is probably less than that caused by the procedure itself. As noted earlier, transient increases in ICP in patients undergoing BBBD do not seem to be associated with an adverse neurologic outcome.

The BBB excludes charged molecules with molecular weights >180 daltons[25] unless their transport is facilitated by a specific carrier system. The neuromuscular blocking agents are charged at physiologic pH, have MW ranging from 397 (succinylcholine) to 1243 (atracurium), and are thus excluded from the brain by the BBB in normal subjects.[14,15,19,128,129] The ratio of CSF to plasma concentration of D-tubocurarine (D-Tc), for example, is 10^{-5} in normal subjects.[14] When a nondepolarizing agent, such as D-Tc, is injected into a cerebral cistern or ventricle of a normal, lightly anesthetized animal, clinical and electrophysiologic evidence of seizure activity is observed.[9,64] Lumbar subarachnoid injection of D-Tc in cats results in a strychnine-like effect on spinal reflexes, progressing to frank convulsions.[123] Intrahippocampal injection of D-Tc and other neuromuscular blocking agents also leads to EEG activation and evidence of seizure activity.[1,21] An intubating dose of D-Tc in neurosurgical patients with an abnormal BBB results, however, in a markedly increased CSF/plasma ratio (10^{-2}; CSF concentrations as high as 25 ng/ml) without apparent adverse neurologic sequelae.[62] A histamine-related increase in cerebral blood flow has been reported in animals receiving a 1 to 5 mg/kg IV dose of curare after urea-induced BBBD.[121] EEG effects were not reported in that study. Whether epileptic thresholds for nondepolarizing neuromuscular blocking agents would be reached with intubating doses administered just before osmotic BBBD is uncertain. CSF concentrations of vecuronium and pancuronium are significantly elevated when administered intravenously with osmotic BBBD.[130] These considerations may be moot because the direct CNS effects of the newer relaxants and their metabolites have not yet been established. Nonetheless, the practice at this institution is to avoid the use of nondepolarizing muscle relaxants shortly before osmotic BBBD.

Topical application of succinylcholine to the cortical surface also results in EEG seizure activity.[117,118] When succinylcholine is administered intravenously 3 minutes after osmotic BBBD in the dog, there is no significant difference in EEG activity, hemispheric cerebral blood flow, and cerebral metabolic rate when compared with saline-injected BBBD animals.[57] A likely explanation for the discrepancy between the effects of topical application and intravenous injection is that the local concentration of succinylcholine is higher with topical application. The rapid metabolism of succinylcholine[27,46] makes it extremely unlikely that significant plasma levels of the drug are present at the time of BBBD, generally 20 to 30 minutes after induction of anesthesia.

The CNS pharmacokinetics of most anesthetic agents, which readily cross the BBB, should not be significantly altered by BBBD. On the other hand, CNS clearance of normally excluded agents, such as the neuromuscular blockers, metoclopramide, ranitidine, glycopyrrolate, and some sympathomimetic agents, could be prolonged, particularly after closure of the transiently opened BBB. The direct CNS effects of such agents should therefore be examined before their use with BBBD in patients.

Interactions between anesthetic agents and the chemotherapeutic agents used with BBBD are also possible. For example, the combination of cyclophosphamide (CTX), an alkylating agent, and halothane is lethal in rabbits and mice.[7,120] This lethal effect was not present if CTX was discontinued 12 hours before halothane exposure or CTX was administered 2 hours after halothane exposure.[120] A group of 23 halothane-anesthetized patients undergoing osmotic BBBD and receiving intravenous CTX, however, had no apparent complications.[58] The increased lethality of the halothane/CTX combination in mice and rabbits is neither understood nor is it of apparent clinical significance in humans. Adverse interactions between isoflurane, the anesthetic agent currently used during osmotic BBBD at this institution, and CTX have not been observed.

High doses of CTX also significantly decrease plasma cholinesterase activity[135,138] and may result in prolonged apnea in patients receiving succinylcholine.[135] High-dose alkylating-agent–related inhibition of plasma cholinesterase activity lasts for days to weeks.[126] This effect, however, is not clinically significant because twitch recovery times ranging from 6 to 9 minutes are routinely observed in BBBD patients receiving CTX and succinylcholine.

Anesthetic drugs and physiologic variables may also affect the BBB and the quality of the osmotic BBBD. Isoflurane, pentobarbital, ketamine, and fentanyl all significantly reduce the blood-brain transfer coefficient (K_i) for alpha-aminoisobutyric acid, a small hydrophilic molecule.[10,11,114] In spite of this effect on K_i, isoflurane, pentobarbital, and ketamine did not adversely affect blood-to-brain transfer of ^{125}I-albumin and ^{99m}Tc-gluheptonate after osmotic BBBD in animals.[36] Fentanyl administered with droperidol, however, completely prevented osmotic BBBD.[36] Methoxyflurane, which resulted in a lower blood pressure after mannitol infusion, also prevented osmotic BBBD. This effect was reversed by administration of phenylephrine in the postinfusion period and suggests that blood pressure rather than anesthetic choice is a critical determinant of osmotic BBBD. This is not surprising because acute hypertension is known to increase the permeability of the BBB.[104]

Although the cerebral vasculature is very sensitive to changes in arterial CO_2 tension, its effect on BBBD is modest. Hypocarbic ($Paco_2$ of 28 mm Hg) subjects had a blood-to-brain MTX transfer 34% and 69% greater than that observed in hypercarbic (56 mm Hg) and normocarbic (38 mm Hg) subjects, respectively.[77]

A significant number of patients scheduled for osmotic BBBD experience seizures either before or during the procedure. Potentially epileptogenic anesthetic agents, such as methohexital, ketamine, etomidate, and enflurane[68] are therefore avoided. In addition, antiseizure medications, including dilantin, valium, and phenobarbital, are given prophylactically to patients undergoing BBBD to minimize the incidence of seizures.

PROCEDURE

The patient scheduled for osmotic BBBD (Box 22-1) is premedicated with 0.1 to 0.2 mg/kg diazepam PO and delivered to the angiography suite. Before induction, ECG, pulse oximeter, blood pressure cuff, and a precordial stethoscope are applied to the patient. Intravenous fluids are connected to the patient, often via a Portacath or Hickman catheter, in a sterile manner. Phenobarbital, 1 mg/kg IV, is administered just before induction.

After preoxygenation, anesthesia is induced with a 3 to 5 mg/kg IV dose of sodium thiopental. Muscle relaxation is obtained with succinylcholine, 1 mg/kg IV, and the patient is intubated and mechanically ventilated during and immediately after the procedure. Although others have reported no adverse effects associated with the use of other intravenous agents, such as fentanyl and pancuronium,[132] we prefer to keep the medications administered before the BBBD to a minimum. Anesthesia is subsequently maintained with 0.5 to 1.0 vol% isoflurane and 50% nitrous oxide in oxygen. Patients are hyperventilated to an E_tco_2 of 25 to 28 mm Hg, both to decrease cerebral blood volume in a setting of decreased intracranial compliance and be-

cause moderate hypocapnia significantly increases MTX transfer into the brain during osmotic BBBD.[77]

A Foley catheter is inserted in anticipation of the brisk diuresis that occurs after osmotic BBBD, typically on the order of 1 to 2 L in the first hour after intraarterial injection of 25% mannitol. The drug regimen that follows is the one used for BBBD treatment of CNS lymphoma and is only a cursory description of the procedure. Furosemide, 10 mg IV, is administered to establish a diuresis before the BBBD. Cyclophosphamide, an alkylating chemotherapeutic agent converted by the hepatic cytochrome P-450 system into active metabolites (aldophosphamide, acrolein, and phosphoramide mustard)[119] is administered (15 mg/kg IV) at least 10 minutes before BBBD. The femoral artery is percutaneously cannulated with a 6.5 French catheter, which is then guided with fluoroscopy to the vessel of interest, one of the vertebral or internal carotid arteries.

In canine studies, excessively high flow rates during intraarterial injection of 25% mannitol resulted in diffuse and severe cerebral edema, elevations of ICP as high as 140 mm Hg, and hemorrhagic lesions characteristic of emboli.[83] Flow rates that are too low decrease the success rate for barrier disruption. It is critical to determine a flow rate that does not damage the brain yet ensures that the BBB will be disrupted. In patients this was initially determined to be the minimum flow rate of intraarterially injected mannitol that caused blanching of the cortical surface, as viewed through a burr-hole craniotomy.[103] The optimum flow rate for intraarterial injection of mannitol is currently determined angiographically. Contrast material is injected into the vessel of interest, and the flow rate is increased until significant reflux, flow across the circle of Willis, or flow into the contralateral vertebral artery occurs. The maximum flow at which significant reflux or cross flow does not occur, typically 6 to 12 ml/sec, is taken as the optimal flow rate for BBBD[78] and correlates well with values determined by cortical blanching. Immediately after the flow rate is determined, 0.4 to 0.8 mg atropine is administered to prevent bradycardia and hypotension during osmotic BBBD, an effect that may be related to carotid sinus stimulation.[132] A second dose of thiopental, 1 to 3 mg/kg, and of diazepam, 10 mg, is administered as seizure prophylaxis just before intraarterial injection of the mannitol. Osmotic BBBD is then accomplished with injection of 250 to 300 ml of warmed, crystal-free 25% (1.4 M) mannitol into either an internal carotid or vertebral artery over 25 to 30 seconds. As the mannitol is injected, the patient is observed for ipsilateral pupillary dilation and blanching of the ipsilateral medial forehead. Additional treatment with atropine is instituted should the patient become bradycardic during the mannitol injection. The position of the intraarterial catheter is reestablished because infusions at these rates occasionally result in movement of the catheter tip. MTX, 2.5 g in 200 ml warmed normal saline, is delivered as a 15- to 20-minute intraarterial infusion starting 5 minutes after the mannitol injection. To establish the extent and intensity of

---

BOX 22-1

CLINICAL OSMOTIC BLOOD-BRAIN BARRIER DISRUPTION PROTOCOL

1. Preoperative medication: diazepam 10 mg PO
2. Induction of anesthesia/intubation/controlled ventilation
3. Phenobarbital 1 mg/kg IV, furosemide 10 mg IV
4. Catheterization of selected artery (carotid or vertebral)
5. Determination of flow rate for injection of mannitol
6. Cyclophosphamide 15-30 mg/kg IV
7. Hyperventilation to E_tco_2 25-28 mm Hg
8. Atropine (0.4 mg), diazepam (10 mg), and thiopental (1-3 mg/kg)
9. 25% Mannitol infusion 180-300 ml over 30 seconds
10. Observation of pupillary dilation and facial blanching
11. 150 ml Isovue 300 IV immediately after mannitol infusion
12. Methotrexate 1-5 g intraarterially over 10-15 minutes
13. Propofol infusion to maintain anesthesia
14. CT scan to document extent of blood-brain barrier disruption
15. Recovery from anesthesia/procedure and removal of catheter in postanesthetic care unit

the osmotic BBBD, either ^{99m}Tc gluheptonate (740 MBq) or 150 ml iopamidol (Isovue 300) is administered intravenously immediately after IC mannitol infusion.

After completion of the MTX infusion, the volatile anesthetic is discontinued and propofol is intravenously infused to maintain anesthesia, typically at a rate of 80 to 160 $\mu g/kg^{-1}/min^{-1}$. The patient is then transferred to the CT scanning suite, where a CT of the head is obtained. Significant contrast enhancement of the brain parenchyma by the normally excluded contrast agent occurs in the areas in which osmotic BBBD is the most pronounced, as shown in Fig. 22-2, A. Similarly, a radionuclide brain scan, obtained 3 hours after BBBD, shows significantly increased radioactivity in the treated hemisphere (Fig. 22-2,B). Upon completion of the CT scan, the propofol infusion is stopped and the spontaneously ventilating patient is taken to the postanesthesia care unit (PACU). When the patient is able to follow commands, breathes without difficulty, and has a sustained head lift, the endotracheal tube is removed, usually 10 to 15 minutes after arriving in the PACU. The introducer for the 6.5 Fr femoral arterial catheter is then removed and the site compressed for 10 minutes. The patient is closely monitored for seizure activity, fluid status, complications related to the femoral artery catheter site, and changes in neurologic signs. If the patient remains in stable condition, he/she is sent to the ward 4 hours after admission to the PACU. The entire process from the time the patient arrives at the angiography suite to the time he/she is admitted to the PACU is typically 90 minutes. A complete course of therapy for primary CNS lymphoma includes eight treatments in each of the internal carotid arteries and in the vertebrobasilar system for a total of 24 osmotic BBBD procedures over a 1-year period.

RESULTS

More than 3000 osmotic BBBD procedures have been performed at this institution in more than 200 patients. Phase II clinical trials (efficacy) are underway for a number of CNS tumors, including glioblastoma multiforme, malignant astrocytoma, germinoma, primitive neuroectodermal tumors, and metastatic lung and breast cancer. Patients with primary CNS lymphoma, however, have a significantly improved median survival with preservation of cognitive function after chemotherapy with osmotic BBBD.[85]

The incidence of CNS lymphoma has tripled in the nonimmunosuppressed population in the last decade and continues to increase for unclear reasons.[45] CNS lymphoma patients treated with a combination of surgery and surgery with postoperative cranial radiation have a short median survival, 4.6 and 15.2 months, respectively, with no long-term survivors.[42,45] Patients treated with BBBD with and

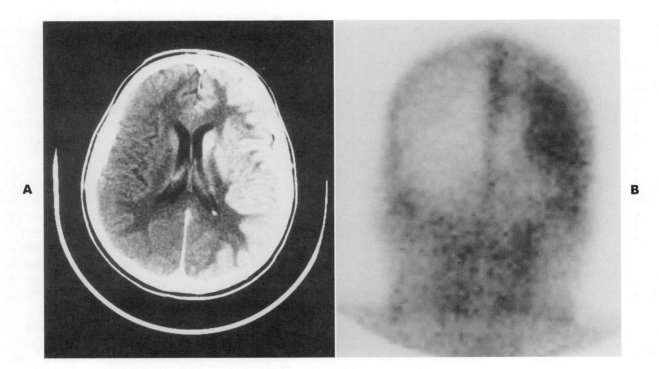

FIG. 22-2   **A,** Contrast enhancement in the distribution of mannitol perfusion (right internal carotid artery), indicating increased BBB permeability. Brain drug levels correlate with the degree of contrast enhancement. **B,** Brain scan obtained 3 hours after perfusion also shows ipsilateral increased BBB permeability but with a lower resolution than that obtained with CT.

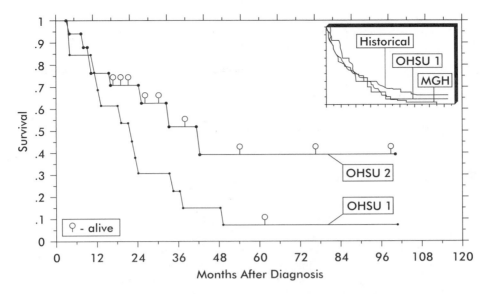

FIG. 22-3 Survival curves in CNS lymphoma patients treated with MTX/CTCX/BBBD with (OHSU 1) and without (OHSU 2) cranial radiation. Note the plateau at 40% survival in the OHSU 2 group. *Inset:* Survival curves in CNS lymphoma patients compiled from historical series, the OHSU 1 group, and a previously published Massachusetts General Hospital (MHG) series. Median survival in OHSU 2 patients (44.5 months) was significantly better (p. <0.039) than in OHSU 1 patients (17.8 months). OHSU, Oregon Health Sciences University. *(From Neuwelt EA, Goldman DL, Dahlborg SA et al: J Clin Oncol 9:1580-1590, 1991.)*

without cranial radiation, on the other hand, have a median survival of 17.8 and 44.5 months, respectively.[85] BBBD-treated CNS lymphoma patients usually had normal CT and MR brain images after a complete (1-year) course of chemotherapy. Cranial radiation is of survival benefit in biopsy-proved CNS lymphoma patients but provides no benefit and may actually be deleterious in patients receiving chemotherapy with BBBD. Thus, in addition to improving median survival in patients with CNS lymphoma, BBBD with appropriate chemotherapy obviates the need for cranial radiation, which has known adverse long-term cognitive effects.[50,51] The survival curve for patients receiving only chemotherapy with BBBD has a plateau at 40% (Fig. 22-3), suggesting that a significant number of these patients may be cured of their disease.[85] Although these data suggest that chemotherapy with BBBD is of significant benefit in patients with CNS lymphoma, a multicenter randomized trial comparing outcome results for this chemotherapy regimen with and without BBBD is needed to clarify whether the improved outcome is due to choice of chemotherapy or to method of administration.

COMPLICATIONS

Both neurologic and nonneurologic complications occur in patients undergoing osmotic BBBD. In a recent series, no patient died within 1 week of a BBBD procedure,[85] however, there were three deaths within 30 days of the proce-

TABLE 22-1

Complications of Chemotherapy Administered After BBBD in a Series of 471 Treatments in 30 Patients

Complication	Number	Percent
Neurologic		
Seizures	34	7.2
Stroke	2	0.4
Subdural hygromas	1	0.2
Obtundation >24 hr	3	0.6
Nonneurologic		
Sepsis	5	1.1*
Febrile with granulocytopenia	31	6.6
Deep venous thrombosis	4	1.3
Pulmonary thrombosis	2	0.4
Pseudoaneurysm	2	0.4
Arterial injury	5	1.1
Pneumothorax	1	0.2
Interstitial pneumonitis	1	0.2
Hemorrhagic cystitis	2	0.4
Hip fractures	2	0.4
Avascular necrosis, femur	1	0.2
Ocular toxicity	0	0.0
Mortality (within 30 days)	3	0.6
Total morbidity	97	21

*Resulted in two deaths within 30 days.

dure, two of sepsis and one of disease progression. The most frequent neurologic side effect (Table 22-1) was seizure activity, which occurred in 7% of the procedures (47% of patients). Most seizures were focal motor, occurring in the anesthetized patient and resolving within 15 to 30 seconds. Seizures most commonly occurred shortly after IC infusion of hypertonic mannitol, during IC infusion of MTX, or during IV infusion of contrast agent. The incidence of seizures rapidly declined in the 24 hours immediately after BBBD, and no patient had uncontrolled seizures. Two patients had CT evidence of cerebral infarction (6.7% of patients and 0.4% of procedures), which may be due to the angiography procedure and not necessarily to BBBD. These CT findings were incidental and were not associated with neurologic deficits. Three patients had episodes of prolonged obtundation lasting several days after osmotic BBBD. Two of these patients recovered to baseline neurologic function, and one patient, who underwent a BBBD procedure while on a neuroleptic drug and lithium for treatment of a psychiatric disorder, recovered over several weeks. None of the patients in this series had clinical evidence of visual impairment, but several patients were noted to have changes in retinal pigmentation, an effect that has been previously reported.[66] Neuropsychologic summary scores were stable or showed some degree of improvement in the majority of BBBD treated patients without cranial radiation in this series. Neurogenic diabetes insipidus has been observed after osmotic BBBD in one patient with a pineal tumor and panhypopituitarism. This patient responded well to the vasopressin analog, desmopressin acetate (DDAVP), and has continued to receive chemotherapy during BBBD without complication.

Complications associated with chemotherapy made up most of the nonneurologic morbidity and mortality reported in the same series of patients (see Table 22-1). The most frequent nonneurologic complication was a febrile episode in a granulocytopenic patient, occurring in 31 of 471 procedures (6.6%). Other chemotherapy-related complications included five episodes of sepsis, which resulted in two deaths, deep venous thrombosis, hemorrhagic cystitis, and interstitial pneumonitis.[85] These complication rates are comparable with those observed in the treatment of systemic lymphoma using chemotherapy.[16] Other nonneurologic complications were associated with angiography, in-cluding arterial injury and hematoma. The total morbidity and mortality for the procedure were 21% and 0.6%, respectively.

SUMMARY

Osmotic BBBD reliably increases blood-to-brain and blood-to-tumor transfer of systemically administered agents that do not normally traverse the BBB. Although the clinical application of this technique is debated in the literature[26,105] and is practiced in relatively few centers,[34] chemotherapy with osmotic BBBD is proving to be of benefit in patients with some CNS tumors. Whether the technique proves to be effective with other chemotherapeutic regimens and other brain tumor types remains to be determined. The physiologic effects of this procedure in patients have been established such that side effects can be anticipated and prophylactically treated. With the demonstration that osmotic BBBD can be routinely performed with relatively low morbidity and mortality, use of the technique to deliver other therapeutic agents that do not appreciably cross the BBB is likely. Examples of such agents include monoclonal antibodies to brain-tumor-specific antigens, which are not likely to reach all tumor cells even with direct surgical application. Blood-to-brain transfer of large IgG and IgM antibodies is significantly increased by osmotic BBBD.[76,88,91] One of the more exciting developments in molecular biology is the ability to introduce a gene that is either missing or malfunctioning in a population of cells. Gene therapy for a variety of CNS metabolic diseases is currently under investigation in animals. The vectors for CNS gene therapy will possibly be replication-defective viruses. The blood-to-brain transfer of an ultraviolet-light–inactivated virus is also significantly increased by osmotic BBBD,[90] suggesting its possible utility in future CNS gene therapy.

References

1. Baker WW, Benedict F: Local electrographic responses to intrahippocampal D-tubocurarine and related neuromuscular blocking agents, *Proc Soc Exp Biol Med* 124:607-611, 1967.

2. Barry DI, Hemmingsen R, Westergaard E: Cerebrovascular vasodilation, vesicular transport, and a protective effect of halothane during osmotic disruption of the blood-brain barrier, *Acta Neurol Scand* 60 (suppl 72):76-77, 1979.

3. Blasberg RG, Groothuis DR: Blood-tumor barrier disruption controversies (letter), *J Cereb Blood Flow Metab* 11:165-168, 1991.

4. Bradbury M: *The concept of a blood-brain barrier*, New York, 1979, Wiley.

5. Brightman MW, Hori M, Rapoport SI et al: Osmotic opening of tight junctions in cerebral endothelium, *J Comp Neurol* 152:317-25, 1973.

6. Broman T, Lindberg-Broman AM: An experimental study of disorders in the permeability of the cerebral vessels ("the blood-brain barrier") produced by chemical and physicochemical agents, *Acta Physiol Scand* 10:102-125, 1945.

7. Bruce DL: Anesthetic-induced increase in murine mortality from cyclophosphamide, *Cancer* 31:361-363, 1973.

8. Bullard DE, Bourdon M, Bigner DD: Comparison of various methods for delivering radiolabeled monoclonal antibody to normal rat brain, *J Neurosurg* 61:901-911, 1984.

9. Chang H-T: Similarity in action between curare and strychnine on cortical neurons, *J Neurophysiol* 16:221-233, 1953.

10. Chi OZ, Anwar M, Sinha AK et al: Effects of isoflurane on transport across the blood-brain barrier, *Anesthesiology* 76:426-431, 1992.

11. Chi OZ, Wei HM, Anwar M et al: Effects of fentanyl on a-aminoisobutyric acid transfer across the blood-brain barrier, *Anesth Analg* 75:31-36, 1992.

12. Chiueh CC, Sun CL, Kopin IJ et al: Entry of [^{3}H] norepinephrine, [^{125}I] albumin and Evan's Blue from blood into brain following unilateral osmotic opening of the blood-brain barrier, *Brain Res* 145:291-301, 1978.

13. Cottrell JE, Hartung J, Giffin JP et al: Intracranial and hemodynamic changes after succinylcholine administration in cats, *Anesth Analg* 62:1006-1009, 1983.

14. Dal Santo G: Kinetics and distribution of radioactive-labeled muscle relaxants. I Investigations with ^{14}C-dimethyl-D-tubocurarine, *Anesthesiology* 25:788-800, 1964.

15. Dal Santo G: Kinetics of distribution of radioactive labeled muscle relaxants: III. Investigations with ^{14}C-succinyldicholine and ^{14}C-succinylmonocholine during controlled conditions, *Anesthesiology* 29:435-443, 1968.

16. Dana BW, Dahlberg S, Miller TP et al: m-BACOD treatment for intermediate- and high-grade malignant lymphomas: a Southwest Oncology Group phase II trial, *J Clin Oncol* 8:1155-1162, 1990.

17. Drayer BP, Schmeckel DE, Hedlund LW et al: Radiographic quantitation of reversible blood-brain barrier disruption in vivo, *Radiology* 143:85-89, 1982.

18. Ehrlich P: *Das sauerstoff bedürfnis des organismus. Eine farbenanalytische studie,* Berlin, 1885, Hirschwald.

19. Fahey MR, Sessler DI, Cannon JE et al: Atracurium, vecuronium, and pancuronium do not alter the minimum alveolar concentration of halothane in humans, *Anesthesiology* 71:53-56, 1989.

20. Farrell CL, Shivers RR: Capillary junctions of the rat are not affected by osmotic opening of the blood-brain barrier, *Acta Neuropathol* 63:179-189, 1984.

21. Feldberg W, Lotti VJ: Direct and indirect activation of the hippocampus by tubocurarine, *J Physiol* 210:697-716, 1970.

22. Fenstermacher JD: Current models of blood-brain transfer, *Trends Neurosci* 8:449-453, 1985.

23. Fenstermacher JD: Pharmacology of the blood-brain barrier. In Neuwelt EA, editor: *Implications of the blood-brain barrier and its manipulation,* vol 1, New York, 1989, Plenum.

24. Fenstermacher JD, Cowles AL: Intraarterial infusions of drugs and hyperosmotic solutions as ways of enhancing brain tumor chemotherapy, *Cancer Treatm Rep* 61:519-526, 1981.

25. Fenstermacher JD, Johnson JA: Filtration and reflection coefficients of the rabbit blood-brain barrier, *J Physiol (Lond)* 211:341-346, 1966.

26. Fishman RA: Is there a therapeutic role for osmotic breaching of the blood-brain barrier? (editorial), *Ann Neurol* 22:298-299, 1987.

27. Foldes FF, Vandervort RS, Shanor SP: The fate of succinylcholine in man, *Anesthesiology* 16:11-21, 1955.

28. Goldman EE: Die aussere und innere sekretion des gesunden und kranken organismus im lichte der "vitalen farbung", *Beitr Klin Chirurg* 64:192-265, 1909.

29. Goldman EE: Vitalfarbung am zentralnervensystem. Abh preuss akad wiss, *Phys Math Kl* 1:1-60, 1913.

30. Greig NH: Optimizing drug delivery to brain tumors, *Cancer Treat Rev* 14:1-28, 1987.

31. Groothuis DR, Fischer JM, Lapin G et al: Permeability of different experimental brain tumor models to horseradish peroxidase, *J Neuropathol Exp Neurol* 41:164-185, 1982.

32. Groothuis DR, Fischer JM, Vick NA et al: Comparative permeability of different glioma models to horseradish peroxidase, *Cancer Treat Rep* 2:13-18, 1981.

33. Groothuis DR, Warnke PC, Molnar P et al: Effect of hyperosmotic blood-brain barrier disruption on transcapillary transport in canine brain tumors, *J Neurosurg* 72:441-449, 1990.

34. Gumerlock MK, Belshe BD, Madsen R et al: Osmotic blood-brain barrier disruption and chemotherapy in the treatment of high grade glioma: patient series and literature review, *J Neurooncol* 12:33-46, 1992.

35. Gumerlock MK, Neuwelt EA: Principles of chemotherapy in brain neoplasia. In Jellinger K, editor: *Malignant brain tumors,* Vienna, 1987, Springer-Verlag.

36. Gumerlock MK, Neuwelt EA: The effects of anesthesia on osmotic blood-brain barrier disruption, *Neurosurgery* 26:268-277, 1990.

37. Habeshaw JA, Lauder I: *Malignant lymphomas,* New York, 1988, Churchill-Livingstone.

38. Halldin M, Wahlin A: Effect of succinylcholine on intraspinal fluid pressure, *Acta Anaesthesiol Scand* 38:155-161, 1980.

39. Hansson HA, Johansson BB: Induction of pinocytosis in cerebral vessels by acute hypertension and by hyperosmolar solutions, *J Neurosci Res* 5:183-190, 1980.

40. Hasegawa H, Allen JC, Mehta BM et al: Enhancement of CNS penetration of methotrexate by hyperosmolar intracarotid mannitol or carcinomatous meningitis, *Neurology* 29:1280-1286, 1979.

41. Hawkey CJ, Toghill PJ: The need for prophylactic treatment to the central nervous system in patients with aggressive non-Hodgkins lymphoma, *Postgrad Med J* 59:283-287, 1983.

42. Henry JM, Heffner RJ, Dillard SH et al: Primary malignant lymphomas of the central nervous system, *Cancer* 34:1293-1302, 1974.

43. Hicks JT, Albrecht P, Rapoport SI: Entry of neutralizing antibody to measles into brain and cerebrospinal fluid of immunized monkeys after osmotic opening of the blood-brain barrier, *Exp Neurol* 53:768-779, 1976.

44. Hiesiger EM, Voorhies RM, Basler GA et al: Opening the blood-brain and blood-tumor barriers in experimental rat brain tumors: the effect of intracarotid hyperosmolar mannitol on capillary permeability and blood flow, *Ann Neurol* 19:50-59, 1986.

45. Hochberg FH, Miller DC: Primary central nervous system lymphoma, *J Neurosurg* 68:835-853, 1988.

46. Holst-Larsen H: The hydrolysis of suxamethonium in human blood, *Br J Anaesth* 48:887-892, 1976.

47. Houtoff HJ, Go KG, Gerrits PO: The mechanisms of blood-brain barrier impairment by hyperosmolar perfusion. An electron cytochemical study comparing exogenous HRP and endogenous antibody to HRP as tracers, *Acta Neuropathol (Berlin)* 56:99-112, 1982.

48. Hryniuk WM, Bertino JR: Treatment of leukemia with large doses of methotrexate and folinic acid: clinical-biochemical correlates, *J Clin Invest* 48:2140-2155, 1969.

49. Johansson B, Strandgaard S, Lassen NA: On the pathogenesis of hypertensive encephalopathy: the hypertensive "breakthrough" of autoregulation of cerebral blood flow with forced vasodilatation, flow increase, and blood-brain barrier damage, *Circ Res* 34(suppl 1):I-167–I-171, 1974.

50. Johnson BE, Becker B, Goff WB et al: Neurologic, neuropsychologic, and computed cranial tomography scan abnormalities in 2- to 10-year survivors of small-cell lung cancer, *J Clin Oncol* 3:1659-1667, 1985.

51. Johnson BE, Patronas N, Hayes W et al: Neurologic, computed cranial tomographic, and magnetic resonance imaging abnormalities in patients with small-cell lung cancer: further follow-up of 6- to 13-year survivors, *J Clin Oncol* 8:48-56, 1990.

52. Karnofsky DA, Burchenal JH: The clinical evaluation of chemotherapeutic agents in cancer. In MacLeod CM, editor: *Evaluation of chemotherapeutic agents,* New York, 1949, Columbia University Press.

53. Karnovsky MJ: The ultrastructural basis of capillary permeability studied with peroxidase as a tracer, *J Cell Biol* 35:213-236, 1967.

54. Karnovsky MJ, Shea SM: Transcapillary transport by pinocytosis, *Microvasc Res* 2:353-360, 1970.

55. Lanier WL, Iaizzo PA, Milde JH: Cerebral function and muscle afferent activity following intravenous succinylcholine in dogs anesthetized with halothane: the effects of pretreatment with a defasciculating dose of pancuronium (published erratum appears in *Anesthesiology* 17:482, 1989), *Anesthesiology* 71:87-95, 1989.

56. Lanier WL, Milde JH, Michenfelder JD: Cerebral stimulation following succinylcholine in dogs, *Anesthesiology* 64:551-559, 1986.

57. Lanier WL, Milde JH, Sharbrough FW: Effects of suxamethonium on the cerebrum following disruption of the blood-brain barrier in dogs, *Br J Anaesth* 65:708-712, 1990.

58. Lee JT, Erbguth PH, Stevens WC: Failure to detect toxicity with the concomitant use of cyclophosphamide and halothane in humans, *Anesthesiology* 64:810-811, 1986.

59. Levin VA, Freeman DM, Landahl HD: Permeability characteristics of brain adjacent to tumors in rats, *Arch Neurol* 32:785-791, 1975.

60. Levin VA, Landahl HD, Freeman DM: The application of brain capillary permeability coefficient measurements to pathological conditions and the selection of agents which cross the blood-brain barrier, *J Pharmacokinet Biopharm* 4:499-519, 1976.

61. Marsh ML, Dunlop BJ, Shapiro HM et al: Succinylcholine-intracranial pressure effects in neurosurgical patients, *Anesth Analg* 59:550-551, 1980.

62. Matteo RS, Pua EK, Khambatta HJ et al: Cerebrospinal fluid levels of d-tubocurarine in man, *Anesthesiology* 46:396-399, 1977.

63. Mayhan WG, Heistad DD: Permeability of blood-brain barrier to various sized molecules, *Am J Physiol* 235:H712-H718, 1985.

64. McGuigan H: The central action of curare, *J Pharmacol Exp Ther* 8:471-477, 1916.

65. Mendenhall NP, Thar TL, Agee OF et al: Primary lymphoma of the central nervous system. Computerized tomography scan characteristics and treatment results for 12 cases, *Cancer* 52:1993-2000, 1983.

66. Millay RH, Klein ML, Shults WT et al: Maculopathy associated with combination chemotherapy and osmotic opening of the blood-brain barrier, *Am J Ophthalmol* 102:626-632, 1986.

67. Minton MD, Grosslight K, Stirt JA et al: Increases in intracranial pressure from succinylcholine: prevention by prior nondepolarizing blockade, *Anesthesiology* 65:165-169, 1986.

68. Modica PA, Templehoff R, White PF: Pro- and anticonvulsant effects of anesthetics (part 1), *Anesth Analg* 70:303-315, 1990.

69. Nagy Z, Brightman MW: Cerebral vessels cryofixed after hyperosmosis or cold injury in normothermic and hypothermic frogs, *Brain Res* 440:315-327, 1988.

70. Nagy Z, Pappius HM, Mathieson G et al: Opening of tight junctions in cerebral endothelium. I. Effect of hyperosmolar mannitol infused through the internal carotid artery, *J Comp Neurol* 185:569-578, 1979.

71. Neuwelt EA, Barnett P: Blood-brain barrier disruption in the treatment of brain tumors: animal studies. In Neuwelt EA, editor: *Implications of the blood-brain barrier and its manipulation,* vol 2, New York, 1989, Plenum.

72. Neuwelt EA, editor: *Implications of the blood-brain barrier and its manipulation: clinical aspects,* vol 2, New York, 1989, Plenum.

73. Neuwelt EA, Barnett PA, Bigner DD et al: Effects of adrenal cortical steroids and osmotic blood-brain barrier opening on methotrexate delivery to gliomas in the rodent: the factor of the blood-brain barrier, *Proc Natl Acad Sci U S A* 79:4420-4423, 1982.

74. Neuwelt EA, Barnett PA, Frenkel EP: Chemotherapeutic agent permeability to normal brain and delivery to avian sarcoma virus-induced brain tumors in the rodent: observations on problems of drug delivery, *Neurosurgery* 14:154-160, 1984.

75. Neuwelt EA, Barnett PA, Glasberg M et al: Pharmacology and neurotoxicity of cis-diamminedichloroplatinum, bleomycin, 5-fluorouracil, and cyclophosphamide administration following osmotic blood-brain barrier mod-

ification, *Cancer Res* 43:5278-5285, 1983.

76. Neuwelt EA, Barnett PA, Hellstrom I et al: Delivery of melanoma-associated immunoglobulin monoclonal antibody and Fab fragments to normal brain utilizing osmotic blood-brain barrier disruption, *Cancer Res* 48:4725-4729, 1988.

77. Neuwelt EA, Barnett PA, McCormick CI: Osmotic blood-brain barrier disruption: parameters affecting drug delivery. *Proceedings of the Fifth International Meeting of the International Society for Developmental Neuroscience,* Amsterdam, 1984, Elsevier, pp 173-179.

78. Neuwelt EA, Dahlborg SA: Blood-brain barrier disruption in the treatment of brain tumors: clinical implications. In Neuwelt EA, editor: *Implications of the blood-brain barrier and its manipulation,* vol 2, New York, 1989, Plenum.

79. Neuwelt EA, Diehl JT, Vu LH et al: Monitoring of methotrexate delivery in patients with malignant brain tumors after osmotic blood-brain barrier disruption, *Ann Intern Med* 1981.

80. Neuwelt EA, Frenkel EP, D'Agostino AN et al: Growth of human lung tumor in the brain of the nude rat as a model to evaluate anti-tumor agent delivery across the blood-brain barrier, *Cancer Res* 45:2827-2833, 1985.

81. Neuwelt EA, Frenkel EP, Diehl J et al: Reversible osmotic blood-brain barrier disruption in humans: implications for the chemotherapy of malignant brain tumors, *Neurosurgery* 7:44-52, 1980.

82. Neuwelt EA, Frenkel EP, Rapoport S et al: Effect of osmotic blood-brain barrier disruption on methotrexate pharmacokinetics in the dog, *Neurosurgery* 7:36-43, 1980.

83. Neuwelt EA, Glasberg M, Diehl J et al: Osmotic blood-brain barrier disruption in the posterior fossa of the dog, *J Neurosurg* 55:742-748, 1981.

84. Neuwelt EA, Glasberg M, Frenkel E et al: Neurotoxicity of chemotherapeutic agents after blood-brain barrier modification: neuropathological studies, *Ann Neurol* 14:316-324, 1983.

85. Neuwelt EA, Goldman DL, Dahlborg SA et al: Primary CNS lymphoma treated with osmotic blood-brain barrier disruption: prolonged survival and preservation of cognitive function, *J Clin Oncol* 9:1580-1590, 1991.

86. Neuwelt EA, Maravilla KR, Frenkel EP et al: Use of enhanced computerized tomography to evaluate osmotic blood-brain barrier disruption, *Neurosurgery* 6:49-56, 1980.

87. Neuwelt EA, Maravilla KR, Frenkel EP et al: Osmotic blood-brain barrier disruption. Computerized tomographic monitoring of chemotherapeutic agent delivery, *J Clin Invest* 64:684-688, 1979.

88. Neuwelt EA, Minna J, Frenkel E et al: Osmotic blood-brain barrier opening to IgM monoclonal antibody in the rat *Am J Physiol* 250:R873-R883, 1986.

89. Neuwelt EA, Pagel M, Barnett P et al: Pharmacology and toxicity of intracarotid adriamycin administration following osmotic blood-brain barrier modification, *Cancer Res* 41:4466-4470, 1981.

90. Neuwelt EA, Pagel MA, Dix RD: Delivery of ultraviolet-inactivated 35S-herpesvirus across an osmotically modified blood-brain barrier, *J Neurosurg* 74:475-479, 1991.

91. Neuwelt EA, Specht HD, Barnett PA et al: Increased delivery of tumor-specific monoclonal antibodies to brain after osmotic blood-brain barrier modification in patients with melanoma metastatic to the central nervous system, *Neurosurgery* 20:885-895, 1987.

92. Neuwelt EA, Specht HD, Howieson J et al: Osmotic blood-brain barrier modification: clinical documentation by enhanced CT scanning and/or radionuclide brain scanning, *AJNR* 4:907-913, 1983.

93. Ohata M, Fredericks WR, Neuwelt EA et al: [^{3}H] Methotrexate loss from the rat brain following enhanced uptake by osmotic opening of the blood-brain barrier, *Cancer Res* 45:1092-1096, 1985.

94. Ohno K, Fredericks WR, Rapoport SI: Lower limits of cerebrovascular permeability to nonelectrolytes in the conscious rat, *Am J Physiol* 253:H299-H307, 1978.

95. Ohno K, Fredericks WR, Rapoport SI: Osmotic opening of the blood-brain barrier to methotrexate in the rat, *Surg Neurol* 12:323-328, 1979.

96. Okisaka S, Kuwabara T: Selective destruction of the pigmented epithelium in the ciliary body of the eye, *Science* 184:1298-1299, 1974.

97. Okisaka S, Kuwabara T, Rapoport SI: Effect of hyperosmotic agents on the ciliary epithelium and trabecular meshwork, *Invest Ophthalmol* 15:617-625, 1976.

98. Pagani JJ, Hayman LA, Bigelow RH et al: Prophylactic diazepam in prevention of contrast media-associated seizures in glioma patients undergoing cerebral computed tomography, *Cancer* 54:2200-2204, 1984.

99. Pagani JJ, Hayman LA, Bigelow RH et al: Diazepam prophylaxis of contrast media-induced seizures during computed tomography of patients with brain metastases, *Am J Roentgenol* 140:787-792, 1983.

100. Pappius HM, Savaki HE, Fieschi C et al: Osmotic opening of the blood-brain barrier and local cerebral glucose utilization, *Ann Neurol* 5:211-219, 1979.

101. Posner JB: Management of central nervous system metastases. *Semin Oncol* 4:81-91, 1977.

102. Rapoport SI: Effect of concentrated solutions on the blood-brain barrier, *Am J Physiol* 219:270-274, 1970.

103. Rapoport SI: *Blood-brain barrier in physiolology and medicine,* New York, 1976, Raven Press.

104. Rapoport SI: Opening of the blood-brain barrier by acute hypertension, *Exp Neurol* 52:467-479, 1976.

105. Rapoport SI: Osmotic opening of the blood-brain barrier, *Ann Neurol* 24:677-684, 1988.

106. Rapoport SI, Bachman DS, Thompson HK: Chronic effects of osmotic opening of the blood-brain barrier in the monkey. *Science* 176:1243-1245, 1972.

107. Rapoport SI, Fredericks WR, Ohno K et al: Quantitative aspects of reversible osmotic opening of the blood-brain barrier, *Am J Physiol* 238:R421-R431, 1980.

108. Rapoport SI, Hori M, Klatzo I: Reversible osmotic opening of the blood-brain barrier, *Science* 173:1026-1028, 1971.

109. Rapoport SI, Hori M, Klatzo I: Testing of a hypothesis for osmotic opening of the blood-brain barrier, *Am J Physiol* 223:323-331, 1972.

110. Rapoport SI, Matthews K, Thomp-

son HK et al: Osmotic opening of the blood-brain barrier in the rhesus monkey without measurable brain edema, *Brain Res* 136:23-29, 1977.

111. Rapoport SI, Robinson PJ: Tight-junctional modification as the basis of osmotic opening of the blood-brain barrier, *Ann NY Acad Sci* 481:250-267, 1986.

112. Rapoport SI, Thompson HK: Osmotic opening of the blood-brain barrier in the monkey without associated neurological deficits, *Science* 180, 1973.

113. Robinson PJ, Rapoport SI: Size selectivity of blood-brain permeability at various times after osmotic opening, *Am J Physiol* 22:R459-R466, 1987.

114. Saija A, Princi P, DePasquale R et al: Modifications of the permeability of the blood-brain barrier and local cerebral metabolism in pentobarbital- and ketamine-anaesthetized rats, *Neuropharmacology* 28:997-1002, 1989.

115. Steinwall O: An improved technique for testing the effect of contrast media and other substances on the blood-brain barrier, *Acta Radiol* 49:281-284, 1958.

116. Steinwall O, Klatzo I: Selective vulnerability of the blood-brain barrier in chemically induced lesions, *J Neuropathol Exp Neurol* 25:542-559, 1966.

117. Tan U: Electrocorticographic changes induced by topically applied succinylcholine and biperiden, *Electroencephalogr Clin Neurophysiol* 42:252-258, 1977.

118. Tan U, Marangoz C, Senyuva F: The effects of topical succinylcholine on single unit and electrocorticographic activity, *Experientia* 33:1333-1335, 1977.

119. Torkelson AR, LaBudde JA, Weikel JGJ: The metabolic fate of cyclophosphamide, *Drug Metab Rev* 3:131-165, 1974.

120. Van Dyke RA, Powis G: Lethal effects of co-administration of halothane and cyclophosphamide in mice, *Anesthesiology* 64:810-811, 1983.

121. Vesely R, Hoffman WE, Gil KS et al: The cerebrovascular effects of curare and histamine in the rat, *Anesthesiology* 66:519-523, 1987.

122. Vick NA: Chemotherapy of brain tumors: the blood-brain barrier is not a factor, *Arch Neurol* 34:123-125, 1977.

123. Von Euler US, Wahlund H: Über zentrale Kurarewirkungen, *Acta Physiol Scandinav* 2:327-333, 1941.

124. Wagner RC, Casley-Smith JR: Endothelial vesicles, *Microvasc Res* 21:267-298, 1981.

125. Walker MD, Weiss H: Chemotherapy in the treatment of malignant brain tumors, *Adv Neurol* 13:149-191, 1975.

126. Wang RIH, Ross CA: Prolonged apnea following succinylcholine in cancer patients receiving AB-132, *Anesthesiology* 24:363-367, 1963.

127. Warnke PC, Blasberg RG, Groothuis DR: The effect of hyperosmotic blood-brain barrier disruption on blood-to-tissue transport in ENU-induced gliomas, *Ann Neurol* 22:300-305, 1987.

128. Waser PG: Localization of ^{14}C-pancuronium by histo- and wholebody-autoradiography in normal and pregnant mice, *Naunyn Schmiedebergs Arch Pharmacol* 279:399-412, 1973.

129. Waser PG, Wiederkehr H, Sin RA et al: Distribution and kinetics of 14C-vecuronium in rats and mice, *Br J Anaesth* 59:1044-1051, 1987.

130. Werba A, Gilly H, Weindlmayr-Goettel M et al: Concentration of pancuronium and vecuronium in cerebrospinal fluid before and after blood-brain barrier disruption in the pig, *J Neurosurg Anesthesia* 3:A247, 1990.

131. Wientraub S, Mesulam MM: Mental status assessment of young and elderly patients in behavioral neurology. In Mesulam MM, editor: *Principles of behavioral neurology,* Philadelphia, 1985, FA Davis, pp 71-123.

132. Williams WT, Lowry RL, Eggers GWN: Anesthetic management during therapeutic disruption of the blood-brain barrier, *Anesth Analg* 65:188-190, 1986.

133. Witten DM: Reactions to urographic contrast media, *JAMA* 231:974-977, 1975.

134. Witten DM, Hirsch FD, Hartman GW: Acute reactions to urographic contrast medium: incidence, clinical characteristics and relationship to history of hypersensitivity states, *Am J Roentgenol Radium Ther Nucl Med* 119:832-840, 1973.

135. Wolff H: The inhibition of serum cholinesterase by cyclophosphamid, *Klin Wochenschr* 43:819-824, 1965.

136. Ziylan YZ, Robinson PJ, Rapoport SI: Differential blood-brain barrier permeabilities to [14C] sucrose and [3H] inulin after osmotic opening in the rat, *Exp Neurol* 79:845-857, 1983.

137. Ziylan YZ, Robinson PJ, Rapoport SI: Blood-brain barrier permeability to sucrose and dextran after osmotic opening, *Am J Physiol* 247:R634-R638, 1984.

138. Zsigmond EK, Robins G: The effect of a series of anti-cancer drugs on plasma cholinesterase activity, *Can Anaesth Soc J* 19:75-82, 1972.

23

Occlusive Cerebrovascular Disease: Medical and Surgical Considerations

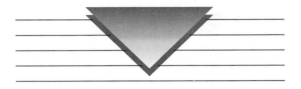

HUGH A. GELABERT
WESLEY S. MOORE

HISTORICAL PERSPECTIVE
PATHOPHYSIOLOGY OF
  CEREBROVASCULAR DISEASE
  Theories of pathogenesis
  Flow reduction theory
  Embolic theory
  Atherosclerotic plaque
  Growth of plaque
  Cerebral susceptibility to ischemia
PRESENTATIONS OF
  CEREBROVASCULAR DISEASE
  Asymptomatic presentations
  Symptomatic presentations
  Syndromes
  Stroke, transient ischemic attack,
    reversible ischemic neurologic deficit
DIAGNOSIS OF CEREBROVASCULAR
  DISEASE: HISTORY
  Physical examination
  Laboratory examination
  Cerebral imaging
  Angiography

NATURAL HISTORY OF
  CEREBROVASCULAR DISEASE
  SYNDROMES
  Stroke
  Transient ischemic attacks
  Asymptomatic high-grade stenosis
  Ulcerations
MEDICAL MANAGEMENT OF
  ISCHEMIC CEREBROVASCULAR
  DISEASE
  Risk factor control
  Measures to reduce thromboembolism
  Anticoagulants
  Antiplatelet drugs
THE ROLE OF SURGERY
  Accepted indications
  Controversial indications
RESULTS OF CAROTID
  ENDARTERECTOMY
  Asymptomatic patients
  Symptomatic patients (stroke and TIA)
  Randomized studies
SURGICAL TECHNIQUE OF

CAROTID ENDARTERECTOMY
  Anesthesia
  Positioning
  Carotid exposure
  Preparation for endarterectomy
  Use of carotid shunt
  Monitoring cerebral perfusion and
    function
  Endarterectomy
  Patch closure vs. primary closure
  Arterial closure
  Assessment of carotid repair
  Operation completion
  Recovery from anesthesia
COMPLICATIONS
  Stroke
  Duplex scan
  Angiography
  Reexploration
  Cranial nerve lesions
  Cardiac morbidity
SUMMARY

In the 38 years since DeBakey first performed a carotid endarterectomy, the indications and results of this operation have changed greatly. Perhaps the most notable development is the intense debate that has grown around the operation itself. Opponents have cited dismal results and varying surgical complication rates in different parts of the country. A myriad of alternative therapies have been proposed and tested; some have been found to yield modest benefit. Despite this, the need for carotid endarterectomy persists. It is thought to be one of the best methods of reducing the risk of stroke in those populations suffering from atherosclerotic occlusive disease of the carotid arteries. Understanding the range of issues involved in this topic is difficult. The operation has been clearly described, the complications from surgery are well known, the general indications have been outlined, and still there is much controversy and debate. However, the same set of data may be viewed from several perspectives, and the conclusions will differ accordingly. This chapter provides a basis for understanding how, when, and why carotid endarterectomy is performed.

HISTORICAL PERSPECTIVE

The series of observations and discoveries that led to carotid endarterectomy dates back over 150 years. The earliest accounts of carotid arterial disease derive from the dissections of John Hunter, whose specimens of sclerotic carotid arteries are still preserved in the Hunterian Museum of the Royal College of Surgeons in England.[5]

The initial association between disease of the carotid artery and the manifestations of cerebrovascular disease is attributed to William Savoy, who correlated clinical symptoms with a pathologic specimen.[64] He surmised the probable relationship between deficient carotid artery flow and the neurologic symptoms of his patient. In 1905, Chiari[13] described the pathogenic mechanism whereby thrombi from an ulcerated plaque in the carotid artery bifurcation caused cerebral emboli. Hunt,[39] in 1914, drew an analogy between intermittent claudication and cerebral symptoms of a vascular nature. He observed that the circle of Willis is not always sufficient to allow adequate collateral flow and concluded that some cases of cerebral insufficiency would result from restricted cerebral circulation. In 1951 and 1954, Fischer[23,24] reported autopsy findings that established the relationship between carotid artery bifurcation plaque and cerebral embolization. Milikan and Seikert in 1955[48] defined the syndromes of carotid artery and vertebrobasilar insufficiency.

With the establishment of the pathologic association between arterial obstruction and cerebral dysfunction, the stage was set for the modern era of carotid artery surgery. Carrell[11] developed the techniques of vascular suturing and Moniz refined the techniques of arteriography. In 1954, Eascott et al.[18] reported one of the first surgical approaches. Their patient, who had been suffering from repetitive transient ischemic attacks (TIA), underwent resection of the carotid artery bulb with reanastomosis of the carotid artery to the internal carotid artery. The first carotid endarterectomy was performed by DeBakey and associates in 1953.[15]

PATHOPHYSIOLOGY OF CEREBROVASCULAR DISEASE

Although several factors contribute to the pathophysiology of cerebrovascular disease, the predominant lesion is the atherosclerotic plaque. Stroke or TIA is the end point of events that begin with the genesis of plaque at the carotid artery bifurcation and terminate as complications of a degenerative plaque. Several theories have been formulated to account for the development of cerebral symptoms from carotid artery plaques.

Theories of Pathogenesis

There are two major theories relating carotid artery disease and neurologic damage. Proponents of the flow reduction theory hypothesize that the arterial lesion reduces the flow through the internal carotid artery, thus depriving the brain of adequate perfusion. In contrast, the major concept of the embolic theory is that emboli arising from the carotid artery bifurcation obstruct the perfusion of regions of the brain by occluding distal vessels.

Flow Reduction Theory

The flow reduction theory was the first to be generally accepted. In cases where the carotid artery was thrombosed, stroke followed because of loss of blood flow.[39,48] Similarly, individuals with flow-limiting lesions suffered effects of reduced perfusion and were at risk of complete occlusion and stroke. The analogy to intermittent claudication of the legs suggested that a stenotic lesion could account for intermittent cerebral ischemia. Stroke that occurred in the presence of a stenosis was due to a reduction of cerebral blood flow (CBF) below the brain perfusion threshold. The role of endarterectomy in correcting this situation is evident.

However, the flow reduction theory had difficulty explaining several observations. If the stenotic lesion is a fixed lesion such as a carotid artery plaque, how does it account for intermittent ischemic events? In addition, how could it account for delayed stroke after carotid artery ligation? Finally, how could it account for Hollenhorst plaques (retinal cholesterol emboli) and subsequent stroke?

Several explanations were invoked. Intermittent TIAs could be the summation of several events, such as postural changes or cardiac dysrhythmias, along with the carotid artery stenosis. Delayed stroke after carotid ligation could simply be the result of the slow strangulation of the hypoperfused brain. Ultimately, the relationship of retinal lesions and stroke overwhelmed the flow reduction theory.

Embolic Theory

The embolic theory suggested that embolization of debris from the atherosclerotic plaque would account for both intermittent and permanent cerebrovascular symptoms.[47] This theory suffers from doubts regarding the central hypothesis that recurrent embolic episodes would cause repeated, stereotypic TIAs. For example, how these emboli would direct themselves to the same location to produce the stereotypic deficits of a TIA was unclear. This question was answered by Milikan,[47] who used small ball bearings to produce embolism from a point source in the carotid artery.

These bearings were later discovered to have been directed by the arterial flow to the same cortical artery branches. Thus emboli from a fixed point source in the arterial wall could embolize to the identical point, given constant flow dynamics.

The current view of the pathogenesis of cerebrovascular disease is that both mechanisms operate to produce cerebrovascular accidents. The embolic events are considered the principal cause of TIAs and most strokes. Flow reduction is considered a significant cause of carotid artery occlusion and an important coprocess in the development of embolic disease. It is also a marker of significant atherosclerotic disease. As a consequence of insight developed during the elucidation of these theories, researchers have recognized the vital role of the endothelium as well as the growth and degeneration of atherosclerotic plaques.

Atherosclerotic Plaque

Atherosclerotic plaque is composed principally of matrix and cellular elements.[62] The matrix is the product of the cellular elements and lipid deposition in the subendothelial layers of the arterial wall. The principal components of matrix are deposits of lipid and cholesterol esters and collagenous protein extruded from the cells. In addition, degenerative byproducts of senescent cells add to the matrix.

The principal importance of matrix is that it forms the bulk of a plaque. Furthermore, the composition of the matrix significantly determines the behavior of the plaque. Some plaques are characterized by homogeneous matrix that is thought to be principally fibrous and firm, others have heterogeneous matrices incorporating both calcific and fibrous elements, and some plaques are principally calcific. Some matrix is predominantly composed of cholesterol deposits along with disorganized collagenous strands and cellular debris, and these tend to be "soft." Softer plaques are more likely to generate emboli than firm fibrous plaques.

The cellular elements of the plaque are responsible for the growth of the plaque and the composition of the matrix. The principal cellular elements are monocytes and smooth muscle cells, neither of which are indigenous to the subendothelial space. The presence of both suggests the action of mitogens and chemotactic factors. Monocytes are recruited from blood. They pass between the endothelial cells and enter the subendothelial space. Smooth muscle cells are attracted from the medial layers of the arterial wall. Initially, the monocytes become macrophages and ingest the cholesterol particles. As they ingest cholesterol, they grow and extrude matrix. Ultimately they become giant cells, which are characterized by the foamy appearance of their cytoplasm, leading to the description "foam cells." The smooth muscle cells are also transformed into these foam cells.

The factors that stimulate plaque to form are still unclear. The most common assumption is that plaque development is the result of localized arterial trauma.[28] One theory proposes that hemodynamic stress traumatizes endothelial cells and leads to plaque deposition. According to this theory, shear stress develops at arterial bifurcations, and this shear stress is thought to damage the endothelium and facilitate the deposition of plaque. Alternative theories incriminate genetic factors, ingested toxins, and aberrant lipid metabolism. The etiologic agent remains unproved, but most researchers agree that atherosclerosis is a multifactorial disease.

Growth of Plaque

The growth of plaque explains its protean manifestations. The earliest stage of growth is the fatty streak.[62] This subendothelial accumulation of lipids appears as yellow streaks within the arterial lumen and is visible to the unaided eye. These streaks are smooth and flat, and offer no obstruction to the flow of blood. Histologically, these lesions are characterized by the deposition of cholesterol and monocytes, and the presence of foam cells. Fatty streaks are frequently found in arteries of young individuals.

Mature plaques are firm, elevated lesions and represent the second stage of plaque growth.[62] On inspection, they appear yellow, often with white encrustations. Their surface is often relatively smooth and covered with endothelium. Histologically, these lesions are composed of smooth muscle cells plus most of the same elements as the fatty streak. The most notable change from the fatty streak to mature plaque is the tremendous accumulation of matrix. Furthermore, the matrix may display evidence of calcification, which occurs as a consequence of passive deposition of calcium salts within the plaque. Although calcium salts are deposited in all arterial walls, the matrix appears to display an increased affinity for calcium.

Complex or degenerative plaque is responsible for most of the manifestations of vascular disease and is the final step in plaque evolution. Complex plaque forms as the consequence of degeneration of mature plaque. Three primary events may occur to produce symptoms: plaque hemorrhage, endothelial denudation, and plaque erosion.

Plaque hemorrhage is one of the principal mechanisms accounting for rapid plaque growth, disruption of plaque structure,[44] and is the consequence of an ischemic event leading to the necrosis of the center of a plaque. The ischemic event occurs when the expanding plaque outgrows its nutrient supply. With insufficient nutrients, the cellular elements at the center of the plaque die, and the necrosis may lead to hemorrhage within the plaque from one of the investing vessels. When the intraplaque hemorrhage occurs, a hematoma may force rapid expansion of the plaque, which may lead to abrupt occlusion of the arterial lumen or fracture of the plaque leaving an irregular exposed surface, or it may expel the contents of the plaque into the bloodstream.

Denudation of the endothelium on a mature plaque exposes the underlying plaque to the flow of the blood. The loss of the endothelial surface eliminates the antithrombotic and vasodilatory effects of the endothelium and exposes the collagenous elements of the plaque to the bloodstream. This allows an interaction between the collagen and platelets that may stimulate the deposition of both platelet and fibrin aggregates. Fragmentation of these aggregates generates platelet and fibrin emboli.

Plaque erosion occurs if soft plaque is exposed to the flowing blood, which may occur with endothelial denudation or hemorrhagic fracture of the plaque. The exposed soft matrix may be eroded by the flowing blood, the plaque becomes excavated, and small emboli can be released into the cerebral vessels.

After they are formed, plaque ulcers may undergo several modifications: They may be further excavated, becoming larger ulcers; they may be resurfaced with endothelial tissue, becoming small quiescent ulcers or "pits"; or they may persist as a nidus for further deposition of fibrin and platelets, causing persistent embolic symptoms.[44]

Cerebral Susceptibility to Ischemia

Because the brain lacks significant reserves energy and is unable to sustain itself under anaerobic conditions, several mechanisms have developed to ensure continued adequate cerebral circulation. First, regional CBF regulation allows the cerebral circulation to adjust to a wide range of perfusion pressures.[43] Second, collateral circulatory pathways represent a homeostatic mechanism that helps assure continued flow of oxygen and nutrients to the brain in the event of an arterial occlusion. The cerebral pathway circuits may be broadly grouped into those that are ordinarily present and those that develop in response to flow restriction.

The circle of Willis is a vascular ring that is formed as a consequence of the anastomosis of the principal vessels at the base of the brain. It receives contributions from both internal carotids directly and from the two vertebral arteries by means of their common trunk, the basilar artery. When intact, the circle of Willis may allow perfusion of all cerebral territories from a single arterial trunk. Thus instances of asymptomatic occlusion of both right and left carotid arteries have been reported. Anatomic studies of the circle of Willis have revealed that the circulatory collateral is incomplete or insufficient in a large fraction of the population. Depending on what is considered abnormal, the circle of Willis has been reported to bear some abnormality in 50% to 80% of people.[37] Although this is usually not a problem, it may be critical in event of transient or permanent occlusion of one of the cerebral vessels.

A second group of collaterals is formed in response to chronic circulatory insufficiency. These collaterals are most common in the region of the face. The predominant collateral is that between the external and internal carotid arteries across the orbit of the eye and forms in the presence of a significant stenosis or occlusion of the internal carotid artery. The collateral flow is from the external carotid artery to the superficial temporal artery, across the orbital rim to behind the eye to the ophthalmic artery. The ophthalmic artery is the first major branch of the internal carotid artery and is the most common recipient of collateral flow. Alter-

native connections may be established between the facial and maxillary arteries through their ethmoid branches to the ophthalmic artery. The collection of facial vessels serving as collateral circulatory pathways has led to the concept of a facial collateral vascular unit.

PRESENTATIONS OF CEREBROVASCULAR DISEASE

The spectrum of presentation of cerebrovascular disease is explained by the anatomic characteristics of the central nervous system. Because of the variety of collateral circulatory pathways, not all cerebral emboli or occlusions become symptomatic. Because of the redundancy of the neuronal network, small events may pass undetected. Stereotypic symptoms are best explained by the remarkable consistency of cerebral architecture; neuroanatomic features do not vary much between individuals.

Asymptomatic Presentations

Asymptomatic lesions are most commonly discovered in the course of evaluation of other problems. A patient with symptomatic cardiac or peripheral vascular disease should be screened for concomitant carotid artery disease because of the high concordance between these lesions. The presence of a cervical bruit also serves as a sign calling for further evaluation in neurologically asymptomatic patients.

A second form of asymptomatic presentation includes patients who are discovered to have suffered "silent" cerebral infarcts on CT scan performed for an unrelated indication. The presence of a silent stroke has led to the creation of a new category of patients, those who are signomatic (having a sign but no symptom). Although many lesions may be detected by detailed neurologic examination, it is accepted that a significant number of silent strokes do not manifest clinical symptoms. It is suspected that progressive senile dementia may, in part, be explained by multiple silent strokes.[32]

Symptomatic Presentations

Symptomatic presentations have been grouped by the arterial territories involved, by the affected cerebral region, and by the duration and persistence of symptoms. The arterial territories may be used to describe a lesion as belonging to either the anterior or the posterior circulation. Anterior circulatory lesions are those that are located in the distribution of the carotid arteries; and posterior symptoms are those that are located in the distribution of the vertebral and basilar arterial systems.

A focal or lateralizing symptom is readily assigned to either the right or left hemisphere and frequently may be further localized to a particular lobe or region of the brain. They are more typical of anterior circulatory events. Cortical events typically produce focal symptoms, a neurologic deficit that stems from a lesion in the cerebral cortex. Typically these lesions involve functions such as motor control, sensory recognition, speech, cognition, or emotion.

Basilar or posterior events commonly present with symptoms of ataxia, vertigo, dizziness, incoordination, and syncope. They also may present with global symptoms that are difficult to place within the definitions of cerebral region. Typically, these symptoms include loss of consciousness, dizziness, or obtundation, and are more often associated with events of the posterior circulation. These symptoms are distinguished from the focal symptoms in that they may be difficult to localize to one hemisphere or one region.

Syndromes

A more precise definition of these lesions is based on the affected cerebral territory and the neurologic manifestations of a cerebrovascular event that allow determination of the territory involved.

Amaurosis fugax is a syndrome in which a transient loss of vision occurs as the result of occlusion of the retinal arteries and is characterized by the sudden progressive loss of vision, usually in one eye. The visual loss occurs in a pattern that is described as a shade being lowered in front of the eye and is due to occlusion in the arteriolar distribution within the retina where the central retinal artery branches in a craniocaudad orientation. An occasional variation of this symptom occurs when the retinal arterioles branch in a horizontal pattern. In such patients, the shade appears to be drawn across the visual field from one side to the other.

A syndrome of contralateral paresis and sensory deficit is produced by an embolus to the anterior cerebral artery (ACA). The paresis usually involves the lower extremity, with relative sparing of the arm. Finally, frontal lobe symptoms may be noted. These include slowing of mentation, abnormal emotional response, and difficulty in concentration. Additional symptoms may include sucking of fingers and incontinence.

A syndrome of combined sensory and motor deficits on the contralateral side of the body is produced by occlusion of the middle cerebral artery (MCA). Involvement of the dominant hemisphere may produce aphasia, and a lesion in the nondominant hemisphere may result in amorphosynthesis (the inability to name objects). Involvement of the inferior division may result in a homonymous hemianopsia (loss of vision from the same side visual field in both eyes). This may frequently be associated with a hemineglect-type syndrome where the patient acts as if the affected arm or leg is nonexistent.

As mentioned previously, the posterior cerebral artery (PCA) may be fed by either the carotid artery or the basilar systems. In the event of a PCA occlusion, the patient will suffer a homonymous hemianopsia, with macular sparing because of a dual blood supply from the MCA and the PCA to the macular region. The hemianopsia of the occipital lobe is different from that of the MCA lesion so that patients are often disturbed by the hemianopsia, and they may also suffer symptoms such as neglect and optikokinetic nystagmus.

One final syndrome of arterial occlusion is due to a choroidal arterial lesion. These vessels supply the internal capsule, and their manifestations may be difficult to characterize. Typically these lesions produce contralateral hemiplegia, hypesthesia, and even hemianopsia. Other associated symptoms include constructional aphasia, alexia, and motor impersistence. That many of these symptoms may be confused with PCA lesions is, in part, explained by the fact that the anterior choroidal artery supplies the posterior internal capsule and adjacent white matter.

Stroke, Transient Ischemia Attack, Reversible Ischemic Neurologic Deficit

The most common grouping of symptomatic patients is according to the duration and persistence of symptoms. Patients whose symptoms persist, creating a permanent neurologic deficit, are said to have suffered a stroke. Patients whose symptoms are brief, lasting between a few minutes and 24 hours, are said to have suffered a TIA. There is some variation between these two extremes. Symptoms may last longer than 24 hours yet not persist, and these patients are said to have suffered a reversible ischemic neurologic deficit (RIND) if their symptoms resolve within 72 hours. Some physicians consider a lesion an RIND if it resolves within 3 weeks.

Within these major groupings, the neurologic presentations are subclassified according to severity, persistence, and repetition. Strokes are sometimes designated as either major or minor, depending on the degree of disability. A stroke in evolution is one that demonstrates progressive deterioration with the development of increasingly profound neurologic deficits.

TIAs are classified as single or multiple. Multiple TIAs are considered more significant than a single event, yet both are of concern. Crescendo TIAs are rare events in which multiple TIAs occur in rapid succession. The TIAs may fall into one of two patterns. The first pattern is characterized by a decreasing time between the TIAs so that they occur in increasingly rapid succession. The second pattern is one in which the degree of disability caused by each successive TIA is greater, so that the patient becomes progressively more incapacitated. Crescendo TIAs are considered signs of impending stroke and should be treated urgently.

DIAGNOSIS OF CEREBROVASCULAR DISEASE: HISTORY

A complete and thorough history of events leading to the patient's consultation provides at least 90% of the data required for formulating the diagnosis and therapeutic plan. Any neurologic events that the patient may have experienced must be carefully delineated, and specific questions should be asked to establish the timing, concordance, and repetitive nature of any cerebral symptoms. Patients may not be aware of the significance of repeated episodes of paresthesia or clumsiness; these should be sought. Because not all neurologic events represent cerebrovascular accidents, it is important to try to identify other possible causes of a patient's symptoms. Accordingly, diseases such as migraine, arthropathies, autoimmune problems, and vasculitis must be considered. One must also obtain a clear idea of specific risk factors, such as hypertension, cigarette smoking, diabetes, cardiovascular disease, peripheral vascular disease, and cardiac dysrhythmias. Questions regarding family history may reveal particularly virulent forms of atherosclerosis, hyperlipidemia, or cardiac or cerebrovascular disease.

Physical Examination

The physical examination is directed toward establishing the patient's neurologic function at the time of the visit. Neurologic deficits need to be carefully delineated so that any progression may be clearly documented. In addition, patients may not be aware of certain neurologic deficits, such as small areas of paresthesia, loss of minor segments of the visual fields, or proprioceptive deficits, such as loss of vibratory or position sense. Although not routinely incorporated into clinical practice, laryngoscopy (for the visualization of vocal cord mobility) is recommended in patients who are to undergo bilateral carotid endarterectomy or who present with recurrent carotid stenosis. In the former group, bilateral vocal cord palsy may be a serious problem. In the latter group, there is a high incidence of cranial nerve injury.

Laboratory Examination

Two areas of noninvasive testing of particular importance are the use of cerebral imaging (computed tomography [CT] or magnetic resonance imaging [MRI]), and tests directed at identifying and categorizing carotid arterial stenosis. The latter category includes duplex scans, oculoplethysmography (OPG), and transcranial Doppler.

The duplex scan, the most commonly employed test, is the combined application of B-mode imaging and pulse Doppler spectral analysis for surveying the carotid artery bifurcation. The B-mode image provides a rough two-dimensional image of the arterial contour. The quality and sensitivity of the B-mode image may vary from one examination to another, and although some authors have used this image to identify carotid ulcers and stenosis, it is not yet an ideal test. The pulse-Doppler is a device that uses the Doppler shift phenomenon to evaluate the velocity of blood flow in a specific portion of the arterial lumen. The velocity of flow and the degree of turbulence serve as indices of the degree of stenosis within the artery. In the case of duplex scanning the accuracy compared with angiography has been estimated at as high as 95% to 98%.[56]

OPG is a measure of retinal arterial blood pressure, but its use has considerably diminished with the advent of the duplex scanner. By comparing the results of right and left eye examinations, one may draw conclusions regarding the hemispheric perfusion. It is now used primarily in instances where duplex scanning may be inconclusive and further information is warranted.

Cerebral Imaging

CT scanning of stroke patients being considered for carotid endarterectomy allows confirmation of the presence, extent, and age of the cerebral infarct. The use of CT scanning during evaluation of asymptomatic patients before endarterectomy has been debated, and it has been generally rejected on the basis that it provides little benefit despite significant cost.[59] The phenomenon of asymptomatic cerebral infarction exists, but its prevalence and its significance with regard to surgical morbidity are unknown. The incidence of these lesions in stroke patients has been found to be as high as 10%, but the lesions apparently do not affect the prognosis of surgery and serve principally as indicators of possible further strokes.[41]

The value of MR scans, as opposed to CT scans, is also a subject of debate. The MR scan provides enhanced sensitivity, but the significance of many of the lesions identified on MR images is unknown. Thus the added information may be of relatively little benefit.[7]

Angiography

Angiography remains the single best method of evaluating a carotid lesion,[26] despite the fact that it is an invasive procedure and carries a low risk of stroke, renal dysfunction, or other complications.

Regular, cut-film angiography is important in assessing carotid ulcers. This technique enables one to measure the size of the ulcer and accordingly assign a relative risk.[17] This cannot be done using any of the other imaging techniques, so it is not possible to grade the various ulcer types using other methods. Digital subtraction angiography uses image processing and enhancement to produce an image of carotid lesions with less angiocontrast dye. Although the reduced dye contrast load is an advantage, it is counterbalanced by limitations in the quality of some images.

The introduction of magnetic resonance angiography has been enthusiastically adopted as a substitute for conventional angiography or even digital angiography. The proposed advantages include the absence of invasive catheters or toxic angiographic contrast drugs. The principal drawback is that accuracy in evaluating carotid plaques is unproved. Initial experience has revealed a significant incidence of false-positive tests. Radiologists recognize that the magnetic characteristics of turbulent flow may sometimes cause these aberrations, although this has not been generally acknowledged in the medical literature. Until these tests are validated, they should be considered adjunctive.

NATURAL HISTORY OF CEREBROVASCULAR DISEASE SYNDROMES

For therapy to be of benefit, it must improve the natural course of the disease. Establishing the natural history of cerebrovascular disease is difficult. First, the definitions of various syndromes have changed over time. Second, the advances of technology have rendered much of the historical data irrelevant. Third, the methodology by which much of the current data has been generated is not what would currently be considered optimal. Finally, most patients receive some form of treatment, and thus the course of the disease without treatment is difficult to define contemporaneously.

Any discussion of the natural history of cerebrovascular disease is best organized in terms of three large patient groups: those who have suffered stroke, those who present with a history of TIAs, and those with asymptomatic high-grade (70% to 99%) carotid artery stenosis. Symptomatic patients are further subdivided according to the extent of carotid stenosis and the presence of ulceration. Patients in each of these groups have remarkably different characteristics, and the progression of their disease is significantly different. Surgical indications and the expected results vary dramatically between these groups.

Stroke

Stroke is a relatively common disease, and, if not fatal, may severely disable a person. About 500,000 strokes occur annually, and it is the third leading cause of death in the United States.[69] In 1976, the cost of stroke was estimated at $7 billion.[1] An accurate estimate of the current cost is difficult, but some authors have postulated that this figure has quadrupled. Adding to this cost is evidence suggesting that the death rate from acute stroke has decreased, but the incidence of stroke has not.[10,68] Although this trend has not been clearly established, the implication is that patients are surviving their stroke and requiring increased care. When combined with the demographic trends of our population, the effect of stroke is enormous. The mortality from acute stroke ranges from 15% to 30%.[69] The associated deaths from myocardial disease further elevate this figure. The leading cause of late death in victims of stroke is another stroke.

The risk of recurrent stroke in patents who have suffered a stroke is estimated to range from 4.8% to 20% each year, and this risk appears to be relatively constant over a period of up to 5 years. Thus the cumulative risk of a second stroke in stroke patients is thought to be as high as 50% over a 5-year period. Most authors believe that the rate of recurrent stroke is about 9% per year and that the generally accepted 5-year repeat stroke rate is about 45%.[63]

Transient Ischemic Attacks

Patients who present with TIAs demonstrate a 10% risk of stroke during the first year after their initial attack. This risk falls during subsequent years to a constant yearly rate of 6%.[31] The cumulative 5-year stroke rate for TIA patients is estimated to be about 35% although higher stroke rates have been reported. In a population study by Mayo Clinic, the 1-year stroke rate in untreated patients was as high as 23% and the 5-year stroke rate was 45%.[67]

Asymptomatic High-Grade Stenosis

The natural history of asymptomatic high-grade stenosis is particularly difficult to estimate for several reasons. First, the indices of the disease have changed over the past decade. For example, patients were once diagnosed by cervical bruit, but this is no longer considered a valid indicator of advanced cerebrovascular disease. Second, the definition of "significant stenosis" has gradually advanced from 50% to 70% occlusion. Occlusion of 75% was once considered significant. Now 80% occlusion is considered the accepted threshold for significance in asymptomatic patients.

Despite these variations in methodology and analysis, several persistent themes appear in the natural history of asymptomatic carotid stenosis. First, these lesions are associated with a higher than normal risk of stroke. In studies where the criterion used to identify the high-risk group was an arterial stenosis of 50% or more, threat of stroke in untreated patients ranged up to 7.5% yearly.[49] In a more recent series where the high-risk lesion was defined as 75% stenosis or greater, the yearly risk of stroke was found to be 5%. The 1-year risk of stroke and TIA was 22%. What is more significant is that about 50% of these patients were taking aspirin while suffering these events.[12] In a study that compared the incidence of stroke with the degree of arterial stenosis, the progression of a plaque to 80% stenosis or greater was found to signal a high risk of neurologic event or arterial thrombosis. The progression of a plaque to this degree of stenosis carried a 46% risk of ischemic symptoms or occlusion at 1 year.[60] Another more recent series combined the criteria of 75% lesion and plaque characteristics as recorded by duplex scanning. In this report, the risk of stroke was associated with both plaque consistency and lumen reduction. These factors combined to produce a spectrum of risk from less than 1% (dense plaque with stenosis less than 75%) up to 16% per year (soft plaque with stenosis greater than 75%).[57]

Ulcerations

An unusual subgroup of asymptomatic patients have carotid plaque ulcers. The potential for stroke in these patients may be considerable and is directly related to the size of the ulcer. In a study of patients with asymptomatic plaque ulcers, those with large, complex ulcers had a 7.5% yearly stroke rate, and those with intermediate-size ulcers had a yearly stroke rate of 4.5%. Those with the smallest ulcers had a yearly stroke rate of 0.9%.[17] Although the prognosis of the intermediate ulcers has been debated,[42] the recommendation that large complex ulcers be repaired by means of carotid endarterectomy is widely accepted.

MEDICAL MANAGEMENT OF ISCHEMIC CEREBROVASCULAR DISEASE

Management of ischemic cerebrovascular disease is principally directed along two distinct lines: reduction of risk factors and therapy directed at reducing thromboemboli.

Risk Factor Control

The principal risk factors are age, hypertension, cigarette smoking, diabetes, cardiovascular disease, atrial fibrillation, and hyperlipidemia. Regression analysis allows development of a stroke risk profile for a given individual. In this profile the various risk factors assume their proportional effect in determining the stroke risk. Hypertension is the strongest risk factor, followed by cardiac disease (left ventricular hypertrophy, atrial fibrillation, cardiovascular disease) and smoking. Both systolic and diastolic hypertension are associated with increased stroke rates, and the incidence of stroke is directly proportional to the degree of the blood pressure elevation.[69] The result of controlling risk factors is a dramatic reduction in the stroke risk for any age and gender. The results of a prospective trial of controlling systolic hypertension are still pending, but this study is expected to document the effectiveness of risk factor control.[69]

Measures to Reduce Thromboembolism

Identification of the embolic mechanisms leading to stroke have afforded an opportunity to attempt to reduce the incidence of stroke. This has been attempted by intervening in the events that form emboli: fibrin deposition and platelet aggregation. Researchers reason that inhibiting these processes will reduce the incidence of thromboembolic events and consequently the rate of stroke.

Anticoagulants

Chronic anticoagulation has been used under the supposition that it may reduce the likelihood of intravascular thrombotic events, and in turn, also reduce the number of strokes. More than 14 trials of anticoagulants in patients presenting with minor stroke or TIA have been published.[69] The results of these trials are, at best, mixed. Many of the trials have employed different durations of treatment. Most have used the same drug (warfarin) in similar doses. Although the results of some trials have been encouraging, this has not been the general rule.[27] Some studies have reported an increase in mortality in patients taking anticoagulants.[27] The general conclusion is that there is no therapeutic benefit to the use of anticoagulants in patients with completed stroke. Furthermore, it may result in an increased mortality caused by complications of the anticoagulation.

Antiplatelet Drugs

At least seven major prospective randomized studies have been published reporting the results of using a variety of antiplatelet drugs to reduce the risk of stroke.* These studies generally reveal a significant decrease in the incidence of TIAs within treatment groups (Table 23-1 to 23-3). The effect on the incidence of stroke has been more varied, but these drugs are believed to reduce the rate of stroke by 15% to 30%. However, the effectiveness of these drugs has not

---

*References 8, 9, 22, 29, 31, 33, 66.

always been statistically significant. Furthermore, a decrease in mortality has not been statistically significant unless death from cardiac disease is included. The overall impression from these studies is that the use of antiplatelet drugs reduces the incidence of TIAs and slightly reduces the rate of stroke. The most impressive effect is the reduction of cardiac mortality, an effect that is more pronounced in men than in women.

THE ROLE OF SURGERY

The role of surgery in the management of ischemic cerebrovascular disease is the prevention of stroke. The operation attempts to remove the carotid bifurcation plaque because it is the principal cause of symptoms and stroke by virtue of its ability to progress to occlusion and its propensity to generate cerebral emboli. By removing the cause, one hopes to prevent future occurrence. The operation does not produce recovery from a stroke. After a stroke has occurred, the affected tissues of the brain are permanently damaged by the ischemic insult. Reestablishing the normal contour of the carotid bulb by removing an atherosclerotic plaque will not directly affect residual cerebral function, although carotid endarterectomy may result in functional improvement in a few, unusual instances. The most clearly documented of these instances are flow-limiting lesions causing transient ischemic events, such as bright-light amaurosis.

The degree to which a patient will benefit from a carotid endarterectomy is directly proportional to the risk of stroke from the carotid lesion. A second important consideration is the risk of the operation. If the risk of stroke in the course of a carotid endarterectomy is so great that it exceeds the risk of the lesion itself, the surgery should not be performed.

Accepted Indications

Certain indications for carotid endarterectomy are generally well established because the natural course of these syndromes presents a considerable risk of stroke. Included in this group are patients with repeated TIAs, both hemispheric and amaurosis. A hemispheric stroke with good recovery is also a reasonable indication for operation, provided the patient is neurologically stable. Asymptomatic patients with high-risk lesions, such as large carotid ulcers or preocclusive stenosis, might also be included in this group.

Controversial Indications

Controversy still surrounds the role of carotid endarterectomy for asymptomatic high-grade stenosis, stroke in evolution, acute stroke, and global or vertebrobasilar symptoms in the face of multiple stenosis.[50] The repair of a carotid lesion in the face of a stroke in evolution with waxing and waning symptoms has not been clearly demonstrated to be beneficial.

Endarterectomy for an acute stroke should be undertaken

TABLE 23-1
Summary of Randomized Controlled Trials of Antiplatelet Agents

Year	Study	Patients	Months	Drugs Used (Daily Dose)
1977	Aspirin-TIA[22]	178	37	Aspirin 1.3 g vs. placebo
1978	Canadian Coop[31]	585	26	Aspirin 1.3 g vs. sulfinpyrazone 800 mg
1983	Danish Coop[66]	203	25	Aspirin 1 g vs. placebo
1983	AICLA[8]	604	36	Aspirin 1 g vs. aspirin 1 g plus dipyridamole 225 mg vs. placebo
1985	American-Canadian[29]	890	48	Aspirin 325 mg vs. aspirin 325 mg plus dipyridamole 75 mg
1987	Swedish Coop[9]	505	24	Aspirin 1.5 g vs. placebo
1989	Ticlopidine vs. aspirin[33]	3069	36	Aspirin 1.3 g vs. ticlopidine 500 mg

TABLE 23-2
Cumulative Stroke Rate (%) for Antiplatelet Trials

Study	Placebo	Aspirin	Aspirin/ Sulfinpyrazone	Sulfinpyrazone	Aspirin/Dipyridamole	Ticlopidine	Statistical Significance*
Aspirin-TIA[22]	15.5	12.5					5
Canadian Coop[31]	14.4	15.2	9.5	18.5			4
Danish Coop[66]	10.8	16.8					3
AICLA[8]	18	10.5			10.5		1
American-Canadian Coop[29]		13.6			11.8		3
Swedish Coop[9]	13	12					3
Ticlopidine vs. aspirin[33]		13				10	2

*Statistical significance: *1* = p < 0.01; *2* = p < 0.05; *3* = No statistical significance; *4* = this statistic not calculated; *5* = attained statistical significance by excluding patients.

TABLE 23-3
Cumulative Stroke and Death Rate (%) for Antiplatelet Studies

Study	Placebo	Aspirin	Aspirin/ Sulfinpyrazone	Sulfinpyrazone	Aspirin/Dipyridamole	Ticlopidine	Statistical Significance*
Aspirin-TIA[22]	21	14.7					5
Canadian Coop[31]	21.5	18	13.6	24.3			2
Danish Coop[66]		20.8					3
AICLA[8]	18.6	13.6			12.8		4
American-Canadian Coop[29]		19			18.9		3
Swedish Coop[9]	23	22					3
Ticlopidine vs. aspirin		19				17	2

*Statistical significance: *1* = p < 0.01; *2* = p < 0.05; *3* = no statistical significance; *4* = this statistic not calculated; *5* = attained statistical significance by excluding patients.

only under very specific circumstances. The stroke should be the result of an acute occlusion, and it should be a very recent event (the time between the onset of the stroke and surgical repair must be less than 4 hours). Such instances are exceedingly rare.

Endarterectomy for global symptoms may result in a patient who claims relief or improvement, but the benefit has not been clearly demonstrated in repeated studies. Similarly, patients whose complaint is gradual deterioration of mentation, in the absence of multiple small cerebral infarctions, should be carefully evaluated for other diseases, which are more likely the cause. Another controversial in-

dication is asymptomatic stenosis in the face of symptomatic coronary artery disease. Not only is the indication for endarterectomy itself debated, but the timing and sequence of the operations is not clearly established.

RESULTS OF CAROTID ENDARTERECTOMY

Reported results for carotid endarterectomy demonstrate a stratification of outcomes according to the indications for surgery. Patients with asymptomatic stenosis usually have the best outcomes, followed by patients with recurrent TIAs.[51] Patients who undergo surgery after a stroke with good recovery have a slightly higher risk of perioperative morbidity than patients with TIAs.

Analysis of the results of carotid endarterectomy has suffered from a profusion of classifications, terminology, and analytic methods. This provides impetus for several attempts at standardizing the cataloging and reporting of cerebrovascular disease and its management. Toward this end, the Society for Vascular Surgery and the International Society for Cardiovascular Surgery has proposed reporting standards that are becoming widely adopted.[3] In evaluating reports of carotid surgery, it is important to remember that these standard reporting criteria have not been adopted until recently and that centers with a large experience may have different results from institutions where the operation is done infrequently.

The Stroke Council of the American Heart Association has proposed a set of standards for the upper acceptable limit of morbidity and death in the various patient categories.[6] For asymptomatic patients this is 3%; for TIA patients 5%; for stroke patients 7%; and for recurrent carotid stenosis patients it should be no greater than 10%. These standards serve as guidelines by which to gauge the results of surgery.

Asymptomatic Patients

Based on the best historical data and nonrandomized studies, carotid endarterectomy for asymptomatic patients has effectively reduced the risk of stroke in patients with high-grade stenosis. In experienced hands, the operation carries minimal morbidity and mortality. Although some reports have emphasized dismal perioperative complication rates, the best series have complication rates well below the recommended 3% limit. Long-term duration of the protection against stroke has been reported, with the annual stroke rate reduced to as low as 0.3%.[52] On the average, the yearly stroke rate is about 1% to 2%, and the cumulative 5-year stroke rate, after carotid endarterectomy, ranges from 0% to 6%.[51]

Symptomatic Patients (Stroke and TIA)

Results of carotid endarterectomy in symptomatic patients have revealed an impressive reduction in the long-term risk of stroke. This has been noted despite a slightly increased risk of perioperative complications. The stroke rate during the first year after surgery for TIA has been reported to range from 1.6% to 4.8%.[25,55] This includes both perioperative complications and those arising in the course of the year. The cumulative 5-year stroke rate, after carotid endarterectomy, has been reported to be between 6% and 13%.[51]

When the indication for surgery is a completed stroke with recovery of function, the operative stroke rate has been recorded as 0% to 4.9%,[46,61] and the yearly stroke rate has been reduced to the range of 0.7% to 2.2%. The 5-year incidence of stroke in the territory of the repaired artery is as low as 3.2%.[49] However, if all strokes are counted, then the 5-year cumulative stroke rate may be as high as 24%.[34]

Randomized Studies

Because of the debate regarding the benefit of carotid endarterectomy, several multicenter prospective randomized trials have been initiated with the goal of comparing "best medical care alone" to "best medical care plus carotid endarterectomy." Two of the studies are being supported by

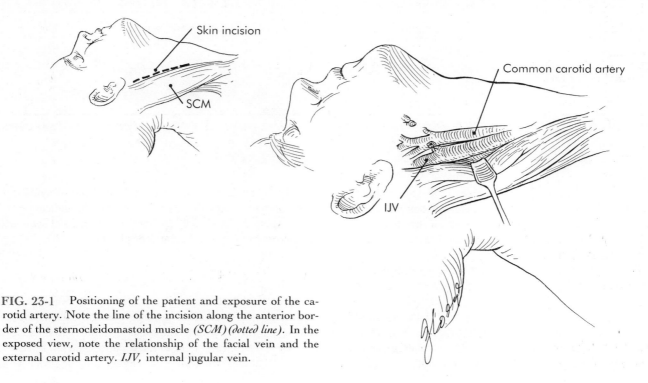

FIG. 23-1   Positioning of the patient and exposure of the carotid artery. Note the line of the incision along the anterior border of the sternocleidomastoid muscle *(SCM)(dotted line)*. In the exposed view, note the relationship of the facial vein and the external carotid artery. *IJV,* internal jugular vein.

the Veteran's Administration, one is a study of symptomatic patients and one is of asymptomatic patients.[38] Similarly, the two NIH studies focus on symptomatic (North American Symptomatic Carotid Endarterectomy Trial, NASCET[14]) and asymptomatic (Asymptomatic Carotid Atherosclerosis Study, ACAS[30]) patients with significant carotid disease (60% or greater carotid artery stenosis) and no symptoms of stroke.

A segment of the NASCET study was terminated early because of a significant difference between the surgical and medical groups. Symptomatic patients with stenosis of 70% or greater derived a very significant benefit from surgical intervention. The rates of perioperative stroke and death were 5.8%. The stroke rate alone was 5.5%. At a follow-up period of 2 years, surgery reduced the risk of any ipsilateral stroke from 26% to 9%, which represents a 17% absolute reduction in the risk of stroke. In addition, surgery reduced the rate of major ipsilateral or fatal stroke from 13% to 2.5%. Finally, the rate of all strokes or death was reduced from 32% to 15%.

Almost simultaneously with the NASCET report, a multicentered cooperative European[20] study reported almost identical results. In symptomatic patients with stenosis ranging from 70% to 99%, there was a sixfold reduction in the risk of stroke over a period of 3 years. The cumulative risk of all stroke was reduced from 21.9% to 12.3%. The combination of these reports has provided the clearest evidence regarding the benefit of carotid endarterectomy in symptomatic patients with higher grade (>70%) stenosis. The indication for surgery in other categories of symptomatic patients remains unanswered, and a study is in progress to determine whether symptomatic patients with low-grade lesions (30% to 69% stenosis) can benefit from surgery.

SURGICAL TECHNIQUE OF CAROTID ENDARTERECTOMY
Anesthesia

Carotid endarterectomy may be accomplished safely under either general or regional anesthesia. Most surgeons prefer general anesthesia because it allows for a quieter operating environment and better control of the patient's airway. Regional anesthesia for carotid endarterectomy offers the advantage of direct assessment of the patient's neurologic function during the course of the operation. This is particularly useful when the carotid artery is clamped because it allows an estimate of the need for a shunt. The cardiac depressant effects of general anesthesia are also avoided by the use of regional block, which is especially helpful in instances of patients with borderline cardiac function who are not candidates for coronary artery bypass grafting.

Positioning

The position of the patient for carotid artery surgery is important because it improves exposure of the distal internal carotid artery and greatly facilitates the conduct of the op-

eration. The patient should be supine, with the head comfortably turned away from the side of surgery. The neck should be mildly extended by placing a rolled sheet under the patient's shoulders. This has the effect of raising the patient's chin as if he/she were looking up and over his/her shoulder (Fig. 23-1).

The operating table position should provide a comfortable posture for the patient and the surgeon. One should first place the operating table in a slightly head-up position by raising the back of the table (some surgeons prefer configuring the table into a chairlike position). Next, the table should be raised to proper height for the surgeon and rotated slightly away from the side of surgery.

Carotid Exposure

The vertical incision is preferred. This incision should follow a line extending from the tip of the mastoid process to the jugular notch, directly in front of the anterior border of the sternocleidomastoid muscle (SCM). The length of the incision should be sufficient to comfortably perform the endarterectomy, and it should be centered directly over the carotid bifurcation. In most cases, this means that it will reach from the middle third of the neck to just below the level of the pinna of the ear (see Fig. 23-1).

After the skin is incised, attention is paid to obtaining hemostasis of the dermal vessels. The platysma muscle is incised and the SCM exposed. The SCM is mobilized to allow visualization of the jugular vein. The investing connective tissues are divided so that the length of the jugular vein is visible (see Fig. 23-1). The bifurcation of the facial vein is an important landmark because it is an indicator of the approximate level of the carotid bifurcation (Fig. 23-2).

The facial vein is divided. The jugular vein is retracted laterally as its investing loose areolar tissues are divided. Beneath the jugular vein lies the carotid artery, ensheathed by its adventitial tissues and nerves. At this point one should note the position of the vagus nerve as well as the cervical ansa. The vagus usually runs behind the carotid artery but may occasionally encircle the artery. In the latter position, the vagus nerve may be inadvertently damaged in the course of dissecting the carotid periadventitial tissues.

The carotid investment is opened longitudinally. Proximal and distal extension of the dissection leads to exposure of the internal and external carotid arteries. While dissection of the internal carotid is proceeding, the surgeon must carefully watch for the hypoglossal nerve, which crosses in front of the internal carotid in its course toward the base of the tongue. It should be identified and carefully preserved.

It is not uncommon at this point in the dissection to have a sudden fluctuation in the patient's blood pressure and bradycardia. This may be caused by dissection in the vicinity of the carotid body. Should the pulse rate fall, carotid body block should be performed by injecting xylocaine into the

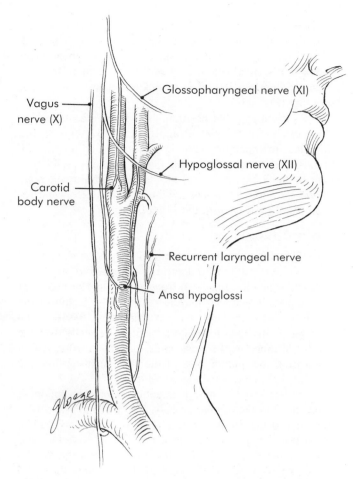

Vagus nerve (X)

Glossopharyngeal nerve (XI)

Hypoglossal nerve (XII)

Carotid body nerve

Recurrent laryngeal nerve

Ansa hypoglossi

FIG. 23-2   Anatomic study of the neck, illustrating position of major arteries and principal nerves.

tissue at the carotid bifurcation. This is almost always effective and lasts for the duration of the operation.

After the anterior surface of the carotid artery has been exposed, the surgeon first sees the distribution of disease in the artery. This is important because it will help determine whether further extension of the incision is necessary. Next, the lateral and posterior surfaces of the carotid artery are cleared to allow for safe control of the artery. The distal extent of the plaque in the internal carotid artery is then gently palpated to gain a clear appreciation of the extent of the plaque. The exposure should allow the arteriotomy to clearly pass beyond the end point of the plaque.

Should an extended exposure be required, several maneuvers will satisfy the majority of cases. First, the hypoglossal nerve should be gently mobilized by ligating and dividing the small vessels that tether the nerve. A second maneuver involves division of the posterior belly of the digastric muscle to expose an additional 5 or 10 mm of the distal internal carotid artery. In the course of dividing this muscle, one must exercise care to avoid injury to the hypoglossal and glossopharyngeal nerves, which are in proximity. Should further exposure be required, three maneuvers may be employed: removal of the styloid process, anterior distraction of the mandible, and a partial mastoidec-

tomy. In most instances where these maneuvers are required, this is recognized before surgery and plans are made accordingly.

Preparation for Endarterectomy

After exposure requirements have been satisfied, the next steps lead to opening of the artery. Preliminary control of the three principal vessels is established by passing surgical tapes around the external, internal, and common carotid arteries. Depending on whether a shunt is to be used and how it is to be secured, some surgeons place umbilical tape around the common and internal carotid arteries with the intention of using these with a Rumel-type tourniquet. The patient must be heparinized (5000 units IV) before the arteries are clamped so that deposition of intraluminal thrombus or thromboembolization is prevented.

Use of Carotid Shunt

The use of shunts in carotid surgery is an issue that has generated considerable debate.[4] Some surgeons use this technique routinely; others prefer to use shunts selectively. The routine use of shunts is recommended in instances where the patient has suffered an ipsilateral stroke because periinfarction tissues are thought to be more sensitive to reductions in cerebral flow (Fig. 23-3).

The principal advantage of shunting is that it allows for continued blood flow to the brain while the endarterectomy is underway. On the basis of EEG monitoring and observations of patients under regional anesthesia, about 10% to 15% of patients will not have adequate cross-filling to support cerebral function.[53,54] Without a shunt, these patients would suffer ischemic infarctions.

One places a shunt by first clamping all carotid branches. Next, the artery is opened. The clamps are removed from the internal carotid artery, and, as it backbleeds, the distal limb of the shunt is placed into the arterial lumen. One should take care to ensure that the arteriotomy extends beyond the atherosclerotic plaque so that the shunt is placed into normal arterial lumen. Blood is allowed to backbleed through the shunt to flush out both emboli and bubbles. The shunt is clamped with a hemostat, and then the proximal end is placed into the lumen of the common carotid artery and secured through clamping of the Rumel tourniquets. The common carotid clamp is removed. Finally, one slowly removes the hemostat from the shunt while observing for bubbles or emboli within the shunt tube. If any bubbles or emboli are seen, the shunt should be immediately occluded with the hemostat, the common carotid artery clamped, and the shunt flushed again before repositioning. If no debris is sighted in the shunt, the endarterectomy may proceed.

The use of shunts is not without risk. Although the incidence of shunt-related complications is low, they have been well documented.[4] Malfunction, with occlusion of the lumen and cessation of flow, eliminates the intended benefit of the shunt. Complications may arise in placement. As it is introduced into the arterial lumen, the shunt may dissect the intima from the arterial wall so that blood may not

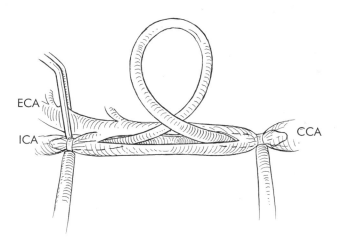

FIG. 23-3   Positioning of a Javid shunt in the carotid artery.

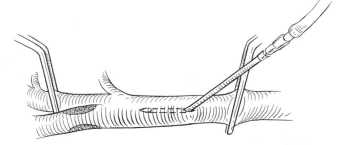

FIG. 23-4   Technique of back pressure measurement.

be able to flow through the shunt or a flap valve within the vessel lumen may be created, causing the lumen to occlude. Embolization is another risk. As the shunt is placed, it may excavate atherosclerotic material, and this in turn may be delivered through the shunt into the distal cerebral circulation, causing a stroke. A similar complication is the development of thrombus on the shunt and embolization of this thrombus into the distal cerebral arterial bed.

Monitoring Cerebral Perfusion and Function

Because of these risks, some surgeons prefer to use shunts only when necessary. This determination of need is made on the basis of one of three tests: communication with an awake patient, determination of the carotid artery back pressure, or continuous EEG monitoring.

Communicating with a patient who is under regional anesthesia may be accomplished by means of a prearranged signaling system. Some surgeons ask their patients to press a button or some such signaling device held in their hand. The patient is able to hear questions and respond with the signaling device. Should there be a failure to respond, the surgeon assumes that the patient has not tolerated carotid clamping and proceeds to place the shunt. Placement of a shunt in these instances leads to the prompt recovery of the patient's mentation, and the surgery may proceed.

One determines carotid artery back pressure, "stump pressure," by placing a needle connected to a pressure transducer into the carotid artery while the common and external carotid arteries are clamped (Fig. 23-4). In this manner, the pressure reading reflects the pressure within the internal carotid and thus the cerebral circulation of the ipsilateral hemisphere. If the pressure is above 25 mm Hg, shunting should not be necessary.[40,53,54] Some surgeons advocate using a slightly higher pressure as the cutoff point to provide a margin of safety. If the back pressure is below the cutoff point, shunting is necessary. In such instances, the internal carotid artery is clamped, opened, and the shunt is placed. The stump pressure is a poor predictor of adequacy of collateral flow and as such has been largely aban-

doned in favor of continuous monitoring of the EEG.

Intraoperative EEG monitoring provides a continuous assessment of the cortical function during the course of the operation. The gold standard of EEG monitoring is the use of a 12-lead EEG under the supervision of a trained neurologist or an experienced technician who has immediate access to a trained neurologist. Technical variations include the use of 2 to 16 channels and computer analysis of the recordings. These techniques allow a comparison of tracings from the ipsilateral and contralateral hemispheres. By noting the changes in the EEG at the time of carotid cross-clamping, one can determine whether the cross-circulation is adequate or if a shunt is needed.

A convenient variation of the EEG monitor is the brain map system. This consists of an expanded 32-lead EEG that provides both the EEG readout and a computer-generated, color-coded image of the two hemispheres. It facilitates the identification and interpretation of changes between the hemispheres.[2]

Endarterectomy

After all clamps are applied, the common carotid artery is pierced and the resulting opening is enlarged. The incision should be made on the side of the artery opposite the external carotid artery. This avoids injuring the flow divider at the bifurcation of the external and internal carotid arteries. The artery is opened along its length, exposing the carotid plaque. If a shunt is to be placed, it is placed at this point.

The endarterectomy itself involves removing plaque from within the artery. The level of dissection should be sufficiently deep to remove the bulk of the plaque yet not destroy the artery. A level that is too deep creates significant problems in establishing a smooth end point in the internal carotid artery. Another problem with a plane of dissection that is too deep is that the remnant artery may be very thin and thus more difficult to close. If the endarterectomy plane is too shallow, it will not effectively remove all of the plaque. Ideally, the endarterectomy plane is entered in the common carotid artery at a point where the plaque has greatest bulk. The dissection should follow the plane of the internal elastic lamina, between the diseased intima and the circular medial fibers.

After the plaque has been freed from the common and

internal carotid arteries, it may be necessary to follow it into the external carotid artery. Removal of the plaque from the external carotid artery is most readily accomplished by gently pulling the plaque off the arterial wall while using a dissector or a fine mosquito forceps to supplement this action. If the plaque extends beyond the point where the clamp occludes the external carotid artery, one may need to remove the clamp to accomplish the plaque removal.

Upon completion of the endarterectomy, the arterial lumen is thoroughly irrigated and loose tissue fragments are removed. The proximal and distal end points should be inspected and revised if necessary. Simultaneously one should decide whether a patch is required for closure of the artery.

Patch Closure vs. Primary Closure

Primary closure consists of suturing the arterial walls directly together. Patch angioplasty is a technique that uses a small portion of a patch material (vein, Dacron, or polytetrafluoroethylene [PTFE]) to allow for a slight expansion of the arterial diameter in the course of suturing the artery closed (Fig. 23-5).

The primary indications for the use of a carotid patch are presence of a small internal carotid artery or recurrent carotid stenosis. In the event of a small internal carotid artery, the use of a patch allows safe closure of the arteriotomy without compromising the depth and spacing of the sutures or reducing the arterial lumen. The use of a patch

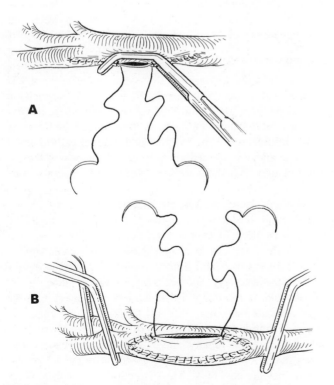

FIG. 23-5 Two methods of closing the arteriotomy: a primary closure **(A)** and a patch closure **(B)**.

is thought to provide the secondary benefit of reducing the incidence of recurrent carotid stenosis. In instances of recurrent carotid stenosis, the rationale behind the use of a patch is that it allows an angioplastic remodeling of the artery to provide a normal diameter. This is necessary because recurrent stenosis is frequently caused by myointimal hyperplasia and is not amenable to repeated endarterectomy.

The use of patches, however, has several drawbacks. If not tailored correctly, the patch may create a pseudoaneurysmal artery with a bulbous configuration. This is thought to create a risk of platelet and thrombus accumulation on the patch, causing embolization and a stroke. A second concern is that the expanded diameter of the artery will serve to increase the wall stress on the segment treated by endarterectomy. Much as an aneurysm's growth is compounded by its enlarging size, an overly large arterial lumen may promote disruption of the arterial closure.

Arterial Closure

Arterial closure is accomplished from the most distal point of the internal carotid artery with a continuous running suture carried toward and onto the common carotid artery. A second suture may be started at the common carotid end of the arteriotomy and carried toward the internal carotid artery. If a shunt is in place, one must remove this before the suture line is completed. When the shunt is removed, the arteries should be flushed by transiently removing the clamps in sequential order. All vessels are transiently occluded while the final sutures are placed. A technical alternative is to use a Satinsky-like clamp to exclude the open arteriotomy from the arterial lumen and allow partial resumption of perfusion. With this method, blood flow is restored while the suture line is completed.

Arterial flow should be reestablished expeditiously in the following order:

- The common carotid artery should be allowed to flow into the external carotid artery while the internal carotid artery is kept clamped so that any debris or thrombi in the common carotid artery will be initially carried into the external carotid arterial bed, thus preventing emboli entry to the brain.
- All clamps are removed and the common carotid artery is allowed to perfuse both the internal and external carotid arteries.

Assessment of Carotid Repair

After restoration of blood flow, the patient should be carefully monitored for significant physiologic alterations that may be indicators of a problem with cerebral circulation. The carotid repair should be assessed for patency and absence of flow impediments by sonographic techniques or preferably by intraoperative angiography.

Sonography may be employed using intraoperative duplex scanning, which allows visualization of the arterial lumen by means of a B-mode imaging device. Simultaneously, the pulse Doppler provides an estimate of the flow velocities. Alternatively, the hand-held Doppler may be used to insonate the artery. The characteristic flow patterns of the common, external, and internal carotid arteries should be clearly identified. An aberrance in the flow pattern requires further investigation either with angiography or by reopening of the artery.

Routine use of completion angiography is the best method for assessment of the adequacy of the carotid repair.[65] In this procedure, a plate of radiographic film is placed beneath the patient's head and exposed while contrast is injected directly into the common carotid artery. The image should reveal luminal defects. If any are found, the artery should be reopened and the defect removed. Although some surgeons routinely reverse the heparin effect by administering protamine sulfate, it does carry a slight risk of a protamine reaction. Routine administration of protamine is best avoided.

Operation Completion

The wound is closed after adequate hemostasis is achieved. If there is fear of fluid accumulation within the wound, the surgeon may elect to place a small drain. The wound is then closed by approximating the platysma muscle layer with interrupted absorbable sutures. The skin is then closed with appropriate sutures or clips.

Recovery From Anesthesia

The patient should be allowed to awaken from the anesthetic in the operating room, and sufficient time should be allowed so that the surgeon may determine whether any significant neurologic alterations are present. If a profound neurologic deficit is encountered, one should consider immediately reexploring the carotid artery for possible occlusion.

A second concern is the problem of blood pressure control. It is not uncommon for patients to display significant shifts in blood pressure as they are extubated. Should the arterial pressure rise sufficiently, it could produce an arterial suture line leak and a cervical hematoma. In a worst case, the suture line could become disrupted, producing a rapidly expanding neck hematoma. This is a serious problem and is best managed by prompt reintubation, reopening of the wound, and repair of the arterial defect.

Hypotension is another common problem during the immediate postoperative period because it may compromise brain oxygen delivery. This needs to be promptly corrected. Major alterations in blood pressure during the postoperative period are thought to be associated with significant neurologic morbidity.

COMPLICATIONS

There are three principal postoperative complications: stroke, cranial nerve injury, and myocardial infarction. Recurrent carotid stenosis, although not clearly a postoperative problem, does raise concerns about the durability of the carotid repair and is a possible cause of recurrent symptoms. Other significant problems that have been noted after the operation are rare but include carotid artery thrombosis, disruption of the arterial repair, and wound complications.

Stroke

Neurologic dysfunction after carotid endarterectomy may exhibit a range of presentations and severities comparable to those of the naturally occuring disease. Although some of these lesions may be subtle and escape detection, most are readily apparent. As with any event, one should perform an examination with the intention of discovering the extent of the deficit and to document progression or resolution.

The incidence of stroke after carotid endarterectomy is quite variable and reflects the experience of the individual center. The actual incidence may also vary as a reflection of the surgical indications. Patients who undergo carotid endarterectomy for asymptomatic stenosis have the lowest stroke rates, and those who undergo surgery because of a prior stroke have the highest stroke rates.[51] Patients whose indication was TIA have an intermediate stroke rate.

The cause of most postoperative strokes is thought to be intraoperative embolization, traditionally attributed to manipulation of the carotid artery before cross-clamping. Other possible sources include embolization of plaque, fibrin, or platelets from the shunt or the treated surfaces. Roughly one third of events may be related to hypoperfusion of the ipsilateral cortex during endarterectomy, failure to shunt, shunt malfunction, or a prolonged period of hypotension. Some postoperative strokes may be caused by technical problems such as intimal flaps; others may be the result of accumulation of fibrin or platelet thrombi on the endarterectomy surface. One should immediately investigate to determine whether the carotid repair remains patent and unobstructed. This may be accomplished by direct surgical examination, angiography, or duplex scanning. Should a correctable lesion be identified, immediate reoperation is necessary to prevent stroke progression.

Duplex Scan

In many hospitals, duplex scanning is the quickest, simplest, and safest means of screening for carotid artery occlusion or stenosis. In certain institutions, duplex scanning has attained a degree of reliability that is equivalent to angiography. If doubt persists about the result, angiography should be performed.

Angiography

If duplex scanning is not available or is less than satisfactory, angiography is essential for evaluating the postendarterectomy neurologic deficit. The timing of the angiogram in this setting is clear. If a deficit has been identified, it requires urgent evaluation. If the deficit is identified in the operating room, the patient should be observed for a few minutes. If there is not rapid improvement, the patient should be reintubated, the wound reopened, and an angiogram performed.

If the patient is out of the operating room when the deficit is identified, the question arises as to where and when to do an angiogram. This decision must be individualized to the institution and depends on whether the hospital facilities allow for efficient and safe transfer of patients between intensive care, radiology, and surgery suites. In certain circumstances, the most expedient location for performing the angiogram is in the operating room itself, so that the arterial repair may be performed immediately.

Reexploration

Reexploration for a postoperative neurologic deficit should be based on the results of duplex scanning or angiography. In the absence of these two examinations, exploration itself may be the best means of ascertaining the patency of the carotid artery. In the course of reexploration, the carotid artery should be approached in the same manner as the initial operation.

If a platelet or fibrin plug is identified, the artery is opened, the plug removed, the artery irrigated, and the lumen inspected for features that might have served as a nidus. If a flap of intima is discovered, the artery is reopened (the endarterectomy may require extension). The end point may require suture-fixation to prevent further dissection. In both instances, a patch closure should be considered because it may serve the beneficial purpose of improving hemodynamics of the repair and at the same time it may allow for added fixation of the intima to the arterial wall.

Cranial Nerve Lesions

The most common postoperative nerve deficits are the result of traction or compressions on cranial nerves. Rarely is injury secondary to inadvertent division of the nerves. The incidence of cranial nerve injuries has varied widely among reports. Principally this discrepancy reflects the diligence with which these lesions are sought. In retrospective reviews, the incidence of cranial nerve injury ranges from 7.9% to 17%.[16, 45] If routine laryngoscopy and detailed neurologic examination are employed, the incidence of postoperative cranial nerve injury may be as high as 16%.[36]

It is thought that the majority of these cranial nerve lesions are essentially asymptomatic and would not be detected but for the special efforts made to identify them.[21] In another study, however, Hertzer[36] estimated that about 60% of such lesions were symptomatic. The most commonly identified injury was to the vagus or the recurrent laryngeal nerve (about 7%). Hypoglossal injuries accounted for 5.8% of injuries. Superior laryngeal and marginal mandibular nerve injuries occurred in 1.8% of the cases. These authors noted that most of these cranial nerve deficits were

transient and resolved within 3 months. The incidence of cranial nerve injury in the event of reoperation for recurrent carotid stenosis is significantly higher (16%)[58] than during the primary procedures because scar tissue invests both nerves and the carotid artery, making the safe identification and preservation of the nerves more difficult. In this situation the hypoglossal nerve was the most commonly injured.[58]

Cardiac Morbidity

Myocardial infarction is the leading cause of death after carotid endarterectomy. In a series comparing the mortality of patients with angina with mortality of patients without cardiac symptoms, Ennix et al.[19] noted mortality rates of 18% and 1.5% respectively.

The concordance of coronary and carotid artery disease has been well documented by Hertzer et al. at the Cleveland Clinic.[35] In a series of 1000 vascular patients evaluated with preoperative coronary angiography, they studied a subset of 506 patients with cerebrovascular disease. Of this group, only 7% had normal coronary arteries, and 28% had mild-to-moderate coronary lesions. Well-compensated, advanced coronary disease was noted in 30% of these patients. Probably most significant was the size of the group of patients who were considered to be at increased risk of myocardial infarction. These patients represented 35% of the cerebrovascular population. Of these, 7% were inoperable, and 28% required preoperative coronary artery bypass grafting. These data emphasize the close correlation between carotid and cardiac disease. This further emphasizes the importance of thorough cardiac evaluation in this patient population.

▼

SUMMARY

In the time since the first carotid endarterectomy, the field of cerebrovascular disease has matured into one of considerable complexity. Seemingly self-evident questions are now recast in a confusion of fact and opinion. A new era of surgery for cerebrovascular disease has been launched by the systematic questioning of basic beliefs. The adoption of randomized studies as the standard by which we identify the best treatment should resolve long-standing questions regarding the proper indications, acceptable outcome, and adjuvant pharmacotherapy for these patients. The new era of treating cerebrovascular disease will be based on a clear understanding of pathogenesis and scientifically procured data supporting the role of surgical intervention.

References

1. Adelman SM: Economic impact. In McDowell FM, editor: Report on the National Survey of Stroke (American Heart Association monograph number 75), *Stroke* 12:1, 1981.
2. Ahn S, Jordan S, Newer M et al: Computerized electroencephalographic topographic brain mapping. A new and accurate monitor of cerebral circulation and function for patients having carotid endarterectomy, *J Vasc Surg* 8:247-254, 1988.
3. Baker JD, Rutheford RB, Bernstein EF et al: Suggested standards for reports dealing with cerebrovascular disease, *J Vasc Surg* 8:721-729, 1988.
4. Baker W, Littooy F, Hayes A et al: Carotid endarterectomy without a shunt: the control series, *J Vasc Surg* 1:50-56, 1984.
5. Barker W: The history of surgery for cerebrovascular disease. In Moore W, editor: *Surgery for cerebrovascular disease,* New York, 1987, Churchill-Livingstone, pp 11-15.
6. Beebe HG, Clagett GP, DeWeese JA et al: Assessing the risk associated with carotid endarterectomy. A statement for health professionals by an ad hoc committee on carotid surgery standards for the Stroke Council, American Heart Association, *Circulation* 79:472-473, 1989.
7. Black A, Helpern J, Kertesz A et al: Nuclear magnetic resonance imaging and spectroscopy in stroke. In WS Moore, editor: *Surgery for cerebrovascular disease,* New York, 1987, Churchill-Livingstone, pp 217-253.
8. Bousser MG, Eschwege E, Haugenau M et al: AICLA: controlled trial of aspirin and dipyridamole in the secondary prevention of atherothrombotic cerebral ischemia, *Stroke* 14:5-14, 1983.
9. Britton M, Helmers C, Samuelsson K: High-dose acetylsalicylic acid after cerebral infarction, *Stroke* 18:325-334, 1987.
10. Broderick J, Phillips S, Whisnant J et al: Incidence rates of stroke in the eighties: the end of the decline in stroke? *Stroke* 20:577-582, 1989.
11. Carrel A: Les anastomoses vasculaire et leur technique operatoire, *Un Med Can* 33:521-526, 1904.
12. Chambers BR, Norris JW. Outcome in patients with asymptomatic neck bruits, *N Engl J Med* 315:860-865, 1986.
13. Chiari M. Ueber das verhalten des tei lungs-winkels der carotis communis bei der endarteritis chronica deformans, *Verh Dtsch Ges Pathol* 9:326-336, 1905.
14. Collaborators NASCET: Beneficial effect of carotid endarterectomy in symptomatic patients with high-grade carotid stenosis, *N Engl J Med* 325:445-453, 1991.
15. De Bakey M, Creech O, Cooley D: Occlusive disease of the aorta and its treatment by resection and homograft replacement, *Ann Surg* 140:290, 1954.
16. De Weese JA, Rob CG, Satran R et al: Results of carotid endarterectomies for transient ischemic attacks five years later, *Ann Surg* 178:258-264, 1973.
17. Dixon S, Pais SO, Raviola C et al: Natural history of nonstenotic, asymptomatic ulcerative lesions of the carotid artery. A further analysis, *Arch Surg* 117:1493-1498, 1982.
18. Eastcott HHG, Pickering GW, Robb C: Reconstruction of internal carotid artery in a patient with intermittent attacks of hemiplegia, *Lancet* 2:994-996, 1954.
19. Ennix CL, Lawrie GM, Morris GC et al: Improved results of carotid endarterectomy in patients with symptomatic coronary disease: an analysis of 1546 consecutive carotid operations, *Stroke* 10:122-125, 1979.
20. European Carotid Surgery Trialists' Collaborative Group: MRC European Carotid Surgery Trial: interim results for symptomatic patients with severe (70-99%) or with mild (0-29%) carotid stenosis, *Lancet* 337:1235-1243, 1991.
21. Evans WE, Mendelowitz DS, Liapis C et al: Motor speech deficit following carotid endarterectomy, *Ann Surg* 196:461-464, 1982.
22. Fields WS, Lemak NA, Frankowski RF et al: Controlled trial of aspirin in cerebral ischemia, *Stroke* 8:301-315, 1977.
23. Fischer M: Occlusion of the internal carotid artery, *Arch Neurol* 65:346, 1951.
24. Fischer M: Occlusion of the carotid arteries, *Arch Neurol Pathol* 72:187, 1954.
25. Forsell C, Takolander R, Berquist D et al: Long term results after carotid artery surgery, *Eur J Vasc Surg* 2:93, 1988.
26. Gelabert HA, Moore WS: Carotid endarterectomy without angiography, *Surg Clin North Am* 70:213-223, 1990.
27. Genton E, Barnett HJM, Fields WS et al: Cerebral ischemia: the role of thrombosis and of antithrombotic therapy, *Stroke* 8:150-175, 1977.
28. Gordon T, Kannel WT: Predisposition to atherosclerosis, in the head, heart, and legs: the Framingham Study, *JAMA* 221:661-666, 1972.
29. Group A-CCS: Persantine aspirin trial in cerebral ischemia. Part II: endpoint results, *Stroke* 16:406-415, 1985.
30. Group ACAS: Study design for randomized prospective trial of carotid endarterectomy for asymptomatic atherosclerosis, *Stroke* 20:844-849, 1989.
31. Group CCS: A randomized trial of aspirin and sulfinpyrazone in threatened stroke, *N Engl J Med* 299:53-59, 1978.
32. Hachinski VC, Lassen NA, Marshall MJ: Multi infarct dementia. A cause of mental deterioration in the elderly, *Lancet* 2:207-210, 1974.
33. Hass WK, Easton JD, Adams HP et al: A randomized trial comparing ticlopidine hydrochloride with aspirin for the prevention of stroke in high-risk patients, *N Engl J Med* 321:501-507, 1989.
34. Healy DA, Clowes AW, Zierler RE et al. Immediate and long-term results of carotid endarterectomy, *Stroke* 20:1138-1142, 1989.
35. Hertzer NR, Beven EG, Young JR et al: Coronary artery disease in peripheral vascular surgery patients. A classification of 1000 coronary angiograms and the results of surgical management, *Ann Surg* 199:223-233, 1984.
36. Hertzer NR, Feldman BJ, Beven EG et al: A prospective study of the incidence of injury to the cranial nerves during carotid endarterectomy, *Surg Gynecol Obstet* 151:781-784, 1980.
37. Hillen B: The variability of the circle of Willis: univariate and bivariate analysis, *Acta Morphol Neerl-Scand* 24:87-101, 1986.
38. Hobson RW, Fields WS, Gage A et al: Role of carotid endarterectomy in

asymptomatic carotid stenosis, *Stroke* 17:534-539, 1986.

39. Hunt JR: The role of carotid arteries in the causation of vascular lesions of the brain with remarks on certain special features of the symptomatology, *Am J Med Sci* 147:704-713, 1914.

40. Hunter GC, Seifert G, Malone JM et al: The accuracy of carotid back-pressure as an index for shunt requirements—a reappraisal, *Stroke* 13:319-326, 1982.

41. Kase CS, Wolf PA, Chodosh EH et al: Prevalence of silent stroke in patients presenting with initial stroke: the Framingham study, *Stroke* 20:850-852, 1989.

42. Kroerner JM, Dorn PL, Shoor PM et al: Prognosis of asymptomatic ulcerated carotid lesions, *Arch Surg* 115:1387-1392, 1980.

43. Lassen NA: Cerebral blood flow and oxygen consumption in man, *Physiol Rev* 39:183-238, 1959.

44. Lusby RJ, Ferrel LD, Wylie E: The significance of intraplaque hemorrhage in the pathogenesis of carotid arteriosclerosis. In Bergan J, Yao J, editors: *Cerebrovascular insufficiency,* New York, 1983, Grune & Stratton, pp 41-51.

45. Matsumoto GH, Cossman D, Callow AD: Hazards and safeguards during carotid endarterectomy. Technical considerations, *Am J Surg* 133:458-462, 1977.

46. McCullough JL, Mentzer RM, Harman PK et al: Carotid endarterectomy after a completed stroke: reduction in long-term neurologic deterioration, *J Vasc Surg* 2:7-14, 1985.

47. Milikan CH: The pathogenesis of transient focal cerebral ischemia, *Circulation* 32:438-450, 1965.

48. Milikan CH, Siekert RG: Studies in cerebrovascular disease. II. The syndrome of intermittent insufficiency of the carotid arterial system, *Mayo Clin Proc* 30:186-191, 1955.

49. Moore DL, Miles RD, Gooley NA et al: Noninvasive assessment of stroke risk in asymptomatic and nonhemi-spheric patients with suspected carotid disease. Five-year follow-up of 294 unoperated and 81 operated patients, *Ann Surg* 202:491-504, 1985.

50. Moore W. Indications for carotid endarterectomy. In Moore W, editor: Surgery for cerebrovascular disease, New York, 1987, Churchill Livingstone, pp 439-442.

51. Moore W, Quinones-Baldrich W: Extracranial cerebrovascular disease—the carotid artery. In Moore W, editor: *Vascular surgery. A comprehensive review,* Philadelphia, 1991, WB Saunders, pp 434-472.

52. Moore WS, Boren C, Malone JM et al: Asymptomatic carotid stenosis: immediate and long-term results after prophylatic endarterectomy, *Am J Surg* 138:228-233, 1979.

53. Moore WS, Hall AD: Carotid artery back pressure. A test of cerebral tolerance to temporary carotid occlusion, *Arch Surg* 99:702-710, 1969.

54. Moore WS, Yee JM, Hall AD: Collateral cerebral blood pressure. An index of tolerance to temporary carotid occlusion, *Arch Surg* 106:520-523,1973.

55. Nunn DB: Carotid endarterectomy in patients with territorial transient ischemic attacks, *J Vasc Surg* 8:447-459, 1988.

56. O'Donnell TF, Erdoes L, Mackey WC et al: Correlation of B-mode ultrasound imaging and arteriography with pathologic findings at carotid endarterectomy, *Arch Surg* 120:443-449, 1985.

57. O'Holleran LW, Kennelly MM, McClurken M et al: Natural history of asymptomatic carotid plaque, *Am J Surg* 154:659-662, 1987.

58. Rapp J, Stoney RW: Recurrent carotid stenosis. In Bernhard VM, Towne JB, editors. *Complications in vascular surgery,* ed 2, Orlando, 1985, Grune & Stratton, pp 763-770.

59. Ricotta J, Ouriel K, Green R et al: Use of computerized tomography in selection of patients for elective and urgent carotid endarterectomy, *Ann Surg* 202:783-787, 1985.

60. Roederer GO, Langlois YE, Jager KA et al: The natural history of carotid arterial disease in asymptomatic patients with cervical bruits, *Stroke* 15:605-613, 1984.

61. Rosenthal D, Borrero E, Clark MD et al: Carotid endarterectomy after reversible ischemic neurologic deficit or stroke: is it of value? *J Vasc Surg* 8:527-534, 1988.

62. Ross R: The pathogenesis of atherosclerosis—an update, *N Engl J Med* 20:488-500, 1986.

63. Sacco RL, Wolf PA, Kannel WB et al: Survival and recurrence following stroke—the Framingham study, *Stroke* 61:1183-1187, 1982.

64. Savoy WS: Case of a young woman in whom both arteries of the upper expremities and of the left side of the neck were thought completely obliterated, *Med Chir Trans (London)* 39:205, 1956.

65. Scott S, Sethi G, Bridgman A: Perioperative stroke during carotid endarterectomy: the value of intraoperative angiography, *J Cardiovasc Surg* 23:363-364, 1982.

66. Sorensen PS, Pedersen H, Marquardsen J et al: Acetylsalicylic acid in the prevention of stroke in patients with reversible cerebral ischemic attacks. A Danish cooperative study, *Stroke* 14:15-22, 1983.

67. Whisnant JP, Matsumoto N, Elveback LR: The effect of anticoagulant therapy on the prognosis of patients with transient ischemic attacks in a community. Rochester, Minnesota, 1955 through 1969, *Mayo Clin Proc* 48:844-847, 1973.

68. Wolf P, O'Neil A, D'Agostino R et al: Declining mortality not declining incidence of stroke: the Framingham study, *Stroke* 20:158, 1989.

69. Wolf PA, D'Agostino RB, Belanger AJ et al: Probability of stroke: a risk profile from the Framingham study, *Stroke* 22:312-318, 1991.

24

Occlusive Cerebrovascular Disease: Anesthetic Considerations

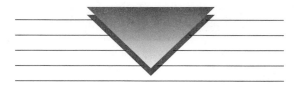

IAN A. HERRICK
ADRIAN W. GELB

PHYSIOLOGIC CONSIDERATIONS	ANESTHETIC MANAGEMENT	Complications
Carbon dioxide tension	Preanesthetic assessment	EXTRACRANIAL/INTRACRANIAL
Blood pressure	Monitoring	(EC/IC) BYPASS
Cerebral protection	Choice of anesthetic technique	SUMMARY
	Postoperative care	

Surgical procedures to prevent stroke have been the subject of considerable controversy for much of the past decade. For example, the surgical creation of an anastomosis between an extracranial and an intracranial artery (EC/IC bypass) enjoyed considerable popularity until 1985 when the EC/IC Bypass Study Group[6] failed to demonstrate that this procedure was superior to medical therapy for the prevention of stroke. In recent years EC/IC bypass has faded into relative obscurity as a treatment modality for occlusive cerebrovascular disease.

Carotid endarterectomy (CEA) has also experienced a marked increase in popularity since it was first described in the early 1950s. By 1984, despite the absence of properly designed prospective studies supporting the efficacy of the procedure,[24] CEA had become the third most common operation performed in the United States.[1] However, since 1985 the number of CEAs performed appears to have declined because of concerns related to the paucity of evidence supporting its efficacy, wide variation in the reported

rates of morbidity and mortality, particularly in the face of a rising frequency of CEA for inadequately validated indications, and evidence that the overall incidence of stroke is declining. Unlike the EC/IC bypass study, the results of two large, prospective, multicenter studies have recently demonstrated CEA to be superior to the best available medical therapy alone for the prevention of stroke in symptomatic patients with high-grade carotid stenosis (>70%).[25,87] These results will likely revive interest in CEA for this group of patients.

Several large, randomized, prospective studies are currently in progress designed to evaluate the efficacy and safety of CEA in the spectrum of symptomatic and asymptomatic patients with varying degrees of carotid stenosis .[54] In addition to the results previously mentioned, the European Carotid Surgery Trial (ECST) has reported no benefit from CEA in patients with symptomatic low-grade (<30%) stenoses.[25] Both the ECST and the North American Symptomatic Carotid Endarterectomy Trial (NASCET) continue to enroll patients with symptomatic moderate carotid stenosis (30% to 70%).[25,87] Data available from studies involving asymptomatic patients with carotid stenosis are currently inadequate to definitively evaluate the utility of CEA in this group of patients.[17,69,128] Two multicenter, prospective studies in asymptomatic patients are still in progress.[54]

The patient presenting for CEA is often elderly and has advanced cerebrovascular disease. Frequently, these patients also have significant coexisting disease involving other organ systems. Finally, the surgical procedure involves disruption of the major cerebral hemispheric blood supply for a significant period of time. Thus the anesthetic challenge presented by these patients is formidable. This chapter will review the anesthetic management of the patient undergoing surgery for occlusive cerebrovascular disease, with major emphasis on the principles of anesthesia for CEA.

PHYSIOLOGIC CONSIDERATIONS

The brain is highly active metabolically but is essentially devoid of oxygen and glucose reserves, making it dependent on the continual delivery of oxygen and glucose by the cerebral circulation. Cerebral blood flow (CBF) is provided by the internal carotid arteries (approximately 80%) and the vertebral arteries (approximately 20%). These major arteries anastomose at the base of the brain to form the circle of Willis, which provides the primary collateral vascular channel between the cerebral hemispheres. However, other collateral channels between the intracranial and extracranial circulations (e.g., through the orbit) may become well developed in patients with occlusive disease of the internal carotid artery.

Under normal circumstances, CBF is varied to match the brain's metabolic requirements; this autoregulation is a process common to many specialized vascular beds. The purpose of autoregulation is to maintain CBF at levels consistent with normal neuronal function. CBF is a function of cerebral perfusion pressure (CPP) and cerebral vascular resistance (CVR) according to the equation:

$$CBF = CPP \div CVR$$

CPP equals mean arterial blood pressure (MAP) minus intracranial pressure (ICP) or central venous pressure (CVP), whichever is greater. CVR is a function of blood viscosity and the diameter of the cerebral vessels. Clearly the physiology of cerebral autoregulation is far more complex than implied by these simple relationships. The anesthesiologist attempting to optimize CBF during CEA is hampered by the fact that the only factors readily amenable to intraoperative manipulation are arterial blood pressure and arterial carbon dioxide tension (Pa_{CO_2}), which affect CPP and CVR. In addition, current understanding of the physiology of CBF is incomplete, particularly with respect to the effect of various interventions on the distribution of CBF under pathologic conditions.

Carbon Dioxide Tension

CBF is exquisitely sensitive and directly related to Pa_{CO_2}. Within the range of Pa_{CO_2} from 20 to 80 mm Hg, CBF changes 1 to 2 ml/100 g/min for every 1 mm Hg change in Pa_{CO_2}. The most appropriate level of Pa_{CO_2} during CEA has been the subject of considerable debate. It was originally believed that deliberate *hypercapnia* was appropriate because it would produce an increase in global CBF.[133] This concept was criticized on the grounds that in areas of ischemia, the cerebral blood vessels are already maximally dilated. Thus increasing Pa_{CO_2} will cause vasodilation in normal brain and potentially "steal" blood from ischemic zones. Others have suggested that *hypocapnia* is beneficial because vasoconstriction in areas of normal (CO_2 responsive) brain will potentially divert blood flow toward ischemic regions, the "Robin Hood" syndrome.[31,65]

Despite these considerations, studies of regional cerebral blood flow (rCBF) during carotid cross-clamping under hypercapnic conditions have demonstrated that the rCBF response is not entirely predictable.[15] Although most of the patients studied experienced an increase in rCBF on the occluded side, 23% demonstrated a "steal" response to increased Pa_{CO_2}. Cerebral autoregulation was completely lost during carotid cross-clamping under hypercapnic conditions and partially lost during hypocapnia, illustrating the relatively greater importance of blood pressure control during CEA surgery. In addition, hypercapnia has been found to be associated with a higher incidence of cardiac dysrhythmias during CEA,[5] and the sympathomimetic response often associated with hypercarbia may adversely affect myocardial oxygen balance in patients with coronary artery disease.

Comparisons of CBF during carotid cross-clamping under conditions of normocapnia and hypocapnia have not demonstrated any advantage with hyperventilation.[14] Similarly, animal experiments have yielded conflicting results with regard to the neurologic effect of hypercapnia or hypocapnia during cerebral ischemia.[75,111,121] In view of these contradictions and the absence of clear clinical benefit associated with either hypercapnia or hypocapnia, the most prudent approach to the ventilatory management of patients undergoing CEA appears to be maintenance of normocapnia. This is accomplished by reference to preoperative arterial blood gas measurements or, if these are not available, by ventilating to a Pa_{CO_2} that produces a normal pH in a patient who does not have a coexisting metabolic acidosis. Based on this approach, one attempts to achieve a balance between the optimization of CBF and the avoidance of "cerebral steal."

Blood Pressure

Normally, CBF is maintained remarkably constant within the range of MAP from 50 to 150 mm Hg. Beyond this range the limit of vasomotor activity is exceeded and CBF becomes directly dependent on changes in CPP. In patients with preexisting chronic hypertension, both the upper and lower limits of autoregulation are shifted toward higher pressures.

A deliberate increase in intraoperative blood pressure has been advocated[133] as part of the care of these patients. This is based on the assumption that autoregulation will maintain normal CBF in areas of healthy brain while flow will be increased in areas of the brain that are hypoperfused because of vasomotor paralysis or atherosclerotic vascular narrowing. Patients with cerebrovascular disease have been shown to have a relative depression of the CBF response to changes in Pa_{CO_2}, suggesting that blood vessels distal to regions of atherosclerotic narrowing are operating near the limits of autoregulatory vasodilation.[135] Under these conditions, improvement in CBF is likely to largely depend on increases in CPP. Indeed, higher stump pressures and reversal of ischemic electroencephalographic (EEG) recordings after cross-clamping have been reported in some patients in response to induced hypertension.[31,46]

Deliberate hypertension is not devoid of risk, because it may produce cerebral hemorrhage and can increase edema formation in regions of the brain that have lost the ability to autoregulate. In addition, the patients most at risk of developing cerebral ischemia, those with the poorest collateral blood flow, have been shown to have the poorest response to induced hypertension.[14] In patients with ischemic heart disease, systemic vasoconstriction associated with drugs commonly used to induce hypertension may lead to an adverse myocardial oxygen balance. This premise is supported by evidence that the incidence of myocardial ischemia is significantly higher in patients who receive phenylephrine infusions[110] or metaraminol[99] to support blood pressure during CEA.

The advantages of induced hypertension during CEA remain controversial, but there is general agreement that hypotension is detrimental[19,59,114] because it can promote intravascular thrombosis and may render marginally adequate collaterals inadequate. Based on the available evidence, we do not recommend the routine intraoperative elevation of blood pressure above the patient's normal level but advocate careful maintenance of blood pressure within the normal preoperative range. Spontaneous increases in systolic blood pressure of up to 20% above normal at the time of cross-clamping are acceptable.

Cerebral Protection

In addition to efforts to delineate the appropriate management of physiologic parameters to optimize CBF, the possibility of anesthetic-induced cerebral protection has generated considerable interest. Patients undergoing CEA are at risk for the development of cerebral ischemia; thus the possibility of providing an additional margin of safety through the administration of anesthetic drugs that potentially protect the brain from ischemic injury is appealing.

Barbiturates have long been advocated as useful anesthetic agents for CEA.[133] Considerable experimental data, largely from animal models, document the ability of pro-

phylactic barbiturates to reduce the size of cerebral infarction under conditions of focal ischemia.[73,104] Although a variety of theories have been proposed to explain the efficacy of barbiturates to prevent or treat cerebral ischemia, a definitive explanation has not emerged.

Clinical evidence supporting the efficacy of barbiturate protection during periods of focal cerebral ischemia is largely anecdotal. In humans, there are no prospective, controlled trials. The administration of barbiturates during CEA, either continuously or as a prophylactic bolus before cross-clamping, has been advocated as a means of providing brain protection.[42,113] However, evidence available to date has not demonstrated a beneficial effect associated with this practice.[35,80] In addition, the potential adverse hemodynamic effect of thiopental may compromise maintenance of adequate CPP although evidence suggests that when thiopental is administered in repeated small boluses, EEG burst suppression can be achieved with minimal hemodynamic effect.[113,137] Barbiturate coma may also significantly delay emergence from anesthesia and thus compromise neurologic assessment in the immediate postoperative period.

Each of the volatile anesthetic agents, halothane, enflurane, and isoflurane, produce a decrease in the cerebral metabolic rate (CMR) and an increase in CBF. The ability of isoflurane to depress CMR to the point of EEG burst-suppression combined with the fact that the vasodilatory effects of this agent can be effectively attenuated with mild hyperventilation has made isoflurane the most popular volatile agent for neurosurgical anesthesia. Early speculation that isoflurane-induced suppression of CMR might be associated with a cerebral protective effect similar to the barbiturates has not, despite considerable research effort, been adequately substantiated.*

Similarly, in humans undergoing CEA, conflicting evidence surrounds the issue of a potential cerebroprotective effect associated with isoflurane. Based on retrospective comparisons,[72,74] the incidence of ischemic EEG changes has been reported to be lower in patients who receive isoflurane during CEA compared with enflurane and halothane, and critical CBF during CEA (the level of CBF at which EEG evidence of ischemia occurs in 50% of patients) has been reported to be lower (approximately 10 ml/100 g/min) in the presence of isoflurane compared with halothane and enflurane (approximately 20 and 15 ml/100 g/min respectively). This evidence suggests that isoflurane may provide some "protection" by decreasing the CBF threshold for EEG change and thereby possibly increasing the severity of insult that can be tolerated or increasing the period of time before the critical CBF threshold is breached. However, other investigators have failed to demonstrate an advantage associated with isoflurane compared with halothane in metabolic suppression during light levels of anesthesia for CEA.[136]

The benzodiazepines, etomidate, and propofol have also been shown to produce dose-related decreases in CMR and

---

*References 34, 62, 71, 86, 129, 130.

CBF. Although each of these drugs has properties that may make it useful during CEA,† available data based on animal models have yet to establish a definitive cerebroprotective advantage associated with the administration of these agents.[26,52,77,131] Despite these considerations, some anesthesiologists prefer to administer additional intravenous anesthetic drugs or increase the depth of anesthesia before carotid cross-clamping based on the assumption, as yet unsubstantiated, that some degree of cerebral protection may be realized.

ANESTHETIC MANAGEMENT
Preanesthetic Assessment

The preoperative visit should include an assessment of the patient's state of health based on history, pertinent physical examination, and chart review. The head and neck should be examined to identify potential problems associated with airway management and, by placing the head in the operative position, to elicit evidence of positional ischemia.

Special attention should be directed toward the assessment of other potentially diseased organ systems. Patients presenting for CEA commonly have significant coexisting coronary artery disease, arterial hypertension, peripheral vascular disease, chronic obstructive pulmonary disease, diabetes mellitus, and/or renal insufficiency. Examples of medical problems, based on the histories of patients eligible (randomized and nonrandomized) for enrollment in the North American Symptomatic Carotid Endarterectomy Trial (NASCET), are shown in Table 24-1.[88] These statistics were based on symptoms at the time of enrollment; thus asymptomatic patients with significant coexisting disease would not be detected and patients with evidence of valvular heart disease, significant dysrhythmias, and organ failure were excluded. Although these figures are consistent with data reported by other investigators,[25,99,100,125] it is likely that the overall incidence of coexisting disease in patients presenting for CEA is considerably higher than these recent statistics suggest.

Cardiac complications have been reported to be the primary source of mortality associated with CEA.[51,89,125] A variety of preoperative factors have been postulated to correlate with increased perioperative cardiac morbidity and mortality, the most ominous and well documented being the presence of congestive heart failure, recent myocardial infarction, and/or malignant ischemia-induced dysrhythmias, such as frequent or multifocal premature ventricular contractions.[68] A risk stratification scheme has been proposed for patients undergoing CEA that appears to correlate with the incidence of perioperative complications (Table 24-2).[83,116,118]

Cognizant of the high incidence of coronary artery disease in patients undergoing CEA, some investigators have advocated routine coronary angiography.[51] Based on the results of angiography, high-risk patients, such as those with severe coronary artery disease, left main coronary artery

†References 10, 26, 32, 40, 98, 126.

TABLE 24-1
Medical Characteristics of NASCET-Eligible Patients

Medical Condition (Based on History)	Symptomatic Patients (%) (n = 2256)
Angina	24
Previous myocardial infarction	20
Hypertension	60
Claudication	15
Smoking: current	37
previous	40
Diabetes	19

Modified from North American Symptomatic Carotid Endarterectomy Trial (NASCET) Steering Committee: *Stroke* 22:711-720, 1991.

TABLE 24-2
Preoperative Risk Stratification For Patients Undergoing CEA

Risk Group	Characteristics	Total Morbidity and Mortality (%)
1	Neurologically stable, no major medical or angiographic risk	1
2	Neurologically stable, significant angiographic risk, no major medical risk	2
3	Neurologically stable, major medical risk, ± major angiographic risk	7
4	Neurologically unstable, ± major medical or angiographic risk	10

Type of Risk	Risk Factors
Medical risk	Angina Myocardial infarction (<6 months) Congestive heart failure Severe hypertension (>180/110 mm Hg) Chronic obstructive pulmonary disease Age >70 years Severe obesity
Neurologic risk	Progressing deficit New deficit (<24 hours) Frequent daily TIAs Multiple cerebral infarcts
Angiographic risk	Contralateral internal carotid artery occlusion Internal carotid artery siphon stenosis Proximal or distal plaque extension High carotid bifurcation Presence of soft thrombus

Modified from Sundt TM Jr, Sandok BA, Whisnant JP: *Mayo Clinic Proc* 50:301-306, 1975.

stenosis, or poor left ventricular function, can be selected for CEA staged or combined with a coronary artery bypass graft (CABG) procedure.[23,51] The risk of cardiac and neurologic complications appears to be higher in patients undergoing CEA and CABG as a combined procedure although this may reflect a selection bias toward high-risk patients.[23,30,89] The sequence of staged procedures is controversial and, if staged procedures are used, the sequence is probably best decided on an individual basis.[23] We rarely perform coronary angiography as a prelude to CEA but, if performed, we operate on the "presenting" lesion first.

Several studies have documented a positive correlation between uncontrolled or inadequately controlled preoperative arterial hypertension (systolic blood pressure greater than 150 to 170 mm Hg) and an increased risk of postoperative hypertension and adverse neurologic outcome following CEA.[4,36,57,124] Aggressive perioperative control of blood pressure in patients undergoing CEA, including adequate preoperative treatment of hypertension, has been associated with improved outcome.[109]

If feasible, coexisting medical conditions should be made optimal before surgery. Other preoperative considerations include a review of the patient's blood pressure record to establish a baseline range of blood pressures to aid with intraoperative hemodynamic management. Cerebral angiograms should also be reviewed to identify patients at increased risk caused by the presence of significant contralateral carotid disease or poor collateral circulation.

The administration of a preoperative sedative-anxiolytic drug may be beneficial for some patients. A small preoperative dose of oral diazepam (5 to 10 mg) is usually effective. Lorazepam or midazolam are reasonable alternatives. Antihypertensive and antianginal medications should be continued preoperatively.

Monitoring
Cardiovascular

Careful management of the cardiovascular system is crucial to the outcome of surgery because adequate cerebral perfusion must be maintained without compromising myocardial performance. In view of the high incidence of coronary artery disease in these patients, the ECG is monitored with an emphasis on the detection of ischemia. Use of a modified chest lead such as CM5 may facilitate detection of ST segment changes. Alternatively, in higher risk patients a five-lead ECG with continuous monitoring of leads II and V_5 can be used. Oxygenation is monitored continuously with a pulse oximeter in all patients. Placement of an esophageal stethoscope after induction of general anesthesia facilitates monitoring of both ventilation and heart sounds when the chest is not readily accessible after the commencement of surgery. An intraarterial cannula, placed under local analgesia before the induction of anesthesia (regional or general), permits the continuous monitoring of systemic blood pressure throughout the perioperative period and facilitates the sampling of arterial blood for blood gas

analyses. Alternatively, in low-risk patients, a rapidly cycling (1-minute intervals) noninvasive blood pressure device can be used during induction and the arterial cannula placed before commencement of surgery. Central venous pressure, pulmonary capillary wedge pressure, cardiac output, and/or urine output are not routinely monitored, but such measurements are performed on patients who are especially high cardiac risks, such as those who have had a recent myocardial infarction or those with significantly compromised left ventricular function.

End-tidal CO_2 ($ETCO_2$), checked against an arterial blood gas sample obtained after induction of anesthesia, facilitates the continuous maintenance of $Paco_2$ within the patient's normal range. In patients who undergo CEA under regional anesthesia or local infiltration, the use of nasal prongs with a CO_2 sampling port enables the provision of supplemental oxygen and the detection of expired CO_2. The CO_2 measurements provided by these nasal prongs do not consistently correlate with $ETCO_2$, but detection of expired CO_2 provides a useful aid in monitoring respiratory rate and rhythm in situations where the patient's face and chest may be partially obscured by surgical drapes.

Neurologic

A variety of techniques have been advocated for monitoring neurologic function during CEA, including electroencephalography (EEG), somatosensory evoked potential responses (SSEP), CBF measurement, and carotid artery stump pressure.* The application of neurologic monitoring techniques to patients undergoing CEA is based on two premises: (1) that the monitor is able to accurately identify patients at risk for developing intraoperative neuronal injury and (2) that, with identification, interventions can be instituted (e.g., placement of an internal shunt) to prevent irreversible neuronal injury and thereby improve outcome. Despite intense interest, these premises remain controversial regarding both the reliability of currently available monitoring modalities, including EEG, to accurately predict outcome and the utility of interventions, particularly the use of internal shunts, to favorably influence neurologic outcome after CEA.†

The utility of a neurologic monitor is intimately linked to the efficacy of available interventions. A perfectly accurate monitor in the absence of an effective intervention does little to improve outcome other than to inform the operator that something has happened. In contrast, the availability of a 100% effective intervention that carries no inherent risk mitigates the need for monitoring because the intervention can be used in everyone, even those at no risk. Unfortunately, currently available interventions are neither fully effective nor totally safe, and current monitoring modalities are neither perfectly sensitive nor specific. Advocates of intraoperative monitoring believe, on the basis of ethical and/or medicolegal concerns, that the application of inter-

---

*References 18, 50, 64, 79, 81, 82, 117, 119, 134.
†References 12, 27-29, 41, 60, 83, 138.

ventions based on the results of available monitoring modalities is associated with a favorable, or at least an acceptable, risk-benefit ratio. Contrasting opinion, based on rationale similar to those applied to the introduction of new drugs, cautions that the accuracy of monitoring modalities and the efficacy and safety of associated interventions need to be clearly established before they are enshrined as a standard of practice.

In centers where neurologic monitoring is routinely employed during CEA, the EEG remains the most extensively used indicator[18,64] despite the absence of convincing prospective studies demonstrating the ability of EEG to accurately predict outcome. Extensive data is available documenting a correlation between EEG changes and alterations in CBF.[117,119,120] Unfortunately this correlation does not necessarily predict neurologic outcome, which is the clinically relevant end point. Overall, most available evidence[12,41,64,119,134] suggests that EEG is a reasonably sensitive predictor of adverse hemodynamic and embolic complications associated with CEA; most patients who experience an adverse neurologic outcome will be identified as being at high risk (low false-negative rate). However, EEG appears to lack specificity because many patients who are identified as being at high risk do not experience an adverse outcome (high false-positive rate). Data from the few prospective studies available in which intervention was not initiated in response to EEG changes, suggest either that EEG fails to consistently predict outcome[83,138] or that it identifies only a small group of patients at high risk for adverse neurologic outcome.[12,27] Further prospective studies are necessary to confirm and delineate the ability of EEG to accurately identify this group of high-risk patients and then to evaluate the efficacy and safety of applying therapeutic interventions such as internal shunting or the pharmacologic treatment of ischemia to this patient subgroup.

The measurement of SSEP responses during CEA remains inadequately validated as a means of identifying patients at risk for adverse neuologic outcome. Most of the available data suggest that SSEP monitoring yields results similar to EEG monitoring.[43,56,60,103]

The intraoperative measurement of CBF using intraarterial xenon has not been widely used primarily because of the high costs associated with the equipment. The utility of this technique as a predictor of outcome after CEA remains controversial. Advocates of this technique, reporting experience with large numbers of patients, have tended to intervene when abnormally low measurements of CBF are documented.[117,119,120] In contrast, the few studies, involving small numbers of patients, in which intervention was not performed in response to low CBF measurements have failed to demonstrate a consistent correlation with outcome.[29,83,138] Because cerebral ischemia represents an imbalance between blood flow and metabolism, failure of CBF measurements to accurately predict outcome likely reflects the fact that blood flow techniques measure only one component of this relationship and the duration of cerebral tolerance to low flow states during CEA is likely markedly influenced by metabolic factors. The increasing availability of transcranial Doppler sonography (TCD)[8,45,91,112,132] may stimulate a resurgence of interest in intraoperative blood flow measurement, particularly as an adjuvant to other monitoring modalities such as EEG, although the utility of this technique requires adequate validation.

Stump pressure represents the mean arterial pressure measured in the carotid stump (the internal carotid artery cephalad to the common carotid cross-clamp) after cross-clamping of the common and external carotid arteries. This measurement thus represents pressure transmitted retrograde along the ipsilateral carotid artery from the vertebral and contralateral carotid arteries and has been postulated to provide a useful indicator of the adequacy of collateral circulation.[50,81] However, stump pressure measurements have fallen into disrepute because of (1) failure of available data to validate this technique as a useful predictor of outcome, (2) controversy related to the level of stump pressure that reflects inadequate collateral circulation, and (3) evidence that the pressure measurements are influenced by the choice of anesthetic technique.[29,64,70,79,115] Although this technique is no longer considered adequate as the sole monitor of the adequacy of cerebral perfusion during CEA, some surgeons consider it a useful adjuvant technique when combined with another modality such as EEG.[27]

Although the use of an accurate neurologic monitor during CEA is both intuitively appealing and logical, obtaining convincing evidence that available monitoring techniques can accurately identify patients who will experience an adverse outcome is confounded by several factors. First, the incidence of neurologic complications associated with CEA is low; thus data from large numbers of patients are required to convincingly demonstrate the sensitivity and specificity of a particular technique. This requires many years of data collection at any single institution (a process complicated by changes in patient management over time) or the need for multicenter studies (which have not been performed in relation to monitoring during CEA). Second, the availability of some of these modalities is limited by the high cost of equipment or the need for experienced personnel with specific expertise to interpret results. Although some progress has been made developing less expensive technologies and simplifying monitoring and data analysis (e.g., TCD and processed EEG), these techniques also require confirmation of their accuracy as predictors of outcome. Finally, much of the available monitoring data is based on studies that use end points other than outcome or include causes of adverse outcome that are equivocally influenced by the use of intraoperative monitoring and/or intervention (e.g., stroke in the early postoperative period). Thus the fundamental question of whether these modalities can usefully predict outcome remains largely unanswered.

Choice of Anesthetic Technique

General anesthesia represents the most common anesthetic technique for CEA although regional anesthesia, using a cervical plexus block, is popular in some centers. Other techniques have been reported, such as local anesthetic infiltration[44] and cervical epidural,[55] but these have not become popular. The safety, in terms of morbidity and mortality, of CEA performed under regional block has been well documented,[20,21,33,66,97] and advocates of this technique cite as a major advantage the superior neurologic monitoring afforded by an awake patient.[20,66] Conversely, advocates of general anesthesia endorse airway security, the ability to control $Paco_2$ and ensure adequate oxygenation, and the avoidance of potential problems should a patient become agitated or emotionally distraught, or experience an intraoperative neurologic complication such as a seizure (circumstances in which advocates of a regional technique generally convert to general anesthesia).[28,29] There is no convincing evidence that overall outcome is better with one form of anesthesia than with the other.

Regional Anesthesia

Monitors should be applied and an arterial cannula placed under local anesthetic infiltration. The patient's head can be placed on a padded ring and turned to the side opposite to the surgical site, and the neck can be moderately extended, ensuring that no evidence of positional ischemia develops. Techniques for performing superficial and deep cervical plexus blocks are well described.[84]

An attentive, reassuring anesthesiologist, gentle surgical technique, supplemental local anesthetic infiltration by the surgeon as required, and carefully titrated sedation using small, repeated, intravenous doses of fentanyl (10 to 20 μg) and/or midazolam (0.5 to 2 mg) should ensure a comfortable and cooperative patient during the operation. Even with a successful deep cervical plexus block, supplemental local anesthetic applied to the carotid sheath is often needed to alleviate discomfort associated with manipulation of the artery. Each patient should receive supplemental oxygen via nasal cannula, oxygen saturation should be monitored, and adequate tenting of the surgical drapes should be provided to allow observation of the patient. Provisions should be immediately available to convert to a general anesthetic if intraoperative conditions warrant.

Potential complications associated with deep cervical plexus blocks include inadvertent injection of local anesthetic into the subarachnoid space, either directly or via puncture of a dural sheath, resulting in total spinal anesthesia. Inadvertent intraarterial injection, typically involving the vertebral artery, which courses in close proximity to the site of the block as it passes through the foramena transversaria of the transverse processes, results in rapid local anesthetic toxicity. Puncture of the vertebral artery can also produce an embolic TIA or stroke in patients with atherosclerotic involvement of the vertebral artery. Deep cervical plexus blockade can also be associated with phrenic nerve block, brachial plexus block, recurrent laryngeal nerve block, and stellate ganglion block.

General Anesthesia

The key consideration during induction of anesthesia is the provision of adequate anesthesia to ensure stable hemodynamic conditions during intubation and positioning while avoiding hypotension that can accompany the relatively unstimulating period of surgical preparation and draping. Thiopental is the most commonly used induction agent. The potential adverse hemodynamic effect of thiopental can be effectively attenuated by administering an opioid such as fentanyl (2 to 5 μg/kg), sufentanil (0.5 to 1.0 μg/kg) or alfentanil (10 to 25 μg/kg) intravenously before thiopental. Thiopental is administered by slow intravenous injection (typically 2 to 5 mg/kg), with the dose titrated to the patient's response. Other induction regimens using midazolam, propofol, or etomidate are reasonable alternatives based on individual preferences.

Tracheal intubation is facilitated with a nondepolarizing neuromuscular blocking drug. Atracurium and vecuronium are popular choices because of the absence of cardiovascular side effects. Pancuronium is also commonly used. Although potentially associated with tachycardia and hypertension, these responses appear to be readily attenuated with induction doses of opioids and in our experience are rarely of clinical significance. Succinylcholine also is a reasonable alternative and may be advantageous in some clinical circumstances; however, use of this agent is contraindicated in patients who have experienced a recent paretic cerebral infarct.

The hemodynamic response to tracheal intubation can be attenuated by administration of intravenous lidocaine (1 to 1.5 mg/kg), additional opioid, or supplemental thiopental (1 to 2 mg/kg), or the addition of a volatile agent such as isoflurane before intubation. An armored endotracheal tube, although not essential, may be of benefit because its flexibility facilitates positioning of the tube without impinging on the surgical field.

Anesthesia is maintained with nitrous oxide (50%), oxygen, isoflurane, and supplemental opioid. We prefer to establish a relatively light level of general anesthesia, with neuromuscular blockade maintained throughout the procedure, and blood pressure maintained at preoperative levels. As discussed previously, the patient is ventilated mechanically to maintain $ETco_2$ (checked against an arterial blood gas sample) at normocapnic levels.

Intravenous fluids should be administered to meet maintenance requirements. Blood loss during CEA is typically minimal although the potential for hemorrhage exists. Some evidence suggests that cerebral ischemia may be aggravated in the presence of hyperglycemia[61,63,105] although the evidence is conflicting in some animal models of focal ischemia.[38,58] Because there is concern over administering glucose, and there is no compelling reason, in most patients, for it,[105] it is our practice to avoid dextrose-containing solutions.

Some controversy has surrounded the use of isoflurane in patients with coronary artery disease (which likely includes a substantial proportion of patients undergoing CEA) because of reports that this agent is potentially capable of inducing myocardial ischemia via coronary steal in a minority of patients with a specific pattern of coronary arterial occlusions.[95] The use of isoflurane does not appear to pose a significant problem in patients undergoing CEA, probably because inspired concentrations are kept relatively low (typically 1.0 % by volume or less), and coronary perfusion pressure is carefully maintained along with cerebral perfusion pressure. This impression is supported by retrospective data, which suggest that, in patients undergoing CEA, the incidence of myocardial infarction is not significantly different regardless of the volatile anesthetic agent used.[22]

The use of nitrous oxide in neurosurgical patients has recently come under scrutiny after reports that it may cause an increase in CBF and CMR and that it may reduce the cerebroprotective effects associated with thiopental in animal models of cerebral ischemia.* These issues remain controversial because studies have yielded conflicting results.[2,76,78,107] For patients undergoing anesthesia for CEA, there is no evidence that the use of nitrous oxide adversely affects outcome, nor is data available demonstrating that these potential neurophysiologic effects are necessarily detrimental under the clinical conditions associated with CEA (e.g., concomitant use of thiopental, narcotics, and/or isoflurane). Thus concerns related to its use in this procedure remain conjectural. Evidence derived from the North American Symptomatic Carotid Endarterectomy Trial (NASCET) anesthesia data indicates that the use of nitrous oxide as a component of general anesthesia for CEA remains very popular (78% in United States, 92% in Canada) among neurosurgical centers across North America.[21a]

During the operation, episodes of hypertension are treated initially by increasing the depth of anesthesia, usually achieved by increasing the concentration of inhalational anesthetic. When this is inadequate, intravenous antihypertensive drugs such as esmolol, propranolol, labetalol, sodium nitroprusside, and nitroglycerine are used. Hypotension is treated by reducing the concentration of inhalational anesthetic, by infusing intravenous fluid, or, if necessary, by administering a vasopressor such as phenylephrine, prepared before induction, in boluses of 0.5 to 1.0 μg/kg to maintain blood pressure. Ephedrine (5 to 10 mg IV) may represent a reasonable alternative to phenylephrine, particularly for hypotension associated with bradycardia. However, the short duration of action associated with phenylephrine is often advantageous in light of the rapid

---

*References 2, 3, 47-49, 76, 78, 93, 107.

changes in hemodynamic parameters commonly associated with CEA.

Hypotension and/or bradycardia often occur with manipulation of the carotid artery during surgical dissections and at the time of carotid cross-clamping because of parasympathetic reflexes associated with stimulation of the carotid sinus. This can be attenuated by blockade of the carotid sinus nerve with local anesthetic injected by the surgeon. Hypertension may also occur, probably reflects a response to visceral pain associated with traction or distortion of the carotid artery or surrounding structures, and typically responds to injection of local anesthetic into the carotid sheath or deepening of the level of anesthesia.

Before carotid cross-clamping, heparin (75 to 100 units/kg) is administered intravenously. Application of the carotid clamps is often associated with an increase in blood pressure. Mild increases in arterial pressure are acceptable (up to approximately 20% above preoperative levels), but excessive increases should be controlled.

Heparin is typically not reversed after closure of the artery. In the rare event that the surgeon is unsatisfied with hemostasis at the time of wound closure, a small dose of protamine (0.5 mg/kg) intravenously may occasionally be given. Depth of anesthesia is adjusted so that at the end of surgery the patient can be promptly extubated to avoid prolonged coughing and straining. A small dose of opioid (e.g., fentanyl 0.5 to 1.0 μg/kg or alfentanil 5 to 10 μg/kg) or lidocaine (1 to 1.5 mg/kg) given before emergence often attenuates coughing but temporarily deepens the level of anesthesia. Hemodynamic responses associated with emergence and extubation should be anticipated and treated. Several drugs have been used effectively to control perioperative hypertension, including propranolol, hydralazine, trimethaphan, nitroglycerine, and sodium nitroprusside. Newer drugs such as esmolol and labetolol are currently popular, and considerable evidence supports their effectiveness for control of hemodynamics during emergence and in the early postoperative period.[37,39,85,90]

Postoperative Care

The intraarterial cannula is maintained during the initial postoperative period to permit continuous blood pressure monitoring and blood sampling for arterial blood gas analyses. All patients receive supplemental oxygen, and the adequacy of oxygenation is monitored by pulse oximetry. Bilateral carotid endarterectomy is associated with changes in the chemical control of ventilation.[127] Resting $Paco_2$ rises by about 5 mm Hg, and the ventilatory and cardiovascular responses to hypoxemia are abolished. Provision of supplemental oxygen and close monitoring of ventilatory status thus is particularly important in these patients.

Postoperative hemodynamic instability is common (incidence >40%)[4,13] after CEA and is postulated to be related to carotid baroreceptor dysfunction. CEA performed using a technique that spares the carotid sinus nerve is associated with a higher incidence of postoperative hypotension, which is postulated to be due to increased exposure of the carotid sinus to the higher arterial pressure occurring after removal of the atheromatous plaque.[16,94,122] This hypotension has also been shown to be associated with a marked decrease in systemic vascular resistance.[96] The hypotension can be prevented or treated with local anesthetic blockade of the carotid sinus nerve.[16,94] Hypotension is also responsive to intravenous fluid administration or, if necessary, the administration of vasopressor drugs, such as phenylephrine.[96,122]

Hypertension after CEA is less well understood and has been reported to be more common in patients with preoperative hypertension, particularly poorly controlled or uncontrolled hypertension,[4,13,124] and in patients who undergo CEA in which the carotid sinus is denervated. Hypertension after CEA in which the sinus nerve is preserved has been postulated to be due to temporary dysfunction of the baroreceptors or nerve caused by intraoperative trauma.[13] Mild increases in postoperative blood pressure are acceptable (up to approximately 20% above preoperative normotensive levels), but marked increases are treated with antihypertensive drugs.

Other causes of hemodynamic instability after CEA include myocardial ischemia/infarction, dysrhythmias such as atrial fibrillation, hypoxia, hypercarbia, pneumothorax, pain, confusion, and distention of the urinary bladder.

Complications

Major postoperative complications after CEA include stroke, myocardial infarction, and hyperperfusion syndrome. The majority of strokes complicating CEA have been reported to occur in the postoperative period and appear to be primarily related to surgical factors involving carotid thrombosis (occlusion) or emboli originating at the surgical site rather than hemodynamic factors.[59,106,108,114,123] Researchers have suggested that, beyond the meticulous application of currently recommended anesthetic techniques, the anesthesiologist has little ability to further affect the outcome of stroke during carotid endarterectomy.[106]

The incidence of stroke complicating CEA varies among institutions,[7] but, based on available data, the Ad Hoc Committee on Carotid Surgery Standards of the Stroke Council of the American Heart Association[9] has suggested that the 30-day mortality from all causes for CEA should not exceed 2%, and combined morbidity and mortality caused by stroke associated with CEA should not exceed 3% for asymptomatic patients. This limit is increased to 10% for patients with recurrent disease in the same artery after previous endarterectomy (Table 24-3). Numerous reports confirm that these limits are achievable.*

Given the high incidence of concomitant coronary artery

---

*References 20, 27, 100, 118, 119, 125.

TABLE 24-3

Recommended Risk Limits for Adverse Neurologic Outcome following CEA

Indication for CEA	Maximum Acceptable Risk for Neurologic Morbidity and Mortality
Asymptomatic	3%
Transient ischemic attack	5%
Ischemic stroke	7%
Recurrent disease in the same artery after CEA	10%
Total 30-day mortality (all cases, all causes)	2%

Adapted from Beebe HG, Clagett GP, DeWeese JA et al: *Stroke* 20:314-315, 1989.

disease in patients undergoing CEA, it is not surprising that myocardial infarction represents the principal cause of mortality after CEA.[30,123,125] In general, the reported incidence of fatal postoperative myocardial infarction is 0.5% to 4%,[30,51,89,97,100] and the proportion of total perioperative mortality (within 30 days of operation) attributed to cardiac causes is estimated to be at least 40%,[51,89,100] with some studies attributing 80% to 100% of perioperative mortality to cardiac causes.[89,125] In addition, myocardial infarction has been reported to be responsible for slightly more than one third of the mortality among CEA patients within 5 and 11 years.[51]

An increase in CBF has been reported to occur frequently after CEA.[101,102] Typically the magnitude of this increase is relatively small (<35%)[101]; however, in severe cases, increases in CBF can exceed 200% of preoperative levels and can be associated with increased morbidity and mortality.[119,120] Clinical features of this hyperperfusion syndrome include headache (usually unilateral), face and eye pain, cerebral edema, seizures, and intracerebral hemorrhage.[67,101] Patients at greatest risk include those with reduced preoperative hemispheric CBF caused by bilateral high-grade carotid stenoses, unilateral high-grade carotid stenosis with poor collateral cross-flow, or unilateral carotid occlusion with contralateral high-grade stenosis.[67] The syndrome is postulated to develop after restoration of perfusion to an area of the brain that has lost its ability to autoregulate because of a chronic state of decreased CBF and thus chronic maximal vasodilation. Restoration of blood flow after CEA thus leads to a state of hyperperfusion until autoregulation is reestablished, which occurs over a period of days.[11,101] Histologically, the hyperperfusion syndrome has features very similar to hypertensive encephalopathy.[11] Patients at risk for this syndrome should be monitored closely in the perioperative period, and blood pressure should be meticulously controlled. In treating hypertension in these patients, one should probably avoid drugs that cause cerebral vasodilation, such as hydralazine.[101,102]

Therapies aimed at blocking pathophysiologic mechanisms associated with this syndrome remain under investigation.[67]

Other complications associated with CEA include hematoma formation and cranial nerve palsies. Hematoma formation may lead to airway compromise caused by mass effect and may cause cranial nerve dysfunction. Cranial nerve palsies are typically temporary and may manifest as vocal cord paralysis and/or altered gag reflex.[28,108]

EXTRACRANIAL/INTRACRANIAL (EC/IC) BYPASS

The creation of a microvascular anastomosis between the superficial temporal and middle cerebral arteries was initially described as a means of preventing stroke. Since its first use, indications for EC/IC bypass have been expanded to include revascularization of the posterior circulation and the creation of surgical collaterals as a component of the treatment of certain complex aneurysms.[92] In 1986, the results of the EC/IC Bypass Study failed to demonstrate a superior outcome in the prevention of stroke among patients randomized to EC/IC bypass compared with medical treatment alone.[6] Although these results were controversial, this study represents the only large, randomized, prospective study available.[7,53] As a result, the popularity of this procedure has declined markedly from an estimated 2000 operations per year in 1985 (in the United States) to less than 500 procedures annually.[7] EC/IC bypass continues to be used occasionally for patients with cerebral ischemia caused by occlusive cerebrovascular disease and somewhat more frequently for the creation of collaterals as a prelude to the Hunterian ligation of an artery supplying an aneurysm, where the aneurysm itself is not amenable to surgical clip obliteration.

Hemispheric blood flow is not interrupted during EC/IC bypass. However, an intracranial artery is temporarily occluded, so anesthesia considerations are, in essence, the same as those for CEA. Anesthetic management is modified in only a few ways. The intracranial anastomosis is performed through a small burr hole. Intravenous volume expansion and maintenance of normal or mildly increased Paco$_2$ facilitate surgery by ensuring that the surface of the brain remains in close proximity to the site of surgical exposure and that the vessels being anastomosed remain dilated and therefore easier to manipulate. In a patient with a recent ischemic episode, the brain may be edematous. If this becomes obtrusive, mannitol rather than hyperventilation can be used to reduce brain bulk.

The operation is performed under magnification that amplifies the normal cardiac and respiratory pulsations, which may be distracting for the surgeon. Respiratory pulsations are due to transmission of changes in intrathoracic pressure through the veins of the neck and head and can be attenuated by head-up positioning, a reduction in tidal volume, and/or a reduction in the inspiratory flow rate. Cardiac pulsations can be minimized by head-up positioning and by ensuring that head position does not obstruct venous outflow. When these measures are inadequate, heart rate, blood pressure, and/or cardiac contractility can be reduced by the administration of intravenous esmolol or propranolol or by the introduction of an inhalational anesthetic agent, such as halothane, that depresses myocardial contractility.

After the completion of surgery, emergence and postoperative management are essentially the same as described for CEA. Coughing is minimized to avoid straining the fresh anastomosis, and, because vessel patency and anastomotic integrity depend in part on blood pressure, hypertension and hypotension are avoided.

▼ SUMMARY

The past decade has witnessed the results of a major commitment by the neuroscience community to answer longstanding questions about the safety and efficacy of surgical procedures to prevent stroke. As a result, EC/IC bypass has declined markedly in popularity although it will likely continue to be employed in the management of some patients with complex cerebral aneurysms. In contrast, initial data related to CEA suggests that this procedure will continue to play an important role in the treatment of patients with symptomatic high-grade carotid stenosis. Additional results from several ongoing multicenter studies are anticipated to further delineate the role of CEA for the prevention of stroke. One hopes the future will include a similar research commitment directed at other areas of controversy, such as the application of neurologic monitors, modalities for the prevention and/or treatment of cerebral ischemia, and the development and evaluation of effective interventions to reduce the high cardiac morbidity and mortality that continues to plague this patient population.

This chapter has focused on the anesthetic management of patients undergoing surgery for cerebrovascular occlusive disease, with an emphasis on CEA. Current recommendations related to the choice of anesthetic technique, drugs, monitoring, and hemodynamic and ventilatory management have been reviewed. The neurophysiologic concepts that form the basis for current management have also been discussed, areas of consensus have been defined, and areas of controversy have been highlighted. The management of patients undergoing EC/IC bypass has also been reviewed, emphasizing differences in surgical objectives that mandate a difference in anesthetic technique compared with CEA.

References

1. Alpert JN: Extracranial carotid artery—current concepts of diagnosis and management, *Tex Heart Inst J* 18:93-97, 1991.
2. Algotsson L, Messeter K, Rosen I et al: Effects of nitrous oxide on cerebral haemodynamics and metabolism during isoflurane anaesthesia in man, *Acta Anaesthesiol Scand* 36:46-52, 1992.
3. Archer DP, Labrecque P, Tyler JL et al: Cerebral blood volume is increased in dogs during administration of nitrous oxide or isoflurane, *Anesthesiology* 67:642-648, 1987.
4. Asiddao CB, Donegan JH, Whitesell RC et al: Factors associated with perioperative complications during carotid endarterectomy, *Anesth Analg* 61:631-637,1982.
5. Baker WH, Rodman JA, Barnes RW et al: An evaluation of hypocarbia and hypercarbia during carotid endarterectomy, *Stroke* 7:451-454, 1976.
6. Barnett HJ, Peerless SJ, Fox AJ et al: Failure of extracranial-intracranial arterial bypass to reduce the risk of ischemic stroke: results of an international randomized trial. Report of the EC/IC Bypass Study Group, *N Engl J Med* 313:1191-1200, 1985.
7. Barnett HJM: Evaluating methods for prevention in stroke, *Ann RCPSC* 24:33-42, 1991.
8. Baughman VL: The transcranial Doppler, *J Neurosurg Anesth* 3:71-72, 1991.
9. Beebe HG, Clagett GP, DeWeese JA et al: Assessing risk associated with carotid endarterectomy, *Stroke* 20:314-315, 1989.
10. Bendriss P, Stoiber HP, Bendriss-Brusset AC et al: Propofol effects on EEG and relationship with plasma concentration during neurosurgery (abstract), *Anesthesiology* 73:A203, 1990.
11. Bernstein M, Fleming JFR, Deck JHN: Cerebral hyperperfusion after carotid endarterectomy: a cause of cerebral hemorrhage, *Neurosurgery* 15:50-56, 1984.
12. Blume WT, Ferguson GG, McNeill K: Significance of EEG changes at carotid endarterectomy, *Stroke* 17:891-897, 1986.
13. Bove EL, Fry WJ, Gross WS et al: Hypotension and hypertension as consequences of baroreceptor dysfunction following carotid endarterectomy, *Surgery* 85:633-637, 1979.
14. Boysen G, Engell HC, Henriksen H: The effect of induced hypertension on internal carotid artery pressure and regional cerebral blood flow during temporary carotid clamping for endarterectomy, *Neurology* 22:1133-1144, 1972.
15. Boysen G, Ladegaard-Pedersen HJ, Henriksen H et al: The effects of Paco2 on regional cerebral blood flow and internal carotid arterial pressure during carotid clamping, *Anesthesiology* 35:286-300, 1971.
16. Cafferata HT, Merchant RF, DePalma RG. Avoidance of postcarotid endarterectomy hypertension, *Ann Surg* 196:465-472, 1982.
17. CASANOVA Study Group: Carotid surgery versus medical therapy in asymptomatic carotid stenosis, *Stroke* 22:1229-1235, 1991.
18. Chemtob G, Kearse LA: The use of electroencephalography in carotid endarterectomy, *Int Anesth Clin* 28:143-146, 1990.
19. Cole DJ, Drummond JC, Shapiro HM et al: Influence of hypotension and hypotensive technique on the area of profound reduction in cerebral blood flow during focal cerebral ischaemia in the rat, *Br J Anaesth* 64:498-502, 1990.
20. Corson JD, Chang BB, Shah DM et al: The influence of anesthetic choice on carotid endarterectomy outcome, *Arch Surg* 122:807-812, 1987.
21. Corson JD, Chang BB, Leopold PW et al: Perioperative hypertension in patients undergoing carotid endarterectomy: shorter duration under regional block anesthesia, *Circulation* 74(suppl 1):I 1-4, 1986.
21a. Craen RA, Gelb AW, Eliasziw M et al: Anesthesia for carotid endarterectomy. The North American practice at 50 centres. NASCET Study Results, *Anesth Analg* 76:S61, 1993.
22. Cucchiara RF, Sundt TM Jr, Michenfelder JD: Myocardial infarction in carotid endarterectomy patients anesthetized with halothane, enflurane, or isoflurane, *Anesthesiology* 69:783-784, 1988.
23. Dunn EJ: Concomitant cerebral and myocardial revascularization, *Surg Clin North Am* 66:385-395, 1986.
24. Dyken ML: Carotid endarterectomy studies: a glimmering of science, *Stroke* 17:355-357, 1986.
25. European Carotid Surgery Trialists' Collaborative Group: MRC European carotid surgery trial: interim results for symptomatic patients with severe (70-99%) or with mild (0-29%) carotid stenosis, *Lancet* 337:1235-1243, 1991.
26. Farling PA: Intravenous anaesthetics, *Curr Opin Anaesthesiol* 3:689-693, 1990.
27. Ferguson GG: Carotid endarterectomy—to shunt or not to shunt? *Arch Neurol* 43:615-617, 1986.
28. Ferguson GG: Extracranial carotid artery surgery, *Clin Neurosurg* 29:543-574, 1982.
29. Ferguson GG, Gamache FW Jr: Cerebral protection during carotid endarterectomy: intraoperative monitoring, anesthetic techniques, and temporary shunts. In Smith RR, editor: *Stroke and the extracranial vessels,* New York, 1984, Raven Press, pp 187-201.
30. Fode NC, Sundt TM Jr, Robertson JT et al: Multicenter retrospective review of results and complications of carotid endarterectomy in 1981, *Stroke* 17:370-376, 1986.
31. Fourcade HE, Larson P, Ehrenfeld WK et al: The effects of CO2 and systemic hypertension on cerebral perfusion pressure during carotid endarterectomy, *Anesthesiology* 33:383-390, 1970.
32. Fox A, Gelb AW, Manninen PH et al: Human CBF-CO2 responsiveness is maintained during propofol-nitrous oxide anesthesia (abstract), *Anesthesiology* 75:A169, 1991.
33. Gabelman CG, Gann DS, Ashworth CJ et al: One hundred consecutive carotid reconstructions: local versus general anesthesia, *Am J Surg* 145:477-482, 1983.
34. Gelb AW, Boisvert D, Tang C et al: Primate brain tolerance to temporary focal cerebral ischemia during isoflurane- or sodium nitroprusside-induced hypotension, *Anesthesiology* 70:678-683, 1989.
35. Gelb AW, Floyd P, Lok P et al: A prophylactic bolus of thiopentone does not protect against prolonged focal cerebral ischaemia, *Can Anaesth Soc J* 33:173-177, 1986.
36. Gelb AW, Herrick IA: Preoperative hypertension does predict postcarotid endarterectomy hypertension, *Can J Neurol Sci* 17:95-96, 1990.
37. Gibson BE, Black S, Maass L et al:

Esmolol for the control of hypertension after neurologic surgery, *Clin Pharmacol Ther* 44:650-653, 1988.

38. Ginsberg MD, Prado R, Dietrich WD et al: Hyperglycemia reduces the extent of cerebral infarction in rats, *Stroke* 18:570-574, 1987.

39. Goldberg ME, Seltzer JL, Azad SS et al: Intravenous labetalol for the treatment of hypertension after carotid endarterectomy, *J Cardiothorac Anesth* 3:411-417, 1989.

40. Gooding JM, Weng JT, Smith RA et al: Cardiovascular and pulmonary responses following etomidate induction of anesthesia in patients with demonstrated cardiac disease, *Anesth Analg* 58:40-41, 1979.

41. Green RM, Messick WJ, Ricotta JJ et al: Benefits, shortcomings and costs of EEG monitoring, *Ann Surg* 201:785-792, 1985.

42. Grundy BL, Heros R: Ischemic cerebrovascular disease. In Matjasko J, Katz J, editors: *Clinical controversies in neuroanesthesia and neurosurgery*. Orlando, 1986, Grune & Stratton, pp 20-21.

43. Gugino V, Chabot RJ: Somatosensory evoked potentials, *Int Anesth Clin* 28:154-164, 1990.

44. Hafner CD, Evans WE: Carotid endarterectomy with local anesthesia: Results and advantages, *J Vasc Surg* 7:232-239, 1988.

45. Halsey JH, McDowell HA, Gelmon S et al: Blood velocity in the middle cerebral artery and regional cerebral blood flow during carotid endarterectomy, *Stroke* 20:53-58, 1989.

46. Hansebout RR, Blomquist G, Gloor P et al: Use of hypertension and electroencephalographic monitoring during carotid endarterectomy, *Can J Surg* 24:304-307, 1981.

47. Hansen TD, Warner DS, Todd MM et al: Effects of nitrous oxide and volatile anesthetics on cerebral blood flow, *Br J Anaesth* 63:290-295, 1989.

48. Hartung J, Cottrell JE: Nitrous oxide reduces thiopental-induced prolongation of survival in hypoxic and anoxic mice, *Anesth Analg* 66:47-52, 1987.

49. Hartung J, Cottrell JE: On hot mice, cold facts and would-be replication, *Anesth Analg* 69:408-410, 1989.

50. Hayes RJ, Levinson SA, Wylie EJ: Intraoperative measurement of carotid back pressure as a guide to operative management for carotid endarterectomy, *Surgery* 72:953-960, 1972.

51. Hertzer NR, Lees CD: Fatal myocardial infarction following carotid endarterectomy, *Ann Surg* 194:212-218, 1981.

52. Hoffman WE, Prekezes C: Benzodiazepines and antagonists: effects on ischemia, *J Neurosurg Anesth* 1:272-277, 1989.

53. Holohan TV. Extracranial-intracranial bypass to reduce the risk of ischemic stroke, *Can Med Assoc J* 144:1457-1465, 1991.

54. Howard VJ, Grizzle J, Diener HC et al: Comparison of multicenter study designs for investigation of carotid endarterectomy efficacy, *Stroke* 23:583-593, 1992.

55. Kainuma M, Shimada Y, Matsuura M: Cervical epidural anaesthesia in carotid artery surgery, *Anaesthesia* 41:1020-1023, 1986.

56. Kearse LA Jr, Brown EN, McPeck K: Somatosensory evoked potentials sensitivity relative to electroencephalography for cerebral ischemia during carotid endarterectomy, *Stroke* 23:498-505, 1992.

57. Kirshner DL, O'Brien MS, Ricotta JJ: Risk factors in a community experience with carotid endarterectomy, *J Vasc Surg* 10:178-186, 1989.

58. Kraft SA, Larson P Jr, Shuer LM et al: Effect of hyperglycemia on neuronal changes in a rabbit model of focal cerebral ischemia, *Stroke* 21:447-450, 1990.

59. Krul JMJ, van Gijn J, Ackerstaff RGA et al: Site and pathogenesis of infarcts associated with carotid endarterectomy, *Stroke* 20:324-328, 1989.

60. Lam AM, Manninen PH, Ferguson GG et al: Monitoring electrophysiologic function during carotid endarterectomy: a comparison of somatosensory evoked potentials and conventional electroencephalogram, *Anesthesiology* 75:15-21, 1991.

61. Lam AM, Winn HR, Cullen BF et al: Hyperglycemia and neurologic outcome in patients with head injury, *J Neurosurg* 75:545-551, 1991.

62. Lam AM: Isoflurane and brain protection: lack of clear-cut evidence is not clear-cut evidence of lack, *J Neurosurg Anesth* 2:315-318, 1990.

63. Lanier WL, Stangland KJ, Scheithauer BW et al: The effects of dextrose and head position on neurological outcome after complete cerebral ischemia in primates: examination of a model, *Anesthesiology* 66:39-48, 1987.

64. Lanier WL: Cerebral function monitoring during carotid endarterectomy, *J Neurosurg Anesth* 1:207-210, 1989.

65. Lassen NA, Palvolgyi R: Cerebral steal during hypercapnia and the inverse reaction during hypocapnia observed by the ^{133}xenon technique in man, *Scand J Lab Clin Invest* 22(Suppl 102):13D, 1968.

66. Lee KS, Davis CH, McWhorter JM: Low morbidity and mortality of carotid endarterectomy performed with regional anesthesia, *J Neurosurg* 69:483-487, 1988.

67. MacFarlane R, Moskowitz MA, Sakas DE et al: The role of neuroeffector mechanisms in cerebral hyperperfusion syndromes, *J Neurosurg* 75:845-855, 1991.

68. Mangano DT: Perioperative cardiac morbidity, *Anesthesiology* 72:153-184, 1990.

69. Mayo Asymptomatic Carotid Endarterectomy Study Group: Results of a randomized, controlled trial of carotid endarterectomy for asymptomatic carotid stenosis, *Mayo Clin Proc* 67:513-518, 1992.

70. McKay RD, Sundt TM, Michenfelder JD et al: Internal carotid artery stump pressure and cerebral blood flow during carotid endarterectomy: modification by halothane, enflurane and Innovar, *Anesthesiology* 45:390-399, 1976.

71. Messeter K: Inhalation anaesthetics, *Curr Opin Anaesthesiol* 3:694-698, 1990.

72. Messick JM, Casement B, Sharbrough FW et al: Correlation of regional cerebral blood flow (rCBF) with EEG changes during isoflurane anesthesia for carotid endarterectomy: critical rCBF, *Anesthesiology* 66:344-349, 1987.

73. Messick JM, Milde LN: Brain protection, *Adv Anesth* 4:47-88, 1987.

74. Michenfelder JD, Sundt TM Jr, Fode N et al: Isoflurane when compared to enflurane and halothane decreases the frequency of cerebral ischemia during carotid endarterectomy, *Anesthesiology* 67:336-340, 1987.

75. Michenfelder JD, Sundt TM Jr: The effect of $Paco_2$ on the metabolism of ischemic brain in squirrel monkeys, *Anesthesiology* 38:445-453, 1973.

76. Michenfelder JD: Nitrous oxide. In Michenfelder JD, editor: *Anesthesia and the brain*, New York, 1988, Churchill-Livingstone, pp 51-59.

77. Milde LN, Milde JH: Preservation of cerebral metabolites by etomidate during incomplete ischemia in dogs, *Anesthesiology* 65:272-277, 1986.

78. Milde LN: The hypoxic mouse model for screening cerebral protective agents: a re-examination, *Anesth Analg* 67:917-922, 1988.

79. Modica PA, Tempelhoff R: A comparison of computerized EEG with internal carotid artery stump pressure for detection of ischemia during carotid endarterectomy, *J Neurosurg Anesth* 1:211-218, 1989.

80. Moffat JA, McDougall MJ, Brunet D et al: Thiopental bolus during carotid endarterectomy—rational drug therapy? *Can Anaesth Soc J* 30:615-622, 1983.

81. Moore WS, Hall AD: Carotid artery back pressure: a test of cerebral tolerance to temporary carotid occlusion, *Arch Surg* 99:702-710, 1969.

82. Moorthy SS, Markand ON, Dilley RS et al: Somatosensory-evoked responses during carotid endarterectomy, *Anesth Analg* 61:879-883, 1982.

83. Morawetz RB, Zeiger HE, McDowell HA Jr et al: Correlation of cerebral blood flow and EEG during carotid occlusion for endarterectomy (without shunting) and neurologic outcome, *Surgery* 96:184-189, 1984.

84. Murphy TM. Somatic blockade of head and neck. In Cousins MJ, Bridenbaugh PO, editors: *Neural blockade in clinical anesthesia and management of pain,* ed 2, Philadelphia, 1988, JB Lippincott, pp 551-557.

85. Muzzi DA, Black S, Losasso TJ et al: Labetalol and esmolol in the control of hypertension after intracranial surgery, *Anesth Analg* 70:68-71, 1990.

86. Nehls D, Todd M, Spetzler R et al: A comparison of the cerebral protective effects of isoflurane and barbiturates during temporary focal ischemia in primates, *Anesthesiology* 66:453-464, 1987.

87. North American Symptomatic Carotid Endarterectomy Trial (NASCET) Investigators: Clinical alert: benefit of carotid endarterectomy for patients with high-grade stenosis of the internal carotid artery, *Stroke* 22:816-817, 1991.

88. North American Symptomatic Carotid Endarterectomy Trial Steering Committee: North American Symptomatic Carotid Endarterectomy Trial. Methods, patient characteristics, and progress, *Stroke* 22:711-720, 1991.

89. O'Donnell TF, Callow AD, Willet C et al: The impact of coronary artery disease on carotid endarterectomy, *Ann Surg* 198:705-712, 1983.

90. Orlowski JP, Shiesley D, Vidt DG et al: Labetalol to control blood pressure after cerebrovascular surgery, *Crit Care Med* 16:765-768, 1988.

91. Padayachee TS, Bishop CCR, Gosling RG et al: Monitoring cerebral perfusion during carotid endarterectomy, *J Cardiovasc Surg* 31:112-114, 1990.

92. Peerless SJ, Mervart JM: Extracranial-intracranial arterial anastomosis: indications and surgical aspects, *Int Anesth Clin* 22:77-87, 1984.

93. Pelligrino DA, Miletich DJ, Hoffman WE et al: Nitrous oxide markedly increases cortical metabolic rate and blood flow in the goat, *Anesthesiology* 60:405-412, 1984.

94. Pine R, Avellone JC, Hoffman M et al: Control of postcarotid endarterectomy hypotension with baroreceptor blockade, *Am J Surg* 147:763-765, 1984.

95. Priebe H: Isoflurane and coronary hemodynamics, *Anesthesiology* 71:960-976, 1989.

96. Prough DS, Scuderi PE, McWhorter JM et al: Hemodynamic status following regional and general anesthesia for carotid endarterectomy, *J Neurosurg Anesth* 1:35-40, 1989.

97. Prough DS, Scuderi PE, Stullken E et al: Myocardial infarction following regional anesthesia for carotid endarterectomy, *Can Anaesth Soc J* 31:192-196, 1984.

98. Renou AM, Vernhiet J, Macrez P et al: Cerebral blood flow and metabolism during etomidate anaesthesia in man, *Br J Anaesth* 50:1047-1050, 1978.

99. Riles TS, Kopelman I, Imparato AM: Myocardial infarction following carotid endarterectomy: a review of 683 operations, *Surgery* 85:249-252, 1979.

100. Rubin JR, Pitluk HC, King TA et al: Carotid endarterectomy in a metropolitan community: the early results after 8535 operations, *J Vasc Surg* 7:256-260, 1988.

101. Schroeder T, Sillesen H, Sorensen O et al: Cerebral hyperperfusion following carotid endarterectomy, *J Neurosurg* 66:824-829, 1987.

102. Schroeder T: Hemodynamic significance of internal carotid artery disease, *Acta Neurol Scand* 77:353-372, 1988.

103. Schweiger H, Kamp H-D, Dinkel M: Somatosensory-evoked potentials during carotid artery surgery: experience in 400 operations, *Surgery* 109:602-609, 1991.

104. Shapiro HM: Barbiturates in brain ischemia, *Br J Anaesth* 57:82-95, 1985.

105. Sieber FE, Smith DS, Traystman RJ et al: Glucose: a reevaluation of its intraoperative use, *Anesthesiology* 67:72-81, 1987.

106. Sieber FE, Toung TJ, Diringer MM et al: Factors influencing stroke outcome following carotid endarterectomy (abstract), *Anesth Analg* 70:S370, 1990.

107. Skaredoff MN: Implications of nitrous oxide administration, *Adv Anesth* 8:177-208, 1991.

108. Skillman JJ: Neurological complications of cardiovascular surgery: procedures involving the carotid arteries and abdominal aorta, *Int Anesth Clin* 24:135-157, 1986.

109. Skudlarick JL, Mooring SL: Systolic hypertension and complications of carotid endarterectomy, *South Med J* 75:1563-1565, 1982.

110. Smith JS, Roizen MF, Cahalan MK et al: Does anesthetic technique make a difference? Augmentation of systolic blood pressure during carotid endarterectomy: effects of phenylephrine versus light anesthesia and of isoflurane versus halothane on the incidence of myocardial ischemia, *Anesthesiology* 69:846-855, 1988.

111. Soloway M, Nadel W, Albin MS et al: The effect of hyperventilation on subsequent cerebral infarction, *Anesthesiology* 29:975-980, 1968.

112. Spencer MP, Thomas GI, Nicholls SC et al: Detection of middle cerebral artery emboli during carotid endarterectomy using transcranial Doppler ultrasonography, *Stroke* 21:415-423, 1990.

113. Spetzler RF, Martin N, Hadley MN et al: Microsurgical endarterectomy under barbiturate protection: a prospective study, *J Neurosurg* 65:63-73, 1982.

114. Steed DL, Peitzman AB, Grundy BL et al: Causes of stroke in carotid endarterectomy, *Surgery* 92:634-641, 1982.

115. Sublett JW, Seidenberg AB, Hobson RW: Internal carotid artery stump pressures during regional anesthesia, *Anesthesiology* 41:505-508, 1974.

116. Sundt TM Jr, Sandok BA, Whisnant JP: Carotid endarterectomy. Complications and preoperative assessment of risk, *Mayo Clin Proc* 50:301-306, 1975.

117. Sundt TM Jr, Sharbrough FW, Anderson RE et al: Cerebral blood flow measurements and electroencephalograms during carotid endarterectomy, *J Neurosurg* 41:310-320, 1974.

118. Sundt TM Jr, Whisnant JP, Houser OW et al: Prospective study of the effectiveness and durability of carotid endarterectomy, *Mayo Clin Proc* 65:625-635, 1990.

119. Sundt TM Jr, Sharbrough FW, Piepgras DG et al: Correlation of cerebral blood flow and electroencephalographic changes during carotid endarterectomy: with results of surgery and hemodynamics of cerebral ischemia, *Mayo Clin Proc* 56:533-543, 1981.

120. Sundt TM Jr: The ischemic tolerance of neural tissue and need for monitoring and selective shunting during carotid endarterectomy, *Stroke* 14:93-98, 1983.

121. Symon L: Regional cerebrovascular responses to acute ischaemia in normocapnia and hypercapnia. An experimental study in baboons, *J Neurol Neurosurg Psychiatry* 33:756-762, 1970.

122. Tarlov E, Schmidek H, Scott RM et al: Reflex hypotension following carotid endarterectomy: mechanisms and management, *J Neurosurg* 39:323-327, 1973.

123. Toronto Cardiovascular Study Group: Risks of carotid endarterectomy, *Stroke* 17:848-852, 1986.

124. Towne JB, Bernhard VM: The relationship of postoperative hypertension to complications following carotid endarterectomy, *Surgery* 88:575-580, 1980.

125. Towne JB, Weiss DG, Hobson RW: First phase report of cooperative Veterans Administration asymptomatic carotid stenosis study—operative morbidity and mortality, *J Vasc Surg* 11:252-259, 1990.

126. Van Hemelrijck J, Tempelhoff R, Jellish WS et al: Comparison of thiopental-isoflurane-N$_2$O, propofol-N$_2$O, and propofol alone for neuroanesthesia (abstract), *Anesthesiology* 73:A167, 1990.

127. Wade JG, Larson CP, Hickey RF et al: Effect of carotid endarterectomy on carotid chemoreceptor and baroreceptor function in man, *N Engl J Med* 15:823-829, 1970.

128. Walker MD: Carotid endarterectomy: a little more light at the end of the tunnel, *Mayo Clin Proc* 67:597-600, 1992.

129. Warner DS: Isoflurane: more than an anesthetic? *J Neurosurg Anesth* 2:319-321, 1990.

130. Warner DS: Volatile anesthetics and the ischemic brain, *J Neurosurg Anesth* 1:290-294, 1989.

131. Weir DL, Goodchild CS, Graham DI: Propofol: effects on indices of cerebral ischemia, *J Neurosurg Anesth* 1:284-289, 1989.

132. Werner C: Transcranial Doppler sonography: trend monitor of cerebral hemodynamics? *J Neurosurg Anesth* 3:73-76, 1991.

133. Wells BA, Keats AS, Cooley DA: Increased tolerance to cerebral ischemia produced by general anesthesia during temporary carotid occlusion, *Surgery* 54:216-223, 1963.

134. Whittemore AD, Kauffman JL, Kohler TR et al: Routine electroencephalographic (EEG) monitoring during carotid endarterectomy, *Ann Surg* 197:707-713, 1981.

135. Yamamoto M, Meyer JS, Sakai F et al: Aging and cerebral vasodilator responses to hypercarbia. Responses in normal aging and in persons with risk factors for stroke, *Arch Neurol* 37:489-496, 1980.

136. Young WL, Prohovnik I, Correll JW et al: Cerebral blood flow and metabolism in patients undergoing anesthesia for carotid endarterectomy. A comparison of isoflurane, halothane and fentanyl, *Anesth Analg* 68:712-717, 1989.

137. Young WL, Prohovnik I, Correll JW et al: Thiopental effect on cerebral blood flow during carotid endarterectomy, *J Neurosurg Anesth* 3:265-269, 1991.

138. Zampella E, Morawetz RB, McDowell HA et al: The importance of cerebral ischemia during carotid endarterectomy, *Neurosurg* 29:727-731, 1991.

25

Anesthesia for Epileptic Patients and for Epilepsy Surgery

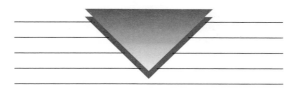

W. Andrew Kofke
René Tempelhoff
Richard M. Dasheiff

The first surgical resection for epilepsy was performed in 1886 by Horsley.[39,111] In the intervening century, the procedure has evolved extensively. Although it is now technically straightforward, this operation must be done with precision to ensure an optimal outcome. Before a patient is accepted for surgery, drug therapy is attempted. If this fails to improve the condition, the patient undergoes extensive diagnostic evaluation to determine the presence of a resectable seizure focus or an interruptable seizure pathway. These tests are most successful when performed in a center with an epilepsy program.[39,159] The pathophysiology of epilepsy is complex, and this complexity justifies a detailed, specialized evaluation. Thus epileptics compose a unique subset of patients in the practice of neurosurgical anesthesiology. This chapter will review the effect and classification of epilepsy, therapeutic options, diagnostic procedures, specific surgical procedures, important concomitant medical problems, specific concerns for the anesthetic management of patients undergoing seizure surgery and related procedures, and anesthetic considerations in patients experiencing status epilepticus.

ROLE OF THE NEUROANESTHESIOLOGIST

Traditionally, the anesthesiologist's role in the management of the epilepsy patient has been to provide an anesthetic that does not trigger seizures. Over the years, the neuroanesthesiologist has become involved in developing anesthetic techniques that are safe and consistent with the needs of the operating neurosurgeon. Presently, this may entail providing appropriate sedation or monitored anesthetic care for awake craniotomy, administering anesthetic drugs to provoke seizures for intraoperative electrocorticography, or providing a technique that has anticonvulsant properties. Moreover, anesthesiologists are increasingly involved in neuroscience research and intensive care. Neuroanesthesiologist-intensivists are helping to determine the cerebral depressants most appropriate for stopping seizures, proconvulsant and anticonvulsant properties of anesthetics, and the important interactions between anesthetic therapy and epilepsy or antiepileptic drugs. Finally, neurologists and neurosurgeons consult with anesthesiologists to determine the optimal management of refractory status epilepticus.

EFFECT OF EPILEPSY

Epilepsy has a profound effect on each individual diagnosed with this disease and, as a consequence, on society.[36,305] Patients with poorly controlled epilepsy cannot maintain a normal lifestyle. Virtually all aspects of a patient's life are adversely affected. Relatives and friends may be anxious about the individual's disease. In addition, ignorance and prejudice in the general population are an onerous burden.[28] Children with epilepsy have been reported to have a poor self-image as a result of parental nonacceptance, misunderstanding, and frustration.[218] As they mature, some patients develop intellectual and social deficits resulting from the brain-damaging effects of uncontrolled recurrent seizures, the negative attitudes society has exhibited toward them,[28] or, possibly, the side effects of treatment.[75] Although studies suggest an association between emotional problems and epilepsy,[28,218] this association has been refuted.[148] Nonetheless, people with epilepsy marry less often, have more sexual difficulties, have greater levels of unemployment or underemployment, have poor self-esteem, and tend to be reluctant to disclose their disability to others. Moreover, patients with epilepsy have difficulty getting a driver's license, which further adversely affects their lifestyle.[194]

Approximately 300,000 people have medically uncontrolled epilepsy in the United States. About 13% of these are thought to be candidates for surgery, but only about 1% actually undergo surgery.[240] Most studies estimate the incidence of epilepsy to be 0.5% to 2% of the total population,[28,126,234] with about 25% to 30% of epileptics having seizures more frequently than once per month.

CLASSIFICATION OF EPILEPSY

The classification of seizures (both epileptic and nonepileptic) has changed during the last several decades. Specialized epilepsy centers have facilitated more precise delinea-

---

BOX 25-1
CLASSIFICATION OF SEIZURES

I. Partial seizures
   A. Simple
   B. Complex
   C. Partial onset with generalization
II. Generalized seizures
   A. Inhibitory
      1. Absence
      2. Atonic
   B. Excitatory
      1. Myoclonic
      2. Clonic
      3. Tonic
III. Pseudoseizures
IV. Unclassified

---

tions. These centers have used closed-circuit monitoring combined with scalp or intracranial electroencephalography (EEG) to record and review in detail the components of seizures. The most recent and widely accepted classification of epileptic seizures was published in 1981.[51] In addition to spontaneous epileptic seizures, alcohol withdrawal and exogenous toxins can also induce seizures. Finally, there are "pseudoseizures," which have no EEG correlate and represent either conscious malingering or, more frequently, a psychiatric condition such as a conversion disorder. Differentiation among epileptic seizures, toxin-evoked seizures, and pseudoseizures may require expert skills and sophisticated resources.

Box 25-1 combines the international classification of epileptic seizures with nonepileptic seizures and is a more practical classification for general use. Epilepsies are much more difficult to classify than seizures and will not be discussed here. Interested readers are referred to a recent textbook, *Seizures in Epilepsy*, by Engel.[78]

Partial Seizures

The term *partial seizure* implies a local or focal onset within the brain. These partial seizures can occur in silent areas of the brain, have no clinical manifestations, and cannot be diagnosed without the aid of intracranial EEG recordings. One type of clinically relevant partial seizure is the simple partial seizure. Here *simple* implies an undetectable alteration in consciousness during the seizure. Electrographically, these seizures have a limited distribution in the brain, consistent with the understanding that bilateral cerebral involvement is required to alter consciousness. Simple partial seizures have frequently been termed *auras*. When seizures spread into multiple areas of the brain and alter consciousness (no matter how slightly), they are classified as complex partial seizures. Also termed *psychomotor* or *temporal lobe seizures,* they produce automatisms, varying degrees of unresponsiveness, and amnesia after the seizure.

Another seizure in this category is the partial onset seizure with generalization. This seizure starts focally in one part of the brain and then spreads to involve much of the brain and brainstem, producing a convulsive seizure. Convulsive seizures are usually either clonic or tonic, and after they occur, the type of onset, partial or generalized, cannot be determined. A simple partial seizure can progress to a complex partial seizure and then to a convulsion.

Generalized Seizures

A generalized seizure occurs when the EEG shows simultaneous involvement of both cerebral hemispheres. The term *generalized seizures* implies no focal onset; however, some types are multifocal or have a partial onset that cannot be resolved by present diagnostic technology. Therefore, operationally, it is best to simply categorize these seizures as generalized. This group can be divided into two major categories: (1) inhibitory generalized seizures, which produce predominantly negative phenomena and include absence seizures (petit mal seizures) and atonic seizures (during which the patient loses muscle tone and falls down), and (2) excitatory seizures, which produce positive phenomena and include myoclonic, clonic, and tonic seizures.

Pseudoseizures

Pseudoseizures may mimic any of the previously mentioned partial or generalized seizures. If a patient's behavior is clearly outside the range of that expected for a true seizure,

this differentiation may be important. Of aggressively treated cases of status epilepticus, 5% turn out to be pseudoseizures.

Unclassified Epilepsy

Nonepileptic seizures caused by alcohol withdrawal or other exogenous toxins usually occur as generalized tonic or clonic seizures. However, some patients may have underlying brain damage that produces an area of decreased seizure threshold so that a partial onset may occur. Consequently, such patients may have multifocal seizures or focal motor seizures without having true epilepsy. Status epilepticus of these different types can occur in people who do not have epilepsy.

THERAPY FOR EPILEPSY
Medical Therapy

This is the first line of therapy. A variety of antiepileptic drugs are available to neurologists and epileptologists to treat epilepsy on an outpatient basis. These drugs include phenytoin, phenobarbital, primidone, carbamazepine, valproic acid, and benzodiazepines. Optimal management generally involves maximizing therapy with one drug before resorting to multiple drug therapy.[20,300] The choice of the appropriate drug entails consideration of pharmacokinetics (Table 25-1), clinical toxicity (Table 25-2), and efficacy. Different types of epilepsy respond differently to antiepileptic drugs (Table 25-3).

TABLE 25-1
Pharmacokinetic Variables of Antiepileptic Drugs

Generic Drug Name	Dose (mg/kg)	Dosage Interval (hr)	Oral Availability (%)	Peak Time of Effect (hr)	Plasma Protein Binding (%)	Plasma Half-life (hr)	Therapeutic Plasma Concentration Range (μg/ml)	Toxic Plasma Concentration (μg/ml)
Carbamazepine	10-20	8	80	5-15	51	96-144	10-30	30
Clonazepam*	0.1-0.2	8	98	1-3	80	20-40†	0.02-0.07	—
Clorazepate	0.52-0.66	12		0.5-1	97	Very fast	Not detectable	—
Diazepam	0.1-1.8	8	75	1-2	96-98	10-25‡	0.15-0.25§	—
Ethosuximide	15-30	8	100	1-4	0	30-40	40-100	120
Mephenytoin	3-10	8		2-4	40	24-48	2-3.2	50‖
Mephobarbital	3-7	8		~5		Short	6	
Methsuximide	20-60	6-24		1-4	0	1.4	0.04	—
Phenobarbital	2-5	8-12	80	5-15	51	96-144	10-30	30
Phensuximide	30-100	6-12		0.5-1.5	0	7.8	3.9-7.9	—
Phenytoin	4-8	6-8	80-95	4-8	89	24¶	10-20	20
Primidone	10-20	8	92	2-4	19	8-12	5-12	10
Valproic acid	15-40	6	100	1-4	93	7-16	45-100	120

*Occurrence of side effects is not correlated with the plasma concentration of clonazepam or its metabolites. It is recommended that lower starting doses should be used to minimize sedation. Effects are transient due to development of tolerance.
†Half-life decreases after chronic administration to 8-15 hr because of enzyme induction.
‡Half-life of diazepam is dependent on age.
§Sum total of diazepam and dimethyldeazepam plasma concentrations is probably the most meaningful figure, as both are pharmacologically active.
‖Sum total of parent compound and metabolites.
¶Phenytoin dosage adjustments should be in small (25 mg) increments when in the upper range of therapeutic blood concentrations because the drug shows saturation kinetics. It is advisable not to change brands because bioavailability varies markedly with different preparations.
Modified from Aird RB, Masland RL, Woodbury DM: *The epilepsies: a critical review*. New York. 1984. Raven Press.

TABLE 25-2
Major Antiepileptic Drugs and Side Effects

Generic Name	Proprietary Name	Dose-Related Side Effects	Toxic Effects
Carbamazepine	Tegretol	Double vision, dizziness, lethargy, leukopenia, anorexia	Skin rash, blood dyscrasia, hepatitis, fluid retention
Clonazepam	Clonopin	Lethargy, depression, tremor, headache	Hair loss, nephritis, glaucoma
Clorazepate	Tranxene	Lethargy, depression, tremor, headache	None
Diazepam	Valium	Lethargy, depression, tremor, headache	None
Ethosuximide	Zarontin	Anorexia, nausea, fatigue, headache	Blood dyscrasia, lupus, hepatitis
Mephenytoin	Mesantoin	Ataxia, diplopia, tremor	Rash, blood dyscrasia, hepatitis
Mephobarbital	Mebaral	Lethargy, headache, irritability, anorexia	Facial edema, skin rash
Methsuximide	Celontin	Nausea, ataxia, dizziness, weakness	Rash, blood dyscrasia, nephritis
Phenobarbital		Lethargy, irritability	Rash
Phensuximide	Milontin	Nausea, lethargy, ataxia	Blood dyscrasia, rash, lupus, hepatitis
Phenytoin	Dilantin	Ataxia, gum hypertrophy, hirsutism, altered facies	Neuropathy, blood dyscrasia, rash, lupus (Stevens-Johnson), Dupuytren's contracture
Primidone	Mysoline	Lethargy, irritability, impotence	Rash
Valproic acid	Depakene	Nausea, weight gain, tremor	Loss of hair, hepatitis

TABLE 25-3
Antiepileptic Drugs Used for Specific Epilepsy Syndromes

Epilepsy Syndrome	Drug
Simple and complex partial seizures, clonic-tonic seizures	Phenytoin, carbamazepine, primidone, phenobarbital, mephenytoin, clonazepam, methsuximide, valproic acid, phenacemide
Absence seizures	Ethosuximide, valproic acid, clonazepam, acetazolamide
Myoclonic seizures	Valproic acid, phenobarbital, clonazepam
Infantile spasms	ACTH, corticosteroids, valproic acid, clonazepam, nitrazepam
Myoclonic epilepsy of early childhood	Valproic acid, ethosuximide, methsuximide, valproic acid, clonazepam, nitrazepam
Myoclonic-astatic epilepsy of childhood	ACTH, corticosteroids, valproic acid, clonazepam nitrazepam, ethosuximide, ketogenic diet

Surgical Therapy

Although surgical management of epilepsy has been used for approximately 100 years, only in the past 10 to 20 years has it been subjected to critical scrutiny. This resulted in a recent National Institutes of Health Consensus Conference that addressed the issue of surgery for epilepsy.[186,258,259] This conference involved neurologists, neurosurgeons, psychologists, and other health care providers. It addressed issues regarding epilepsy surgery, including patient selection and management, localization of the site of seizure onset, diagnostic techniques, postoperative outcome, and future research. The panel concluded that surgery is a reasonable alternative treatment when medication fails to control sei-

zures. In deciding whether surgery is appropriate, the panel recommended that physicians evaluate the frequency, severity, and type of seizure, possible brain damage or injury, and the overall effect on a given patient's quality of life. Areas of disagreement remain and include (1) the optimal combination of preoperative tests, (2) the need to preoperatively identify areas of the brain that control speech, (3) the optimal surgical procedure for different types of epilepsy, and (4) the precise definition of intractable epilepsy.

The types of surgery usually employed are divided into two categories. The first category entails resection of a specific seizure focus, most typically represented by an anterior temporal lobectomy. The second entails interruption of seizure circuits to prevent generalization, as with a corpus callosotomy.

STATUS EPILEPTICUS

Status epilepticus is defined as "epileptic seizures that are so frequently repeated or so prolonged as to create a fixed and lasting epileptic condition."[65] Generalized convulsive status epilepticus is considered to be a neurologic emergency. To prevent brain damage,[56] seizures should be stopped as soon as possible, optimally within 30 minutes but certainly within 60 minutes of onset.[65, 66] However, treatment to secure the airway, provide oxygen, and maintain circulation must be initiated within the first few minutes to prevent complications such as hypoxemia, systemic hypertension, tachydysrhythmias, rhabdomyolysis, hyperthermia, and trauma. In addition, an urgent approach to seizure control is further supported by observations of seizure-associated brain damage in humans[56] and by animal studies showing that uncontrolled status epilepticus for 20 minutes or longer is associated with neuronal damage.[188,195,276]

TABLE 25-4
Management of Tonic-Clonic Status Epilepticus

Time from Initiation of Observation and Treatment (min)	Procedure
0	Assess cardiorespiratory functions as the presence of tonic-clonic status is verified. If unsure of diagnosis, observe one tonic-clonic attack and verify the presence of unconsciousness after the end of the tonic-clonic attack. Insert oral airway and administer O_2 if necessary. Insert an indwelling intravenous catheter. Draw venous blood to determine anticonvulsant levels, glucose, BUN, electrolytes, and CBC stat. Draw arterial blood for stat pH, Po_2, Pco_2, Hco_3. Monitor respiration, blood pressure, and electrocardiograph. If possible, monitor electroencephalograph.
5	Start intravenous infusion through indwelling venous catheter with normal saline containing vitamin B complex. Give a bolus injection of 50 ml of 50% glucose.
10	*Infuse diazepam intravenously* no faster than 2 mg/min until seizures stop or to total of 20 mg. *Also start infusion of phenytoin* no faster than 50 mg/min to a total of 18 mg/kg. If hypotension develops, slow the infusion rate. (Phenytoin 50 mg/ml in propylene glycol may be placed in a 100-ml volume-control set and diluted with normal saline. The rate of infusion should be watched carefully). Alternatively, phenytoin may be injected slowly by intravenous push.
30-40	If seizures persist, two options are available: phenobarbital or diazepam as an IV drip. The two infusions should not be given to the same patient. An endotracheal tube should be inserted. Phenobarbital IV: Start infusion of phenobarbital no faster than 100 mg/min until seizures stop or to a loading dose of 20 mg/kg. Diazepam IV drip: 100 mg of diazepam is diluted in 500 ml of 5% dextrose in water and infused at 40 ml/hr. This ensures diazepam serum levels of 0.2 to 0.8 μg/ml.
50-60	If seizures continue, general anesthesia with isoflurane or pentobarbital is instituted.
80	If status epilepticus reappears when general anesthesia is stopped, a neurologist who has expertise in status epilepticus should be consulted. Advice from a regional epilepsy center on the management of intractable status epilepticus also should be sought.

Modified from Delgado-Excueta AV, Wasterlain C, Treiman DM et al: *N Engl J Med* 306:1337-1340, 1982.

The management of convulsive status epilepticus remains controversial. One of many approaches to treatment is shown in Table 25-4. This protocol was published before the widespread use of lorazepam titrated to effect (0.03 to 0.22 mg/kg[92])as a substitute for diazepam.

There are other approaches besides that given in Table 25-4. The initial drug choices include phenobarbital,[97] phenytoin,[297] or a benzodiazepine.[263] A recent study compared diazepam plus phenytoin with phenobarbital and concluded that phenobarbital was rapidly effective and comparable in safety, and had a shorter latency and a shorter median cumulative convulsion time although both regimens had similar frequencies of side effects such as need for tracheal intubation, hypotension, and dysrhythmias.[232] Phenytoin, although generally effective, is sometimes awkward to administer and requires 15 to 20 minutes to effectively control seizures in most patients.[297] Other studies comparing phenobarbital or phenytoin with diazepam have shown diazepam to be effective but short-lived[191] and more often associated with the requirement for endotracheal intubation.[201]

When phenytoin and phenobarbital are ineffective, a benzodiazepine is often suggested. The primary advantage of the benzodiazepines is that they are usually effective.* In addition, some evidence in animals suggests that post-

seizure maturation of damage in the substantia nigra pars reticulata may be favorably altered with benzodiazepines although the clinical relevance of this to temporal lobe epilepsy is unclear.[132] Many considerations influence the choice of benzodiazepine. Midazolam and diazepam have a shorter onset time than lorazapam although lorazapam generally has a longer duration of action with a lower likelihood of severe respiratory depression, making it the preferred agent of some authors.[48] Diazepam has been reported to be effective rectally,[6,230] and midazolam has been reported to be effective intramuscularly[171]; both have been used effectively as continuous infusions.[22,58]

If seizures continue to be refractory to treatment with the previously noted drugs, a barbiturate, usually pentobarbital* but sometimes thiopental,[31,249] titrated to EEG effect can be used. Alternatively, volatile anesthetics can also be used.[133,197] The anesthetic approach to status epilepticus is described in more detail later in this chapter.

EVALUATION OF PATIENTS FOR SEIZURE SURGERY
General Procedures

A patient progresses through several phases from initial presentation for seizure disorder, to diagnosis, and finally to

*References 6, 22, 58, 92, 171, 277, 278.

*References 35, 84, 97, 156, 262, 287, 307.

full rehabilitation.[29,160,246,258] In phase I, patients undergo noninvasive evaluation, including a medical history interview, physical examination, neuropsychiatric evaluation, brain structural and functional imaging, psychosocial evaluation, and video camera monitoring with surface electrode EEG.[219] Some patients enter phase II, which includes intracranial EEG monitoring. Patients in this phase usually undergo manipulations in their antiepileptic drug therapy and may undergo procedures to increase their tendency to have seizures (e.g., sleep deprivation or electrical stimulation). In some centers patients also undergo thiopental tests (see following discussion) to further localize the origin of seizures. Most patients have an intracarotid amobarbital (WADA) test to ascertain the dominant cerebral hemisphere. In phase III, surgery is performed. In phase IV, outcome is evaluated.

Radiologic Evaluation

Neuroimaging techniques provide important additional information that can supplement EEG data and increase confidence in seizure focus localization based on electrophysiologic observations. Computed tomography (CT) and magnetic resonance imaging (MR) are the two most commonly used tests. MR can help identify low-grade, occult intracranial neoplasms not visualized on a CT scan, precisely localize depth electrode recordings, and evaluate the extent of surgical resection during phase IV.[170] MR has also been used to provide supporting information to localize a seizure focus.[225] When carefully done, MR may show the site of hippocampal sclerosis, which frequently correlates with the seizure focus.[41]

Functional imaging is done with positron emission tomography (PET), single-photon emission computed tomography (SPECT), and other methods that detect cerebral blood flow. PET has been reported to be helpful in localizing seizure foci[2,77,208] and evaluating the metabolic effects of seizure focus resection.[60] Interictally, patients with partial seizures show pronounced hypometabolism in the region of seizure foci.[2,208] Occasionally the physical extent of interictal hypometabolic zones is substantially greater than the extent of overt neuropathologic changes. Some authors believe PET to be superior to other diagnostic methods in localizing seizure foci.[208] Others have suggested that SPECT may be useful to identify epileptic foci by determining regions of aberrant blood flow.[258] Ictal SPECT studies appear to be superior to interictal studies but require significantly more resources. The details of radiologic imaging, seizure monitoring, magnetoencephalography, neuropsychiatric assessment, and amobarbital testing are beyond the scope of this chapter. The interested reader is referred to several references detailing these methods used to evaluate epilepsy surgery.* Thiopental testing and intraoperative electrocorticography will be discussed in some detail here and later in the chapter.

---

*References 18, 43, 118, 119, 169, 180, 222, 258, 292.

Thiopental Test

A thiopental test is performed to assist in EEG localization of seizure foci. The technique is to produce a gradual increase in blood levels of thiopental, thereby producing electrographic beta activity. Such beta activity will occur in normally functioning neural tissue, whereas seizure foci will not show a normal response.[131,151,152] The abnormal response may take the form of absent beta activity or activation of interictal epileptic activity.

Intraoperative Electrocorticography

This procedure is used intraoperatively to further guide the surgeon in increasing precision of the excision. Drugs such as methohexital and enflurane are given to activate seizure foci, making the concomitant anesthetics an extremely important aspect of patient management.

SURGICAL PROCEDURES

Procedures used for seizure surgery generally are intended to resect a specific epileptogenic focus or interrupt a seizure pathway. The specific procedures include various methods of temporal lobectomy, amygdalohippocampectomy, extratemporal/extrafrontal cortical excision, hemispherectomy, corpus callosotomy, or stereotactic excision.* The surgical results of such procedures are reported to be generally favorable, with combined morbidity and mortality rates below 5% for epileptogenic focus resection, 20% for corpus callosotomy, and 50% for "functional" hemispherectomy.[258] Either no seizures or a substantial decrease in seizure frequency is reported in 50% to 90% of patients.† (Table 25-5). A larger excision is associated with greater success with respect to seizures although a larger resection is associated with significant morbidity, such as visual difficulties, memory problems, or speech difficulties.‡ In addition to stopping seizures, early surgery for epilepsy is thought to improve later psychosocial status and adaptive function by preventing brain damage resulting from the adverse effects of antiepileptic drugs and by avoiding the cumulative effects of the negative attitudes of family and friends.[71,107]

A retrospective study compared surgical and nonsurgical treatment for epilepsy.[101] No significant difference in survival between the two groups was reported although the data indicated that surgical treatment for partial epilepsy is more successful at reducing the frequency of seizures than nonsurgical treatment. Surgical treatment of epilepsy seldom provides a cure. Most of these patients continue to require antiepileptic drugs and continue to carry the diagnosis of epilepsy although they may have an improvement in lifestyle. The cost of diagnostic evaluation and surgery in

---

*References 165, 181, 196, 206, 240, 246, 258.
†References 2, 11, 12, 20, 27, 50, 64, 100, 101, 113, 118, 125, 142, 165, 176, 240, 244, 246-248, 258, 292, 298.
‡References 11, 12, 43, 105, 117, 118, 122, 248.

TABLE 25-5
Results of the Surgical Treatment of Epilepsy Reported by Four Treatment Groups

Interval	Number of Patients	Seizure Free (%)	Occasional Seizures (%) (<3/yr)	Marked Reduction (%) (<50%)	Moderate or No Improvement (%)	Mortality
1928-1971	1267	36.0	11	17.0	36.0	1.7
?-1975	143	21.0	18.4	21.1	28.9	1.3
1971-1975	53	71.0		18.0	11.0	?
?-1977	220	54.2	19.1	14.5	9.1	3.1
1973-1977	74	59.4	21.6	13.5	4.1	1.4
1973-1977	36	69.4	28.0	0	2.6	0

Modified from Aird RB, Masland RL, Woodbury DM: *The epilepsies: a critical review,* New York, 1984, Raven Press.

1991 was $25,000 to $100,000, with a median charge of $40,000 to $60,000.[258]

ANESTHETIC CONCERNS IN THE PATIENT WITH EPILEPSY

The primary concerns for the neuroanesthesiologist are (1) the ability of anesthetics to suppress or potentiate seizure activity, (2) the interactions of anesthetic drugs with antiepileptic drugs, and (3) concomitant medical problems.

Proconvulsant and Anticonvulsant Properties of Anesthetics

Opitz et al.[197] reported on the use of general anesthesia in 1172 epileptic patients. Induction of anesthesia was achieved with methohexital (913 patients), etomidate (39 patients), ketamine (20 patients), and thiopental (5 patients). Anesthesia was maintained with halothane (642 patients), enflurane (345 patients), regional anesthesia (132 patients), intravenous anesthesia (43 patients), and balanced anesthesia with droperidol and fentanyl (10 patients). They observed epileptiform activity on EEG after administration of methohexital and etomidate, and in one patient under spinal anesthesia with mepivacaine (serum concentration was 10% of toxic level). In none of the patients were motor manifestations of convulsions observed. Nonetheless, there are situations where anesthetics have been reported to produce seizure patterns on EEG with accompanying manifestations such as convulsions, hypermetabolism, or, in animals, brain damage. Thus, to plan the anesthetic management of a given patient with epilepsy, one must appreciate the specific conditions and doses under which some anesthetics can promote seizure activity while others tend to inhibit it. Some anesthetics can, paradoxically, exhibit both proconvulsant and anticonvulsant properties with different doses or under different physiologic situations. This topic has been reviewed in detail by Modica et al.[178,178a] Salient aspects and examples of these phenomena are summarized here.

Volatile Anesthetics
Nitrous Oxide

In rodents, withdrawal of nitrous oxide has been reported to be associated with induction of seizures.[21] However, this is an uncommon observation in humans and many other animal models. Nitrous oxide had little effect when administered as an adjunct to other anesthetic drugs in a human with status epilepticus.[221]

Halothane

Although, anecdotally, halothane has been suggested as the primary agent to stop status epilepticus,[84] such recommendations generally were made before the availability of isoflurane and without justification from clinical studies. Halothane does appear generally to be an effective anticonvulsant.[197,221] It does not appear to have proconvulsant effects.[251] Nonetheless, convulsions associated with halothane anesthesia have been reported.[139,242]

Enflurane

Seizures in humans during or after enflurane have been frequently reported.[62,106,116,192] Moreover, enflurane reproducibly activates the human electrocorticogram.[116] Controlled studies have demonstrated that higher concentrations (1 to 2 MAC) of enflurane are associated with motor manifestations of seizures,[37,80,192] which are accentuated by hyperventilation and auditory, visual, and tactile stimulation.[37,146,183] When given in doses sufficient to produce seizures in rodents, metabolic activity increases in the hippocampus and in the intercortical and corticothalamic pathways.[185] The hippocampus and related limbic system structures are thought to be the epileptogenic foci for seizures induced by enflurane in rats.[183] No neuropathologic studies on the effects of enflurane-induced seizures have been reported. However, in animal studies enflurane has been shown to suppress amygdaloid-kindled and bicuculline- and penicillin-induced seizures at subconvulsive and convulsive doses.[202] In humans, temporal lobe seizures have been stopped with enflurane,[90,198] and it has been used successfully to treat convulsive status epilepticus.[197] When used for surgery in epileptic patients, it produces less epileptiform activity on EEG than does physiologic sleep.[197]

Isoflurane

In two animal models, isoflurane was shown to be an effective anticonvulsant although it had no effect on postseizure maturation of nigral brain damage.[132] It has not been shown to be a proconvulsant in animals although reports are conflicting. There appears to be a tendency for occasional idiosyncratic seizures during or after isoflurane in humans.[19,104,114,124,215] However, isoflurane has been demonstrated to suppress seizure activity in very difficult cases of status epilepticus[133,174,221] and intraoperatively to suppress epileptogenic tissue as demonstrated by electrocorticogram recordings.[116]

Nonopioid Intravenous Anesthetics
Barbiturates

In animals, thiopental stopped seizures in two different generalized status epilepticus models although it did not reduce postseizure maturation of nigral brain damage.[132] Thiopental also inhibited cortical and subcortical epileptic activity resulting from penicillin-induced focal seizures.[67] Many clinical reports provide evidence that anesthetic doses of barbiturates are effective anticonvulsants.* Nonetheless, when given in the appropriate (low) dose, even thiopental can produce evidence of clinical seizure activity (Goldberg and McIntyre[97] and personal observations). Depth EEG recordings have also demonstrated seizure activity during thiopental tests.[128a] In humans, methohexital, in doses as small as 25 mg, produced seizure spike activation on the intraoperative electrocorticogram. This was selective to an epileptogenic focus and was seen during both local and general anesthesia.[299] Methohexital has also been reported to produce seemingly new foci in 43% of the patients[83] and can produce epileptiform activity with induction of anesthesia.[197] In addition, it has been reported to induce convulsions.[16,163] Amobarbital, in doses sufficient for the WADA (Amytal) test, and methohexital were both observed to produce hippocampal-depth electrode activation in humans.[1]

Etomidate

This drug can produce seizures[140,145,197] and has been associated with postoperative seizures.[99,102,141] Such reports have been attributed to spinal cord disinhibition and reduced supraspinal control of motor neurons,[13,175] however, etomidate possibly has the potential to produce cortical seizures. Intraoperatively, it has been useful for activating the electrocorticogram recorded from epileptogenic foci.[74,91,140] Nonetheless, in at least one report, etomidate was used to stop status epilepticus;[305] however for delirium tremens

caused by alcohol withdrawal it was ineffective and actually potentiated the tremors.[190]

Benzodiazepines

Convulsive seizure activity has not been produced or augmented by benzodiazepines in intact animal preparations or humans. However, in one report, nonconvulsive status epilepticus occurring in a patient with Lennox-Gastaut syndrome was exacerbated with a benzodiazepine.[154] In the same report, five other patients with nonconvulsive status epilepticus did not exhibit cessation of electrographic seizure activity with benzodiazepine therapy. The reports of other investigators describe 13 patients with status epilepticus refractory to benzodiazepine therapy.[154,287] Nonetheless, numerous reports demonstrate the efficacy of midazolam, diazepam, lorazepam, and clonazepam as anticonvulsants.* One animal study[132] showed that midazolam, when used to stop seizures, lessened postseizure maturation of damage in the substantia nigra. The limbic system was not severely damaged in this model. Thus protective aspects of benzodiazepine use were not assessed in this brain region, making the relevance of these results to clinical temporal lobe epilepsy unclear.

Ketamine

Epileptogenic foci recorded by depth electrode recordings have been activated by ketamine in epileptic patients.[82,23] However, ketamine has been used to stop status epilepticus in humans.[85] It is a noncompetitive antagonist of the N-methyl-D-aspartate subtype of the glutamate receptor.[8] It has been tested in animals for efficacy as an anticonvulsant and as a drug that might protect the brain against ischemic damage. Ketamine administered during kainic-acid–induced seizures reduced behavioral seizure activity and electrographic seizures in the neocortex. However, ketamine did not reduce seizures in the limbic system although it did prevent seizure-related brain damage.[52] In another animal model, ketamine prevented seizure-induced thalamic damage although it did not eliminate persistent electrographic seizure activity.[53] Given to rodents with flurothyl- or mercaptopropionic-acid–induced seizures, ketamine effectively stopped seizures recorded with subdermal electrodes. Evidence of reduced nigral brain damage was statistically insignificant.[132] This last study measured effects primarily in the substantia nigra, whereas the two former studies measured effects in the limbic system. These two brain regions may sustain damage via unrelated biochemical mechansims.[269,270]

Propofol

Seizure activity has been reported in humans receiving propofol, prompting a warning from the United King-

*References 35, 84, 97, 156, 262, 287.

*References 6, 22, 48, 92, 171, 201, 232, 277, 278.

dom Committee on the Safety of Medicine.[204,239,291] Significantly, seizures have been reported to occur after propofol use.[33,204,268] However, when given as an anesthetic for electroconvulsive therapy, and, compared with methohexital, seizure time is shortened.[238] Propofol has been found to effectively stop seizures in humans and animals.[47,157,161,302]

Althesin

This drug is reported to decrease penicillin-induced focal seizures in rodents.[67] In humans, althesin was used effectively in a patient with status epilepticus.[284]

Droperidol

When given with fentanyl for surgery, droperidol was not observed to produce epileptiform activity on EEG.[197]

Opioid Intravenous Anesthetics

Opioid drugs represent a class of anesthetic agents with endogenous peptidergic neurotransmitter analogs that appear to have both inhibitory and excitatory effects.* Given intracerebroventricularly to animals, they produce opiate-receptor–specific stereotypic seizure patterns that can be stopped with intravenous administration of mu opioids.[286] They are thought to have a disinhibitory effect on hippocampal interneurons.[236,309] In immunohistochemistry studies, high concentrations of endogenous opioid peptides have been identified in those limbic structures known to be prone to seizure.[55,236] Indeed, a primary function of limbic opioids may be to regulate limbic system excitability.[108,272,275] Thus some have suggested that endogenous peptidergic opiate systems have a role in the pathogenesis of epilepsy.[46,89,217,236,275] Studies supporting this theory include reports of higher affinity binding of opioids in the human temporal lobe as determined by PET scanning[89] and epileptic patients with high levels of cerebrospinal fluid enkephalin who responded to therapy with opioid antagonist treatment.[46,149,182] The potential proconvulsant effect of exogenously administered opioid anesthetics in humans remains controversial.

Reports of opioid-induced or augmented seizures† and opioid-induced kindled seizures[40,110] in animals have been published. Apparently, the specific pattern of seizure activation and spread is opiate-receptor specific.[40,49,243,257,274] Mu-agonist seizures originate in the limbic system, most likely the ventral hippocampus or amygdala.[49,55,108,129,243] Researchers have demonstrated that (1) opioids are involved in kindling via increased levels of endogenous enkephalin[110] or antagonism of inhibitory neurons,[236] (2) opioids potentiate kainic-acid–induced kindled limbic seizures,[261] (3) opioids also potentiate pentylenetetrazole-induced seizures,[87] and (4) in vitro opioids have been reported to aug-

ment the electrophysiologic effects of glutamate.[45] Seizures produced by intracerebroventricular opioids can be suppressed by parenteral opioids,[286] and electroconvulsive-shock–induced seizures in mice can be blunted with morphine.[216]

Seizures in the absence of hypoxia or other systemic abnormalities can produce brain damage.[54,65,188,195,276] Relevant to this is research demonstrating that 1-2 hours of high-dose alfentanil-, fentanyl-, or sufentanil-induced seizures produced limbic system brain damage in rats, with the most sensitive area being the amygdala.[129,129a]

However, applicability of animal data to humans is unclear. Numerous reports without EEG monitoring describe apparent mu-opioid–induced convulsions in humans.* However, in studies during which scalp EEG recordings were made to determine whether the seizurelike movements actually represented seizures, no seizure activity was indicated,[32,229,241] although such data may be falsely negative. If opioids produce seizures in humans, they undoubtedly do so in the limbic system, with seizures being generated deep in the brain within the medial temporal lobes or amygdala. These are areas where dramatic seizure activity may be missed on scalp EEG. An example of this is depicted in Fig. 25-1.[82] Despite these caveats regarding scalp EEG recordings, Kearse et al.[123] have shown an association between high-dose opioid use and the occurrence of epileptiform patterns on scalp EEG in humans undergoing carotid or cardiac surgery. Tempelhoff et al.[265] have observed an epileptiform pattern on depth electrode temporal lobe recordings in the nonepileptic hemisphere in epileptic humans given moderate doses (20 to 52 μg/kg) of fentanyl (Fig. 25-2); Sharbrough has observed alfentanil-induced interictal spikes on depth electrode hippocampal recordings during epilepsy surgery.[232a] Thus opioids apparently can produce limbic system epileptiform activity in epileptic patients. Whether this occurs with sufficient duration and intensity to be dangerous and whether it occurs in the limbic system of nonepileptic humans is not known.

Opioids and some neurotoxins may have similar effects in both rats and humans. Opioids produce a limbic system hypermetabolism in rats that is virtually identical to that produced by kainic acid.[54,129,129a,271,306] Glutamic acid, kainic acid (a structural analog of glutamic acid), and domoic acid are potent excitatory neurotoxins.[63,172,252] In rats, domoic acid produces a pattern of damage observed by light microscopy that is similar to that produced by alfentanil.[129,129a,281,283] Moreover, domoic acid, given to mice, results in a spectrum of sterotypic behavior similar to that seen in humans, such as stereotypic nasopharyngeal movements, sedation, rigidity, and convulsions.[255] Domoic acid, a toxin derived from seaweed-contaminated mussels in Canada, produced an epidemic of human intoxication in

---

*References 55, 108, 129, 236, 286, 309.
†References 40, 49, 70, 87, 129, 129a, 173, 257, 261, 273, 274, 285.

*References 14, 24, 136, 143, 179, 223, 229, 256, 295.

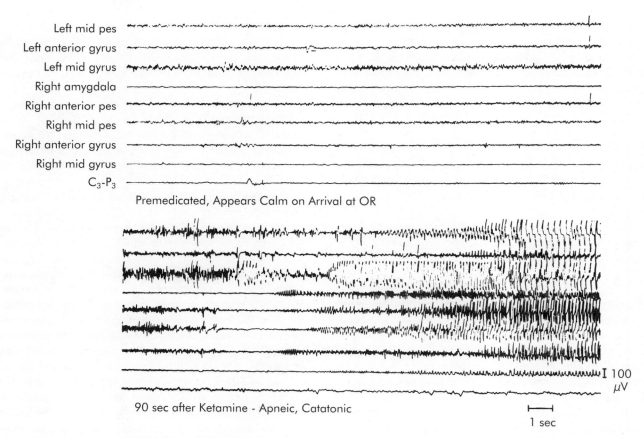

Left mid pes
Left anterior gyrus
Left mid gyrus
Right amygdala
Right anterior pes
Right mid pes
Right anterior gyrus
Right mid gyrus
C_3-P_3

Premedicated, Appears Calm on Arrival at OR

90 sec after Ketamine - Apneic, Catatonic

I 100 μV

1 sec

FIG. 25-1   Scalp electrodes can miss hippocampal epileptiform activity. EEG evidence of seizure is apparent in the depth electrodes but not in scalp electrodes (C_3-P_3) after administration of ketamine 2 to 4 mg/kg IV to an epileptic patient. *(From Ferrer-Allado T, Berchme VL, Dymond A et al: Anesthesiology 38:333-344, 1973.)*

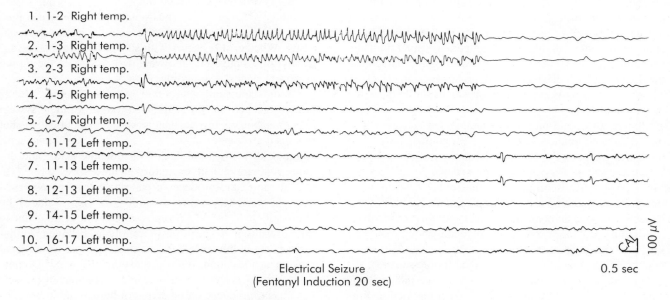

1. 1-2 Right temp.
2. 1-3 Right temp.
3. 2-3 Right temp.
4. 4-5 Right temp.
5. 6-7 Right temp.
6. 11-12 Left temp.
7. 11-13 Left temp.
8. 12-13 Left temp.
9. 14-15 Left temp.
10. 16-17 Left temp.

100 μV

Electrical Seizure
(Fentanyl Induction 20 sec)

0.5 sec

FIG. 25-2   Temporal lobe EEG recording after fentanyl administration to an epileptic patient with a left-sided seizure focus.

1987.[211,264] These patients initially exhibited a variety of neurologic symptoms ranging from headache to seizures and coma.[211] Many of the survivors of this domoic acid ingestion subsequently sustained permanent neuropsychiatric deficits.[264,308] On PET scanning, these patients exhibited decrements in glucose utilization in the hippocampus and amygdala.[96,264] Moreover, on neuropathologic examination, nonsurvivors were found to have lesions in the amygdala and hippocampus, areas where alfentanil and domoic acid produce brain damage in rats. This pattern of domoic-acid–induced damage was confirmed under controlled conditions in monkeys.[282]

The clinical relevance of this information is currently speculative because the propensity for opioids to produce sustained, intense seizures with consequent brain damage in humans has not been demonstrated. However, the data do suggest a need for awareness regarding the possibility of opioid-mediated effects. If high doses of opioids are indicated, coadministration of anticonvulsant anesthetics, such as isoflurane, thiopental, or benzodiazepines, might be helpful.

Muscle Relaxants

There is concern that atracurium could decrease the seizure threshold as a result of accumulation of the metabolite laudanosine.[19,304] However, this is not thought to be a clinically important phenomenon.[115,144,178,178a]

Antiepileptic Drug Therapy and Anesthesia

Patients receiving antiepileptic drugs have resistance to the effects of neuromuscular blocking agents.[73,199,200,224,266] In addition, epileptic patients also require higher doses of fentanyl to maintain a comparable depth of anesthesia.[267] The data suggest a relation between the number of anticonvulsants a patient receives and the maintenance dose of fentanyl required during a balanced anesthetic technique.[267] The cause or causes of this resistance to opioids and neuromuscular blocking agents are unknown. However, possibilities include changes in the number of receptors, alterations in drug metabolism, and interactions with endogenous neurotransmitters.

CONCOMITANT MEDICAL PROBLEMS
Psychiatric Disorders

Various psychiatric disorders have been associated with epilepsy. Neuroses in the form of anxiety and personality disorders have been reported.[127,237] Affective disorders also have been associated with epilepsy and are manifested primarily in increased suicide rates. The risk of suicide seems to be higher with temporal lobe epilepsy, epilepsy with a greater degree of handicap, and in the early years of the condition.[17,279] Finally, cognitive dysfunction also can occur as a psychosis.[187,279]

Rare Syndromes

Many rare syndromes are associated with epilepsy (see appendix at end of Chapter). These syndromes may include disturbances in other major organ systems, which may affect anesthetic management.

Tuberous Sclerosis

With a gene frequency of approximately 1 in 30,000, tuberous sclerosis accounts for up to 33% of infantile seizures.[5] Surgery has been reported to be helpful with this syndrome.[38,212] However, such patients pose a problem to the neuroanesthesiologist because tuberous sclerosis is associated with cardiac dysrhythmias,[57,93,120] cardiac ventricular tumors,[93,233,294] and other medical problems. One study of 60 patients found an incidence of cardiac tumor in adults of 18% and in children of 58%.[294] In addition, tuberous sclerosis has also been associated with renal dysfunction,[25,68,193,253,290] cerebral embolism resulting from cardiac tumor,[121,135] cerebral tubers,[193,213] pulmonary dysfunction,[147,150,158] hepatic tumors,[86,220] cerebral aneurysms,[30] and aortic aneurysms.[189] In patients with tuberous sclerosis undergoing neurosurgery for epilepsy, anesthetic-related mortality was not reported.[38,212] Nonetheless, it seems prudent to evaluate these patients preoperatively for the presence of cardiac neoplasia, possible cardiac rhythm abnormalities, adequacy of pulmonary function, and perhaps adequacy of renal and hepatic function.

Neurofibromatosis

Von Recklinghausen's disease is an autosomal dominant trait occurring in 1 in 3000 births, with epilepsy being a common concomitant condition.[5,10] It involves tumor growth from Schwann cells and thus has protean manifestations. Problems relevant to anesthetic management[26] include a 66% incidence of tumors in the central nervous system,[167] increased incidence of meningioma and gliomas, cranial nerve dysfunction, pituitary dysfunction, and spinal cord dysfunction. The following have also been reported: airway compromise,[42,155,254] fibrosing alveolitis (in as many as 20% of patients) with cor pulmonale,[214,226] visceral hypertrophy, pheochromocytoma (in 1%),[138] genitourinary obstruction,[34] renal arterial stenosis,[138] prolonged neuromuscular blockade,[15,162,177,184,301] hydrocephalus,[231] cerebral aneurysms,[245] hypophosphatemic osteomalacia,[109,134] achalasia of the esophagus,[88,166] and atlantoaxial instability.[81]

Multiple Endocrine Adenomatosis

Problems relevant to anesthetic management that may be encountered with the three multiple endocrine adenomatosis syndromes include adrenocortical hyperplasia, insulinoma of the pancreas, medullary carcinoma of the thyroid with hypercalcitoninemia, pheochromocytoma, and parathyroid adenoma.[209]

Jervell and Lange-Nielsen Syndrome

Patients with this disease have deafness and a prolonged QTc interval in association with microcytic-hypochromic anemia and epilepsy. One patient was reported to have developed polymorphous ventricular tachycardia during induction of anesthesia with halothane.[3]

Sudden Death Syndrome

A significant cause of mortality in people with epilepsy is sudden death syndrome. Seven patients who were being studied in a large epilepsy surgery program died suddenly and unexpectedly without prior evidence of cardiac disease.[61] The incidence of sudden, unexpected death in this epilepsy program was five times higher than that reported in the general population. Unfortunately, little is presently known that will identify this high-risk subset of epileptic patients or prevent these deaths. The etiology presumably is a seizure-mediated cardiac dysrhythmia, most likely ventricular fibrillation. The pathogenesis most likely involves autonomic neural impulses secondary to seizures. This is supported by observations that seizures can be manifest as autonomic dysfunction.[137,293] When actually observed, seizure discharges have been noted to occasionally produce various manifestations including cardiac dysrhythmias, angina, neurogenic pulmonary edema, symptoms of pheochromocytoma, and sudden death. Although these manifestations could occur during anesthesia with potentially significant effects on patient stability during surgery, no cases have been reported.

Trauma History

Many patients who develop epilepsy have a history of trauma at a younger age. Part of the evaluation of such patients includes consideration of other injuries that may have occurred and the important subsequent sequelae.

Hypoglycemia and Hyperglycemia

The effects of fasting that resulted in hypoglycemia were studied in 22 patients with medically refractory epilepsy. Healthy individuals with similar serum glucose conentrations showed a diffuse background slowing of the EEG, whereas one third of the epileptic patients developed focal temporal lobe changes, including focal spike and slow wave activation. Hypoglycemic activation of EEG has been suggested as a technique for predicting the presence of abnormalities in patients considered for anterior temporal lobectomy[250]; however, it poses excessive risk because it has a low level of sensitivity.

Substantial data suggest that deleterious effects occur with hyperglycemia in association with cerebral lactic acidosis during ischemia.[235] Although seizures also produce cerebral lactic acidosis,[112] hyperglycemia in animals has not been shown to exacerbate the neuropathologic effects of seizures.[128,260] On the contrary, some evidence has been reported of metabolic[72] and morphologic[128] protection conferred by hyperglycemia during seizures.

Sleep Deprivation

Sleep deprivation appears to have an independent activating effect on local epileptogenicity.[59,76,180] It has been known for centuries that sleep and epilepsy have strong reciprocal influences.[180] This property has been advantageously used in epilepsy-monitoring programs. The pattern of seizure activity can provide helpful information about the localization of seizures and overall characteristics of the patient's epilepsy.[59,76] Thus epileptic patients who, for whatever reason, are sleep deprived might have an increased risk of seizure activation perioperatively.

ANESTHETIC CONSIDERATIONS IN STATUS EPILEPTICUS

After all standard therapy has failed or has been determined to have unacceptable side effects, most neurology textbooks recommend consulting an anesthesiologist for administration of general anesthesia to manage status epilepticus. Under these circumstances, what anesthetic should the neuroanesthesiologist administer? Unfortunately, there are no controlled clinical studies to adequately answer this question. However, several clinical series report experience with different anesthetic approaches. Anesthetic drugs that have been used successfully to stop status epilepticus include pentobarbital,[89,97,156,287] thiopental,[35,262] benzodiazepines,* isoflurane,[130,133,153,174,221] etomidate,[305] propofol,[161,302] ketamine,[85] enflurane,[197] halothane,[197,221] and althesin.[284] However, administration of volatile anesthetics outside the operating room is fraught with logistic problems.[130,133,221]

When general anesthesia is required to manage status epilepticus, a patient's outcome is thought to correlate more with the underlying disease than with success in stopping seizures.[133,287] One factor in this is the delay in initiating general anesthesia caused by the need to first try less potent drugs and the logistic problems in getting an anesthetic started in an ICU. Prolonged use of high-doses of barbiturates (i.e., for days or weeks) has been associated with barbiturate tolerance,[130,203] which may exacerbate the underlying seizure problem. In one case report, isoflurane was used to facilitate the withdrawal of barbiturates.[130] In addition, the neurochemical effects of such prolonged anesthetic use have never been evaluated. One study using animals suggests that prolonged anesthetic use can result in substantial increases in brain glycogen after only a few hours.[36] Moreover, the potential for prolonged volatile anesthesia to be organotoxic or to induce tolerance is unknown.

To help answer the question of whether anesthetic choice may alter seizure-induced brain damage,[132] the effects of isoflurane, thiopental, ketamine, and midazolam were assessed in rats undergoing mercaptopropionic-acid–induced or flurothyl-induced seizures. Midazolam resulted in less

---

*References 6, 22, 48, 58, 92, 171, 230, 278.

damage in the substantia nigra after seizures. No protective effect was suggested with isoflurane or thiopental, and, although a protective effect was suggested with ketamine, it was statistically insignificant. Unfortunately, this study revealed nothing about the anesthetic effects on seizure-induced damage in the limbic system. The ketamine data, however, are supported by other reports of the anticonvulsant or neuroprotective effects of ketamine in the limbic system during seizures in rodents.[52,227,288,289]

For the reasons previously given, the therapeutic approach in choosing an anesthetic agent for status epilepticus should first involve increasing doses of benzodiazepines or barbiturates. Only after this therapy fails should volatile anesthetic drugs be considered. Volatile anesthetics have the advantage of allowing continuous "real-time" titration to maintain a specific blood anticonvulsant level based on end-tidal gas monitoring. They are the only anticonvulsants with which this can be done. In one patient,[133] the monitoring of end-tidal volatile anesthetic concentration facilitated titration of the anticonvulsant anesthetic against EEG. In another patient, isoflurane use facilitated withdrawal of a prolonged barbiturate infusion on which the patient was suspected to be dependent.[130] Thus volatile anesthetics may have a role in closely titrating anticonvulsant therapy for seizures in situations where the duration of use can reasonably be expected to be short.

The standard approach to managing seizures with a general anesthetic is to use as little anesthetic as possible, while observing the patient closely for cessation of seizure and for hemodynamic compromise. Such patients must be tracheally intubated and mechanically ventilated. Optimally, continuous EEG should be monitored throughout anesthetic administration. If thiopental is used, 50 to 500 mg IV can be given as a loading dose (in an adult), followed by an intravenous infusion. The pharmacokinetic properties of thiopental suggest that the infusion rate initially should be higher and then should be decreased as indicated by EEG. Thus, after the loading dose, the infusion rate could be initially set at 500 to 1000 mg/hr and then slowly decreased to the lowest rate feasible. Repeated boluses, 100 to 500 mg, might be needed initially to maintain close titration. If isoflurane is used, it should be started at 0.2% to 0.3% inspired concentration and increased over 10 to 20 minutes as indicated by EEG and hemodynamic toleration. Determining the end point to guide drug titration can be difficult; for example, bursts occurring within a burst-suppression pattern on EEG can resemble epileptiform discharges. The decision about seizure control and EEG interpretation should be made jointly with the referring neurologist or epileptologist. After seizures are controlled and if the etiology is still unclear, reversible causes should be sought and corrected, after which anesthesia should be stopped. Otherwise, the anesthetic dose should be decreased periodically to permit assessment. If seizures continue to recur on anesthetic discontinuation, the next decision is whether to continue anesthesia, considering the many unknown effects, bioethical concerns, and the logistic and economic issues of prolonged anesthetic adminstration, compared with the effects of allowing seizures to continue or withdrawing life support.

ANESTHESIA FOR PREOPERATIVE PROCEDURES AND SEIZURE SURGERY
Radiologic Procedures

Patients being evaluated for seizure surgery may be required to undergo a variety of radiologic procedures, including CT, MR, or PET scans. Ordinarily, adult patients require no involvement of neuroanesthesiologists during these procedures. However, immobility is a requirement, and, for anxious or claustrophobic adults or for children, heavy sedation or general anesthesia may be required.

Preoperative Medication

For radiologic procedures, seizure activity is not provoked. Accordingly, a benzodiazepine is a suitable choice because of its anticonvulsant properties. Moreover, intravenous diazepam given before injection of contrast media has been reported to reduce the incidence of contrast-media–associated seizures in glioma patients.[205] Presumably, this effect would also occur with other benzodiazepines, such as midazolam or lorazepam. The exception is the amytal test, which is preceded by cerebral angiography. In this case no (or minimal) sedative drugs are used.

Monitoring

The patient's medical problems and the specific anesthetic chosen determine the type of monitoring required. Generally, EEG monitoring is not required.

Anesthetic Technique

Many anesthetic methods can be applied to facilitate acquisition of suitable neuroanatomic images, including no sedation, local anesthesia only (for invasive procedures), monitored anesthetic care with sedation, or general anesthesia.

Anesthetic Management

When choosing specific drugs, one should consider their proconvulsant or anticonvulsant properties. Generally, anticonvulsant anesthetics are preferred, because seizure-induced movement or nonconvulsive seizure activity compromise the study. Otherwise, the major issues in anesthetic management concern anesthetic administration outside the operating room, as discussed in detail elsewhere in this text.

Intracranial Electrode Insertion

Intracranial electrodes are used to maximize sensitivity and specificity in electrographic identification and localization of a seizure focus. There are two types of intracranial electrode techniques. One involves stereotactic insertion of electrodes through burr holes. The other involves craniotomy with application of strip or grid electrodes.

Preoperative Medication

Anticonvulsant medications are usually continued at the discretion of the epileptologist. Benzodiazepines can be reasonably included with preoperative sedative drugs. If electrocorticography is planned with epidural grid electrode placement, preoperative sedation is usually omitted.

Anesthetic Approaches

For stereotactic depth electrode insertion, at least four burr holes must be drilled, a stereotactic frame is applied, CT scan is obtained, and immobilization is maintained. Thus, although a local anesthetic approach theoretically is possible, this procedure is usually performed under general anesthesia. Epidural electrodes or grids are placed under general anesthesia.

Monitoring

Invasive monitoring techniques are generally not required for stereotactic electrode insertion unless indicated by other medical conditions. These patients usually require monitoring by sphygmomanometer, electrocardiogram (ECG), precordial stethoscope, and pulse oximeter. A Foley catheter generally is unnecessary. During electrode insertion, the EEG of each depth electrode can be monitored. For epidural electrode or grid placement, which involves a craniotomy, an arterial catheter also is usually inserted.

Anesthetic Management

The anesthetic technique used depends on the need for electrocorticographic monitoring in the operating room or after surgery. If intraoperative electrocorticography (ECoG) is planned, anesthetic induction is carried out with an ultrashort-acting barbiturate followed by maintenance based on a nitrous oxide/narcotic technique supplemented as required with a low dose of isoflurane or enflurane. Neuromuscular blockade is used. When stimulation of epileptogenic foci is requested, methohexital in 10 to 25 mg increments is administered intravenously.

If postoperative monitoring is planned, two operative procedures are performed: electrode insertion followed by craniotomy and resection of an epileptogenic focus. These procedures are separated by a period of observation with the patient awake.[98] In such cases, electrodes are removed outside of the OR and, when infection risk has decreased, the patient is electively scheduled for resective surgery.

Stereotactic depth electrode placement does not require intraoperative EEG monitoring. Thus an anesthetic with anticonvulsant properties is used. An ultrashort-acting thiobarbiturate is suitable for induction, followed by isoflurane, nitrous oxide, and/or moderate fentanyl doses, with neuromuscular blockade as needed.

Epidural electrodes are placed often with the use of intraoperative ECoG. No barbiturate or sedative agents are used during the first operative stage. Induction of anesthesia is carried out with fentanyl and droperidol only, and intubation is facilitated by a medium-acting nondepolarizing muscle relaxant. Muscle relaxants have a shorter duration of action in patients on chronic anticonvulsant medication,[255,342] and their effects usually subside before skin incision, thereby allowing a baseline to be established for sensorimotor response to stimulation. Anesthesia is maintained with a fentanyl infusion (2 to 8 μg/kg/min), nitrous oxide, and 0.25% end-tidal isoflurane. The cortical somatosensory and motor areas are defined intraoperatively. As muscle relaxants are not being used and coughing is to be avoided, the anesthesiologist must be aware that fentanyl requirements are increased up to fourfold in patients on chronic anticonvulsant therapy, as compared with nonepileptic patients.[267] An epidural Silastic patch with multiple ECoG electrodes is left in situ so that the eloquent (speech, memory) areas of the brain and their relationship to the seizure foci can be defined postoperatively when the patient is awake and there is no pharmacologic interference.

Postoperatively, both the patient's behavior and the ECoG or EEG are recorded continuously, displayed on the split screen of a television monitor in a specially designed room. The resection, if any, is carried out during a second surgical procedure with the usual general anesthesia suitable for craniotomy.

Thiopental Test

This procedure is performed in some epilepsy programs to provide further data regarding localization of seizure focus.[61a,128a] The procedure entails gradually increasing thiopental levels in the blood with continuous monitoring of the intracranial electrode EEG until a uniform neurologic end point (loss of corneal reflex) is attained. Thus the anesthetic administration is guided by specific protocol. The neuroanesthesiologist's primary contribution is to ensure that it is performed safely, to report when adverse effects mandate aborting a given test, and to devise appropriate methods to deal with concomitant medical problems.

Preoperative Medication

No preoperative medication is given for this procedure. The administration of anticonvulsant drugs is primarily at the discretion of the epileptologist.

Monitoring

Invasive monitoring is not required, and the procedure is done in the epilepsy suite. Patients require monitoring by sphygmomanometer, ECG, and pulse oximeter. The procedure is brief (30 minutes), and therefore a Foley catheter is unnecessary. Depth or scalp-electrode EEG can also be used. Esophageal pH monitoring has been suggested to be of value in patients with hiatal hernia although it has not been tested in a large series of patients.[131]

Anesthetic Technique and Management

A general anesthetic is inherent in the thiopental test although patients gradually progress from very light sedation to mild excitation to a deeper plane of anesthesia. This procedure requires the simultaneous attendance of and close cooperation between the epileptologist and neuroanesthesiologist. Patients are given increasing doses of intravenous thiopental. A suggested treatment protocol is thiopental 25 mg, every 30 seconds to a maximum dose of 1 g. In children weighing less than 40 kg, 0.3 to 0.4 mg/kg every 20 seconds is given to a maximum dose of 15 mg/kg. Thiopental is infused until an adverse side effect occurs (e.g., apnea or hypotension) or the patient sustains bilateral loss of corneal reflexes. The physiologic results of this procedure are summarized in Table 25-6. This procedure has proved to be safe with no serious morbidity observed and provides valuable information to assist the epileptologist and neurosurgeon in identifying a seizure focus.

During thiopental testing, patients cannot undergo endotracheal intubation because local anesthetic or high doses of thiopental would be required, thus preventing the procedure. If the patient requires intubation because a hiatal hernia prevents safe administration of the anesthetic, the neuroanesthesiologist has three choices: (1) not to perform the test, (2) have the patient intubated 24 hours before the test and monitored in an intensive care unit as the effects of local or general anesthetic agents needed for intubation subside, or (3) perform the test with compromise of the conflicting therapeutic priorities. One suggested approach to this dilemma is to pretreat the patient and then monitor esophageal pH during administration of thiopental with cricoid pressure, while being prepared to rapidly anesthetize, paralyze, and intubate the well-oxygenated patient in the event of a sustained decrease in esophageal pH.[131]

Seizure Surgery

Patients scheduled for seizure surgery generally undergo seizure focus resection, which usually involves a temporal lobectomy or interruption of the seizure pathway. Less frequently, surgery may involve a hemispherectomy or resection of an extratemporal focus.

Preoperative Medication

These patients are extensively evaluated, having undergone the previously described first two evaluation phases in an epilepsy surgery program. By the time they arrive at the operating room, substantial neurologic and psychosocial information is available to the neuroanesthesiologist. Anticonvulsants are generally given preoperatively, but the doses are usually decreased by 50% or more at the discretion of the epileptologist or neurosurgical team (most antiepileptic drugs are not available in intravenous forms). If stimulation of epileptogenic foci is unnecessary, a benzodiazepine[197] or a moderate dose of narcotic or other similar agent may be preferred. If awake craniotomy or stimulation of epileptogenic foci under general anesthesia is anticipated, premedication is limited to an antacid and an antiemetic. In these instances, the preoperative visit becomes extremely important. The neuroanesthesiologist should attempt to create a good rapport with the patient, alleviating fears through an explanation of the anticipated events.

Monitoring

Before the patient presents for the operation, the intracranial EEG electrodes are generally removed to decrease the risk of infection. Monitors required include the sphygmomanometer, ECG, precordial Doppler, arterial catheter, and Foley catheter. The use of a central venous catheter for management of air embolism is controversial because patients usually are supine or have minimal head elevation during surgery. Venous air embolism has not been reported as a significant problem. Thus a central venous catheter may be inserted, but only after careful consideration of its risks in a given patient in the context of a relatively low chance of needing it. Monitoring for awake craniotomies has to be as limited as possible to avoid adding to the obvious stress inherent in this technique. ECG, automatic sphygmomanometer, oxygen saturation, and end-tidal carbon dioxide are standard. An apnea monitor is useful. Invasive devices

TABLE 25-6
Thiopental Tests at the University of Pittsburgh Epilepsy Center*

| | Age (yr) | Weight (kg) | Dose Thiopental (mg) | Systolic Pressure (mm Hg) | | Heart Rate (min^{-1}) | | | Lowest Sao$_2$[†] (%) |
				Pre-Thiopental	Minimum Post-Thiopental	Pre-Thiopental	Minimum	Maximum	
Mean	29.9	73	568	118	107	75	73	81	98
Standard deviation	6.5	16	201	12	11	12	10	11	4
Minimum	17	36	200	88	80	52	50	60	67
Maximum	43	114	1000	150	136	110	98	110	100

Incidence of Sao$_2$ < 95%[†]	9/65	Incidence of nausea	0/72
Incidence of airway intervention[‡]	31/72	Incidence of emesis	0/72

*The study retrospectively reviewed 72 anesthetic records to determine anesthesia-related morbidity.
†Where recorded, all but one patient maintained Sao$_2$ >90%. The patient with the minimum Sao$_2$ of 67% became apneic and responded to bag-valve-mask 100% oxygen ventilation. A repeat thiopental test 9 days later was uneventful.
‡Two patients required brief bag-valve-mask ventilation. All others required opening of an obstructed airway with the jaw-lift maneuver.

such as arterial catheter or Foley catheter are often omitted initially but can be inserted when sedation-analgesia has been initiated.

Anesthetic Technique

The choice of anesthesia depends on two main requirements of the neurosurgical team. First is the need for intraoperative ECoG and second is the intention to perform a craniotomy, either with general anesthesia and tracheal intubation or with local anesthesia and conscious sedation.

If general anesthesia is used without electrocorticography, the anesthetic regimen is designed to maintain suppression of seizure activity and provide optimal operating conditions. Thus an ultrashort-acting barbiturate followed by isoflurane, a moderate dose of an opioid, and possibly nitrous oxide is one preferred anesthetic technique. If a general anesthetic is used with intraoperative electrocorticography, the method of induction may be the same, but the maintenance anesthetic should generally consist of nitrous oxide and a narcotic with or without a lower supplemental dose of isoflurane or enflurane. When stimulation of epileptogenic foci is planned, a common, reasonably dependable approach is to use methohexital, not as an induction agent, but intraoperatively in 10 to 25 mg increments given during nitrous oxide–narcotic anesthesia with neuromuscular blockade.

The usual and, in the author's opinion, only valid reason for awake craniotomy (i.e., craniotomy with local anesthesia and conscious sedation) is to facilitate electrocorticography (ECoG). The neuroanesthesiologist should be involved in deciding the appropriateness of this procedure. One must assess the ability of an individual patient to tolerate the procedure awake. There is significant associated discomfort and possibly pain, which must be explained very clearly to the patient. Inability to comprehend this (e.g., in mentally retarded patients or children) is a relative contraindication to awake craniotomy. The upper airway should be assessed; a patient in whom difficulty with tracheal intubation is predicted may not be a suitable candidate for awake craniotomy because intubation occasionally is required emergently, even with the patient in the awkward position required for surgery. Another factor is the anesthesiologist's experience; local anesthesia with conscious-sedation analgesia for craniotomy should not be used without proper training.[280]

The optimal anesthetic approach to seizure surgery is still controversial. No prospective controlled trials have conclusively demonstrated the superiority of awake craniotomy vs. general anesthesia in the management of these patients. In one retrospective review of 354 patients undergoing craniotomy for surgical treatment of epilepsy with conscious-sedation analgesia,[9] no perioperative morbidity or mortality could be attributed to the anesthetic. However, that technique proved unsuitable for seven patients, and general anesthesia had to be used. During conscious-sedation analgesia, the intraoperative problems encountered

included convulsions (16%) and nausea and vomiting (8%). Other less frequent problems included excessive sedation (3%), "tight brain" (1.4%), and local anesthetic toxicity (2%). The authors concluded that local anesthesia with conscious sedation provides suitable conditions for accurate ECoG recording. However, the potential for pharmacologic interference with the intraoperative ECoG tracings recently has been demonstrated, such as beta activity triggered by propofol.[69]

Anesthetic Management—General Anesthesia

Ultrafast-acting thiobarbiturates are generally recommended for induction. If electrocorticography is planned, either etomidate or methohexital is a suitable alternative.

If electrocorticography is not planned, an anticonvulsant anesthetic maintenance regimen such as isoflurane with or without nitrous oxide or a moderate-dose opioid should be used. Consideration in anesthetic management must be given to the effects of long-term anticonvulsant therapy that increase the dosage requirements for opioids[267] and neuromuscular blocking agents.[200,266] Hyperventilation can produce or potentiate seizure activity[44,79,146,168]; therefore, unless required for surgical exposure, it should not be used. During intraoperative electrocorticography, patients should be maintained with a nitrous-oxide–based or enflurane-based technique with added methohexital as indicated.

If electrocorticography is planned, nitrous-oxide–narcotic techniques are preferable, and both isoflurane and halothane should be avoided.[228] Enflurane has been observed to produce paroxysms of synchronous high-voltage spikes although both isoflurane and enflurane might distort the electrocorticogram and confound accurate identification of the seizure focus.[116] When used judiciously, enflurane may effectively synchronize and activate an epileptogenic focus, making it easier to identify.[116] Methohexital and alfentanil have also been used as activating agents.[232a,299] Methohexital has been used both preoperatively and intraoperatively and was observed in 87% of cases to cause selective activation of the epileptogenic focus during acute electrocorticography. As little as 25 mg of methohexital was required to induce activation.[299] Although methohexital is reported to be a safe, reliable agent for activating epileptogenic foci during electrocorticography, additional reports from other centers are required to confirm this. Methohexital can also be used for intraoperative electrocorticography under general anesthesia.[83,299] However, methohexital can induce seemingly "new" spike foci in nonepileptogenic tissue in 43% of patients.[83] In another report[103] 34 patients underwent preoperative and perioperative EEG activation with methohexital. Preoperative spike localization with methohexital was congruent with perioperative recordings in most cases. Two of these patients received methohexital in doses large enough to render the EEG nearly isoelectric in normal tissue. Areas of abnormal spiking activity were refractory to the effects of methohexital.

In positioning these patients, special attention should be

given to the facial nerve because idiopathic peripheral facial nerve palsy was reported in 4 of 110 patients undergoing temporal lobe resection.[7] Peripheral nerve or geniculate ganglion injury during resection was suspected.

Emergence after craniotomy for seizure surgery is similar to that for other types of intracranial surgery and involves prevention of postoperative hypertension, facilitation of rapid emergence, and prevention of excessive coughing. In planning for the completion of the procedure, the sometimes dramatic antiepileptic-drug–induced decrease in the duration of neuromuscular blocking agents and opioid drugs should be anticipated.

Anesthetic Management—Conscious Analgesia

This approach has been described in detail by Trop et al.[280] and by others.* Patients position themselves on the operating table so they are as comfortable as possible. Although they need to be restrained, a small amount of movement should be allowed to maintain comfort throughout this long procedure. Careful attention is paid to the protection of pressure points, which should be padded. Oxygen is delivered through nasal prongs while capnography can be performed via an 18 to 20 g Teflon catheter in one nasal prong. Before the surgeon starts skin preparation and application of the drapes, fentanyl 0.5 to 0.75 μg/kg and droperidol 0.15 mg/kg are administered intravenously. At this time, an indwelling urinary catheter is inserted although some prefer to limit the amount of IV fluids and withhold the catheter. Before surgical incision, local anesthesia is injected subcutaneously into the scalp. Some patients do not require further sedation at incision. However, the painful parts of the procedure should be anticipated; they mostly occur early during surgical exposure. Immediately before these episodes, the patient needs reassurance and, possibly, supplementation of sedation-analgesia with fentanyl in 25 to 100 μg IV boluses, titrated to maintain a comfortable level of analgesia and a respiratory rate of 12 breaths/min. In addition, the technique can be varied by using a continuous infusion of fentanyl titrated to a respiratory rate of 12 breaths/min.[164] More recently, propofol has been used; initially a bolus of 1 mg/kg is given, and this is usually followed by an infusion at 75 μg/kg/min. In case of insufficient sedation, supplementary boluses of 0.5 mg/kg are added, and the infusion rate is gradually increased to 125 μg/kg/min.[69]

Most patients tolerate the procedure, especially when the anesthesiologist has been able to establish good rapport and is able to predict and control painful stimulation. However, there may be complications: some patients become increasingly uncooperative and agitated, objecting to the continuation of the procedure. A low dose of methohexital or propofol is indicated for this situation to produce loss of consciousness that is brief enough not to interfere with planned electrocorticography. More commonly, patients experience nausea or vomiting, which may be exacerbated

*References 9, 94, 95, 164, 207, 210, 251, 296.

by surgical stimulation, such as stripping of the dura or temporal lobe or meningeal vessel manipulation, or by insufficient analgesia combined with hypovolemia. Nausea and vomiting can be controlled with metoclopramide, 5 to 10 mg, or droperidol, 1.25 to 2.5 mg, and deepening of the analgesia. Obviously, these epileptic patients are at risk for sudden onset of seizures. This may be due to decreased levels of anticonvulsant and/or direct stimulation of specific cortical or subcortical structures. The seizures can be focal or general and are usually self-limiting or stop when the electrical stimulation is discontinued, but, if prolonged, they should be controlled with intravenous methohexital in increments of 0.5 to 1 mg/kg. If the seizures occur near the end of the procedure after the completion of the ECoG, benzodiazepines may be used. During the postictal period, if airway control is in jeopardy, tracheal intubation may become necessary. To achieve a slack brain required for intracranial surgery, the patient should be kept moderately hypovolemic; IV fluid is kept to a minimum, being limited to 50 ml/hr (especially if no Foley catheter has been inserted). Careful attention also should be paid to replacing blood loss; IV fluid or blood products must be administered before the usual signs of tachycardia or hypotension develop.

The intracranial components of this procedure, that is, ECoG, brain resection, and repeat ECog (to confirm extent of surgical resection), are not painful. However, when closure of the craniotomy is started, the patient has been in the same position on the operating table for many hours and is exhausted. The airway may become compromised and may need to be controlled, or the patient may become restless and titration of intravenous benzodiazepine may be required during this final stage. Anticonvulsant medications usually are resumed before wound closure to achieve therapeutic levels before the end of the procedure.

POSTOPERATIVE CONSIDERATIONS

Blood levels of an antiepileptic drug can be significantly affected by anesthetics and the changes in body physiology resulting from the surgery itself. These effects include changes in the volume of distribution of the antiepileptic drug, enzyme saturation, binding competition (both at the neuroreceptor level and with carrier substances such as albumin), pharmacokinetics, and, rarely, pharmacodynamics. The blood level of carbamazepine, the most notorious drug, frequently doubles after surgery and returns to normal after 7 to 10 days. The level of phenytoin can also increase substantially, and other drugs produce more complex problems such as bound and unbound levels moving in opposite directions. The blood levels of antiepileptic drugs should be obtained before surgery and followed closely after surgery. Increasing levels of antiepileptic drugs may cause clinical toxicity, which may be confused with an intracranial complication. Conversely, if the antiepileptic drug levels decrease unexpectedly, seizures could be precipitated, which would complicate postoperative management.

SUMMARY

Epilepsy is a common disease that has a major effect on both individuals carrying the diagnosis and society as a whole. A substantial research effort is striving to develop effective antiepileptic drugs. Unfortunately, results are occasionally unsatisfactory or the side effects are sometimes unacceptable. Accordingly, surgical management of this disease, particularly when the epilepsy focus can be localized, continues to evolve. Neuroanesthesiologists can help improve strategies for managing epilepsy using a wide array of drugs. Each of these drugs has important effects on seizure genesis or suppression and interacts with epilepsy and with concurrently administered antiepileptic drugs in unique ways. Consequently, neuroanesthesiologists are in an important position to make suggestions regarding the pathogenesis of epilepsy and methods of evaluation and treatment.

The fields of epilepsy and epilepsy surgery continue to be somewhat controversial. One of the more impor-

tant of these concerns is the most appropriate anesthetic approach for seizure surgery, that is, whether to use general anesthesia or conscious analgesia with local anesthesia. Other disputed areas include the optimal anesthetic technique, whether anesthetic-induced seizure activity can cause brain damage, and the appropriateness of inducing a seizure with an anesthetic drug during electrocorticography. In addition, substantial laboratory research still is needed on neurotransmitter involvement in epilepsy, electrophysiology of epilepsy, clinical applicability of kindling and other methods used in animal models of epilepsy, and choice of anesthetics in the management of status epilepticus. With increasing numbers of epilepsy centers, neuroanesthesiologists are likely to have greater involvement in clinical programs, contribute to the determination of optimal clinical protocols, and participate in efforts to answer some of these important questions about epilepsy.

Acknowledgments

The secretarial assistance of Charlotte Dietrich and the editorial assistance of Nancy Arora in preparing this chapter are gratefully acknowledged.

References

1. Aasly J, Blom S, Silfvenius H et al: Effects of amobarbital and methohexital on epileptic activity in mesial temporal structures in epileptic patients. An EEG study with depth electrodes, *Acta Neurol Scand* 70:423-431, 1984.

2. Ackermann RF, Engel J Jr, Phelps ME: Identification of seizure-mediating brain structures with the deoxyglucose method: studies of human epilepsy with positron emission tomography, and animal seizure models with contact autoradiography, *Adv Neurol* 44:921-934, 1986.

3. Adu-Gyamfi Y, Said A, Chowdhary UM et al: Anaesthetic-induced ventricular tachyarrhythmia in Jervell and Lange-Nielsen syndrome, *Can J Anaesth* 38:345-346, 1991.

4. Aird RB, Masland RL, Woodbury DM: *The epilepsies: a critical review,* New York, 1984, Raven Press, pp 201-243.

5. Aird RB, Masland RL, Woodbury DM: *The epilepsies: a critical review,* New York, 1984, Raven Press, pp 117-134.

6. Albano A, Reisdorff EJ, Wiegenstein JG: Rectal diazepam in pediatric sta-

tus epilepticus, *Am J Emerg Med* 7:168-172, 1989.

7. Anderson J, Awad IA, Hahn JF: Delayed facial nerve palsy after temporal lobectomy for epilepsy: report of four cases and discussion of possible mechanisms, *Neurosurgery* 28:453-456, 1991.

8. Anis NA, Berry SC, Burton NR et al: The dissociative anesthetics, ketamine and phencyclidine, selectively reduce excitation of central mammalian neurons by N-methyl-aspartate, *Br J Pharmacol* 79:565-575, 1983.

9. Archer DP, McKenna JM, Morin L et al: Conscious-sedation analgesia during craniotomy for intractable epilepsy: a review of 354 consecutive cases, *Can J Anaesth* 35:338-344, 1988.

10. Arkhipov BA, Sadovskaia IuE: Epileptic paroxysms in Recklinghausen's neurofibromatsis, *Zh Nevropatol Psikhiatr* 90:20-23, 1990.

11. Awad IA, Katz A, Hahn JF et al: Extent of resection in temporal lobectomy for epilepsy. I. Interobserver analysis and correlation with seizure outcome, *Epilepsia* 30:756-762, 1989.

12. Awad IA, Rosenfeld J, Ahl J et al: Intractable epilepsy and structural lesions of the brain: mapping, resection strategies, and seizure outcome, *Epilepsia* 32:179-186, 1991.

13. Baiker-Heberlein M, Kenins P, Kikillus H et al: Investigations on the site of the central nervous action of the short-acting hypnotic agent R-(+)-ethyl-l-(a-methyl-benzyl) imidazole-5-carboxylate (etomidate) in cats, *Anaesthesist* 28:78-84, 1979.

14. Baraka A, Haroun S: Grand mal seizures following fentanyl- lidocaine (letter), *Anesthesiology* 62:206, 1985.

15. Baraka A: Myasthenic response to muscle relaxants in von Recklinghausen's disease, *Br J Anaesth* 46:701-703, 1974.

16. Barra D, Dru M, Truffa-Bachi J: Generalized seizure induced by methohexital, *Ann Fr Anesth Reanim* 6:120-121, 1987.

17. Barraclough BM: The suicide rate of epilepsy, *Acta Psychiatr Scand* 76:339-345, 1987.

18. Baumgartner C, Deecke L: Magnetoencephalography in clinical epilep-

tology and epilepsy research, *Brain Topogr* 2:203-219, 1990.

19. Beemer GH, Dawson PJ, Bjorksten AR et al: Early postoperative seizures in neurosurgical patients administered atracurium and isoflurane, *Anaesth Intens Care* 17:504-509, 1989.

20. Beghi E, Di Mascio R, Tognoni G: Drug treatment of epilepsy. Outlines, criticism and perspectives, *Drugs* 31:249-265, 1986.

21. Belknap JK, Laursen SE, Crabbe JC: Ethanol and nitrous oxide produce withdrawal-induced convulsions by similar mechanisms in mice, *Life Sci* 41:2033-2040, 1977.

22. Bell HE, Bertino JS Jr: Constant diazepam infusion in the treatment of continuous seizure activity, *Drug Intell Clin Pharm* 18:965-970, 1984.

23. Bennett DR, Madsen JA, Jordan WS et al: Ketamine anesthesia in brain-damaged epileptics: electroencephalographic and clinical observations, *Neurology* 23:449-460, 1973.

24. Benthuysen JL, Stanley TH: Concerning the possible nature of reported fentanyl seizures (letter), *Anesthesiology* 62:205, 1985.

25. Bernstein J, Robbins TO: Renal involvement in tuberous sclerosis, *Ann NY Acad Sci* 615:36-49, 1991.

26. Berryhill RE: Skin and bone disorders. In Katz J, Benumof J, Kadis LB, editors: *Anesthesia and uncommon diseases,* Philadelphia 1981, WB Saunders, pp 562-587.

27. Bidzinski J: Temporal lobectomy, *Acta Neurochir Suppl (Wien)* 50:119-121, 1990.

28. Bjrnaes H: Consequences of severe epilepsy: psychosocial aspects, *Acta Neurol Scand Suppl* 117:28-33, 1988.

29. Blume WT: Principles of clinical investigation of surgical patients, *Int Anesthesiol Clin* 24:47-73, 1986.

30. Blumenkopf B, Huggins MJ: Tuberous sclerosis and multiple intracranial aneurysms: case report, *Neurosurgery* 17:797-800, 1985.

31. Bonati M, Marraro G, Celardo A et al: Thiopental efficacy in phenobarbital-resistant neonatal seizures, *Dev Pharmacol Ther* 15:16-20, 1990.

32. Bowdle TA: Myoclonus following sufentanil without EEG seizure activity, *Anesthesiology* 67:593-595, 1987.

33. Bredhal C: Seizures and opistotonus after propofol anesthesia. A possible connection, *Ugeskr Laeger* 52:748-749, 1990.

34. Brooks PT, Scally JK: Bladder neurofibromas causing ureteric obstruction in von Recklinghausen's disease, *Clin Radiol* 36:537-538, 1985.

35. Brown A, Horton J: Status epilepticus treated by intravenous infusion of thiopentone sodium, *Br Med J* 1:27-28, 1967.

36. Brunner EA, Passonneau JV, Molstad C: The effect of volatile anesthetics on levels of metabolites and on metabolic rate in rat brain, *J Neurochem* 18:2301-2316, 1971.

37. Burchiel KJ, Stockard JJ, Myers RR et al: Metabolic and electrophysiologic mechanisms in the initiation and termination of enflurane-induced seizures in man and cats, *Electroencephalogr Clin Neurophysiol* 38:555, 1975.

38. Bye AM, Matheson JM, Tobias VH et al: Selective epilepsy surgery in tuberous sclerosis, *Aust Paediatr* 25:243-245, 1989.

39. Cahan LD, Engel J Jr: Surgery for epilepsy: a review, *Acta Neurol Scand* 73:551-560, 1986.

40. Cain DP, Corcoran ME: Epileptiform effects of met-enkephalin beta-endorphin and morphine: kindling of generalized seizures and potentiation of epileptiform effects by handling, *Brain Res* 338:327-336, 1985.

41. Cascino GD, Jack CR, Parisi JE et al: Magnetic resonance imaging based on volume studies in temporal lobe epilepsy: pathological correlations, *Ann Neurol* 30:31-36, 1991.

42. Chang-lo M: Laryngeal involvement in von Recklinghausen's disease: a case report and review of the literature, *Laryngoscope* 87:435, 1977.

43. Channon S, Daum I, Polkey CE: The effect of categorization on verbal memory after temporal lobectomy, *Neuropsychologia* 27:777-785, 1989.

44. Chater SN, Simpson KH: Effect of passive hyperventilation on seizure duration in patients undergoing electroconvulsive therapy, *Br J Anaesth* 60:70-73, 1988.

45. Chen L, Huang L-YM: Sustained potentiation of NMDA receptor mediated glutamate responses through activation of protein kinase C by a mu

opioid, *Soc Neurosci Abstr* 17:957, 1991.

46. Cheng JG, Xie XK: A study on opioid peptides in CSF of patients with epilepsy, *Epilepsy Res* 6:141-145, 1990.

47. Chilvers CR, Laurie PS: Successful use of propofol in status epilepticus (letter), *Anaesthesia* 45:995-996, 1990.

48. Chiulli DA, Terndrup TE, Kanter RK: The influence of diazepam or lorazepam on the frequency of endotracheal intubation in childhood status epilepticus, *J Emerg Med* 9:13-17, 1991.

49. Chugani HT, Ackermann RF, Chugani DC et al: Opioid-induced epileptogenic phenomena: anatomical, behavioral, and electroencephalographic features, *Ann Neurol* 15:361-368, 1984.

50. Chung MY, Walczak TS, Lewis DV, et al: Temporal lobectomy and independent bitemporal interictal activity: what degree of lateralization is sufficient? *Epilepsia* 32:195-201, 1991.

51. Commission on Classification and Terminology of the International League Against Epilepsy: Proposal for revised clinical and electroencephalographic classification of epileptic seizures, *Epilepsia* 22:489-501, 1981.

52. Clifford DB, Olney JW, Benz AM et al: Ketamine phencyclidine, and MK-801 protect against kainic acid-induced seizure-related brain damage, *Epilepsia* 31:382-390, 1990.

53. Clifford DB, Zormuski CF, Olney JW: Ketamine and MK-801 prevent degeneration of thalamic neurons induced by focal cortical seizures, *Exp Neurol* 105:272-279, 1989.

54. Collins RC, Lothman EW, Olney JW: Status epilepticus in the limbic system: biochemical and pathological changes, *Adv Neurol* 34:277-288, 1983.

55. Corrigall WA: Opiates and the hippocampus: a review of the functional and morphological evidence, *Pharmacol Biochem Behav* 18:255-262, 1983.

56. Corsellis JAN, Bruton CJ: Neuropathology of status epilepticus in humans, *Adv Neurol* 34:129-140, 1983.

57. Cosnett JE, Gibb GH: Tuberous sclerosis and cardiac arrhythmias in three Zulu patients, *Br Med J* 2:672, 1969.

58. Crisp CB, Gannon R, Knauft F: Continuous infusion of midazolam hydrochloride to control status epilepticus, *Clin Pharm* 7:322-324, 1988.

59. Dahl M, Dam M: Sleep and epilepsy, *Ann Clin Res* 17:235-242, 1985.

60. Dasheiff RM, Rosenbek J, Matthews C et al: Epilepsy surgery improves regional glucose metabolism on PET scan. A case report, *J Neurol* 234:283-288, 1987.

61. Dasheiff RM: Sudden unexpected death in epilepsy: a series from an epilepsy surgery program and speculation on the relationship to sudden cardiac death, *J Clin Neurophysiol* 8:216-222, 1991.

61a. Dasheiff RM, Kofke WA: Evaluation of the thiopental test in epilepsy surgery patients, *Epilepsy Res* 15:253-258, 1993.

62. DeWolf AM, Chang JL, Larson CE et al: Enflurane-induced grand mal seizures during otic microsurgery, *Anesth Prog* 31:136-137, 1984.

63. Debonnel G, Beauchesne L, de Montigny C: Domoic acid, the alleged "mussel toxin," might produce its neurotoxic effect through kainate receptor activation: an electrophysiological study in the dorsal hippocampus, *Can J Physiol Pharmacol* 67:29-33, 1989.

64. Delgado-Escueta AV, Walsh GO: Type I complex partial seizures of hippocampal origin: excellent results of anterior temporal lobectomy, *Neurology* 35:143-154, 1985.

65. Delgado-Escueta AV, Wasterlain C, Treiman DM et al: Management of status epilepticus, *N Engl J Med* 306:1337-1340, 1982.

66. Delgado-Escueta AV, Wasterlain C, Trieman DM et al: Status epilepticus: summary, *Adv Neurol* 34:537-541, 1983.

67. De Riu PL, Mameli O, Tolu E: Comparison of the effect of althesin with diazepam and thiopental sodium on cortical and subcortical epileptic activity in the rat, *Pharmacol Res Commun* 19:59-68, 1987.

68. Dossi F, Marconi AM, Riegler P et al: Renal involvement in tuberous sclerosis, *Adv Exp Med Biol* 252:65-71, 1989.

69. Drummond JC, Iragui-Modoz VJ, Alksne CJ et al: Masking of epileptiform activity by propofol during seizure surgery, *Anesthesiology* 76:652-654, 1992.

70. Dua AK, Pinsky C, LaBella FS: Mu- and delta-opioid receptor-mediated epileptoid responses in morphine-dependent and non-dependent rats, *Electroencephalogr Clin Neurophysiol* 61:569-572, 1985.

71. Duchowny MS: Surgery for intractable epilepsy: issues and outcome, *Pediatrics* 84:886-894, 1989.

72. Dwyer BE, Wasterlain CG: Neonatal seizures in monkeys and rabbits: brain glucose depletion in the face of normoglycemia, prevention by glucose loads, *Pediatr Res* 19:992-995, 1985.

73. Ebrahim Z, Bulkley R, Roth S: Carbamazepine therapy and neuromuscular blockade with atracurium or vecuronium, *Anesth Analg* 67:S55, 1988.

74. Ebrahim ZY, DeBoer GE, Luders H et al: Effect of etomidate on the electroencephalogram of patients with epilepsy, *Anesth Analg* 65:1004-1006, 1986.

75. Eich E: Epilepsy and state specific memory, *Acta Neurol Scand Suppl* 109:15-21, 1986.

76. Ellingson RJ, Wilken K, Bennett DR: Efficacy of sleep deprivation as an activation procedure in epilepsy patients, *J Clin Neurophysiol* 1:83-101, 1984.

77. Engel J Jr: The role of neuroimaging in the surgical treatment of epilepsy, *Acta Neurol Scand Suppl* 117:84-89, 1988.

78. Engel J Jr: *Seizures in epilepsy,* Philadelphia, 1989, FA Davis.

79. Esquivel E, Chaussain M, Plouin P et al: Physical exercise and voluntary hyperventilation in childhood absence epilepsy, *Electroencephalogr Clin Neurophysiol* 79:127-132, 1991.

80. Fariello RG: Epileptogenic properties of enflurane and their clinical interpretation, *Electroencephalogr Clin Neurophysiol* 48:595-598, 1980.

81. Ferner RE, Honavar M, Gullan RW: Spinal neurofibroma presenting as atlanto-axial subluxation in von Recklinghausen neurofibromatosis, *Neurofibromatosis* 2:43-46, 1989.

82. Ferrer-Allado T, Berchnre VL, Dymond A et al: Ketamine-induced electroconvulsive phenomena in the human limbic and thalamic regions, *Anesthesiology* 38:333-344, 1973.

83. Fiol ME, Torres F, Gates JR et al: Methohexital (Brevital) effect on electrocorticogram may be misleading, *Epilepsia* 31:524-528, 1990.

84. Fischer JH, Raineri DL: Pentobarbital anesthesia for status epilepticus, *Clin Pharm* 6:601-602, 1987.

85. Fisher MMcD: Use of ketamine hydrochloride in the treatment of convulsions, *Anaesth Intens Care* 2:266-268, 1974.

86. Fleury P, Smits N, van Baal S: The incidence of hepatic hamartomas in tuberous sclerosis. Evaluation by ultrasonography, *Fortschr Geb Rontgenstr Nuklearmed* 146:694-696, 1987.

87. Foote F, Gale K: Proconvulsant effect of morphine on seizures induced by pentylenetetrazol in the rat, *Eur J Pharmacol* 105:179-184, 1984.

88. Foster PN, Stewart M, Lowe JS et al: Achalasia like disorder of the oesophagus in von Recklinghausen's neurofibromatosis, *Gut* 28:1522-1526, 1987.

89. Frost JJ, Mayberg HS, Fisher RS et al: Mu-opiate receptors measured by positron emission tomography are increased in temporal lobe epilepsy, *Ann Neurol* 23:231-237, 1988.

90. Gallagher TJ, Galindo A, Richey ET: Inhibition of seizure activity during enflurane anesthesia, *Anesth Analg* 57:130-132, 1978.

91. Gancher S, Laxer KD, Krieger W: Activation of epileptogenic activity by etomidate, *Anesthesiology* 61:616-618, 1984.

92. Giang DW, McBride MC: Lorazepam versus diazepam for the treatment of status epilepticus, *Pediatr Neurol* 4:358-361, 1988.

93. Gibbs JL: The heart and tuberous sclerosis. An echocardiographic and electrocardiographic study, *Br Heart J* 54:596-599, 1985.

94. Girvin JP: Neurosurgical considerations and general methods for craniotomy under local anesthesia, *Int Anesth Clin* 24:89-114, 1986.

95. Girvin JP: Resection of intracranial lesions under local anesthesia, *Int Anesth Clin* 24:133-155, 1986.

96. Gjedde A, Evans AC: PET studies of domoic acid poisoning in humans: excitotoxic destruction of brain glutamatergic pathways, revealed in measurements of glucose metabolism by positron emission tomography, *Can Dis Wkly Rep* 16 (suppl 1E):105-109, 1990.

97. Goldberg MA, McIntyre HB: Barbi-

turates in the treatment of status epilepticus, *Adv Neurol* 34:499-503, 1983.

98. Goldring S, Gregorie EM, Tempelhoff R: Surgery of epilepsy. In Symon L, Thomas DGT, Clarke K, consulting editors: Neurosurgery. In Dudley H, Carter D, Russell RCG, general editors: *Rob and Smith's operative surgery,* London, 1989, Butterworths, pp 427-442.

99. Goroszeniuk T, Albin M, Jones RM: Generalized grand mal seizure after recovery from uncomplicated fentanyl-etomidate anesthesia, *Anesth Analg* 65:979-981, 1986.

100. Green RC, Adler JR, Erba G: Epilepsy surgery in children, *J Child Neurol* 3:155-166, 1988.

101. Guldvog B, Lyning Y, Hauglie-Hanssen E et al: Surgical versus medical treatment for epilepsy. I. Outcome related to survival, seizures, and neurologic deficit, *Epilepsia* 32:375-388, 1991.

102. Hansen HC, Drenck NE: Generalized seizures after etomidate anaesthesia (letter), *Anaesthesia* 43:805-806, 1988.

103. Hardiman O, Coughlan A, O'Moore B et al: Interictal spike localisation with methohexitone: preoperative activation and surgical follow-up, *Epilepsia* 28:335-339, 1987.

104. Harrison JL: Postoperative seizures after isoflurane anesthesia, *Anesth Analg* 65:1235-1236, 1986.

105. Helgason CM, Bergen D, Bleck TP et al: Infarction after surgery for focal epilepsy: manipulation hemiplegia revisited, *Epilepsia* 28:340-345, 1987.

106. Helmy ES, Tripplet R: Phenytoin syndrome developing after administration of dilantin for an enflurane-induced seizure, *J Oral Maxillofac Surg* 46:52-58, 1988.

107. Henriksen O: Surgical treatment of epilepsy. Clinical aspects in children, *Acta Neurol Scand Suppl* 117:47-51, 1988.

108. Henriksen SJ, Bloom FE, McCoy F et al: b-Endorphin induces nonconvulsive limbic seizures, *Proc Natl Acad Sci USA* 75:5221-5225, 1978.

109. Hogan DB, Anderson C, MacKenzie RA et al: Hypophosphatemic osteomalacia complicating von Recklinghausen's neurofibromatosis: increase in spinal density on treatment, *Bone* 7:9-12, 1986.

110. Hong JS, McGinty JF, Grimes L et al: Seizure-induced alterations in the metabolism of hippocampal opioid peptides suggest opioid modulation of seizure-related behaviors, *Natl Inst Drug Abuse Res Monogr Ser* 82:48-66, 1988.

111. Horsley V: Brain surgery, *Br Med J* 2:670-675, 1886.

112. House DC: Metabolic response to status epilepticus in the rat, cat, and mouse, *Can J Physiol Pharmacol* 57:205-212, 1978.

113. Huber Z: The critical evaluation of the late results after temporal lobectomy performed because of medically refractory complex partial epilepsy (CPE), *Zentralbl Neurochir* 51:78-81, 1990.

114. Hymes JA: Seizure activity during isoflurane anesthesia, *Anesth Analg* 64:367-368, 1985.

115. Ingram MD, Sclabassi RJ, Cook DR et al: Cardiovascular and electroencephalographic effects of laudanosine in "nephrectomized" cats, *Br J Anaesth* 58:14S-18S, 1986.

116. Ito BM, Sato S, Kufta CV et al: Effect of isoflurane and enflurane on the electrocorticogram of epileptic patients, *Neurology* 38:924-928, 1988.

117. Ivnik RJ, Sharbrough FW, Laws ER Jr: Anterior temporal lobectomy for the control of partial complex seizures: information for counseling patients, *Mayo Clin Proc* 63:783-793, 1988.

118. Ivnik RJ, Sharbrough FW, Laws ER Jr: Effects of anterior temporal lobectomy on cognitive function, *J Clin Physiol* 43:128-137, 1987.

119. Jack CR Jr, Nichols DA, Sharbrough FW et al: Selective posterior cerebral artery Amytal test for evaluating memory function before surgery for temporal lobe seizure, *Radiology* 168:787-793, 1988.

120. Jayakar PB, Stanwick RS, Seshia SS: Tuberous sclerosis and Wolff-Parkinson-White syndrome, *J Pediatr* 108:259-260, 1986.

121. Kandt RS, Gebarski SS, Goetting MG: Tuberous sclerosis with cardiogenic cerebral embolism: magnetic resonance imaging, *Neurology* 35:1223-1225, 1985.

122. Katz A, Awad IA, Kong AK et al: Extent of resection in temporal lobectomy for epilepsy. II. Memory changes and neurologic complications, *Epilepsia* 30:763-771, 1989.

123. Kearse LA, McPeck K: Prevalence of epileptiform activity of narcotic anesthesia during carotid endarterectomy (abstract), *Anesthesiology* 75:A1029, 1991.

124. Keats AS: Seizures from isoflurane? (letter), *Anesth Analg* 64:1225-1226, 1985.

125. Kelly PJ, Sharbrough FW, Kall BA et al: Magnetic resonance imaging-based computer-assisted stereotactic resection of the hippocampus and amygdala in patients with temporal lobe epilepsy, *Mayo Clin Proc* 62:103-108, 1987.

126. Keranen T, Riekkinen P: Severe epilepsy: diagnostic and epidemiological aspects, *Acta Neurol Scand Suppl* 117:7-14, 1988.

127. Koch-Weser M, Garron DC, Gilley DW et al: Prevalence of psychologic disorders after surgical treatment of seizures, *Arch Neurol* 45:1308-1311, 1988.

128. Kofke WA, Barmada MA, Rudy TE: Effects of hyperglycemia on seizure induced brain damage in the rat, *Neurol Res* (in press).

128a. Kofke WA, Dasheiff RM, Dong M-L et el: Anesthetic care during thiopental tests to evaluate epileptic patients for surgical therapy, *J Neurosurg Anes* 5:164-170, 1993.

129. Kofke WA, Garman RH, Tom WC et al: Alfentanil-induced hypermetabolism, seizure, and histopathology in rat brains, *Anesth Analg* 75:953-964, 1992.

129a. Kofke WA, Garman RH, Garman R et al: High-dose narcotics cause seizures and brain damage in ventilated rats, *Soc Neurosci Abstr* 19, 1993 (in press).

130. Kofke WA, Snider MT, Young RS et al: Prolonged low flow isoflurane anesthesia for status epilepticus, *Anesthesiology* 62:653-656, 1985.

131. Kofke WA, Thayer T: Induction of thiopental anesthesia without tracheal intubation in a patient with hiatal hernia: use of esophageal pH monitoring, *Anesthesiology* 72:950-951, 1990.

132. Kofke WA, Towfighi J, Garman RH: Effects of anesthetics on neuropathologic sequelae of status epilepticus in rats, *Anesth Analg* 77:330-337, 1993.

133. Kofke WA, Young RSK, Davis P et al: Isoflurane for refractory status ep-

ilepticus: a clinical series, *Anesthesiology* 71:653-659, 1989.

134. Konishi K, Nakamura M, Yamakawa H et al: Hypophosphatemic osteomalacia in von Recklinghausen neurofibromatosis, *Am J Med Sci* 301:322-328, 1991.

135. Konkol RJ, Walsh EP, Power T et al: Cerebral embolism resulting from an intracardiac tumor in tuberous sclerosis, *Pediatr Neurol* 2:108-110, 1986.

136. Koren G, Butt W, Pape K et al: Morphine-induced seizures in newborn infants, *Vet Hum Toxicol* 27:519-520, 1985.

137. Kothari SS: When epilepsy masquerades as heart disease. Awareness is key to avoiding misdiagnosis, *Postgrad Med* 88:167, 170-171, 1990.

138. Kremen AF, Hill E, Kremen AJ: Pheochromocytoma, renal artery stenosis, and lymphocytic lymphoma associated with von Recklinghausen's neurofibromatosis. Case report and literature review, *Minn Med* 68:99-101, 1985.

139. Krenn J, Porges P, Steinbereithner K: Case of anesthesia convulsions under nitrous oxide-halothane anesthesia, *Anaesthetist* 16:83-85, 1967.

140. Krieger W, Cooperman J, Laxer KD: Seizures with etomidate anesthesia (letter), *Anesth Analg* 64:1226-1227, 1985.

141. Krieger W, Koerner M: Generalized grand mal seizure after recovery from uncomplicated fentanyl-etomidate anesthesia (letter), *Anesth Analg* 66:284-285, 1987.

142. Kuzniecky R, Faught E, Morawetz R: Surgical treatment of epilepsy: initial results based upon epidural electroencephalographic recordings, *South Med J* 83:637-639, 1990.

143. Landow L: An apparent seizure following inadvertent intrathecal morphine (letter), *Anesthesiology* 62:545-546, 1985.

144. Lanier WL, Sharbrough FW, Michenfelder JD: Effects of atracurium, vecuronium or pancuronium pretreatment on lignocaine seizure thresholds in cats, *Br J Anaesth* 60:74-80, 1988.

145. Laughlin TP, Newberg LA: Prolonged myoclonus after etomidate anesthesia, *Anesth Analg* 64:80-82, 1985.

146. Lebowitz MH, Blitt CD, Dillon JB: Enflurane-induced central nervous system excitation and its relation to

carbon dioxide tension, *Anesth Analg* 51:355-363, 1972.

147. Lenoir S, Grenier P, Brauner MW et al: Pulmonary lymphangiomyomatosis and tuberous sclerosis: comparison of radiographic and thin-section CT findings, *Radiology* 175:329-334, 1990.

148. Levin R, Banks S, Berg B: Psychosocial dimensions of epilepsy: a review of the literature, *Epilepsia* 29:805-816, 1988.

149. Li WW, Lombroso CT, Stephenson JBP: Eradication of incapacitating self-induced ischemic seizures by opioid receptor blockade (abstract), *Epilepsia* 30:679, 1989.

150. Lie JT: Cardiac, pulmonary, and vascular involvements in tuberous sclerosis, *Ann NY Acad Sci* 615:58-70, 1991.

151. Lieb JP, Babb TL, Engel J Jr: Quantitative comparison of cell loss and thiopental-induced EEG changes in human epileptic hippocampus, *Epilepsia* 30:147-156, 1989.

152. Lieb JP, Sperling MR, Mendius JR et al: Visual versus computer evaluation of thiopental-induced EEG changes in temporal lobe epilepsy, *Electroencephalogr Clin Neurophysiol* 63:395-407, 1986.

153. Lipert MM: Isoflurane anaesthesia for status epilepticus (letter), *S Afr Med J* 75:350-351, 1989.

154. Livingston JH, Brown JK: Nonconvulsive status epilepticus resistant to benzodiazepines, *Arch Dis Child* 62:41-44, 1987.

155. Lossos IS, Breuer R, Lafair JS: Endotracheal neurofibroma in a patient with von Recklinghausen's disease, *Eur Respir J* 1:464-465, 1988.

156. Lowenstein DH, Aminoff MJ, Simon RP: Barbiturate anesthesia in the treatment of status epilepticus: clinical experience with 14 patients, *Neurology* 38:395-400, 1988.

157. Lowson G, Gent JP, Goodchild CS: Anticonvulsant properties of propofol and thiopentone: comparison using two tests in laboratory mice, *Br J Anaesth* 64:59-63, 1990.

158. Luna CM, Gene R, Jolly EC et al: Pulmonary lymphangiomyomatosis associated with tuberous sclerosis. Treatment with tamoxifen and tetracycline-pleurodesis, *Chest* 88:473-475, 1985.

159. Lyning Y: Surgical treatment of epilepsy. Organization (localization,

staff, referral procedures), *Acta Neurol Scand Suppl* 117:129-135, 1988.

160. MacKenzie SJ, Kapadia F, Grant IS: Propofol infusion for control of status epilepticus, *Anaesthesia* 45:1043-1045, 1990.

161. MacKenzie R, Smith JS, Matheson J et al: Selection criteria for surgery in patients with refractory epilepsy, *Clin Exp Neurol* 24:67-76, 1987.

162. Magbagbeola JAO: Abnormal responses to muscle relaxants in patients with von Recklinghausen's disease, *Br J Anaesth* 42:710, 1970.

163. Male CG, Allen EM: Methohexitone-induced convulsion in epileptics, *Anaesth Intens Care* 5:226-230, 1977.

164. Manninen P, Contreras J: Anesthetic considerations for craniotomy in awake patients, *Int Anesth Clin* 24:157-173, 1986.

165. Marino JR: Surgery for epilepsy. Selective partial microsurgical callosotomy for intractable multiform seizures: criteria for clinical selection and results, *Appl Neurophysiol* 48:404-407, 1985.

166. Marshall JB, Ravendhran N, Diaz-Arias AA: Esophageal achalasia associated with von Recklinghausen's neurofibromatosis (letter), *J Clin Gastroenterol* 12:710-711, 1990.

167. Mashiyama S, Mori T, Seki H et al: Multiple brain tumors with von Recklinghausen's disease, *Acta Neurochir* 84:29-35, 1987.

168. Mattson RH: Closed-circuit-televised videotape recording and electroencephalography (CCTV/EEG) in convulsive status epilepticus, *Adv Neurol* 34:37-46, 1983.

169. Mattson RH, Heninger GR, Gallagher BB et al: Psychophysiologic precipitants of seizures in epilepticus, *Neurology* 20:407, 1970.

170. Maxwell RE, Gates JR, McGeachie R: Magnetic resonance imaging in the assessment and surgical management of epilepsy and functional neurological disorders, *Appl Neurophysiol* 50:369-373, 1987.

171. Mayhue FE: Midazolam for status epilepticus in the emergency department, *Ann Emerg Med* 17:643-645, 1988.

172. McGeer RG, Olney JW, McGeer PL: *Kainic Acid as a tool in neurobiology*, New York, 1978, Raven Press.

173. McGinty JF, Kanamatsu T, Obie J et al: Modulation of opioid peptide me-

tabolism by seizures: differentiation of opioid subclasses, *Natl Inst Drug Abuse Res Monogr Ser* 71:89-101, 1986.

174. Meeke RI, Soifer BE, Gelb AW: Isoflurane for the measurement of status epilepticus, *DICP* 23:579-581, 1989.

175. Meinck H-M, Mohlenhof O, Kettler D: Neurophysiological effects of etomidate, a new short-acting hypnotic, *Electroencephalogr Clin Neurophysiol* 50:515-522, 1980.

176. Meyer FB, Marsh WR, Laws ER Jr et al: Temporal lobectomy in children with epilepsy, *J Neurosurg* 64:371-376, 1986.

177. Mitterschiffthaler G, Maurhard U, Huter O et al: Prolonged action of vecuronium in neurofibromatosis (von Recklinghausen's disease), *Anaesthesiol Reanim* 14:175-178, 1989.

178. Modica PA, Tempelhoff R, White PF: Pro- and anticonvulsant effects of anesthetics (part I), *Anesth Analg* 70:303-315, 1990.

178a. Modica PA, Tempelhoff R, White PF: Pro- and anticonvulsant effects of anesthetics (part II), *Anesth Analg* 70:433-444, 1990.

179. Molbegott LP, Flashburg MH, Karasic HL et al: Probable seizures after sufentanil, *Anesth Analg* 66:91-93, 1987.

180. Montplaisir J, Laverdiere M, Saint-Hilaire JM et al: Nocturnal sleep recording in partial epilepsy: a study with depth electrodes, *J Clin Neurophysiol* 4:383-388, 1987.

181. Morrell F, Whisler WW, Bleck TP: Multiple subpial transection: a new approach to the surgical treatment of focal epilepsy, *J Neurosurg* 70:231-239, 1989.

182. Myer EC, Trepathi HL, Dewey WL: Cerebrospinal fluid b-endorphin immunoreactivity in epilepsy and the response to naltrexone (abstract), *Epilepsia* 31:611, 1990.

183. Myers RR, Shapiro HM: Local cerebral metabolism during enflurane anesthesia: identification of epileptogenic foci. *Electroencephalogr Clin Neurophysiol* 47:153-162, 1979.

184. Naguib M, Al-Rajeh SM, Abdulatif M et al: The response of a patient with von Recklinghausen's disease to succinylcholine and atracurium, *Middle East J Anesthesiol* 9:429-434, 1988.

185. Nakakimura K, Sakabe T, Funatsu N et al: Metabolic activation of intercortical and corticothalamic pathways during enflurane anesthesia in rats, *Anesthesiology* 68:777-782, 1988.

186. National Institute of Health Consensus Conference: Surgery for epilepsy, *JAMA* 264:729-733, 1990.

187. Neppe VM, Tucker GJ: Modern perspectives on epilepsy in relation to psychiatry: behavioral disturbances of epilepsy, *Hosp Community Psychiatry* 39:389-396, 1988.

188. Nevander G, Ingvar M, Auer R et al: Status epilepticus in well-oxygenated rats causes neuronal necrosis, *Ann Neurol* 18:281-290, 1985.

189. Ng SH, Ng KK, Pai SC et al: Tuberous sclerosis with aortic aneurysm and rib changes: CT demonstration, *J Comput Assist Tomogr* 12:666-668, 1988.

190. Nickel B, Schmickaly R: Increased tendency to seizures as affected by long-term infusions of etomidate in delirium tremens, *Anaesthetist* 34:462-469, 1985.

191. Nicol CF, Tutton JC, Smith BH: Parenteral diazepam in status epilepticus, *Neurology* 19:332-343, 1969.

192. Nicoll JM: Status epilepticus following enflurane anaesthesia, *Anaesthesia* 41:927-930, 1986.

193. Nishimura M, Takashima S, Takeshita K et al: Immunocytochemical studies on a fetal brain of tuberous sclerosis, *Pediatr Neurol* 1:245-248, 1985.

194. O'Brien SJ: The controversy surrounding epilepsy and driving: a review, *Public Health* 100:21-27, 1986.

195. O'Connell BK, Towfighi J, Kofke WA et al: Neuronal lesions in mercaptopropionic acid-induced status epilepticus, *Acta Neuropathol* 77:47-54, 1988.

196. Olivier A: Surgery of epilepsy: methods, *Acta Neurol Scand Suppl* 117:103-113, 1988.

197. Opitz A, Marschall R, Degan R et al: General anesthesia in patients with epilepsy and status epilepticus, *Adv Neurol* 34:531-535, 1983.

198. Opitz A, Oberwetter WD: Enflurane or halothane anaesthesia for patients with cerebral convulsive disorders? *Acta Anesthesiol Scand* 71(suppl):43-47, 1979.

199. Ornstein E, Matteo RS, Schwartz AE et al: The effect of phenytoin on the magnitude and duration of neuromuscular block following atracurium or vecuronium, *Anesthesiology* 67:191-196, 1987.

200. Ornstein E, Matteo RS, Young WL et al: Resistance to metocurine-induced neuromuscular blockade in patients receiving phenytoin, *Anesthesiology* 63:294-298, 1985.

201. Orr RA, Dimand RJ, Venkataraman ST et al: Diazepam and intubation in emergency treatment of seizures in children, *Ann Emerg Med* 20:1009-1013, 1988.

202. Oshima E, Urabe N, Shingu K et al: Anticonvulsant actions of enflurane on epilepsy models in cats, *Anesthesiology* 63:29-40, 1985.

203. Osorio I, Reed RC: Treatment of refractory generalized tonic-clonic status epilepticus with pentobarbital anesthesia after high-dose phenytoin, *Epilepsia* 30:464-471, 1989.

204. Paech MJ, Storey JM: Propofol and seizures (letter), *Anaesth Intens Care* 18:585, 1990.

205. Pagani JJ, Hayman LA, Bigelow RH et al: Prophylactic diazepam in prevention of contrast media-associated seizures in glioma patients undergoing cerebral computed tomography, *Cancer* 54:2200-2204, 1984.

206. Papo K, Del Pesce M, Provinciali L et al: Commissurotomy in intractable epilepsy: clinical and surgical comment, *Ital J Neurol Sci* 8:571-577, 1987.

207. Pasquet A: Combined regional and general anesthesia for craniotomy and cortical exploration. Part II. Anesthetic considerations, *Int Anesthesiol Clin* 24:12-20, 1986.

208. Pawlik G, Holthoff VA, Kessler J et al: Positron emission tomography findings relevant to neurosurgery for epilepsy, *Acta Neurochir Suppl (Wien)* 50:84-87, 1990.

209. Pender JW, Basso LV: Diseases of the endocrine system. In Katz J, Benumof J, Kadis L, editors: *Anesthesia and uncommon diseases,* Philadelphia, 1981, WB Sanders, pp 155-220.

210. Penfield W: Combined regional and general anesthesia for craniotomy and cortical exploration. Part I: neurosurgical considerations, *Int Anesthesiol Clin* 24:1-11, 1986.

211. Perl TM, Bedard L, Kosatsky T et al: An outbreak of toxic encephalopathy caused by eating mussels contami-

nated with domoic acid, *N Engl J Med* 322:1775-1780, 1990.

212. Perot P, Weir B, Rasmussen T: Tuberous sclerosis: surgical therapy for seizures, *Arch Neurol* 15:498-506, 1966.

213. Pinto-Lord MC, Abroms IF, Smith TW: Hyperdense cerebral lesion in childhood tuberous sclerosis: computed tomographic demonstration and neuropathologic analysis, *Pediatr Neurol* 2:245-248, 1986.

214. Porterfield JK, Pyeritz RE, Traill TA: Pulmonary hypertension and interstitial fibrosis in von Recklinghausen neurofibromatosis, *Am J Med Genet* 25:531-535, 1986.

215. Poulton TJ, Ellingson RJ: Seizure associated with induction of anesthesia with isoflurane, *Anesthesiology* 61:471-476, 1984.

216. Puglisi-Allagra S, Castellano C, Csanyl V et al: Opioid antagonism of electroshock-induced seizures, *Pharmacol Biochem Behav* 20:767-769, 1984.

217. Ramabadran K, Bansinath M: Endogenous opioid peptides and epilepsy, *Int J Clin Pharmacol Ther Toxicol* 28:47-62, 1986.

218. Renier WO: Learning disabilities and behavioural problems in children with epilepsy, *Wien Klin Wochenschr* 102:218-222, 1990.

219. Report of the American Academy of Neurology, Therapeutics and Technology Assessment Subcommittee: Assessment: intensive EEG/video monitoring for epilepsy, *Neurology* 39:1101-1102, 1989.

220. Robinson JD, Grant EG, Haller JO et al: Hepatic angiomyolipomas in tuberous sclerosis. Report of two cases, *J Ultrasound Med* 8:575-578, 1989.

221. Ropper AH, Kofke WA, Bromfield EB et al: Comparison of isoflurane, halothane, and nitrous oxide in status epilepticus (letter), *Ann Neurol* 19:98-99, 1986.

222. Rose DF, Smith PD, Sato S: Magnetoencephalography and epilepsy research, *Science* 238:329-335, 1987.

223. Rosman EJ, Capan LM, Turndorf H: Another case of probable seizure after sufentanil (letter), *Anesth Analg* 66:922, 1987.

224. Roth S, Ebrahim ZY: Resistance to pancuronium in patients receiving carbamazepine, *Anesthesiology* 66:691-693, 1987.

225. Rougier A, Biset JM, Kien P et al: MRI and surgery of epilepsy, *Neurochirurgie* 34:188-193, 1988.

226. Sagel SS, Foreest JV, Askin FB: Interstitial lung disease in neurofibromatosis, *South Med J* 68:647, 1975.

227. Sagratella S, Niglio T, Scotti de Carolis A: An investigation on the mechanism of anticonvulsant action of ketamine and phencyclidine on convulsions due to cortical application of penicillin in rabbits, *Pharmacol Res Commun* 17:773-786, 1985.

228. Schachter SC: Electroencephalography for epilepsy surgery, *Int Anesth Clin* 28:139-142, 1990.

229. Scott JC, Sarnquist FH: Seizure-like movements during a fentanyl infusion with absence of seizure activity in a simultaneous EEG recording, *Anesthesiology* 62:812-814, 1985.

230. Seigler RS: The administration of rectal diazepam for acute management of seizures, *J Emerg Med* 8:155-159, 1990.

231. Senveli E, Altinors N, Kars Z et al: Association of von Recklinghausen's neurofibromatosis and aqueduct stenosis, *Neurosurgery* 24:99-101, 1989.

232. Shaner DM, McCurdy SA, Herring MO et al: Treatment of status epilepticus: a prospective comparison of diazepam and phenytoin versus phenobarbital and optional phenytoin, *Neurology* 38:202-207, 1988.

232a. Cascino GD, Sharbrough FW, Elson LS et al: Intraoperative alfentanil hydrochloride in temporal lobe epilepsy: correlation with MRI-based volume studies (abstract), *Epilepsia* 33:85, 1992.

233. Shiraishi H, Yanagisawa M, Kuramatsu T et al: Cardiac tumour in a neonate with tuberous sclerosis: echocardiographic demonstration and magnetic resonance imaging, *Eur J Pediatr* 148:50-52, 1988.

234. Shorvon SD: Epidemiology, classification, natural history, and genetics of epilepsy, *Lancet* 336:93-96, 1990.

235. Sieber FE, Traystman RJ: Special issues: glucose and the brain, *Crit Care Med* 20:104-114, 1992.

236. Siggins GR, Henriksen SJ, Chavkin C et al: Opioid peptides and epileptogenesis in the limbic system: cellular mechanisms, *Adv Neurol* 44:501-512, 1986.

237. Silfvenius H: Pre- and postoperative rehabilitation related to epilepsy sur-

gery, *Acta Neurochir Suppl (Wien)* 50:100-106, 1990.

238. Simpson KH, Halsall PJ, Carr CM et al: Propofol reduces seizure duration in patients having anaesthesia for electroconvulsive therapy, *Br J Anaesth* 61:343-344, 1988.

239. Simpson PJ: Adverse drug reactions, *Curr Opin Anaesthesiol* 2:725-729, 1989.

240. Smith JR, Flanigin HF, King DW et al: Surgical managment of epilepsy, *South Med J* 82:736-742, 1989.

241. Smith NT, Benthuysen JL, Bickford RG et al: Seizures during opioid anesthetic induction—are they opioid-induced rigidity? *Anesthesiology* 71:852-862, 1989.

242. Smith PA, MacDonald TR, Jones CS: Convulsions associated with halothane anaesthesia. Two case reports, *Anaesthesia* 21:229-233, 1966.

243. Snead OC III, Bearden LF: The epileptogenic spectrum of opiate agonists, *Neuropharmacology* 21:1137-1144, 1982.

244. So N, Olivier A, Andermann F et al: Results of surgical treatment in patients with bitemporal epileptiform abnormalities, *Ann Neurol* 25:432-439, 1989.

245. Sobata E, Ohkuma H, Suzuki S: Cerebrovascular disorders associated with von Recklinghausen's neurofibromatosis: a case report, *Neurosurgery* 22:544-549, 1988.

246. Spencer DD, Spencer SS: Surgery for epilepsy, *Neurol Clin* 3:313-330, 1985.

247. Spencer SS, Katz A: Arriving at the surgical options for intractable seizures, *Semin Neurol* 10:422-430, 1990.

248. Spencer SS: Surgical options for uncontrolled epilepsy, *Neurol Clin* 4:669-695, 1986.

249. Sperling MR, Brown WJ, Crandall PH: Focal burst-suppression induced by thiopental, *Electroencephalogr Clin Neurophysiol* 63:203-208, 1986.

250. Sperling MR: Hypoglycemic activation of focal abnormalities in the EEG of patients considered for temporal lobectomy, *Electroencephalogr Clin Neurophysiol* 58:506-512, 1984.

251. Stefan H, Quesney LF, Abou-Khalil B et al: Electrocorticography in tem-

poral lobe epilepsy surgery, *Acta Neurol Scand* 83:65-72, 1991.

252. Stewart GR, Zorumski CF, Price HT et al: Domoic acid: a dementia-inducing excitotoxic food poison with kainic acid receptor specificity, *Exp Neurol* 110:127-138, 1990.

253. Stillwell TJ, Gomez MR, Kelalis PP: Renal lesions in tuberous sclerosis, *J Urol* 138:477-481, 1987.

254. Stines J, Rodde A, Carlous JM et al: CT findings of laryngeal involvement in von Recklinghausen disease, *J Comput Assist Tomogr* 11:141-143, 1987.

255. Strain SM, Tasker RAR: Hippocampal damage produced by systemic injections of domoic acid in mice, *Neuroscience* 44:343-352, 1991.

256. Strong WE, Matson M: Probable seizure after alfentanil, *Anesth Analg* 68:692-693, 1989.

257. Stutzmann JM, Bohme GA, Roques BP et al: Differential electrographic patterns for specific mu- and delta-opioid peptides in rats, *Eur J Pharmacol* 123:23-29, 1986.

258. *Surgery for epilepsy. National Institute of Health Consensus Statement,* 8:1-20, 1990, National Institutes of Health, Bethesda, MD.

259. Surgery for epilepsy: summary of a consensus statement, *Can Med Assoc J* 144:145-146, 1991.

260. Swan JH, Meldrum BS, Simon RP: Hyperglycemia does not augment neuronal damage in experimental status epilepticus, *Neurology* 36:1351-1354, 1986.

261. Sztriha L, Lelkes Z, Benedek G et al: Potentiating effect of morphine on seizures induced by kainic acid in rats. An electroencephalographic study, *Naunyn Schmiedebergs Arch Pharmacol* 333:47-51, 1986.

262. Tasker RC, Boyd SG, Harden A et al: EEG monitoring of prolonged thiopentone administration for intractable seizures and status epilepticus in infants and young children, *Neuropediatrics* 20:147-153, 1989.

263. Tassinari CA, Daniels O, Michelucci R et al: Benzodiazepines: efficacy in status epilepticus, *Adv Neurol* 34:465-475, 1983.

264. Teitelbaum JS, Zatorre RJ, Carpenter S et al: Neurologic sequelae of domoic acid intoxication due to the ingestion of contaminated mussels, *N Engl J Med* 322:1781-1787, 1990

265. Tempelhoff R, Modica PA, Bernardo KL et al: Fentanyl-induced electrocorticographic seizures in patients with complex partial epilepsy, *J Neurosurg* 77:2, 1992.

266. Tempelhoff R, Modica PA, Jellish WS et al: Resistance to atracurium-induced neuromuscular blockade in patients with intractable seizure disorders treated with anticonvulsants, *Anesth Analg* 71:665-669, 1990.

267. Tempelhoff R, Modica PA, Spitznagel EL Jr: Anticonvulsant therapy increases fentanyl requirements during anaesthesia for craniotomy, *Can J Anaesth* 37:327-332, 1990.

268. Thomas JS, Boheimer NO: An isolated grand mal seizure 5 days after propofol anaesthesia (letter), *Anaesthesia* 46:508, 1991.

269. Tombaugh GC, Sapolsky RM: Mechanistic distinctions between excitotoxin and acidotic hippocampal damage in an in vitro model of ischemia, *J Cereb Blood Flow Metab* 10:527-535, 1990.

270. Tombaugh GC, Sapolsky RM: Mild acidosis protects hippocampal neurons from injury induced by oxygen and glucose deprivation, *Brain Res* 506:343-345, 1990.

271. Tommasino C, Maekawa T, Shapiro HM: Fentanyl-induced seizures activate subcortical brain metabolism, *Anesthesiology* 60:283-290, 1984.

272. Tortella FC, Long JB, Holaday JW: Endogenous opioid systems: physiological role in the self-limitation of seizures, *Brain Res* 332:174-178, 1985.

273. Tortella FC, Robles L, Mosberg HI et al: Electroencephalographic assessment of the role of delta receptors in opioid peptide-induced seizures, *Neuropeptides* 5:213-216, 1984.

274. Tortella FC, Robles L, Mosberg HI: Evidence for mu opioid receptor mediation of enkephalin-induced electroencephalographic seizures, *J Pharmacol Exp Ther* 240:571-577, 1987.

275. Tortella FC: Endogenous opioid peptides and epilepsy: quieting the seizing brain? *Trends Pharmacol Sci* 9:366-372, 1988.

276. Towfighi J, Kofke WA, O'Connell BK et al: Substantia nigra lesions in mercaptopropionic acid induced status epilepticus: a light and electron microscopic study, *Acta Neuropathol* 77:612-620, 1989.

277. Treiman DM: Pharmacokinetics and clinical use of benzodiazepines in the management of status epilepticus, *Epilepsia* 30(suppl 2):S4-S10, 1989.

278. Treiman DM: The role of benzodiazepines in the management of status epilepticus, *Neurology* 40:32-42, 1990.

279. Trimble MR: Psychiatric aspects of epilepsy, *Psychiatr Dev* 5:285-300, 1987.

280. Trop D: Conscious-sedation analgesia during the neurosurgical treatment of epilepsies—practice at the Montreal Neurological Institute, *Int Anesth Clin* 24:175-184, 1986.

281. Tryphonas L, Iverson F: Neuropathology of excitatory neurotoxins: the domoic acid model, *Toxicol Pathol* 18:165-169, 1990.

282. Tryphonas L, Truelove J, Iverson F: Acute parenteral neurotoxicity of domoic acid in cynomolgus monkeys (M. fascicularis), *Toxicol Pathol* 18:297-303, 1990.

283. Tryphonas L, Truelove J, Nera E et al: Acute neurotoxicity of domoic acid in the rat, *Toxicol Pathol* 18:1-9, 1990.

284. Tzeng JI, Lu CC, Chan TH et al: Status epilepticus controlled by althesin infusion (a case report), *Ma Tsui Hsueh Tsa Chi* 24:229-232, 1986.

285. Urca G, Frenk H, Liebeskind JC et al: Morphine and enkephalin: analgesia and epileptic properties, *Science* 197:83-86, 1977.

286. Urca G, Frenk H: Systemic morphine blocks the seizures induced by intracerebroventricular (i.c.v.) injections of opiates and opioid peptides, *Brain Res* 246:121-126, 1982.

287. Van Ness PC: Pentobarbital and EEG burst suppression in treatment of status epilepticus refractory to benzodiazepines and phenytoin, *Epilepsia* 31:61-67, 1990.

288. Velisek L, Mikolasova R, Blankova-Vankova S et al: Effects of ketamine on metrazol-induced seizures during ontogenesis in rats, *Pharmacol Biochem Behav* 32:405-410, 1989.

289. Veliskova J, Velisek L, Mares P et al: Ketamine suppresses both bicuculline- and picrotoxin-induced generalized tonic-clinic seizures during ontogenesis, *Pharmacol Biochem Behav* 37:667-674, 1990.

290. Verdura G, Lupi G, Contardi I et al: Clinical aspects (especially nephropathologic) and genetic counseling in

tuberous sclerosis. Presentation of a case with polycystic kidney, *Pediatr Med Chir* 9:351-359, 1987.

291. Victory RA, Magee D: A case of convulsion after propofol anaesthesia (letter), *Anaesthesia* 43:904, 1988.

292. Walczak TS, Radtke RA, McNamara JO et al: Anterior temporal lobectomy for complex partial seizures: evaluation, results, and long-term follow-up in 100 cases, *Neurology* 40:413-418, 1990.

293. Wannamaker BB: Autonomic nervous system and epilepsy, *Epilepsia* 26(suppl 1):S31-S39, 1985.

294. Watson GH: Cardiac rhabdomyomas in tuberous sclerosis, *Ann NY Acad Sci* 615:150-157, 1991.

295. Webb MD: Seizure-like activity during fentanyl anesthesia. A case report, *Anesth Prog* 37:306-307, 1990.

296. Welling EC, Donegan J: Neuroleptanalgesia using alfentanil for awake craniotomy, *Anesth Analg* 68:57-60, 1989.

297. Wilder BJ: Efficacy of phenytoin in treatment of status epilepticus, *Adv Neurol* 34:441-446, 1983.

298. Wyler AR, Hermann BP, Richey ET: Results of reoperation for failed epilepsy surgery, *J Neurosurg* 71:815-819, 1989.

299. Wyler AR, Richey ET, Atkinson RA et al: Methohexital activation of epileptogenic foci during acute electrocorticography, *Epilepsia* 28:490-494, 1987.

300. Wyllie E, Rothner AD, Luders H: Partial seizures in children: clinical features, medical treatment, and surgical considerations, *Pediatr Clin North Am* 36:343-364, 1989.

301. Yamashita M: Anaesthetic considerations in von Recklinghausen's disease (multiple neurofibromatosis). Abnormal response to muscle relaxants, *Anaesthetist* 26:317, 1977.

302. Yanny HF, Christmas D: Propofol infusion for status epilepticus (letter), *Anaesthesia* 3:514, 1988.

303. Yaqoob M, Saffman C, Mohamed AS et al: Acute urate nephropathy due to partial hypoxanthine-guanine phosphoribosyl transferase deficiency, *Nephrol Dial Transplant* 5:383-384, 1990.

304. Yate PM, Flynn PJ, Arnold RW et al: Clinical experience and plasma laudanosine concentrations during the infusion of atracurium in the intensive therapy unit, *Br J Anaesth* 59:211-217, 1987.

305. Yeoman P, Hutchinson A, Byrne A et al: Etomidate infusions for the control of refractory status epilepticus, *Intens Care Med* 15:255-259, 1989.

306. Young ML, Smith DA, Greenburg J et al: Effects of sufentanil on regional cerebral glucose utilization in rats, *Anesthesiology* 61:564-568, 1984.

307. Young RS, Ropper A, Hawkes D et al: Pentobarbital in refractory status epilepticus, *Pediatr Pharmacol* 3:63-67, 1983.

308. Zatorre RJ: Memory loss following domoic acid intoxication from ingestion of toxic mussels, *Can Dis Wkly Rep* 16(suppl 1E):101-103, 1990.

309. Zieglgansberger W, French ED, Siggins GR et al: Opioid peptides may excite hippocampal pyramidal neurons by inhibiting adjacent inhibitory interneurons, *Science* 205:415-417, 1979.

Genetic Syndromes Associated with Seizures

Phenotypes	Concerns for Anesthesia*
Autosomal Dominant	
Alopecia, psychomotor epilepsy, pyorrhea, and mental subnormality	
Basal cell nevus syndrome (multiple basal cell nevi, odontogenic keratocysts and skeletal anomalies)	Laryngeal carcinoma,[68] congenital hydrocephalus,[43] medulloblastoma,[6] osteolytic lesions[9]
Centralopathic epilepsy	
Convulsions, benign familial neonatal	
Convulsive disorder and mental retardation	
Craniometaphyseal dysplasia	Secondary hyperparathyroidism,[22] nasal obstruction,[72] deafness,[72] cervical spine deformity,[82] hydrocephalus[33]
Endocrine adenomatosis, multiple (Werner syndrome; multiple endocrine neoplasia, type I)	See text
Epilepsy, photogenic	Hyperprolinemia[80]
Fibromatosis, gingival with hypertrichosis	
Flunn-Aird syndrome	
Hemifacial atrophy, progressive (Parry-Romberg syndrome)	Facial deformity,[26] scleroderma,[38,41] cerebral hemiatrophy,[41] microsomia,[58] hypertrophic cardiomyopathy[7]
Huntington's chorea	Abnormal response to thiopental[19,23]
Hyperostosis frontalis interna (Morgangi-Stewart-Morel syndrome)	Acromegaly,[27] hypoparathyroidism[48]
Kok disease	
Myoclonic epilepsy, Hartung type	
Myoclonus and ataxia	
Myoclonus, cerebellar ataxia, and deafness	
Myoclonus, hereditary essential	
Neurofibromatosis	See text
Neuronal ceroid-lipofuscinosis, dominant or Parry type	Phenothiazine-induced tardive dyskinesia[28]
Noonan syndrome	Pulmonary hypertension,[74] renal anomalies,[18] pulmonic stenosis,[18,56] atrial septal defect,[18,56] potential airway difficulty,[18] neurofibromatosis,[52] syringomyelia,[39] coagulopathy,[25] hypertrophic cardiomyopathy,[56] malignant hyperthermia[40,46]
Photomyoclonus, diabetes mellitus, deafness, nephropathy, and cerebral dysfunction	
Porphyria, acute intermittent (Swedish type of prophyria)	
Porphyria, varigata	Chronic hypertension/tachycardia, bulbar dysfunction, prophyria induced by barbiturates, benzodiazepines, althesin, ethanol, phenytoin, pentazocine (and others)[35]; anesthesia†[54]
Sturge-Weber syndrome	Renal hemangioma,[84] vena caval anatomic abnormality,[84] hypoplastic larynx,[44] hydrocephalus,[51,84] surgery[13]
Telangiectasia of brain	
Tuberous (or tuberose) sclerosis	See text
Autosomal Recessive	
Alopecia-epilepsy-oligophrenia syndrome of Moynahan (familial congenital alopecia, epilepsy, mental retardation, and unusual EEG)	

*Concerns for anesthesia indicate major systemic or neurologic effects of a syndrome that have been reported that may affect anesthesia. Such notation does not connote incidence of a cited concomitant condition only that it has been reported. Absence of a notation indicates only that no such reports were found. References to neurologic presentation, motor disturbances, and epilepsy are not included. This is not a comprehensive list of syndromes and their manifestations.
†Anesthetic management issues discussed.
Modified from Aird RB, Masland RL, Woodbury DM: *The epilepsies: a critical review,* New York, 1984, Raven Press.

Phenotypes	Concerns for Anesthesia*
Alpers diffuse degeneration of cerebral gray matter (poliodystrophia cerebri progressive) with hepatic cirrhosis	Liver failure[30]
Amautrotic family idiocy, juvenile type (Batten disease in England, Vogt-Spielmeyer disease in Europe)	Similar to neuronal ceroid-lipofuscinosis,[34] hypertrophic cardiomyopathy[5]
Amaurotic idiocy, adult type (Kuf disease)	
Amaurotic idiocy (congenital form)	
Amaurotic idiocy, late infantile, with multilamellar cytosomes	
Angiomatosis, diffuse corticomeningeal, of Divry and Van Bogaert	Multiple cerebral ischemic events[21]
Argininemia	Valproate intolerance[16]
Argininosuccinicaciduria	
Ataxi with myoclonus epilepsy and presenile dementia	
Carnosinemia	
Cerebelloparenchymal disorder V (CPA V; spinodentate atrophy; dyssynergia cerebellaris myoclonic of Hunt)	
Cerebral calcification, nonarteriosclerotic	
Cerebral gigantism (Sotos syndrome)	Congenital heart defects,[37] scoliosis surgery[+70]
Citrullinuria (citrullinemia)	
Convulsive disorder, familial, with prenatal or early onset	
Cornelia de Lange syndrome	Suprasellar germinoma with diabetes insipidus,[69] esophageal reflux,[15] pulmonary aspiration,[59] anesthesia,†[65,71] endocrinopathy[87]
Corpus callosum, agenesis of, with neuronopathy (Charlevoix disease)	
Craniodiaphyseal dysplasia	
Crome syndrome	
Cystathioninuria	Abnormal liver function[32]
Deaf-mutism and familial myoclonus epilepsy	
Deaf-mutism and onychodystrophy, recessive form	
Dermochondrocorneal dystrophy of Francois	
Dysmyelination with jaundice	
Epilepsy and yellow teeth	
Epilepsy, photogenic, with spastic diplegia and mental retardation	
Epilepsy telangiectasis	
Folic acid, transport defect	
Fructose intolerance, hereditary (fructosemia)	
Galactosemia	
Gaucher disease type III (juvenile and adult, cerebral)	Splenomegaly, anemia, neutropenia, thrombocytopenia[2]
Goldberg syndrome	
Hallervorden and Spatz syndrome	Liver and pituitary abnormalities,[81] Parkinsonism[1]
"Happy puppet" syndrome	
Hemihypertrophy	Airway compromise,[67] adrenal adenoma,[75] genitourinary anomalies[79]
Homocystinuria	Thromboembolism,[8,77] arterial occlusions,[49] hypercoagulation,[53] megaloblastic anemia,[61] cor pulmonale,[12] postoperative dystonia,[4] anesthesia†[17]
Hydroxlysinuria	
Hyper-beta-alaninemia	
Hyperglycinemia, isolated	
Hyperlysinemia	
Hyperphosphatasia with mental retardation	
Hyperphosphatemia, polyuria, and seizures	
Hyperprolinemia, type II	
Hypoadrenocorticism, with hypoparathyroidism and superficial moniliasis	
Hypomagnesemia, primary	Hypocalcemia and hyperphosphatemia[50,83]
Krabbe disease (globoid cell sclerosis)	
Lactic acidosis, congenital infantile	Cardiomyopathy[76]
Lipidosis, juvenile dystonic	
Lipid proteinosis of Urbach and Wiethe (lipoproteinosis; hyalinosis cutis et mucosae)	
Lissencephaly syndrome	Apnea[31]

Phenotypes	Concerns for Anesthesia*
Mercaptolactate-cysteine disulfiduria	
Metachromatic leukodystrophy, late infantile (metachromatic leukoencephalopathy; metachromatic form of diffuse cerebral sclerosis; sulfatide lipidosis)	
Methionine malabsorption syndrome	
Mucolipidosis I (lipomucopolysaccharidosis)	Atlantoaxial instability[14]
Mucolipidosis II (I-cell disease)	Hyperparathyroidism,[55] cardiomyopathy[86]
Myoclonic epilepsy of Unverricht and Lundberg	
Neuraminidase deficiency	Nephrotic syndrome[62]
Neuroaxonal dystrophy, infantile (Seitelberger)	Diencephalic syndrome[47]
Neuroectodermal melanolysosomal disease	
Neuronal ceroid-lipifuscinosis, infantile Finnish type	
Neimann-Pick disease (sphingomyelin lipidosis)	Anesthesia†,[36] hepatosplenomegaly,[11] pulmonary dysfunction,[10,57] hepatic dysfunction[24]
Phenylketonuria	Cardiac dysrhythmia,[29] low blood catecholamine concentration,[35] fasting-induced hyperphenylalanemia,[35] anesthesia,†[35] hypoglycemia[35]
Pseudohypoparathyroidism, type II	
Pryidoxine dependency with seizures	Anemia[45]
Spastic diplegia, infantile type	
Tachycardia, hypertension, microphthalmos, hyperglycinuria	
Tay-Sachs disease: GM2-gangliosidosis, type I	Anesthesia†[35]
Theroninemia	
Xylosidase deficiency	
X-Linked	
Borjeson syndrome (mental deficiency, epilepsy, endocrine disorders)	Abnormal airway[20]
Corpus callosum, parital agenesis of	
FG syndrome	Subvalvular aortic stenosis[85]
Hereditary hemihypotrophy hemiparesis hemiathetosis (HHH) syndrome	
Hyperphenylalaninemia, X-linked	Similar to phenylketonuria[73]
Hypoxanthine guanine phosphoribosyl transferase deficienty; Lesch-Nyhan syndrome	Urate nephropathy,[3,89] aspiration pneumonia,[42] anesthesia†[42]
Infantile spasms (X-linked)	
Menkes syndrome (kinky hair disease)	Copper deficiency,[78] hypothermia,[78] sepsis[78]
Mental deficiency (Martin-Bell or Renpenning type) X-linked mental retardation	Mitral valve prolapse,[60] pulmonic and tricuspid valvular regurgitation[60]
Methylmandelicaciduria	
Paine syndrome (microencephaly with spastic diplegia)	
Pallister W syndrome	
Pelizaeus-Merzbacher disease	Laryngeal abnormalities[89]

References:

1. *J Neurol Neurosurg Psychiat* 50:1665, 1987.
2. Katz J, Benumof J, Kadis LB, editors: *Anesthesia and uncommon diseases,* Philadelphia, 1981, Saunders, p 313.
3. *Nephron* 46:179, 1987.
4. *J Pediatr* 113:863, 1988.
5. *Br Heart J* 51:674, 1984.
6. *Med Cutan Ibero Lat Am* 13:5, 1985.
7. *J Assoc Physicians India* 36:394, 1988.
8. *Br J Ophthalmol* 74:696, 1990.
9. *Skeletal Radiol* 12:196, 1984.
10. *Rev Mal Respir* 7:267, 1990.
11. *Neurol Clin* 7:75, 1989.
12. *Am J Med Genet* 36:167, 1990.
13. *Aust Pediatr J* 25:103, 1989.
14. *Spine* 16:215, 1991.
15. *J Pediatr Surg* 24:248, 1989.
16. *Rev Neurol (Paris)* 146:764, 1990.
17. *Br J Anaesth* 43:96, 1971.
18. *Anesthesiology* 68:636, 1988.

19. *Br J Anaesth* 38:490, 1966.
20. *Clin Genet* 29:317, 1986.
21. *Rev Neurol (Paris)* 143:798, 1987.
22. *J Pediatr* 112:587, 1988.
23. *Br J Anaesth* 49:1167, 1977.
24. *Neurology* 39:1040, 1989.
25. *Am J Clin Pathol* 95:739, 1991.
26. *Ann Plast Surg* 20:140, 1988.
27. *Postgrad Med J* 66:16, 1990.
28. *Pediatr Neurol* 2:236, 1986.
29. *Acta Paediatr Scand* 79:1259, 1990.
30. *J Child Neurol* 5:273, 1990.
31. *Brain Dev* 6:331, 1984.
32. *J Ment Defic Res* 31(3):299, 1987.
33. *Neurosurgery* 20:617, 1987.
34. *Neuropathol Appl Neurobiol* 11:475, 1985.
35. Katz J, Benumof J, Kadis LB, editors: *Anesthesia and uncommon diseases,* Philadelphia, 1981, Saunders, p 1.
36. Katz J, Benumof J, Kadis LB, editors: *Anesthesia and uncommon diseases,* Philadelphia, 1981, Saunders, p 485.

37. *Am J Med Genet* 26:569, 1987.
38. *Ann Pediatr (Paris)* 36:123, 1989.
39. *Jpn J Psychiat Neurol* 40:101, 1986.
40. *Birth Defects* 21:111, 1985.
41. *J R Soc Med* 77:138, 1984.
42. *Anesthesiology* 63:197, 1985.
43. *Can Med Assoc J* 132:1037, 1985.
44. *Clin Exp Dermatol* 13:128, 1988.
45. Stein JH et al, editors: *Internal medicine,* Boston, 1990, Little Brown, p 1074.
46. *Am J Med Genet* 21:493, 1985.
47. *Neurology* 35:735, 1985.
48. *Rinsho Shinkeigaku* 30:1114, 1990.
49. *Q J Med* 53:251, 1984.
50. *Endocrinol Jpn* 35:159, 1988.
51. *Can J Neurol Sci* 16:78, 1989.
52. *Am J Med Genet* 21:477, 1985.
53. *J Pediatr* 109:1001, 1986.
54. *Anaesthesia* 45:594, 1990.
55. *Eur J Pediatr* 148:553, 1989.
56. *G Ital Cardiol* 17:800, 1987.
57. *Arch Fr Pediatr* 47:373, 1990.
58. *Acta Chir Plast* 30:194, 1988.
59. *J Pediatr* 63:1000, 1963.
60. *Cardiologia* 35:857, 1990.
61. *Am J Med Genet* 26:377, 1987.
62. *Clin Genet* 34:185, 1988.
63. *South Med J* 68:647, 1975.
64. *Pharmacol Res Commun* 17:773, 1985.
65. *Anesthesiology* 74:1162, 1991.
66. *Int Anes Clin* 28:139, 1990.
67. *Head Neck Surg* 8:124, 1985.
68. *Z Hautkr* 63:113&117, 1988.
69. *Brain Dev* 8:541, 1986.
70. *Br J Anaesth* 66:728, 1991.
71. *Anesth Prog* 34:63, 1987.
72. *Australas Radiol* 33:84, 1989.
73. Stein JH et al, editors: *Internal medicine,* Boston, 1990, Little Brown, p 2301.
74. *Br Heart J* 62:74, 1989.
75. *Br J Radiol* 61:851, 1988.
76. *Am J Cardiol* 61:193-194, 1988.
77. Vaughn VC et al, editors: *Nelson textbook of pediatrics,* ed 10, Philadelphia, 1975, Saunders, p 1689.
78. Vaughn VC et al, editors: *Nelson textbook of pediatrics,* ed 10, Philadelphia, 1975, Saunders, p 1433.
79. *Clin Genet* 26:81, 1984.
80. *Clin Genet* 37:485, 1990.
81. *J Neurol Neurosurg Psychiatry* 52:1410, 1989.
82. *Surg Neurol* 27:284, 1987.
83. *Magnesium* 4:153, 1985.
84. *J Urol* 136:442, 1986.
85. *G Ital Cardiol* 15:349-353, 1985.
86. *Monatsschr Kinderheilkd* 135:708, 1987.
87. *J Pediatr* 117:920, 1990.
88. *Arch Otolaryngol Head Neck Surg* 116:613, 1990.
89. *Nephrol Dial Transplant* 5:383, 1990.

26

Anesthesia for Pediatric Neurosurgery

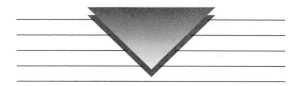

Philippa Newfield

Anesthetic management and perioperative care significantly affect the prognosis of the pediatric patient undergoing a neurosurgical procedure. The interaction between pharmacologic and mechanical maneuvers and intracranial pathophysiology also critically influences the outcome of therapeutic intervention. The increased understanding of these relationships developed over the past decade has fostered sophisticated advances in the practice of neurosurgery and neuroanesthesia, enabling neurosurgeons to perform more intricate operations on sicker children, with decreased mortality and improved results.

INTRACRANIAL DYNAMICS

Although the skull sutures have not fused in infants, in most pediatric patients the cranium is a rigid, bony structure containing brain and water (80%), blood (12%), and cerebrospinal fluid (CSF) (8%). In maturity, the total cerebral blood flow (CBF), supplied by the internal carotid and basi-lar arterial systems, is 50 ml/100 g of brain/min, and blood flow to individual areas of brain, the regional cerebral blood flow (rCBF), varies between 20 and 80 ml/100 g/min. CBF in children is 100 ml/100 g of brain/min.

The regulation of cerebral arteriolar tone and thereby CBF is determined by metabolic, neurogenic, and myogenic factors.[55] CBF in infants and children is affected by the same drugs and maneuvers that produce alterations in adults, but there may be quantitative differences in response. The normal cerebral metabolic rate for oxygen consumption is 3 to 3.5 ml/100 g of brain/min in adults, and 5 ml/100 g of brain/min in children. As the concentration of hydrogen ions increases with the accumulation of lactate and pyruvate from increased metabolism or decreased oxygen supply, vessels dilate and CBF increases. The elevation of the arterial carbon dioxide tension ($Paco_2$) causes a similar accumulation of hydrogen ions, vasodilation, and increased CBF. This response may be blunted in neonates when $Paco_2$ is less than 30 mm Hg. In addition, sympathetic and parasympathetic innervation of cerebral vessels contributes to the coarse and fine adjustments of CBF.

The cerebral vascular resistance varies with the muscle tone of the vessel wall in response to changes in the cerebral perfusion pressure (CPP), the difference between the mean arterial pressure (MAP) and the intracranial pressure (ICP). Autoregulation is the process by which vascular dilation or constriction causes the CBF to remain constant, despite variations in CPP from 50 to 150 mm Hg. Beyond these lower and upper limits, CBF is affected by the systemic blood pressure such that it decreases as the MAP falls below 50 mm Hg, and increases as the MAP rises about 150 mm Hg. Autoregulation in children occurs at different absolute values from adults. MAP may not reach 60 mm Hg until months after birth.

The anesthetic drugs affect CBF and thus cerebral blood volume (CBV) by changing the cerebral vascular resistance and the cerebral metabolic oxygen requirement. Because the volume of the brain, the lesion, and the CSF cannot be altered before the induction of anesthesia, the CBV is the only intracranial component that is readily controllable by the anesthesiologist through choice of anesthetic and manipulation of head position, systemic blood pressure, and Pa_{CO_2}.

PATHOPHYSIOLOGY

Separate but related insults cause injury to the brain after trauma or operation. The "primary" injury involves the biomechanical effects of trauma or surgical manipulation. The "secondary" injury is a series of events, often preventable or treatable, including systemic hypotension, hypoxemia, hypercapnia, mass effect, intracranial hypertension, and infection, that exacerbate and compound the initial damage. Because the sequelae of the secondary injury may seriously compromise survival and recovery, it is essential that these disorders be prevented or treated vigorously if they occur. Intracranial hypertension figures prominently among the complications of intracerebral disorders, including trauma, tumors, and hydrocephalus.

Normal individuals respond to small, acute increases in intracranial volume with a rapid readjustment to normal levels of ICP through extracranial translocation of blood and CSF. Other methods of compensation include a decrease in the production of CSF and the distortion of brain parenchyma. With progressive expansion of intracranial volume, however, compensatory mechanisms are exhausted, and the ability to restore or maintain the normal ICP is progressively impaired. As the intracranial volume expands, each new increment in volume causes a more marked elevation in ICP. This hyperbolic pressure response is clinically significant because the patient's position on the pressure-volume curve is usually unknown, and the response to any increase in intracranial volume (whether from hypertension, hypercarbia, or anesthetic drugs) is therefore unpredictable.

The presence of intracranial hypertension may not be ap-

parent on clinical examination. Pupillary dilation, increasing blood pressure, and bradycardia are usually late and ominous signs. Even papilledema may be absent in children who die as a result of intracranial hypertension. Rather, an abnormal level of consciousness and abnormal motor responses to painful stimuli are frequently associated with increased ICP.

Abrupt and marked increases in systemic blood pressure will also cause a sudden expansion of intracranial volume, owing to a breakthrough in the upper limit of autoregulation. The resultant increase in CBF in focal areas of the brain with disruption of the blood-brain barrier is accompanied by the transudation of plasma and protein from overdistended capillaries and the formation of cerebral edema. Autoregulation can thus be impaired in the presence of cerebral ischemia, trauma, infection, hypoxia, tumor, edema, and abscess. The dose-dependent vasodilatory effects of volatile anesthetic drugs on the cerebral resistance vessels also interfere with autoregulation.[20]

The normal value for ICP is less than 15 mm Hg. Before the sutures have closed, ICP can remain in the normal range while significant increases in head circumference occur. Intracranial hypertension can also exist without bulging fontanelles, especially if ICP increases slowly. The occurrence of frequent pressure waves despite a low baseline ICP is hazardous in children who have intracranial disorders.[16]

PREOPERATIVE EVALUATION

The preoperative evaluation includes special attention to age, associated medical problems (seizures, asthma), allergies, previous drug reactions, medication, and family history of adverse reactions to anesthetics. The weight and vital signs are important because they vary with age (Table 26-1).). The neurologic assessment includes level of consciousness, presence of intracranial hypertension, motor weakness, sensory changes, pupillary responsiveness and equality, and cranial nerve function.

Patients usually have a contracted blood volume immediately before operation because of poor fluid intake, prolonged vomiting, deliberate fluid restriction, intravenous administration of osmotic or contrast agents, disordered se-

TABLE 26-1
Vital Signs (Mean)

Age	Weight (kg)	Blood Pressure (mm Hg)	Heart Rate (per min)	Respiratory Rate (per min)
Premature	<2.5	50/30	140	35-80
Term neonate	>2.5	60/40	140	35-60
1 year	10	90/65	120	20-40
6 years	20	100/60	100	20-25
12 years	40	115/60	90	18-20

cretion of antidiuretic hormone, or occult bleeding in the presence of multisystem trauma. Significant blood loss can also occur from scalp lacerations. Consequently, patients will not tolerate anesthetic drugs, changes in position, or induced hypotension very well. In addition, hypovolemia leads to hypotension, which might decrease CBF—especially when combined with positive-pressure ventilation, barbiturates, and hypoxia.[100] Volume replacement is therefore indicated and is accomplished with intravenous administration of crystalloid solution (normal saline or lactated Ringer's) before the induction of anesthesia and positioning for surgery. In children, skin turgor, moistness of the mucous membranes, and urine output are more reliable indications of volume status than are blood pressure and heart rate.

Preoperative Medication

The premedication of children requiring neurosurgical procedures offers the double challenge of dealing with a group of "repeaters" (ventriculoperitoneal shunt malfunction, sequelae of spina bifida, frequent neurodiagnostic studies) who relish each additional trip to the operating room even less than the last but who also are intolerant of any degree of respiratory depression and resultant CO_2 retention. The possibility of narcotic-induced dysfunction and hypoventilation contraindicates the use of narcotics, especially via the newer "ouchless" routes. The administration of oral transmucosal fentanyl citrate (OTFC), 20 μg/kg, was reported to slow the respiratory rate by 10 minutes after administration[101] and to induce hemoglobin desaturation below 90% in 12% of the patients receiving OTFC as measured by pulse oximetry.[36] Likewise, the administration of intranasal sufentanil, 1.5 or 3.0 μg/kg, was associated with marked decreases in ventilatory compliance when the patients subsequently received inhalational anesthetic drugs.[48] In another report, all children who had received sufentanil, 1.5 μg/kg intranasally, developed respiratory depression, and 45% had hemoglobin saturations of less than 88%.[53]

Although the combination of a benzodiazepine and a narcotic can cause respiratory depression and even arrest in children,[7] benzodiazepines alone may be suitable for children undergoing neurosurgical procedures in that they induce sedation without respiratory depression. Neither oral midazolam, 0.5 to 0.75 mg/kg,[34] nor intranasal midazolam, 0.2 or 0.3 mg/kg, in preschool-aged children[115] caused apnea or changes in respiratory rate or oxyhemoglobin saturation during induction of anesthesia with halothane. Children who received intramuscular midazolam, 0.1 or 0.2 mg/kg, demonstrated a slight decrease in minute ventilation and respiratory rate but had an adequate ventilatory response to CO_2.[18]

Rectal thiopental, 30 mg/kg, and methohexital, 20 or 30 mg/kg, elevated the mean Pa_{CO_2} in infants, placing them at increased risk for hypoventilation when they subsequently received halothane.[54] Several children in another group who had received rectal thiopental, 30 mg/kg, were noted

to have reduced oxyhemoglobin saturations on arrival in the operating suite.[82] Therefore rectal barbiturates may be inadvisable as the premedicant in a child who has increased ICP or a decrease in intracranial compliance.

Because ketamine increases CBF and cerebral metabolic oxygen requirements, it has no role in the premedication, sedation, or anesthetic regimen of children whose intracerebral compliance is compromised. If ketamine is used as a "premedicant" at all, it should be with the understanding that it is actually the beginning of the anesthetic induction and therefore should be administered with immediate access to a source of positive-pressure ventilation and suction.

Patients who have altered levels of consciousness receive no premedication. Corticosteroids and anticonvulsants are continued in the perioperative period.

Preoperative Fasting

Infants and children possess several risk factors that predispose them to aspiration, including shorter esophagus, higher resting intragastric pressure owing to smaller stomachs and impingement of intraabdominal viscera, incoordination of neonatal breathing and swallowing mechanisms, and facilitation of regurgitation by angulation of the vocal cords during laryngoscopy. The highest-risk groups are children who have had previous esophageal surgery and premature infants who have persistent pulmonary disease, neurologic sequelae, or previous episodes of aspiration pneumonitis. Nonetheless, the incidence of aspiration in children has been reported to be as low as 2 in 40,000,[108] despite the fact that many children have a gastric-content pH of less than 2.5 and a volume greater than 0.4 ml/kg.[62,63]

The H_2-receptor antagonists inhibit histamine-mediated production of hydrochloric acid by parietal cells in the stomach and reduce gastric pH. Cimetidine[41] and ranitidine[61] have been given preoperatively to neonates, infants, and children. Caution is indicated, however because intravenous administration of cimetidine has been associated with hypotension and cardiac dysrhythmias including bradycardia; chronic administration may cause cerebral toxicity.[107] Goudsouzian et al.[41] determined the dose of cimetidine required to raise gastric pH to greater than 2.5. The ED_{50} was 3.0 mg/kg and the ED_{95} was 7.5 mg/kg. Based on these data, they suggest a single-dose preoperative regimen of 7.5 mg/kg of cimetidine given orally 1 to 3 hours before surgery as prophylaxis for acid aspiration in infants and children.

Ranitidine is also effective in children and has fewer side effects than cimetidine[35,121] because of decreased binding at androgen receptors, the hepatic mixed-function oxidase system, and peripheral lymphocytes. Although bradycardia has been reported after intravenous administration, the decreased binding reduces the serum concentrations of propranolol, lidocaine, and diazepam to a greater extent than with concurrent cimetidine therapy. Ranitidine may be administered to children intravenously (1.25 mg/kg), intramuscularly (1 to 2 mg/kg), or orally (2.5 mg/kg). Because the incidence of clinically significant aspiration of gastric contents in healthy children undergoing elective surgery is very low, routine prophylaxis is not necessary.[21]

For decreasing gastric fluid volume, metoclopramide, 0.1 mg/kg orally, intravenously, or subcutaneously, speeds gastric evacuation in children.[61] Glycopyrrolate, 7.5 to 10 μg/kg, reduces the volume of gastric secretions more effectively than either atropine or scopolamine but less so than cimetidine.[62]

Recent studies have addressed the optimal fasting period before elective induction of anesthesia in children. Schreiner et al. noted no significant differences in gastric fluid pH or volume in children undergoing outpatient surgery, regardless of whether they had ingested unlimited clear liquids up to 2 hours before induction of anesthesia or had fasted for 6 to 8 hours before induction of anesthesia.[92] Crawford also concluded that children could drink 2 ml/kg of water up to 2 hours before surgery without decreasing gastric pH or increasing gastric fluid volume beyond the pHs and volumes noted after 6 hours of fasting.[28] Infants and children, however, tolerate prolonged fasting and fluid restriction without hypoglycemia although neonates do not.[19]

For children who require emergency surgery under general anesthesia, it is difficult to determine how long to wait after oral intake because the severity of the trauma and its occurrence in relation to the last oral intake affect gastric emptying to a greater extent than the actual duration of fasting.[76] There may therefore be little advantage to waiting an arbitrarily predetermined length of time between the last oral intake and anesthesia, although 6- to 10-year-old children appear to be at higher risk for aspiration than younger children in that a higher percentage had a pH less than 2.5 and a gastric fluid volume greater than 0.4 ml/kg.[94]

MONITORING

Because of the possibility of significant blood loss, cardiac dysrhythmias, blood pressure fluctuations, venous air embolism, and voluminous urinary output, extensive monitoring is necessary. Monitoring includes: continuous measurement and display of intraarterial blood pressure, central venous pressure (with position verified by chest x-ray, transduced pressure-wave form, or p-wave configuration on ECG), cardiac rate and rhythm by ECG, esophageal stethoscope, nasopharyngeal or tympanic temperature (to approximate brain temperature), end-tidal CO_2 tension, and blood oxygen saturation; and intermittent measurement of arterial blood gases, hematocrit, serum electrolytes and osmolality, and urinary output. Detection of venous air embolism is accomplished with the use of the precordial ultrasonic Doppler device and with measurement of end-tidal CO_2 and nitrogen.

The rapid respiratory rate, small tidal volume, high rate of fresh gas flow, and high sampling rate all contribute to the underestimation of end-tidal gas concentrations in small children. The increased dead-space volume introduced by the sensors may also be detrimental in spontaneously-breathing infants. In-line and infrared CO_2 analyzers are more accurate in small children than devices that aspirate gas samples from the lines, but they weigh more and present the risk of displacement of the endotracheal tube.

POSITIONING

To achieve adequate and minimally traumatic exposure during the neurosurgical procedure, patients are placed in one of several operative positions. Common to all of these positions is elevation of the head to decrease bleeding and ICP and to promote gravitational drainage of CSF. The protection of all pressure points is crucial during positioning in children, as is the maintenance of the neck in a neutral position.

The sitting position provides excellent access to the brain, improves venous and CSF drainage, and facilitates hemostasis. There is, however, an increased incidence of venous air embolism, depression of cardiac output, hypotension,[3] cerebral ischemia secondary to a reduction in CPP, and postoperative quadriplegia.[51] To avoid hypotension with the change of position, patients must have an adequate circulating blood volume, the legs must be wrapped from toes to groin; the new position must be achieved slowly, and there must be continuous, direct monitoring of blood pressure and heart rate. The sitting position may be justified with proper monitoring when such use poses an equal or reduced overall patient risk compared with the supine or lateral position.[9] This position is usually avoided, however, in sicker patients because postural hypotension is positively correlated with poor physical condition.[3]

TEMPERATURE CONTROL

Lowering the body temperature decreases the brain's metabolic demands and oxygen consumption and is protective against ischemia, but it has deleterious effects. Shivering raises the ICP and oxygen consumption, metabolic acidosis can depress cardiac output, and dysrhythmias occur when the temperature falls below 30° C. To maintain normothermia in children, it is important to warm the operating room before the induction of anesthesia, provide a heated water mattress, limit the time and extent of body exposure, warm the cleansing solutions, cover the uninvolved areas of the body, heat and humidify the inspired gases, and warm all intravenous solutions and blood products.

BRAIN VOLUME

The hyperosmotic drugs, mannitol, urea, and glycerol, reduce brain volume by increasing plasma osmolality.

This serves to move water from the brain to the intravascular compartment down a concentration gradient, thus shrinking the brain and facilitating surgical manipulation. Although mannitol is excluded from the brain in the presence of an intact blood-brain barrier and may be given to patients who have a renal disease, it does cause an initial transient increase in intravascular volume, CBF, and ICP.

The maintenance of a mild fluid deficit or the use of a loop diuretic such as furosemide (0.15 to 0.30 mg/kg)[27] may help reduce the increase in ICP, which may occur after the use of mannitol. The osmotic diuresis from mannitol also increases urinary losses of sodium and potassium. Because this may be exacerbated by the addition of furosemide,[91] it is necessary to monitor the electrolytes intraoperatively and replace potassium as indicated. Mannitol (0.25 mg/kg) is given 30 minutes before the skin incision. Its action begins within 10 to 15 minutes, and it remains effective for 2 hours.

Corticosteroids reduce cerebral edema by reducing CSF formation, decreasing membrane permeability, and improving intracranial compliance. Dexamethasone is most effective in treating patients who have perifocal edema surrounding malignant brain tumors[44] and brain abscesses. Prospective, double-blinded studies have failed, however, to demonstrate any beneficial effect of corticosteroids in improving the outcome after head injury.[10,89] Corticosteroids may also have increased the incidence of intracranial infections[80] and pneumonia[10] in these patients.

Hyperventilation to a $Paco_2$ of 25 to 30 mm Hg reduces brain volume by decreasing CBF through cerebral vasoconstriction. Impaired responsiveness to changes in CO_2 tension associated with extensive intracranial disease (ischemia, trauma, tumor, infection) may interfere with the effectiveness of this measure. There is also evidence that a $Paco_2$ of less than 20 mm Hg impairs oxygenation and causes an increase in brain lactate secondary to severe restriction of CBF.

BLOOD, COLLOID, AND CRYSTALLOID ADMINISTRATION

The intraoperative administration of fluids is governed by the patient's maintenance fluid requirement, blood loss, insensible loss, third-space loss, and urine output. For maintenance, most children require 100 ml/kg for the first 10 kg for 24 hours, 50 ml/kg for the next 11 to 20 kg for 24 hours, and 20 ml/kg for each kilogram above 20 kg for 24 hours. In the operating room, this translates to 4 ml/kg/hr for the first 10 kg, 2 ml/kg/hr for the next 10 kg, and 1 ml/kg/hr for each kilogram above 20 kg.

Crystalloid solutions are administered as necessary to maintain cardiac filling pressure, cardiac output, and urine output. Although the administration of glucose had been recommended for all pediatric patients in the past, recent studies have revealed that the average healthy pediatric patient does not develop intraoperative or postoperative hypoglycemia, despite extended fasting.[6] Rather, the serum glucose levels actually rose during most operations owing to the catechol response to surgery and anesthesia.[98] Excessive glucose is also avoided because of evidence of exacerbation of damage from cerebral ischemia in patients who have a high blood glucose level at the time of the hypoxic insult.[33,81]

Consequently, it is recommended that glucose-free solutions such as lactated Ringer's be used for all blood loss, third-space loss, and deficit-fluid replacement. Because lactated Ringer's solution is relatively hypotonic to plasma (and thus may exacerbate cerebral edema formation), normal saline may be preferable for treatment of hypovolemia in children who have an intracranial space-occupying lesion or damage to the blood-brain barrier. Dextrose 2.0% in lactated Ringer's or half-normal saline may be given as a constant infusion for the maintenance fluid replacement.[67] For infants weighing less than 10 kg who have debilitating diseases and those undergoing long operations, blood glucose should be measured to determine the need for administration of exogenous glucose. All neonates require a constant infusion of glucose.

The replacement of blood depends on the amount of operative loss and the patient's age, hematocrit, and clinical condition. Estimation of the child's blood volume and the minimal acceptable hematocrit facilitates determination of the maximal allowable blood loss and the blood products necessary for the planned surgical procedure. The blood volume of the premature infant is 90 to 100 ml/kg; the term infant, 80 to 90 ml/kg; children 3 months to 1 year of age, 70 to 80 ml/kg; and children older than 1 year of age, approximately 70 ml/kg. Most healthy pediatric patients tolerate a hematocrit of 20% to 25%, providing the circulating blood volume is maintained. Patients requiring a higher hematocrit are premature infants, infants less than 3 months of age, and children who have cyanotic congenital heart disease and severe pulmonary disease.

Maximum allowable blood loss (MABL) may be calculated as a proportion[23] using the patient's starting hematocrit and the lowest acceptable hematocrit (25%):

$$\frac{\text{Estimated blood volume} \times (\text{starting patient hematocrit} - 25)}{\text{Starting patient hematocrit}}$$

For example, the maximum allowable blood loss to reach a hematocrit of 25% for a 20 kg child whose starting hematocrit is 35% is:

$$\frac{(70 \text{ ml/kg})(20 \text{ kg}) \times (35-25)}{35} = \frac{(1400)(10)}{35} = 400 \text{ ml}$$

The maximum allowable blood loss may be replaced, in addition to the administration of fluids for deficit, maintenance, and third-space losses, with either 5% albumin on a milliliter-for-milliliter basis or 2 to 3 ml of balanced salt solution (normal saline or lactated Ringer's) for each milliliter of blood lost. For neurosurgical patients, neonates, and patients in whom extensive blood loss is anticipated, 5% albumin may be the better choice because the larger fluid load from the balanced salt solution can be problematic.

After the blood loss exceeds the calculated maximum allowable blood loss, packed red blood cells (PRBC) and balanced salt solution are used for replacement by transfusing 0.5 ml PRBCs for each milliliter of blood lost beyond the maximum allowable blood loss. For the pediatric population, frozen PRBCs, although expensive, offer the advantages of less blood-group sensitization, better preservation of 2,3 diphosphoglycerate (2,3 DPG), less potential for transmission of viral illnesses, a smaller citrate load, and less leakage of potassium from the red blood cells.

Fresh frozen plasma (FFP) contains all the clotting factors but no platelets. It also has the highest proportion of citrate per unit volume of any blood product and may cause citrate toxicity or acute ionized hypocalcemia when large amounts are administered rapidly to pediatric patients.[26] For this reason, FFP is reserved for use when there is evidence of inadequacy of hemostasis intraoperatively. This has been noted to occur in children when the blood loss exceeds 1.5 blood volume, and the PT and PTT are prolonged to 1.5 times control, which may times warrant correction with FFP.[11]

Platelets may be required in patients who have massive surgical blood loss or drug-induced thrombocytopenia. When pediatric patients who have a prolonged bleeding time require emergent neurosurgical procedures in which complete hemostasis is mandatory, it is important to administer the platelets just before the operation to achieve the highest levels at the time hemostasis is most essential. A transfusion of 0.1 to 0.3 U of platelets/kg will increase the platelet count by 20,000 to 70,000/mm^3. In the face of massive ongoing blood loss, the higher dose of 0.3 U/kg is more effective than the lower dose of 0.1 U/kg.[24] For most surgical situations, however, prophylactic platelet transfusions are not indicated without clinical evidence of microvascular bleeding and ongoing blood loss.[85]

The starting platelet count correlates with the need for and timing of platelet transfusion. A low initial count suggests the need for early exogenous platelet transfusion, whereas a high initial platelet count indicates that exogenous platelets may not be required until several blood volumes have been lost. Therefore a baseline platelet count must be obtained before patients undergo procedures in which extensive blood loss is anticipated to ascertain the need for, and timing of, exogenous platelet administration.[24]

In addition to coagulopathy from dilutional thrombocytopenia and dilution of clotting factors, massive blood transfusion is associated with a number of other problems, including abnormalities of potassium and calcium homeostasis, hypothermia, acid-base imbalance, and shifts of the oxygen-hemoglobin dissociation curve.

The incidence of hyperkalemia is greatest after transfusion with whole blood, particularly if the blood is not absolutely fresh. If neonates or infants receive whole blood, even when fresh, the potassium content should be measured before transfusion. Citrated or frozen PRBCs may also have high potassium concentrations in the supernatant, but clinically significant hyperkalemia has not been observed after routine transfusion.[23] Rapid transfusion has been implicated in the development of serious hyperkalemia, however.[12] In addition, the longer the delay between thawing and administration, the higher the potassium concentration in the supernatant. Furthermore, transfusion, even with component therapy, may lead to hyperkalemia if the rate of administration is sufficiently rapid.[32]

Citrate toxicity is the ionized hypocalcemia caused by the binding of ionized calcium by the sodium citrate preservative in blood products, most notably in whole blood and FFP. Ionized hypocalcemia has been implicated in the depression of cardiac function[103] seen most commonly in infants who receive enough FFP that it composes a significant proportion of their circulating blood volume. Further, the myocardial-depressant effects of ionized hypocalcemia and halothane anesthesia are synergistic; the combined effects are greater than the sum of each effect individually.[22]

In the treatment of ionized hypocalcemia, Coté et al. found that the rates of ionization of calcium gluconate and calcium chloride were equivalent, and the cardiovascular responses were similar. The administration of frequent small doses is equally efficacious and, in all likelihood, safer than the administration of single large doses of calcium.[25] FFP should be administered through a peripheral catheter rather than a central venous catheter to avoid the delivery of high concentrations of citrate to the coronary circulation, and exogenous calcium should be administered during the transfusion of FFP whenever the rate of infusion is 1.0 ml/kg/min or greater, especially in neonates and small infants.[23]

Hypothermia, a further potential hazard of extensive blood transfusion, causes a leftward shift of the oxygen/hemoglobin dissociation curve whereby oxygen is more tightly bound to hemoglobin and consequently less available for delivery to tissues. Blood products should be warmed and measures taken to maintain body temperature, including the use of warming blankets, in-line heated humidifiers, artificial noses, head covering, and plastic wrap of extremities. Metabolic alkalosis will cause a further leftward shift of the oxygen/hemoglobin dissociation curve, but exogenous bicarbonate should be withheld unless there is a clearly documented lactic acidosis. The low 2,3 DPG associated with the transfusion of large volumes of citrated whole blood and FFP will also shift the oxygen/hemoglobin dissociation curve to the left. Because frozen PRBCs do not contain citrate and the concentration of 2,3 DPG is preserved, they may offer some advantage in minimizing the leftward shift of the curve.

ANESTHETIC PHARMACOLOGY AND TECHNIQUE

Of utmost importance in anesthetizing patients who are at risk for the development of or who already have intracranial hypertension is the maintenance of CPP in the presence of disordered autoregulation, impaired response of CBF to changes in $Paco_2$, abnormal regional CBF, and decreased intracranial compliance. The inhalation anesthetics, halothane, enflurane, and isoflurane, decrease cerebral vascular resistance, inducing vascular dilation and dose-dependent increases in CBF, cerebral blood volume, and ICP.[2] At the same time, they reduce the cerebral metabolic oxygen requirement, causing an excess of oxygen supply over demand. In addition, enflurane stimulates the production of CSF,[5] and halothane prevents the uptake of the CSF from the arachnoid villi. Although isoflurane is a less potent cerebral vasodilator than halothane or enflurane,[30] isoflurane increases ICP in patients who have brain tumors large enough to cause a shift of the midline structures on computed tomographic scan[43] despite the presence of hypocapnia. The volatile anesthetics also impair autoregulation in a dose-dependent fashion.[56]

INHALATION ANESTHETICS

Cerebral blood flow velocity in children varies directly with the end-tidal CO_2 partial pressure during halothane anesthesia.[59] CBF velocity increases as the concentration of halothane increases[57] but does not change significantly with increasing concentrations of isoflurane. Because enflurane may precipitate seizure activity, especially in the presence of hypocapnea, it is advisable to avoid enflurane in children who have a history of epilepsy. Neither desflurane nor sevoflurane initiates seizures,[90] and both decrease CBF in proportion to their effects on the cerebral metabolic rate for oxygen consumption, as does isoflurane.

In terms of cardiovascular stability during administration of inhalation anesthetics to neonates and infants, studies in newborn swine demonstrated that halothane depressed the circulation to the same extent as isoflurane; sevoflurane depressed the circulation less than either halothane or isoflurane at equipotent anesthetic concentrations.[60] Halothane also may cause bradycardia, particularly in newborns, presumably because vagal influences predominate over the limited sympathetic innervation of the myocardium in this age group. The effect can be reversed with atropine. Halothane also sensitizes the myocardium to catecholamines so that serious dysrhythmias may occur if epinephrine is used in patients anesthetized with halothane. Isoflurane, desflurane, and sevoflurane do not sensitize the myocardium to catecholamines to the same extent.[113]

In view of the fact that inhalation anesthetics cause a decrease in heart rate and systolic blood pressure, atropine, 0.02 mg/kg IV, must be included at induction. The concentration of the anesthetic must be increased slowly and in small increments, and normal saline or 5% albumin, 10 to 15 ml/kg, must be administered to maintain the systolic blood pressure above 40 mm Hg as the concentration of the inhaled anesthetic is increased.

Although an inhalation induction may not be appropriate for infants and children who have a decrease in intracranial compliance, other children undergoing surgery for spinal cord problems (excluding mass lesions) and orthopedic and urologic complications of spina bifida (in the presence of a functioning ventriculoperitoneal shunt) may undergo an inhalation induction. Halothane remains the favored drug for induction of anesthesia because it carries a lower incidence of breath holding, coughing, salivation, excitement, laryngospasm, and arterial oxygen desaturation than isoflurane.[78] Induction of unpremedicated infants and children up to 12 years of age with desflurane was marked by breath holding, laryngospasm, coughing, and arterial oxygen desaturation. The MAC of desflurane in infants and children depends on the age, although the difference in the MAC of neonates and older infants is smaller than with halothane and isoflurane. The hemodynamic responses to 1 MAC of desflurane are similar in neonates, infants, and children to age 12 and approximate those of halothane.[106]

In contrast, induction with sevoflurane in healthy children does not irritate the upper airway.[72] There is a report, however, of malignant hyperthermia during sevoflurane anesthesia in a child who had central core disease,[77] indicating that sevoflurane can trigger malignant hyperthermia in a susceptible patient. The episode was successfully treated with intravenous dantrolene.

The addition of nitrous oxide to the anesthetic regimen of patients who have space-occupying lesions causes an increase in ICP, which can be attenuated in patients who have been previously hyperventilated.[49] The prior administration of thiopental or diazepam also has been demonstrated to blunt this response.[73] In normal human volunteers, CBF increases with the breathing of 60% nitrous oxide.[88] This effect may be due to cerebrovasodilation.

Fentanyl, used with oxygen, nitrous oxide, muscle relaxant, low-dose inhalation anesthesia, and controlled ventilation, reduces the CBF and cerebral metabolic rate when the $Paco_2$ is maintained at normal to hypocapneic levels.[66] CPP is not reduced, nor is ICP increased in patients receiving fentanyl who have space-occupying lesions.[73]

Fentanyl and sufentanil also offer the advantage of hemodynamic stability when used with oxygen and pancuronium to anesthetize neonates and infants.[40,86,117] Hypotension and bradycardia are rare, as long as vagolytic drugs (pancuronium, atropine) are given as well. In the newborn-lamb model, fentanyl did not significantly affect the heart rate, blood pressure, cardiac output, or regional distribution of blood flow to the major organs, including the brain and gastrointestinal tract, in doses ranging from 30 to 3000 µg/kg.[118] This stability may be compromised, however, by the concomitant administration of nitrous oxide, barbiturates, or benzodiazepines.[119]

The dose of fentanyl in newborns and infants varies and depends on postnatal age, type of surgery, and the presence or absence of acidosis, hypoxia, and hemodynamic stability. Fentanyl also is highly bound in the blood to alpha acid glycoprotein, a protein present in low concentrations in the neonate's blood. The fraction of free unbound sufentanil in neonates and children less than a year of age is greater than in older children and adults, which correlates with age-related differences in the concentration of alpha acid glycoproteins in blood. The total-body clearance of fentanyl in 3- to 12-month-old infants is also greater than in children above 1 year of age and in adults, and the elimination half-life is longer. Fentanyl's prolonged elimination half-life may lead to respiratory depression with frequent repeated doses, but older infants may tolerate more fentanyl without respiratory depression because the enhanced clearance of fentanyl will reduce the plasma concentration.[50]

Barbiturates increase cerebral vascular resistance and reduce cerebral metabolic rate, CBF, cerebral blood volume, and ICP. In spite of the effectiveness of thiopental in reducing acute elevations of ICP and improving CPP after the administration of vasodilating drugs (ketamine, halothane) or noxious stimuli (tracheal intubation, skin incision), the administration of pentobarbital prophylactically after head trauma not only failed to improve the outcome, but also increased the complications from hypotension.[112] There was no difference in the mean ICP, the incidence of elevated ICP, the duration of elevated ICP, the doses of mannitol required to control the ICP, or the number of patients who died from uncontrollable increases in ICP between the patients who received pentobarbital and those who did not.

In addition to reducing ICP, the barbiturates also improve the brain's tolerance for focal ischemia. The possible mechanisms for this effect include metabolic suppression, a decrease in cerebral edema formation, and the creation of a reverse steal effect, increasing CBF to ischemic regions. During barbiturate-induced anesthesia, when the electroencephalogram becomes isoelectric, there is a 50% decrease in oxygen utilization by the brain and an increase in glycogen and high-energy phosphate content, probably secondary to the decrease in neuronal activity. Barbiturates may provide brain protection for young patients by reducing the hyperemic response to head injury.[2,99] In addition, patients undergoing cardiopulmonary bypass for open-heart procedures (valve replacement, aneurysmectomy) who received barbiturates were reported to have fewer neuropsychiatric complications than those who did not.[75] This effect was not substantiated, however, in patients undergoing coronary artery bypass grafting with hypothermic cardiopulmonary bypass.[120] There is no benefit derived from barbiturate therapy in complete ischemia (cardiac arrest) either, whether given before, during, or after the event, in animals[39] or in humans.[1]

Midazolam[65] and etomidate induce rapid loss of consciousness, reduce CBF, cerebral metabolic rate, and ICP; and maintain reasonable cardiovascular stability. Etomidate, if injected rapidly, may produce severe pain and myoclonus. A single intravenous bolus as well as a continuous infusion have been associated with suppression of the adrenal cortex.[58] Diazepam also decreases CBF, cerebral metabolic rate, and ICP in head-injured patients and in patients who have a decrease in intracranial compliance from other causes: tumor, abscess, hydrocephalus, or subarachnoid hemorrhage.[105] Respiratory depression with diazepam and midazolam has been reported, particularly when narcotics are given simultaneously.

Propofol is a new intravenous sedative-hypnotic drug useful for both induction of anesthesia when administered as a bolus and for maintenance when administered as a continuous infusion. Emergence from anesthesia with propofol is fairly rapid. Because propofol is available as an emulsion in lecithin, it has the potential for bacterial contamination. To avoid infection, the drug is handled using sterile precautions, and the unused portion is discarded after each case.

Propofol produces a dose-dependent reduction in CBF[109,110] and a smaller decrease in cerebral metabolic rate. The uncoupling of CBF and cerebral metabolic rate is not of the same magnitude or direction as that caused by the inhalation anesthetics, but neither does the effect of propofol resemble the strictly-coupled decrease in CBF and cerebral metabolic rate caused by thiopental. For this reason, intravenous anesthesia with propofol by infusion has been used successfully in the anesthetic management of craniotomy for a penetrating craniocerebral air-rifle missile injury.[116] Large doses of propofol, however, have caused documented decreases in the CPP to less than 50 mm Hg.[79]

The ED_{50} and ED_{95} for propofol for induction of anesthesia in unpremedicated children are 1.5 (1.3 to 1.7) mg/kg and 2.3 (2.1 to 3.0) mg/kg, respectively.[47] Mild to moderate pain on induction was reported in 6.6% of children, involuntary movement in 12.7%, and apnea in 21%. The systemic blood pressure decreased more than 20% of baseline in 48% of patients who received halothane after the propofol. With a dose of 2.5 to 3.0 mg/kg for induction, the children experienced a loss of lash reflex within 50 seconds of injection.

Westrin reported the ED_{50} of propofol to be 3.0 ± 0.2 mg/kg in infants 1 to 6 months of age and 2.4 ± 0.1 mg/kg in children 10 to 16 years of age.[114] In this study, 50% of infants and 18% of children had pain on injection, but there was no bradycardia or clinically relevant decrease in blood pressure. In addition, 18% of patients experienced more than 15 seconds of apnea.

Ketamine increases ICP, interferes with autoregulation, and can reduce CPP despite normal or elevated blood pressure.[96] Consequently, ketamine has no place in neurosurgical anesthesia or in sedation for neurodiagnostic procedures. Lidocaine, on the other hand, reduces the cerebral metabolic rate, increases cerebrovascular resistance, and reduces CBF and cerebral blood volume. Intravenous lidocaine, 1.5 mg/kg, in combination with thiopental, muscle relaxant, and narcotic, given 1 minute before laryngoscopy and intubation, can prevent intracranial hypertension and limit the intensity and duration of cardiovascular changes.[46]

None of the commonly used muscle relaxants is known to cross the blood-brain barrier or to affect the neurovasculature directly. The major advantages of vecuronium and atracurium are their cardiovascular stability and failure to increase ICP in the presence of reduced intracranial compliance.[38,70] Laudanosine, a metabolite of atracurium, has been associated with an arousal pattern on the electroencephalogram and an increase in the minimum alveolar concentration of experimental animals.[97] Pipercuronium and doxacurium combine long duration of action with cardiovascular stability.

Succinylcholine, on the other hand, has been shown to raise ICP after the effects of thiopental have dissipated when anesthesia is maintained with nitrous oxide and oxygen, and controlled ventilation has produced normocarbia.[71] Consequently, rapid-sequence induction for emergency surgery requires adequate anesthesia before laryngoscopy and intubation if succinylcholine is used. Succinylcholine is contraindicated in patients who have spinal cord injury, major trauma, muscle wasting (such as from prolonged coma or paralysis), and burns, because release of potassium has caused cardiac arrest.

Alternatively, intubation can be accomplished by pretreating the patient with a small dose of nondepolarizing muscle relaxant (atracurium, 0.1 mg/kg, or vecuronium, 0.015 mg/kg) during preoxygenation. This is then followed by a larger dose (atracurium, 0.7 mg/kg, or vecuronium, 0.1 mg/kg) given right after the sleep dose of thiopental. Intubating conditions obtain in 60 to 90 seconds.[64]

The induction of anesthesia for elective craniotomy is accomplished smoothly and quickly with the intravenous administration of thiopental. Anesthesia may be induced in children who do not have an intravenous catheter in place by mask with nitrous oxide, oxygen, and halothane in sufficient concentrations to permit the insertion of an intravenous catheter. As soon as this is accomplished, nitrous oxide and halothane are discontinued, and the intravenous induction sequence is instituted. Alternatives to a mask induction include rectal methohexital (20 to 30 mg/kg) or the nasal administration of midazolam, both of which need to be given by the anesthesiologist in an area where full resuscitation equipment is available.

Fentanyl, 3 to 6 µg/kg, and either vecuronium, 0.1 mg/kg, or atracurium, 0.5 mg/kg, are added to thiopental after institution of controlled hyperventilation with 100% oxygen. The larynx is intubated after the abolition of laryngeal reflexes, paralysis of skeletal muscles, and intravenous administration of additional thiopental, 2 mg/kg, to prevent systemic and intracranial hypertension during laryngoscopy and intubation. For patients who have a full stomach, anesthesia may be induced with thiopental and succinylcholine in rapid sequence. Patients who are hypovolemic and hypotensive from multisystem injury may benefit from the substitution of either midazolam or etomidate for thiopental.

Anesthesia is maintained with the continuous administration of oxygen and either nitrous oxide or air; intermittent doses or infusions of narcotic, muscle relaxant, and a barbiturate; and low concentrations of isoflurane. Ventilation is controlled to keep the arterial Pa_{CO_2} between 25 and 30 mm Hg.

Smooth emergence from anesthesia requires that the patient neither cough nor strain on the endotracheal tube, as this will elevate systemic pressure and ICP and endanger hemostasis. Muscle relaxation is reversed with neostigmine and either glycopyrrolate or edrophonium and atropine. The trachea of the stable, responsive patient who has adequate spontaneous ventilation is extubated in the operating room. Naloxone is indicated for the treatment of persistent respiratory depression after the reversal of muscle relaxation and reaccumulation of CO_2 to normal levels. Patients who will be ventilated postoperatively because of trauma, cerebral edema, poor preoperative status, or a catastrophic intraoperative event remain asleep and paralyzed.

Oxygen and portable ECG and blood pressure monitoring equipment accompany the patient from the operating suite to the recovery unit, where complete monitoring is continued. Diagnostic tests, including the determination of arterial blood gases, hematocrit, serum glucose, electrolytes, and osmolality; urine specific gravity; chest roentgenogram; and ECG, are performed in the recovery unit as soon as the patient's vital signs have stabilized.

HEAD INJURY

The majority of deaths in children are caused by accidents, and head injury is the leading cause of these fatalities. Of the 12,000 head injuries per 100,000 children that occur each year, 230 per 100,000 per year receive some type of hospitalization.[4] For children less than 2 years of age, the most frequent cause of fatal head trauma is child abuse or carelessness on the part of the custodian.[8] Beyond this age, most of the mortality from trauma is caused by falls and automobile accidents; 80% of these deaths are associated with head trauma, and the mortality in children who have multisystem trauma plus a head injury is two to three times greater than for children who sustain head trauma alone.[111]

Children who sustain severe head trauma have a mortality equal to a quarter of that of older patients.[15] The overall mortality rate for severe head injury in children varies from 9% to 38%.[111] The ultimate outcome and risk of death correlate with the Glascow Coma Scale score and the duration of coma. The mortality rate for children who have a Glascow Coma Scale score of 5 or greater varies from 0% to 20%, but for those who have a Glascow Coma Scale score of 8 or less, the overall mortality rate is 15% to 25%. When spontaneous ventilation is preserved, recovery to a moderately disabled state from a Glascow Coma Scale score of 3 may occur in up to 40% of patients. With early resuscitation and intensive care, it is estimated that close to 90% of children who have Glasgow Coma Scale score of 8 or less who survive their head injury will make a good recovery or be moderately disabled. Not a few will have cognitive defects and behavioral problems as well.

Head injury is considered in terms of primary and secondary damage. Primary damage is produced by the impact to the skull and brain at the time of the traumatic event. Primary arterial damage causes vessel disruption and epidural, subdural, and intracerebral hemorrhage. Acute subarachnoid hemorrhage occurs in up to 70% of children who have a Glasgow Coma Scale score of 7 or less.[122]

Three degrees of injury to the brain parenchyma have been described[37]: (1) stretching, which produces physiologic dysfunction, but no gross structural damage, with recovery; (2) disruption of the myelin sheaths with intact axons, which results in physiologic dysfunction and anatomic disruption, probably reversible with repair of the myelin; and (3) complete anatomic disruption of axons, which produces permanent irreversible loss of function in these fibers. Focal injury results from the impact itself and is associated with either skull fracture or brain contusion, but diffuse injury is produced by the sheering stresses arising from the forces of acceleration and deceleration. Thus recovery after head injury depends on the type of injury sustained.

Secondary brain injury after trauma refers to the pathophysiologic changes initiated by the primary injury, which do not cause damage for minutes, hours, or days after the initial injury. Secondary injury is produced by hypoxia, hypercarbia, intracranial hypertension, increased cerebral metabolic oxygen requirements,[104] systemic hypotension, cerebral herniation, cerebral edema and swelling,[52,74] and brain distortion. Although only prevention can eliminate the effects of the primary injury, either prevention or prompt diagnosis and treatment will reverse the effects of secondary injury, limit the resultant ischemia, and improve the outcome after head trauma.

Victims of head trauma become hypoxic because of mechanical and pathophysiologic reasons. Obstruction of the airway can occur with loss of consciousness, decreased muscle tone of the tongue and pharyngeal structures, and flexion of the neck. Apnea also can accompany loss of consciousness and, if prolonged, will cause secondary anoxic injury to neuronal structures. Hypoxia caused in this way is exacerbated by aspiration of blood, teeth, saliva, and vomitus after injury. Damage to the upper cervical spine also may cause secondary anoxic ischemic injury from apnea, diaphragmatic impairment, or neurogenic pulmonary edema. In addition, direct trauma to the face or neck may compromise the upper airway completely. Injury to the lungs will impair gas exchange because of contusion, hemothorax, pneumothorax, or bronchial rupture.

The hypercarbia that accompanies hypoxia is detrimental because it increases CBF, cerebral blood volume, and ICP. The decrease in arteriolar tone from the hypercarbia-induced vasodilation is associated with higher end-capillary pressure, which increases the likelihood of intracerebral hemorrhage and the rate of formation of cerebral edema.

Systemic hypotension as the direct result of head injury in children is secondary to scalp laceration or evulsion with extensive blood loss or cervicomedullary injury with damage to the vasopressor centers in the medulla. High cervical-cord injury may also cause hypotension because of the ensuing sympathectomy. More commonly, however, because 20% to 50% of children who sustain serious head injury also have other injuries, system hypotension in the severely injured child is caused by the associated injuries, usually abdominal and thoracic. The addition of shock markedly worsens the expected outcome for any given Glasgow Coma Scale score.[111] In the child, tachycardia, tachypnea, bradypnea, and depressed level of consciousness all may be signs of hypovolemia, so a child's neurologic status should not be considered permanent until fluid resuscitation is accomplished. Early intervention to prevent or reverse shock is crucial for good neurologic recovery.

Children may experience an initial period of sodium retension for the first 2 to 4 days after injury. The inappropriate secretion of antidiuretic hormone (ADH) associated with cerebral injury will also cause hyponatremia. Therefore fluid should be administered at 50% of the child's normal requirement during the first 2 to 4 days.

The destruction of brain tissue in children may also impair coagulation because of the release of thromboplastin, activation of the clotting pathways, and an attendant decrease in fibrinogen, platelets, and factors V and VIII. Disseminated intravascular coagulation was reported to occur in one third of children seen within 2 hours of sustaining a major head injury.[68] The treatment of coagulopathies is replacement of the necessary hemostatic factors.

Neurogenic pulmonary edema also has been reported in children[69] and is associated with focal brainstem lesions in the region of the nucleus tractus solitarius. The mechanism involves an increase in the pulmonary artery pressure with an attendant increase in capillary permeability. The treatment includes positive-pressure ventilation, positive end-expiratory pressure, and diuretics.

Aside from the intracranial hypertension caused by epidural, subdural, and intracerebral hemotomas, the most common cause of an increase in ICP after head injury in children is cerebral swelling. This results from an increase in CBF and cerebral blood volume, and can lead to ischemia and herniation if not controlled promptly.[45,52] Such hyperemic congestion has a good prognosis, as opposed to the diffuse low-density appearance of the cerebrum on computed tomographic scan. This is an indication of severely elevated ICP and very low cortical CBF, and is associated with a very poor outcome. Cerebral edema rarely occurs in children in the first 24 hours after injury, except around intracerebral hematomas. The elevation of ICP from mass lesions, brain swelling, or brain edema can cause secondary damage from the decrease in CBF, concomitant ischemia, and transalar, subfalcine, uncal, or tonsillar herniation. These herniation syndromes compress cerebral arteries, impair regional CBF, and cause focal ischemia.

Hematomas occur in 20% to 30% of children after head injury. If surgically significant, they must be removed as quickly as possible because good recovery depends on the rapidity with which a hematoma is evacuated. Epidural hematomas, the result of injury to the branches of the middle meningeal artery in the dura mater, occur most frequently in the parietal and parietotemporal areas in children. Venous epidural hematomas, which may not become evident for several days after injury, are caused by fracture across a major venous sinus. Acute subdural hematomas in children result from disruption of either cortical tissue, with arterial hemorrhage and bleeding into the subdural and subarachnoid space, or bridging veins, with bleeding in the subdural and subarachnoid space. The incidence of surgically treatable subdural hematomas varies from 5% to 30% of pediatric head injuries.[45] In children under 1 year of age, acute subdural hematomas occur most frequently after impact injury.[122] Although they rarely require surgical intervention, aspiration of 10 ml of CSF has helped to lower ICP, at least transiently. Subacute and chronic subdural hematomas and intracerebral hematomas are rare in children, although their occurrence should prompt concern about child abuse.

The skull fractures that require operative correction include: compound skull fractures, displaced skull fractures where the fractured segment is displaced below the inner table of the surrounding skull, fractures associated with an intracranial hematoma that produces a mass effect, and fractures that cause disfigurement.

Hemodynamic instability results most commonly from the preload deficit caused by hemorrhage from the associated multisystem trauma. The most useful initial intervention involves prompt infusion of electrolyte-containing solutions with or without colloid, blood products, or whole blood. If the augmentation of preload fails to produce hemodynamic stability in terms of adequate cardiac output and CPP, the need to adjust afterload and contractility may require the insertion of a pulmonary artery catheter for measurement of cardiac output and calculation of systemic and pulmonary vascular resistance.

The initiation of monitoring of ICP in the emergency room will facilitate diagnosis and treatment of the dynamic pathophysiology of pediatric head injury. The current indications for ICP monitoring in children include a Glasgow Coma Scale score of 3, 4, or 5 or a Glasgow Coma Scale score of 7 or less plus systemic hypotension.[14] The presence of an open fontanel is no protection against intracranial hypertension. The ICP can equal the blood pressure just as readily in an infant as it can in an older child whose sutures have closed. The features of ICP that suggest a decrease in intracranial compliance and therefore indicate the need for active therapy are: ICP greater than 15 mm Hg for 30 minutes; ICP greater than 20 mm Hg for 3 minutes;

CPP less than 50 mm Hg for 3 minutes; and pupillary dilation and bradycardia.

The initial control of intracranial hypertension is best achieved by hyperventilation to a $Paco_2$ of 20 to 25 mm Hg, maintenance of blood pressure within the normal range, adequate oxygenation to a Pao_2 of 80 to 100 mm Hg, alignment of the head and neck in a neutral midline position to facilitate cerebral venous drainage, and elevation of the head 15 to 20 degrees (systemic arterial pressure permitting).

These early maneuvers to control ICP are compatible with the needs of the spinal-cord-injured child. Although spinal and cranial injury do occur together, spinal-cord injury is rare: 1.8/100,000 children per year vs. 230/100,000 per year for head injury require hospitalization. In small children, cervical injuries occur at C1-C2. Most vehicular accidents do not cause spinal-cord injury in children; the majority rather result from falls and diving accidents. The history of the head injury thus is important in determining the probability of associated spinal-cord injury.

Hyperventilation is extremely effective in controlling intracranial hypertension from cerebral swelling caused by an increase in CBF. There is little clinical indication that hyperventilation will decrease cerebral perfusion to the point of ischemia.[13] Despite the evidence that prolonged hyperventilation loses its effectiveness in normal animals,[83] this is not the case in head-injured humans. Hyperventilation in children is also associated with sustained reductions in CBF beyond 6 hours, possibly for as long as 24 to 48 hours,[17] and the chronic respiratory alkalosis is well-tolerated in children without cardiac compromise. Although muscle paralysis itself does not decrease ICP, the use of muscle relaxants prevents the unconscious child from breathing against the ventilator and raising the ICP.

Adjunctive measures to reduce the ICP after head trauma, including barbiturates (thiopental and pentobarbital) and diuretics, are indicated. Barbiturates reduce cerebral metabolism and constrict cerebral blood vessels, thus decreasing CBF and cerebral blood volume. As such, they help counteract the cerebral swelling phase, but should only be used when ICP and arterial pressure are being monitored because the negative inotropic and vasodilator effects of the barbiturates cause hemodynamic depression. The augmentation of preload and contractility are frequently necessary to avoid hypotension, which occurs in 50% of patients who have barbiturate levels of 25 to 30 mg/L.[84] The presence of a burst-suppression pattern on the electroencephalogram indicates maximal cerebral metabolic depression. When either burst suppression or isoelectricity has been achieved, no further reduction in cerebral metabolic oxygen requirement is produced by increasing the blood level of the barbiturate. There is no evidence that the barbiturates have any protective effect against global cerebral ischemia, nor does their use improve outcome after head injury.

The osmotic diuretic mannitol is used to keep the ICP between 15 and 20 mm Hg. The greatest benefit from mannitol is derived when the CPP is less than 70 mm Hg and autoregulation is intact.[87] The initial dose in children is 0.5 to 1.0 g/kg. There is no evidence that mannitol is effective as a routine medication in the emergency room immediately after head injury in children.[17] Indeed, this may cause an acute electrolyte imbalance, and the attendant vasodilation can also reduce the systemic pressure abruptly in a child who is already hypovolemic. Osmotic diuretics have been used in the first 24 hours, to small effect, when the combination of hyperventilation, barbiturates, CSF drainage, and head-up position has failed to control ICP. The loop diuretics, furosemide, 0.5 to 1 mg/kg, and ethacrinic acid, reduce CSF production but do not decrease ICP reliably. They may be useful in the presence of the overhydration occasionally seen after fluid resuscitation from hypovolemic shock.

Steroids have not been of benefit in head injury, either for control of ICP or for improvement in outcome.[31] Their use has been associated, in fact, with an increase in the incidence of infection, particularly pneumonias. Methylprednisolone has been effective in attenuating the severity of neurologic deficit after spinal-cord injury.

Hypothermia, which decreases cerebral metabolism and CBF, may be efficacious in controlling the intracranial hypertension caused by an increase in CBF. The reduced temperature also may exert some protective effect against cerebral ischemia. The core temperature of children receiving barbiturates to control ICP may drift down to 34° C because the barbiturates interfere with the central mechanism for heat control and produce peripheral vasodilation.

The removal of CSF is also an effective way to reduce ICP. In children who have sustained severe head injury, the amount of CSF is reduced, but the removal of CSF from the ventricles will still lower the ICP. CSF may be withdrawn safely only from the ventricular system and not the lumbar subarachnoid space. Even this method becomes ineffective as the ventricles collapse and no more CSF is available.

The ability to diagnose and control intracranial hypertension is crucial because acute deterioration in children is most often caused by either generalized brain swelling and increased ICP or by seizure activity rather than surgically correctable lesions. Radiologic study such as CT scan elucidates the etiology of the deterioration and should be performed before surgery. Because a swollen, congested brain rather than cerebral edema is observed, hyperventilation and head-up tilt are appropriate. Mannitol is indicated if the presence of an epidural hematoma is strongly suspected.[15]

The immediate treatment of the head-injured child is predicated on attention to the ABCs of airway, breathing, and circulation. The patency of the airway should be assured, oxygen administered, and the mouth cleared of vomitus and traumatic debris. Ventilation is maintained by means of a bag and mask. Comatose patients benefit from endotracheal intubation if they cannot maintain a patent airway or if there is evidence of alveolar hypoventilation. The level of spinal cord injury also dictates airway management, because lesions below the sixth cervical vertebra preserve diaphragmatic function but paralyze intercostal muscles. Injury at the fifth cervical level maintains partial diaphragmatic function, but lesions at or above the fourth cervical vertebra cause major impairment of the movement of the diaphragm.

In intubating the trachea of a head-injured child, the attending physician must consider a number of factors. There may be cervical spine injury and instability. Hyperextension or flexion of the neck and the presence of either a cervical fracture or a dislocation can exacerbate the initial spinal-cord injury. The patient is also at risk for regurgitation and aspiration of stomach contents, so the physician must reduce the likelihood of these events during intubation. The ICP-elevating effect of laryngoscopy must be mitigated by the use of thiopental, diazepam, or lidocaine in conjunction with muscle relaxation. Ventilation must be maintained to prevent hypoxia and hypercarbia while the drugs are reaching their peak effect. During laryngoscopy, an assistant maintains the head in a neutral position. After the airway has been established, ventilation is adjusted to keep the Pa_{CO_2} between 30 and 35 mm Hg. In the presence of intracranial hypertension, the Pa_{CO_2} is maintained between 20 and 25 mm Hg.

SPINAL DYSRAPHISM

Meningomyelocele and encephalocele are dysraphic conditions of the spine and cranium, respectively, that result from defects in the formation of the neural tube. They are often associated with neurologic deficits and hydrocephalus.[29,93] Meningomyelocele may occur in the lumbar, thoracic, or cervical regions of the cord, with concomitant damaging effects on the function of the bowel, bladder, and lower limbs. Because infection is the primary risk associated with meningomyelocele, most neurosurgeons repair the defect within the first week of life.

Closure of the identifiable defects requires attention during the anesthetic period to blood and evaporative fluid loss, neonatal fluid requirements, temperature maintenance, prone positioning, and securing of the endotracheal tube. If the surgeon plans to use a nerve stimulator, neuromuscular blockade should be carefully monitored or avoided altogether. The presence of both meningomyelocele and encephalocele may complicate ventilation with bag and mask and endotracheal intubation in the supine position, requiring ingenious padding arrangements under the child's back and head.

The Arnold-Chiari malformation, a developmental anomaly frequently associated with meningomyelocele, involves a downward displacement of the inferior cerebellar structures into the upper cervical spinal canal. The accompanying elongation of the medulla and fourth ventricle causes obstructive hydrocephalus, which may require early ventriculostomy or the placement of a ventriculoperitoneal shunt. The Arnold-Chiari malformation may also be associated with bradycardia and stridor secondary to unilateral or bilateral paresis or paralysis of the vocal cords. Endotracheal intubation may be necessary.

Patients who have the Arnold-Chiari malformation may require decompression of the posterior fossa to relieve pressure on the brainstem. When there is a functioning CSF shunt in place before the decompressive operation, the intracranial compliance most likely will be normal. Assessing the adequacy of the airway preoperatively is crucial; securing the airway may require endotracheal intubation before the induction of anesthesia. The patient's ability to maintain a patent airway at the conclusion of surgery must be evaluated carefully with the ready capability of reintubation. Elective tracheotomy is indicated when the decompression of the brainstem fails to relieve the vocal cord paresis.

CRANIOSYNOSTOSIS

Premature fusion of the skull sutures requires operative intervention to enable the brain to grow and develop normally. Although the procedure is extradural, the blood loss may be considerable and also sudden if the surgeon enters a major venous sinus. Intracranial hypertension may be present if multiple sutures have fused. There is also a risk of venous air embolism because of the dissection around bone and sinuses; monitoring of the end-tidal carbon dioxide tension and the use of the Doppler ultrasound device for detection of intracardiac air are recommended. Surgery is also frequently performed in the prone position, necessitating attention to securing of the endotracheal tube and free excursion of the thorax and abdomen.

CRANIOFACIAL DEFORMITIES

The repair of craniofacial deformities, such as Apert's syndrome, Crouzon's syndrome, hypertelorism, and hypotelorism, requires extensive cranial surgery. The preoperative evaluation is crucial for establishing rapport with the child and for determining the presence of intracranial hypertension and of coexisting medical problems, which most often involve the cardiovascular system.

Because of the certainty of extensive blood loss, the monitoring of intraarterial and central venous pressure, urinary output, and brain temperature (with tympanic or nasopharyngeal thermistor) is essential, as is securing intravenous access for the replacement of blood. An adequate volume of blood and blood products should be typed and crossmatched preoperatively, although controlled hypotension, autologous blood transfusion, hemodilution, and red-cell saving devices may be used to reduce blood loss and limit reliance on bank blood. Clotting abnormalities may also develop if the patient requires replacement of more than one blood volume.

The reduction of intracranial volume also is necessary to facilitate intracranial access to facial structures and to re-

duce the compression to which the frontal lobes are subjected in the process. Techniques include the use of hyperventilation, osmotic or loop diuretics, barbiturates, narcotics, and limited concentrations of inhalation anesthetics. Prolonged retraction of the frontal lobes may cause cerebral edema postoperatively. Fluid and electrolyte disorders, including inappropriate secretion of antidiuretic hormone and diabetes insipidus, also may result from the retraction.

Because endotracheal intubation may be difficult in children who have facial anomalies, the anesthesiologist should have the fiberoptic bronchoscope available, and the surgeon should be prepared to perform a tracheotomy during induction of anesthesia if endotracheal intubation cannot be accomplished. After the larynx is intubated, the endotracheal tube should be secured by wire or suture to nonmobile facial structures (mandible, alveolar ridge, nasal alae) that will not move during the procedure. The trachea is also not extubated at the conclusion of the procedure until the patient is alert and breathing adequately. Wire cutters, drugs, and equipment for securing the airway should be at the bedside during the postoperative period.

HYDROCEPHALUS

Hydrocephalus is caused by obstruction to the flow of CSF, which leads to an increase in the size of the ventricles and in the intracranial volume of CSF. Although the condition of normal-pressure hydrocephalus is described in adults, most children who have hydrocephalus have either intracranial hypertension or, at the least, a decrease in intracranial compliance. The causes of hydrocephalus include tumors of the posterior fossa, congenital obstruction, infection and resultant stenosis of the CSF pathways, meningomyelocele, Arnold-Chiari malformation, neonatal intraventricular hemorrhage, subarachnoid hemorrhage, and trauma.

The treatment of hydrocephalus requires the insertion of a drainage system to shunt the CSF from the ventricular system to another site in the body, from which the CSF may be absorbed. The most common shunt in children is the ventriculoperitoneal shunt, although ventriculopleural, ventriculoatrial, ventriculojugular, and lumboperitoneal shunts are used as well. Besides the effect of anesthetic drugs on the child who has a decrease in intracranial compliance, each shunt procedure has its own attendant problems. Enough CSF may accumulate in the pleural cavity to compromise respiration and require thoracentesis or the insertion of a chest tube. The insertion of a ventriculoatrial shunt through the jugular vein may be complicated by venous air embolism, which can be avoided by minimizing the duration of the venotomy and by clamping the previously fluid-filled shunt tube after it is inserted into the vessel. Although the use of longer, nonreactive tubing for ventriculoperitoneal shunts has reduced the need for frequent replacement of the shunt as the child grows, the tubing still may perforate the bowel and cause either intestinal obstruction or intracranial infection by the cephalad migration of enteric organisms through the tubing.

The major difficulties encountered in children who have shunts in place are shunt malfunction and infection with attendant failure of CSF drainage, enlargement of the ventricles, either immediately or as a late and ominous sign, and increase in the volume of CSF and the ICP. The diagnosis of shunt malfunction is relatively straightforward in the child who is lethargic, vomits frequently, and has enlarged ventricles on magnetic resonance image or computerized tomographic scan. Neurosurgeons, neurologists, pediatricians, family practitioners, and anesthesiologists must recognize that behavioral changes, deterioration in school performance, and headaches in the *absence* of enlarged ventricles can also be associated with shunt malfunction. These children require shunt revision to prevent further neurologic damage, as do the children who have a change in level of consciousness; all require the attendant anesthetic precautions. It is just more difficult to make the diagnosis.

Anesthesia for correction of hydrocephalus through the insertion of a shunt or for treatment of either shunt obstruction or displacement is designed to improve intracranial compliance, even in infants whose cranial sutures are not yet fused. The sequence of an intravenous induction with thiopental, narcotic, nondepolarizing muscle relaxant, and hyperventilation with 100% oxygen in the prepared patient is optimal. In an emergency, preoxygenation, cricoid pressure, and intravenous induction with thiopental and a depolarizing muscle relaxant are indicated to secure the airway rapidly and safely. An inhalation induction and endotracheal intubation with a high concentration of halothane are contraindicated, because children who have untreated hydrocephalus or a malfunctioning shunt, regardless of whether their cranial sutures are fused, should not be exposed to the concentration of halothane necessary to accomplish endotracheal intubation. If an inhalation induction is necessary because the child does not have intravenous access, this should be secured as quickly as possible, the halothane discontinued, and the intravenous sequence instituted. After the trachea is intubated, hyperventilation is continued until a functioning shunt is inserted, the ventricles are drained, and the compliance is improved.

CAVERNOUS ANGIOMAS

Cavernous angiomas of the CNS in children can present in a variety of ways: acute or progressive neurologic deficit, seizures, irritability, or headaches. The occurrence of multiple lesions as well as a family history of vascular malformations of the central nervous system is described. The pathology of the lesions includes closely approximated cavernous vessels with areas of marked proliferation of granulation tissue and partially re-endothelialized hemorrhage.

Despite the possibility of a long hemorrhage-free clinical course after subtotal resection, residual malformation is present on late follow-up studies.[95] Subtotal resection thus does not eliminate the occurrence of rebleeding in the residual malformation. Seemingly innocuous lesions (1 cm) should be excised because they can cause serious hemorrhage. Because lesions do bleed frequently and silently with hemorrhages of small volume and low pressure, surgical exploration should be considered when the patient's clinical course is one of repetitive and progressive neurologic deficits. The gamma knife may be an alternative if the malformation is inaccessible. Improvement in preexisting neurologic deficits can be apparent postoperatively.

NEURORADIOLOGIC PROCEDURES

The complexity and challenge of anesthetizing children for neuroradiologic procedures increased greatly with the advent of magnetic resonance imaging. Heretofore, anesthesia for computerized tomographic scanning, myelography, spinal-cord and intracranial angiography, and endovascular neurointerventional procedures, which may require phlebotomy in infants, was complicated by the need for anesthesia in remote locations not designed for pediatric anesthesia, and by the use of intravenous contrast drugs, which could cause an osmotic diuresis as well as allergic reactions. On the plus side, however, was the fact that standard anesthesia and monitoring equipment could be used, and the anesthesiologist had direct and immediate access to the child.

Because of the high-energy magnetic fields generated for magnetic resonance imaging, however, the use of ferromagnetic materials in the immediate vicinity of the magnet is impossible; they degrade and distort the magnetic resonance image, and they impose the danger of injury from flying projectiles. The magnet also is never turned off, although the sequence can be interrupted if necessary. Consequently, new equipment manufactured from nonferromagnetic materials has been designed for the monitoring and administration of anesthesia.

The useful monitoring modalities range from the sophisticated to the prosaic, and include the finger plethysmograph, electrocardiograph by means of a telemetry signal, apnea monitor by nasal sensor or chest-movement sensor, and aluminum precordial stethoscope. The pulse oximeter was modified so that the signal does not degrade the magnetic resonance image. Caution is necessary to avoid loops in the cable, however, because contact of the loop with the child's skin can cause a third-degree burn. The use of fiberoptic cable has obviated this problem. A blood pressure cuff with a Doppler device also has proved satisfactory. Currently available from a single company (In Vivo, Seattle) is MR-compatible equipment for monitoring blood pressure, ECG, pulse oximetry, end-tidal CO_2, and respiratory rate.

As with computed tomographic (CT) scanning, the patient undergoing magnetic resonance (MR) imaging must remain perfectly still, but for a longer period of time (on the average of 40 minutes). Because the majority of children requiring magnetic resonance evaluation have brain tumors, hydrocephalus, or spinal-cord compromise, the choice of drugs and anesthetic technique must be governed by the patient's decrease compliance. Rectal methohexital,[42] oral chloral hydrate (25 to 50 mg/kg), intravenous or intramuscular pentobarbital (5 to 6 mg/kg),[102] the combination of intravenous pentobarbital and morphine (0.1 mg/kg), and propofol by bolus or infusion have been recommended because they confer sleep without causing significant respiratory depression. Children who take diphenyl hydantoin, Tegretol, or phenobarbital may require higher doses or may require general endotracheal anesthesia and controlled ventilation with nitrous oxide, oxygen, narcotic, and muscle relaxant—the same technique used to improve intracranial compliance when these patients require surgery. There is no place in this setting for the use of either ketamine, which increases CBF and cerebral metabolic oxygen requirement, or the combination of halothane and spontaneous ventilation, which also will increase CBF in children who have a decrease in intracranial compliance.

General anesthesia is usually required for arteriography, myelography, and polytomography to prevent movement and to eliminate the possibility of excessive sedation. When there is a decrease in intracranial compliance, controlled hyperventilation and the use of minimal concentrations of halogenated drugs are indicated. The intraarterial injection of contrast drug may produce systemic hypotension from vasodilation and also may increase ICP in patients who have poor intracranial compliance. Because the water-soluble contrast drug metrizamide can cause seizures, drugs that reduce the seizure threshold, such as phenothiazines and butyrophenones, should be avoided when metrizamide is used in conjunction with CT scanning.

SUMMARY

Pediatric patients undergoing neurosurgical procedures require the same anesthetic and monitoring considerations as adults and deserve the same care. The major difference is that pediatric patients are more susceptible to hypoxia and hypovolemia because of limited reserves. Consequently, all pediatric neurosurgical patients require excellent intravenous access and comprehensive monitoring, including intraarterial pressure, urinary output, and CVP when necessary.

Because inhalation anesthetics increase CBF and impair autoregulation, induction of anesthesia is accomplished with IV drugs (pentothal/propofol, narcotic, muscle relaxant) and ventilation with 100% oxygen until endotracheal intubation is accomplished in children who have decreased intracranial compliance from tumor, hematoma, abcess, hydrocephalus, or cerebral hyperemia.

Premedication in children who have intracranial pathology may cause respiratory depression that can further impair intracranial compliance. Therefore, creative solutions to the smooth induction of anesthesia are necessary, including the presence of parents in the operating room. Where posssible, children should be given a choice: IV catheter now or later, flavor for the mask, presence of parents. Their active involvement enhances the therapeutic process.

References

1. Abrahamson NS, Safar P, Detre K et al: Randomized clinical study of thiopental loading in comatose survivors of cardiac arrest, *N Engl J Med* 314:397-403, 1986.
2. Aitkenhead AR: Do barbiturates protect the brain? *Br J Anaesth* 53:1011-1013, 1981.
3. Albin MS, Babinski M, Maroon JC et al: Anesthetic management of posterior fossa surgery in the sitting position, *Acta Anaesth Scand* 20:117-128, 1976.
4. Anderson DW, McLaurin RL: The national head and spinal cord injury survey, *J Neurosurg* 53:606-610, 1980.
5. Artru AA: Enflurane causes a prolonged and reversible increase in the rate of CSF production in the dog, *Anesthesiology* 57:255-260, 1982.
6. Aun CST, Panesar NS: Paediatric glucose homeostasis during anesthesia, *Br J Anaesth* 64:413-418, 1990.
7. Bailey P, Pace N, Asburn M et al: Frequent hypoxemia and apnea after sedation with midazolam and fentanyl, *Anesthesiology* 73:826-830, 1990.
8. Billmire RE, Myers PA: Serious head injury in infants: accident and abuse, *Pediatrics* 75:340-342, 1985.
9. Black S, Ockert DB, Oliver WC Jr et al: Outcome following posterior fossa craniotomy in patients in the sitting or horizontal positions, *Anesthesiology* 69:49-56, 1988.
10. Braakman R, Schouten HJA, Dishoeck MB et al: Megadose steroids in severe head injury—results of a prospective double-blind clinical trial, *J Neurosurg* 58:326-330, 1983.
11. Braunstein AH, Oberman HA: Transfusion of plasma components, *Transfusion* 24:281-286, 1984.
12. Brown KA, Bissonnette B, Mac Donald M et al: Hyperkalemia during massive transfusion in paediatric craniofacial surgery, *Can J Anaesth* 37:401-408, 1990.
13. Bruce DA: Effects of hyperventilation on cerebral blood flow and metabolism, *Clin Perinatol* 11:673-680, 1984.
14. Bruce DA: Central nervous system injuries. In KS Welch, JG Randolph, MM Ravitch et al, editors: *Pediatric neurosurgery*, Chicago, 1986, Year Book Medical Publishers, p. 214.
15. Bruce DA: Head trauma: management. In Newfield P, Cottrell JE, editors: *Neuroanesthesia. Handbook of clinical and physiological essentials,* ed 2, Boston, 1991, Little, Brown, pp 282-300.
16. Bruce DA, Berman WA, Schut L: Cerebrospinal fluid pressure monitor-

ing in children: physiology, pathology and clinical usefulness, *Adv Pediatr* 24:233-290, 1977.

17. Bruce DA, Alavi A, Bilaniuk L et al: Diffuse cerebral swelling following head injuries in children: the syndrome of "malignant brain edema," *J Neurosurg* 54:170-178, 1981.

18. Charlton A, Hatch D, Lindahl S et al: Ventilation, ventilatory carbon dioxide and hormonal response during halothane anesthesia and surgery in children after midazolam premedication, *Br J Anaesth* 50:1234-1241, 1986.

19. Cheshey RW, Zelikovic I: Pre- and postoperative fluid management in infancy, *Pediatr Rev* 11:153-158, 1989.

20. Christensen MS, Moedt-Rasmussen K, Lassen NA: Cerebral vasodilation by halothane anesthesia in man and its potentiation by hypotension and hypercapnia, *Br J Anaesth* 39:927-934, 1967.

21. Coté C: NPO after midnight for children—a reappraisal, *Anesthesiol* 72:589-592, 1990.

22. Coté CJ: Depth of halothane anesthesia potentiates citrate-induced ionized hypocalcemia and adverse cardiovascular events in dogs, *Anesthesiology* 67:676-680, 1987.

23. Coté CJ: Blood, colloid and crystalloid therapy. In Lerman J, editor: New developments in pediatric anesthesia, *Anesthesiol Clin North Am* 9:865-884, 1991.

24. Coté CJ, Liu LMP, Szyfelbein SK et al: Changes in serial platelet counts following massive blood transfusion in pediatric patients, *Anesthesiology* 62:197-201, 1985.

25. Coté CJ, Drop LJ, Daniels AL et al: Calcium chloride versus calcium gluconate: comparison of ionization and cardiovascular effects in children and dogs, *Anesthesiology* 66:465-470, 1987.

26. Coté CJ, Drop LJ, Hoaglin DC et al: Ionized hypocalcemia after fresh frozen plasma administration to thermally-injured children: effects of infusion rate, duration, and treatment with calcium chloride, *Anesth Analg* 67:152-160, 1988.

27. Cottrell JE, Robustelli A, Post K et al: Furosemide- and mannitol-induced changes in intracranial pressure and serum osmolarity and electrolytes, *Anesthesiology* 47:28-30, 1977.

28. Crawford M, Lerman J, Christensen S et al: Effects of duration of fasting on gastric fluid pH and volume in healthy children, *Anesth Analg* 71:400-403, 1990.

29. Creighton RE, Relton JES, Meridy HW: Anaesthesia for occipital encephalocoele, *Can Anaesth Soc J* 21:402-406, 1974.

30. Cucchiara RF, Theye RA, Michenfelder JD: The effects of isoflurane on canine cerebral metabolism and blood flow, *Anesthesiology* 40:571-574, 1974.

31. Dearden NM, Gibson JS, McDowell DG et al: Effect of high-dose dexamethasone on outcome from severe head injury, *J Neurosurg* 64:88-98, 1986.

32. Driscoll DF, Bistrian BR, Jenkins RL et al: Development of metabolic alkalosis after massive transfusion during orthotopic liver transplantation, *Crit Care Med* 15:905-908, 1987.

33. Drummond JC, Moore SS: The influence of dextrose administration in the rabbit, *Anesthesiology* 70:64-70, 1989.

34. Feld L, Negus J, White P: Oral midazolam preanesthetic medication in pediatric outpatients, *Anesthesiology* 73:831-834, 1990.

35. Finley A, Bissonnette B, Goresky G et al: The effect of oral ranitidine and preoperative oral fluids on gastric fluid pH and volume in children, *Can J Anaesth* 36:595, 1989.

36. Friesen R, Lichtor J: Cardiovascular depression during halothane anesthesia in infants: a study of three induction techniques, *Anesth Analg* 61:42-45, 1982.

37. Gennarelli TA, Thibault LF, Adams JH et al: Diffuse axonal injury and traumatic coma in the primate, *Ann Neurol* 12:564-574, 1982.

38. Giffin JP, Cottrell JE, Shwiry B et al: Intracranial pressure after ORG NC 45 (Norcuron) in cats, *Anesth Analg* 63:218-221, 1984.

39. Gisvold SE, Safar P, Hendrick HHL et al: Thiopental treatment after global ischemia in pigtail monkeys, *Anesthesiology* 60:88-96, 1984.

40. Greeley WJ, deBruijn NP: Changes in sufentanil pharmacokinetics within the neonatal period, *Anesth Analg* 67:86-90, 1988.

41. Goudsouzian N, Cote C, Liu LMP et al: The dose-response effects of oral cimetidine on gastric pH and volume in children, *Anethesiology* 55:533-536, 1981.

42. Griswold JD, Liu LMP: Rectal methohexital for CT and MRI scans, *Anesthesiology* 67:A494, 1987.

43. Grosslight K, Colohan A, Bedford RF: Isoflurane and anesthesia-risk factors for increased ICP, *Anesthesiology* 63:533-536, 1985.

44. Gutin PW: Corticosteroid therapy in patients with brain tumors, *Natl Cancer Inst Monograph* 46:151-156, 1977.

45. Hahn YS, Raimondi AS, McLone DG et al: Traumatic mechanisms of head injury in child abuse, *Child Brain* 10:229-241, 1983.

46. Hamill JF, Bedford RF, Weaver DC et al: Lidocaine before endotracheal intubation: intravenous or laryngotracheal? *Anesthesiology* 55:578-581, 1981.

47. Hannallah RJ, Baker SB, Casey W et al: Propofol effective dose and induction characteristics in unpremedicated child, *Anesthesiology* 74:217-219, 1991.

48. Henderson JM, Brodsky BA, Fisher DM et al: Pre-induction of anesthesia in pediatric patients with nasally administered sufentanil, *Anesthesiology* 68:671-675, 1988.

49. Henriksen HT, Jorgensen PB: The effect of nitrous oxide on intracranial pressure in patients with intracranial disorders, *Br J Anaesth* 45:486-491, 1973.

50. Hertzka RE, Gauntlett IS, Fisher DM et al: Fentanyl-induced ventilatory depression: effects of age, *Anesthesiology* 70:213-218, 1989.

51. Hitselberger WE, House WSA: Warning regarding the sitting position for acoustic tumor surgery, *Arch Otolaryngol* 106:69, 1980.

52. Ito V, Tomita H, Yamazaki Y et al: Brain swelling and brain edema in acute head injury, *Acta Neurochirurgica (Wein)* 79:120-124, 1986.

53. Jordan W: Nasal sufentanil 1.5 μg/kg: effectiveness and complications as an induction agent for pediatric orthopedic surgery [abstract 12], *American Academy of Pediatrics Spring Meeting,* 28, 1989.

54. Larsson L, Nilsson K, Andreasson S et al: Effects of rectal thiopentone

and methohexitone on carbon dioxide tension in infant anesthesia with spontaneous ventilation, *Acta Anaesth Scand* 31:227-230, 1987.

55. Lassen N: Control of the cerebral circulation in health and disease, *Circ Res* 34:749-760, 1974.

56. Lassen NA, Christensen MS: Physiology of cerebral blood flow, *Br J Anaesth* 48:719-734, 1976.

57. Lazzell V, Bissonnette B, Lerman J: Effect of halothane on the cerebral circulation in infants and children: a hysteresis phenomenon, *Anesthesiology* 71:A327, 1989.

58. Ledingham IM, Watt I: Influence of sedation on mortality in critically ill multiple trauma patients, *Lancet* 1:1270, 1983.

59. Leon J, Bissonnett B, Lerman J: Cranial duplex sonography: does halothane affect the cerebrovascular response to carbon dioxide in anesthetized children? *Can J Anaesth* 37:524, 1990.

60. Lerman J, Burrows FA, Oyston JP et al: The minimum alveolar concentration (MAC) and cardiovascular effects of halothane, isoflurane and sevoflurane in newborn swine, *Anesthesiology* 73:717-721, 1990.

61. Lerman J, Christensen S, Farrow-Gillespie A: Effects of metoclopramide and ranitidine on gastric fluid pH and volume in children, *Br J Anaesth* 65:456-460, 1990.

62. Manchikanti L, Hawkins J, McCracken J et al: Effects of preanaesthetic glycopyrrolate and cimetidine on gastric fluid acidity and volume in children, *Eur J Anaesth* 1:123-131, 1984.

63. Meakin G, Dingivall A, Addison G: Effects of fasting and oral premedication on the pH and volume of gastric aspirate in children, *Br J Anaesth* 59:678-682, 1987.

64. Mehta MP, Choi WW, Geralis SD et al: Facilitation of rapid endotracheal intubation with divided doses of neuromuscular blocking drugs, *Anesthesiology* 62:392-395, 1985.

65. Michenfelder JD: Midazolam: uses in neurosurgery, *Anesth Rev* 13:45-46, 1986.

66. Michenfelder JD, Theye RA: Effects of fentanyl, droperidol, and Innovar on canine cerebral metabolism and blood flow, *Br J Anaesth* 43:630-635, 1971.

67. Mikawa K, Maekawa N, Goto R et al: Effects of exogenous intravenous glucose on plasma glucose and lipid homeostasis in anesthetized children, *Anesthesiology* 74:1017-1022, 1991.

68. Miller ME: Disseminated intravascular coagulation fibrinolytic syndrome following head injury in children: frequency and prognostic implications, *J Pediatr* 100:687-694, 1982.

69. Milley JR, Nugent SK, Rogers MD: Neurogenic pulmonary edema in childhood, *J Pediatr* 94:700-709, 1979.

70. Minton MD, Stirt JA, Bedford RF: Intracranial pressure after atracurium in neurosurgical patients, *Anesth Analg* 64:113-116, 1985.

71. Minton MD, Stirt JA, Bedford RF: Increased intracranial pressure from succinylcholine: prevention by prior nondepolarizing blockade, *Anesthesiology* 63:165-169, 1986.

72. Morisaki H, Suzuki G, Miyazawa N et al: A clinical trial of sevoflurane in children for herniorrhaphy, *Can J Anaesth* 2:94-97, 1988.

73. Moss E, Powell D, Gibson RM et al: Effects of fentanyl on intracranial pressure and cerebral perfusion pressure during hypocapnia, *Br J Anaesth* 50:779-784, 1978.

74. Muizellaar JP, Marmorou A, De-Salles AAF et al: Cerebral blood flow and metabolism in severely head injured children. Part I: relationship with GCS score outcome, ICP, and PVI, *J Neurosurgery* 71:63-71, 1989.

75. Nussmeier NA, Arlend C, Slogoff S: Neuropsychiatric complications after cardiopulmonary bypass: cerebral protection by a barbiturate, *Anesthesiology* 64:165-170, 1986.

76. Olsson G, Hallen B: Pharmacological evaluation of the stomach with metoclopramide, *Acta Anaesthesiol Scand* 26:417-420, 1982.

77. Otsuka H, Komura Y, Mayumi T et al: Malignant hyperthermia during sevoflurane anesthesia in a child with central core disease, *Anesthesiology* 75:699-701, 1991.

78. Phillips AJ, Brimacombe JR, Simpson DL: Anaesthetic induction with isoflurane or halothane: oxygen saturation during induction with isoflurane or halothane in unpremedicated children, *Anaesthesia* 43:927-929, 1988.

79. Pinaud M, Lelausque JN, Chetanneau A et al: Effects of propofol on cerebral hemodynamics and metabolism in patients with brain trauma, *Anesthesiology* 74:404-409, 1990.

80. Pitts LH: Medical complications of head injury. In Cooper PR, editor: *Head injury,* Baltimore, 1982, Williams & Wilkins, pp 327-342.

81. Pulsinelli WA, Levy DE, Sigsbee B et al: Increased damage after ischemic stroke in patients with hyperglycemia with or without established diabetes mellitus, *Am J Med* 74:540-544, 1983.

82. Raftery S, Warde D: Oxygen saturation during inhalation induction with halothane and isoflurane in children: effect of premedication with rectal thiopentone, *Br J Anaesth* 64:167-169, 1990.

83. Raichle HE, Posner JB, Plum F: Cerebral blood flow during and after hyperventilation, *Arch Neurol* 23:394-397, 1970.

84. Raphaely RC: Central nervous system trauma in children. In Rogers MC, editor: *Current practice in anesthesiology,* Toronto, 1982, BC Decker, p 272.

85. Reed RL II, Ciavarella D, Heimbach DM et al: Prophylactic platelet administration during massive transfusion: a prospective, randomized, double-blind clinical study, *Ann Surg* 203:40-48, 1986.

86. Robinson S, Gregory GA: Fentanyl air-oxygen anesthesia for patent ductus arteriosus in preterm infants, *Anesth Analg* 60:331-334, 1981.

87. Rosner MJ, Coley I: Cerebral perfusion pressure: a hemodynamic mechanism of mannitol and the post mannitol hemogram, *Neurosurgery* 21:147-156, 1987.

88. Sakabe T, Kuramoto T, Kumagae S et al: Cerebral responses to the addition of nitrous oxide to halothane in man, *Br J Anaesth* 48:957-961, 1976.

89. Saul TG, Ducker TB, Salcman M et al: Steroids in severe head injury—a prospective randomized clinical trial, *J Neurosurg* 54:596-600, 1981.

90. Scheker MS, Tateishi A, Drummond JC et al: The effects of sevoflurane on cerebral blood flow, cerebral metabolic rate for oxygen, intracranial pressure, and the electroencephalogram are similar to those of isoflur-

ane in the rabbit, *Anesthesiology* 68:548-551, 1988.

91. Schettini A, Stahurski B, Young HF: Osmotic and osmotic-loop diuresis in brain surgery. Effects on plasma and CSF electrolytes and ion excretion, *J Neurosurg* 56:677-684, 1982.

92. Schreiner M, Treibwasser K, Keon T: Ingestion of liquids compared with preoperative fasting in pediatric outpatients, *Anesthesiology* 72:593-597, 1990.

93. Schroeder HG, Williams NE: Anaesthesia for menigomyelocoele surgery, *Anaesthesia* 21:57-65, 1966.

94. Schurizek K, Rubro L, Beggild-Madsen N et al: Gastric volume and pH in children for emergency surgery, *Acta Anaesthesiol Scand* 30:404-409, 1986.

95. Scott RM, Barnes P, Krupsky W et al: Cavernous angiomas of the central nervous system in children, *J Neurosurg* 76:38-46, 1992.

96. Shapiro HM, Wyte SR, Harris AB: Ketamine anesthesia in patients with intracranial pathology, *Br J Anaesth* 44:1200-1204, 1972.

97. Shi WZ, Fahey MR, Fisher DM et al: Laudanosine (a metabolite of atracurium) increases the minimum alveolar concentration of halothane in rabbits, *Anesthesiology* 63:584-588, 1985.

98. Sieber FE, Smith DS, Crosby L et al: The effects of intraoperative glucose on protein metabolism and serum glucose levels in patients with supratentorial tumors, *Anesthesiology* 64:453-459, 1986.

99. Smith AL: Barbiturate protection in cerebral hypoxia, *Anesthesiology* 17:285, 1977.

100. Smith DS: Fluid management of the neurosurgical patient, *ASA Refresher Course Lecture* 122:1-7, 1986.

101. Stanley T, Leiman B, Rawal N et al: The effects of oral transmucosal fentanyl citrate premedication on preoperative behavioral responses and gastric volume and acidity in children, *Anesth Analg* 69:328-335, 1989.

102. Strain JD, Campbell JB, Harvey LA et al: IV Nembutal: safe sedation for children undergoing CT, *Ann J Neuroradiol* 9:955-959, 1988.

103. Stulz PM, Scheidegger D, Drop LJ et al: Ventricular pump performance during hypocalcemia, *J Thoracic Cardiovasc Surg* 78:185-194, 1979.

104. Swedlow D, Frewein T, Watcha W et al: Cerebral blood flow, $AJDo_2$ and $CMRo_2$ in comatose children. In Go KG, Baethmann A, editors: *Brain Edema* New York, 1984, Plenum Press, pp 365-372.

105. Tateishi A, Maekawa T, Takeshita H et al: Diazepam and intracranial pressure, *Anesthesiology* 54:335-337, 1981.

106. Taylor RH, Lerman J: Minimum alveolar concentration of desflurane and hemodynamic responses in neonates, infants and children, *Anesthesiology* 75:975-979, 1991.

107. Thompson J, Lilly J: Cimetidine-induced cerebral toxicity in children (Letter), *Lancet* 1:725, 1979.

108. Tiret L, Nivoche Y, Hatton F et al: Complications related to anaesthesia in infants and children—a prospective survey of 40,240 anaesthetics, *Br J Anaesth* 61:263-269, 1988.

109. Vandesteene A, Trempont V, Engelman E et al: Effects of propofol on cerebral blood flow and metabolism in man, *Anesthesia* 34(suppl):42-43, 1988.

110. Van Hemelrijck J, Fitch W, Matteussen M et al: Effect of propofol on cerebral circulation and autoregulation in the baboon, *Anesth Analg* 71:49-54, 1990.

111. Walker ML, Storrs BB, Mayer T: Factors affecting outcome in the pediatric patient with multiple trauma, *Concepts Pediatr Neurosurg* 4:243-252, 1983.

112. Ward JD, Becker DP, Miller JD et al: Failure of prophylactic barbiturate coma in the treatment of severe head injury, *J Neurosurg* 62:383-388, 1985.

113. Weiskopf RB, Eger E II, Holmes MA et al: Epinephrine-induced premature ventricular contractions and changes in arterial blood pressure and heart rate during I-653, isoflurane, and halothane anesthesia in swine, *Anesthesiology* 70:293-298, 1989.

114. Westrin P: The induction dose of propofol in infants 1-6 months of age and in children 10-16 years of age, *Anesthesiology* 74:455-458, 1991.

115. Wilton N, Leigh J, Rosen D et al: Preanesthetic sedation of preschool children using intranasal midazolam, *Anesthesiology* 69:972-975, 1988.

116. Wright PJ, Murray RJ: Penetrating craniocerebral airgun injury: anaesthetic management with propofol infusion and review of recent reports, *Anaesthesia* 44:219-221, 1989.

117. Yaster M: The dose response of fentanyl in neonatal anesthesia, *Anesthesiology* 66:433-435, 1987.

118. Yaster M, Koehler RC, Traystman RJ: Effects of fentanyl on peripheral and cerebral hemodynamics in neonatal lambs, *Anesthesiology* 66:524-530, 1987.

119. Yaster M, Koehler RCX, Traystman RJ: Interaction of fentanyl and pentobarbital on peripheral and cerebral hemodynamics in newborn lambs, *Anesthesiology* 70:461-469, 1989.

120. Zaiden JR, Klochany A, Martin WM et al: Effect of thiopental on neurologic outcome following coronary artery bypass grafting, *Anesthesiology* 74:406-411, 1991.

121. Zeldis JB, Friedman LS, Isselbacher KJ: Ranitidine: a new H_2-receptor antagonist, *N Engl J Med* 309:1368-1373, 1983.

122. Zimmerman RA, Bilaniuk LT, Bruce DA et al: Computed tomography of craniocerebral injury in the abused child, *Radiology* 130:687-690, 1979.

27

Neurosurgical Diseases of the Spine and Spinal Cord: Surgical Considerations

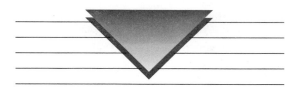

JOHN I. MILLER
ANDREW T. PARSA

Elsberg's 1925 description of the surgical treatment of spinal cord tumors is among the first extensive series on surgery of the spine.[34] The series illustrated the limitations of that time in delineating tumor size and location. These limitations were associated with long surgical procedures and a significant mortality rate. Today, excellent results can be anticipated with all but the most malignant of spinal cord tumors. This progress has been fostered by significant advances in disciplines that are essential to safe and efficacious surgery of the bony elements of the spine and the neural structures of the spinal cord.

Spinal cord tumors, disk disease, stenosis, and cervical spine instability are among the many disease processes treated by the neurosurgeon. In this chapter we present surgical considerations for physicians administering anesthetic care. These considerations include a constellation of eval-

uations that are performed before, during, and after the surgical procedure. In understanding the disease process that affects the spine or spinal cord, the neurosurgeon draws on knowledge of the pertinent neuroanatomy. Imaging studies serve to place the disease process and neuroanatomy within the context of the patient's history and physical findings. The preoperative evaluations culminate in a differential diagnosis and determination of the best surgical approach.

PLAIN FILM ASSESSMENTS

Plain radiographs of the vertebral column remain essential to all cases despite substantial progress in spine-imaging techniques. The bony landmarks of the spine can have both local and remote responses to pathology affecting the spine, spinal cord, or nerve roots. Plain films allow a rapid re-

543

view of bony landmarks and alignment. The anteroposterior (AP) projection can reveal an abnormal curvature of scoliosis that usually involves the thoracic spine. Causes of scoliosis include neuromuscular imbalances of paraspinal muscle tone, unilateral irritation or pain, and structural abnormalities of the vertebral bodies and facets. The AP projection can also detect vertebral body abnormalities, erosion of the pedicles, and the presence of paraspinal masses.

With respect to neoplastic disease, the vertebral bodies often reveal specific patterns of bony destruction that suggest the aggressiveness of the tumor involved. A slowly expanding or benign lesion causes a regional or scalloping pattern of destruction. Conversely, a rapidly growing tumor produces a lytic or permeative pattern of bone destruction that may lead to vertebral body collapse. The pedicle adjoins the vertebral body to the posterior neural arch, which consists of the spinous process and paired laminae (Fig. 27-1). An AP projection may demonstrate pedicle erosion from either spinal cord expansion or tumor emanating from the vertebral body itself.[64] Widening of the vertebral canal occurs in response to chronic neoplastic or cystic expansions within or adjacent to the spinal cord.

Lateral radiographic projections of the spine may be used to evaluate conditions involving malalignment or instability. A lateral plain film can demonstrate the anterior slipping of one vertebral body over another. In the lumbosacral segments, this is referred to as a spondylolisthesis, and at other spinal levels this is often termed subluxation. Insidious instability occurs with an occult fracture or ligamentous failure. It can be accentuated by changes in head and body position or by dynamic fluoroscopy.

A lateral projection demonstrates the normal spinal curvatures of an open "S" with a mild lordosis in the cervical and lumbar regions. A loss of normal curvature suggests underlying pathology. An abnormal anterior angulation of the vertebral column over many segmental levels is known as a *kyphosis,* and an acute angulation is termed a *gibbus deformity.* The causes of the angulation are similar to those of scoliosis, and, with progression, surgical planning must make allowances for operative stabilization. Degenerative and bony irregularities along the vertebral canal, such as osteophytes (bone spurs), loss of disk space, and facet hypertrophy, are indicative of a stenosis or spondylosis that may impinge on neural elements. Prevertebral soft tissue swelling along the anterior longitudinal ligament can be caused by infectious or traumatic injury to a vertebral level that otherwise looks radiographically normal. Lateral projections of the vertebral column offer initial and crucial triage for malalignment after trauma. In the absence of fractures, ligamentous injury may account for the instability. The cervical spine warrants first priority, and the lateral projection must extend from the craniocervical junction to C7.

Oblique projections of the spine allow direct viewing of the foramina, through which nerve roots must exit. Enlargement or constriction of foraminal outlets is caused by neoplasms involving the nerve roots and degenerative vertebral changes, respectively (Fig. 27-2). These radiographic observations are often associated with the clinical findings of a radiculopathy. In trauma, the suspicion of a jumped facet on lateral viewing may be clarified by an oblique projection revealing distortion of the neural foramina. A loss of height or spontaneous fusion within the intervertebral disk space can be assessed and may relate to nerve root and/or spinal cord compression.

After the more global plain-film assessments, axial or horizontal radiographic slices with sagittal or vertical reconstruction can be obtained using computed tomography (CT scan). Through selective radiographic sectioning, CT scans elaborate any focal abnormalities evident on plain films. Polytomography retains its value in revealing fractures, extent of bone healing or fusion, and focal disruption of functional components of the vertebral column. Plain-film assessments of the targeted vertebral level fulfill a critical need for accurate intraoperative localization using either anatomic landmarks or radiopaque markers on the patient. Precise localization assures a direct approach, exposure of the pathology, and an overall economy to surgical efforts.

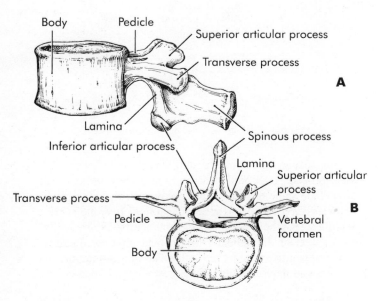

FIG. 27-1   Lateral and axial views of a thoracic vertebra. **A,** On the lateral view, the lamina is obscured by both the transverse process and facets. The pedicle adjoins the vertebral body to the neural arch. **B,** On the axial view, the vertebral body, paired pedicles, transverse processes, facets, lamina, and spinous process are clearly demonstrated. These structures circumscribe the vertebral canal.

ASPECTS OF NEURORADIOLOGY PERTINENT TO SURGICAL PLANNING

Certain aspects of neuroradiology deserve emphasis because they are particularly pertinent to planning surgery of the spine. Imaging of the neural elements in proximity to the vertebral column is facilitated by the use of myelogra-

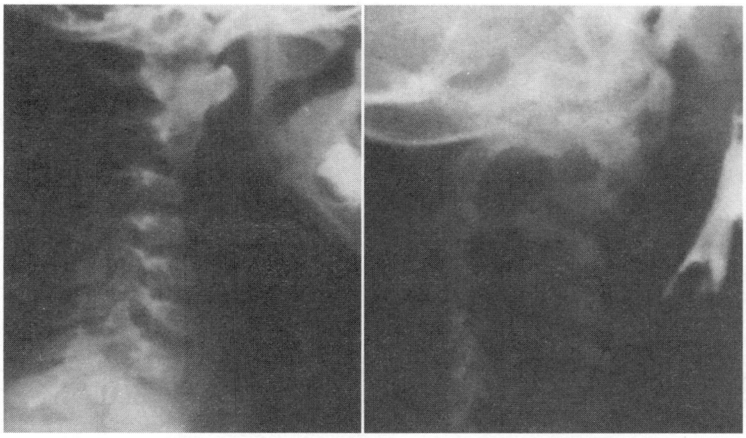

Fig. 27-2   Lateral cervical radiograph of a child with neurofibromatosis demonstrating an enlarged neural foramina from C1 through C3.

phy, CT scanning, and magnetic resonance (MR) imaging. Abnormalities are categorized according to distortion of the anatomic spaces that surround the spinal cord. The arachnoid membrane is closely approximated to the dura, leaving a capacious subarachnoid space that surrounds the spinal cord and its proximal nerve roots. Aberrations in the normal patency of the subarachnoid space reveal the level of impingement on the spinal cord and/or nerve roots.

The extent of pressure on neural structures can be dynamically assessed with myelography. Myelographic images are facilitated by the administration of nonionic, water-soluble contrast agent into the thecal sac by lumbar or C1-C2 puncture. The contrast agent highlights the subarachnoid space in a radioopaque fashion and permits a dynamic assessment of regions of spinal cord impingement. Specific patterns of impingement include the intramedullary type, caused by intrinsic expansion of the spinal cord; the extramedullary type, which is external to the cord but intradural; and the epidural type, which is external to both the cord and the dura. The spinal cord normally appears enlarged at levels C5-C6 and T10-T11. Definitive pressure can appear as a high-grade (near complete) or complete block of the subarachnoid space (Fig. 27-3). Intraoperative myelography can be used to confirm surgical decompression, allowing the surgeon to monitor the achievement of operative goals. Multiple sites of neural impingement, such as in diffuse spondylosis or multiple-disk disease, lead to a confusing picture for targeting surgical decompression. In this situation, myelography may demonstrate the site of maximum impingement and the bony elements of a spondylotic spur.

A high-grade block that impedes the rostral flow of contrast during myelography makes it difficult to discern the upper limits of a compressive lesion. In these cases, the CT scan can be used as a noninvasive method to detect small amounts of contrast above the site of compression.

Alternatively, an invasive C1-C2 puncture can be done to show the rostral extent of a block. When combined with myelography, CT studies help discern the relationship between bony pathology and neural impingement. MR demonstrates deformation of a neural structure without showing the offending bone. Patients who require metallic hardware for skeletal traction and mechanical ventilation represent a cumbersome obstacle for MR imaging. These patients are better served with myelography followed by CT imaging. In the presence of a high-grade block, further neurologic deterioration may follow myelography. This is secondary to a shift in the intrathecal compartment after lumbar puncture and warrants urgent decompressive, surgical intervention.

CT imaging is more sensitive than plain radiographs to changes in bone mineralization. In the vertebral column, neoplasms greater than one third of the bony trabeculae can be lost to detection by plain radiography.[86] The CT scan detects bone loss at a much earlier interval in the disease course. The axial (horizontal) sections of the CT scan allow the surgeon to assess the patency of the spinal canal and thecal sac. This is particularly useful in evaluating degenerative processes that constrict the spinal canal, such as spondylotic spurs, facet hypertrophy, and other components of spinal stenosis. In trauma, the CT scan can readily demonstrate hyperdense acute blood or retropulsed vertebral body fragments within the spinal canal.

The use of intravenous contrast infusion during CT scanning can improve visualization of neoplastic and inflammatory tissue. This maneuver helps to distinguish between postoperative scarring and recurrent disk or fragments of disk in the epidural space. After injection of intrathecal contrast, delayed CT scanning has the capacity to define a syrinx in the posttraumatic spinal cord and other conditions that predispose to syrinx formation.

CT imaging of the spine provides important extraspinal

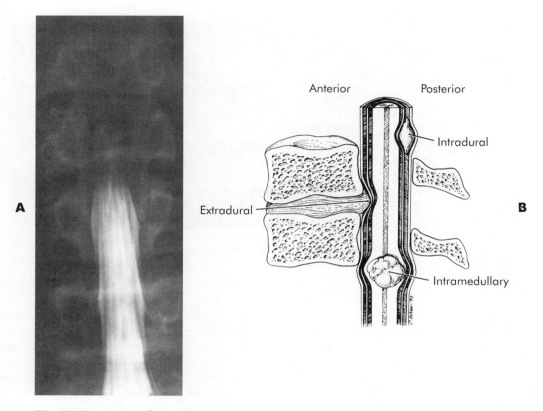

Fig. 27-3   **A,** AP radiographic projection of a contrast myelogram showing a high-grade epidural block secondary to a pathologic fracture of L1 vertebral body. The patient is positioned head down; note the "sawtooth" pattern where the dye terminates. **B,** Sagittal section of the spinal cord being circumscribed by closely approximated arachnoid and dural coverings. Surrounding vertebral segments are demonstrated, showing a herniated intervertebral disk causing epidural compression, attenuation of the subarachnoid space, and cord compression. Also note intradural extramedullary and intramedullary masses. Intramedullary lesions enlarge the cord, attenuating subarachnoid space bilaterally, whereas extramedullary lesions displace the cord with dilatation of subarachnoid space on the side of the lesion and attenuation on the side opposite the lesion.

information about abnormalities of paraspinal structures, the chest, and the abdomen that may influence surgical planning. Axial images can be reconfigured by computer software to enhance and display sagittal, coronal, and three-dimensional images. The multiplanar viewing of osseous elements can detect abnormalities such as chance fractures that are obscured in the horizontal plane. A chance fracture is a horizontal fracture that traverses the posterior neural arch and vertebral body.[17] It typically occurs in the thoracolumbar region as a high-velocity, flexion injury (Fig. 27-4).

Unlike CT scanning and myelography, MR can directly image the parenchyma of the spinal cord. MR can be used for evaluating a variety of spinal diseases, of which some are nonsurgical, such as the demyelinating process in multiple sclerosis. MR is noninvasive and well tolerated by the patient and does not require intrathecal contrast or ionizing radiation.

MR permits direct multiplanar imaging without loss of resolution. A coronal or sagittal image provides an overview of many segmental levels. This feature localizes the upper and lower borders of cord compression and/or lesions. Such information is crucial to plan the extent of surgical exposure and to target postoperative radiotherapy for spinal neoplasms. Spinal curvatures, as in scoliosis and kyphosis, disrupt the continuity of any single image and limit the utility of sagittal and coronal sectioning.

MR uses a strong magnetic field (1 tesla or more) to deliver a pulse sequence that induces a transient alignment of tissue protons. Perturbations of proton alignment emit detectable signals or echoes that reflect the composition and motion of tissue and fluid. The echoes are detected over a

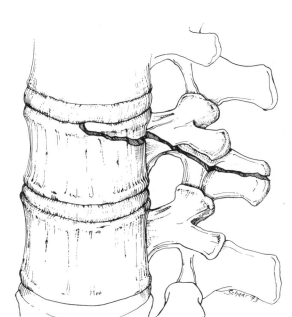

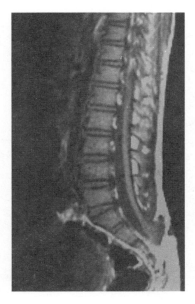

FIG. 27-5   Sagittal MR projection of a tethered spinal cord secondary to a lipomeningocele in a 5-year-old child. This T_1-weighted image demonstrates spinal cord elements to be present below L1 and tethered at the sacral segmental level.

FIG. 27-4   Lateral schematic illustration of vertebral segment demonstrating a chance fracture that traverses both the posterior neural arch and vertebral body.

time sequence that is indicated by the repetition time (TR) and the echo time (TE). Tissue signals can be processed or T_1 weighted for short TR and TE intervals to optimize spatial resolution. T_1-weighted images depict the distribution of gray-matter and white-matter structures, with the fluid compartments appearing dark or hypointense. Components of fluid include the cerebrospinal fluid (CSF) of the subarachnoid space, tissue edema, syrinxes, and arachnoid cysts of the spinal column. Long TR and TE intervals refer to a T_2-weighted image that intensifies the hydrogen elements of water, which appear white or hyperintense. Tissue edema appears white and is a sensitive indicator of parenchymal injury or blood-brain barrier (BBB) dysfunction within the cord.[8] A spin-echo study requires more time to process its increased number of echoes. A gradient-echo study is faster, although less detailed, and serves to minimize patient motion artifact. The effects of physiologic motion can also be limited with flow compensation techniques, such as cardiac gating. This may be important in assessing the attenuations of subarachnoid space at levels of normal cord enlargement. Various surface coils can cone down on a region of interest to optimize resolution. Any ferromagnetic material in proximity to the magnetic field will impose image artifacts and may also be hazardous. The epidural and subarachnoid spaces can be clearly delineated when MR is used. The anterior and posterior longitudinal ligaments course along the front and back of the vertebral bodies. Elevation of the ligaments may be secondary to traumatic disruption or disk herniation, or result from a

spondylotic spur. MR is very sensitive to tumor infiltration of vertebral bone marrow and helps to distinguish between tumor and infection. Infectious processes infilitrate the disk space; in the case of tumor, the disk space is spared.

The diagnostic accuracy of MR approaches 90% with cervical disk disease and is greater when combined with CT/myelography.[58] These three modalities offer the best in soft-tissue, subarachnoid space, and osseous imaging when used in the context of multiplanar viewing. MR also is particularly beneficial for noninvasive assessments of the pediatric age group. In this age group, MR can discern the presence of spinal cord tethering, establish the etiology, and thus contribute significantly to the plan of surgical treatment (Fig. 27-5).

SPINAL CORD SYNDROMES: NEUROANATOMY AND CLINICAL PRESENTATION

Vertebral column abnormalities may clinically present with trauma, pain, neurologic symptoms, and abnormal posture. Neurologic symptoms suggest the involvement of neural elements and require neuroradiologic imaging of soft tissues to include the spinal cord and nerve roots. The neurologic symptoms associated with vertebral column abnormalities may result from a myelopathy, a radiculopathy, or a combination of both. Often, pain precludes any definitive neurologic findings and prompts further neuroradiologic investigation. An understanding of spinal-cord neuroanatomy and related cord syndromes allows the surgeon to recog-

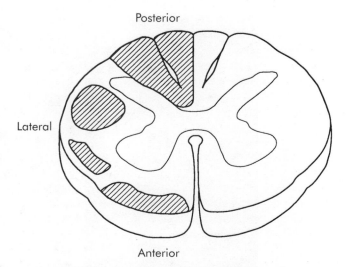

Posterior

Lateral

Anterior

FIG. 27-6 Cross section of the spinal cord demonstrating the distribution of the major spinal tracts within the three funiculi.

nize the need for neuroimaging within an appropriate region of interest.

The cross-sectional anatomy of the spinal cord consists of three funiculi, with one posterior and the other two anterolateral in location (Fig. 27-6). The lateral attachments of the dentate ligaments to the cord define the anterior (ventral) and posterior (dorsal) halves of the spinal cord. Motor symptoms are caused by damage to the descending corticospinal or pyramidal tract in the posterior portion of the anterolateral funiculus. Chronic disruption along this anatomic course causes upper motor neuron (UMN) or long-tract findings that include a segmental level of paralysis or weakness, muscle atrophy, hyperactive deep-tendon reflexes, spasticity, a disturbance of fine movements, and a pathologic extensor response of the toes to plantar stimulation. Acute disruptions may evoke a flaccid paralysis or weakness that ultimately progresses to spasticity. In both acute and chronic disruptions, motor symptoms are ipsilateral to the pathology. Bilateral symptoms herald more diffuse spinal cord involvement.

Lower motor neuron (LMN) deficits can originate from the anterior horn cell, nerve root, and any point along the peripheral nerve. LMN findings may occur jointly with a myelopathy and are otherwise associated with anterior horn-cell diseases, radiculopathies, and peripheral neuropathies. The clinical picture may overlap with pyramidal signs, but its distinguishing features include hypoactive or absent deep tendon reflexes, decreased tone or flaccidity, fasciculations, and the absence of a pathologic extensor response of the toes.

Within the descending motor tract, the cervical or arm axons are more centrally located, exiting through the ventral gray matter and ventral nerve roots first. This is the anatomic basis of a central cord syndrome, which leaves the arms weaker than the legs.[71] A similar clinical picture is observed with a brachial cruciate paralysis.[10] In this deficit, the odontoid tip of the second cervical vertebra injures the lower decussating or crossing motor axons of the pyramids on the ventral surface of the lower medulla.

The ascending sensory nerves traverse the dorsal root ganglia and dorsal nerve root to enter the dorsal-horn gray matter of the spinal cord. A portion of these sensory fibers carry position, tactile (deep touch), and vibratory axons. They run directly to the ipsilateral half of the posterior funiculi or columns and ascend in the posterior portion of the cord. The remaining sensory fibers subserve pain (sharp, dull), temperature, and light touch. These fibers synapse over several spinal levels in the dorsal horns before crossing to the opposite anterolateral funiculus, where they begin an ascent as the lateral spinothalamic tract. The spinothalamic tracts are located anterior to the dentate ligaments. In acute central cord injuries, the more centrally located cervical axons of the spinothalamic tract are disrupted. The remaining lateral axons account for the sacral sparing of perianal sensation.

Because pain and temperature synapses occur in the dorsal horns over several spinal levels, localization of a spinal cord lesion can only be approximated to within three spinal segments. For localization, cord pathology is often dynamic and may ascend to include higher levels of motor, sensory, and autonomic dysfunction. It is crucial to define and follow the disparity between an osseous level of pathology shown radiographically and the actual neurologic level of cord function. An ascending level of neurologic loss should prompt a rapid reassessment of the patient's clinical status and vertebral alignment and warrants reimaging of the cord itself.

The crossing of pain and temperature axons through the central cord to the opposite side is an anatomic correlate for two neurologic findings. First, unilateral pain and temperature sensory levels or deficits are opposite the spinal cord lesion. Second, central cord disruption impairs the sensation for pain and temperature axons, with preservation of posterior column sensory modalities. Clinically, the second finding constitutes a dissociated sensory disorder.[11]

A myelopathy may impair motor, sensory, or autonomic function and can vary in severity. A partial or incomplete myelopathy will present as one of several major spinal-cord syndromes, each having a certain propensity for recovery, depending on the duration and extent of the spinal cord insult. The etiology can include congenital, degenerative, traumatic, infectious, or neoplastic disease processes.

The anterior cord syndrome results from damage to the anterior two thirds of the spinal cord, which includes the anterior horn cells of the ventral gray matter (LMN) and the axons or white-matter tracts of the anterolateral funiculi (UMN) (Fig. 27-7, A). The anterior cord syndrome occurs more commonly in the cervical region and is characterized by LMN paralysis of the arms and UMN paralysis of the legs. Below the level of injury there is motor paral-

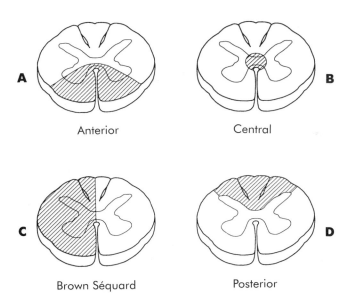

Anterior

Central

Brown Séquard

Posterior

FIG. 27-7   Cross section of the spinal cord depicting distribution of injury for the major partial myelopathies relevant to surgical assessments (**A** to **D**).

ysis with complete deficits of pain (sharp/dull), temperature, and light-touch sensory modalities. The partial myelopathy that presents as an anterior-cord syndrome is often due to ventral compression from retropulsed bone or disk, a flexion injury, or interruption of anterior spinal artery blood flow. The variable sparing of the posterior columns accounts for residual tactile, vibration, and position sense in the lower extremities.

The central cord syndrome is a common myelopathy (Fig. 27-7, *B*). Acute central-cord syndromes are distinguished from chronic syndromes by the sacral sparing of pain (sharp/dull) and temperature sensory modalities and by a more dense motor weakness in the arms vs. the legs. In trauma, the acute central-cord syndrome presents with a central-cord contusion and/or hematoma (hematomyelia). This is often seen in the more rigid and spondylitic spines of older patients with extension injuries. Motor, sensory, and bladder functions have good prospects for recovery, with earlier improvements noted in the legs. Presentations of a chronic central-cord syndrome can be caused by cysts, such as in syringomyelia, or by intrinsic cord tumors. A dissociated sensory disorder, LMN-type flaccid paralysis, and muscle atrophy of the upper extremities are typically associated with a chronic central-cord syndrome. Progressive disruption of the dorsal horns accounts for the trophic disorders that may involve the arms and fingers.[9]

A cord syrinx can present as an incomplete myelopathy and may extend rostrally to the medulla (syringobulbia) to impair various lower cranial nerve functions, such as phonation and swallowing. It is not uncommon for abnormalities at the foramen magnum level to predispose patients to syringomyelia.[9] This is frequently observed in the congen-

ital Chiari malformations, which include a constricted volume in the posterior fossa, cerebellar tonsillar impaction, obliteration of local CSF cisterns, and abnormal local CSF dynamics. The concurrence of hydrocephalus and a rostral spinal cord syrinx is termed *hydromyelia* and often responds to treatment of the hydrocephalus with ventriculoperitoneal shunting.[56] Syringomyelia can also be the consequence of prior cord trauma, tumor, arachnoiditis, and compressive spondylosis.

The Brown-Séquard syndrome is less prevalent than the previously mentioned incomplete myelopathies (Fig. 27-7. *C*). The lesion impairs one half of the spinal cord and spares the opposite half. Clinically, there is a UMN paralysis and a loss of position sense ipsilateral to the lesion. This is consistent with unilateral disruption of both the corticospinal tract and the posterior columns, neither of which cross during their course through the cord. Opposite the lesion, there is a level of sensory deficit for pain and temperature. Disruption of the spinothalamic tract impairs ascending pain and temperature axons, which have crossed from the side opposite the lesion. This syndrome may be observed with unilateral encroachment of epidural tumor through the neural foramina or intradural tumor from the nerve root. Because of compression, a complete transverse myelopathy may supervene, with a worse prognosis for recovery. Penetrating or contusive injuries can impair one lateral half of the cervical or thoracic cord to produce the Brown-Séquard presentation. The prognosis for motor recovery is better than that of other incomplete myelopathies but remains influenced by the nature of the insult, rapidity of diagnosis, and, when appropriate, expeditious decompression.[21]

For surgical considerations, the posterior-cord syndrome is a rare presentation of an incomplete myelopathy (Fig. 27-7, *D*). A level of sensory loss for posterior column modalities coincides with preservation of motor function. Its rare occurrence limits the value of prognostic assessments. Of greater relevance is posterior column damage caused by disease not treated surgically, including multiple sclerosis, subacute combined degeneration (B_{12} deficiency), Freiderich's ataxia, tabes dorsalis, and pure sensory neuropathies. Pure sensory neuropathies may be observed in paraneoplastic syndromes and can be caused by the idiopathic synthesis of antibodies to the dorsal root ganglia.[25] The posterior column axons, within the dorsal root ganglia, are the principle targets in pure sensory neuropathies.

Rarely, a dorsal extramedullary tumor may present as a posterior cord syndrome. Tumors situated within the dura and outside the cord are termed *extramedullary,* and those occurring within the cord are termed *intramedullary.* Disruption of posterior column function impairs position sense at the spinal-cord level and leads to an ataxic gait disturbance. The patient can partially compensate for this by using visual cues as cortical input to improve balance. During neurologic examination, eye closure will exacerbate spinal ataxia and provoke more imbalance to indicate a positive Romberg's sign. Impaired position sense of the toes combined with a positive Romberg's sign localizes the cause of ataxia to a lesion in the spinal cord.

Posterior to the T12 to L1 vertebral bodies, within the vertebral canal, the spinal cord attenuates in diameter to form the conus medullaris. A lesion or injury at this level may produce impotence and a loss of bowel and bladder control. Any corticospinal (UMN) or motor lesion above the conus medullaris spares local lumbar and sacral bladder innervation. The result is a spastic bladder that will empty automatically or by reflex action at reduced volumes. An LMN lesion at or below the conus level (below L1) disrupts local lumbar and sacral innervation, leaving the bladder flaccid. The bladder's extent of neurologic impairment can be accurately evaluated using cystometrics. Other physical findings of a conus medullaris syndrome include an anesthesia of the saddle region, reduced anal sphincter tone during rectal examination, and variable sparing of the lower extremities.[67] The prognosis for recovery of bowel and bladder control is poor. Below the T9 level, a greater percentage of the spinal cord is occupied by gray matter. Accordingly, there is a greater vulnerability to neurologic morbidity during surgical manipulation or with the progression of a lesion caudal to T9.

Below L1 the conus medullaris or cord proper divides into the multiple lumbar and sacral nerve roots of the cauda equina (L1-L5). The conus is anchored by a thin (2 mm) filum terminale that extends caudally through the cauda equina and the lumbar thecal sac. The thecal sac ends at the mid-S1 vertebral level. UMN findings that are associated with the spinal cord proper are not present in the cauda equina. Typical physical findings include variable LMN sensory and motor loss to the lower extremities, and sphincteric disturbances. The prognosis for motor recovery is excellent, and this region is associated with good postoperative neurologic results.[4]

During axial growth of the vertebral column, the conus may tether and remain below L1. Tethering is associated with congenital abnormalities of the posterior neuropore, such as a thickened filum terminale or spinal dysraphisms. Dysraphic conditions include meningoceles, myelomeningoceles, and occult lesions, as seen in presentations of diastematomyelia, lipomyelomeningocele, and dermal sinus tracts. A lipoma, sinus tract, nevus, or tufts of hair are typical cutaneous findings along the caudal midline that facilitate the early detection of occult lesions. Early detection mandates surgical release to avoid irreversible neurologic sequelae. Protracted tethering may result in progressive scoliosis, disruption of gait, and sphincteric disturbances.[52]

A complete myelopathy over a protracted interval or after an acute and completed injury offers little hope for neurologic recovery. After an acute injury, spinal cord shock may halt all cord functions, including motor, sensory, and reflex activity. During this interval, an accurate neurologic evaluation cannot be made, and hemodynamic support may be required. Usually within 24 to 72 hours, a return in reflex function (i.e., the bulbocavernosus reflex and/or priapism) indicates a receding sequelae of spinal shock and permits the validation of a neurologic level.[59] Genital stimulation induces a reflex contraction of the anal sphincter and indicates the presence of a bulbocavernosus reflex. An accurate determination of a neurologic level after a complete cord injury is critical in discerning improvement vs. an ascending loss of function. The latter warrants a prompt reevaluation of the patient.

HEMODYNAMIC EFFECTS OF SPINAL CORD SHOCK: IMPORTANCE OF PERFUSION PRESSURES

During spinal cord shock, the loss of sympathetic tone in a patient results in a generalized hemodynamic instability characterized by bradycardia, peripheral arterial and venous vasodilation, and hypotension. Hypovolemia in patients with spinal cord shock should be treated with prompt blood replacement for any blood loss and with crystalloid. Central venous pressure (CVP) and pulmonary arterial pressure (PAP) monitoring is helpful in following the patient's status. Substantial hypotension despite normovolemia will require vasopressors, such as phenylephrine, and bradycardia may require atropine, either with or without phenylephrine. Multiple-trauma patients who are hypotensive, hypovolemic, and yet bradycardic should be highly suspect for spinal cord shock.[89] Operative intervention for spinal injury should await an improved hemodynamic status and accurate assessment of the segmental level of neurologic deficit.

In both acute cord injuries and spine surgery, adequate spinal cord perfusion pressures are necessary for maintenance of neurologic function. In experiments, recovery of cord function after injury was unlikely in simulated clinical situations where the systemic diastolic pressure was less than 70 mm Hg.[32] Conversely, systemic perfusion above a diastolic pressure of 70 mm Hg can adequately sustain cord function. Adequate perfusion pressures are likely to be more important when autoregulation and CO_2 reactivity are attenuated because of cord injury or in association with anesthesia during spine surgery. During surgical exposures, continuous surface monitoring of spinal cord blood flow in the microcirculation now may be feasible with laser Doppler flowmetry.[14] This modality may shed more light on the hemodynamic behavior of the human spinal cord.

USE OF STEROIDS

The use of steroids remains controversial for cord injuries because the improvement is minimal, is difficult to document, and involves a limited number of cord injuries. Most recently, a suggested protocol for traumatic cord injuries includes the use of high-dose methylprednisolone with an intravenous bolus of 30 mg/kg followed by a 5.4 mg/kg/hr infusion for 23 hours. Studies describing the effectiveness of this protocol in 164 patients declared a motor improvement of 3 points (out of 70 possible points) over a naloxone-treated group and approximately 6 points over a placebo group. However, follow-up testing at 6 weeks and 6 months gave little insight into what, if any, functional improvement occurred as a final outcome.[15] Steroids must be used within 8 hours of the cord insult to be of any benefit.[84] The surgeon should realize that steroids may nearly double the incidence of postoperative wound infections, approaching 7%.[27] The administration of steroids is short term, especially when no improvement is discerned. Some of the partial cord syndromes have been reported to respond favorably and prompted the maintenance of steroids through a subacute interval of 1 week, followed by weaning.[15] Serious cord injuries predispose patients to latent stress ulcers and gastrointestinal bleeding, and this risk is exacerbated by steroids.[36] The short interval of administration after cord injury serves to minimize the risks associated with steroids. It is interesting to note that in recent years the administration of steroids for cranial components of central nervous system (CNS) injuries has decreased.

SURGERY
Stability

Good preoperative planning avoids an approach that has the possibility of iatrogenically destabilizing the spine. The ver-

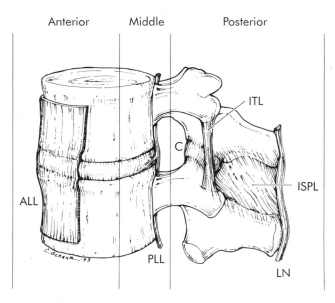

FIG. 27-8   Schematic representation of the vertebral columns with supportive ligamentous structures. Note that the three columns of stability are anterior, middle, and posterior. The anterior column includes the anterior longitudinal ligament *(ALL)* and the anterior annulus of the intravertebral disk space. The middle column includes the annulus of the posterior disk space and the posterior longitudinal ligament *(PLL)*. The posterior column includes the capsular *(C)* attachments of the facet joint, intertransverse ligament *(ITL)*, interspinous ligament *(ISPL)*, and ligamentous nuchae *(LN)*. Compromise of two of the columns of spinal stability imparts spinal instability.

tebral spine and its ligamentous support can be divided into three columns of stability. The anterior half of the vertebral body is part of the anterior column, which includes the anterior half of the intervertebral disk and the anterior longitudinal ligament. The middle column consists of the posterior half of the vertebral body and the intervertebral disk, with ligamentous support provided by the posterior longitudinal ligament. The posterior column includes the paired facets, which are superior and inferior to the pars interarticularis (pillars), the transverse and spinous processes, and the paired laminae. The capsule over the facet joints, intertransverse ligaments, interspinous ligaments, and ligamentum flavum are structures of ligamentous support specific to the posterior column.[28]

A normal spine remains stable unless two of the three columns have been disrupted. However, prior trauma, neuromuscular paralysis, and deformity can compromise spinal stability. Prophylactic fusion is a consideration for all spine-surgery patients who have a documented destabilizing predisposition (Fig. 27-8).[28]

Posterior Approaches
Operative Considerations

A posterior approach to the vertebral column requires that the patient be placed in a prone position. To avoid painful neck positions, the surgeon should assess the patient's cervical range of motion preoperatively. Such an evaluation may reveal an incomplete range of motion, local neck pain, dysesthesia, or a sudden brief electric-shock–like sensation radiating down the spine (L'hermitte's sign). Head positions that manifest any symptoms of discomfort are contraindicated intraoperatively. An awareness of discomfort associated with specific head positions is especially relevant when treating patients undergoing posterior approaches for degenerative lumbar disease. These patients are likely to have cervical disease, which may become symptomatic after stressful positioning of the head for a protracted interval.[35] When one is in doubt, the neck can remain in neutral position (face-down) while prone using a cushioned horseshoe headrest. The orbits require an occlusive covering. Pressure is to be avoided over the orbits and malar region of the face.

A preoperative neuromonitoring study is advised if the patient is to be monitored intraoperatively. Data obtained during the preoperative assessment will assist the neurophysiologist or technician in configuring the optimal stimulus-response routine, given the site of spinal-cord deficit and the intended surgical approach. Sufficient electrical grounding for both electrocautery and neuromonitoring is obtained through the return pad of an electrocautery unit. To prevent the patient from conducting current between grounding sources, the surgeon confirms that no more than one source is attached to the patient. The location of cables and electronic instrumentation is configured to minimize AC (60 cycles) interference with the neuromonitoring.

It is advisable for the surgical team to determine the necessity of any additional venous access and arterial lines based on the medical condition of the patient as well as the duration and nature of the procedure. Any substantial hemodynamic fluctuation after anesthetic induction may be exacerbated by prone positioning. Volume supplementation, vasoactive amines, central venous access, and arterial line monitoring serve to counteract possible repercussions of this hemodynamic fluctuation. Certain preoperative maneuvers can induce acute dysrhythmias and hypertension in patients with chronic paralysis from a complete cord lesion (autonomic hyperreflexia). Intubation, suctioning, prone positioning, and bladder catheterization can each induce autonomic dysreflexia the treatment of which requires optimal hemodynamic monitoring and the availability of sympatholytic agents.[46] Patients with a high, complete cord lesion of greater than 1 week's duration may experience massive hyperkalemia after muscle relaxation with succinylcholine.[77] The hyperkalemia is typically a result of extensive denervation and an abnormal response of the muscle cell membrane to depolarizing agents. Compressive thigh-length stockings help to counteract venous pooling in the lower extremities. In addition, segmental compression boots can be used since they also serve as a preventive measure for deep venous thrombosis during long procedures. Bladder catheterization is indicated for most spinal procedures and certainly for those involving cord manipulation. In addition, the use of epidural or intradural analgesics for control of early postoperative pain requires bladder catheterization.

Any condition that reduces space in the cervical spinal canal precludes hyperextension of the neck during intubation. Patients with cervical spinal canal impingement are best served by fiberoptic, laryngoscopic intubation while the patient is awake. Alternatively, having assessed neck mobility preoperatively, the anesthesiologist in the presence of the surgeon can conduct a simple laryngoscopic viewing with the cervical spine in a neutral position. An obstructed view of the larynx, cervical instability, or radiographic evidence of cervical cord impingement mandates fiberoptic intubation of an awake patient with a locally anesthetized pharynx. An armored endotracheal (ET) tube will assure patency with any surgical positioning of the cervical spine. Given the difficulty associated with reintubating a patient in the prone position, securing the ET or nasotracheal (NT) tube is of paramount importance. Prone positioning of infants mandates even greater vigilance in securing the cuffless ET. The thin-caliber ET tube may kink with cervical flexion, requiring that the neck be repositioned. Before prone positioning, abdominal relaxation can be increased by using oral or nasogastric catheter suction to decompress trapped air in the stomach.

Frequently, after anesthetic induction, a headholder with pin fixation to the skull is applied to optimize control of cervical positioning. Patients with cervical instability require the maintenance of skeletal traction throughout the surgical procedure, including the period of intubation and any repositioning, such as when the patient is turned. The traction is supported by a horseshoe headrest. While turning the patient, the surgeon uses one hand to pull the skeletal tongs that are attached to the skull by pin fixation. This distracts the unstable cervical spine to maintain alignment. The opposite hand or a rigid cervical collar can be used for counter support. The head and body are rotated in unison, maintaining a neutral neck position. The anesthesiologist disconnects and reconnects the airhose allowing safe passage of the face and endotracheal tube into the horseshoe headrest. Radiographic confirmation of alignment should be obtained. In addition, a wake-up test can be performed to assure that there is no loss of preoperative neurologic function.[84]

Skeletal tongs are available that provide two-point (Gardner-Wells) or four-point (halo or Trippi-Wells) skull fixation. The latter provides more complete control of cervical flexion/extension and can be interfaced with a four-post body vest for external fixation. With external fixation, patients can undergo intubation, positioning, and surgery for both posterior and anterior approaches to the cervical spine. However, the maintenance of acceptable alignment must be radiographically confirmed preoperatively. Metal skeletal tongs could potentially conduct and focus charge densities from transcranial magnetic motor evoked potential (tcMMEP) stimulations to the skeletal pins in the skull, thereby exposing the cortical surface to current. The risk of exposure to current is minimized by using nonparamagnetic skeletal fixation devices and nonconductive ceramic-tipped skeletal pins. Fixation pins need not penetrate the inner table of the calvarium for secure fixation. Nonparamagnetic tongs and halos are available, given the need for follow-up MR imaging.

Neuromonitoring should be performed both before and after turning the patient. The operating room table is prepared with paired, anterior, axillary cushioned rolls or bolsters that extend along the anterolateral chest to the anterior iliac crests. The bolsters elevate the prone surface of the body off the table, allowing for abdominal relaxation. There are padded laminectomy frames that may be used for the same purpose, but they generally do not suffice for obese patients. Abdominal relaxation will optimize hemostasis by reducing pressure on the vena cava, thus limiting distension of the epidural and paravertebral veins (Batson's plexus). Good hemostasis is also facilitated by the preoperative discontinuance of antiinflammatory agents that impede platelet function. Bladder catheterization avoids bladder distension and maintains low intraabdominal pressure. Pressure on the groin is to be avoided to spare both the femoral nerve and artery. Distal pulses can be checked for verification. Rarely, in proximity to the anterior iliac crest, the lateral femoral cutaneous nerve can sustain a compressive injury as it traverses the inguinal ligament. The compression can cause a syndrome termed *meralgia paresthetica*, which is characterized by dysesthesias over the lateral thigh.[33]

Patient Positioning

Unimpeded head-side access to the posterior cervical spine is facilitated by pin fixation or the horseshoe headrest. The head is face down and slightly flexed to expand both the interspinous and interlaminar spaces. The back of the neck faces the surgeon, parallel to the floor, and the patient's body is placed straight prone or in a semi-kneeling position. Both arms are pronated and secured by the patient's side to permit the surgeons to stand adjacent to the posterior neck. A footboard and restraining belt secure the patient for any necessary tilts of the operating room table. Slight angulation of the body in a reverse Trendelenburg position, below the shoulder level, further reduces venous pressure in the cervical spine. Proximal to sites of neural impingement, the epidural veins may remain compressed and engorged. Local epidural bleeding is usually controlled through low-wattage, bipolar electrocautery and hemostatic adjuvants. Under the microscope, even a minimal amount of bleeding will obscure the surgeon's view. The tilt of the patient can be altered to meet the needs of the surgeon and to suit the hemodynamic status of the patient.

Posterior approaches to the cervical spine can also be accomplished by placing the patient in a sitting position. Advocates cite better exposure, improved venous drainage, and easier hemostasis as some of the incentives for placing the patient in this position.[18] There are several disadvantages to the sitting position, especially with regard to the fragile hemodynamic status in patients with cardiac disease and the elderly. In addition, the sitting position increases the risk of air embolus and limits the ability of the surgeon to tilt the operating table during the course of the procedure.[11] The principles of prone positioning remain consistent for all levels of the spine. The face-down, prone position is also optimal for posterior approaches to the cervicothoracic spine. At this level, avoidance of neck rotation helps to maintain midline alignment of the spinous processes. As in cervical posterior approaches, the arms remain at the patient's side. Thoracic and lumbar approaches are facilitated by moving the arms up into a semireaching position on arm boards. Each elbow is cushioned to prevent pressure-induced injury of the ulnar nerve at the olecranon. For the thoracic spine, the operating table can be slightly flexed to optimize both the interspinous and interlaminar spaces.

Posterior approaches to the lumbar spine benefit from specially equipped operating tables. The prone patient can be flexed both at the hips and the knees after the head extension is removed (Fig. 27-9). The patient remains on cushioned bolsters and can assume a semikneeling to kneeling position, with the padded head extension now supporting the anterior tibial regions. In the kneeling position, the buttocks and lateral thighs are supported by extensions with cushioned plates. In the male patient, the scrotum remains free of any compression. This flexed position maintains abdominal relaxation, reduces traction on both the femoral and sciatic nerves, and opens the interspinous and interlaminar spaces. The weight-bearing points must be evenly distributed to avoid compressive injuries.

Hyperflexion at the hip and knee levels beyond 90 degrees brings the patient into a tucked or knee-chest position, and several factors require caution. Abdominal relaxation is often compromised, especially in the obese patient. Myoglobinuria has been associated with this position and attributed to reduced perfusion of the lower extremities.[44] Further extrusion of a prolapsed lumbar disk could provoke postoperative, radicular discomfort and/or neurologic sequelae.

A minority of neurosurgeons prefer the patient to be in a lateral decubitus position for posterior approaches to both the thoracic and lumbar spine (Fig. 27-10). An axillary roll between the patient and table permits unimpeded excursions of the chest with mechanical ventilation. Additional padding protects the weight-bearing points of the iliac crest, fibular head, and lateral malleolus. The arms are placed in

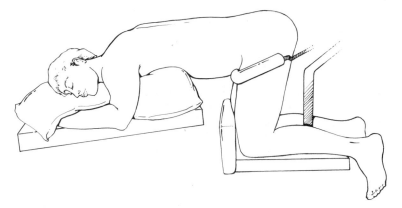

Fig. 27-9   Schematic illustration of a patient in semi-kneeling position for posterior lumbar approach. Abdomen remains free of compression and weight is evenly distributed over well-cushioned anterior tibial surfaces. Cushioned support is provided for the anterior axillary regions and elbows.

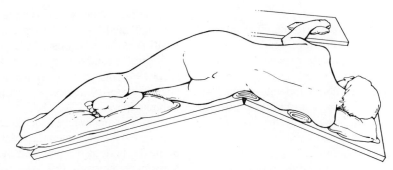

Fig. 27-10 Schematic illustration of the lateral decubitus position for posterior approaches to both the thoracic and lumbar spine. Note the axillary roll on the dependent side and padded protection of iliac crest, dependent fibular head, and lateral malleolus. The arm opposite the dependent side is supported by a cushioned Mayo stand.

front of the patient, with the up-side arm supported either by a pillow or a padded table extension. For disk removal, the patient's flank, on the dependent side, can be aligned above the flexion break of the table. Table flexion will elevate the adjacent flank and open the opposite side of the targeted disk space.

Operative Procedures

In posterior approaches, targeting the lesion remains a potent source of surgical confusion and wasted anesthesia time. A combination of radiographs and topographic examination allows appropriate placement of the incision. Lesions that are targeted by myelography should be marked, with a member of the surgical team confirming the aspect of the lesion (top, middle, or bottom) to which the marking refers. Radiographs are more useful surgically when they include the targeted lesion and a bony landmark that functions as a reference point for segmental counting. Coned-down views do not fulfill this purpose. In the operating room, radiographic views are best displayed in the same orientation as the patient position.

Most posterior approaches are midline, with the initial surgical goal being the exposure of normal anatomy above and below any targeted lesion. On the patient, segmental counting of the spinous processes puts the surgeon in proximity to the target, and a needle is placed into the interspinous ligament with a cephalad angle. An image intensifier or plain x-ray locates the needle in reference to landmarks, which can include the foramen magnum for cervicothoracic localization in the lateral projection, the first rib for thoracic localization in the anteroposterior (AP) projection, and the top of the iliac crest and sacrum for thoracolumbar localization in the lateral projection. The needle is either on target or serves as a second reference from which an accurate incision can be made. Alternatively, when the surgical exposure incorporates known points of reference, the targeted level can be determined by segmental counting in the operative field. This is often the case for cervical and lum-

bar exposures with C2 as the first spinous process and S1 as the last.

When counting spinous processes, the surgeon can encounter anomalies that mandate radiographic imaging to confirm the segmental level. Sacralization of the L5 vertebra or lumbarization of the S1 vertebra and missing spinous processes can make accurate determination of the caudal cord level difficult. From 20 % to 30% of the general population has spina bifida occulta within the lumbar region of the spine.[88] In spinal neoplasms, especially metastatic tumors, a whole vertebral body can be missing (Fig. 27-11). This may be capricious in the thoracic spine, and careful segmental counting will substantiate the missing link and assure an accurate identification of the targeted level.

During posterior approaches, the midline is incised to detach and mobilize the paraspinous muscles through a subperiosteal technique. Removal of the posterior neural arch in a piecemeal fashion is termed a *laminectomy*. Beneath the posterior neural arch is the ligamentum flavum (yellow ligament), which extends laterally to the facet. The epidural fat and veins lie between the ligamentum flavum and dura. For reconstructive purposes, multiple levels of the posterior neural arch can be elevated as one segment by drilling bilateral troughs in the lamina *(laminoplasty)*. This method preserves the interspinous and interlaminar ligaments of the mobilized segment (Fig. 27-12).

During intradural explorations and nerve root decompressions, laminectomies may require more lateral exposure. This is accomplished by undercutting the medial one third of the facet. The facet or apophyseal joints overlay the lateral recess, which contains the nerve root and neural foramina. Ventral to the nerve root and cord is the disk space.

A *laminotomy* is a partial resection of the laminae for two adjacent segmental levels. It provides access for disk removals and nerve-root decompressions. Extension of the laminotomy to the lateral recess with partial removal of the

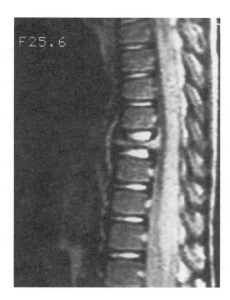

FIG. 27-11   MR study shows a sagittal section of thoracic spine with pathologic compression and near complete loss of vertebral body segment secondary to eosinophilic granuloma.

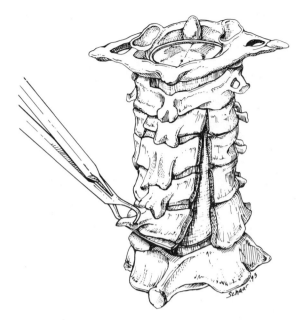

FIG. 27-12   Schematic illustration demonstrating the posterior cervical neural arch undergoing a laminoplasty for posterior exposure. This maneuver allows for reconstruction of the posterior neural arch at the completion of the procedure.

facet (facetectomy) is termed a *foraminotomy*. This procedure decompresses the nerve root and provides access for posterior removal of a disk with lateral herniation in the cervical spine. With extreme lateral retraction of the paraspinal muscles, the transverse process can be visualized lateral to the superior facet. The pedicle is anterior to the junction of the lamina, superior facet, and transverse process. The pedicle is the posterior entry point for transpedicular screw fixation. Removal of the lamina and superior facet permits a transpedicular approach to the vertebral body, with exposure of the lateral spinal cord. Disruption of the posterior neural arch is compatible with retained spinal stability as long as the facets are preserved. The facets, facet capsule, and intertransverse ligament remain mostly intact for residual posterior column stability. Posterior approaches do not require instrumentation, provided that the anterior and middle columns of stability are intact.

Spinal Tumors

An extensive discussion of spinal cord tumor pathology is beyond the scope of this chapter. However, several issues pertinent to surgical considerations can be addressed by discussing generalities of spinal-cord tumors and by emphasizing specific examples of lesions.

The spinal cord and surrounding dura provide a simple anatomic classification of spinal cord tumors as epidural, intradural and extramedullary, or intramedullary. Patients can experience neurologic symptoms as a result of compromised spine stability, compression of nerve roots and the cord proper, or interference with vasculature. Benign lesions generally present insidiously in the posterior spine of children and young adults. Malignant neoplasms tend to occur in older patients, presenting as back pain that progresses to neurologic deficit localized to the anterior structures of the spine.

The majority of epidural neoplasms are metastatic, with 66% of these disseminating from the breast, prostate, hematopoietic system, or lung.[78] Myelography of epidural lesions can reveal a characteristic saw-tooth pattern of partial to complete blockage, which, in conjunction with corroborating plain films and bone scans, constitutes a diagnosis of epidural metastasis. The decision to surgically treat epidural metastasis should consider the general medical condition of the patient. A recent scoring system employing various clinical parameters has been published in an attempt to more uniformly advise neurosurgeons.[80] The system rates patients according to six variables, including Karnofsky status and number of metastases. Patients who score low are unlikely to survive more than 3 months postoperatively (Box 27-1). Those who score high have a reasonable chance of surviving more than a year postoperatively. In general, the surgical approach for removal of a spinal metastasis depends on the anterior or posterior location of the tumor.

The most common spine tumors of middle-to-late adulthood are metastatic. These tumors are the result of hematogenous spread through the venous system of Batson's plexus into the vertebral elements of the spine. The spine is the most common bony segment to acquire metastases.

The vertebral body retains its red marrow longer than most other bony structures, and the microemboli of metastasis has a predilection for red marrow. Metastatic tumors invade the epidural space and infiltrate the epidural fat from the surrounding bony spine.[5]

The dura is resistant to tumor invasion and thereby confines metastatic tumor and cord compression to the epidural compartment. Intradural metastasis is rare, less than 2%, and is metastatic rather than invasive.[19] Tumors with the greatest propensity for spine metastasis include multiple myeloma, followed by prostatic and renal cell carcinoma.[13] The thoracic spine is more commonly involved.

The vertebral body and bony elements of the spine give rise to paravertebral tumor, which tends to both circumscribe the vertebral column and invade the epidural compartment. The paravertebral tumor often can be targeted for posterior percutaneous biopsy under CT or fluoroscopic control, with a local anesthetic and sedation. With local anesthesia, inadvertent contact with the nerve root can be immediately detected and avoided. Because 10% of spinal metastasis presents with no known primary tumor, biopsies can play an important role.[57]

Cord compression is most often anterior and results from both bony fragments and epidural tumor.[39] With appropriate surgical indications, anterior decompression requires an anterior or anterolateral surgical approach. Conversely, paravertebral tumor can invade the posterolateral epidural compartment through the neural foramina and compress the cord. A decompressive laminectomy is the most common procedure for relieving cord compression induced by posterolateral epidural tumor.

Spinal metastasis commonly presents with local pain of several months' duration before any neurologic deficit. Radiation therapy is the treatment of choice, and it will often alleviate the pain. Factors favoring primary radiation therapy include a radiation-responsive tumor, neural impingement from tumor exclusive of bone, life expectancy of less then 4 months, complete neurologic deficit below the compressed cord for more than 24 hours, and multilevel metastatic spine disease.[20] Stable and unstable pathologic fractures can be treated with external bracing and radiation if appropriate alignment is maintained and in the absence of neural impingement. Radiation reduces tumor burden, which may allow the fracture to heal. In addition, osteoblasts are radioresistant up to approximately 4000 rad (40 Gy).[72]

Factors favoring surgical intervention include rapid progression of neurologic deficit, histologic diagnosis of a radioresistant tumor, cord compression from bone fragments and/or malalignment, spinal instability, and failure of radiation therapy.[20]

Patients with spinal metastases harbor the effects of chemotherapy, radiation therapy, tumor burden, and various inappropriate secretions of hormones from their tumors. They are often anemic, immunocompromised, osteoporotic, hypercalcemic, hypercoagulable, and deficient at wound healing. A diligent preoperative evaluation is mandated, and the scope of the surgery must be concise and expeditious. In the case of progressive neurologic deficit, low-dose dexamethasone should be prescribed. There are no consistent data from clinical and prospectively controlled trials suggesting that high-dose dexamethasone is of any further benefit.[38] For those spinal metastases known to be hypervascular, preoperative angiography and embolization are advisable.[20] This preparation minimizes intraoperative blood loss. As in all decompressive procedures of the spine, four units of packed red blood cells should be available.

A decompressive laminectomy should extend at least one and often two levels above and below the tumor-induced cord compression. Resected bone should be sent for histopathologic evaluation as it may harbor neoplasm. Resected bone cannot be used for reconstructive laminoplasty nor as graft for fusion. Epidural tumor is debulked from the dorsum of the cord and the lateral gutters. Ideally, a decompressive procedure concludes with the surgeon observing epidural space above and below the formerly compressed segment, reappearance of epidural fat, and the possible resumption of cord pulsation. With posterolateral epidural tumor only, decompressive laminectomy is appropriate. Through MR, the stability of the anterior and middle columns can be scrutinized and may prompt a laminectomy followed by posterior spinal instrumentation.

The commonly involved thoracic spine benefits from the additional stability afforded by the rib cage. Most patients undergoing thoracic spinal surgery remain stable after laminectomy. Instability can be treated by inserting pedicle screws in combination with plating and fusion. The pedicle is considered the strongest part of the vertebra, and effective fixation is achieved using a limited number of healthy segments above and below the affected vertebrae.[2,82] With radiographic assessment, transpedicular fixation requires well-defined pedicles and viability of the vertebral body at the affected segment. Because of their larger size, the pedicles of the lower thoracic vertebrae are best suited for transpedicular fixation. Several universal, internal-fixation systems are available with requisite instrumentation for various methods of fixation, including pedicle screws. C-arm fluoroscopy is necessary for accurate placement of the pedicle screws. All operating room personnel should wear lead aprons. The operating room table and sterile draping should be configured to accommodate the use of the C-arm unit in both the AP and lateral projection. The goal of surgical therapy is to improve the quality of life by fostering painless ambulation coupled with bowel and bladder continence.

Primary tumors of the spine can be either benign or malignant and tend to occur in the younger patient who is otherwise healthy.[86] Pediatric spine tumors are uncommon, and nearly 70% of primary bone tumors are benign. Tumors emanate from each of the tissue components of the spine, which include fibrous tissue, cartilage, bone, vascular tissue, fat, hematopoietic cells from the bone marrow, neural tissue, leptomeninges, notochord remnants, and histiocytes. The location of these tissue components determines the spinal compartment from which the tumor arises. Tumors of the bone and cellular elements contained therein can involve the vertebral body, posterior neural arch, or both. The location of the tumor determines the operative approach. Typically, the more benign spectrum of bony tumors are posterior.[86] Neurologic symptoms are caused by epidural cord compression. More than 40% of benign tumors are from bone and cartilage, including osteoid osteomas, osteoblastomas, osteochrondromas, and aneurysmal bone cysts. The most frequent primary malignancy is Ewing's sarcoma.[86] Unlike the metastatic lesions of adulthood, pediatric metastases result from contiguous invasion; the more frequent lesions include neuroblastoma from the paraspinal sympathetic ganglion chain, embryonal carcinoma, and the sarcomas.[79] After treatment of the neoplasm, the immature spine might sustain deformities that require intervention. Orthotic and/or corrective surgery can be used to manage the effects of both radiotherapy and prior tumor surgery.

Intradural tumors involve any tissue element that is contained within the dura. The leptomeninges, nerve sheaths, fat cells, and neural and vascular tissue can each give rise to tumor. Most intradural tumors are approached through a posterior laminectomy. Tumors of the leptomeninges, such as meningiomas, often have an anterolateral location. It is more difficult, confining, and destabilizing to attempt an anterior exposure by removing a vertebral body (corpectomy). Intradural tumors situated in an anterolateral position require a modified posterolateral approach. Intradural explorations require more exposure and complete control of the dural closure to avoid a CSF fistula. Most intradural tumors require the use of a microscope, microinstrumentation, and fiberoptic illumination. The source of illumination is distant from the head of the microscope to minimize heating near the operative field. The principles are uniform for posterior laminectomy and intradural exposures of all extramedullary or intramedullary lesions of the cervical, thoracic, and lumbosacral regions.

Intradural exposures after laminectomy benefit from intraoperative ultrasound for accurate determination of caudal and rostral extent of exposure. After initial laminectomy, the wound is filled with saline and the ultrasound probe is used to image the intradural anatomy. The examination will determine whether the laminectomy should be extended for adequate exposure of the lesion. Often, a syrinx is associated with an intramedullary tumor, and the exposure can be centered to arrive at the lesion, with part of the syrinx above and below the lesion. The patient's clinical findings usually correlate with the intramedullary tumor site and not the associated syrinx.

The most common intradural lesions of childhood are metastases through the seeding of CSF pathways by primary intracranial tumors.[74] As previously discussed, intradural metastases from malignancies outside the CNS are rare in all age groups. Intradural drop metastases can result in extramedullary growths on both the pia and arachnoid membranes involving the spinal cord surface, nerve roots, and cauda equina. These lesions are detected by MR imaging or myelography and are often treated nonsurgically with radiation therapy and/or chemotherapy.

More than half of adult extramedullary tumors are benign and consist of meningiomas and nerve-sheath tumors.[45] The latter include neurofibromas and schwannomas, which have a predilection for the dorsal or sensory nerve root. These tumors often assume a dumbbell configuration on each side of the neural foramen. This includes an extradural, paravertebral, and intradural-extramedullary component. The intradural component is surgically mobilized first to relieve the spinal cord compression. Within a neurofibroma, the nerve fibers course through the tumor, requiring sectioning of the nerve root for excision. Schwannomas displace nerve fibers, allowing excision without disruption of the remaining nerve root.[76] Meningiomas and nerve-sheath tumors occur most frequently along the thoracic segments, followed by the cervical segments, and rarely the lumbosacral segments. The sex occurrence is equal, except for an increased incidence of meningiomas in females.[76]

Intramedullary tumors of childhood are infrequent. They compose 6% of pediatric CNS tumors and occur rostrally toward the cervicothoracic cord, with more than half being astrocytomas.[29] Adult intramedullary tumors occur more caudal toward the thoracic region; approximately half are ependymomas, and the remaining half are mostly astrocytomas.[7] The ependymomas have a predilection for the conus region of the cord.[51] Dermoids, epidermoids, lipomas, and teratomas are in the differential diagnosis for intradural tumors. These tumors can assume an intramedullary and/or extramedullary position and have a propensity to occur on either end of the cord.[76] This propensity may be the result of retained epithelial (inclusion) cells after closure of the anterior (rostral cord) and posterior (caudal cord) neuropores.[60]

Cervicomedullary Junction, Chiari Malformations, and Syringomyelia

Posterior intradural exposures of the cervicomedullary junction include a suboccipital craniectomy with removal of the posterior rim of the foramen magnum, removal of the posterior arch of the atlas (C1), and a posterior cervical laminectomy to the caudal extent of the targeted pathology. This exposure is frequently used to treat the Chiari malformations and associated syrinxes. The posterior intradural exposure is also used for cytoreduction or resection of intramedullary glial tumors and to excise extramedullary meningiomas and nerve sheath tumors.

The Chiari II malformation is almost always associated with a myelomeningocele and involves an array of anomalies of the hindbrain, cervical spinal cord, and craniovertebral junction.[66] These anomalies are not as extensive in the Chiari I malformation. The Chiari II patients with myelodysplasia may have an increased risk for anaphylactic reactions to latex-related antigens.[66] This can occur in the anesthetic setting, and in the event of cardiovascular collapse, treatment requires 100% oxygen with an established airway, intravenous epinephrine, and volume resuscitation, followed by aminophylline, steroids, and inhalational beta-agonists. Common to the Chiari malformations is variable caudal displacement of the inferior cerebellar vermis, tonsils, lower brainstem, and fourth ventricle. There is crowding through an enlarged foramen magnum with platybasia (flat subocciput). The tentorial septum, between the cerebellar hemispheres, is hypoplastic, with caudal displacement of both the transverse and torcular dural venous sinuses to within 2 cm of the foramen magnum[66] (Fig. 27-13).

In the Chiari II malformations of early life, most symptoms referable to the cervicomedullary junction, such as stridor, can be ameliorated by shunting to reduce the associated hydrocephalus. Within the ensuing years, the Chiari malformations are prone to develop symptoms of syrinx formation and/or cervicomedullary compression.[56] Before surgery, the craniovertebral junction must be evaluated to ascertain that the odontoid process of C2 has a normal anatomic relationship with the atlas and foramen magnum. Occasionally, the odontoid may be projecting rostral to the anterior foramen magnum (basion), indicating basilar impression.[66] Posterior bony and ligamentous disruption for decompressive exposures could increase the degree of basilar impression, leading to ventral brainstem impingement. Preoperatively, the degree of basilar impression and evidence of neural impingement can be assessed on MR and may require craniovertebral stabilization after decompressive maneuvers (Fig. 27-14). Posterior stabilization around the decompression site can be achieved through autologous

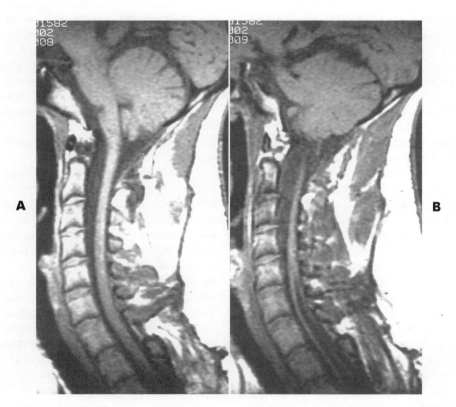

Fig. 27-13   **A,** Midline parasagittal MR (T_1-weighted) image of the neural axis of a Chiari II malformation. The fourth ventricle is attenuated in size, and both the medulla and cerebellar tonsils are caudally displaced within the region of the foramen magnum. **B,** Right parasagittal MR (T_2-weighted) image of the neural axis in the same patient with a Chiari II malformation demonstrates a syrinx within the spinal cord with rostral extension to the C5-C6 segmental level.

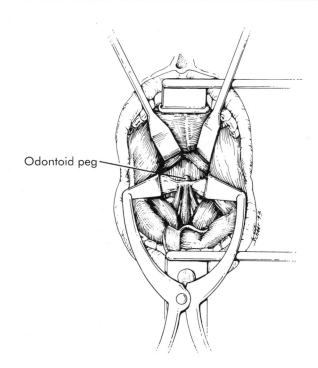

Odontoid peg

FIG. 27-14 Schematic illustration of the anterior, transoral approach to the odontoid process of C2. Note the anterior arch of C1 in front of the odontoid. Neural compression from the odontoid process can be approached in this manner.

rib strut grafts or contoured titanium loops and wiring.[65] Atlantoaxial (C1-C2) stability also requires preoperative confirmation by viewing the odontoid's position with respect to the anterior arch of C1, termed the atlantodental distance. Lateral cervical radiographs for both flexion and extension should show that the atlantodental distance remains less than 3 mm. Preoperative brainstem auditory evoked potential (BAER) and SSEP evaluations will assist the interpretation of intraoperative neuromonitoring. Tolerance of cervical flexion should be confirmed preoperatively. A flexed neck position will simplify access to the foramen magnum in patients with platybasia. In all posterior exposures of the craniovertebral junction, the paired vertebral arteries are vulnerable to surgical injury at the lateral extent of the exposure. The vertebral arteries traverse the transverse foramina from C6-C7 up through the atlas, circumscribe the top of the posterior arch of the atlas and atlantooccipital membrane in a medial direction, and pierce the dura for posterior fossa entry. Vertebral arterial bleeding can be troublesome because of the surrounding osseous structures. To counter bleeding, the surgeon can slightly increase the reverse Trendelenburg tilt, apply local hemostatic adjuvants and pressure.

The goals of surgical intervention for symptomatic Chiari malformations remain controversial, as seen in the variety of suggested maneuvers and the uncertainty of clinical results. Often an associated spinal cord syrinx is located at a considerable distance below the Chiari malfor-

mation, with syrinx-free cord interposed.[56] MR imaging can demonstrate the syrinx, and assuming appropriate neurologic findings, the surgical intervention can be limited to decompression of the syrinx.[53] Surgical treatment entails radiographic localization of the involved segmental levels, a posterior laminectomy or laminoplasty over the rostral extent of the syrinx, ultrasound imaging to confirm the target, and a midline opening of the dura. An enlarged spinal cord will be apparent with attenuation of the surrounding subarachnoid space. A portion of the syrinx may appear at the cord surface, often near the dorsal root entry zone. The proximal limb of a diversionary shunt can be placed into the apparent dome of the syrinx and secured to the leptomeninges, followed by dural closure. A midline dorsal myelotomy can be performed to enter the syrinx for shunt placement if the syrinx is not apparent at the spinal-cord surface. A myelotomy is a dorsal midline incision into the cord between the paired posterior columns.

At this juncture, the opposite end of the shunt could be placed in the adjacent subarachnoid space to create a syringosubarachnoid shunt.[83] However, the subarachnoid space remains blocked rostrally at the foramen magnum level because of the impacted anatomy of the Chiari malformation. Traditionally, the other end of the shunt is routed to a distant body cavity that includes the pleura (syringopleural shunt)[63] or the peritoneum (syringoperitoneal or lumboperitoneal shunt).[49,61] Alternatively, the shunt catheter can be routed through a continuous exposure or tunneled to a separate exposure of the suboccipital bone. Lateral burr-hole placement, incision of the dura, and a separate incision of the arachnoid allow passage of the shunt into a patent cerebellopontine CSF cistern above the Chiari malformation.[53] Often, an immediate deflation of the cord can be observed. This diversion is above the subarachnoid block, represents an internal CNS shunt, and is termed a *syringocisternostomy*. An internal CNS shunt may require fewer revisions than shunting to distant body cavities.

The traditional approach to the symptomatic Chiari malformation is a posterior fossa or craniovertebral decompression. Many additional steps have been recommended and include lysis of adhesions, resection of the cerebellar tonsils, plugging of the obex, draining of the fourth ventricle, and duraplasty.[11] A series of patients studied for outcome indicates that only 50% had significant improvement in symptoms and reduction of syrinx size.[63] Successful shunting of the syrinx is a preferred option.[53] However, symptoms may be compelling in the absence of a sizable syrinx and warrant direct decompression. Such symptoms can include weakness and spasticity of the extremities, neck pain, radicular pain, progressive scoliosis, nystagmus, dysphagia, stridor, torticollis, and other lower-cranial-nerve palsies.[37]

Direct decompression uses the previously discussed bony exposure of the cervicomedullary junction. The cervical laminectomy extends one segmental level below the caudal extent of the descended cerebellar tonsils. The dura is opened with caution because of the caudally displaced dural venous sinuses. Beneath the dura, the surgeon observes extreme crowding of the cervicomedullary junction and obliteration of the normal cisterns, subarachnoid space, and a lack of CSF patency. Dorsally, the cerebellar tonsils are caudally displaced, hypoplastic, flattened, and matted to the inferior or calamus scriptorius portion of the fourth ventricle. The caudal loop of the posterior inferior cerebellar artery (PICA) also adheres to this region and requires protection. The medulla may descend against an upper cervical cord segment that is anchored by the stretched dentate ligaments. The result is a dorsal medullary kink at about the C2 level that augments the fullness and crowding of the region.

The surgical goal is to establish some evidence of CSF patency. The microscope is used to remove the cerebellar tonsils from the dorsum of the calamus and roof of the aperture to the central canal of the cervical cord (the obex). The lateral gutters of the cervicomedullary junction adhere to the dura and require delicate lysis of arachnoid adhesions. The dorsal cervical nerve roots show an ascending rather than descending course into their respective neural foramina. If the upper dentate ligaments can be visualized, they can be released. Manipulations of this region may induce brief bradycardic episodes, and the surgeon must be immediately alerted so he/she can cease the ongoing maneuver. A duraplasty is completed using autogenous fascia or cadaveric dura to effect a capacious closure.

Several prior hypotheses about the etiologic basis of syrinx formation have a common theme. At the foramen magnum level or Chiari malformation site, the outlets of the fourth ventricle and their respective cisterns have been obliterated by caudal displacement and crowding. CSF pulsations are then forced into the central canal of the spinal cord, which undergoes distension and dissection into the cord substance.[37] Alternatively, a pressure differential has been suggested at the foramen magnum level that draws CSF into the central canal from the fourth ventricle or surrounding subarachnoid space.[6,87] Implicit in these hypotheses is that a syrinx should evolve from and be continuous with the caudally displaced fourth ventricle.

However, MR imaging of Chiari malformations shows that fewer than 10% of syrinxes communicate directly with the fourth ventricle and most syrinxes are at a considerable distance below the foramen magnum.[61] Furthermore, syrinxes have been associated with a variety of other conditions, such as posterior fossa cysts, basilar impression, foramen magnum tumors, extramedullary cysts and tumors, intramedullary tumors, arachnoiditis, spinal cord trauma, transverse myelitis, multiple sclerosis, cervical spondylosis, degenerative disk disease, Paget's disease, and hydrocephalus (Box 27-2). With the exceptions of intramedullary tumors and spinal cord trauma, syrinx formation usually occurs caudal to the disease process.[56] When a syrinx is discovered, spinal cord imaging must encompass remote segmental levels to determine a cause.

BOX 27-2
CONDITIONS THAT CAN RESULT IN SYRINX FORMATION

Arachnoiditis
Basilar impression
Cervical spondylitis
Degenerative disk disease
Extramedullary cysts and tumors
Foramen magnum tumors
Hydrocephalus
Intramedullary tumors
Multiple sclerosis
Paget's disease
Posterior fossa tumor
Spinal cord trauma
Transverse myelitis

The observation that syrinxes form caudal to the disease process, as seen in recent experimental evidence, suggests two plausible hypotheses.[54,55] First, the interstitial fluid of the cord may have a special relationship to the central canal that is similar to that of the cerebrum and ventricles. Second, both the central canal and subarachnoid space may have a rostral flow that is impeded at the diseased site.

The pattern of syrinx formation may be dictated by the pattern of central canal involution that results during adult life.[56] The tumor vasculature of intramedullary tumors exudes edema and leads to syrinx formation both above and below the tumor. After trauma, a latent syrinx can occur and usually extends above the site of injury. This may result from the rostral clearance of red blood cells and other byproducts of injury through the central canal with eventual rostral impedance.[54] The impedance may follow inflammatory scarring of the ependymal lining. The term *hydromyelia* refers to distension of the central canal, and *hydrosyringomyelia* includes dissection of the cavity into the cord. These terms often defy histologic definition and may be confusing. Syringomyelia is sufficient to describe a pathologic cavity in the cord substance.

Anterolateral Approaches
Anterior Atlantoaxial

At the atlantoaxial junction, the odontoid process may require a transoral resection to relieve or avert impingement of the cervicomedullary junction. Frequent indications include trauma, basilar impression, rheumatoid arthritis, and congenital dysgenesis of the odontoid. Down's, Klippel-Feil, and achondroplastic syndromes represent some congenital conditions with associated anomalies of the craniovertebral junction. Patients with rheumatoid arthritis have surgical and anesthetic problems related to a recessed mandible, subluxed cervical spine, lung disease, decreased chest excursion, anemia, increased bleeding time, and delicate skin.[75] Susceptibility to infection, operative fractures, and bleeding has been documented.[43]

In many circumstances, the posterior or rostral displacement of the odontoid process can be corrected with skeletal traction. In the absence of any residual neural impingment, a posterior approach can be used to provide atlantoaxial or atlantooccipital fixation. However, failing the recovery of normal alignment, or given the persistence of ventral neural impingement, the odontoid process can be removed using the transoral approach.

Fiberoptic nasotracheal intubation with an armored cuffed tube is preferred. Tracheostomy is an option that may be advantageous, but the process of insertion requires intubation for airway control. The patient can remain in the supine position with cranial fixation maintaining a neutral neck position. Skeletal traction can also be maintained in this position to effect distraction. The traction lowers the tip of the odontoid in relation to the clivus and simplifies the surgical exposure. If traction is not needed, some surgeons advocate a lateral position with a dependent axillary roll.[22] The table can be put into a side-tilt away from the surgeon so that the patient is facing 45 degrees up toward the surgeon. This position allows the surgeon to sit, and after odontoid resection, the patient can be tilted in the opposite direction for posterior atlantooccipital fixation in a one-stage procedure, thus avoiding the hazardous movement of a patient with craniovertebral instability to the prone position.[24] Alternatively, most surgeons opt for posterior fixation as a second procedure, using external bracing or skeletal traction to maintain stability. The lateral position also pools secretions and blood on the dependent tonsillar pillar. Regardless of the position, radiographic confirmation of the odontoid process position should be obtained.

Before the transoral procedure, the oral cavity is prepared and intravenous antibiotics are given. Steroid cream has been cited as effective for limiting postoperative swelling. The cream is applied to both the lips and tongue.[23] Intravenous steroids can also limit postoperative swelling. Unstable dentition must be protected and secured. A portion of the lateral thigh should be prepared and draped in case autogenous fascia lata is needed to cover an inadvertent CSF fistula. A transoral retractor is placed to retract both the mandible and tongue caudally. A self-retaining palatal extension allows the soft palate to be retracted up and laterally. The nasotracheal and nasogastric tubes are pushed laterally by the palatal extension. The posterior pharynx is inspected, and the midline must be identified through the bony tubercle of the anterior arch of C1. Midline location is particularly important in congenital craniovertebral anomalies, where there is often a component of atlantoaxial rotary luxation and hypoplasia of the odontoid process. The midline approach avoids contact with the lateral mass and the adjacent vertebral artery (see Fig. 27-14).

With dural compression, neuromonitoring is advisable, but many surgeons rely exclusively on changes in spontaneous respiration, heart rate, and blood pressure. These changes should be immediate with excessive contact or pressure on the ventral brainstem. After the posterior pharyngeal incision, a microscope is used. The anterior arch of C1 is cleared of ligamentous attachments, which include the longus colli muscles and the anterior longitudinal ligament. Part of the clivus, basion, and anterior arch of C1 can be variably resected for adequate exposure and removal of the odontoid process. In rheumatoid arthritis, there is often a pannus of inflammatory synovial tissue that requires debulking. Behind the odontoid process are the transverse ligament, posterior longitudinal ligament, and then dura. The odontoid tip contains suspensory ligaments that insert on the basion or clivus. An intraoperative x-ray can be used to substantiate the anatomy and degree of bony resection.

The patient should remain intubated after closure. This will prevent airway obstruction from oral and pharyngeal swelling. After 8 to 24 hours, a lateral cervical spine x-ray can show the extent of prevertebral swelling before extubation. Early postoperative steroids can be maintained either topically or intravenously for 2 days.

Anterior Cervical Approaches

The anterior cervical approach permits extensive access to levels ranging from C2 to C7. The approach is formally anterolateral and uses a bloodless, direct fascial plain within the anterior triangle of the neck.[68] The most frequent indication for the anterior cervical approach is degenerative disease; however, it is also efficacious in the treatment of tumor, infection, and trauma.

An advantage of the anterior cervical approach is that the patient remains supine with a near-neutral neck position after cautious intubation. The mandibular angle approximates the C3 level and requires slight hyperextension of the neck to simplify access. A small roll behind the neck facilitates the exposure and supports the vertebral column. Other localizing landmarks include the hyoid bone for C4, cricoid cartilage for C5, the first tracheal ring for C6, and two finger breadths above the suprasternal notch for C7. A right-sided approach is more practical for the right-handed surgeon. The left side warrants consideration when the pathology is primarily on the left.

Gardner-Wells skeletal tongs and weighted traction can be applied after induction of anesthesia. This provides steady distraction during muscle relaxation to optimize the height of the disk space and can obviate the need for vertebral spreading retractors. With single-level approaches, a horizontal incision heals with good cosmesis. However, an oblique medial sternocleidomastoid incision affords improved exposure for multilevel inspection, exerts less resistance to retraction, and is parallel to the surgical plane. The anterior approach retracts the carotid artery laterally, the esophagus and trachea medially, and the omohyoid muscle and recurrent laryngeal nerve inferiorly. The diagastric muscle and superior laryngeal and hypoglossal nerves are retracted superiorly. Careful retraction avoids distractive or perforation-type injuries to the nonmuscular structures. Bradycardic responses may result from excessive carotid retraction or heightened carotid sinus sensitivity, and the surgeon should be alerted. Neuromonitoring is most important with multilevel, distractive fixation that changes the cervical curvature. Radiographic verification of the targeted vertebral level is mandatory, and an image intensifier may prove useful during the procedure. A microscope is used during disk removal and drilling of the vertebral body. A sandbag is used to elevate the right anterior iliac crest as a donor site for autogenous graft. Within the disk space or vertebral body, excessive lateral or angulated drilling can injure the vertebral artery. Any bleeding should be controlled with light pressure and hemostatic adjuvants. After prolonged retraction or extensive bone work, the endotracheal tube can remain in place for 8 to 24 hours. This allows time to ascertain a stable, hemostatic wound site. Postoperative x-rays can check for appropriate alignment, dislodgment of a bone plug, tracheal deviation, and prevertebral swelling.

Cervical radiculopathy is commonly the result of compression and irritation of a nerve root by a bony or spondylotic spur. Although soft-disk herniation can induce a radiculopathy, this is less frequent in the neck and more common at the lumbar level. With advancing age, the cervical disk degenerates and primarily leads to anterior osteophyte formation.[40]

The top of the vertebral body has a slight raised prominence on each side (the uncinate processes). With disk degeneration, the uncinate process flattens, thus increasing the translational motion. The back of the uncus approximates the lateral recess of the spinal canal and the neural foramen. In addition, the increased translational motion can induce both facet and ligamentous hypertrophy. Both the facet and uncinate process encroach on the lateral recess and neural foramen as osteophytes.[81]

The lower cervical spine bears the brunt of degenerative changes. The most common levels for radiculopathy include C5-C6 affecting the C6 root; and C6-C7, affecting the C7 root. A radiculopathy of C5 or C8 is less frequent and requires differentiation from shoulder disease and thoracic-outlet syndrome or ulnar neuropathy, respectively.[70] Patients with single or multilevel unilateral disease with radiculopathy that has failed conservative measures can undergo a posterior foraminotomy and possible resection of a lateral herniated disk. An anterior diskectomy and fusion is deferred because it may accelerate spondylotic changes at the levels immediately above and below the fusion site. Osteophytes will not enlarge or recur at the successfully fused site because of the cessation of motion.

A central herniated disk, central spur, degenerative hypermobility or subluxation, arthrogenic neck pain, unilateral or bilateral radiculopathy with bilateral neural foraminal stenosis, loss of AP diameter of the spinal canal (<12 mm), compressive myelopathy, and degenerative kyphosis are all indications for anterior diskectomy and fusion. When this procedure includes more than two cervical levels, the risk of nonunion or pseudarthrosis increases. Autogenous iliac-crest graft is optimal for fusion. Cadaveric bone grafts can be used successfully but take longer to fuse. Other concurrent medical conditions can prolong the rate of fusion and warrant autogenous graft.[16] There are various opinions about the need to use an interposed plug of bone for a single-level, soft cervical disk.[40,69] With exclusion of a bone graft, there is a lack of long-term follow-up with radiographic correlation, the potential for loss of height in both the disk space and neural foramen, and the occurrence of osteophytes at the nonfused segments.

Diffuse spondylotic disease and ligamentous hypertrophy may lead to both anterior and posterior compression or cervical stenosis. A posterior decompressive laminectomy may destabilize the diseased segments further, and neurologic deficit could result from anterior impingement during surgery. The clinical experience is more favorable with anterior decompression for prominent foci of impingement.[41] Anterior internal fixation with an H-shaped plating system and cancellous screws can be used to fortify the bone graft after extensive osteophyte resections (osteophytectomy). This obviates the need for a halo brace. External fixation with a rigid collar suffices until fusion is documented by flexion/extension films at 12 weeks. Assuming no improvement, posterior decompression could then be safely carried out over the fused spinal segments.

Anterolateral Approaches of the Thoracic Spine

The posterior laminectomy poses significant neurologic risks with attempts to access or decompress anteriorly situated lesions of the thoracic vertebrae. Anterior access through a posterior laminectomy requires retraction of the thoracic cord, and decompression constricts the posteriorly displaced cord at the rostral and caudal extents of the laminectomy. Either manipulation can lead to neurologic deficit in the case of a thoracic disk herniation.[62] For anteriorly situated vertebral tumors, anterolateral approaches have a superior outcome compared with radiotherapy alone or in combination with laminectomy, and stability of the posterior column remains undisturbed.[20]

Anterolateral access to the thoracic spine includes the transpedicular, costotransverse, and transthoracic approaches. The transpedicular approach involves prone positioning and a posterior laminectomy after radiographic confirmation of the segmental level. On one side, drilling is used to remove the facet, which exposes the neural foramen and nerve root. The nerve root can be protected and retracted or occasionally sectioned so one can continue removing the overlying pedicle leading to the vertebral body. The lateral convexity of the dura and disk space is exposed. Further exposure can be obtained by removing the transverse process laterally to reveal the costovertebral junction. The head of the adjacent rib can also be resected for further vertebral access or for use as an autograft for an evacuated disk space. The intercostal artery, vein, and nerve root, termed the neurovascular bundle, courses beneath the underside of the rib. The transpedicular approach can be useful for the T1 to T5 segments. Transthoracic and costotransverse approaches are encumbered in this region by the overlying scapula on the rib cage and mediastinal anatomy. The scapula can be mobilized but requires considerable muscle sectioning. Any violation of the pleura warrants placement of a small chest tube during closure. Mobilization of the rib requires an early postoperative AP chest x-ray to check for a pneumothorax or hemothorax.

The costotransverse approach can be accomplished with the prone position.[42] A right-sided approach is preferred unless the pathology is on the left side. A semicircular incision is made with the apex toward the surgeon and over the designated ribs for resection. As an example for localization, the seventh rib has its costovertebral junction at the T7 pedicle, which is in front of the corresponding transverse process. This location approximates the T6-T7 interspace, and the corresponding neural foramen is above the rib and pedicle. The T6 root traverses the T6-T7 neural foramen. After radiographic confirmation, the table can be tilted such that the targeted side of the vertebral column faces up toward the surgeon. The paraspinal muscles are reflected toward the midline and away from the surgeon to expose the posterior rib cage and overlying transverse process. Resection of the transverse process and head of the rib exposes the pleura, sympathetic trunk, neurovascular bundle, neural foramen, pedicle, and disk space. The neurovascular bundle guides the surgeon to the corresponding neural foramen. Usually two rib resections are required for adequate exposure, but more than three may destabilize the ipsilateral rib cage.

The exposure permits a diskectomy, osteophytectomy, ventral epidural decompression, partial corpectomy (vertebral body resection) above and below the disk space, and bone graft insertion for fusion. With this approach, a sympathectomy can be conducted for a causalgic sympathetic dystrophy involving the ipsilateral arm.[30] In contrast to the transthoracic approach, the costotransverse approach has limited exposure for anterior instrumentation but is well tolerated, with postoperative recovery being fairly simple and rapid. The costotransverse approach is well suited for targets caudal to T9 and for laterally situated disk protrusions and/or osteophytes. Rarely, an extradural myelographic block may prompt a posterior decompressive laminectomy for spinal epidural metastasis. After a negative exploration for epidural tumor and review of the radiographs, a suspected thoracic disk herniation can be pursued in the same sitting by converting to a transpedicular or costotransverse approach.[47]

The transthoracic approach provides the most expansive exposure of the thoracic vertebrae with anterolateral viewing.[62] Vertebral body resection, reconstruction, and anterior column instrumentation are best accomplished through

this approach. Anterior epidural impingement from tumor, trauma, and infection can be directly decompressed without neural manipulation. Kyphotic deformities can be stabilized and/or corrected with distractive instrumentation. For degenerative disease, a centrally located disk or osteophyte is best viewed through the transthoracic approach.

Many patients with significant thoracic cord pathology will have concurrent conditions that adversely affect pulmonary function. Both paralysis and advanced spinal deformities require pulmonary assessment. A forced vital capacity of less than 1 L, an arterial blood gas indicating elevated Pco_2 levels, and dyspnea are findings that may require postoperative mechanical ventilation, aggressive respiratory therapy, and early mobilization of the patient. Upper thoracic and cervical-cord deficits include neuromuscular compromise of intercostal thoracic excursions. The patient is left with diaphragmatic breathing and is prone to atelectasis and pneumonia. Tracheostomy may allow more effective pulmonary care, avoid infectious complications, and hasten an end to full-time mechanical ventilatory support.

Transthoracic approaches require that the patient be placed in a lateral decubitus position. A double-lumen ET tube allows selective deflation of the lung to optimize exposure of the thoracic vertebrae. During surgery, the collapsed lung is periodically reinflated to minimize atelectasis. A right-sided, intrapleural exposure of the upper thoracic vertebrae (T2-T5) avoids hindrance from the left carotid and subclavian arteries and aortic arch in the upper mediastinum. At the midthoracic levels (T5-T9), a left-sided approach takes advantage of the larger thoracic cavity. For further vertebral access, it is simpler to mobilize the segmental arteries and aorta on the left rather than the azygos vein and branches on the right. The intercostal incision circumscribes the rib cage and should be made about two rib levels above the targeted vertebrae. This is due to the downward obliquity of the rib cage. An axillary roll supports the dependent side and avoids protracted compression of neurovascular structures in the axilla, and flexion of the operating table opens the contralateral disk spaces of the thoracic vertebrae (Fig. 27-15). The up-side arm must be supported in a semireaching position to elevate the scapula away from the operative site. A cross-table radiograph or fluorscopy will yield an AP view of the chest for localization.

A left-side approach avoids the liver and inferior vena cava when one is targeting the lower thoracic or thoracolumbar (T9-L2) levels. This approach requires an incision followed by repair of the diaphragm and incorporates a retroperitoneal approach to the vertebrae. The ureter elevates with the peritoneum. Routine preoperative angiography can be used to identify the dominant segmental artery of Adamkiewicz. Excluding angiography, several points help to avoid a vascular insult to the cord. First, the paired segmental arteries of the aorta have excellent collateral circulation as they circumscribe each side of the vertebrae. Sec-

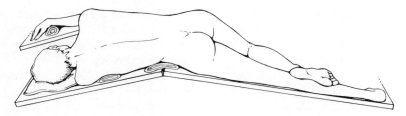

Fig. 27-15   Schematic illustration showing the lateral decubutis position for an anterolateral approach to the thoracic spine through an intercostal incision and exposure. Note the table break to open the thoracic interspaces opposite the dependent side.

ond, the least number of segmental vessels are ligated to access a vertebral body. Third, segmental vessels are ligated in proximity to the aorta and left undisturbed when viewed as end-arteries in the neural foramen.

The resection of a vertebral body for neural decompression mandates replacement with a bony strut graft. Disruption of both the anterior and middle columns of stability requires anterior instrumentation.[28] The exposed lateral surfaces of the vertebral bodies above and below the corpectomy site serve as fixation points for anterior instrumentation. Several fixation systems are available that include transverse insertions of paired cancellous screws with lateral plating for each vertebra.[3] Screw placement requires multiplanar fluoroscopic verification to assure optimal placement and to avoid vascular and neural injury. Unilateral, paired, and parallel rods can be attached to the screws and aligned with the long axis of the vertebral column. Cross-linkage fixation between the paired rods provides rotational stability. The instrumentation has versatility in configuring the amount of distraction and compression that is optimal to correct a spinal deformity. The long-term success of spinal instrumentation depends upon adequate bony fusion. The instrumentation allows early mobilization of the patient and provides an interval of stability pending bony fusion. Inadequate fusion ultimately leads to fatigue and failure of the instrumentation. Thoracolumbosacral orthosis (TLSO) is commonly used to supplement spinal stability with early mobilization. In cases with poor prospects for adequate fusion, such as those involving spinal metastases, corpectomy, or spinal instrumentation, acrylic polymers can be used as a substitute for strut grafts.

Thoracic disk herniation represent less than 1% of disk operations.[3] It tends to occur in the young-to-middle-age patient population and usually involves the middle-to-lower thoracic levels. Achondroplastic conditions, as in dwarfism, involve increased susceptibility to thoracic disk herniation.[12] The disk can herniate centrally or laterally and may accompany degenerative changes, such as osteophytes. Trauma is rarely involved, and symptoms usually include local back and radicular pain. Cord compression can induce additional symptoms, such as heavy and stiff legs, bowel and bladder dysfunction, and unsteadiness. Neurologic findings include gait disturbances, hyperreflexia, sensory

level deficits, and Brown-Séquard presentations. The differential diagnosis includes metastatic neoplasms, diseases affecting the mediastinum and retroperitoneal regions, ankylosing spondylitis, and possibly normal-pressure hydrocephalus. Plain films show a loss of disk space, and MR or CT/myelography can demonstrate the lesion. Conservative therapy and posterior surgical approaches have no role in the treatment of a herniated thoracic disk.

Vertebral fractures and collapse can be secondary to neoplasia, osteoporosis, congenital conditions affecting the vertebral endplates, infection, autoimmune disease (ankylosing spondylitis), and trauma. Axial loading is the principal mechanism behind wedge compression fractures of the vertebral bodies. All three columns of spinal stability can remain intact in the presence of a wedge compression fracture, alleviating the need for corrective surgery and instrumentation. The involvement of two or more vertebral segments and a progressive kyphosis requires anterolateral surgical approaches for distractive instrumentation. The T1-T4 region is particularly prone to latent cervicothoracic kyphosis with wedge compression fractures.[31,50]

Burst fractures of the vertebral body usually involve the thoracolumbar segments (T12-L2) and can be managed conservatively with TLSO for 3 to 6 months. Typically the posterior column is intact, and both the middle and anterior columns are disrupted.[50] Slight retropulsion of vertebral fragments toward the spinal canal, significant loss of vertebral height, slight kyphosis, and the absence of neurologic deficit permits a posterior approach to the lamina for pedicle screw insertions, distractive plating, and fusion maneuvers. Posterior distraction often reduces vertebral fragments that are moderately retropulsed.

The thoracolumbar segments have thick pedicles that provide an additional measure of safety and stability for screw placements. Pedicle screw fixation and plating can provide adequate stability, using only one segmental level above and below the lesion site. Alternatively, segmental spinal instrumentation (SSI) can be used. This involves distractive rodding that is segmentally secured to at least two spinal segments above and below the burst fracture site. Posterior segmental attachments include the use of sublaminar wiring, drummond buttons, and/or various hooks at each end of the paired rods. Sublaminar wiring requires passage under the lamina, which can be hazardous. Alternatively, drummond buttons allow wire fixation of the rods to each side of the spinous processes. Anterolateral decompression may be necessary (in conjunction with anterior instrumentation and fusion) when more than one third of the spinal canal is occupied by retropulsed bone and/or neurologic sequelae.[50]

Thoracic flexion injuries involve posterior ligamentous disruption with the possibility of jumped facets and an anterior wedge compression fracture.[50] Neurologic deficit is common. Posterior approaches are used for open internal reduction, compressive plating or rodding, and fusion. Anterolateral approaches may be required, given the same indications as discussed for burst fractures. Thoracic translational injuries disrupt all three columns of spinal stability and result from high-velocity, shearing forces.[50] There is discontinuity of the spinal column, and the neurologic deficit is usually complete. SSI is useful to permit early mobilization of the patient. With multiple trauma, spinal operative procedures are delayed until the patient is stabilized hemodynamically.

▼

Summary

Surgical considerations for the treatment of neurosurgical diseases of the spine and spinal cord include evaluations that are performed before, during, and after the procedure. Physicians administering anesthetic care should be aware of these evaluations and their relevance to the anesthetic process. The progression starts with general preoperative diagnostics and includes the specific operative procedures used to treat disease. The disease often dictates particular approaches some of which have distinctive risks of intraoperative ischemia and a requirement of spinal cord function monitoring. Other approaches entail special anesthetic considerations for control of airway and hemodynamic status. An understanding of the surgical considerations should help improve anesthetic approaches. We hope this overview may facilitate an excellent working relationship between the neurosurgeon and the anesthesia team.

References

1. Adams RD, Victor M: *Principles of neurology,* New York, 1989, McGraw-Hill, p 130.

2. Allison RE, Amundson G: Spinal fixation using the Steffee pedicle screw and plate system, *AORN J* 49:1016, 1989.

3. An HS, Cotler JM: *Spinal instrumentation,* Baltimore, 1992, Williams & Wilkins, pp 127-456.

4. Apple DF: Spinal cord injury rehabilitation. In Rothman RH, Simeone FA, editors: *The spine,* Philadelphia, 1992, WB Saunders, p 1233.

5. Askin GH, Webb JK: The management of spinal neoplasia. In Torrens MJ, Dickson RA, editors: *Operative spinal surgery,* Edinburgh, 1991, Churchill-Livingstone, pp 242-267.

6. Ball MJ, Dayan AD: Pathogenesis of syringomyelia, *Lancet* 2:799-801, 1972.

7. Banna M, Gryspaerat GL: Review article: Intraspinal tumors in children (excluding dysraphism), *Radiology* 22:17, 1971.

8. Barnes PD, Mulkern RV: Physical and biological principles of MRI. In Walpert SM, Barnes PD, editors: *MRI in pediatric neuroradiology,* St. Louis, 1992, Mosby–Year Book, pp 3-40.

9. Barnett HGM, Foster JB, Hudgson D: *Syringomyelia,* London, 1973, WB Saunders, pp 1-318.

10. Bell HS: Paralysis of birth arms from injury of the upper portion of the pyramidal decussation: "cruciate paralysis," *J Neurosurg* 33:376-380, 1970.

11. Bedford RF: Posterior fossa procedures. In Newfield P, Cottrell JE, editors: *Neuroanesthesia: handbook of clinical and physiologic essentials,* Boston, 1991, Little, Brown, pp 251-252.

12. Bethem D, Winter RB, Lutter L et al: Spinal disorders of dwarfism. Review of the literature and report of eighty cases, *J Bone Joint Surg* 63A:1412-1425, 1981.

13. Black P: Spinal metastasis: current status and recommended guidelines for management, *Neurosurgery* 5:726-746, 1979.

14. Bolognese P, Miller JI, Heger IM et al: Laser Doppler flowmetry in neurosurgery, *J Neurosurg Anesth* 5:151-158, 1993.

15. Bracken MS, Shepard MJ, Collins WF et al: A randomized, controlled trial of methylprednisolone or naloxone in the treatment of acute spinal cord injury: results of the Second National Acute Spinal Cord Injury Study, *N Engl J Med* 322:1405-1411, 1990.

16. Brown MD, Malinin TI, Davis PB: A roentgenographic evaluation of frozen allografts versus autografts in anterior cervical fusions, *Clin Orthop* 119:231-236, 1976.

17. Chance GQ: Note on a type of flexion fracture of the spine, *Br J Radiol* 21:452-453, 1948.

18. Collins JC, Roberts MP: Posterior operations for cervical disc herniation and spondylotic myelopathy. In Schmidek HH, Sweet WH, editors: *Operative neurosurgerical techniques: indications, methods, and results,* Philadelphia, 1988, WB Saunders pp 1352-1353.

19. Constans JP, de Divitis E, Donelli R et al: Spinal metastasis with neurological manifestations: review of 600 cases, *J Neurosurg* 59:111-118, 1983.

20. Cooper PR, Errico TJ, Martin R et al: A systematic approach to spinal reconstruction after anterior decompression for neoplastic disease of the thoracic and lumbar spine, *Neurosurgery* 32:1-8, 1993.

21. Crandall PH, Batsdorf U: Cervical spondylotic myelopathy, *J Neurosurg* 25:37-66, 1966.

22. Crockard HA: Anterior approaches to lesions of the upper cervical spine, *Clin Neurosurg* 34:389-416, 1988.

23. Crockard HA: Atlantoaxial subluxation: anterior and posterior approaches. In Torrens MJ, Dickson RA, editors: *Operative spinal surgery,* Edinburgh, 1991, Churchill-Livingstone, pp 10-26.

24. Crockard HA, Galder I, Ransford AD:

One stage transoral decompression and posterior fixation in rheumatoid atlanto-axial subluxation: a technical note, *J Bone Joint Surg* 72B;682-685, 1990.

25. Croft PB, Hensen RA, Rich H: Sensory neuropathy with bronchial carcinoma: a study of 4 cases showing serological abnormalities, *Brain* 88:501, 1965.

26. DeBarros ML, Farias W, Atride L et al: Basilar impression and Arnold-Chiari malformation: a study of 66 cases, *J Neurol Neurosurg Psychiatry* 1:596, 1968.

27. Demaria EJ, Reichman W, Kenney PR et al: Septic complications of corticosteroid administration after severe nervous system trauma, *Ann Surg* 202:248-252, 1985.

28. Denis F: The three column spine and its significance in the classification of acute thoracolumbar spine injuries, *Spine* 8:817-831, 1983.

29. DeSousa AL, Kalsbeck JE, Mealey J Jr et al: Intraspinal tumors in children: a review of 81 cases, *J Neurosurg* 51:437-445, 1979.

30. Dohn DF, Sava GM: Sympathectomy for vascular syndromes and hyperhidrosis of the upper extremities, *Clin Neurosurg* 25:637-650, 1978.

31. Ducker TB, McAfee PC: Thoracic and thoracolumbar spine fracture. In Long DM, editor: *Current therapy in neurological surgery—2,* Toronto, 1989, BC Decker, pp 221-223.

32. Ducker TB, Salcman M, Perot PL et al: Experimental spinal cord trauma. I: correlations of blood flow, tissue oxygen and neurologic status in the dog, *Surg Neurol* 10:60-63, 1978.

33. Ecker AD, Woltman HW: Meralgia paresthetica: a report of one hundred and fifty cases, *JAMA* 110:1650, 1938.

34. Elsberg, CA: *Tumors of the spinal cord and the symptoms of irritation and compression of the spinal cord and nerve roots: pathology, symptomatology, diagnosis and treatment,* New York, 1925, Paul B Hoeber, pp 206-239.

35. Epstein N, Epstein J, Carras R et al: Co-existing cervical and lumbar spinal stenosis: diagnosis and management, *Neurosurgery* 10:489-496, 1984.

36. Epstein N, Hood DC, Ransonoff J: Gastrointestinal bleeding in patients with spinal cord trauma. Effects of steroids, cimetidine, and mini-dose heparin, *J Neurosurg* 54:16-20, 1981.

37. Gardner WJ, Goodall RJ: The surgical treatment of Arnold-Chiari malformation in adults. An explanation of its mechanism and importance of encephalograph in diagnosis, *J Neurosurg* 7:199-206, 1950.

38. Greenberg HS, Kim J, Posner JB: Epidural spinal cord compression from metastatic tumor: results with a new treatment protocol, *Ann Neurol* 8:361-366, 1980.

39. Harrington KD: Anterior decompression and destabilization of the spine as a treatment for vertebral collapse and spinal cord compression from metastatic malignancy, *Clin Orthop* 233:177-197, 1988.

40. Herkowitz HN: Surgical management of cervical radiculopathy: anterior fusion. In Rothman RH, Simeone FA, editors: *The spine,* ed 3, Philadelphia, 1992, WB Saunders, pp 597-606.

41. Herkowitz KN: A comparison of anterior cervical fusion, cervical laminectomy and cervical laminoplasty for the surgical management of multiple level spondylotic radiculopathy, *Spine* 13:774-780, 1988.

42. Hulme A: The surgical approach to thoracic intervertebral disc protrusions, *J Neurol Neurosurg Psychiatry* 23:133-137, 1960.

43. Katz W: Modern management of rheumatoid arthritis, *Am J Med* 79:24, 1985.

44. Keim H, Weinstein JD: Acute renal failure: a complication of spine fusion in the tuck position, *J Bone Joint Surg* 50A:1248-1250, 1970.

45. Klein DM: Extramedullary spinal tumors. In McLaurin RL, Scaut L, Venes J et al, editors: *Pediatric neurosurgery,* Philadelphia, 1989, WB Saunders, pp 443-452.

46. Kurnick NB: Autonomic hyperreflexia and its control in patients with spinal cord lesions, *Ann Intern Med* 44:678, 1956.

47. Long DM: Herniated thoracic disc. In Long DM, editor: *Current therapy in neurological surgery—2,* Toronto, 1989, BC Decker, pp 267-268.

48. MacKinnon SE, Dellon AL: *Surgery of the peripheral nerve,* New York, 1988, Thieme, pp 535-549.

49. Matsumoto T, Symon L: Surgical management of syringomyelia—current results, *Surg Neurol* 32:258-265, 1989.

50. McAfee PC, Yuan HA, Frederickson BE et al: The value of computed tomography in thoracolumbar fractures.

An analysis on one hundred consecutive cases and a new classification, *J Bone Joint Surg* 65A:461-473, 1983.

51. Milhorat TH: *Pediatric neurosurgery, contemporary neurology series,* vol 16, Philadelphia, 1979, FA Davis, pp 295-296.

52. Milhorat TH: *Pediatric neurosurgery, contemporary neurology series,* vol 16, Philadelphia, 1979, FA Davis, pp 154-164.

53. Milhorat TH, Johnson WD, Miller JI: Syrinx shunt to posterior fossa cisterns (syringocisternostomy) for bypassing obstructions of upper cervical theca, *J Neurosurg* 77:871-874, 1992.

54. Milhorat TH, Adler DE, Heger IM et al: Histopathology of experimental hematomyelia, *J Neurosurg* 75:911-915, 1991.

55. Milhorat TH, Johnson RW, Johnson WD: Evidence of CSF flow in rostral direction through the central canal of spinal cord in rats. In Matsumoto S, Tamaki N, editors: *Hydrocephalus. Pathogenesis and treatment,* Tokyo, 1991, Springer-Verlag, pp 207-217.

56. Milhorat TH, Johnson WD, Miller JI et al: Surgical treatment of syringomyelia based on magnetic resonance imaging criteria, *Neurosurgery* 31:231-245, 1992.

57. Miller CA: Spinal metastasis with and without neurological deficit. In Long DM, editor: *Current therapy in neurological surgery—2,* Philadelphia, 1989, BC Decker, pp 234-236.

58. Modic MT, Masaryk TJ, Mulopuous GP et al: Cervical radiculopathy prospective evaluation with surface coil MR imaging, CT with metrizamide, and metrizamide myelography, *Radiology* 161:753-759, 1986.

59. Ogilvy CS, Heros RC: Spinal cord compression. In Ropper AH, editor: *Neurological and neurosurgical intensive care,* New York, 1993, Raven Press, pp 437-441.

60. Okazaki H: *Fundamentals of neuropathology,* New York, 1983, Igaku-Shoin, p 232.

61. Park TS, Gail WS, Broaddus WC et al: Lumboperitoneal shunt combined with myelotomy for treatment of syringohydromyelia, *J Neurosurg* 70:721-727, 1989.

62. Perot PL Jr, Munro DD: Transthoracic removal of midline thoracic disc protrusions causing spinal cord compression, *J Neurosurg* 31:452-458, 1969.

63. Pillay PK, Awad IA, Little JR et al: Symptomatic Chiari malformation in

adults: a new classification based on magnetic resonance imaging with clinical and prognostic significance, *Neurosurgery* 28:639-645, 1991.

64. Ramsey RG: *Neuroradiology with computer tomography,* Philadelphia, 1981, WB Saunders, p 740.

65. Ransford AB, Crockard HA, Pozo JL et al: Craniocervical instability treated by contoured loop fixation, *J Bone Joint Surg* 68:173-177, 1986.

66. Rekate HL: *Comprehensive management of spina bifida,* Boca Raton, 1991, CRC Press, pp 67-92.

67. Rengachary SS: Examination of the motor and sensory systems and reflexes. In Wilkins RH, Rengachary SS, editors: *Neurosurgery,* New York, 1985, McGraw-Hill, p 141.

68. Robinson RA, Smith GW: Anterolateral cervical disc removal and interbody fusion for cervical disc syndrome, *Bull Johns Hopkins Hosp* 96:223-224, 1955.

69. Rosenorn J, Hansen E, Rosenorn M: Anterior cervical discectomy with and without fusion, *J Neurosurg* 59-252-255, 1983.

70. Rybock JD: Cervical disc and spur. In Long DM, editor: *Current therapy in neurological surgery—2,* Toronto, 1989, BC Decker, pp 261-263.

71. Schneider RC, Cherry G, Pantak H: The syndrome of acute central cervical spinal cord injury: special reference to the mechanisms involved in hyperextension injuries of cervical spine, *J Neurosurg* 11:546-577, 1954.

72. Shepstone BJ: The radiobiology of bone, *Curr Orthop* 2:168-172, 1988.

73. Slater JE, Mostello LA, Shaer C: Rubber-specific IgE in children with spina bifida, *J Urol* 146:578-579, 1991.

74. Stanley P, Senal MO, Segall HD: Intraspinal seeding from intracranial tumors in children, *AJR* 144:157, 1985.

75. Stark DC, Miller R: Anesthesia for patients with rheumatoid arthritis, *Orthop Rev* 7:21, 1978.

76. Stein BM: Spinal intradural tumors. In Wilkins RH, Rengachery SS, editors: *Neurosurgery,* vol 1, New York, 1985, McGraw-Hill, pp 1048-1061.

77. Stone WA, Beach TP, Hamelberg W: Succinylcholine-induced hyperkalemia in dogs with transected sciatic nerves or spinal cords, *Anesthesia* 32:515, 1970.

78. Sundaresan N, Galicich J, Lane J et al: Treatment of neoplastic epidural cord compression by vertebral body resection and stabilization, *J Neurosurg* 63:676-684, 1985.

79. Tachdjiian MO, Matson DD: Orthopedic aspects of intraspinal tumors in infants and children, *J Bone Joint Surg* 47A:223-248, 1965.

80. Tokuheshi Y, Matsuzaki H, Toriyama S et al: Scoring system for the preoperative evaluation of metastatic spine tumor prognosis 1990, *J Neurosurg* 15:1110-1113, 1990.

81. Tondury G: Morphology of the cervical spine. In Jung A, Kehr P, Magerl F et al, editors: *The cervical spine,*

Bern, Switzerland, 1974, Hans Huber, pp 14-35.

82. Vaccaro NR, An HS, Cotler JM: Transpedicular fixation of the spine using the variable screw placement system. In An HS, Cotler JM, editors: *Spinal instrumentation,* Baltimore, 1992, Williams & Wilkins, pp 197-217.

83. Vaquero J, Martiner R, Salazar J et al: Syringosubarachnoid shunt for treatment of syringomyelia, *Acta Neurochir* 84:105-109, 1987.

84. Vauzelle C, Stagnara P, Louvinroux P: Functional monitoring of spinal cord activity during spinal surgery, *Clin Orthop* 93:173-178, 1973.

85. Weinstein JH, McLain RF: Primary tumors of the spine, *Spine* 12:843-851, 1987.

86. Weinstein JN, McLain RF: Tumors of the spine. In Rothman RK, Simeone FA, editors: *The spine,* Philadelphia, 1992, WB Saunders, pp 1279-1314.

87. Williams B: On the pathogenesis of syringomyelia: a review, *JR Soc Med* 73:798-806, 1980.

88. Yamada S, Zinke DE, Sanders D: Pathophysiology of "tethered cord syndrome," *J Neurosurg* 54:494-503, 1981.

89. Yashon D: Surgical management of trauma to the spine. In Schmidek HH, Sweet WH, editors: *Operative neurosurgical techniques: indications, methods, and results,* Philadelphia, 1988, WB Saunders, pp 1451-1452.

28

Neurosurgical Diseases of the Spine and Spinal Cord: Anesthetic Considerations

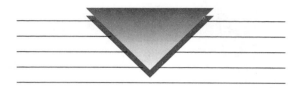

Wayne K. Marshall
James L. Mostrom

This chapter explores the anesthetic management of patients undergoing surgery for diseases of the bony spine and spinal cord. An overview of anatomy and physiology is provided as background, but emphasis is placed on the preservation of spinal cord function.

ANATOMY

The anatomy of the spine can be divided into that pertaining to the bony spine and that pertaining to the spinal cord.[123] The two structures are intimately related, and surgical operations on either one will generally affect the other.

For this reason, the division of procedures into either orthopedic or neurosurgical is somewhat artificial.

Vertebral Column

The vertebral column is a bony structure composed of 33 vertebrae. In adult life this number is functionally reduced to 24 presacral vertebrae, one sacrum, and one coccyx. The presacral vertebrae consist of 7 cervical, 12 thoracic, and 5 lumbar bones. The 5 sacral and 4 coccygeal vertebrae fuse early in development (Fig. 28-1). The vertebral column normally exhibits four curves in the anteroposterior plane. There are two forward curves or lordoses, one in the cervical and one in the lumbar area. There are two posterior curves or kyphoses as well, one in the thoracic and one in the sacral area. The combination of these curves gives the normal bony spine the characteristic S shape when viewed from the side (Fig. 28-1).

The individual vertebrae that make up the vertebral col-

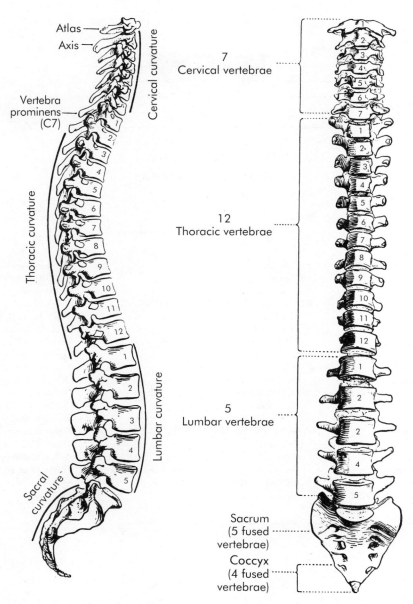

FIG. 28-1   The vertebral column showing the 24 presacral vertebrae, the sacrum, the coccyx, and the curvatures of the adult vertebral column. Note that the first coccygeal vertebra has fused with the sacrum. Most vertebral columns are 72 to 75 cm long; about one fourth of this length is contributed by the fibrocartilaginous intervertebral disks. The vertebral column supports the skull and transmits the weight of the body through the pelvis to the lower limbs. *(From Moore KL: Clinically oriented anatomy, ed 2, Baltimore, 1985, Williams & Wilkins, p 566.)*

umn are each a single bony structure consisting of a large body, bilateral pedicles, bilateral lamina, bilateral transverse processes, a spinous process, and four articular processes (Fig. 28-2). The two pedicles laterally, the two lamina posteriorly, and the body anteriorly together form the vertebral canal in which lies the spinal cord. The segmental nerves exit between the vertebrae through the intervertebral foramen. The four articular processes mate with corresponding processes on the vertebrae above and below to form the facet joints. The facet joint articulations provide posterior stability, and the body articulations provide anterior and vertical stability to the spinal column as a unit. In addition, the facet joints provide flexion, extension, and lateral rotation of the spine.

The anterior longitudinal ligament and the posterior longitudinal ligament are placed anterior to and posterior to the vertebral column, respectively (Fig. 28-3). They extend from the base of the skull and atlas to the sacrum. The anterior ligament is attached to the anterior surface of the vertebrae and intervertebral disks. The posterior ligament is attached to the posterior surface of the vertebrae and the intervertebral disks and lies within the vertebral canal. These two ligaments provide extension and flexion stability to the vertebral column. The posterior elements of the bony spine are joined together by several lesser ligaments (Fig. 28-3). The supraspinal and interspinal ligaments unite the spinous processes at each level, providing additional flexion stability. The ligamentum flavum unites the vertebral laminae at

each level and forms part of the posterior border of the intervertebral foramen.

The intervertebral disks are fibrocartilaginous joints composed of an interior nucleus pulposus surrounded and enclosed by a tough annulus fibrosus (Fig. 28-4). Together, these two components act to provide a strong attachment between adjacent vertebrae but allow for some movement. In addition, the disks act as a very efficient shock absorber during movement and activity.

The facet joints are synovial joints between adjacent vertebrae posterior to the vertebral canal, and thus compose part of the posterior elements of the vertebral column (Fig. 28-5). These joints are paired at each level, one on each side of the spine. With the intervertebral disks they form the remaining articulations of the vertebrae with each other. As posterior elements, the facet joints allow for flexion of the spine. The facet joints of the cervical region are less rigid, thus allowing greater flexion of the neck. Each facet joint has a capsule of fibrous tissue and is innervated by the dorsal primary ramus of each segmental spinal nerve as it exits the intervertebral foramen (Fig. 28-5). To reach the joint, this nerve branch must traverse the transverse process and lamina of each respective vertebra.

Spinal Cord

The spinal cord[41] is contained within the confines of the vertebral canal, which affords protection to this very important and complex structure. The spinal cord is contigu-

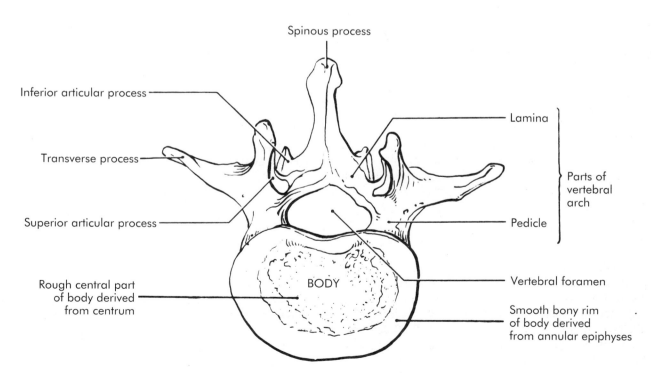

FIG. 28-2   Parts of the second lumbar vertebra, superior view. *(From Moore KL:* Clinically oriented anatomy, *ed 2, Baltimore, 1985, Williams & Wilkins, p 574.)*

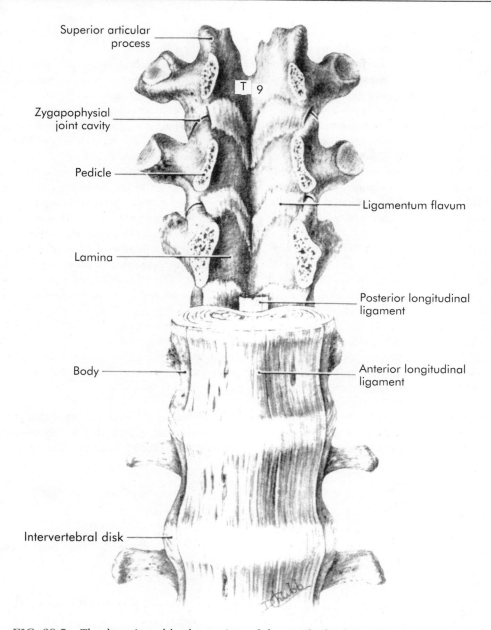

Superior articular process

Zygapophysial joint cavity

Pedicle

Lamina

Body

Intervertebral disk

T 9

Ligamentum flavum

Posterior longitudinal ligament

Anterior longitudinal ligament

FIG. 28-3   The thoracic and lumbar regions of the vertebral column, showing its joints and ligaments. The pedicles of T9 to T11 vertebrae have been sawed through, and their bodies discarded. Note that the anterior longitudinal ligament is broad whereas the posterior longitudinal ligament is narrow. *(From Moore KL:* Clinically oriented anatomy, *ed 2, Baltimore, 1985, Williams & Wilkins, p 586.)*

ous with the brainstem at the foramen magnum, and in the adult it extends to the conus medullaris at about the level of the first or second lumbar vertebra. The filum terminale attaches the end of the conus to the first coccygeal segment of the bony spine. The spinal cord carries all afferent and efferent information to and from the brain and the rest of the body below the cranium. The segmental spinal nerves enter and exit the cord on either side. Approximately 30 segments are involved. These are made up of 8 cervical,

12 thoracic, 5 lumbar, 5 sacral, and a variable number of coccygeal segments. The corresponding spinal nerves are the same except there is only one coccygeal nerve. The cord exhibits two prominent bulges, in the cervical and lumbar areas, which correspond to the origins of the nerves to the upper and lower extremities, respectively.

A cross-section of the cord reveals a mixture of white and gray matter (Fig. 28-6). The gray matter is in the shape of an H surrounding the central canal and contains the cell

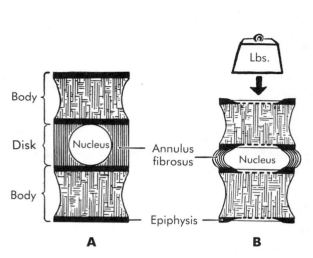

FIG. 28-4 **A,** A fibrocartilaginous intervertebral disk, composed of a ring of fibrous tissue (annulus fibrosus) surrounding an internal semifluid mass (nucleus pulposus). **B,** Illustration of the cushioning value of the nucleus pulposus during weight-bearing. *(From Moore KL: Clinical oriented anatomy, ed 2, Baltimore, 1985, Williams & Wilkins, p 570.)*

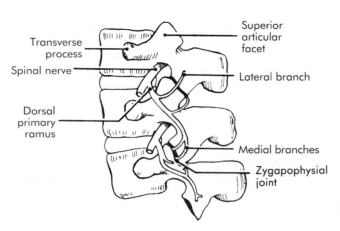

FIG. 28-5 Part of the lumbar region of the vertebral column showing the innervation of the zygapophysial joints. Observe that the dorsal primary ramus arises from the spinal nerve outside the intervertebral foramen and then divides into medial and lateral branches. The medial branch descends in a groove posterior to the transverse process beside the superior articular process. It sends small articular branches to the capsule of the zygapophysial joint beside it and to the subjacent joint as well. *(From Moore KL: Clinically oriented anatomy, ed 2, Baltimore, 1985, Williams & Wilkins, p 591.)*

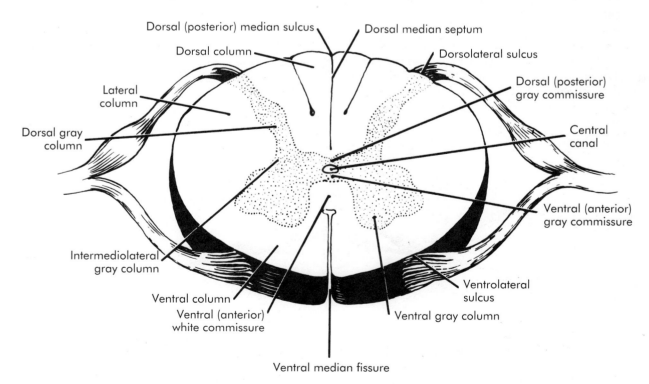

FIG. 28-6 Anatomy of the spinal cord. *(From deGroot JG: Correlative neuroanatomy, ed 20, East Norwalk, Conn, 1988, Appleton & Lange, p 35.)*

bodies of the spinal neurons. The dorsal horns are associated with sensory functions, including pain, position sense, touch, and temperature. The ventral horns contain neurons associated with motor functions and spinal reflexes. The surrounding white matter contains the myelinated and unmyelinated fibers that communicate with higher and lower centers, including the brainstem and cerebral cortex. The descending motor pathways travel in the white matter of the cord in the lateral and ventral areas. The corticospinal tract conducts all primary motor impulses. The vestibulospinal and rubrospinal tracts also participate in motor function and are located in the ventral and lateral white matter, respectively. The dorsal areas of white matter contain the dorsal column tracts, the spinothalamic tracts, and the spinoreticular tracts, among others. These pathways transmit sensory information, including pain, touch, proprioception, temperature, and vibration, to higher cord segments and the brain.

The sympathetic nervous system is also segmental and traverses the length of the vertebral column in two chains anterior to the bony spine (Fig. 28-7). Segmental communication is accomplished at each spinal segment via the communicating ramus of each segmental spinal nerve. The segmental spinal nerves are made up of the confluence of a dorsal and a ventral root at each level. (Fig. 28-7). A nerve emerges from each side of the spinal cord; thus they are paired. The dorsal roots conduct sensory information, including pain. All nerve cell bodies of afferent axons are located in the dorsal root ganglion. The ventral roots conduct primarily motor and efferent information from the cord to the periphery. The two roots combine into the spinal nerve as they traverse the vertebral foramen. The nerve then divides into three rami, dorsal, ventral, and communicating. The ventral ramus continues as the primary spinal nerve. The dorsal ramus innervates the paraspinous muscles of the back and the facet joints at each level. The communicating ramus provides segmental neuronal connections to the sympathetic chains.

The spinal nerves have a particular relationship to the respective spinal vertebrae (Fig. 28-8). The spinal nerves exit the vertebral canal via the intervertebral foramen. These foramen are formed by the juxtaposition of each two vertebrae in the spinal column. Because there are 8 cervical nerves and only 7 cervical vertebrae, the segmental spinal nerves change in relation to the respective vertebrae at the level of the seventh cervical vertebra. Cervical nerves 1 through 7 exit the canal superior to the corresponding vertebra. At the seventh cervical vertebra the eighth cervical nerve exits inferior to it. Thereafter the spinal nerves exit inferior to the corresponding vertebra at each level.

Spinal Cord Blood Supply

The spinal cord is supplied with blood from the aorta via the vertebral and segmental or radicular arteries.[45] This is accomplished through the three main arteries of the cord: the single anterior spinal artery in the anterior or ventral median sulcus, and two posterior spinal arteries located in the area of the posterior or dorsal nerve rootlets (Fig. 28-9). These three arteries usually arise as branches of the vertebral arteries at the base of the brainstem and traverse the entire length of the cord (Fig. 28-10). The blood carried in them is augmented by multiple segmental radicular and medullary arteries that enter at the intervertebral foramen (Figs. 28-9 and 28-10).

The anterior spinal artery supplies the anterior two thirds of the cord, and the posterior spinal arteries supply the posterior one third. Below the level of the cervical cord segments, the blood supply from the three arterial trunks is insufficient to support the metabolic needs of the cord without the additional blood from these segmental arteries. The segmental or radicular arteries arise as branches of the aorta and enter the cord arterial system, although in a variable manner at different levels. The most consistent of these arteries is the artery of Adamkiewicz, which is the largest segmental feeder in the thoracolumbar region of the cord. It usually enters as a single vessel at a single level between

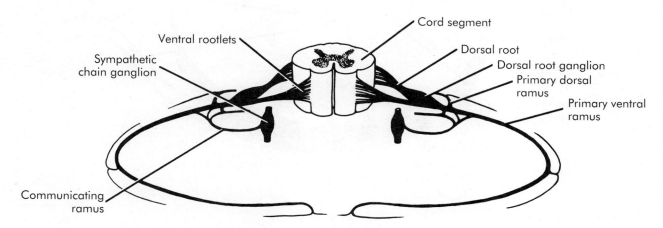

FIG. 28-7   Cord segment with its roots, ganglia, and branches. (*From deGroot J, Chusid JG: Correlative neutoanatomy, ed 20, East Norwalk, Conn, 1988, Appleton & Lange, p 37.*)

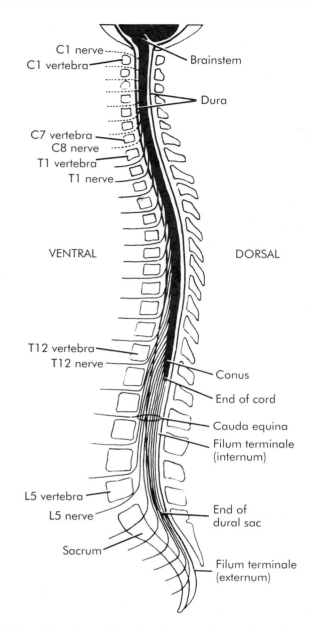

FIG. 28-8   The relationships between the spinal cord, spinal nerves, and vertebral column (lateral view). The termination of the dura (dura mater spinalis) and its continuation as the filum terminale externum are shown. *(From deGroot J, Chusid JG: Correlative neuroanatomy, ed 20, East Norwalk, Conn, 1988, Appleton & Lange, p 54.)*

the ninth and the eleventh thoracic levels and arises on the left side of the aorta in 80% of cases.[45] This arterial feeder vessel is thought to be the principal contributor to the arterial supply of the entire thoracic and lumbar cord distal to its entry. Loss of this artery after operation or trauma to the aorta may produce paraplegia in the thoracic region.

The arterial network of the three main blood vessels supplies blood to the interior of the cord through an extensive

network of arterioles and capillaries. The density of the capillary bed reflects the metabolic demands of the different areas of the cord. Thus the gray matter of the horns contains 15 times the number of capillaries as the white matter because of the relatively high metabolic needs of cells vs. axon bundles. Blood flow through these capillaries is very sensitive to compression of the cord, and ischemia may result.

The distribution of blood supply in the spinal cord is illustrated by a case report from Wolf et al.[183] demonstrating arterial-border-zone necrosis of the spinal cord in a 74-year-old man who suffered prolonged hypotension and aortic dissection. This area of necrosis was localized to the zone between the anterior and posterior spinal arteries in the lower thoracic cord and represents a secondary border between the segmental radicular arteries. The area of necrosis involved both white and gray matter in a symmetric distribution. The fact that this is a relatively rare occurrence suggests that superimposed conditions such as hypotension and compromised circulation are necessary for this to be evident. This is contrasted with the well-documented border-zone necrosis (so-called "watershed infarct") in the cerebral circulation. The vascular anatomy of the spinal cord appears to be an important factor in the development of paraplegia as a complication of aortic surgery.

Venous drainage of the spinal cord is through radial veins serving the parenchyma.[10] These veins feed into the coronal venous plexus or longitudinal veins on the surface of the cord, which are, in turn, drained by medullary veins that penetrate the dura adjacent to the dural penetration of the nerve roots to join the epidural venous plexus (see Fig. 28-9). The epidural or internal vertebral venous system drains into the external vertebral venous system, which communicates with the caval veins. The veins in the epidural system are valveless and therefore subject to engorgement in certain normal and disease states, such as pregnancy and obesity, where there is an increase in the intraabdominal pressure or obstruction to venous flow through the inferior vena cava.

Certain areas of the spinal cord are very susceptible to ischemia resulting from compromise of the arterial blood supply (see Fig. 28-10). For the anterior spinal artery, the areas around the fourth thoracic and first lumbar segments are at risk. For the posterior arteries, the area that surrounds the first to the third thoracic segments of the cord are at most risk.

PHYSIOLOGY
Blood Flow

Spinal cord blood flow (SCBF) has been studied extensively in animal models using various techniques. The values and data obtained from these studies are consistent with values obtained for the brain; average SCBF is about 60 ml/100 g/min.[58,149] Autoregulation in the cord mimics that in the brain, with flow well maintained between a mean arterial

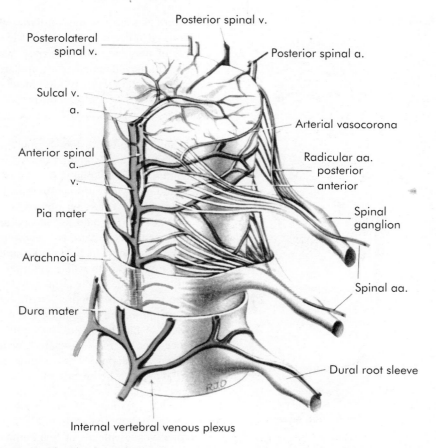

Posterior spinal v.

Posterolateral spinal v.

Posterior spinal a.

Sulcal v.
a.

Arterial vasocorona

Anterior spinal a.

Radicular aa.
posterior
anterior

v.

Pia mater

Spinal ganglion

Arachnoid

Spinal aa.

Dura mater

Dural root sleeve

Internal vertebral venous plexus

FIG. 28-9   The blood supply and venous drainage of the spinal cord. The anterior spinal artery and the paired posterior spinal arteries run longitudinally throughout the length of the spinal cord. Observe that the anterior and posterior radicular arteries run along the dorsal and ventral roots of the spinal nerves to reach the spinal cord. The dura mater evaginates along the dorsal and ventral nerve roots of the spinal nerves and the spinal ganglia to form dural root sleeves (dorsal root sleeves). *(From Moore KL:* Clinically oriented anatomy, *ed 2, Baltimore, 1985, Williams & Wilkins, p 614.)*

blood (MAP) pressure of 60 to 120 mm Hg.[72] Likewise, the effects of arterial blood gas tensions are similar to those in the cerebrum; hypoxemia and hypercarbia cause vasodilation, and hypocarbia causes vasoconstriction.[62]

Autoregulation of SCBF is maintained during hypotension by hemorrhage or by trimethaphan down to a MAP of 50 to 60 mm Hg in a dog model using an anesthetic consisting of 60% N_2O and 0.5% halothane.[53] In the same model, autoregulation was maintained during induced hypertension with norepinephrine to a MAP of 150 mm Hg. The effects of drugs on SCBF are also similar to their effects on the brain. The effect of isoflurane on SCBF in rats is vasodilatory at 1.0 MAC or above.[73] There is no reason to suspect a different response to other inhalation or intravenous drugs in the spinal cord than in the brain. Injury to the spinal cord disturbs the autoregulation of blood flow. As in the brain, trauma to the cord results in a decrease in SCBF and loss of autoregulation function.[60,65]

The nature of the operative procedure itself may also have an effect on SCBF. This is well recognized with spinal distraction and instrumentation but may also occur during other operations, such as simple laminectomy. In a cat model, it was found that with exposure of the dura after laminectomy, there was a depression of SCBF of 22% to 45% along the entire length of the spinal cord.[7] SCBF approached control values within 1 hour after closure of the laminectomy site but decreased again with reexposure. The authors postulated a temperature-induced vasoconstriction as the etiology.

TYPES OF SPINAL SURGERY

Surgery on the spine, spinal cord, or structures adjacent to these or immediately involved with them involves a broad variety of surgical therapies and problems.[175] Usually an operation is performed for stabilization of the spinal col-

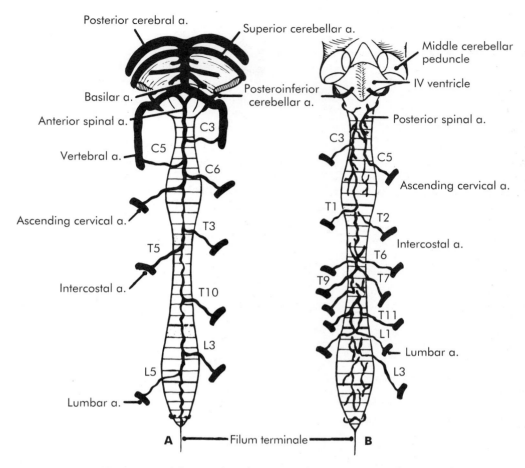

FIG. 28-10 The arteries of the spinal cord. **A,** Ventral aspect. **B,** Dorsal aspect. The regions most vulnerable to vascular deprivation when the contributing arteries are injured are T3 to T5 and T12 to L2 for the anterior spinal artery and C8 to T4 for the dorsal circulation. The levels of entry of the common radicular branches are shown (e.g., C5 and T5). Note that the spinal cord is enlarged in two regions for innervation of the limbs. The cervical enlargement extends from C4 to T1, and the lumbosacral enlargement extends from the L2 to the S3 segments of the spinal cord. *(From Moore KL:* Clinically oriented anatomy, *ed 2, Baltimore, 1985, Williams & Wilkins, p 613.)*

umn, relief of compression of the spinal cord or nerve root, removal of foreign bodies or other masses including tumors, or correction of deformity of the vertebral column. Lesions of the spine, spinal cord, or contents of the spinal canal can be considered to be either congenital or acquired. The pathology of spine lesions leading to surgery varies widely (Box 28-1). The specific pathology and location of the lesion may give an indication of prognosis for recovery and potential complications.[175]

Tumor Resection

Tumor resection is usually undertaken to relieve pressure on the spinal cord and/or to provide stability to the bony spine. Tumors are typically classified according to location along the spine (cervical, thoracic, thoracolumbar, lumbar, lumbosacral, sacral), the relation of the tumor to the dura and/or spinal cord (extradural, intradural-extramedullary, and intramedullary), the pathology of the neoplasm (primary, metastatic, benign, malignant), and the cell type if known.[161] Some nonneoplastic masses (infections, hematoma) may mimic tumors. The nature and location of the tumor indicate the prognosis for complete excision and return of function. Even in cases of malignant or nonresectable tumors, partial removal may be attempted for palliation.

Arteriovenous Malformation

Arteriovenous malformations (AVM) are typically congenital and present with intermittent neurologic findings, often mimicking multiple sclerosis.[129] The disability from these lesions is due to thrombosis of vessels and resulting spinal cord ischemia as well as hemorrhage into and around the

---

BOX 28-1
LESIONS OF THE SPINE AND SPINAL CORD

I. Congenital
  A. Spine
    1. Spondylolisthesis
    2. Klippel-Feil syndrome
  B. Spinal cord
    1. Syringomyelia
    2. Arteriovenous malformations
    3. Arnold-Chiari malformation
    4. Spinal dysraphism/spina bifida
II. Acquired
  A. Spine
    1. Spondylosis
    2. Fracture
    3. Degenrative disk disease
    4. Arthritis
  B. Spinal cord
    1. Infarction
    2. Hematoma
    3. Traumatic injury
    4. Secondary syrinx
    5. Tumors
    6. Arteriovenous malformations
  C. Spinal canal
    1. Herniated nucleus pulposus
    2. Foreign body
    3. Tumors
    4. Abscess
    5. Hematoma

---

spinal cord that produces compression of the neural structures. Anesthesia may be required for resection or for embolization of the vessels supplying the AVM.

AVMs of the spine are classified as either intradural or dural and subclassified as juvenile (analogous to cerebral AVMs), glomus, or a direct arteriovenous fistula. The majority of spinal AVMs are of the intradural type. Generally, intradural AVMs occur in the young, have an acute onset, present with subarachnoid hemorrhage or a bruit, and primarily involve the cervical and thoracic cord. These lesions are usually approached posteriorly; therefore positioning is usually prone. Induced hypotension may be necessary to minimize blood loss during operation before the surgeon has control of the feeding vessels. Because the surgical approach is posterior, monitoring of somatosensory evoked potentials is essential. It has been suggested that observation of the effects of test injections of short-acting barbiturates or lidocaine into AVM feeder vessels (a spinal Wada test) preoperatively may predict the effect of embolization.[129] A classic Wada test is the intracarotid injection of a barbiturate (amobarbital) to determine the laterality of speech. Temporary loss of the power of speech results from injection on the dominant side.

Dural AV fistulas make up a minority of spinal AVMs. These may be acquired lesions, because they tend to occur in older patients with a gradual onset and progressive worsening of symptoms, and they tend to occur in the lower half of the spinal cord, commonly affecting the legs. The surgical approach is similar to that of intradural AVMs. The pathology of dural AVMs is related to venous hypertension. Functional valves in the veins at the level of the dura prevent retrograde flow of blood from the epidural to the medullary veins; however, there are no valves in the intrathecal venous system. For this reason coronal venous hypertension occurs because of retrograde flow from a dural arteriovenous fistula and from anterograde flow from an intradural arteriovenous malformation.[129] This venous engorgement reduces cord blood flow and produces ischemic symptoms.

Trauma Repair/Reconstruction

Surgical intervention for trauma to the spine typically involves procedures for removal of foreign bodies, for decompression of the spinal cord, and for assuring stability of the bony spine to minimize further injury to the surrounding structures, particularly the spinal cord. Trauma to the spinal cord may result in systemic vasomotor and respiratory compromise and complicate the management of anesthesia. Of primary concern, particularly in the presurgical phases of anesthetic management, is prevention of further dislocation of elements of the spine until surgical stability can be obtained. This is of particular concern in cases of cervical injury and necessitates care in moving and positioning the patient for induction of anesthesia and operation. The anesthesiologist should assist the surgeon during this phase. In certain circumstances, it may be beneficial for the patient to assist in performing "awake pronation" (see later discussion).

Discectomy for Herniated Nucleus Pulposus

One of the more common indications for surgery on the spine is discectomy and removal of herniated nucleus pulposus material causing radicular symptoms. Rupture and involvement of the nucleus pulposus in spinal cord and nerve root compression and its relief by surgery was first recognized by Mixter and Barr.[119] They suggested, in contrast to contemporary ideas, that this was a more common etiology for clinical radiculopathy than was neoplasia (chondroma). Surgical intervention is generally deferred until more conservative measures, such as bed rest and antiinflammatory medications, have proved inadequate or a demonstrable neurologic deficit develops. A trial of steroids placed in the epidural space often may be warranted. Spontaneous resolution of symptoms may be related to reduction in the inflammation of the nerve root, change in orientation of the nerve root in relation to the disk fragment, or desiccation and shrinkage of the herniation.[82] Urgent surgery should be considered when cauda equina syndrome or other progressive neurologic deficit is present. Other indications for surgery include:

- Recurrent episodes of pain, especially when sciatica is predominant
- Unrelieved acute attack of sciatica unresponsive to conservative measures.
- Progressive CNS involvement
- Suspected central protrusion
- Diagnosis in doubt

Disks commonly involved with symptomatic herniation include the L4-L5 and L5-S1 levels, involving the L5 and S1 nerve roots respectively. Most disk herniations are lateral and involve the adjacent nerve root; however, central protrusion may lead to a cauda equina syndrome with loss of bowel and bladder function. Excessive flexion should be avoided during positioning and manipulation, especially with central protrusions because this may lead to paraplegia.[82]

Spinal Stenosis

Another common operation on the lower spine is laminectomy for decompression of spinal stenosis when this is associated with pain or neurologic findings. Although spinal stenosis most commonly produces symptoms in the lumbar area, it can also occur in other parts of the spine. Particular care must be exercised in the treatment of patients with cervical spinal stenosis, especially when this is associated with cervical myelopathy, because these patients may be especially prone to develop sudden aggravation of symptoms after hyperextension of the neck, such as during endotracheal intubation.[82]

Fusion

Instability of the spine may result from traumatic or destructive (e.g., neoplastic, degenerative, congenital) disruption of the stabilizing elements (anterior and posterior longitudinal ligaments, pedicles, and articulations). A patient may require 9 to 10 weeks for healing of unstable components after trauma[82]; therefore external or internal fixation is necessary to avoid complications of prolonged immobilization. The decision to fuse the spine is generally based on symptomatology, neuropathy, and demonstration (usually through bracing) that stabilization ameliorates these.

Correction of Scoliosis with Instrumentation

In the younger patient, one of the most common indications for spinal surgery is correction of progressive scoliosis of the spine, either idiopathic or secondary to a concomitant disability such as paraplegia. Management depends on the degree of curvature of the spine and the presence of progression of the disease. Bracing is suggested for curvatures of 20 to 30 degrees, and fusion for curvatures greater than 60 degrees.[28] Progressive scoliosis may cause impairment of ventilation because of development of restrictive pulmonary disease from the abnormal geometry of the rib cage and impaired efficiency of the respiratory musculature. Decrements in total lung capacity generally are evident when the degree of curvature exceeds 65 degrees. There is greater impairment of vital capacity at curvatures greater than 90 degrees.[28] This may lead to secondary pulmonary hypertension and right ventricular hypertrophy. Pulmonary function testing should be performed preoperatively in any patient with diminution of exercise tolerance or respiratory symptomatology, or when these cannot be determined. Arterial blood gas measurement and electrocardiography are useful adjuncts in determining preoperative pulmonary status.

Operations for scoliosis may be aimed at either stabilization or correction. When correction of the scoliosis is attempted, tension may be placed on the spinal cord during distraction of the vertebral elements, and neurologic dysfunction may result. This dysfunction is thought to be primarily due to spinal cord ischemia. Monitoring of the spinal cord and the effect of the distraction is therefore advisable. Traditionally, an intraoperative "wake-up" test is performed to assess motor function after distraction (see later discussion). This procedure presents risks to the patient, including awareness, discomfort, and disconnection of monitors and life-support apparatus, and therefore must be done with care. It is also a sporadic form of neurologic assessment. An alternative and complementary method of monitoring the function of the spinal cord is with somatosensory evoked potentials (SSEP). This is a continuous method of monitoring the function of only the posterior sensory spinal tracts and does not involve patient wakefulness. However, the SSEP is affected by anesthetic drugs and hypothermia to various degrees and requires skill in performance and interpretation. In addition, monitoring the function of the posterior sensory pathways does not preclude dysfunction of the anterior motor pathways.[57]

One other complication associated with this operation is a large blood loss caused by the exposure required for the surgery. Techniques to minimize the loss of red cell mass and the use of homologous blood include (1) autologous donation of blood preoperatively, (2) induced hypotension to minimize bleeding, (3) isovolemic hemodilution to conserve red cells for later transfusion, and (4) the use of erythropoietin to boost starting hemoglobin and hematocrit.[145] For these practices to be performed safely and judiciously, invasive monitoring of arterial and central venous pressures is warranted.

Diagnostic Studies

Anesthesia may be necessary for diagnostic studies in patients with spinal cord disease. Some patients may be unable or unwilling to tolerate the sequestration and immobility necessary for such studies as computed axial tomography (CT) or magnetic resonance imaging (MR) because of young age, mental impairment, or psychologic distress. The incidence of claustrophobia associated with MR may be 3% to 7%.[124] Sedation and occasionally general anesthesia then are needed to obtain an adequate study. Appropriate monitoring of the patient, particularly of respiratory and cardiovascular function, must be performed. This is often a challenge in these relatively inconvenient locations, where the anesthesiologist may be physically isolated from the patient. Factors such as lighting, space limitation, isolation from the patient (during exposure to radiation), availability of monitoring equipment, access to emergency equipment and drugs, and presence of intense electromagnetic fields all add to the complexity of the management of these patients. Special nonferromagnetic instruments and monitors may be necessary in the MR scanner to avoid inducing dangerous electric currents, damage to the monitoring equipment, and distortion of the image. Careful attention should be paid to the application of these monitors because coiling of wires may induce current from changes in the magnetic field, which may result in burns.[68]

Placement of Epidural Electrodes for Spinal Cord Stimulation

Spinal cord stimulation using epidural electrodes is sometimes used for the treatment of chronic pain recalcitrant to more conservative therapies,[40,139,141] chronic muscle spasms,[14] vasospastic disease,[142] and reflex sympathetic dystrophy. It has also been demonstrated to be a useful monitor of spinal cord integrity in vascular repair of thoracoabdominal aortic aneurysm.[46] The procedure involves the placement of electrodes either percutaneously or via a limited laminotomy along the spinal cord posterior surface either epidurally or subdurally. Some types of procedures require patient interaction to determine the proper location of the electrode. Therefore it is occasionally useful to have the patient awake and coherent during the placement or manipulation of the electrode. This may be accomplished through the use of local or regional anesthesia with additional light sedation for the initial access and manipulation, and then heavier sedation or general anesthesia for the remainder of the implantation. The electrode may also be placed under general anesthesia using a short-acting intravenous agent such as propofol. The patient may then be awakened during the stimulation phase of the procedure. After satisfactory positioning is attained, the implantation closure can be done with further use of general anesthesia. Propofol provides ideal conditions for this procedure because of its short duration of action and minimal residual effects.

SURGICAL SITE AND APPROACH

The surgical site and choice of approach have an effect on management, particularly in the positioning of the patient, monitoring, and the degree of intraoperative access to the patient that may be expected. This last element may influence the degree of monitoring that may be thought necessary. If access is easily attained, less invasive monitoring may be accepted with the provision that more invasive monitoring may be easily placed if it becomes necessary. Approaches to the spine may be anterior, posterior, or both.

The spinal cord itself is usually approached from the posterior aspect because of the ease of access through the vertebral laminae. Operations on the vertebral bodies may necessitate an anterior approach, regardless of the level along the spine. Each combination of level and approach has a peculiar set of associated considerations.[83]

Cervical

Operations on the cervical spine may pose the greatest limitation to vascular and monitoring access to the patient. The head may be oriented toward the anesthetic area, which results in severe limitation of access to the patient. Or, the head may be oriented away from the anesthetic area 180 degrees, providing access to the lower extremities. Thus in most cases all monitors and vascular catheters using the upper extremities should be placed before final positioning and draping of the patient.

The anterior approach to the cervical spine provides direct access to the vertebral body and transverse processes. The posterior approach provides access to the spinous process, laminae, facet joints, and spinal cord.[83] For stabilization procedures, the posterior elements allow the application of fixation devices that provide immediate stability, whereas anterior fixation depends on the delayed healing of osseous graft elements. Of major concern with operations on the cervical spine is preoperative and postoperative stability of the neck. In these circumstances, flexing and extending movements of the neck are to be avoided. In cases of severe instability, the patient may arrive in the operating room already in an external-fixation device. Under such conditions, securing the airway with an awake intubation, preferably with a flexible fiberoptic instrument, effectively prevents the need to manipulate the neck during induction of anesthesia.[132] The anterior approach to cervical lesions requires the least change in patient position from a standard supine induction position. Posterior approaches necessitate a postintubation turn to the prone position. Postoperatively, patients may still be in cervical fixation. In this situation, the tracheal tube is best left in place until the patient is fully awake and recovered from the anesthetic. The acute need to reintubate in the immediate postoperative period should be avoided if possible because of cervical instability.

Thoracic

Access to the head and neck is generally possible during operations involving the thoracic spine, particularly during operations on the lower thoracic spine. There are three possible approaches to the thoracic spine: anterior, posterior, and posterolateral (combined). The anterior or transthoracic approach provides direct access to the vertebral bodies but requires a thoracotomy. This may result in a greater operative risk from pulmonary complications. The posterolateral approach is used for access to the transverse processes, pedicles, and parts of the vertebral body and involves a costotransversectomy. The posterior approach is used for surgery on the posterior elements of the thoracic spine or the spinal cord. This is the approach generally taken for repair of scoliosis, repair of trauma to the posterior elements, fusion of the spine, and treatment of tumors of the cord. The considerations of positioning the patient as previously described are appropriate. An additional risk is the intentional or unintentional entry into the thoracic cavity, with associated pneumothorax and the proximity of the lung parenchyma and great vessels to the operative site.

Lumbosacral

The lumbosacral spine is approached either through a posterior, anterior, or a combined dissection. The posterior dissection is useful for access to the posterior elements, spinal cord, and nerve roots. This is the most common approach used in disk surgery at this level. The posterior approach may be enlarged to allow access to the transverse processes and mamillary processes of the facets. The anterior approach through a transverse flank incision provides access to the bodies of the lumbar vertebrae. The left flank approach is the desired side because of problems associated with retraction of the liver on the right and the proximity of the vena cava.

PREOPERATIVE EVALUATION AND PREPARATION
Considerations

Preoperative considerations derive from the overall medical condition of the patient and the reason for, type, and site of surgery. Patients presenting for surgery of the spine may already manifest peripheral neuropathy, paraplegia, or quadriplegia, each with its attendant complications and anesthetic considerations. Choice of anesthesia depends on the debility of the patient and the intended surgery. Most spinal surgery, because of considerations of positioning and airway control, require general endotracheal anesthesia. Therefore considerations include premedication, the need for specific and invasive monitoring, the approach to controlling the airway, patient positioning, fluid requirements, special maneuvers such as an intraoperative "wake-up," extubation, and postoperative pain control. Many of these considerations depend on preoperative clinical findings, the past medical history, and the review of systems.

The spinal canal may be considered analogous to the cranium in many respects. Both have a limited and relatively bounded volume and space that is relatively noncompliant. Both contain various tissues including neurons, blood, and cerebrospinal fluid. Changes in these various elements affect the volume contained in the spinal canal, the cerebrospinal fluid pressure, and the blood supply to the neural elements. Normally there is a direct connection between the cerebrospinal fluid contents of the cranium and those of the spinal canal, and continuity of the vessels carrying blood. Many of the principles that are applied to intracranial dynamics (autoregulation, cerebral perfusion pressure, CSF

pressure, volumetric redistribution between compartments) may also be applied to the contents of the spinal canal.*

Airway Evaluation

The airway of the patient for spine surgery should be evaluated in the same manner as for any patient undergoing anesthesia. Particular attention should be paid to the range of motion of the head and neck and to the presence of any neurologic symptoms or pain during this maneuver. The patient with limitation caused by mechanical or neurologic restrictions should be considered for awake intubation under local anesthesia to minimize movement of the head and neck. The patient should be capable of responding to questions or volunteering information about his/her degree of comfort and other symptoms. In the patient with cervical spinal instability, the spine should be stabilized externally before surgery and intubation if at all possible. Several means of intubating the trachea should be available (fiberoptic bronchoscope, transtracheal cannula) if they should prove necessary.

Pulmonary Evaluation

The pulmonary system may be compromised in the patient with thoracic or cervical spine disease that is associated with the loss of intercostal and/or diaphragmatic muscle function. Pulmonary function tests may be warranted if there is a history of shortness of breath, difficulty coughing, or frequent pneumonias. With loss of the intercostal muscles, ventilation depends on diaphragmatic breathing. Tidal volume may be adequate, but forced exhalation and coughing may be weak because of the loss of the accessory musculature. This leads to difficulty in clearing secretions from the airways and frequent pulmonary infections. The patient reliant on diaphragmatic breathing often is more comfortable in the supine position, where the curvature of the diaphragm yields the greatest mechanical advantage for its function. Intraabdominal processes, such as ileus with bloating, fecal impaction, or pregnancy, may limit the excursion of the diaphragm and cause further impairment of pulmonary function. Patients presenting for spinal instrumentation for scoliosis may also present with preoperative pulmonary compromise in the form of restrictive lung disease as a result of mechanical inefficiency of the rib cage caused by the abnormal spine curvature.

Cardiac Evaluation

The cardiovascular system may also be compromised. The patient presenting for urgent spinal cord decompression may be in spinal shock and have loss of sympathetic tone distal to the lesion. This is particularly prevalent in patients with high thoracic lesions. With time, autonomic hyperreflexia may develop, particularly in patients with injury at spinal cord level T7 or above. In this instance, there is un-

*References 60-62, 65, 72, 73, 148, 149.

inhibited spinal cord autonomic discharge with vasoconstriction caused by stimulation of visceral afferent fibers. This is associated with hypertension, reflex bradycardia, and reflex vasodilation in spinal segments proximal to the spinal cord lesion. This may lead to myocardial ischemia, cardiac failure, or intracerebral hemorrhage. The autonomic hyperreflexia response, or mass reflex, may be blunted or ablated by the use of regional or general anesthesia, or by direct-acting vasodilators.

Neurologic Deficit

Patients presenting for spinal surgery should be carefully evaluated for a preexisting neurologic deficit. This should be carefully documented for comparison with postoperative condition. The neurologic deficit, its duration, and its extent may influence other organ systems, as noted previously. It may also alter the choice of anesthetic drugs and adjuncts, such as muscle relaxants. The use of regional anesthesia in the patient with preexisting neurologic deficit should be a considered decision. The risks and benefits should be carefully discussed with the patient. There should be careful documentation in case the deficit worsens.

Pharmacology

Patients with chronic spinal cord injuries may have altered clinical pharmacokinetics with various medications.[153] Such patients generally demonstrate an increased ratio in the size of extravascular to intravascular albumin pools. Total body water is decreased, and body fat content is increased. However, the percentage of body weight that is represented by water can increase with extensive erosion of muscle mass.[153] In addition, endogenous creatinine clearance does not correlate with inulin clearance in paraplegics and therefore should not be used as a measure of glomerular filtration.[153]

One important anesthetic consideration in patients with a preexisting neurologic deficit is the effect of succinylcholine on denervated muscle. Succinylcholine normally causes a muscular depolarization with resultant relaxation. In denervated muscle, motor end plate receptors proliferate and succinylcholine then produces an exaggerated response with a very large release of potassium into the circulation.[64] This acute increase in serum potassium may cause cardiac dysrhythmias, cardiac arrest, or death. Succinylcholine should therefore be avoided in these patients.[64]

In patients with spinal cord injury, gastrointestinal (GI) motility may be impaired, and thus the bioavailability of orally administered drugs that require intact postprandial gastric emptying to be absorbed may be reduced. Gut motility disturbances are related to dyssynergy between the parasympathetic (vagal) and sympathetic innervation of the upper GI tract that may be particularly problematic in patients with high spinal-cord lesions. Therefore the timing of anesthetic induction, the last ingestion of food, and airway management may be affected. Metoclopramide given as a premedication may be effective in improving gastric emptying. Drugs that undergo biotransformation and have relatively small volumes of distribution in the body when given as a single dose, such as lorazepam, are not likely to have disturbed pharmacokinetics. Intramuscular injections may have delayed absorption secondary to decreased blood flow in paralyzed muscles.

Patients with chronic neurologic dysfunction may be receiving low-dose heparin anticoagulation subcutaneously for prophylaxis against deep-vein thrombophlebitis. The decision to use regional anesthetic techniques in this instance must be tempered by the slight risk of hematoma formation and spinal cord or nerve compression and injury. It may be advisable to measure coagulation parameters, particularly a partial thromboplastin time, and to administer the block at least 4 to 6 hours after the last dose of heparin.[76]

Preparation
Patient Education

The patient and family must be educated about the procedures involved in the anesthetic to ensure cooperation. There may be several circumstances during spinal surgery that warrant patient cooperation and effort. If the patient is to be turned prone or if the cervical spine is unstable, an awake intubation may be indicated (see later discussion). Likewise, if an intraoperative wake-up test is to be performed, the patient must be educated about this procedure before anesthesia and surgery begin. What the patient may expect about the need for ventilation and pain therapy post operatively and how these concerns are to be managed should also be addressed.

Laboratory Studies

The laboratory studies obtained for surgery are individualized to each patient. However, certain basic evaluations are applicable to all patients presenting for spinal operation. In addition, specific studies may be indicated (Box 28-2). Basic information usually includes assessments of oxygen carrying capacity and organ perfusion and function, particularly renal function. Laboratory evidence of a preoperative infectious process is also important. If extensive bone surgery is contemplated, measurement of clotting function is helpful. When induced hypotension and hemodilution are anticipated to minimize the need for blood transfusion, evaluation of cardiac status and renal function as well as red blood cell mass is indicated. Examinations of the lungs, arterial blood gases, and pulmonary function are warranted when preoperative symptomatology indicates possible pulmonary disease.

Premedication

The need for premedication and the drugs used largely depend on the perceived or stated level of anxiety of the patient, the medical condition of the patient, and aspects of the operation and anesthetic that may be affected. Other factors, such as time of admission, may also influence this decision. In general, premedication is optional and should be

---

BOX 28-2
PREOPERATIVE LABORATORY VALUES OF INTEREST

Basic Laboratory Values
Hematocrit
Hemoglobin
White blood cell count
Urinalysis

Specific Laboratory Values
Blood urea nitrogen
Serum creatinine
Serum electrolytes
Prothrombin time
Partial thromboplastin time
Fibrinogen
Platelet count
Electrocardiogram
Chest x-ray
Arterial blood gases
Pulmonary function tests (spirometry)

---

prescribed at the discretion of the anesthetsiologist and the patient. A potent intravenous benzodiazepine may be considered desirable if the patient is anxious, and narcotic analgesics may be valuable if the patient is in pain. If awake intubation is anticipated, an antisialagogue will make topical anesthesia more effective and airway visualization easier by reducing the quantity of oral secretions. Finally, an alpha-2 agonist, such as clonidine, may be beneficial if induced hypotension is anticipated. In general, patients prefer oral or intravenous routes. Intramuscular injections may be somewhat unpredictable and uncomfortable. The most reliable route is intravenous injection under the attention of the anesthesiologist.

POSITIONING

Positioning for spinal surgery is most commonly prone, although supine or lateral tilt position may be used for anterior spinal procedures. Most spinal surgery is related to the posterior elements of the bony spine or the spinal cord. Various forms of the prone position with or without additions to the standard operating room table have been advocated and used.* The goals of positioning generally are to:

- Provide adequate surgical exposure of the spine. This usually involves decreasing the lumbar lordotic curvature to increase the site of the interspinous spaces.
- Avoid abdominal compression, allow free movement of the abdomen, and reduce vena caval pressure, thus preventing vertebral venous engorgement and difficulties with bleeding during surgery.

---
*References 8, 49, 94, 122, 140, 165, 172.

- Avoid thoracic compression to allow easier ventilation. Avoid increased airway pressures, because this may worsen vena caval engorgement, and decrease venous return, which in turn may decrease cardiac output.
- Maintain normal positioning of the extremities. Avoid compression or stretching of peripheral nerves or vasculature, or entrapment of digits.
- Support the head. Avoid ocular pressure or pinching of the ears.
- Provide liberal padding, thus avoiding pressure sores that otherwise may occur with long procedures.

Some examples of the prone position are shown in Fig. 28-11. The advantages of the prone position with abdominal freedom have been well demonstrated in a study documenting marked swings in lower vena caval pressure with abdominal compression and tight abdominal musculature.[133] These swings in pressure were postulated to be reflected also in vertebral venous pressure and to possibly contribute to surgical bleeding. Muscle relaxation and the lack of spontaneous respiration also were considered important factors in reducing bleeding.[133]

One of the most commonly used positioning techniques for surgery on the lumbar spine is the Georgia prone position.[165] This position was developed from information on comfort observed in subjects who were awake and placed into the prone position. This represents one of the few prospective studies on the merits of different positioning methods. The findings are interesting and deserve consideration. First, transverse rolls placed anywhere under the prone body except the ankles produced pain from pressure. Second, female subjects could not be made comfortable with longitudinal rolls under the chest. Third, rolls placed under the sternum were poorly tolerated. Fourth, any positioning method that raised the pelvis higher than the chest produced pain in the lower cervical and upper thoracic regions when the head was turned to either side. Fifth, all subjects were intolerant of pressure in the infraclavicular fossae. Sixth, use of armboards produced shoulder pain when the arms were extended and numbness in the hands when the elbows were flexed. Objective measurements revealed that adequate ventilatory compliance could be achieved in any position that allowed free excursion of the abdomen. Venous pressure in the lower extremities was unchanged if the femoral veins and inferior vena cava were unobstructed, and hypotension was not a problem unless the inferior vena cava was obstructed. From this information, the position known as the Georgia prone position was developed. It consists of elevation of the anterior superior iliac spines and chest to allow free abdominal excursion, positioning of the back and neck in the same plane to allow painless rotation of the head, and flexion of the hips with the knees under the anterior superior iliac spines to flatten the lumbar spine. Several modifications of this position currently are in use, although the principles of this position remain the same.[94,140,172]

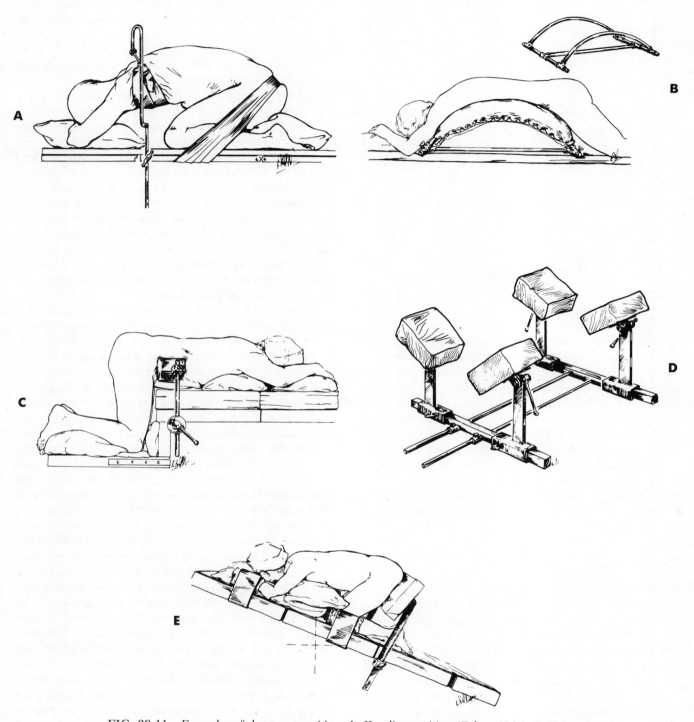

FIG. 28-11   Examples of the prone position. **A,** Kneeling position (Ecker, 1949). **B,** Frame (Moore, 1950). **C,** Georgia prone (Smith, 1961). **D,** Relton-Hall frame (Relton, 1967). **E,** Seated prone (Tarlov, 1967). *(From Anderton JM: Br J Anaesth 67:452-463, 1991).*

These methods of positioning were designed for procedures involving laminectomy and discectomy. On the other hand, patients having spinal surgery for stabilization and instrumentation of spinal deformity such as scoliosis may have difficulty with adequate positioning of supports because of the curvature of the spine. An adjustable four-posted frame has been developed for this purpose.[140] The use of this frame and other conservative techniques to minimize bleeding, including muscle relaxation, low mean airway pressures, infiltration of the wound with epinephrine, and improved surgical technique, have produced a marked decrease in blood loss during scoliosis surgery compared with earlier times.[140]

The significance of proper positioning of the patient with spinal disease cannot be overemphasized, even for nonspinal surgery. Patients with spinal stenosis or small spinal canal resulting from spondylosis may not tolerate hyperextension (hyperlordosis) of the lumbar spine and may suffer paraplegia or cauda equina syndrome as a result.[50,182] Therefore one must inquire into the limitations in positioning or range of motion before surgery, especially if nonanatomic positions may be necessary for the particular operation. Patients with previous coronary-artery-bypass grafting using veins may demonstrate ischemia with prone positioning and anterior chest wall pressure.[180] The ECG should be reviewed for any demonstration of new abnormality after positioning in the prone position in anyone with a previous coronary-artery-bypass graft.

Head Position Control

Compressive lesions of the spinal cord or instability of the spine, especially with neurologic findings that are aggravated or exacerbated by particular positions, warrant consideration of positioning the patient using the technique of "awake pronation" (see later discussion). Patient self-positioning may also be entertained for the very obese individual in whom difficult positioning is anticipated. In the patient in whom the planned surgery will be done in the supine position, after the position is attained general anesthesia may be induced and tracheal intubation performed. If there is any doubt about the ease or difficulty of intubating the trachea, direct laryngoscopy should be performed under topical anesthesia and sedation. After the ease of visualization of the glottic structures is ascertained, anesthesia may be induced for intubation. If there is difficulty in visualizing these structures, one should consider fiberoptic bronchoscopic or other techniques of establishing the airway under sedated but responsive conditions in which the patient may maintain his/her own airway. In the patient without focal neurologic symptoms, compressive lesions, or spinal instability, general anesthesia with intubation may precede positioning. The ability of the patient to tolerate the surgical position without undue discomfort or development of neurologic symptoms should be ascertained at the time of the preoperative interview.

Intraoperative Head Position

The position of the head during operation is usually dictated to some extent by the patient position. Basic principles include avoidance of hyperextension, hyperflexion, or extreme rotation to the side of the cervical spine. In cases where the surgery is for cervical spinal pathology, these considerations are obvious. However, careful positioning of the head and cervical spine during operations on the thoracic and lumbar spine is also important. Hyperextension of the cervical spine is a common complication of the prone position. This can be avoided by placing sufficient padding under the chest. Newer appliances made from soft foam are available that allow midline orientation of the face and head despite the prone position. These pads provide for facial support without pressure on the eyes or nose. If the head is turned to one side, care must be exercised to avoid turning too far and to avoid pressure on the ear. During operations on the anterior cervical spine, it is common for the surgeon to require traction on the head to distract the cervical vertebrae for placement of the bone graft for fusion. This should be performed under the direct supervision of the surgeon because excessive traction may result in stretching and ischemic damage to the cervical cord.

Hyperflexion during cervical laminectomy from the posterior approach is a very common occurrence. This is primarily due to the conflict between the needs of the surgeon and the physical limitations on the cervical spine. To expose the posterior cervical vertebrae high in the neck, the surgeon must often flex the head forward on the chest. This may produce undue strain on the spine itself, but it also results in very restricted venous outflow from the head and face. In addition, the airway may be compromised by sharp bending of the tracheal tube in the posterior pharynx. Restriction of venous outflow from the face and head produces macroglossia and intracranial hypertension, respectively. To prevent this complication, sufficient space must be retained between the anterior angle of the mandible and the sternal notch. This may be ascertained by the comfortable placement of at least two finger widths in this space at peak inspiration after positioning.

MONITORING
Physiologic

Monitoring during spinal surgery consists of two components, routine and specialized (Box 28-3).

Electrocardiographic monitoring may reveal abnormalities specific to patients with spinal cord injury. Altered ventricular repolarization may result from central sympathetic dysfunction associated with chronic spinal cord injury.[97] Multiple-lead ST elevation may be noted in these patients. This is due to the fact that ST-segment height is influenced by activity of the central sympathetic nervous system, which may be altered in patients with high levels of injury.[97]

> **BOX 28-3**
> INTRAOPERATIVE MONITORING TECHNIQUES FOR
> SPINAL SURGERY
>
> **Routine Monitoring**
> Auscultation of heart and lungs
> Electrocardiography
> Blood pressure measurement (noninvasive)
> Pulse oximetry
> End-tidal carbon dioxide
> Temperature
>
> **Invasive Monitoring**
> Arterial blood pressure
> Central venous pressure
> Pulmonary artery pressure
> Urine output
> Cardiac output temperature
> Mixed venous oxygen saturation
> Neurophysiologic monitoring

Hemodynamic conditions may require more intensive monitoring. For long procedures, monitoring urine output by means of a bladder catheter may be a useful indicator of renal perfusion and provide decompression of the bladder. Invasive monitoring of arterial blood pressure is advisable in cases where intentional induced hypotension is planned to minimize bleeding or in patients in whom strict control of blood pressure is desirable. Central venous or pulmonary artery monitoring may be indicated for procedures associated with large amounts of blood loss or fluid shifts, or in patients with a history of congestive heart failure. More invasive monitoring of left ventricular function with pulmonary artery catheterization should be considered, especially for patients in the more acute stages of quadriplegia, when spinal shock and left ventricular dysfunction may be present but their effects unpredictable.[108] The ability to place invasive monitoring lines intraoperatively, should the need arise, may also influence the decision of whether to place them preoperatively. Anticipated responses of the patient to induction of anesthesia also may dictate whether to place invasive monitoring before or after induction.

There is still some debate over the need to monitor patients for venous air embolism when surgery takes place in a position other than the seated position.[5] However, air embolism may occur any time the incision is elevated above the level of the heart, and posterior approaches using the prone position result in a wound located above that level. Although it may be acceptable practice to allow simple lumbar disk surgery without a central venous catheter in place in otherwise healthy patients, more extensive procedures requiring larger incisions and more extensive bone dissection do warrant strong consideration of central venous line

placement. Venous air embolism is particularly likely if bone is involved in the dissection.

Determining adequacy of ventilation through end-tidal carbon dioxide and arterial blood gas monitoring may be of particular importance in that SCBF has been shown to be responsive to changes in arterial Pco_2 in the same way as cerebral blood flow.[62] In the majority of cases, the use of end-tidal carbon dioxide measurement is considered adequate for intraoperative monitoring purposes. However, new data suggest a lack of correlation of end-tidal values and arterial Pco_2.[147] Therefore, in cases where fine control of arterial Pco_2 is desirable, intermittent sampling of arterial blood for direct gas determination to assess the degree of correlation with end-tidal values should be performed.

Neurophysiologic

Monitoring of neurologic function may be indicated for particular types of spinal surgery.[106,179] The usual circumstance involves operations that place the spinal cord or nerve roots at risk of injury. Some examples are surgery for correction of scoliosis of the spine, surgery for removal of a spinal cord tumor, or surgery to fuse an unstable spine.

Three basic methods are used to monitor the spinal cord during operation or manipulation of the spine: an intraoperative wake-up test of motor function, somatosensory evoked potentials, and motor evoked potentials. In addition, one group reports the use of local anesthesia in awake patients for cervical spinal fusion.[187] Also affecting the choice of neurophysiologic monitoring technique are the facts that somatosensory evoked potentials monitor only sensory pathways, and motor evoked potentials monitor only motor pathways.[34,107]

Intraoperative Wake-up Test

The intraoperative wake-up test has been used for many years and is considered the best way to assess the integrity of the spinal anterior motor tracts during spine surgery.[179] The use of this technique began as an attempt to avoid one of the most devastating complications of spinal surgery for scoliosis, postoperative paraplegia. There are many techniques for accomplishing the wake-up test, but all have in common an anesthetic technique that allows for rapid, calm awakening and rapid return to the anesthetized state.[1] This monitoring technique has proven very effective in preventing postoperative paraplegia. (See later discussion of the wake-up test.)

Somatosensory Evoked Potentials

Somatosensory evoked potentials (SSEP) are a modification of the basic electroencephalogram recorded repeatedly in response to time-locked stimuli applied to the peripheral sensory nervous system. This technology intermittently determines the integrity of the posterior spinal sensory pathways and large peripheral nerves. An intact cerebral cortex also is necessary. For spinal operations, typically the posterior tibial nerve at the ankle is stimulated with an electric current, and the resulting sensory activity of the cortex is recorded by scalp electrodes.[51,126] Some variations include median nerve stimulation for cervical surgery, lower-cord stimulation,[125,171] recording from spinous processes or interspinous ligaments, and cervical cord recording directly from the surface of the dura.*

Characteristics of the SSEP wave used in clinical practice include the wave amplitude, wave latency, and wave morphology. The amplitude is a measure of the intensity of the cortical electrical response generated by peripheral stimulation and the latency is the time between the application of the stimulus and the appearance of the cortical response. Morphology is the usual appearance of typical standing waves (Fig. 28-12). Changes in SSEP waves that indicate possible disruption of the sensory pathway include an increase in the latency of constant standing waves and a decrease in the amplitude of those waves. These changes occur when the neural structures of the cord become ischemic or have pressure exerted on them.* This can occur when the cord is stretched during distraction for scoliosis correction (Fig. 28-13), when retraction on the cord is too great, when the spinal cord blood vessels are compromised,

---

*References 2, 29, 35, 55, 84, 128, 134.
*References 3, 19, 39, 88, 156, 178.

thus reducing blood flow, when systemic hypotension occurs, or from hypoxia or hypothermia.[69,178]

One problem with SSEP technology is the confounding effects of systemic changes on the wave forms. These effects can be seen with anesthetic drugs (Fig. 28-14), changes in blood pressure (Fig. 28-15), changes in body temperature, and technical difficulties with the equipment. Anesthetic drugs may affect the SSEP in various ways (Table 28-1).[91]

Evoked potentials measured cortically seem to represent predominantly afferent activity through the posterior columns.[103] Therefore damage to motor pathways may occur without evidence of disturbance in the sensory pathways.[57] However, this appears to occur infrequently, because most dysfunction seems to represent relative ischemia with more general effects on cord function. Other factors, such as loss of the stimulating electrode placement, may also affect

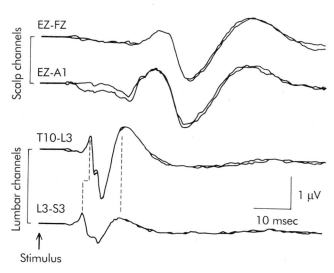

FIG. 28-12 Typical spinal and early cortical SSEPs produced by posterior tibial nerve stimulation. The bipolar lumbar channels show three upgoing, negative peaks. The earliest is in the L3-S3 channel (third lumbar to third sacral vertebral levels). The second is in the T10-L3 channel and is seen as a downgoing peak in the L3-S3 channel. This is followed by a bifid positive peak and then a third, broad negative potential. The scalp channels both show the negative and positive potentials at 35 and 40 ms. The EZ-A1 channel also shows an early subcortical positive potential around 27 to 30 ms. *(From Nuwer MR: Evoked potential monitoring in the operating room, New York, 1986, Raven Press, p 51.)*

TABLE 28-1
Drug Effects on Evoked Potentials

Drug	SSEP
Barbituate	↑ Latency →, ↓ Amplitude
Etomidate	↑ Latency N_{20}, P_{23} → Latency N_{10}, N_{14} ↑ Amplitude N_{20}, P_{23} → Amplitude N_{10}
Ketamine	→ Latency ↑ Amplitude
Droperidol	↑ Latency ↓ Amplitude
Fentanyl	↑ Latency ↓ Amplitude
Sufentanil	→ Lantency ↓ Amplitude
Propofol	↑ Latency ↓ Amplitude
Meperidine	↑ Latency ↓ Amplitude
Morphine	↑ Latency ↓ Amplitude
Nitrous oxide	↓ Amplitude → Latency
Halothane	↑ Latency ↓ Amplitude
Enflurane	↑ Specific activity ↓ Latency ↓ Amplitude
Isoflurane	↑ Latency ↓ Amplitude
Midazolam	↑ Latency ↓ Amplitude
Diazepam	↑ Latency ↓ Amplitude

Modified from Lake CL: Evoked potentials. In Lake CL, editor: *Clinical monitoring*, Philadelphia, 1990, WB Saunders, p 773.

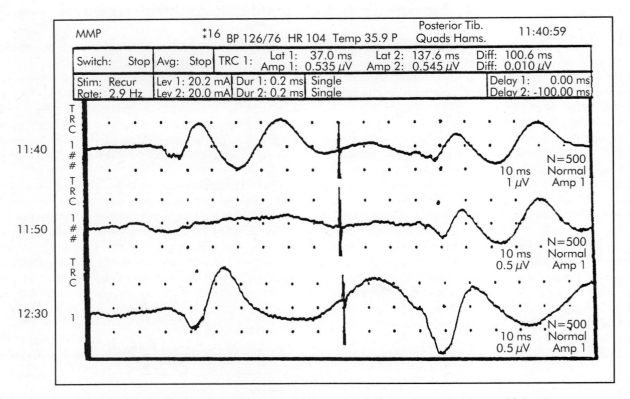

FIG. 28-13 Surgical effects. Posterior tibial nerve evoked potential in a 12-year-old female undergoing posterior spinal fusion with instrumentation. The left SSEP disappears during distraction *(left panel, middle trace)* and returns promptly when pressure is released *(left panel, bottom trace).* The patient was neurologically intact postoperatively.

Trace	Name	Scale (μV)	Filter (Hz)	Range (μV)	Date	Time	Comment
1	FPZ-CZ′	2.0	Hardware	1.40	05-21-91	08:44:17	"BP 97/66 HR 74 I
A	FPZ-CZ′	2.0	Hardware	0.17	05-21-91	09:41:10	"
B	FPZ-CZ′	2.0	Hardware	1.01	05-21-91	10:01:07	"

Stim SOML   Rate 2.9 Hz-20%
Sweeps 1800/1000   Artlev 15 μV
Amplifier 320000X   Filter 30-1067 Hz
Window 0.0-80.0 ms

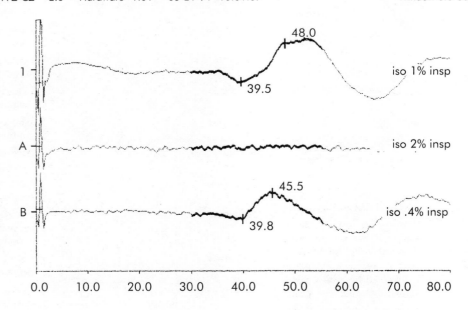

Peak	ms	μV	Peak	ms	μV
1 39.5	39.5	-0.42	B 39.8	39.8	-0.26
1 48.0	48.0	0.84	B 45.5	45.5	0.59

FIG. 28-14 Anesthetic effects. Left tibial nerve evoked response in a 16-year-old male during spinal fusion. The SSEP disappeared with an increase in isoflurane concentration to 2% *(A)* and recovered with a decrease in isoflurane to 0.4% *(B).*

evoked potentials; recording at several points along the conduction pathway is recommended. An alternative to cortically recorded evoked potentials is recording from the epidural space.[103] There is evidence that subcortical or spinal evoked potential recordings are well maintained despite the use of potent anesthetics.[48,152,184] This type of monitoring appears to be less sensitive to the depressant effects of anesthetics[84] and may represent more of the spinal cord activity at the level of measurement.

Disappearance of the SSEP, loss in amplitude of more than 50%, or increase in latency are considered to correlate with significant decreases in neurologic function and if uncorrected lead to neurologic sequelae.[103] If steps are taken to improve perfusion and the waveform abnormalities resolve, typically there are no neurologic sequelae. If the waveform remains diminished, there is a high likelihood of neurologic injury.[128] In the event that there is loss of the SSEP waveform, measures must be taken to rule out technical failure, improve blood supply to the spinal cord, and possibly minimize the depressant effects caused by the anesthetics. When the possible technical causes of a de-pressed SSEP wave have been resolved, attention should focus on a surgical reason for the change and the corrective steps to be taken.

Motor Evoked Potentials

Motor evoked potentials (MEP) are electrical impulses measured in the peripheral nerves and muscles in response to stimulation of the cortex or spinal cord (Fig. 28-16).[130] This monitoring technique measures the functional integrity of the spinal motor tracts, as opposed to the sensory tracts. There are two basic techniques for stimulating the cerebral motor cortex to generate the appropriate waveform: (1) direct transcutaneous electrical stimulation and (2) transcutaneous electromagnetic stimulation.[13,99-101,117] Although this monitoring technique shows promise in possibly eliminating the need to assess motor tract integrity with the intraoperative wake-up test, it does not assess sensory function and is still not in very wide use. The MEPs may be recorded from the peripheral nerves or the spinal cord. The potentials recorded from the periphery are more sensitive to nerve injury and ischemia than are the spinal cord sig-

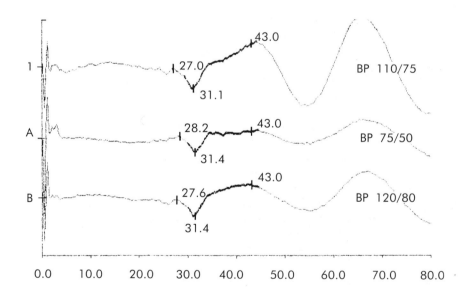

Trace	Name	Scale (μV)	Filter (Hz)	Range (μV)	Date	Time	Comment
1	FPZ-CZ'	2.0	Hardware	1.63	07-10-91	11:05:40	"
A	FPZ-CZ'	2.0	Hardware	0.78	07-10-91	11:45:53	"
B	FPZ-CZ'	2.0	Hardware	1.09	07-10-91	12:17:02	"

Stim SOMR   Rate 2.9 Hz-20%
Sweeps 1000/1000   Artlev 1560
Amplifier 320000X   Filter 30-1067 Hz
Window 9.0-80.0 ms

Peak	ms	μV		Peak	ms	μV
1 27.0	27.0	-0.06		A 43.0	43.0	0.23
1 31.1	31.1	-0.74		B 27.6	27.6	-0.10
1 43.0	43.0	0.80		B 31.4	31.4	-0.62
A 28.2	28.2	0.10		B 43.0	43.0	0.43
A 31.4	31.4	-0.50				

FIG. 28-15 Blood pressure effects. Right tibial nerve recording at the scalp in an 11-year-old female during posterior spinal fusion. The amplitude of the major wave at point 43 decreased with a fall in blood pressure to 75/50 mm Hg *(A)* but returned with normotension *(B)*.

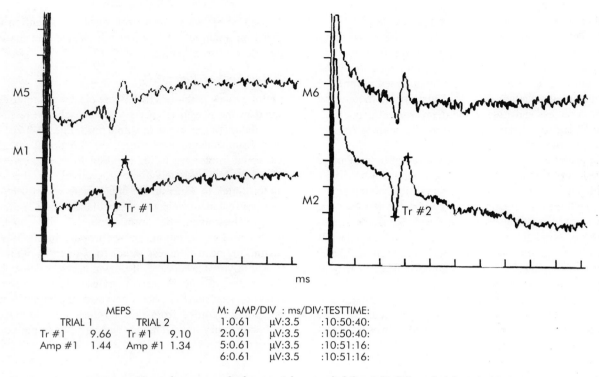

MEPS		M:	AMP/DIV	: ms/DIV	:TESTTIME:
TRIAL 1	TRIAL 2	1:0.61	μV:3.5		:10:50:40:
Tr #1 9.66	Tr #1 9.10	2:0.61	μV:3.5		:10:50:40:
Amp #1 1.44	Amp #1 1.34	5:0.61	μV:3.5		:10:51:16:
		6:0.61	μV:3.5		:10:51:16:

FIG. 28-16 Normal motor evoked potentials recorded from the left and right sciatic nerves. *(From Owen JH: Motor evoked potentials. In Salzman SK, editor,* Neural monitoring — the prevention of intraoperative injury, *Clifton, NJ, 1990, The Humana Press, p 222.)*

nals.[101] Mongan and Peterson[120] found that a greater-than 12.5-minute loss of neurogenic MEPs monitored at the L4 level in swine was sensitive, specific, and accurate in predicting postoperative neurologic dysfunction after aortic cross-clamping and reperfusion of the distal spinal cord. They demonstrated that CSF drainage and intrathecal papavertum extended the interval between aortic cross-clamping and loss of the L4 MEP and that preservation of the MEP was associated with a better neurologic outcome.

MEPs may be influenced by the same drugs as influence SSEPs. Intravenous anesthetic agents such as propofol, midazolam, droperidol, and sodium thiopental by either infusion or bolus dose may cause a significant decrease in the amplitude and/or latency of MEPs.[56,86,102,135] Ketamine and narcotic analgesics such as fentanyl produce less prominent changes.[56,86,135] The inhalation anesthetic drugs, including nitrous oxide, have been shown to depress MEPs in a variety of circumstances.[33,66,85,186]

Kalkman et al.[86] found similar MEP responses with propofol in human volunteers using transcranial electrical (Tce) and magnetic-induced muscle action potentials. Sustained depression of the Tce-MEP amplitude was observed after a dose of propofol sufficient to induce anesthesia or a sedating dose of midazolam (0.05 mg/kg). On the other hand, an anesthetic induction dose of etomidate and a 3 μg/kg dose of fentanyl resulted in no significant change. Therefore they recommended that

etomidate may be preferable as an induction agent and fentanyl as a supplement when monitoring transcranially induced MEPs. Neuroleptanalgesia may prove detrimental to MEP monitoring done with transosseous cortical magnetic stimulation.[56] In primates, droperidol (0.3 mg/kg) caused a significant elevation in threshold, a depression in amplitude, and an increase in latency. The addition of 6 μg/kg of fentanyl caused a slight but additional deterioration in the response.

ANESTHETIC APPROACHES
Regional

Although local[187] and regional anesthetic techniques may be used successfully in spinal surgery,[44,144] local, spinal and epidural anesthesia do not enjoy widespread use. This is due to a combination of reasons, including patient acceptance, particularly during prolonged procedures in the prone position, and avoidance of medicolegal questions concerning the influence of the anesthetic on outcome. However, regional anesthesia may be the method of choice in certain circumstances, such as local anesthesia for the placement of a spinal cord stimulator.

General

An opiate analgesic in combination with N_2O and a muscle relaxant is a technique that allows for an intraoperative wake-up.[1] Using this drug combination alone, however, may lead to a 25% incidence of intraoperative awareness and recall of the awakening[1]; in this study, however, this recall was not regarded as unpleasant. The addition of low doses of a potent inhalational anesthetic prevents any recall of intraoperative events and potentiates the hypotensive effects of drugs used for deliberate hypotension.[15] This potentiation leads to use of less hypotensive drug, a factor of some importance when using sodium nitroprusside. In addition, beta-adrenergic blocking drugs may be helpful in keeping the blood pressure under control.[111] By using large doses of narcotic analgesics and minimal doses of inhalational anesthetics, one can achieve an easy and controlled wake-up with no patient discomfort. Postoperative pain is also minimized immediately after the surgery when large intraoperative narcotic doses are used.

Induction

Induction of anesthesia for spinal surgery carries the same considerations as those for any other general anesthetic. In addition, there may be concerns specific to the patient. As previously noted, a major issue is frequently whether to intubate the awake patient before positioning. This is advisable when there is either a question about the stability of the cervical spine or concern about spinal integrity after positioning in the prone position. Intubation after induction of anesthesia often necessitates movement of the head and neck to visualize the larynx. Some anesthetists are able to place endotracheal tubes with fiberoptic scopes rapidly enough or with the use of specially designed masks[132] to allow this technique under general anesthesia: however, at least two anesthetists frequently are required to properly manage the airway during laryngoscopy, and intubation may occasionally be difficult. Unless absolutely necessary, this technique should be performed with the patient awake and able to manage his/her own airway.

Concerns arise about neurologic integrity after prone positioning when an area of the bony spine is unstable and prone to movement during positioning.[96] If this instability is in the cervical region, the patient may be externally supported with a collar or halo traction. If the area of instability is in the lower spine, the patient may or may not be in traction. Other circumstances include spinal stenosis, severe root impingement by a disk fragment, and preexisting neurologic deficit. With the use of appropriate local and topical anesthesia of the airway in combination with opiate analgesics and tranquilizers, patients can be intubated with the use of a fiberoptic scope without moving the head, still can follow commands to assist in the turn to the prone position, and can demonstrate muscle movement after positioning.[96] Because access to the head and endotracheal tube are restricted and there is a risk of tube kinking, particularly in the prone position, the use of flexible armored endotracheal tubes has been advocated.[77]

After cervical stability is attained, the airway should be examined to assess anticipated ease of intubation. When the neck is rigidly stabilized, the larynx often cannot be visualized by direct vision with a rigid laryngoscope. Often it is helpful to perform an "awake look" using topical anesthesia to the upper airway and direct laryngoscopy. If the glottis is adequately visualized, one can feel confident in proceeding with induction of anesthesia and subsequent intubation. If the glottis is not easily visualized, awake fiberoptic intubation should be done. An excellent review of management of the airway in the patient with cervical trauma is given by Hastings and Marks.[70] In general, they note that both direct laryngoscopy and fiberoptic laryngoscopy appear to be safe and effective methods of airway control in practiced hands. The method of choice depends on the experience of the anesthesiologist and the urgency of the case, as well as other factors such as facial trauma and soft tissue swelling. Stabilization of the head and neck may reduce but not eliminate movement of the spine and may make direct visualization of the glottis more difficult. In the nonemergent situation, external stabilization, such as halo traction, should be placed, after which direct assessment of the airway under topical anesthesia may be attempted. If direct visualization is difficult or impossible, visualization and intubation via fiberoptic endoscopy is indicated. Finally, one may need to consider cricothyrotomy or tracheostomy if attempts at fiberoptic placement of the endotracheal tube are unsuccessful.[112]

Maintenance

Maintenance of anesthesia generally consists of a continuation of the same basic technique used to induce and intubate the patient. Neurophysiologic monitoring needs and the possibility of a wake-up test intraoperatively suggest that a drug regimen based on N_2O and opiate infusion with minimal use of potent anesthetic agents is most advantageous.[1,179]

The issue of whether the patient should be treated with muscle relaxants depends to some degree on the preferences of the surgeon. Some surgeons prefer the patient not have muscle relaxants so that nerve stimulation may result in movement and an indication that surgeons are near a nerve. However, not all movements of the extremities may be apparent under the drapes, and some movement may occur as a result of the patient responding to other stimulation under conditions of "light" anesthesia. Gross movements of the body may disrupt surgery. Alternatives to movement of the extremities are monitoring of nerve function by SSEPs, MEPs, or EMG analysis. The use of muscle relaxants in the patient with neurologic disease also is a question. Succinylcholine may be contraindicated in this circumstance because of the potential for generating significant hyperkalemia. The option then may be to intubate the patient under very deep anesthesia or to use a short- to medium-duration muscle relaxant (mepivacurium, atracurium, or vecuronium) that may reliably wear off during the beginning of the surgery. We generally allow patients to be less-than-completely paralyzed by muscle relaxants so we can monitor subtle movement that may be an indication of nerve stimulation or less-than-satisfactory depth of anesthesia.

Fluid Management and Blood Transfusion

Fluid management in the context of spinal surgery reflects a balance between maintaining vascular volume to assure an adequate blood pressure for perfusion of vital organs, including the spinal cord, and avoiding the venous congestion that may occur with fluid overload. The issue of whether to give crystalloid solutions or colloid solutions for volume resuscitation is longstanding; however, avoidance of glucose-containing fluids is important.[93,137,158] Drummond and Moore[47] demonstrated worse neurologic outcome in rabbits exposed to temporary spinal cord ischemia when they received doses of glucose that caused modest elevation in the plasma glucose level before the injury. This finding correlates well with data demonstrating the same effect of plasma glucose elevations on brain injury[74,136,157] and spinal cord injury after aortic occlusion.[104]

The type of surgery to be performed influences the approach to fluid replacement. Surgery involving extensive exposure of the spine with denudement of bone, such as scoliosis repair or extensive spinal fusion, may be associated with significant blood loss.[98] With the current concerns about transmission of infectious agents during homologous blood transfusion, measures to minimize the need for bank blood should be considered. Two methods designed to avoid the need for homologous blood are hemodilution and the use of autologous blood.

Hemodilution may be performed in one of two ways: isovolemic hemodilution and in vivo hemodilution. Isovolemic hemodilution is the technique of acutely removing blood intraoperatively and replacing the volume simultaneously with crystalloid or treated-colloid solutions. This results in an acute decrease in the hematocrit. The physiologic response to this procedure is to increase cardiac output.[89,92,143] Oxygen delivery to the tissues is unaffected by hematocrit levels as low as 20%.[89,92,143] Cardiovascular stability does not deteriorate until hematocrit levels reach 15%.[113] When circulating red cell mass is reduced in this manner, fewer red cells are lost during bleeding. The harvested red cells are reinfused after the majority of blood loss has occurred.[168] In vivo hemodilution is simply intraoperative volume replacement with acellular products such as crystalloid, processed albumin, or artificial substances such as hydroxyethel starch. Volume replacement using this technique results in a gradually decreasing hematocrit over the duration of the procedure. Problems with identifying blood units, ensuring sterility of autologous blood in vitro, and meeting the technical needs of isovolemic hemodilution can be avoided. In addition, this technique is applicable in patients with religious proscriptions against receiving blood previously removed from the body. Care should be exercised when hydroxyethyl starch is used because this substance has been implicated in postoperative coagulation

derangements and an increase in homologous transfusion rate.[162]

Autologous blood may be obtained for reinfusion by preoperative donation, acute intraoperative harvest with isovolemic hemodilution (as described previously), or blood salvage techniques.[168] Researchers have claimed that as much as half of the routine intraoperative transfusion requirements could be met by aggressive preoperative autologous blood donation.[127] The only real restriction on autologous blood donors is the presence of an active bacteremia.[177] Even small patients or children may donate blood for their own use.[11,160] Some complications are associated with autologous blood transfusion, with an incidence similar to that of homologous transfusion.[90,109] After acute reactions, the most common complication is anemia,[54] the incidence of which can be reduced by the use of preoperative erythropoietin to boost endogenous red blood cell production.[37,58,59,145,146]

Intraoperative blood salvage may also reduce the need for homologous transfusion. Commercially available blood salvage devices, Cell Savers, thoroughly wash the cells to prevent the infusion of activated clotting factors or tissue thromboplastin from nervous tissue and then concentrate them in saline for reinfusion.[168] A relative contraindication to the use of this technique is blood with bacterial[25] or tumor-cell contamination. The main difficulty with the use of Cell Savers is the need for trained personnel to set up and operate the equipment.

Deliberate or induced hypotension is another means of reducing blood loss and therefore reducing the need for transfusion. In a variety of clinical situations, lowering the arterial blood pressure by means of drugs has been shown to reduce blood loss by as much as 50%.[12,48,87,176] The technique used to lower the blood pressure has varied greatly and includes controlled hemorrhage, neuraxial regional anesthesia, inhalation anesthetics, vasodilators, beta-adrenergic-blocking drugs, and calcium-channel-blocking drugs.[118] Each individual drug or combination of drugs has particular advantages and disadvantages. The important aspects of performing induced hypotension are maintenance of organ perfusion and avoidance of toxic drug effects. An acceptable regimen should produce hypotension rapidly, should be easily titratable to the desired blood pressure, should have no toxic side effects, and should be rapidly dissipated when the need for hypotension is no longer present. For most practical situations, this involves the use of a vasodilator in combination with a beta-adrenergic-blocking drug.[16,111,167] Short-acting drugs are most commonly used. Researchers know well that lower perfusion pressure, not a fall in cardiac output, reduces blood loss in these procedures.[163] To maintain perfusion at a lowered blood pressure, cardiac output must be maintained. This is best accomplished by vasodilating the peripheral vasculature and maintaining cardiac filling pressures with adequate venous return. The degree of induced hypotension varies according to the clinical history of the patient, but, in general, a mean arterial pressure (MAP) of 50 to 65 mm Hg usually is well tolerated in an otherwise healthy young adult.[118]

Careful and continuous monitoring of physiologic parameters and neural function in the spinal cord is essential when either hemodilution or induced hypotension are used. Because of the intense need to monitor organ perfusion with either technique, a Foley catheter for monitoring urine output, an intraarterial catheter for monitoring arterial blood pressure, and a central venous or a pulmonary artery catheter for monitoring central vascular filling pressures and volume status are warranted, in addition to basic monitors. In addition, monitors of neural function, SSEP, MEP, and a wake-up test are advised.

The bleeding during spinal surgery may be from abnormal vasculature and surrounding tissues that prevent normal spasm or collapse of the vessel, vascularized scar tissue, and callus. Bleeding may be classified according to the anatomic source: arterial, capillary, or venous bleeding, or any combination of the three. These sources are important when choosing the method of controlling bleeding. Venous bleeding may be increased in the setting of venous hypertension, such as may be found with restriction of venous return or venous congestion. Therefore techniques to minimize this are important. These include proper positioning with the operative site uppermost to assure adequate venous drainage, assuring of freedom of the abdomen to prevent increased intraabdominal pressure on the vena cava,[133] avoidance of the use of positive end expiratory pressure or prolonged positive inspiratory pressure, and avoidance of fluid overload.

Arterial bleeding is related to surgical factors and arterial hypertension. Deliberate arterial hypotension and assiduous surgical technique go a long way toward reducing this form of bleeding. Finally, capillary bleeding is related to a combination of the effects on the arterial and venous sides and factors that influence local regional blood flow through precapillary mechanisms (sphincters), including elevations in temperature, acidosis, increased CO_2, and prostaglandins and other metabolites of ischemia and injury. Preventing hyperthermia and assuring good tissue perfusion and appropriate ventilation should optimize these factors.

SPECIAL PROCEDURES
Awake Pronation

Lee et al.[96] have described the combination of awake intubation and subsequent self-positioning by a patient under sedation as "awake-pronation." For a procedure in the prone position, this is usually accomplished after intubation under local or topical anesthesia of the airway along with moderate degrees of sedation to blunt airway responses to the endotracheal tube. After the patient has assumed a position that is comfortable and suitable for the surgery, induction of general anesthesia may ensue, provided the necessary support is in place so that the assumed position is main-

tained. Patient self-positioning may also be considered in the very obese individual with whom difficult positioning is anticipated.

The Wake-Up Test

The wake-up test is the classic means of assessing motor function in the intraoperative and immediate postoperative period. This generally involves lightening the anesthetic to a plane wherein the patient is able to follow simple commands (i.e., "wiggle your toes" or "squeeze my fingers") but has not fully emerged from the anesthetic. This allows assessment for major motor deficits and quick resumption of the anesthetic for further surgical intervention or reversal if necessary. If a wake-up test is planned as part of the anesthetic, typically a narcotic-based anesthetic with nitrous oxide and low-dose potent inhalational anesthetic for unconsciousness are used. This allows the patient to awaken with a minimum of discomfort, tolerate the tracheal tube during the command phase, and perform the commands comfortably. After the commands are met to the satisfaction of the surgeon and anesthesiologist, the anesthetic is resumed and the operation concluded. This test is particularly useful in cases such as placement of Harrington rods, where the spine is manipulated with the potential for overcorrection. If a wake up test is planned during the anesthetic, the patient should be informed in advance of the nature of the procedure and what to expect in the event there is recall. The patient should be assured that he/she will be comfortable for the procedure to allay anxiety. Abbott and Bentley[1] found that with a technique based on a standard muscle relaxant and nitrous oxide supplemented by both intramuscular and intravenous morphine, 5 of the 20 patients studied remembered being awakened but did not find it unpleasant. In this group, one patient was found to have impaired motor function by this test, and the wake-up test allowed recognition and immediate correction. Potential complications associated with this procedure include patient discomfort and awareness; overzealous movement of the patient, requiring restraint and possibly resulting in injury to the patient or attendants; and dislodgment of monitors, vascular cannula, or the tracheal tube.[67]

POSTOPERATIVE CARE
Extubation

The questions of whether, when, and how to extubate the patient depend largely on the clinical situation. In the vast majority of cases involving spinal surgery, extubation may be performed immediately upon the awakening of the patient, demonstration of the usual criteria of adequate strength, and demonstration of adequate spontaneous ventilation. Intubation may need to be maintained in certain cases of impaired ventilation caused by high cervical or thoracic lesions, preoperative pulmonary impairment, metabolic derangement, or persistent muscle weakness. Extubation is not necessarily imperative for resumption of consciousness or ability to follow command.

Extubation in the prone position may be considered under controlled conditions in patients with a previously demonstrated normal upper airway who can be easily ventilated. This position allows easy drainage of secretions and results in less reduction in lung volumes, provided the abdomen is free and there is less upper airway compromise in the spontaneously ventilating patient. Extubation in the prone position also is easier on the patient during the transition to the supine position because the tracheal tube would be moved during this maneuver and result in tracheal stimulation that induces reflex responses. On the other hand, if compromise of the airway should occur after extubation in the prone position, further management may be more difficult. It is possible to reintubate the larynx in the patient in the prone position, but it may be difficult. Therefore, in any case where difficulty may be anticipated, the conservative approach of turning the patient onto the bed before extubation is desirable. This allows for easier suctioning of the airway and control if difficulty should arise. It also allows easier reintubation. In either case, the prone position may lead to facial edema if the head has been dependent.

Postoperative Pain Control

Postoperative pain control requires serious consideration in these patients, who often have preoperative pain. Indeed, the primary indication for the surgery may be relief of chronic pain. These patients may have been on long-term narcotic therapy and may have developed a tolerance to narcotics. Therefore an individual assessment of pain and provision of adequate analgesic therapy are essential. The use of the popular patient controlled analgesia (PCA) allows the patient to control the delivery of pain medication and provides superior pain relief. Pediatric patients specifically have pain severity that is underestimated by nursing personnel, and these patients benefit greatly from the use of PCA.[181] This technique has been shown effective in patients as young as 11 years old.[30] Advantages of the addition of a basal opiate rate to the PCA regimen have been documented.[20] The addition of a nonsteroidal antiinflammatory agent, such as ketorolac, may provide additional benefit and reduce the amount of narcotic analgesic necessary for pain relief. This drug is the first injectable agent of this class available in the United States. Ketorolac does depress platelet function.

An alternative to systemic opiate therapy is the use of regional analgesia via an epidural catheter implanted during surgery. Infusions through this catheter may include local anesthetics, narcotics, or a combination of the two. Caution must be exercised with local anesthetic use in that postoperative neurologic deficits may be difficult to assess. In addition, the small risk of infection associated with the catheters may discourage their use in patients with spinal instrumentation. For these reasons, this technique has not seen widespread acceptance.

Persistent pain beyond 1 to 2 weeks after wound healing should generate a closer examination for a persistent surgically approachable cause or evaluation by an experienced chronic pain specialist. There also may be a psychologic component to the pain that may require intervention. These issues may be addressed by someone skilled in the treatment of chronic pain problems.

COMPLICATIONS

Complications of spinal surgery may occur intraoperatively or postoperatively. Intraoperative complications include cardiac arrest from hypoxia while in the prone position or acute spinal-cord injury from either direct trauma to the cord or distraction pressure during instrumentation, pneumothorax, and hemothorax.[28] Postoperative complications include respiratory distress from atelectasis or pulmonary edema,[28] and neurologic deficit.[105]

Neurologic Deficit

MacEwan et al.[105] reported on 7885 operations for corrective surgery for scoliosis for the Scoliosis Research Society. In this large series, 74 major acute neurologic complications involving the spinal cord were reported. Half of these resulted in complete paraplegia, and half resulted in partial paraplegia. With extended follow-up, one third of these paraplegic patients recovered completely, one third recovered partially, and one third had no return of function. The incidence of complications was highest in cases of spinal fusion, especially if instrumentation was used. However, several cases of paraplegia were reported after traction alone. In addition to the operative procedure, traction on the spinal cord also appears to have great potential for cord damage.[105] Surgery for scoliosis may result in postoperative complications.[105] The estimated frequency of new neurologic deficits after this operation is 0.72%. In one series, of the 87 reported complications, the great majority (74 complications) involved the spinal cord. Of these, approximately half (41) resulted in complete paraplegia and half (33) resulted in partial paraplegia in the immediate postoperative period. With long-term follow-up, one third recovered fully, one third had partial recovery, and one third did not recover. Peripheral nerve injury occurred to a much lesser extent (13) and was associated with complete recovery. Of 74 cases of paraplegia, 26 occurred in patients who had posterior spinal fusion without instrumentation, and 6 reported cases occurred with skeletal traction alone. Congenital scoliosis repair involved 21 cases in this series but was associated with a higher frequency of neurologic deficit (10%). The severity of the spinal curvature was found to be important, and severe kyphosis markedly increased the incidence of neurologic complications. When complete paralysis complicates instrumentation during scoliosis surgery, removal of the Harrington rods within 3 hours after surgery is recommended.[105] These data predate the routine use of SSEP monitoring.

Anterior Spinal Artery Syndrome

Anterior spinal artery syndrome results from anterior-central cord ischemia in the distribution of the anterior spinal artery.[95] This typically presents as a motor weakness that is greater than any sensory change.[150] This is due to the more central and ventral location of the motor tracts in the spinal cord, as opposed to the more dorsal and peripheral location of the sensory tracts. This syndrome results from obstruction of the feeder vessels to the anterior spinal artery, as in aortic cross-clamping for repair of thoracolumbar aortic aneurysm or coarctation of the aorta.[150] However, anterior spinal artery syndrome may also result from sustained hypoperfusion,[159] correction of scoliosis,[105] cervical spondylosis,[78,174] disk herniation,[22,71] and vertebral trauma.[56,63,79,80] Treatment is aimed at relieving any existing contributory pathology and providing general support.

Epidural Hematoma

Epidural hematomas may arise spontaneously, as a result of a hypocoagulable state or trauma, or by iatrogenic causes. The hematoma may exert a mass effect with corresponding neuropathy or may be asymptomatic, as is often the case after the intentional epidural hematoma created as a result of epidural blood patching for post-dural puncture headache.

Arachnoiditis

Arachnoiditis is an inflammation of the pia-arachnoid membrane surrounding the spinal cord and nerve roots. The inflammation produces fibroblast and collagen proliferation with resultant nerve root entrapment.[32] This then leads to obliteration of the nerve root sheath as well as matting of the nerve roots of the cauda equina and may produce chronic pain and neurologic impairment.[18] This may occur as a result of initial trauma or infection, after myelography,[138,164] or as a postsurgical complication.[121,166] Symptoms usually appear within 2 days of the inciting event.[9] The majority of cases of arachnoiditis occur in the lower spine, with a small percentage occurring in the cervical and thoracic areas.[121] Therapy is difficult because surgical intervention may make the problem worse. Therapy is usually aimed at pain relief and includes spinal cord stimulation.[14]

Deep-Vein Thrombophlebitis

This complication occurs with varying rates in orthopedic patients.[154] Although most studies have been of series of patients undergoing total joint replacement, deep-vein thrombophlebitis also may occur in spinal surgery patients and neurosurgery patients.[154] In some hospitals, regional anesthetic techniques have been associated with a decreased incidence of thrombophlebitis, but this is not universally true.[154] Deliberate hypotension, hypothermia, decreased cardiac output, and hypovolemia all may possibly predispose to thrombophlebitis.[154] The use of compression stockings for the lower extremities and small doses of heparin in the perioperative period are generally accepted as the preventive measures of choice.[116] The pathophysiology of untreated thrombophlebitis includes acute pulmonary embolus; the treatment is aimed at support of organ perfusion and dissolution of the embolus.

Dural Tear

Interruption of the dura mater during spinal surgery is not uncommon and often a necessary part of the operation, particularly in cases of surgery on the cord itself; it also may occur unintentionally, especially when one is working in an area of previous surgery. The tear is usually sewn shut with no further sequelae. However, occasionally a cerebrospinal fluid leak develops, which may result in a postoperative headache, fluid collections, or leaks. If drainage of CSF persists, reoperation and repair may be necessary.

Cardiovascular Problems

Patients with chronic spinal cord injury presenting for surgery, whether related to the spine or for other procedures (typically urologic, plastic, or orthopedic), have the potential for various cardiovascular complications associated with their disease and with anesthesia. The complications generally fall into three categories: (1) hypertension (including autonomic hyperreflexia), (2) dysrhythmias, and (3) hypotension.[151]

Currently the hypertension from autonomic hyperreflexia may be treated pharmacologically with peripherally acting drugs (ganglionic blockers, alpha-adrenergic blockers, and direct-acting vasodilators), through regional anesthesia and the accompanying chemical sympathectomy, or by (deep) general anesthesia. Schonwald et al.[151] recommend the use of spinal anesthesia when using a regional technique to avoid the hazards of large doses of local anesthetics in a patient unable to give accurate assessment of the neurologic effect. The problem of autonomic hyperreflexia is not limited to the operative period. Of 11 cases described by Schonwald et al.,[151] four occurred postoperatively in the recovery room and occurred in patients recovering from both general and spinal anesthesia.

Up to 75% of patients presenting with autonomic hyperreflexia may have associated dysrhythmias, typically ectopic beats and sinus bradycardia. Schonwald et al.[151] noted an 8% incidence of bradycardia followed by hypotension associated with spinal anesthesia. Each of these occurred well into the operation, were sudden and unpredictable, and followed a period of stable anesthesia. They attribute this to the Bainbridge reflex that relates reduction in the right atrial pressure to a reflex bradycardia. Other ECG abnormalities, such as ST segment elevation in multiple leads, are common in patients with chronic spinal-cord injury and are associated with autonomic nervous system dysfunction and its influence on ventricular repolarization.[97]

Finally, patients with chronic spinal-cord injury are susceptible to postural hypotension. Schonwald's group found an incidence of hypotension (less than 80 mm Hg) of 11%

associated with induction of general anesthesia. They recommend adequate preoperative hydration as a preventive measure.

Pulmonary problems may be important, particularly in the quadriplegic patient. Vital capacity may be reduced as much as 35% because of diminished expiratory reserve volume resulting from a loss of intercostal and abdominal muscle contribution to expiration. This patient also has difficulty in coughing effectively and clearing secretions. Distention of the abdomen (e.g., from bowel gas) may significantly impair the effectiveness of the diaphragm. Patients with traumatic spinal paralysis are much more likely to die from renal, pulmonary (pneumonia), and gastrointestinal causes than are other patients.[43] Patients presenting with acute traumatic quadriplegia and followed over time show a decreased vital capacity initially as well as decreased inspiratory and expiratory pressures. Gradually the vital capacity and inspiratory pressure improve, however, the expiratory pressure remains depressed, indicating a relatively greater compromise of expiratory function over inspiratory function. Consequently, spirometry shows a normal functional residual capacity, elevated reserve volume, and decreased total lung capacity, vital capacity, expiratory reserve volume, and forced expiratory volume at 1 second. McMichan et al.[115] demonstrated the value of vigorous deep breathing exercises, incentive spirometry, and assisted coughing along with early fiberoptic bronchoscopy and bronchial lavage in spinal-cord-injured patients in reducing pulmonary complications and improving survival.

Ascending urinary tract infection from urosepsis is one of the main causes of death in spinal-cord-injured patients. These may also lead to chronic renal failure and are associated with renal and adrenal amyloidosis. Patients with chronic renal failure would be susceptible to electrolyte abnormalities. An anemia of chronic disease may be present in the quadriplegic. Quadriplegic patients may have difficulty with thermal regulation and behave as poikilotherms under anesthesia. They may normally have subnormal temperatures.[43] Muscle atrophy and osteoporosis are common in paraplegic and quadriplegic patients and may be associated with abnormal posture and stature. Therefore particular care is necessary in positioning these patients to avoid injury to the skin and peripheral nerves. These patients are susceptible to developing decubiti and fractures.

Air Embolism

Air embolism may occur in any patient during any operation. The predisposing factor in the development of a venous air embolus is a venous pressure at the level of the wound that is less than the surrounding atmospheric pressure. Venous pressures decrease when the wound is above the level of the right atrium, when the intravascular volume is low, or during spontaneous inspiration. The wound need not be very much higher than the heart for this to occur.[155] Spinal surgery in the prone position may well predispose to the development of an air embolism. Monitoring

for air entrainment includes precordial Doppler, end-tidal carbon dioxide measurement, end-tidal nitrogen measurement, and right atrial and pulmonary artery pressure measurement.[52] Treatment consists of deletion of nitrous oxide from the gas mixture, flooding of the wound with saline to prevent further entrainment, and aspiration of the air through a right atrial or pulmonary artery catheter.[17,31,110] Albin et al.[4] described three cases of air embolism, two massive and fatal, in patients for repeat lumbar laminectomy with fusion and recommend the use of precordial Doppler and multiorifice central venous catheters in these patients.

Major Vascular Injury

Injury to the major vessels may occur at any time during any spinal operation. A particularly hazardous complication occurs during posterior spinal surgery in the lumbosacral area when large pelvic vessels, including the iliac arteries and veins, are damaged.[42] This may initially go unnoticed and only become manifest after closure of the wound. The usual circumstance involves procedures around the lateral spinal elements, transverse processes, vertebral bodies, or during disk surgery.[42] The symptoms are the same as overt blood loss and acute hypovolemia. Volume resuscitation is the immediate treatment, with urgent surgical reexploration for repair of the vessel.

SPINAL CORD PROTECTION
Pathophysiology of Spinal Cord Injury

Spinal surgery may itself result in spinal cord injury. Certainly this has been seen in procedures where traction may be placed on the spinal cord. Patients with unstable spines may sustain injury during movement and positioning. The anesthetic state makes evaluation of the patient difficult, and monitoring of the spinal cord attempts to avoid this complication. Nonetheless, it occurs, and a review of the pathophysiology and emergency treatment is warranted.

The pathogenesis and pathophysiology of spinal cord injury are reviewed by Janssen and Hansebout,[81] Tator and Fehlings,[173] and elsewhere in this book. Injury to the spinal cord involves not only the physical trauma but also the secondary injury mechanisms of ischemia and chemical changes in electrolytes, high-energy phosphorous compounds, oxygen, prostaglandins, free radicals, and neurotransmitters. Reduction in spinal cord blood flow, particularly in the gray matter, can be caused by compression from a mass, traction on the cord, disruption of the anatomic blood supply, severe systemic hypotension, and loss of intrinsic autoregulatory control. This ischemia of the cord is considered to be the common pathway of cord injury in the vast majority of cases.[6] In addition, edema formation can occur and compound the ischemic episode.[6] Ischemia is associated with functional changes in the neurons of the cord, leading to loss of conduction (one manifestation is loss of somatosensory evoked potentials). The extension of injury appears to involve a biochemical cascade that potentiates and exacerbates the anoxia and ischemia in the spinal cord and may involve changes in intracellular calcium concentrations and associated disruptions in intracellular and membrane metabolism as the final common pathway in cell death.[173] Edema formation alone does not appear to be a significant determinant of spinal-cord injury or functional outcome as demonstrated by the lack of effectiveness of normal techniques of edema reduction (osmotic diuretics) and the effectiveness of drugs that have no effect on edema formation (steroids). Techniques of spinal cord protection and resuscitation are aimed at maintaining spinal cord perfusion and limiting or interfering with these biochemical events. So far, only the administration of steroids and local hypothermia have been shown to be beneficial,[81] although the calcium channel blocker nimodipine may also have a place in the treatment of spinal cord injury,[173] primarily through improvement of spinal cord blood flow but also possibly through other cytoprotective effects.

Elements of Cord Protection

Many drugs and modalities have been tried in an effort to avoid one of the most feared complications of spinal surgery, postoperative paraplegia or neurologic deficit. These treatments will be outlined here. First, maintenance of cord blood flow, avoidance of direct trauma to the cord, and use of adequate monitoring techniques designed to identify rapidly any untoward occurrence are the basis for all spinal cord protection.

Glucocorticoids are the only drug therapy so far shown to be of definite benefit in protecting the spinal cord. Bracken et al.[27] demonstrated conclusively that high-dose methylprednisolone (30 mg/kg bolus plus 5.4 mg/kg/hr for 23 hours) when begun within 8 hours of injury yielded significant improvement in motor function and sensation to pinprick and touch compared with placebo or high-dose naloxone in patients with acute spinal injury. Benefit was seen in patients whose injuries were initially complete. In cats, Young and Flamm[185] showed that high-dose methylprednisolone given 45 minutes after spinal cord contusion resulted in improved spinal-cord blood flow compared with placebo therapy, and recovery of evoked potentials, where there was none in the control group.

Anesthetic drugs also may be protective against spinal-cord injury. Cole et al.[36] studied spinal-cord injury in rats induced by inflation of epidural balloons and demonstrated a reduced incidence of clinical spinal cord injury in animals receiving halothane, fentanyl/nitrous oxide, or spinal anesthesia with lidocaine. The time to produce sustained neurologic deficit in 50% of animals in each group was longer in the anesthetized animals, especially in the fentanyl/nitrous oxide group. These results may well be due to the anesthetic effect of maintaining spinal-cord blood flow through vasodilation.

Mannitol may also have a role in the treatment of injury-related spinal-cord edema. Parker et al.,[131] using a dog model of spinal-cord trauma and myelography, demonstrated spinal-cord edema and subsequent reduction in spinal cord diameter by 15% to 25% 2 hours after the administration of mannitol. There was no reduction in spinal-cord diameter in dogs that had not sustained spinal cord injury. The study was limited by its methodology but suggests that this form of therapy, which is used commonly in the treatment of intracranial injury, may have some place in treatment of spinal-cord injury. Surgical approaches to acute spinal-cord injury, such as decompressive laminectomy and myelotomy, generally have yielded disappointing results.[81]

Because spinal-cord ischemia is thought to be one final pathway in developing spinal-cord damage, maintenance of cord blood flow is of paramount importance. One of the feared consequences of thoracic and thoracoabdominal aneurysm repair is paraplegia resulting from spinal cord ischemia.[23,24] This complication is estimated to occur in approximately 6.5% to 40% of patients having repair of thoracoabdominal aneurysms.[114] Placement of a shunt around the section of aortic cross-clamping improves distal aortic blood pressure and lumbar spinal-cord blood flow; however, it may not affect the reduction in lower-thoracic-spinal-cord blood flow seen with cross-clamping.[170] This may be related to the vascular anatomy of the anterior spinal artery, which is smaller above than below the entry of the arteria radicularis magna (artery of Adamkiewicz). Thus even distal aortic shunting may result in decreased distal thoracic blood flow and paraplegia in the baboon.

During spinal surgery, ischemia may also occur. This may be caused by stretching of the cord by distraction, induced hypotension without adequate cardiac output, or direct pressure on the cord. In addition, elevations in cerebrospinal fluid pressure may compromise cord blood flow.[61] To address this concern, attempts to increase cord blood flow have been tried. Cerebrospinal fluid drainage via a catheter[26] and intrathecal papaverine have been used.[169] Drainage of cerebrospinal fluid has been shown to improve spinal cord perfusion pressure and prevent paraparesis in dogs with thoracic aortic cross-clamping without shunt.[114] Shorter duration of cross-clamping (40 vs. 60 minutes) also may somewhat reduce the severity of the neurologic injury. Preliminary data about CSF drainage in patients having elective repair of nondissecting thoracoabdominal aortic aneurysms with reimplantation of intercostal arteries but without shunts seem to demonstrate the usefulness of this technique. No instances of paraplegia or paraparesis were found in 24 patients, nor were there any complications from the use of the intrathecal catheter or the drainage of the CSF.

In a study by Berendes et al.,[21] lumbar spinal fluid pressure was monitored in eight patients having repair of coarctation without shunt or repair of thoracic aneurysm with shunt. One patient having a coarctation repair without a shunt developed paraplegia. This patient also demonstrated marked increases in CSF pressure with the addition of nitroprusside for blood pressure control and with aortic cross-clamping. At the same time, distal aortic pressure was reduced. The high CSF pressures may have caused tamponade of the spinal cord. The cross-clamp time on this patient was also the longest of the group (54 minutes), and this may have influenced the outcome as well.

Spinal-cord CSF pressure generally rises in response to cross-clamping. This may occur even without changes in the CVP.[38] This change does not appear to be necessarily correlated with changes in blood pressure alone, because elevation of blood pressure with phenylephrine did not cause the same elevation in spinal-cord CSF pressure, nor did lowering the blood pressure with sodium nitroprusside alleviate the rise in spinal-cord CSF pressure caused by cross-clamping. Either recruitment of arterial capacitance vessels or a neuroreflex arc appear to be involved, or relative cord ischemia may disrupt normal mechanisms for autoregulation of spinal-cord blood flow.

The role of either systemic or local hypothermia remains unclear. Hollier[75] reports that induced hypothermia of the spinal cord appears to increase the "safe" ischemic time by 5 ½ minutes per degree centigrade reduction. He also suggests rapid surgery to minimize the aortic cross-clamp time to less than 30 minutes (without shunt) and reimplantation of all intercostal arteries. With this and routine CSFP monitoring, he has a rate of neurologic deficit of 6.3% and a mortality of 6.3%.

Recommendations

Spinal-cord protection falls under the topic of good basic physiologic support during anesthesia and spinal surgery and an anesthetic technique that allows for preservation of intraoperative cardiac function, systemic perfusion of organs, and neurophysiologic monitoring of cord function. This allows for immediate correction of any intraoperative occurrences compromising cord function and for easily controllable induced hypotension. In some hospitals and under some conditions, cerebrospinal fluid drainage may be advisable but is problematic during extensive spinal operations. Finally, methylprednisolone may be used when acute trauma to the cord is suspected.

SUMMARY

In caring for patients having surgery on the spine and /or spinal cord, there are three main considerations: patient position for the surgery, blood loss, and preservation of spinal cord integrity. In modern anesthesia practice, careful attention to detail allow for routinely excellent performance of very extensive surgical procedures. The use of fiberoptic intubation techniques, awake patient-assisted pronation, induced hypotension, invasive monitoring, neurophysiologic monitoring, and adequate postoperative pain control all have an impact on the successful outcome of these procedures.

References

1. Abbott TR, Bentley G: Intraoperative awakening during scoliosis surgery, *Anaesthesia* 35:298-302, 1980.
2. Abel MF, Mubarak SJ, Wenger DR et al: Brainstem evoked potentials for scoliosis surgery: a reliable method allowing use of halogenated anesthetic agents, *J Pediatr Orthop* 10:208-213, 1990.
3. Albanese SA, Spadaro JA, Lubicky JP et al: Somatosensory cortical evoked potential changes after deformity correction, *Spine* 16(8 suppl): S371-S374, 1991.
4. Albin MS, Ritter RR, Pruett CE et al: Venous air embolism during lumbar laminectomy in the prone position: report of three cases, *Anesth Analg* 73:346-349, 1991.
5. Albin MS, Newfield P, Pautler S et al: Atrial catheter and lumbar disc surgery, *JAMA* 239(6):496, 1978.
6. Albin MS, White RJ, Acosta-Rua G et al: Study of functional recovery produced by delayed localized cooling after spinal cord injury in primates, *J Neurosurg* 29:113-120, 1968.
7. Anderson DK, Nicolosi GR, Means ED et al: Effects of laminectomy on spinal cord blood flow, *J Neurosurg* 48:232-238, 1978.
8. Anderton JM: The prone position for the surgical patient: a historical review of the principles and hazards, *Br J Anaesth* 67:452-453, 1991.
9. Auld AW: Chronic spinal arachnoiditis, a postoperative syndrome that may signal its onset, *Spine* 3:88-94, 1978.
10. Bagshaw RJ, et al: Anesthetic management of surgery in the vertebral canal, *Anesth Rev* 12:13-32, 1985.
11. Bailey TE Jr, Mahoney OM: The use of banked autologous blood in patients undergoing surgery for spinal deformity, *J Bone Joint Surg* 69-A:329-331, 1987.
12. Barbier-Böhm G, Desmonts JM, Couderc E et al: Comparative effects of induced hypotension and normovolaemic haemodilution on blood loss in total hip arthroplasty, *Br J Anaesth* 52:1039-1043, 1980.
13. Barker AT, Jalinous R, Freeston L: Noninvasive magnetic stimulation of human motor cortex (letter), *Lancet* I:1106-1107, 1985.
14. Barolat G, Myklebust JB, Wenninger W: Effects of spinal cord stimulation on spasticity and spasms secondary to myelopathy, *Appl Neurophysiol* 51:29-44, 1988.
15. Bedford RF: Sodium nitroprusside: hemodynamic dose-response during enflurane and morphine anesthesia, *Anest Analg* 58:174-178, 1979.
16. Bedford RF, Berry FA, Longnecker DE: Impact of propranolol on hemo-

dynamic response and blood cyanide levels during nitroprusside infusion: a prospective study in anesthetized man, *Anesth Analg* 58:466-469, 1979.

17. Bedford RF, Marshall WK, Butler A et al: Cardiac catheters for diagnosis and treatment of venous air embolism, *J Neurosurg* 55:610-614, 1981.

18. Benner B, Ehni G: Spinal arachnoiditis: the postoperative variety in particular, *Spine* 3:40-44, 1978.

19. Bennett MH: Effects of compression and ischemia on spinal cord evoked potentials, *Exp Neurol* 80:508-519, 1983.

20. Berde CB, Yee JD, Lehn BM et al: Patient-controlled analgesia in children and adolescents: a randomized comparison with intramuscular morphine, *Anesthesiology* 73:A1102, 1990.

21. Berendes JN, Bredée JJ, Schipperheyn JJ et al: Mechanisms of spinal cord injury after cross-clamping of the descending thoracic aorta, *Circulation* 66(suppl I):112-116, 1982.

22. Blackwood W: Discussion on vascular disease of the spinal cord, *Proc R Soc Med* 51:543-547, 1958.

23. Blaisdell FW, Cooley DA: The mechanism of paraplegia after temporary thoracic aortic occlusion and its relationship to spinal fluid pressure, *Surgery* 51(3):351-355, 1962.

24. Blumbergs PC, Burne E: Hypotensive central infarction of the spinal cord, *J Neurol Neurosurg Psychiatry* 43:751-753, 1980.

25. Boudreaux JP, Bornside GH, Cohn I: Emergency autotransfusion: partial cleansing of bacteria-laden blood by cell washing, *J Trauma* 23:31-35, 1983.

26. Bower TC, Murray MJ, Gloviczki P et al: Effects of thoracic aortic occlusion and cerebrospinal fluid drainage on regional spinal cord blood flow in dogs: correlation with neurologic outcome, *J Vasc Surg* 9:135-144, 1988.

27. Bracken MB, Shepard MJ, Collins WF et al: A randomized, controlled trial of methylprednisolone or naloxone in the treatment of acute spinal-cord injury, *N Engl J Med* 322:1405-1411, 1990.

28. Bradford DS, Moe JH, Winter RB: Scoliosis and kyphosis. In Rothman RH, Simeone FA, editors: *The spine*,

Philadelphia, 1980, WB Saunders, pp 316-439.

29. Britt RH, Ryan TP: Use of a flexible epidural stimulating electrode for intraoperative monitoring of spinal somatosensory evoked potentials, *Spine* 11:348-351, 1986.

30. Brown RE Jr, Broadman LM: Patient-controlled analgesia (PCA) for postoperative pain control in adolescents, *Anesth Analg* 66:S22, 1987.

31. Bunegin L, Albin MS, Helsel PE et al: Positioning the right atrial catheter: a model for reappraisal, *Anesthesiology* 55:343-348, 1981.

32. Burton CV: Lumbosacral arachnoiditis, *Spine* 3:24-30, 1978.

33. Calancie B et al: Isoflurane-induced attenuation of motor evoked potentials caused by electrical motor cortex stimulation during surgery, *J Neurosurg* 74:897-904, 1991.

34. Chatrian GE, Berger MS, Wirch AL: Discrepancy between intraoperative SSEP's and postoperative function, *J Neurosurg* 69:450-454, 1988.

35. Cohen BA, Major MR, Huizenga BA: Pudenal nerve evoked potential monitoring in procedures involving low sacral fixation, *Spine* 16(8 suppl):S375-S378, 1991.

36. Cole DJ, Shapiro HM, Drummond JC et al: Halothane, fentanyl/nitrous oxide, and spinal lidocaine protect against spinal cord injury in the rat, *Anesthesiology* 70:967-972, 1989.

37. Connor JP, Olsson CA: The use of recombinant human erythropoietin in a Jehovah's Witness requiring major reconstructive surgery, *J Urol* 147:131-132, 1992.

38. DAmbra MN, Dewhirst W, Jacobs M et al: Cross-clamping the thoracic aorta. Effect on intracranial pressure, *Circulation* 78(suppl III):198-202, 1988.

39. Dasmahapatra HK, Coles JG, Taylor MJ et al: Identification of risk factors for spinal cord ischemia by the use of monitoring of somatosensory evoked potentials during coarctation repair, *Circulation* 76(suppl III):III-14–III-18, 1987.

40. De La Porte C, Siegfried J: Lumbosacral spinal fibrosis (spinal arachnoiditis). Its diagnosis and treatment by spinal cord stimulation, *Spine* 8:593-603, 1983.

41. DeGroot J, Chusid J: *Correlative*

neuroanatomy, ed 20, East Norwolk, Conn, 1988, Appleton & Lange, Chapter 4, p 3252; Chapter 5, pp 53-79.

42. DeSaussure RL: Vascular injury coincident to disc surgery, *J Neurosurg* 16:222-229, 1959.

43. Desmond J: Paraplegia: problems confronting the anaesthesiologist, *Can Anaesth Soc J* 17:435-451; 1970.

44. Ditzler JW, Dumke PR, Harrington JJ et al: Should spinal anesthesia be used in surgery for herniated intervertebral disk? *Anesth Analg* 38:118-124, 1959.

45. Dommisse GF: The arteries, arterioles, and capillaries of the spinal cord, *Ann R Coll Surg Engl* 62:369-376, 1980.

46. Drenger B, Parker SD, McPherson RW et al: Spinal cord stimulation evoked potentials during thoracoabdominal aortic aneurysm surgery, *Anesthesiology* 76:689-695, 1992.

47. Drummond JC, Moore SS: The influence of dextrose administration on neurologic outcome after temporary spinal cord ischemia in the rabbit, *Anesthesiology* 70:64-70, 1989.

48. Eckenhoff JE, Rich JC: Clinical experiences with deliberate hypotension, *Anesth Analg* 45:21-28, 1966.

49. Ecker A: Kneeling position for operations on the lumbar spine, *Surgery* 25:112, 1949.

50. Ehni G: Significance of the small lumbar spinal canal. Cauda equina compression syndromes due to spondylosis. Part 4, acute compression artificially induced during operation, *J Neurosurg* 31:507-512, 1969.

51. Engler GL, Spielholz NI, Bernhard WN et al: Somatosensory evoked potentials during Harrington instrumentation for scoliosis, *J Bone Joint Surg* 60A:528-532, 1978.

52. English JB, Westenskow D, Hodges MR et al: Comparison of venous air embolism monitoring methods in supine dogs, *Anesthesiology* 48:425-429, 1978.

53. Fahmy NR, Mossad B, Milad M: Effect of blood pressure on spinal cord blood flow in dogs, *Anesthesiology* 51:S79, 1979.

54. Finch S, Haskins D, Finch CA: Iron metabolism. Hematopoiesis following phlebotomy. Iron as a limiting factor, *J Clin Invest* 29:1078-1086, 1950.

55. Fromme K, Miltner FO, Klawki P et al: Spinal cord monitoring during intraspinal extramedullary tumor operations (peroneal nerve evoked responses), *Neurosurg Rev* 13:195-199, 1990.

56. Ghaly R, Stone J, Kartha R et al: Effect of neuroleptanalgesia on motor potentials evoked by transcranial magnetic stimulation in primates, *Anesthesiology* 75:A595, 1991.

57. Ginsburg HH, Shetter AG, Raudzens PA: Postoperative paraplegia with preserved intraoperative somatosensory evoked potentials, *J Neurosurg* 63:296-300, 1985.

58. Goodnough LT, Rudnick S, Price TH et al: Increased preoperative collection of autologous blood with recombinant human erythropoietin therapy, *N Engl J Med* 321:1163-1168, 1989.

59. Graf H, Watzinger U, Ludvik B et al: Recombinant human erythropoietin as adjuvant treatment for autologous blood donation, *Br Med J* 300:1627-1628, 1990.

60. Griffiths IR: Spinal cord blood flow after acute impact injury. In Harper AM et al, editors: *Blood flow and metabolism in the brain,* New York, 1975, Churchill-Livingstone, pp 4.27-4.29.

61. Griffiths IR, Pitts LH, Crawford RA et al: Spinal cord compression and blood flow: I. The effect of raised cerebrospinal fluid pressure on spinal cord blood flow, *Neurology* 28:1145-1151, 1978.

62. Griffiths IR: Spinal cord blood flow in dogs: II. The effect of the blood gases, *J Neurol Neurosurg Psychiatry* 36:42-49, 1973.

63. Grinker RR, Guy CC: Sprain of cervical spine causing thrombosis of anterior spinal artery, *JAMA* 88:1140-1142, 1927.

64. Gronert GA, Theye RA: Pathophysiology of hyperkalemia induced by succinylcholine, *Anesthesiology* 43:4389-4399, 1975.

65. Guha A, Tator CH, Rochon J: Spinal cord blood flow and systemic blood pressure after experimental spinal cord injury in rats, *Stroke* 20:372-377, 1989.

66. Haghighi SS, Madsen R, Green KD, et al: Suppression of motor evoked potentials by inhalation anesthetics, *J Neurosurg Anesth* 2:73-78, 1990.

67. Hall JE, Levine CR, Sudhir KG et al: Intraoperative awakening to monitor spinal cord function during Harrington instrumentation and spine fusion, *J Bone Joint Surg* 60A:533-536, 1978.

68. Hall SC, Stevenson GW, Suresh S: Burn associated with temperature monitoring during magnetic resonance imaging, *Anesthesiology* 76:152, 1992.

69. Hardy RW, Brodkey JS, Richards DE et al: Effect of systemic hypertension on compression block of spinal cord, *Surg Forum* 23:434-435, 1972.

70. Hastings RH, Marks JD: Airway management for trauma patients with potential cervical spine injuries, *Anesth Analg* 73:471-482, 1991.

71. Henson RA, Parsons M: Ischaemic lesions of the spinal cord: an illustrated review, *Q J Med* 36:205-222, 1967.

72. Hickey R, Albin MS, Bunegin L et al: Autoregulation of spinal cord blood flow: is the cord a microcosm of the brain? *Stroke* 17:1183-1189, 1986.

73. Hoffman WE, Edelman G, Kocks E et al: Cerebral autoregulation in awake versus isoflurane-anesthetized rats, *Anesth Analg* 73:753-757, 1991.

74. Hoffman WE, Harrington SL, Braucher E et al: Brain lactate and neurologic outcome following incomplete ischemia in hypo- and hyperglycemic rats, *Anesth Rev* 15:92-93, 1988.

75. Hollier LH: Protecting the brain and spinal cord, *J Vasc Surg* 5:524-528, 1987.

76. Horlocker TT, Wedel DJ: Anticoagulants, antiplatelet therapy, and neuraxis blockade, *Anesth Clin North Am* 10:1-11, 1992.

77. Horton JM: Anesthesia for surgery of the spine and spinal cord, *Int Anesthesiol Clin* 15:253-263, 1977.

78. Hughes JT, Brownell B: Cervical spondylosis complicated by anterior spinal artery thrombosis, *Neurology* 14:1073-1077, 1964.

79. Hughes JT: The pathology of vascular disorders of the spinal cord, *Paraplegia* 2:207-213, 1965.

80. Hughes JT: Vascular disorders. In: *Pathology of the spinal cord,* ed 2, Philadelphia, 1978, WB Saunders, pp 61-90.

81. Janssen L, Hansebout RR: Pathogenesis of spinal cord injury and newer treatments. A review, *Spine* 14:23-32, 1989.

82. Jennett B, Galbraith S: *Spinal compression and injuries; an introduction to neurosurgery,* Chicago, 1983, Year Book Medical Publishers, pp 267-293; 294-324.

83. Johnson RM, Southwick WO: Surgical approaches to the spine. In Rothman RH, Simeone FA, editors: *The spine,* Philadelphia, 1980, WB Saunders, pp 67-187.

84. Jones SJ, Edgar MA, Ransford AO: Sensory nerve conduction in the human spinal cord: epidural recordings made during scoliosis surgery, *J Neurol Neurosurg Psychiatry* 45:446-451, 1982.

85. Kalkman CJ, Drummond JC, Ribberink AA: Low concentrations of isoflurane abolish motor evoked responses to transcranial electrical stimulation during nitrous oxide/opioid anesthesia in humans, *Anesth Analg* 73:410-415, 1991.

86. Kalkman CJ, Drummond JC, Ribberink AA et al: Effects of propofol, etomidate, midazolam and fentanyl on motor evoked responses to transcranial electrical or magnetic stimulation in humans, *Anesthesiology* 76:502-509, 1992.

87. Khambatta HJ, Stone JG, Matteo RS et al: Hypotensive anesthesia for spinal fusion with sodium nitroprusside, *Spine* 3:171-174, 1978.

88. Kobrine AI, Evans DE, Rizzoli HV: Correlation of spinal cord blood flow, sensory evoked response, and spinal cord function in subacute experimental spinal cord compression, *Adv Neurol* 20:389-394, 1978.

89. Krämer AH, Hertzer NR, Beven EG: Intraoperative hemodilution during elective vascular reconstruction, *Surg Gyn Obstet* 149:831-836, 1979.

90. Kruskall MS, Glazer EE, Leonard SS et al: Utilization and effectiveness of a hospital autologous preoperative blood donor program, *Transfusion* 26:335-340, 1986.

91. Lake CL, Evoked potentials. In Lake CL, editor: *Clinical monitoring,* Philadelphia, 1990, WB Saunders, pp 757-800.

92. Laks H, Pilon RN, Kloverkorn P et al: Acute hemodilution: Its effect on hemodynamics and oxygen transport in anesthetized man, *Ann Surg* 180:103-109, 1974.

93. Lanier WL, Stangland KJ, Scheitnauer BW et al: The effects of dextrose infusion and head position on neurologic outcome after complete cerebral ischemia in primates: examination of a model, *Anesthesiology* 66:39-48, 1987.

94. Laurin CA, Migneault G, Brunet JL et al: Knee-chest support for lumbosacral operations, *Can J Surg* 12:245-250, 1969.

95. Lazorthes G: Pathology, classification and clinical aspects of vascular disease of the spinal cord. In Vinken PJ, Bruyn GW, editors: *Handbook of clinical neurology,* Amsterdam, 1972, North Holland Publishing, pp 492-506.

96. Lee C, Barnes A, Nagel EL: Neuroleptanalgesia for awake pronation of surgical patients, *Anesth Analg* 56:276-278, 1977.

97. Lehmann KG, Shandling AH, Yusi AU et al: Altered ventricular repolarization in central sympathetic dysfunction associated with spinal cord injury, *Am J Cardiol* 63:1498-1504, 1989.

98. Lennon RL, Hosking MP, Gray JR et al: The effects of intraoperative blood salvage and induced hypotension on transfusion requirements during spinal surgical procedures, *Mayo Clin Proc* 62:1090-1094, 1987.

99. Levy WJ, York DH, McCaffrey M et al: Motor evoked potentials from transcranial stimulation of the motor cortex in humans, *Neurosurgery* 15:287-302, 1984.

100. Levy WJ, York DH: Evoked potentials from the motor tracts in humans, *Neurosurgery* 12:422-429, 1983.

101. Levy WJ: Clinical experience with motor and cerebellar evoked potential monitoring, *Neurosurgery* 20:169-182, 1987.

102. Losasso TJ, Boudreaux JK, Muzzi DA et al: The effect of anesthetic agents on transcranial magnetic motor evoked potentials (TMEP) in neurosurgical patients, *Anesthesiology* 75:A1032, 1991.

103. Loughnan BA, Hall GM: Spinal cord monitoring, *Br J Anaesth* 63:587-594, 1989.

104. Lundy EF, Ball TD, Mandell MA et al: Dextrose administration increases sensory/motor impairment and paraplegia after infrarenal aortic occlusion in the rabbit, *Surgery* 102:737-742, 1987.

105. MacEwan GD, Bunnell WP, Krishnaswami S: Acute neurological complications in the treatment of scoliosis. A report of the Scoliosis Research Society, *J Bone Joint Surg* 57A:404-408, 1975.

106. Machida M, Weinstein SL, Yamada T et al: Spinal cord monitoring: electrophysiological measures of sensory and motor function during spinal surgery, *Spine* 10:407-413, 1985.

107. Machida M, Weinstein SL, Yamada T et al: Dissociation of muscle action potentials and spinal somatosensory evoked potentials after ischemic damage of spinal cord, *Spine* 13:1119-1124, 1988.

108. MacKenzie CF, Shin B, Krishnaprasad D et al: Assessment of cardiac and respiratory function during surgery on patients with acute quadriplegia, *J Neurosurg* 62:843-849, 1985.

109. Mann M, Sacks HJ, Goldfinger D: Saftey of autologous blood donation prior to elective surgery for a variety of potentially "high-risk" patients, *Transfusion* 32:229-231, 1983.

110. Marshall WK, Bedford RF: Use of pulmonary-artery catheter for detection and treatment of venous air embolism: A prospective study in man, *Anesthesiology* 52:131-134, 1980.

111. Marshall WK, Bedford RF, Arnold WP et al: Effects of propranolol on the cardiovascular and renin-angiotensin systems during hypotension produced by sodium nitroprusside in humans, *Anesthesiology* 55:277-280, 1981.

112. Marshall WK: Management of the difficult airway, *Anesth Rev* 11:18-22, 1984.

113. Martin E, Ott E: Extreme hemodilution in the Harrington procedure, *Bibl Haemat* 47:322-337, 1981.

114. McCullough JL, Hollier LH, Nugent M: Paraplegia after thoracic aortic occlusion: influence of cerebrospinal fluid drainage. Experimental and early clinical results, *J Vasc Surg* 7:153-160, 1988.

115. McMichan JC, Michel L, Westbrook PR: Pulmonary dysfunction following traumatic quadriplegia, *JAMA* 243:528-31, 1980.

116. Melon E, Keravel Y, Gaston A et al: Deep venous thrombosis prophylaxis by low molecular weight heparin in neurosurgical patients, *Anesthesiology* 75A:214, 1991.

117. Merton PA, Hill DK, Morton HB et al: Scope of a technique for electrical stimulation of human brain, spinal cord, and muscle, *Lancet* II:597-600, 1982.

118. Miller ED Jr: Deliberate hypotension. In Miller RD, editor: *Anesthesia,* ed 3, New York, 1990, Churchill-Livingstone, pp 1347-1367.

119. Mixter JM, Barr JS: Rupture of the intervertebral disc with involvement of the spinal canal, *N Engl J Med* 211:210-214, 1934.

120. Mongan P, Peterson R: Neurogenic motor evoked potentials are predictive of neurologic function in a porcine model of aortic occlusion, *Anesthesiology* 75:A1123, 1991.

121. Mooij JJA: Spinal arachnoiditis: disease or coincidence? *Acta Neurochirurgica* 53:151-160, 1980.

122. Moore DC, Edmonds LH: Prone position frame, *Surgery* 27:276-279, 1950.

123. Moore KL: *Clinically oriented anatomy,* ed 2, Baltimore, 1985, Williams & Wilkins, pp 565-625.

124. Mordis CJ: Anesthesia for magnetic resonance imaging, *Anesth Rev* 18:15-20, 1991.

125. Morioka T, Tobimatsu S, Fujii K et al: Direct spinal versus peripheral nerve stimulation as monitoring techniques in epidurally recorded spinal cord potentials, *Acta Neurochir* 108:122-127, 1991.

126. Nash CL, Lorig RA, Schatzinger LA et al: Spinal cord monitoring during operative treatment of the spine, *Clin Orthop* 126:100-105, 1977.

127. Nicholls MD, Janu MR, Davies VJ et al: Autologous blood transfusion for elective surgery, *Med J Aust* 144:396-399, 1986.

128. Nuwer MR: *Evoked potential monitoring in the operating room,* New York, 1986, Raven Press, pp 49-101.

129. Oldfield EH, Doppman JL: Spinal arteriovenous malformations, *Clin Neurosurg* 34:161-183, 1988.

130. Owen JH: Motor evoked potentials. In Salzman SK, editor: *Neural monitoring: the prevention of intraoperative injury,* New Jersey, 1990, Humana Press, pp 219-241.

131. Parker AJ, Park RD, Stowater JL: Reduction of trauma-induced edema of spinal cord in dogs given mannitol, *Am J Vet Res* 34:1355-1357, 1973.

132. Patil V, Stehling L, Zauder H: *Fiberoptic endoscopy in anesthesia,* Chicago, 1983, Year Book Medical Publishers.

133. Pearce DJ: The role of posture in laminectomy, *Proc R Soc Med* 50:109-112, 1957.

134. Pelosi L, Caruso G, Cracco RQ et al: Intraoperative recordings of spinal somatosensory evoked potentials to tibial nerve and sural nerve stimulation, *Muscle Nerve* 14:253-258, 1991.

135. Peterson R, Mongan P: Effect of intravenous anesthetics on neurogenic motor evoked potentials recorded at the spinal and sciatic level, *Anesthesiology* 75:A179, 1991.

136. Prough DS, Coker LH, Lee S et al: Hyperglycemia and neurologic outcome in patients with closed head injury, *Anesth Rev* 15:94-95, 1988.

137. Pulsinelli WA, Waldman S, Rawlinson D et al: Moderate hyperglycemia augments ischemic brain damage: a neuropathologic study in the rat, *Neurology* 32:1239-1246, 1982.

138. Quiles M, Marchisello PJ, Tsairis P: Lumbar adhesive arachnoiditis, etiologic and pathologic aspects, *Spine* 3:45-50, 1978.

139. Racz GB, McCarron RF, Talboys P: Percutaneous dorsal column stimulator for chronic pain control, *Spine* 14:1-4, 1989.

140. Relton JES, Hall JE: An operation frame for spinal fusion. A new apparatus designed to reduce haemorrhage during operation, *J Bone Joint Surg* 49B:327-332, 1967.

141. Richardson RR, Siqueira EB, Cerullo LJ: Spinal epidural neurostimulation of acute and chronic intractable pain: initial and long term results, *Neurosurgery* 5:344-348, 1979.

142. Robaina FJ, Dominguez M, Diaz M et al: Spinal cord stimulation for relief of chronic pain in vasospastic disorders of the upper limbs, *Neurosurgery* 24:63-67, 1989.

143. Rose D, Coutsoftides T: Intraoperative normovolemic hemodilution, *J Surg Res* 31:375-381, 1981.

144. Rosenburg MK, Berner G: Spinal anesthesia in lumbar disc surgery: review of 200 cases. . .with a case history, *Anesth Analg* 44:419-423, 1965.

145. Rothstein P, Roye D, Verdisco L: Preoperative use of erythropoietin in adolescents undergoing scoliosis surgery: hematologic, cardiovascular and side effects, *Anesthesiology* 75:A959, 1991.

146. Rothstein P, Roye D, Verdisco L et al: Preoperative use of erythropoietin in an adolescent Jehovah's Witness, *Anesthesiology* 73:568-570, 1990.

147. Russell GB, Graybeal JM: The relationship between end-tidal and arterial carbon dioxide in neurointensive care patients, *Anesthesiology* 75:A197, 1991.

148. Sandler AN, Tator CH: The effect of spinal cord trauma on the spinal cord blood flow in primates. In Harper AM et al, editors: *Blood flow and metabolism in the brain,* New York, 1975, Churchill-Livingstone, pp 4.22-4.26.

149. Sandler AN, Tator CH: Effect of acute spinal cord compression injury on regional spinal cord blood flow in primates, *J Neurosurg* 45:660-676, 1976.

150. Sandson TA, Friedman JH: Spinal cord infarction: report of 8 cases and review of the literature, *Medicine* 68:282-292, 1989.

151. Schonwald G, Fish KJ, Perkash I: Cardiovascular complications during anesthesia in chronic spinal cord injured patients, *Anesthesiology* 55:550-558, 1981.

152. Sebel PS, Erwin CW, Nevil WK: Effects of halothane and enflurane on far and near field somatosensory evoked potentials, *Br J Anaesth* 59:1492-1496, 1987.

153. Segal JL, Brunnemann SR: Clinical pharmacokinetics in patients with spinal cord injuries, *Clin Pharmacokinet* 17:109-129, 1989.

154. Sharrock NE, Savarese JJ: Anesthesia for orthopaedic surgery. In Miller RD, editor: *Anesthesia,* ed 3, vol 2, New York, 1964, Churchill-Livingstone, pp 1951-1967.

155. Shenkin HN: Air embolism from exposure of posterior cranial fossa in prone position, *JAMA* 210:726, 1969.

156. Shukla R, Docherty TB, Jackson RK et al: Loss of evoked potentials during spinal surgery due to spinal cord hemorrhage, *Ann Neurol* 24:272-275, 1988.

157. Sieber FE, Derrer S, Saudek CD et al: Effect of hypoglycemia on cerebral metabolism and cerebrovascular responsivity, *Anesth Rev* 14:70-71, 1987.

158. Siemkowicz E, Hansen AJ: Clinical restitution following cerebral ischemia in hypo-, normo- and hyperglycemic rats, *Acta Neurol Scand* 58:1-8, 1978.

159. Silver JR, Buxton PH: Spinal stroke, *Brain* 97:539-551, 1974.

160. Silvergleid AJ: Safety and effectiveness of predeposit autologous transfusion in preteen and adolescent children, *JAMA* 257:3403-3404, 1987.

161. Simeone FA, Lawner PM: Intraspinal neoplasms. In Rothman RH, Simeone FA, editors: *The spine,* Philadelphia, 1980, WB Saunders, pp 1041-1054,

162. Singelyn FJ, Gouverneur JM: Increased homologous blood requirement after isovolemic hemodilution with 6% hydroxyethyl starch during elective total hip replacement, *Anesthesiology* 75:A73, 1991.

163. Sivarajan M, Amory DW, Everett GB et al: Blood pressure, not cardiac output, determines blood loss during induced hypotension, *Anesth Analg* 59:203-206, 1980.

164. Skalpe IO: Adhesive arachnoiditis following lumbar myelography, *Spine* 3:61-64, 1978.

165. Smith RH, Gramlin ZW, Volpitto PP: Problems related to the prone position for surgical operations, *Anesthesiology* 22:189-193, 1961.

166. Smolik EA, Nash FP: Lumbar spinal arachnoiditis: a complication of the intervertebral disc operation, *Ann Surg* 133:490-495, 1951.

167. Spargo PM: The effect of nitroglycerin-induced hypotension on spinal cord blood flow, with and without spinal distraction, in dogs, *Anesthesiology* 63:A46, 1985.

168. Stehling L: Autotransfusion and hemodilution. In Miller RD, editor: *Anesthesia,* ed 3, New York, 1990, Churchill-Livingstone, pp 1501-1513.

169. Svensson IG, Stewart RW, Cosgrove DM et al: Intrathecal papaverine for the prevention of paraplegia after operation on the thoracic or thoracoabdominal aorta, *J Thorac Cardiovsc Surg* 96:823-829, 1988.

170. Svensson LG, Rickards E, Coull A et al: Relationship of spinal cord blood flow to vascular anatomy during thoracic aortic cross-clamping and shunting, *J Thorac Cardivasc Surg* 91:71-78, 1986.

171. Tamaki T, Tsuji H, Inoue S et al: The

prevention of iatrogenic spinal cord injury utilizing the evoked spinal cord potential, *Int Orthop* 4:313-317, 1981.

172. Tarlov IM: The knee-chest position for lower spinal operations, *J Bone Joint Surg* 49A:1193-1194, 1967.

173. Tator CH, Fehlings MG: Review of the secondary injury theory of acute spinal cord trauma with emphasis on vascular mechanisms, *J Neurosurg* 75:15-26, 1991.

174. Taylor AR, Aberd MB: Vascular factors in the myelopathy associated with cervical spondylosis, *Neurology* 14:62-68, 1964.

175. Thiagarajah S: Anesthetic management of spinal surgery, *Anesth Clin North Am* 5:587-601, 1987.

176. Thompson GE, Miller RD, Stevens WC et al: Hypotensive anesthesia for total hip arthroplasty: a study of blood loss and organ function (brain, heart, liver, and kidney), *Anesthesiology* 48:91-96, 1978.

177. Toy PTCY, Straus RG, Stehling LC et al: Predeposited autologous blood for elective surgery: a national multicenter study, *N Engl J Med* 316:517-520, 1987.

178. Uematsu S, Uldarico R: Effect of acute compression, hypoxia, hypothermia and hypovolemia on the evoked potentials of the spinal cord, *Electromyogr Clin Neurophysiol* 21:229-252, 1981.

179. Vauzelle C, Stagnara P, Jouvinroux P: Functional monitoring of spinal cord activity during spinal surgery, *Clin Orthop Rel Res* 93:173-178, 1973.

180. Weinlander CM, Coombs DW, Plume SK: Myocardial ischemia due to obstruction of an aortocoronary bypass graft by intraoperative positioning, *Anesth Analg* 64:933-936, 1985.

181. Weldon BC, Connor M, White PF: Nurse-controlled vs patient-controlled analgesia following pediatric scoliosis surgery, *Anesthesiology* 75:A935, 1991.

182. Wilkes LL: Paraplegia from operating position and spinal stenosis in non-spinal surgery, *Clin Orthop* 146:148-149, 1980.

183. Wolf HK, Anthony DC, Fuller GN: Arterial border zone necrosis of the spinal cord, *Clin Neuropath* 9:60-65, 1990.

184. Wolfe DE, Drummond JC: Differential effects of isoflurane/nitrous oxide on posterior tibial somatosensory evoked responses of cortical and subcorticsal origin, *Anesth Analg* 67:852-859, 1988.

185. Young W, Flamm ES: Effect of high-dose corticosteroid therapy on blood flow, evoked potentials, and extracellular calcium in experimental spinal injury, *J Neurosurg* 57:667-673, 1982.

186. Zenter J, Kiss I, Ebner A: Influence of anesthetics—nitrous oxide in particular—on electromyographic response evoked by transcranial electrical stimulation of the cortex, *Neurosurgery* 24:253-256, 1989.

187. Zigler J, Rockowitz N, Capen D et al: Posterior cervical fusion with local anesthesia: The awake patient as the ultimate spinal cord monitor, *Spine* 12:206-208, 1987.

29

Anesthetic Considerations in Patients With Neuroendocrine Disease

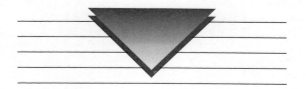

M. JANE MATJASKO

Since neoplastic, postsurgical, and traumatic causes exist for abnormalities in hypothalamic and pituitary function, it is important to be familiar with the anatomy, physiology, and pathophysiology of the hypothalamic-pituitary unit. The specific challenges in the management of patients with actual or potential panhypopituitarism relate to fluid and electrolyte abnormalities (glucocorticoids, mineralocorticoids, antidiuretic hormone) and anesthetic techniques appropriate in the presence of an intracranial mass that will permit early postoperative evaluation of visual acuity, third, fourth, fifth, and sixth cranial nerve function as well as motor strength. This chapter discusses normal pituitary anatomy and physiology, management of the common functioning and nonfunctioning pituitary tumors, and pertinent surgical and anesthetic considerations related to such conditions.

ANATOMY OF THE SELLA AND PERISELLAR REGION

The sella turcica, within the body of the sphenoid, provides bony protection for the pituitary gland. The anterior margin of the sella is the tuberculum; the posterior margin is the dorsum. The clinoids are bilateral anterior and posterior projections. Average dimensions of the sella are length 10 mm, depth 8 mm, width 14 mm, and volume of 600 mm.[3]

The diaphragm sella is a roof of dura pierced by the pituitary stalk with its arachnoid, which extends to the hypothalamus. The cavernous sinus surrounds the walls of the sella and contains the cavernous portion of the internal carotid artery; the oculomotor (III), trochlear (IV), abducens (VI) nerves; and the first division of the trigeminal nerve (V_1) (Fig. 29-1).

604

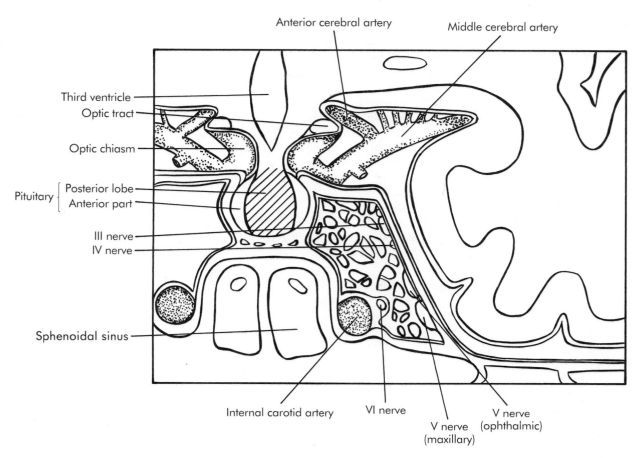

Anterior cerebral artery

Middle cerebral artery

Third ventricle

Optic tract

Optic chiasm

Pituitary { Posterior lobe / Anterior part

III nerve

IV nerve

Sphenoidal sinus

Internal carotid artery

VI nerve

V nerve (maxillary)

V nerve (ophthalmic)

FIG. 29-1 Coronal section through pituitary gland demonstrating perisellar structures and sphenoid sinuses. Cranial nerves: oculomotor nerve (III), trochlear nerve (IV), trigeminal nerve (V), abducens nerve (VI).

The optic nerves converge above the diaphragm to form the chiasm. The pituitary stalk is anterior to the chiasm. The distance between the tuberculum sella and the chiasm varies from 2 to 9 mm (average 4 mm); this distance, if short, is critical in limiting surgical access to the pituitary via the transfrontal approach. In most cases, the chiasm is directly above the diaphragm sella and pituitary. A "prefixed" chiasm overlies the tuberculum (10%) and a "postfixed" chiasm overlies the dorsum sella (15%).[155]

The carotid arteries may indent the lateral surface of the pituitary gland; the distance between the artery and gland ranges from 2 to 7 mm, and the distance between the arteries ranges from 4 to 18 mm (mean 12 mm).[156] Arterial bleeding during transsphenoidal hypophysectomy may be from the carotid artery or its branches (e.g., inferior hypophyseal) while venous bleeding arises from the cavernous sinus. Packing and coagulation maneuvers intraoperatively may result in contralateral hemiparesis or ipsilateral III, IV, VI, and V_1 deficits. Manipulation of the carotid artery may induce spasm, thrombosis, and/or distal

embolism.[197] Aneurysms can develop postoperatively if lacerations of the artery are unrecognized intraoperatively.[24]

Pituitary tumors may outgrow the normal sellar boundaries and invade the suprasellar region, the medial temporal lobes, or invade inferiorly into the sphenoid sinus or laterally into the cavernous sinus.

The sphenoid sinuses vary in size, shape, and symmetry and are often traversed by septae. Preoperative tomography is used to outline the septae-sellar relationships to avoid exposure of structures other than the pituitary (e.g., carotid arteries). For an indepth discussion of otorhinolaryngologic aspects of transsphenoidal surgery, the reader is referred to the review by Pearson and Laws.[145]

ANTERIOR PITUITARY (ADENOHYPOPHYSIS) Physiology

The plasma concentration of anterior pituitary hormones is influenced by the interplay of several factors, including age, emotional factors, sleep-wake cycle, hypothalamic-releasing or inhibiting factors, metabolic degradation, and the presence of functioning or nonfunctioning tumors of the pituitary gland. Pharmacologic agents, including anesthetics, can have marked effects on anterior pituitary function.[142] Preanesthetic medication reduces cortisol output. Adequate depth of anesthesia (volatile or neuroleptanesthesia) or regional anesthesia is not associated with increased cortisol secretion.[57] Growth hormone (GH) release is stimulated during neuroleptanesthesia, while thiopental, spinal anesthesia, and enflurane do not increase GH secretion. Thyroid-stimulating hormone (TSH) plasma levels are variably influenced by anesthesia although halothane increases and thiopental and spinal anesthesia decrease serum thyroxine (T_4) levels. All inhalation and intravenous anesthetics reduce plasma triiodothyronine (T_3) concentration, which remains depressed for up to 7 days postoperatively.[121,134]

In the absence of stress, the secretion of adrenocorticotropic hormone (ACTH), cortisol, prolactin, growth hormone, and gonadotropin is extremely variable and episodic. Central nervous system control is not simply a stimulus-response or feedback loop; it is intimately and temporally related to the 24-hour sleep-wake cycle.[124,196,199]

Secretory cells in the medial basal hypothalamus synthesize and release regulatory hormones that control anterior pituitary function. These regulatory hormones are transported from the median eminence via the portal venous system of the stalk to the anterior pituitary gland cells, which synthesize and release specific hormones (Table 29-1). Radioimmunoassay techniques are available for all hormones.

Pituitary tumors may be functioning or nonfunctioning and may be classified according to the size and extent of sellar involvement. The Hardy[69] classification of pituitary tumors follows:

Grade I: Normal size sella, mild thinning of the floor, less than 10 mm in diameter, microadenoma

Grade II: Sella enlarged but intact, no extrasellar extension

Grade III: Localized erosion of sellar floor, extension into sphenoid sinus or suprasellar space

Grade IV: Diffuse erosion of the sellar floor, "phantom" sella, extension into sphenoid sinus or suprasellar space

It is not clear whether functioning tumors are the result of hypothalamic or pituitary dysfunction or both. Pathologic studies demonstrate extraportal arterial blood supply to microadenomas, supporting the hypothesis that pituitary adenomas arise *de novo* without the influence of hypothalamic factors.[59] Since thyroid-stimulating hormone (TSH), leutinizing hormone (LH), follicle-stimulating hormone (FSH) or pure alpha-producing tumors are rare, they will not be discussed further.* At autopsy, incidental pituitary adenomas are found in as many as 10% of asymptomatic patients. Nearly 1% have multiple adenomas.[99]

TABLE 29-1
Anterior Pituitary and Hypothalamic Regulatory Hormones

	Release	Inhibition
ACTH*	Corticotrophin-releasing factor (CRF)	—
GH*	Growth hormone–releasing factor (GRF)	Growth hormone release–inhibiting hormone (GHRIH, somatostatin)
PRL*	Prolactin-releasing factor (PRF)	Prolactin-inhibiting factor (PIF)
TSH†	Thyrotropin-releasing hormone (TRH)	Somatostatin
LH†	Gonadotropin-releasing hormone (GnRH)	—
FSH†	Gonadotropin-releasing hormone (GnRH)	—

*Polypeptides.
†Glycoproteins with alpha and beta subunits; alpha subunits are serum markers for tumor diagnosis and success of therapy.

Functioning Pituitary Tumors
Adrenocorticotrophin

Corticotrophin-releasing factor (CRF) is a 41 amino acid peptide that stimulates corticotrophic cells of the pituitary.[179] Acetylcholine and serotonin stimulate and norepinephrine inhibits its release at the hypothalamic level. The neural pathways controlling higher cortical or subcortical influences on hypothalamic function have not been elucidated. It is known that the circadian rhythm of cortisol secretion is related to a coincident ACTH pattern. ACTH is secreted episodically and the clustering of such episodes results in the early morning high of cortisol secretion.[196] Serum ACTH values range from 0.1 to 1 mU/ml.

There is an intimate correlation between the sleep-wake cycle and cortisol secretion that is resistant to changes in living habits, including sleep deprivation. A phase shift in the sleep-wake cycle will eventually result in a corresponding shift in peak of cortisol secretion. Periods of stress result in bursts of cortisol secretion superimposed on the normal circadian variations.

ACTH causes cyclic 3-5 adenosine monophosphate (AMP)–mediated adrenal cortical secretion of 17 hydroxycorticosteroid (17 OHCS) (cortisol) and 17 ketosteroids (17 KS) (androcorticoids). Serum cortisol half-life is 60 to 90 minutes and from 5 to 15 mg of 17 OHCS are recovered in the urine per 24 hours. Cortisol inhibits CRF and pituitary ACTH secretion.

The highest serum cortisol levels are observed from 4:00 to 8:00 AM (25 µg/dl), and the lowest levels are observed

*See references 36, 76, 97, 102, 117, 172.

BOX 29-1
CUSHING SYNDROME

Truncal obesity
Moon facies
Abdominal striae
Osteoporosis
Acne
Supraclavicular and posterior cervical fat pads
Easy bruisability
Hirsutism
Hypertension
Hyperglycemia

from 4:00 to 8:00 PM (10 μg/dl). Twenty-four hour urinary free cortisol levels vary greatly and range from 75 to 375 μg in males and 35 to 300 μg in females.

Cushing *syndrome* may occur with adrenal adenoma or carcinoma, and follows ectopic or exogenous ACTH-induced adrenal hyperplasia. Cushing *disease* refers to adrenal hyperplasia secondary to an ACTH-secreting pituitary tumor. The cardinal features are listed in Box 29-1.

There are reported and well-documented cases of the transition of pituitary-dependent to adrenal-dependent Cushing syndrome due to the development of an autonomous macroadenoma of the adrenal gland. Treatment may require both pituitary and adrenal adenectomy.[75] Nelson syndrome refers to the presence of a pituitary tumor in patients who have had a bilateral adrenalectomy for adrenal hyperplasia, most likely from an unrecognized ACTH-secreting pituitary adenoma.

ACTH- or CRF-like peptides produced by extracranial tumors (primarily oat cell carcinoma of the lung) can cause the explosive development of hypercortisolism with hypertension, diabetes mellitus, hyperaldosteronism (hypokalemic alkalosis), and marked pigmentation; obesity and abdominal striae are late developments. Plasma cortisol levels in excess of 50 μg/dl are pathognomonic.

The diagnosis of Cushing disease relies on the measurement of serum cortisol, urinary 17 OHCS, 17 KS, and free cortisol. Serum cortisol levels (usually 75% bound) are influenced by the concentration of transcortin (cortisol-binding globulin), secretory bursts of ACTH, and stress. Urinary 17 KS and 17 OHCS are influenced by hepatic and renal function, body weight, thyroid function, and accuracy of the 24-hour urine collection. The urinary free cortisol is perhaps the single best test for the diagnosis of hypercortisolism, but the level is influenced by glomerular filtration rate and the accuracy of the 24-hour collection.[1] A reliable diagnosis therefore depends on an assessment of the function of the entire hypothalamic-pituitary-adrenal axis.

In Cushing disease, serum ACTH will be high. Most patients will show significant suppression after high-dose dexamethasone administration, and ACTH secretion will increase after metyrapone administration. Metyrapone inhibits 11-β-hydroxylase (an enzyme catalyzing the first step in cortisol biosynthesis), leading to a fall in cortisol secretion, an increase in pituitary ACTH secretion, and increased adrenal secretion of 11-deoxycortisol, which is measured as 17 OHCS in the urine. Maximum response is observed in the 24-hour period after drug administration.

Ectopic ACTH-producing tumors and adrenal tumors are resistant to pharmacologic suppression; in the former, ACTH levels are high, whereas they may be undetectable in the latter.

In Cushing disease, the serum cortisol diurnal variation is lost, with AM and PM levels both elevated. Urinary 17 OHCS will be greater than 12 mg/24 hours, serum ACTH will be high, and urine-free cortisol may be in excess of 550 μg/24 hours. There is substantial evidence that CRF excess is not a pathophysiologic factor in Cushing disease.[59]

Intravenous CRF (1 μg/kg) causes a further increase in ACTH and cortisol.[31] It is uncertain whether the CRF stimulation test will replace other standard tests that differentiate pituitary from ectopic causes of Cushing syndrome.[137]

Plain skull films may show sella enlargement in about one third of patients with microadenomas measuring 10 mm or less in size. Approximately 70% of surgically proved functioning microadenomas can be detected by late generation CT scanners. The most common finding is distortion of the sella walls.[81] There may be no radiographic evidence of tumor; however, resectable microadenomas are usually present when endocrinologic testing is confirmatory. Magnetic resonance (MR) imaging is the method of choice for evaluation of the tumor and its relation to the chiasm, hypothalamus, and cavernous sinus.[138] Gadolinium-enhanced MR studies have improved imaging of the three-dimensional anatomy of most tumors, i.e., location, volume, and relationship to the chiasm, optic nerves, and carotid arteries. Patients with atypical endocrine results indeed may have no adenoma evident at surgery. Peripituitary blood sampling preoperatively and intraoperatively has aided in microadenoma localization and diagnosis and distinction from an ectopic tumor.[112,135]

Growth Hormone

Growth hormone (GH) release from the anterior pituitary is controlled by at least two hypothalamic factors: growth hormone–releasing factor (GHRF) and growth hormone release–inhibiting factor (GHRIF, somatostatin). The molecular structure of somatostatin, but not GHRF, has been identified and the molecule synthesized. Somatostatin inhibits the secretion of virtually every known endocrine and exocrine substance; somatostatin-specific receptors can be radioactively labelled and detected by computerized gamma camera scintigraphy and provide in vivo imaging of somatostatin-receptor positive tumors (including GH tumors) and their metastases (including carcinoid, brain astrocytomas, pancreatic endocrine tumors).[100] GHRF has been found in crude extracts from the hypothalamus and appears to have the dominant hypothalamic effect on pituitary GH. Abrupt increases in secretion occur after the onset of deep sleep and in response to stress and physical exercise. This reflects communication and interaction between suprahypothalamic factors and GHRF. Alpha-adrenergic stimulation increases and beta-adrenergic stimulation decreases GH secretion. Dopamine, acetylcholine, and serotonin increase GH secretion in humans.[35]

GH affects tissue growth in all organ systems through its effects on intermediary metabolism. Linear growth is thought to be mediated by a group of polypeptides (somatomedins) produced in the liver in response to GH stimulation. Somatomedin-mediated cartilage (not bone) proliferation occurs.[187]

The most notable bone and soft tissue changes in acromegaly (GH excess) (Box 29-2) are in the hands, feet, and face, producing the characteristic coarse features. Patients may report increases in glove, ring, and shoe sizes. Skin thickening, connective tissue overgrowth, and interstitial fluid accumulation occur. All major organs increase in size, including heart, lungs, liver, and kidneys, usually accompanied by an increase in function. Patients may also report heat intolerance and excessive perspiration. Serum insulin is increased but hyperglycemia is present as a result of insulin resistance.

Acromegaly is most common in patients from 20 to 60 years of age with equal sex distribution. If untreated, 50% die before the age of 50;[47] the most frequent cause of death is cardiac and may be the result of hypertension, coronary artery disease, compensatory hypertrophy as a result of generalized somatomegaly, or the direct effects of GH on the heart. The existence of "acromegalic cardiomyopathy" (lymphomononuclear cell infiltrate, small vessel disease of the myocardium) may account for the clinical occurrence of congestive heart failure but this has not been proved.[110]

The effects of excess GH on the airway and the anesthetic implications are discussed later in this chapter (see "perioperative and anesthetic considerations").

▼

BOX 29-2
ACROMEGALY

Hypertrophic facial bones
Enlargement of hands, feet, all organs
Hypertension
Cardiomyopathy
Diabetes mellitus

Normal GH levels are less than 5 ng/ml. Most acromegalic patients have random serum GH levels greater than 15 to 35 ng/ml; some may have only borderline elevations difficult to distinguish from high normal values. Oral glucose administration (75 to 100 mg), in normal patients, will result in serum GH levels less than 2 ng/ml 1 to 2 hours later; higher values are suggestive of acromegaly. Insulin, arginine, or TRH administration may produce aberrant responses in patients with acromegaly. The results are sufficiently variable that these tests are not necessary for clinical diagnosis. In the acromegalic patient, 24-hour GH sampling will show marked fluctuations not associated with the usual bursts of secretion observed in the normal patient (e.g., onset of deep sleep). The two most sensitive tests for biochemical confirmation of GH hypersecretion are plasma insulin-like growth factor 1 and the oral glucose test.[119] Hypersecretion of prolactin (PRL) and TSH may also accompany GH overproduction.

The patient with acromegaly may also have hyperprolactinemia as a result of hypothalamic dysfunction from suprasellar extension of the tumor or from a tumor secreting both GH and PRL. Large tumors may cause chiasmatic encroachment and visual field deficits. Hypothyroidism (hypopituitarism) or hyperthyroidism (nontoxic nodular goiter) may be present. Thyroid function should be evaluated preoperatively in all patients with acromegaly.[10] GH or GH-releasing substances may be produced by carcinoid, pancreatic, and islet cell tumors, or gangliocytomas of the hypothalamus. A search for and operative treatment of such tumors should proceed because surgical excision may cause regression of acromegalic symptoms.[173] The cardiovascular manifestations of acromegaly may not progress or regress after therapy; however, diabetes mellitus improves in the majority of patients.[10]

Carpal tunnel syndrome may be the initial complaint in patients with acromegaly and may make radial artery cannulation more hazardous (postcannulation thrombosis)[26] if ulnar flow is compromised as a result of the hypertrophic carpal ligament. Perhaps dorsalis pedis artery cannulation should be considered.

Prolactin

A prolactin-secreting tumor is the most common of the functioning pituitary adenomas. It was described by Forbes et al.[51] in 1954, and a PRL radioimmunoassay[83] developed in 1971 documented the association of the galactorrhea-amenorrhea syndrome with excess serum PRL levels.[54] The amino acid sequence of PRL was reported by Shome and Parlow.[171]

Normal serum PRL is 3 to 20 ng/ml in females and 3 to 15 ng/ml in males. Secretion is regulated by hypothalamic-releasing and inhibiting factors and many physiologic, pharmacologic, and pathologic conditions influence the serum level.[52,115,178] Pregnancy, surgical stress, sleep (3:00 AM to 5:00 AM), breast suckling, exercise, and sexual intercourse in women are associated with increased serum PRL. Decreased metabolic clearance that occurs in chronic renal failure or hypothyroidism tends to increase serum PRL levels.

Prolactin is unusual in that its secretion is controlled by an inhibitory hypothalamic factor (PIF), which is probably dopamine. Prolactin-releasing factors (PRF) have also been identified, e.g., thyrotropin-releasing hormone (TRH), serotonin, estrogens, and opiates.[91,178] Their significance in humans is unclear.

Increased PRL production may occur after loss of inhibition, for example, pituitary stalk section, non-prolactin-secreting pituitary adenomas with suprasellar extension, and hypothalamic infiltrative processes (eosinophilic granuloma, glioma, tuberculosis, histiocytosis X, craniopharyngioma, and sarcoidosis).[113] Drug therapy may increase PRL through dopamine receptor antagonism (metoclopramide, alpha methyldopa, reserpine, phenothiazines) or other unknown mechanisms (opiates, endorphins).[53,74] Anesthesia and surgery are associated with increased PRL. Cimetidine (a histamine H_2 receptor antagonist) causes an abrupt increase in plasma PRL after a 300 mg intravenous dose. PRL returns to near baseline levels in 2 hours.[58] These studies imply that central nervous system histaminergic pathways participate in the control of PRL secretion. Perhaps cimetidine causes a temporary interruption of H_2 receptor–mediated inhibitory tone. The long-term effects of cimetidine administration on fertility and serum PRL levels are unclear.[186]

Estrogens cause release of PRL in vivo and in vitro; however, there is no evidence that prolonged administration of estrogen or oral contraceptives is responsible for the development of prolactinomas in humans.

The diagnostic value of elevated serum PRL levels is related to the clinical and radiologic findings in the patient. The most common etiology of hyperprolactinemia is the prolactin-secreting adenoma. However, craniopharyngiomas and the empty sella syndrome may also result in increased PRL, usually in a moderate range (up to 100 ng/ml).[68,89]

Very high serum PRL values (greater than 1000 ng/ml) are usually observed in patients with sellar and perhaps cavernous sinus destruction caused by an invasive adenoma. PRL levels in the intermediate range of 100 to 1000 ng/ml strongly indicate that a prolactin-secreting tumor rather than hypothalamic invasion or destruction is present.[11,113,166] An increase in the CSF-to-plasma prolactin ratio is a sign of suprasellar extension of the tumor and is valid with or without prior pituitary surgery.[87]

Laboratory studies in rats suggest that damage to hypothalamic dopaminergic neurons may result in the development of prolactin-secreting pituitary adenomas.[162] The signs and symptoms of prolactinoma in males and females are listed in Table 29-2 in descending order of frequency. The development of panhypopituitarism, visual impairment, and intracranial hypertension is more common in males, since tumor size is frequently larger than in females

TABLE 29-2
Prolactinoma

Females	Males
Amenorrhea	Impotence
Galactorrhea	Decreased libido
Anovulation	Infertility
Infertility	Intracranial mass
Decreased libido	Oligospermia
Intracranial mass	Galactorrhea (rare)

because of delay in the recognition of symptoms.[28] The diagnosis of prolactin-secreting tumor is based on elevated serum PRL levels, skull radiographs, sellar tomography, contrast-enhanced computed tomography, magnetic resonance imaging, and the response to PRL provocative (chlorpromazine, thyrotropin-releasing hormone) or suppression tests (L-dopa, bromocriptine).[1,48]

Angiography is not performed routinely but is reserved for patients with symptoms of a pituitary tumor without hormonal hypersecretion or panhypopituitarism, for patients who have undergone previous radiation, or for patients with sellar expansion or suprasellar extension.[157]

Nonfunctioning Pituitary Tumors

The most common nonfunctioning tumors are chromophobe adenoma, craniopharyngioma, meningioma, aneurysm, and, rarely, metastatic or granulomatous lesions. Nonfunctioning pituitary tumors are usually larger than functioning ones because of the delay in presentation and diagnosis; therefore, increased ICP and panhypopituitarism are more common. Because extension of the tumor causes pressure on nearby structures, these patients may have hypothalamic, visual, (most common), and cranial nerve (III, IV, V, VI) symptoms. Epilepsy from medial temporal lobe involvement is rare.

Patients often present with bifrontal or bitemporal headache as a result of the intracranial mass, stretching of the diaphragm sella, or obstruction of the foramina of Monro or the third ventricle. Direct pressure on the anterior chiasm leads to the classic symptom of bitemporal hemianopsia; however, a variety of visual symptoms may occur, depending on the position of the chiasm and its relationship to the gland. Early diagnosis and therapy are essential for preservation and recovery of visual function. Since craniopharyngiomas and meningiomas often have large suprasellar components, inferior visual field deficits and papilledema are more common than with pituitary adenomas, which more often produce superior visual field deficits and, only rarely, papilledema. Aneurysmal "tumors" can lead to a variety of symptoms related to the size and location of the aneurysm.

Panhypopituitarism

Large tumors may exert pressure on adjacent normal pituitary tissue, the portal blood system, or the hypothalamus

---

BOX 29-3
DIAGNOSTIC TESTS FOR PANHYPOPITUITARISM

ACTH-Adrenal Axis

Serum cortisol
Urine 17 hydroxycorticosteroids
Urine 17 hydroxyketosteroids
Provocative tests
   Insulin tolerance
   Propranolol-glucagon
   Metyrapone
   ACTH stimulation

Growth Hormone Axis

Serum GH level
Provocative tests
   Insulin hypoglycemia
   Propranolol-glucagon
   L-dopa
   Arginine
   Clonidine

Prolactin Axis

Serum PRL
Provocative tests
   Chlorpromazine
   TRH

TSH-Thyroid Axis

Serum T_3
Serum T_4
Serum TSH
TRH-provocative tests rarely required

Gonadotropin-Gonadal Axis

Serum FSH, LH
Provocative tests rarely required

---

and produce panhypopituitarism. Radiation of large tumors can lead to delayed panhypopituitarism up to 2 years postoperatively.[132] The patient may not have diabetes insipidus since adrenocortical hormones are necessary to facilitate the renal excretion of a water load.[61] Massive diuresis often begins with steroid replacement therapy. Hyperprolactinemia may be present if the portal system or the hypothalamus is involved and prolactin-inhibiting factor is prevented from reaching normal prolactin-producing cells in the anterior pituitary.

The empty sella syndrome may occur if the dura of the diaphragm sella is incomplete and the arachnoid pulsates into the sella or, secondarily, after surgery or radiation of the sella. With time, the growth of the arachnoid pouch may cause hypopituitarism, visual symptoms, and CSF rhinorrhea.[101] Diagnosis is confirmed by CT scan; response to endocrine testing is quite variable.

An outline of diagnostic tests for panhypopituitarism is provided in Box 29-3. Radioimmunoassay techniques are available for most trophic and pituitary hormones. Differentiation of hypothalamic from pituitary causes for hypopituitarism await the availability of reliable specific assays of the hypothalamic regulatory hormones.

Multiple endocrine neoplasia (MEN), type I, is a syndrome involving growth hormone–producing, prolactin-producing, or chromophobe adenomas of the pituitary, primary hyperparathyroidism, and insulin-producing or gastrin-producing tumors of the pancreas. Primary hyperparathyroidism is also seen in association with acromegaly. These coexisting conditions must be considered in the patient with a pituitary adenoma, particularly in the presence of hypercalcemia and renal calculi. Parathyroidectomy should precede pituitary surgery in these circumstances.[45]

Panhypopituitarism patients are susceptible to water intoxication and hypoglycemia. They are hypersensitive to central nervous system depressants.

Pituitary Apoplexy

Hemorrhagic infarction and necrosis of a pituitary tumor may be an acute or chronic process. Large tumors may compress or outgrow their blood supply; tumors may regress completely and leave an empty sella with or without hypopituitarism.[44,50,191] Spontaneous hemorrhage may occur in small adenomas; pituitary apoplexy may occur following head trauma.[80] Bromocriptine treatment, the dexamethasone suppression test, and the TRH test have been associated with the acute onset of pituitary apoplexy.[170]

In the acute situation, hemorrhagic infarction of a pituitary tumor may produce the signs and symptoms of subarachnoid hemorrhage: sudden loss of consciousness, meningeal symptoms, and xanthochromic CSF. These patients may also present with hypotension (adrenal cortical insufficiency), eye pain, blindness, ophthalmoplegia, and panhypopituitarism. Treatment includes steroid replacement and urgent transsphenoidal or transcranial surgery to decompress the optic nerves and chiasm to preserve visual function.

POSTERIOR PITUITARY (NEUROHYPOPHYSIS) Physiology

The supraoptic and paraventricular nuclei of the hypothalamus synthesize the posterior pituitary hormones, vasopressin (antidiuretic hormone, ADH) and oxytocin. These oc-

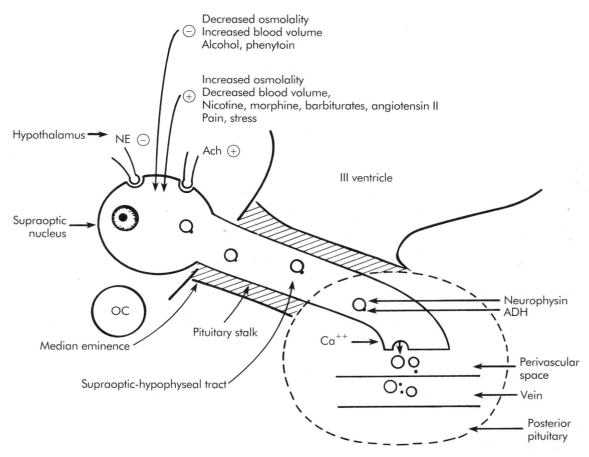

FIG. 29-2   ADH: Synthesis, transport and release. Norepinephrine *(NE)*; acetylcholine *(Ach)*; optic chiasm *(OC)*; calcium ion *(Ca++)*; inhibit *(−)*; stimulate *(+)*.

tapeptide hormones are attached to specific carrier proteins, neurophysines, and are transported along the pituitary stalk in secretory granules. ADH secretion is primarily from the supraoptic nuclei (Fig. 29-2). The secretory granules migrate along the axons of the supraoptic and paraventricular cells through the median eminence and pituitary stalk into the posterior pituitary gland. Axonal transport time has been estimated to be 30 to 60 minutes.[202]

The rate of hormone transport is approximately several hundred millimeters per day, faster than normal axoplasmic flow, suggesting that contractile elements are present in the neurotubules of the axons. The granules are stored in axons that terminate on the basement membranes of capillaries in the posterior lobe. Release into the circulation results from a calcium-facilitated action potential arising in the cell bodies in the hypothalamus and may occur at the median eminence or posterior pituitary. The granules containing ADH and neurophysine are released by an endocytotic process.[42] The commonly known conditions that stimulate, inhibit, or potentiate secretion are listed in Box 29-4.

Anesthetic agents per se, including narcotics, may or may not have a direct stimulating effect on ADH release.

The stress response to surgical stimulation in lightly anesthetized patients is the probable source of the observed increases in ADH in the surgical patient. In addition, other factors (e.g., hypotension, dehydration, and renin-angiotensin release) can cause ADH release and are not infrequent occurrences during anesthesia.[90,140,146,176] Indeed, anesthesia may obtund ADH release.[147] The hypertensive response to skin incision may result from catecholamine and vasopressin release.

Decreased total body water is the prime stimulus for thirst, regardless of the state of cellular hydration.[95] A very slight increase in the serum osmolality (normal 290 mOsm/kg) or a 1% to 2% decrease in total body water will stimulate ADH release as well as the thirst mechanism. For a comprehensive review of the thirst mechanisms the reader is referred to results of symposium held in New York.[192]

The hypothalamic nuclei themselves (the supraoptic primarily) are most likely the "osmoreceptors." The electrical firing rates of these cells increase with an osmotic increase of 2 to 5 mOsm/kg and may be the result of mechanical or osmotic distortion.[71] The mean osmotic threshold is approximately 289 ± 2.3 mOsm/kg.[9]

▼

BOX 29-4
FACTORS CONTROLLING ADH RELEASE AND SUPPRESSION

ADH Release

Hyperosmolality
Hypovolemia
Upright position
Pain
Stress
Morphine
Nicotine
Barbiturates
Tricyclic antidepressants
Angiotensin II
Cholinergic stimulation
Beta-adrenergic stimulation
Positive airway pressure
Head injury
Intracranial hypertension
Vincristine
Cyclophosphamide
Clofibrate
Increased core temperature
Chlorpropamide
Carbamazepine (Tegretol)

ADH Suppression

Hyposmolality
Hypervolemia
Recumbent position
Alpha-adrenergic stimulation
Ethanol
Atropine
Diphenylhydantoin
Reserpine
Glucocorticoids
Chlorpromazine
Decreased core temperature

ADH Potentiation

Chlorpropamide
Acetaminophen
Chlorthiazides

The most potent stimulus to ADH secretion is hemorrhagic shock. The ADH released is in such quantities that peripheral vasoconstriction (primarily direct effect on smooth muscle in splanchnic, coronary, and renal beds) as well as renal water conservation occur. Pulmonary vascular dilatation may occur.[183]

ADH secretion is related to elevated extracellular fluid osmolality detected by osmoreceptors in or around the supraoptic nuclei[95] and to reduced blood volume detected by receptors located in the left atrium and pulmonary veins. The massive sympathetic outflow also activates the renin-angiotensin-aldosterone system. ADH-mediated water retention and aldosterone-mediated sodium retention maintain the response if circulatory instability is prolonged.[165] The thirst mechanism is activated and, in awake patients, leads to increased water intake. Adequate blood volume will be maintained in spite of hyposmolality.

Direct stimulation of the vagus and carotid sinus nerves produces increased firing rates in the supraoptic neurons. Transverse sections through the midbrain abolish the reflex while section at the cervical-medullary level does not. The afferent limb is located in the aortic baroreceptors and in cardiac stretch receptors within the subendocardial portion of the left atrium; the efferent limb (transmission to the neurosecretory neurons of the hypothalamus) has not been elucidated.[169]

ADH circulates unbound in plasma; its half-life is about 15 to 25 minutes. It is removed from the circulation by renal and hepatic metabolic routes. Radioimmunoassay measurements of plasma ADH levels have been made in response to osmotic, water-loading, postural, hemorrhagic, and stressful stimuli. At a plasma osmolality of 287 ± 2.1 mOsm/kg, plasma ADH is about 2.7 ± 1.4 pg/ml. With prolonged fluid deprivation, osmolality may increase to 292 mOsm/kg and ADH levels increase to 5.4 ± 3.4 pg/ml.[158] In addition to osmotic control, ADH secretion is stimulated by intravenous, intracarotid, or direct application of acetylcholine to the hypothalamus, while epinephrine and norepinephrine administered intravenously or into the third ventricle inhibit ADH release. Adrenergic fibers terminate directly on the cell bodies of the supraoptic nuclei.[12]

Neurophysine, a carrier protein with a molecular weight of 10,000, is synthesized in the cell body of the supraoptic nucleus, bound to ADH, transported along the axon, and released into the circulation, at which point it is dissociated from ADH. Stimulation of the median eminence, and paraventricular and supraoptic nuclei causes neurophysine release.[29] The basal serum concentration of neurophysine in adult humans is 2.0 ± 1 ng/ml. The level is elevated during dehydration, in some cases of the syndrome of inappropriate ADH,[159,160] during the last two trimesters of pregnancy, in the presence of ADH-secreting nonendocrine tumors (e.g., oat cell tumors of the lung), and during renal failure. After discrete stimulation, there are several suprahypothalamic areas that cause an increase in ADH secretion (e.g., limbic system [periaqueductal gray, midbrain reticular formation] and hippocampus).[71,200]

In the kidney, ADH attaches to the contraluminal membrane of the distal and collecting tubules, which contain specific vasopressin receptors. The receptor-ADH reaction results in an increase in the rate of cyclic AMP production, which is directly responsible for increased tubular permeability.[109,136]

ADH permits water conservation and concentrated urine by facilitating water movement through aqueous channels from the collecting tubules into the medullary interstitium and systemic circulation.[88] For further discussion of the membrane effects of vasopressin, the reader is referred to several review articles.[72,73,163,177]

ADH increases innermost renal cortical blood flow, and it is possible that inner medullary solute concentration gradients increase through ADH-mediated selective increases in juxtamedullary blood flow and filtration rate, resulting in increase solute delivery to the inner medullary interstitium.[84] In normal subjects, vasopressin increases the net renal tubular reabsorption of sodium and urea and reduces that of potassium.[13]

Diabetes Insipidus

The dilute polyuria of central diabetes insipidus is caused by diminished or absent ADH synthesis or release. Neoplastic or granulomatous infiltration or destruction of the hypothalamic osmoreceptors leads to polyuria with or without loss of thirst.[104,116] Diabetes insipidus may also occur because of the inability to synthesize ADH.[21]

Neurosurgical procedures in the region of the sella result in diabetes insipidus for a variety of reasons: direct hypothalamic injury or ischemia, stalk edema, or high pituitary stalk section.[114] Head trauma can produce direct hypothalamic damage or ischemia secondary to hemorrhagic shock, fat embolization, and interruption of the hypothalamic vascular supply, or the stalk may be compressed on the sharp edge of the diaphragm sella in acute deceleration injuries.

Diabetes insipidus may be permanent or transient, and it may not be evident in the patient with coexistent anterior pituitary insufficiency. Glucocorticoids and, probably, mineralocorticoids are necessary to facilitate the renal excretion of a water load. Diabetes insipidus may become manifest with steroid replacement therapy in such a patient.[61]

Excision of the posterior lobe of the pituitary or stalk section below the median eminence will result in transient diabetes insipidus. Sufficient hormone is released from fibers ending in the median eminence to prevent permanent diabetes insipidus.[114] Axonal disruption above the median eminence results in retrograde degeneration of the supraoptic and paraventricular nuclei and permanent diabetes insipidus.

Diabetes insipidus is common with carcinomatous me-

tastases to the pituitary. Most frequently the site of metastasis is the posterior pituitary, possibly because of its direct arterial blood supply. Panhypopituitarism is rare in these patients, while diabetes insipidus occurs in 6% to 33%.[180]

Transsphenoidal resection of anterior pituitary microadenomas rarely causes permanent diabetes insipidus; however, transient diabetes insipidus may occur on the first-to-third postoperative day as a result of stalk manipulation or edema. Transcranial resection of large pituitary tumors with suprasellar extension can more often lead to permanent diabetes insipidus since the level of stalk section is difficult to control and because of the greater possibility of direct hypothalamic injury or ischemia.

Granulomatous infiltration (sarcoidosis, tuberculosis), meningitides, and aneurysms of the anterior circle of Willis (primarily anterior communicating artery) may cause diabetes insipidus by direct infiltration or rupture and damage to the stalk or hypothalamus.

In the presence of panhypopituitarism, diabetes insipidus may develop after cortisol replacement therapy. Evaluation of anterior pituitary function and necessary steroid replacement therapy should be given prior to testing for diabetes insipidus. A normal subject exposed to water deprivation can reduce urine flow to less than 0.5 ml/min and increase urine osmolality to greater than 800 mOsm/kg. Diagnosis can be confirmed by ADH assay in plasma and urine, correlated with plasma osmolality. Response of the renal tubule is assessed by the administration of aqueous vasopressin. Water deprivation should be discontinued if body weight decreases by 10%.[126,127]

MEDICAL AND SURGICAL THERAPY

Transsphenoidal microsurgical excision is considered the therapy of choice for all pituitary tumors that do not have marked extrasellar extension. Results of surgery are optimal in the presence of microadenomas (≤10 mm). Surgical "cure" is more possible when lesions are discovered early, when there is no extension laterally or into the suprasellar region, and when there has not been prior surgery or radiation therapy. On occasion, second operations (transsphenoidal or transcranial) may be required.

Transsphenoidal surgery offers the advantages of low morbidity and mortality, preservation of normal pituitary function because of direct microscopic visualization of the adenoma and the normal anterior and posterior pituitary gland, a lower incidence of permanent diabetes insipidus, less trauma to the frontal lobes and optic chiasm, less blood loss and no external scar (homograft or allograft fat may be used to pack the tumor cavity), and reconstruction of the floor of the sella with a bone or cartilage homograft. With appropriate attention to nasal and sellar floor reconstruction, postoperative cosmetic and functional abnormalities of the nose and CSF rhinorrhea are lessened or eliminated although life-threatening tension pneumocephalus has occurred.[6,93] Perioperative intravenous antibiotic coverage all but eliminates meningitis.

Tumors of uncertain diagnosis and those that extend into the anterior and middle fossae should be approached transfrontally. Morbidity and mortality are higher when the transfrontal route is used rather than the transsphenoidal route. Permanent diabetes insipidus and absent anterior pituitary function are common operative sequelae. The olfactory nerves may be permanently damaged and the potential for damage to the frontal lobe vasculature, chiasm, and optic nerves is of concern.

Treatment of craniopharyngiomas in young children is controversial and ranges from attempts at total excision to conservative surgery (cyst aspiration, ventricular shunting) plus radiation. In some series, a more conservative approach results in lower mortality and fewer long-term behavioral, developmental abnormalities related to frontal lobe dysfunction.[27,55,82,106] Others believe that aggressive surgical management, i.e., subtotal or total excision results in an acceptable quality of life in the majority of patients.[79]

Cushing Disease

The cure rate for Cushing disease is greater than 90% in many series based on the normalization of 24-hour cortisol output. The surgical results in Nelson syndrome are also improved if the tumor is noninvasive or causes only mild sellar erosion. Since serotonin plays a role in ACTH release, serotonin antagonists (e.g., cyproheptadine) have been used in the medical treatment of Cushing disease; however, they are of limited efficacy.[190] Ketoconazole, an antimycotic agent that is a potent inhibitor of adrenal and gonadal steroidogenesis, rapidly suppresses cortisol and is usually well tolerated. The major side effects are GI symptoms and elevated liver enzymes. Long-term effects are unknown. Patients should be considered for this therapy to control severe hypercortisolism before curative surgery.[98]

Acromegaly

If discovered early, GH-producing microadenomas are best treated by transsphenoidal microsurgical removal. Results are optimal when preoperative GH levels are below 50 ng/ml.[30] This approach offers less morbidity (hypopituitarism, diabetes insipidus) and mortality than radiation or transcranial excision. Controversy exists, however, since reports have been published that support all treatment modalities (medical, surgical and radiotherapeutic). Evaluation of the results of these studies is difficult since tumor size and the criteria used to define "cure" vary. A random postoperative GH level less than 5-10 ng/ml is considered to be evidence of successful treatment;[16] however, other reports indicate that recurrences are less likely if growth hormone is suppressed to less than 2 ng/ml after glucose administration.[98,167]

Transsphenoidal surgery alone can result in remission (normal postoperative GH level) in up to 94% when com-

bined with postoperative radiation. The procedure has very low or no mortality, morbidity is approximately 8%, and 5% develop new hypopituitarism postoperatively. Surgical failures or partial remissions occur in patients with preoperative GH levels greater than 50 ng/ml and suprasellar extension of the tumor. If prior therapy such as radiation or previous unsuccessful surgery has occurred, 74% of the patients have normal postoperative GH levels; 20% are treatment failures.

Conventional radiation has very low morbidity and mortality. However, it may take 2 to 5 years to reduce GH to normal levels with 73% of patients achieving this in 5 years.[43] Hypopituitarism, visual field deficits, and extraocular nerve palsies are reported following proton beam radiation; 94% of patients achieve normal GH levels up to 9 years after treatment.[38,105] Combined surgery and radioactive yttrium implantation have produced cure rates from 46% to 70% within 1 year of treatment.[86]

Bromocriptine[111,128] and L-dopa[190] suppress GH levels and tumor size after oral administration. Both bromocriptine, a dopamine agonist, and L-dopa, which is converted to dopamine, suppress hypothalamic-mediated GH secretion.

Somatostatin analogs, such as octreotide given subcutaneously, will lower GH levels and shrink tumor size in patients with acromegaly. Unfortunately, the drug inhibits gallbladder contraction and gallstones may develop. Pretreatment with octreotide may increase surgery cure rates. Concomitant use of bromocriptine and octreotide is suggested for patients who do not respond to either drug alone.[98,119]

Patients receiving bromocriptine for treatment of acromegaly require larger doses than those with PRL-secreting adenomas, hence the side effects such as dryness of the mouth, hyperkinesis, alcohol intolerance, constipation, and cold-induced transient vasospasm of the fingers may be more troublesome. Nausea, vomiting, and postural hypotension can be reduced by small incremental increases in dosage until therapeutically effective levels are reached. When bromocriptine is discontinued, tumor regrowth occurs.

The advantages and disadvantages of various treatment modalities must be weighed and prescribed according to the individual patient's circumstances. At this time, transsphenoidal surgery for small tumors without suprasellar extension offers the advantages of low morbidity, low mortality, and immediate remission.[16,30]

Prolactinoma

Incidental pituitary adenomas are present in 27% of unselected cadavers and 41% of these are prolactinomas although no evidence of pituitary disease was clinically evident premortem. Sellar polytomography done in unselected cadavers has demonstrated a 20% incidence of false positive and 20% false negatives in relation to histologic data.[22]

The optimal management of patients with prolactinomas is controversial since these tumors may spontaneously regress, remain the same, or enlarge. Each case must be individualized. Rate of growth of the tumor cannot be predicted by PRL levels or radiographic parameters. Pregnancy may be associated with rapid growth, and PRL levels and radiographic criteria are not helpful in prediction.[41] The most sensitive index of tumor enlargement is high resolution CT scan or MR and this has influenced the approach to therapy in patients with prolactinomas. Most prolactinomas grow very slowly or not at all. Spontaneous resolution of the endocrine abnormality has been reported with persistence of the sellar mass.[194]

Some microadenomas may become macroadenomas with time and/or pregnancy, and prolonged hyperprolactinemia (secondary to hyperestrogenemia) is associated with the development of osteoporosis.[96] The long-term consequences of this have not been reported although pathologic fractures could occur.

Microadenomas less than 10 mm in size associated with PRL values of less than 200 ng/ml have been associated with surgical cure rates as high as 90%. Larger tumors with higher PRL levels have much lower cure rates.[15,48,153,164,193] The surgical cure rate in micro- and macroadenomas (>10 mm) is unpredictable; therefore, medical therapy is recommended. Surgery is indicated in patients whose tumors are resistant or in those who are unable to tolerate medical therapy, patients with progressing visual loss, and in those whose tumors grow on dopamine agonist therapy.[98]

Dopamine agonists, including L-dopa, bromocriptine, and apomorphine, reduce PRL serum levels. Bromocriptine, an ergot derivative and a dopamine agonist, reduces prolactin levels in normal patients and patients with prolactin-secreting adenomas.[17,118,150,195] Tumor size decreases, fertility is restored, and visual field defects may resolve. Bromocriptine therapy has not received sufficient clinical trials in patients with nonfunctioning tumors. Reports are conflicting although tumor disappearance has been reported in one patient after 2 years of therapy, perhaps as a result of the antimitotic action of bromocriptine.[14,37,85]

Bromocriptine therapy produces reversible inhibition of protein synthesis in the tumor cell,[154] with resultant tumor shrinkage and reduction of prolactin levels to normal.[175] After prolonged therapy (17 months), total necrosis and fibrosis of an adenoma may occur.[182] This therapy may reduce the size of large tumors, permitting easier surgical excision, or provide a therapeutic alternative if surgery and radiation have failed to achieve remission. Surgical "cure" is achieved in up to 86% of patients, with an operative morbidity of less than 1%.[193] All macroadenomas should be treated surgically with or without prior bromocriptine therapy, particularly if visual field defects are present. Surgery is not recommended as primary therapy when the serum PRL level is over 500 ng/ml because the expected control rates are low. Bromocriptine treatment (2.5 mg three times daily), followed by surgery and irradiation in some cases, is recommended.

Fertility is improved in most patients with adequate bromocriptine administration; however, controversy exists with regard to appropriate therapy in women wishing to conceive since the normal pituitary almost doubles in size during pregnancy. Within 4 to 8 weeks of beginning bromocriptine therapy, ovulatory menstrual cycles occur; mechanical birth control should be used until PRL levels are normal.

Side effects include nausea, vomiting, and orthostatic hypotension. The hypotension is probably related to splanchnic and renal vasodilatation, inhibition of transmitter release at noradrenergic nerve endings, and central inhibition of sympathetic activity.[33,143] Neuropsychiatric symptoms (e.g., hallucinations) occur with increasing dosage, perhaps related to hydrolysis of the lysergic acid diethylamide (LSD) fragment of the bromocriptine molecule. Other side effects are possible but may not become evident until more experience is accumulated.

Because (1) the long-term effects of bromocriptine are not known, (2) discontinuing therapy does not increase the risk of spontaneous abortion, extrauterine pregnancies, or major or minor congenital malformations,[184,201] and (3) the side effects of the drug may preclude its long-term use, the drug should be stopped during pregnancy unless the tumor is quite large initially or expands sufficiently during pregnancy to produce chiasmatic or optic nerve compression. During pregnancy, repeated visual field examinations should be performed; any new defect or the development of headaches should prompt CT scan evaluation of tumor progression. Steroids and bromocriptine may be used to achieve tumor regression in such circumstances. Rarely, surgical excision of the adenoma may be required.[41]

Bromocriptine-induced rapid tumor shrinkage may lead to CSF rhinorrhea. Perhaps tumor shrinkage allows pulsatile extension of the arachnoid into the now partially empty sella with eventual erosion of the sellar floor and resultant rhinorrhea.[3] A surgically created CSF fistula may develop but not become apparent until bromocriptine-induced tumor retraction occurs postoperatively.[8,18,101]

Bromocriptine may be the treatment of choice in patients who have persistent hyperprolactinemia after surgery as a result of pituitary stalk damage. Postoperative PRL levels are usually higher (11.7 ± 1.5 ng/ml) in patients with relapse than in those without (6.4 ± 1.1 ng/ml). Follow-up for as long as 6 years may be necessary to assess the results of surgical therapy.[32,168] Men may have larger tumors and higher PRL levels preoperatively. The cure rate is much lower than in women; combined bromocriptine and radiotherapy may offer curative treatment.[28]

Clearly, microadenomas associated with PRL levels less than 100 ng/ml have the highest cure rate.[131] Bromocriptine may be the treatment of choice for those over 45 years of age, in combination with close assessment of tumor growth or regression and serum PRL levels. Patients in the 30 to 45 age group with microadenomas present a dilemma; therapy must be individualized.[194] Antiserotonergic compounds (e.g., methysergide and cyproheptadine) also lower PRL levels but have not received widespread clinical evaluation.[190]

PERIOPERATIVE AND ANESTHETIC CONSIDERATIONS

Microadenomas of the pituitary gland are extra-arachnoid tumors, while macroadenomas may extend into the sphenoid sinus, the suprasellar intracranial space, and/or the cavernous sinus. The basic principles of neuroanesthesia apply to all these situations. Regional CBF, autoregulation, and carbon dioxide reactivity have been reported to be normal in patients with pituitary tumors (chromophobe, craniopharyngioma, empty sella).[56] Modifications of the basic technique depend on the size and extension of the tumor and the surgical approach chosen. For example, suprasellar tumor extension may require craniotomy rather than transsphenoidal resection. The potential for greater blood loss and necessity for brain retraction will require anticipation of blood transfusion and osmotic and/or loop diuretic administration. During transsphenoidal surgery, the surgeon may wish to monitor the progress of removal of the suprasellar portion of the tumor by the injection of air or nitrous oxide into a previously placed lumbar subarachnoid malleable needle or catheter. Nitrous oxide should be discontinued during and after such an intraoperative air study. The injection of filtered nitrous oxide–oxygen from the inspired gases can be used without changing intracranial dynamics or anesthetic technique.[122,161] Occasionally a Valsalva maneuver (positive end expiratory pressure in the anesthetized patient) may be requested to bring the tumor into the sella. Intraoperative C-arm fluoroscopy of the skull may eliminate the need for the subarachnoid catheter placement.

If there is lateral extension of the tumor into the cavernous sinuses and the patient is positioned in even a slightly head-up position, the anesthesiologist must be prepared for excessive blood loss and/or air embolism. Additional intravenous access routes, precordial Doppler, end-tidal CO_2 and end-tidal N_2 monitoring, and central catheter placement at the superior vena cava–right atrial junction may be indicated.[133] Air embolism is quite rare if the gradient between the heart and operative field is 15 degrees or less. Placing the table in a horizontal position can immediately reduce air entry.

If excessive bleeding from the cavernous sinus occurs, it may be difficult to control. Temporary or permanent packing of the sinus may be necessary. Such pressure may result in partial or complete occlusion of the intracavernous portion of the internal carotid artery and pressure on the third, fourth, fifth, and sixth cranial nerves. Postoperative ophthalmoplegia, facial anesthesia, and contralateral hemiparesis or hemiplegia may result from direct pressure or vasospasm.[25,197] An anesthetic technique that would permit intraoperative EEG or evoked potential monitoring in vulnerable patients is the ideal. There has been no reported experience with the administration or efficacy of protective doses of barbiturates in such circumstances, but they would presumably be most effective if given before carotid occlusion.

The anesthetic technique should also permit gross visual acuity evaluation before patient extubation. If vision is improved or is not worse, extubation can proceed. If acuity is worsened, further diagnostic studies and decompressive surgery may be required on an emergent basis. An anesthetic technique that can be used in a great majority of patients without causing coughing involves the use of narcotic, nitrous oxide, and muscle relaxants. The patient is informed of the planned examination before surgery. Local anesthesia is injected into the sublabial incision just before closure. When the nitrous oxide is discontinued the patient can open the eyes on request and is usually cooperative enough to count fingers; each eye can then be examined separately.

Postoperative CSF rhinorrhea is rare, but some patients with pituitary tumors initially have a CSF leak. Since, in the presence of a CSF leak, there is atmosphere-to-subarachnoid communication and, most probably, nitrogen in the subarachnoid space, nitrous oxide use should be avoided. This also applies to CSF otorrhea secondary to basilar skull fractures. Occasionally, continuous closed system or intermittent CSF drainage via a lumbar subarachnoid catheter or repeated lumbar punctures will allow the leak to seal.

Many surgeons use epinephrine-containing local anesthetics and cocaine as part of their presurgical preparation. The use of these solutions may lead to dysrhythmias in the presence or absence of volatile agents; cocaine may cause greater dysrhythmogenicity since epinephrine reuptake is blocked at the nerve endings. Patients receiving acute or chronic beta-blocker therapy may have alarming and dangerous hypertension as a result of the unopposed alpha action of epinephrine. Total spinal anesthesia may occur if the cribriform plate and arachnoid are penetrated with the local anesthetic mixture. In the anesthetized patient, hypotension, bradycardia, and increased alveolar deadspace would be detected (decreased end tidal CO_2, increased $Paco_2$). Continued ventilatory support, atropine, and fluid volume should be administered.[77]

Hypertension and bothersome bleeding during intrasellar exploration can be effectively controlled with adequate local anesthetic infiltration of the nasal passages combined with appropriate anesthetic depth and, in some instances, intravenous administration of peripheral vasodilators (e.g., nitroglycerin, nitroprusside, hydralazine).[2]

Nasogastric tubes should not be inserted in patients with anterior fossa fractures or pituitary tumors. Large tumors may erode the sella and the sphenoid sinus, permitting direct intracranial penetration by nasogastric and suction catheters with potentially disastrous complications. Placement of such tubes should be avoided entirely or accomplished via the mouth under direct vision; gastrostomy is indicated in patients requiring long-term feeding.[65]

Airway difficulties are discussed in regard to acromegaly later in the text. Rarely, preadolescent GH deficiency and resulting retarded cartilaginous growth may lead to the persistence of a juvenile airway. Preoperative indirect airway evaluation permits selection of an array of endotracheal tubes appropriate for such patients.[189]

Patients are instructed preoperatively that mouth breathing will be required in the postoperative period because of bilateral nasal packs. Prolonged mouth breathing requires airway humidification. Silastic stents or Foley catheters in the nares may permit breathing through the nasal passages but do not obviate the need for humidification, which improves oxygenation.[34,39]

The carotid arteries bulge within the sphenoid sinus in 71% of cases[155] and may approach the midline (as close as 4 mm) or be in the sella. It is important that the approach to the sella be in the midline. Rarely, hemorrhage, delayed development of a carotid cavernous fistula, or intracavernous traumatic aneurysm may require elective or emergency cervical carotid ligation, balloon occlusion, or trapping.[24,123,151]

Endocrinologic Considerations

Under maximal exogenous ACTH stimulation, normal adrenal glands secrete 116 to 185 mg of cortisol per day; maximum stress can lead to excretion of 200 to 500 mg daily. Normally, the maximal plasma cortisol during major surgery varies between 22 and 75 μg/dl, mean 47; the value remains above 26 μg/dl for up to 72 hours postoperatively. During minor surgery, the range is 10 to 44 μg/dl.[23,148,149]

Intramuscular cortisone acetate (100 mg) given to patients with adrenal insufficiency raises plasma cortisol to 10 to 25 μg/dl (mean 19 μg/dl), which is less than half of that required during major surgery in normal patients. Intramuscular or intravenous hydrocortisone (100 mg) produces plasma cortisol concentrations of approximately 30 and 18 μg/dl respectively at 6 hours. Patients with anterior pituitary insufficiency require daily oral prednisone therapy of 5 mg in the AM and 2.5 mg in the PM. If previous adrenalectomy has been done, oral mineralocorticoid replacement (0.1 mg [Florinef] fludrocortisone) is necessary.

Intraoperatively, many methods have been used to replace glucocorticoids in the presence of actual or potential anterior pituitary insufficiency. Hydrocortisone 50 to 100 mg intravenously immediately before the induction of anesthesia may be followed by 10 mg per hour (100 mg in 500 ml normal saline) for the duration of the surgical procedure and continued until oral intake is resumed. The reader is referred to a recent summary for additional therapeutic recommendations.[130] Tapering schedules are individ-

ualized. Patients with Cushing disease may have adrenal insufficiency for several months after pituitary tumor resection. Most patients with microadenomas will not require steroid therapy after the third or fourth postoperative day.

Oral thyroid replacement therapy, levothyroxine (Synthroid) 0.10 to 0.15 mg daily, is indicated in patients with panhypopituitarism. L-thyroxine 500 μg (7-8 μg/kg body weight) may be given intravenously and continued at 1-1.3 μg/kg at 24 hour intervals in patients with severe hypothyroidism. The management of hyperglycemia should follow guidelines recommended for patients with diabetes mellitus.[4,78]

Diabetes Insipidus Treatment

Diabetes insipidus is managed preoperatively by a twice daily intranasal installation of synthetic vasopressin (desmopressin [DDAVP]) 0.0005 ml[107] or with other agents that potentiate endogenous ADH action (chlorpropamide, clofibrate, or carbamazepine). Aqueous vasopressin 0.5 ml (10 U) can be given every 4 to 6 hours subcutaneously intraoperatively. Diabetes insipidus (DI) rarely occurs intraoperatively in previously asymptomatic patients although it has occurred in this and other authors' experience.[121] For this reason, it is advantageous to monitor urine volume, specific gravity, and serum electrolytes during the intraoperative and postoperative periods.

The differential diagnosis includes diuresis from mannitol, glucose, or excessive crystalloid administration, but DI can be suspected if the surgery is in the region of the sella or hypothalamus or if the patient had partial DI preoperatively. In the absence of renal ADH effect, the urine volume may be as high as 1 to 2 L per hour, the urine osmolality will be less than 200 mOsm/L (usually between 50 and 150 mOsm/L) and the specific gravity between 1.001 and 1.005. The urine-to-serum osmolality ratio will be less than 1 because of the pure water diuresis. If salt-containing fluids have been administered during the diuresis, the serum may be severely hyperosmolar (>320 mOsm/L).

If the diuresis is severe, the amount of intravenous glucose in the water replacement leads to hyperglycemia and osmotic diuresis with concomitant sodium loss. Brain edema may occur, since blood glucose falls more rapidly than brain glucose. An osmotic gradient is established, causing net water influx into the brain. In addition, there is concern that elevated blood glucose may cause a worse outcome if cerebral ischemia should occur.

When urinary volumes are excessive and the patient is unable to drink water, the administration of exogenous vasopressin is indicated (aqueous vasopressin 5 to 10 U [0.25 to 0.5 ml] subcutaneously every 4 hours). Fluids are prescribed to include maintenance plus the previous hour's urine output, plus blood and evaporative losses if surgery is still in progress. Serum and urine osmolality, Na$^+$, K$^+$, and glucose determinations will guide therapy. If serum hyperosmolality is already present as a result of water losses and replacement with sodium-containing fluids, the water deficit may be calculated as follows:

- Normal serum sodium = 140 mEq/L
- 60% body weight = Total body water
- Sodium acts as if distributed in total body water
- 70 kg with serum sodium 160 mEq/L
- Total body water = .60 × 70 = 42 L
- Total body sodium predicted = 42 × 140 = 5880 mEq

$$\frac{5880 \text{ mEq}}{160 \text{ mEq/L}} = 36.7 \text{ L}$$

- Water deficit = 42 − 36.7 = 5.3 L

Replacement of half the deficit should proceed, and the need for further therapy should be reevaluated in 1 to 2 hours. Since up to 40% of patients develop transient DI within the first 24 hours postoperatively, aqueous vasopressin (10 U subcutaneously) every 4 to 6 hours is administered, or vasopressin tannate-in-oil (1 ml intramuscularly) every 24 to 48 hours can be used. Water intoxication and hyponatremia may occur if endogenous ADH production resumes before dissipation of the effect of the long-acting drug. When the nasal packing is removed (generally third to fourth day), desmopressin therapy can be prescribed in patients with permanent, partial, or complete DI. Mild DI may be controlled with agents that potentiate the renal effects of ADH—chlorpropamide or clofibrate (Atromid-S).

Acromegaly and the Airway

Airway management difficulties in patients with acromegaly are related to hypertrophy of the facial bones (particularly the mandible), the large bulbous nose, thick tongue and lips, and hypertrophy of the nasal turbinates, soft palate, tonsils, epiglottis, and larynx. These abnormalities may cause difficulties with mask fit and with visualization of the larynx. Glottic stenosis caused by soft tissue overgrowth may cause preoperative hoarseness and dyspnea, and can predispose to postextubation edema. Vocal cord paralysis may be present as a result of stretching of the recurrent laryngeal nerve following laryngeal soft tissue enlargement, impaired mobility of the cricoarytenoid joints, or compression of the recurrent nerves by thyroid enlargement.[20,62,70,94] Only oral intubation can be considered for transsphenoidal surgery since a nasal tube would obstruct the surgical field.

Thorough preoperative evaluation of the airway is mandatory. Patients without hoarseness, dyspnea, or acromegalic stigmata can be managed in the routine manner. Those with glottic abnormalities should be electively intubated with the aid of a fiberoptic laryngoscope. Whether this must be done in the awake or anesthetized state will depend on the degree of laryngeal involvement evaluated by indirect laryngoscopy and by the presence of hypertension and cardiac involvement. If an atraumatic intubation is carried out (conventional or fiberoptic), the need for tracheostomy can be eliminated.[120,139,174,188]

Since bone hypertrophy occurs with acromegaly, patients may present with spinal stenosis as a result of hyper-

trophied laminae and facet joints. This condition has been reported in the lumbar area.[46] The cervical spinal cord may be affected as well, especially if age-related degenerative spondylosis is also present. In some cases, decompressive laminectomy may be necessary if myelopathy, paraparesis, or urinary incontinence occurs. Whether this precedes pituitary adenoma excision will depend on the severity of the myelopathic symptoms and the general condition of the patient.

VISUAL EVOKED RESPONSES

It is not clear whether the visual disturbances caused by pituitary tumors are related to direct compression of the chiasm or its blood supply.[19] Variations in stimulus and recording parameters have led to confusion regarding the clinical usefulness of intraoperative visual evoked responses in conditions other than multiple sclerosis.[67]

Feinsod et al.[49] and others have documented reversible prolongation of visual evoked response latency and deterioration of the waveforms related to manipulation and retraction of the chiasm and optic nerves. In addition, early improvement can be demonstrated with operative decompression of the chiasm and nerves.[49,198] Visual evoked responses also provide earlier evidence of optic nerve or chiasmal involvement than conventional visual testing in patients with pituitary tumors.[60] Fluid aspiration from a cystic craniopharyngioma has caused rapid improvement in visual evoked responses within 3 hours.[66]

Volatile anesthetic agents cause dose-related prolongation of the latency of visual evoked responses in normal patients.[185] Barbiturates enhance and abolish the cortical visual evoked response at low and high doses, respectively. Nitrous oxide has little effect. Premedicant drugs alter visual evoked responses as well.[40] Morphine has little effect, while sedatives tend to produce changes typical of natural sleep. A narcotic-based anesthetic has been shown to permit adequate responses to be measured.

Technical difficulties also preclude routine use of visual evoked responses intraoperatively (e.g., small pupil size, deviation of the eyes [which can be overcome with stimulus delivery through the closed eyelid], and the unavailability of goggles adequate for stimulus delivery but with minimal intrusion into the operative field or potential pressure on or abrasion of the globe).[5,63,152] There is concern that direct pressure on the globe can lead to blindness. Anemia and hypoxia may also adversely effect visual evoked responses and/or somatosensory evoked responses.[64,129]

HYPOPHYSECTOMY AND PAIN

Total hypophysectomy with low stalk section[7,144,181] (to avoid DI), chemical hypophysectomy[92] (stereotactic injection of 100% ethyl alcohol), and pituitary radiation[125] have been used in the therapy of narcotic-refractory pain from metastatic prostatic, renal, breast, and lung cancer. Pain relief and regression of bone metastases can be transient or long-term in these ultimately fatal conditions. Improved life-style and reduced narcotic dependency are advantageous. Pain relief occurs without regression of the primary tumor and occurs immediately or within 24 hours of the hypophysectomy. Successful pain relief is not limited to patients with hormonally dependent tumors.

The pituitary has the highest brain concentration of beta endorphins, which may be released during operative manipulation of the tumor but would not account for the long-term pain relief. Opiate receptor hypersensitivity, perhaps as a result of the absence of pituitary hormonal effect on opiate receptors, has been suggested as a possible mechanism. No prolonged increase in CSF endorphins has been demonstrated and naloxone administration does not reverse the pain relief. Pain relief can occur in the absence of tumor regression or total pituitary ablation.[103]

With total pituitary ablation, there may be no DI if glucocorticoids are not replaced or if stalk section preserves the median eminence. Recent studies have demonstrated that preservation of the posterior pituitary, stalk, and, most importantly, the inferior hypophyseal arteries which supply blood to structures that produce, transport, and store ADH, significantly reduces the incidence of permanent DI following selective anterior hypophysectomy.[108]

▼

SUMMARY

In summary, the anatomy, physiology, pathophysiology, and perioperative management of patients with pituitary tumors needs to be evaluated individually. The resurgence of transsphenoidal surgery, the addition of microsurgical and fluoroscopic controls, and the contribution of modern neuroanesthesia to perioperative management have made a significant impact on the lives and well-being of these patients.

References

1. Abboud CF, Laws ER: Clinical endocrinological approach to hypothalamic-pituitary disease, *J Neurosurg* 51:271-291, 1979.
2. Abou-Madi MN, Trop D, Barnes J: Aetiology and control of cardiovascular reactions during transsphenoidal resection of pituitary microadenomas, *Can Anaesth Soc J* 27:491-495, 1980.
3. Afshar F, Thomas A: Bromocriptine-induced cerebrospinal fluid rhinorrhea, *Surg Neurol* 18:61-63,1982.
4. Alberti KGMM: Diabetes and surgery, *Anesthesiology* 74:209-211, 1991.
5. Allen A, Starr A, Nudelman K: Assessment of sensory function in the operating room utilizing cerebral evoked potentials: a study of fifty-six surgically anesthetized patients, *Clin Neurosurg* 28:457-481, 1981.
6. Altinors N, Arda N, Kars Z et al: Tension pneumocephalus after transsphenoidal surgery. Case report, *Neurosurgery* 23:516-518, 1988.
7. Angell-James J: Transethmosphenoidal hypophysectomy, *Arch Otolaryngol* 86:256-264, 1967.
8. Aronoff SL, Daughaday WH, Laws ER: Bromocriptine treatment of prolactinomas, *N Engl J Med* 300:1391, 1979.
9. Aubry RH, Nankin HR, Moses AM et al: Measurement of the osmotic threshold for vasopressin release in

human subjects and its modification by cortisol, *J Clin Endocrinol Metab* 25:1481-1492, 1965.
10. Balagura S, Derome P, Guiot G: Acromegaly: analysis of 132 cases treated surgically, *Neurosurgery* 8:413-416, 1981.
11. Balagura S, Frantz AG, Housepian EM et al: The specificity of serum prolactin as a diagnostic indicator of pituitary adenoma, *J Neurosurg* 51:42-46, 1979.
12. Barker JL, Crayton JW, Nicoll RA: Noradrenalin and acetylcholine responses of supraoptic neurosecretory cells, *J Physiol* 218:19-32, 1971.
13. Barraclough MA, Jones NF: The effect of vasopressin on the reabsorption of sodium, potassium and urea by the renal tubules in man, *Clin Sci* 39:517-529, 1970.
14. Barrow DL, Tindall GT, Kovacs K et al: Clinical and pathological effects of bromocriptine on prolactin secreting and other pituitary tumors, *J Neurosurg* 60:1-7, 1984.
15. Barrow DL, Mizuno J, Tindall GT: Management of prolactinomas associated with very high serum prolactin levels, *J Neurosurg* 68:554-558, 1988.
16. Baskin DS, Boggan JE, Wilson CB: Transsphenoidal microsurgical removal of growth hormone-secreting pituitary adenomas, *J Neurosurg* 56:634-641, 1982.

17. Baskin DS, Wilson CB: Bromocriptine treatment of pituitary adenomas, *Neurosurgery* 8:741-744, 1981.
18. Baskin DS, Wilson CB: CSF rhinorrhea after bromocriptine for prolactinoma, *N Engl J Med* 306:178, 1982.
19. Bergland R, Ray BS: The arterial supply of the human optic chiasm, *J Neurosurg* 31:327-334, 1969.
20. Bhatia ML, Misra SC, Parkash J: Laryngeal manifestations in acromegaly, *J Laryngol Otol* 80:412-417, 1966.
21. Braverman LE, Mancini JP, McGoldrick DM: Hereditary idiopathic diabetes insipidus: a case report with autopsy findings, *Ann Intern Med* 63:503-508, 1965.
22. Burrow GN, Wortzman G, Newcastle NB et al: Microadenomas of the pituitary and abnormal sella tomograms in an unselected autopsy series, *N Engl J Med* 304:156-158, 1981.
23. Byyny RL: Preventing adrenal insufficiency during surgery, *Postgrad Med* 67:219-225, 1980.
24. Cabezudo JM, Carrillo R, Vaquero J et al: Intracavernous aneurysm of the carotid artery following transsphenoidal surgery, *J Neurosurg* 54:118-121, 1981.
25. Camp PE, Paxton HD, Buchan GC et al: Vasospasm after transsphenoidal hypophysectomy, *Neurosurgery* 7:382-386, 1980.

26. Campkin TV: Radial artery cannulation: potential hazards in patients with acromegaly, *Anaesthesia* 35:1008-1009, 1980.

27. Carazzuti V, Fischer EG, Welch K et al: Neurologic and psychophysiological sequelae following different treatments of craniopharyngioma in children, *J Neurosurg* 59:409-417, 1983.

28. Carter JN, Tyson JE, Tolis G et al: Prolactin-secreting tumors and hypogonadism in 22 men, *N Engl J Med* 299:847-852, 1978.

29. Cheng KW, Martin JB, Friesen HG: Studies of neurophysin release, *Endocrinology* 91:177-184, 1972.

30. Christy NP: Choosing the best treatment for acromegaly, *JAMA* 247:1320, 1982.

31. Chrousos GP, Schuhe HM, Oldfield EH et al: The corticotrophin-releasing factor stimulation test: an aid in the evaluation of patients with Cushing's syndrome, *N Engl J Med* 310:622-626, 1984.

32. Ciric I, Mikhael M, Stafford T et al: Transsphenoidal microsurgery of pituitary macroadenomas with longterm follow up results, *J Neurosurg* 59:395-401, 1983.

33. Clark BJ, Scholtysik G, Fluckiger E: Cardiovascular actions of bromocriptine, *Acta Endocrinol* 216 (suppl):75-81, 1978.

34. Cook TA, Komorn RM: Statistical analysis of the alterations in blood gases produced by nasal packing, *Laryngoscope* 83:1802-1809, 1973.

35. Cryer PE, Daughaday WH: Growth hormone. In Martin L, Besser C, editors: *Clinical endocrinology,* New York, 1977, Academic Press.

36. Danneshdoost L, Gennarelli TA, Bashey HM et al: Recognition of gonadotroph adenomas in women, *N Engl J Med* 324:589-594, 1991.

37. Davies C, Jacobi J, Lloyd HM et al: DNA synthesis and the secretion of prolactin and growth hormone by pituitary gland of the male rate: effects of diethylstilbesterol and 2-bromoergocryptine methane sulphonate, *J Endocrinol* 61:411-417, 1974.

38. Dawson DM, Dingman JF: Hazards of protonbeam pituitary irradiation, *N Engl J Med* 282:1434, 1970.

39. deFigueiredo DG, deCarvalho FFL: Balloon tamponade of the pharynx in transsphenoidal operations: technical note, *Neurosurgery* 8:567-568, 1981.

40. Domino EG: Effects of preanesthetic and anesthetic drugs on visually evoked responses, *Anesthesiology* 28:184-191, 1967.

41. Dommerholt HBR, Assies J, vander-Werf AJM: Growth of a prolactinoma during pregnancy, *Br J Obstet Gyn* 88:62-70, 1981.

42. Douglas W: How do neurons secrete peptides? Exocytosis and its consequences, including "synaptic vesicle" formation in the hypothalamo-neurohypophyseal system, *Prog Brain Res* 39:21-39, 1973.

43. Eastman RC, Gorden P, Roth J: Conventional supervoltage irradiation is an effective treatment for acromegaly, *J Clin Endocrinol Metab* 48:931-940, 1979.

44. Ebersold MJ, Laws ER, Scheithauer BW et al: Pituitary apoplexy treated by transsphenoidal surgery, *J Neurosurg* 58:315-320, 1983.

45. Edis AJ: Prevention and management of complications associated with thyroid and parathyroid surgery, *Surg Clin N Am* 59:83-88, 1979.

46. Epstein N, Whelan M, Benjamin V: Acromegaly and spinal stenosis, *J Neurosurg* 56:145-147, 1982.

47. Evans HM, Briggs JH, Dixon JS: The physiology and chemistry of growth hormone. In Harris GW, Donovan BT, editors: *The pituitary gland,* Berkeley, 1966, University of California Press, pp 439-491.

48. Faria MA, Tindall GT: Transsphenoidal microsurgery for prolactin-secreting pituitary adenomas, *J Neurosurg* 56:33-43, 1982.

49. Feinsod M, Selhorst JB, Hoyt WF et al: Monitoring optic nerve function during craniotomy, *J Neurosurg* 55:29-31, 1976.

50. Findling JW, Tyrrell JB, Aron DC et al: Silent pituitary apoplexy: subclinical infarction of an adrenocorticotropin-producing pituitary adenoma, *J Clin Endocrinol Metab* 52:95-97, 1981.

51. Forbes AP, Henneman PH, Griswold GC et al: Syndrome characterized by galactorrhea, amenorrhea and low urinary FSH: comparison with acromegaly and normal lactation, *J Clin Endocrinol Metab* 14:265-271, 1954.

52. Frantz AG: The assay and regulation of prolactin in humans, *Adv Exp Med Biol* 80:95-133, 1977.

53. Frantz AG: Prolactin, *N Engl J Med* 298:201-207, 1978.

54. Friesen H, Guyda H, Hwang P et al: Functional evaluation of prolactin secretion: a guide to therapy, *J Clin Invest* 51:706-709, 1972.

55. Garcia-Uria J: Surgical experience with craniopharyngioma in adults, *Surg Neurol* 9:11-14, 1978.

56. Gelmers HJ, Beks JWF, Doorenbos H: Regional cerebral blood flow studies in patients with pituitary tumours, *Acta Neurochir* 51:87-90, 1979.

57. Giesecke K, Hamberger B, Jarnberg PO et al: Paravertebral block during cholecystectomy: effects on circulatory and hormonal responses, *Brit J Anaesth* 61:652-656, 1988.

58. Gonzales-Villapando C, Szabo M, Frohman LA: Central nervous system-mediated stimulation of prolactin secretion by cimetidine, a histamine H2-receptor antagonist: impaired responsiveness in patients with prolactin-secreting tumors and idiopathic hyperprolactinemia, *J Clin Endocrinol Metab* 51:1417-1424, 1980.

59. Gorczyca W, Hardy J: Microadenomas of the human pituitary and their vascularization, *Neurosurgery* 22:1-6, 1988.

60. Gott PS, Weiss MH, Apuzzo M et al: Checkerboard visual evoked response in evaluation and management of pituitary tumors, *Neurosurgery* 5:553-558, 1979.

61. Green H, Harrington AR, Valtin H: On the role of antidiuretic hormone in the inhibition of acute water diuresis in adrenal insufficiency and the effects of gluco and mineralocorticoids in reversing the inhibition, *J Clin Invest* 49:1724-1736, 1970.

62. Grotting J, Pemberton J: Fixation of the vocal cords in acromegaly, *Arch Otolaryngol* 52:608-617, 1950.

63. Grundy BL: Monitoring of sensory evoked potentials during neurosurgical operations: methods and applications, *Neurosurgery* 11:556-575, 1982.

64. Grundy BL, Heros RC, Tung AS et al: Intraoperative hypoxia detected by evoked potential monitoring, *Anesth Analg* 60:437-439, 1981.

65. Guerra B, Slade TL, Kelly PJ: Intracranial introduction of a nasogastric tube in a patient with a pituitary tumor, *Surg Neurol* 12:135-136, 1979.

66. Gutin PH, Klemme WM, Lagger RL

et al: Management of the unresectable cystic craniopharyngioma by aspiration through an Ommaya reservoir drainage system, *J Neurosurg* 52:36-40, 1980.

67. Halliday AM, McDonald WI, Mushin J: Delayed visual evoked response in optic neuritis, *Lancet* 1:982-985, 1972.

68. Haney AF, Kramer RS, Wiebe RH et al: Hypothalamic-pituitary function and radiographic evaluation of women with hyperprolactinemia and an "empty" sella turcica, *Am J Obstet Gynecol* 134:917-924, 1979.

69. Hardy J: The transsphenoidal surgical approach to the pituitary, *Hosp Pract* 7:81-89, 1979.

70. Hassan SZ, Matz GJ, Lawrence AM et al: Laryngeal stenosis in acromegaly: a possible cause of airway difficulties associated with anesthesia, *Anesth Analg* 55:57-60, 1976.

71. Hayward JN: Neural control of the posterior pituitary, *Ann Rev Physiol* 37:191-210, 1975.

72. Hays RM: Antidiuretic hormone, *N Engl J Med* 295:659-665, 1976.

73. Hays RM, Levine SD: Vasopressin, *Kidney Int* 6:307-322, 1974.

74. Healy DL, Burger HG: Sustained elevation of serum prolactin by metoclopramide: a clinical model of hyperprolactinemia, *J Clin Endocrinol Metab* 46:709-714, 1978.

75. Hermus AR, Pieters GF, Smals AG et al: Transition from pituitary-dependent to adrenal-dependent Cushing's syndrome, *N Engl J Med* 318:966-970, 1988.

76. Hill SA, Falko JM, Wilson CB et al: Thyrotrophin-producing pituitary adenomas, *J Neurosurg* 57:515-519, 1982.

77. Hill JN, Gershon NI, Gargiulo PO: Total spinal blockade during local anesthesia of the nasal passages, *Anesthesiology* 59:144-146, 1983.

78. Hirsch IB, McGill JB, Cryer PE et al: Perioperative management of surgical patients with diabetes mellitus, *Anesthesiology* 74:346-359, 1991.

79. Hoffman HJ, DeSilva M, Humphreys RP et al: Aggressive surgical management of craniopharyngiomas in children, *J Neurosurg* 76:47-52, 1992.

80. Holness RO, Ogundimu FA, Langille RA: Pituitary apoplexy following closed head trauma, *J Neurosurg* 59:677-679, 1983.

81. Houser OW, Baker HL, Reese DF et al: Radiographic induction of the sella turcica and the pituitary gland. In Laws ER, Randall RV, Kern EB et al, editors: *Management of pituitary adenomas and related lesions,* New York, 1982, Appleton-Century-Crofts, pp 81-109.

82. Humphreys RP, Hoffman HJ, Hendrick EB: A long term postoperative follow up in craniopharyngioma, *Childs Brain* 5:530-539, 1979.

83. Hwang P, Guyda H, Friesen H: A radioimmunoassay for human prolactin, *Proc Natl Acad Sci* 68:1902-1906, 1971.

84. Johnson MD, Park CS, Malvin RL: Antidiuretic hormone and the distribution of renal cortical blood flow, *Am J Physiol* 232:111-116, 1977.

85. Johnston DG, Hall K, McGregor A et al: Bromocriptine therapy for "nonfunctioning" pituitary tumors, *Am J Med* 71:1059-1061, 1981.

86. Joplin GF, Cassar J, Doyle FH et al: Treatment of pituitary tumors by interstitial irradiation. In Derome PJ, Jedynak CP, Peillon F, editors: *Pituitary adenomas: biology, physiopathology, and treatment,* Second European Workshop, La Pitie-Saltpetriere, Paris, 1980, Asclepios Publishers, pp 219-222.

87. Jordan RM, Kendall JW, McDonald SD: CSF prolactin determination in patients following operation for pituitary tumor, *Surg Neurol* 14:387-391, 1980.

88. Kachadorian WA, Wade JB, DiScala VA: Vasopressin induced structural changes in toad bladder luminal membrane, *Science* 190:67-69, 1975.

89. Kapcala LP, Molitch ME, Post KD et al: Galactorrhea, oligo/amenorrhea, and hyperprolactinemia in patients with craniopharyngiomas, *J Clin Endocrinol Metab* 51:798-800, 1980.

90. Kataja J, Viinamaki O, Punnonen R et al: Reni-angiotensin-aldosterone system and plasma vasopressin in surgical patients anaesthetized with halothane or isoflurane, *Eur J Anaesthiol* 5:121-129, 1988.

91. Kato Y, Nakai Y, Imura H et al: Effect of 5-hydroxytryptophan (5-HTP) on plasma prolactin levels in man, *J Clin Endocrinol Metab* 38:695-697, 1974.

92. Katz J, Levin AB: Long-term follow up study of chemical hypophysectomy and additional cases, *Anesthesiology* 51:167-169, 1979.

93. Kern EB, Laws ER: The rationale and technique of selective transsphenoidal microsurgery for the removal of pituitary tumors. In Laws ER, Randall RV, Kern EB et al, editors: *Management of pituitary adenomas and related lesions,* New York, 1982, Appleton-Century-Crofts, pp 219-244.

94. Kitahata LM: Airway difficulties associated with anaesthesia in acromegaly, *Br J Anaesth* 43:1187-1190, 1971.

95. Kleeman CR, Fichman MP: The clinical physiology of water metabolism, *N Engl J Med* 277:1300-1307, 1964.

96. Klibanski A, Neer RM, Beitins IZ et al: Decreased bone density in hyperprolactinemic women, *N Engl J Med* 303:1511-1514, 1980.

97. Klibanski A, Ridgway EC, Zervas NT: Pure alpha sub-unit-secreting pituitary tumors, *J Neurosurg* 59:585-589, 1983.

98. Klibanski A, Zervas NT: Diagnosis and management of hormone-secreting pituitary adenomas, *N Engl J Med* 324:822-831, 1991.

99. Kontogeorgos G, Kovacs K, Horvath E et al: Multiple adenomas of the pituitary, *J Neurosurg* 74:243-247, 1991.

100. Lamberts SWJ, Bakker WH, Reubi JC et al: Somatostatin-receptor imaging in the localization of endocrine tumors, *N Engl J Med* 323:1246-1249, 1990.

101. Landolt AM: Cerebrospinal fluid rhinorrhea: a complication of therapy for invasive prolactinomas, *Neurosurgery* 11:395-401, 1982.

102. Larsen PR: Thyroid-pituitary interaction, *N Engl J Med* 306:23-32, 1982.

103. LaRossa JT, Strong MS, Melby JC: Endocrinologically incomplete transethmoidal trans-sphenoidal hypophysectomy with relief of bone pain in breast cancer, *N Engl J Med* 298:1332-1335, 1978.

104. Lascelles PT, Lewis PD: Hypodipsia and hypernatremia associated with hypothalamic and suprasellar lesions, *Brain* 95:249-264, 1972.

105. Lawrence JH, Chong CY, Lyman JT et al: Treatment of pituitary tumors with heavy particles. In Kohler PO,

Ross GT, editors: *Diagnosis and treatment of pituitary tumors,* International Congress Series 303, New York, 1973, American Elsevier, pp 253-262.

106. Laws ER: Transsphenoidal microsurgery in the management of craniopharyngioma, *J Neurosurg* 52:661-666, 1980.

107. Laws ER, Abboud CF, Kern EB: Perioperative management of patients with pituitary adenomas, *Neurosurgery* 7:566-570, 1980.

108. Leclercq TA, Grisoli F: Avoidance of diabetes insipidus in transsphenoidal hypophysectomy: a modified technique of selective hypophysectomy, *J Neurosurg* 58:682-684, 1983.

109. Levine S, Franki N, Hays RM : Effect of phloretin on water and solute movement in the toad bladder, *J Clin Invest* 52:1435-1442, 1973.

110. Lie JT, Grossman SJ: Pathology of the heart in acromegaly: anatomic findings in 27 autopsied patients, *Am Heart J* 100:41-52, 1980.

111. Lindholm J, Riishede J, Vestergaard S et al: No effect of bromocriptine in acromegaly: a controlled trial, *N Engl J Med* 304:1450-1454, 1981.

112. Ludecke DK: Intraoperative measurement of adrenocorticotropin in peripituitary blood in Cushing's disease, *Neurosurgery* 24:201-205, 1989.

113. Lundberg PO, Osterman PO, Wide L: Serum prolactin in patients with hypothalamus and pituitary disorders, *J Neurosurg* 55:194-199, 1981.

114. Magoun HW, Ranson SW: Retrograde degeneration of the supraoptic nuclei after section of the infundibular stalk in the monkey, *Anat Rec* 75:107-123, 1939.

115. Malarkey WB: Prolactin and the diagnosis of pituitary tumors, *Ann Rev Med* 30:249-258, 1979.

116. Manelfe C, Louvet JP, Boulard C et al: Hypothalamic-pituitary changes in diabetes insipidus demonstrated by computerized tomography, *Lancet* 2:1379-1380, 1978.

117. McCutcheon IE, Weintraub BD, Oldfield EH: Surgical treatment of thyrotropin pituitary adenomas, *J Neurosurg* 73:674-683, 1990.

118. McGregor AM, Scanlon MF, Hall K et al: Reduction in size of a pituitary tumor by bromocriptine therapy, *N Engl J Med* 300:291-293, 1979.

119. Melmed S: Acromegaly, *N Engl J Med* 322:966-977, 1990.

120. Messick JM, Cucchiara RF, Faust RJ: Airway management in patients with acromegaly, *Anesthesiology* 56:157, 1982.

121. Messick JM, Faust RJ, Cucchiara RF: Anesthesia for transsphenoidal microsurgery. In Laws ER, Randall RV, Kern EB et al, editors: *Management of pituitary adenomas and related lesions,* New York, 1982, Appleton-Century-Crofts, pp 253-261.

122. Messick JM, Laws ER, Abboud CF: Anesthesia for transsphenoidal surgery of the hypophyseal region, *Anes Analg* 57:206-215, 1978.

123. Moore D, Budde RB, Hunter CR et al: Massive epistaxis from aneurysm of the carotid artery, *Surg Neurol* 11:115-117, 1979.

124. Moore-Ede MC, Czeisler CA, Richardson GS: Circadian timekeeping in health and disease, *N Engl J Med* 309:469-476, 530-536, 1983.

125. Morales A, Blair DW, Steyn J: Yttrium pituitary ablation in advanced carcinoma of the prostate, *Br J Urol* 43:520-522, 1971.

126. Moses AM, Miller M: Urine and plasma osmolality in differentiation of polyuric states, *Postgrad Med* 52:187-190, 1972.

127. Moses AM, Miller M, Streeten DHP: Pathophysiologic and pharmacologic alterations in the release and action of ADH, *Metabolism* 25:697-721, 1976.

128. Moses AC, Molitch ME, Sawin CT et al: Bromocriptine therapy in acromegaly: use in patients resistant to conventional therapy and effect on serum levels of somatomedin C, *J Clin Endocrinol Metab* 53:752-758, 1981.

129. Nagao S, Roccaforte P, Moody RA: The effects of isovolemic hemodilution and reinfusion of packed erythrocytes on somatosensory and visual evoked potentials, *J Surg Res* 25:530-537, 1978.

130. Napolitano LM, Chernow B: Guidelines for corticosteroid use in anesthetic and surgical stress, *Int Anesthesiol Clin* 26:226-232, 1988.

131. Nelson PB, Goodman M, Maroon JC et al: Factors in predicting outcome from operation in patients with prolactin-secreting pituitary adeno-

mas, *Neurosurgery* 13:634-641, 1983.

132. Nelson PB, Goodman ML, Flickenger JC et al: Endocrine function in patients with large pituitary tumors treated with operative decompression and radiation therapy, *Neurosurgery* 24:398-400, 1989.

133. Newfield P, Albin M, Chestnut JS et al: Air embolism during transsphenoidal pituitary operations, *Neurosurgery* 2:39-42, 1978.

134. Noreng MF, Jensen P, Tjellden NU: Pre- and postoperative changes in the concentration of serum thyreotropin under general anaesthesia, compared to general anaesthesia with epidural analgesia, *Acta Anaesthesiol Scand* 31:292-294, 1987.

135. Oldfield EH, Doppman JL, Nieman LK et al: Petrosal sinus sampling with and without corticotropin-releasing hormone for the differential diagnosis of Cushing's syndrome, *N Engl J Med* 325:897-905, 1991.

136. Orloff J, Handler JS: The cellular mode of action of antidiuretic hormone, *Am J Med* 36:686-697,1964.

137. Orth DN: The old and new in Cushing's syndrome, *N Engl J Med* 310:649-651, 1984.

138. Orth DN: Differential diagnosis of Cushing's syndrome, *N Engl J Med* 325:957-959 1991.

139. Ovassapian A, Doka JC, Romsa DE: Acromegaly: use of fiberoptic laryngoscopy to avoid tracheostomy, *Anesthesiology* 54:429-430, 1981.

140. Oyama T, Taniguchi K, Ishihara H et al: Effects of enflurane anaesthesia and surgery on endocrine function in man, *Br J Anaesth* 51:141-149, 1979.

141. Oyama T, editor: *Endocrinology and the anaesthetist,* New York, 1983, Elsevier.

142. Oyama T, Wakayama S: The endocrine responses to general anesthesia, *Int Anesthesiol Clin* 26:176-181, 1988.

143. Parkes D: Bromocriptine, *N Engl J Med* 301:873-878, 1979.

144. Patterson RH: Hypophysectomy: transfrontal technique and results in the management of metastatic cancer and diabetic retinopathy, *Clin Neurosurg* 21:60-67, 1974.

145. Pearson BW, Laws ER: Anatomical aspects of the transsphenoidal approach to the pituitary. In Laws ER, Randall RV, Kern EB et al, editors:

Management of pituitary adenomas and related lesions, New York, 1982, Appleton-Century-Crofts, pp 65-80.

146. Philbin DM, Coggins CH: Plasma antidiuretic hormone levels in cardiac surgical patients during morphine and halothane anesthesia, *Anesthesiology* 49:95-98, 1978.

147. Philbin DM, Coggins CH: The effects of anesthesia on antidiuretic hormone. In Brown B, editor: *Anesthesia and the patient with neuroendocrine disease,* Philadelphia, 1980, FA Davis, pp 29-38.

148. Plumpton FS, Besser GM, Cole PV: Corticosteroid treatment and surgery I. An investigation of the indications for steroid cover, *Anesthaesia* 24:3-11, 1969.

149. Plumpton FS, Besser GM, Cole PV: Corticosteroid treatment and surgery. II. The management of steroid cover, *Anaesthesia* 24:12-18, 1969.

150. Prescott RWG, Johnston DG, Kendall-Taylor P et al: Hyperprolactinaemia in man: response to bromocriptine therapy, *Lancet* 1:245-248, 1982.

151. Prolo DJ, Hanbery JW: Intraluminal occlusion of a carotid-cavernous sinus fistula with a balloon catheter: technical note, *J Neurosurg* 35:237-242, 1971.

152. Raudzens PA: Intraoperative monitoring of evoked potentials, *Ann NY Acad Sci* 388:308-326, 1982.

153. Rawe SE, Williamson O, Levine JH et al: Prolactinomas: surgical therapy, indications and results, *Surg Neurol* 14:161-167, 1980.

154. Rengachary SS, Tomita T, Jefferies BF et al: Structural changes in human pituitary tumor after bromocriptine therapy, *Neurosurgery* 10:242-251, 1982.

155. Renn WH, Rhoton AL: Microsurgical anatomy of the sellar region, *J Neurosurg* 43:288-298, 1975.

156. Rhoton AL, Harris FS, Renn WH: Microsurgical anatomy of the sellar region and cavernous sinus, *Clin Neurosurg* 24:54-85, 1977.

157. Richmond IL, Newton TH, Wilson CB: Indications for angiography in the preoperative evaluation of patients with prolactin-secreting pituitary adenomas, *J Neurosurg* 52:378-380, 1980.

158. Robertson GL, Mahr EA, Athar S et al: Development and clinical applica-

tion of a new method for the radioimmunoassay of arginine vasopressin in human plasma, *J Clin Invest* S2:2340-2352, 1973.

159. Robinson AG: The neurophysins in health and disease, *Clin Endocrinol Metab* 6:261-275, 1977.

160. Robinson AG, Frantz AG: Radioimmunoassay of posterior pituitary peptides: a review, *Metabolism* 22:1047-1057, 1973.

161. Saidman LJ, Eger EI: Change in cerebrospinal fluid pressure during pneumoencephalography under nitrous oxide anesthesia, *Anesthesiology* 26:67-72, 1965.

162. Sakkar DK, Gottschall PE, Meites J: Damage to hypothalamic dopaminergic neurons is associated with development of prolactin-secreting pituitary adenomas, *Science* 218:684-686, 1982.

163. Scheiner E: The relationship of antidiuretic hormone to the control of volume and tonicity in the human, *Adv Clin Chem* 17:1-52, 1975.

164. Schlechte J, Vangilder J, Sherman B: Predictors of the outcome of transsphenoidal surgery for prolactin-secreting pituitary adenomas, *J Clin Endocrinol Metab* 52:785-789, 1981.

165. Schrier RW: Pathogenesis of sodium and water retention in high output and low output cardiac failure, nephrotic syndrome, cirrhosis, and pregnancy, *N Engl J Med* 319:1065-1072, 1988.

166. Schucart WA: Implications of very high serum prolactin levels associated with pituitary tumors, *J Neurosurg* 52:226-228, 1980.

167. Schuster LD, Bantle JP, Oppenheimer JH et al: Acromegaly: reassessment of the long-term therapeutic effectiveness of transsphenoidal pituitary surgery, *Ann Intern Med* 95:172-174, 1981.

168. Serri O, Rasio E, Beauregard H et al: Recurrence of hyperprolactinemia after selective transsphenoidal adenomectomy in women with prolactinoma, *N Engl J Med* 309:280-283, 1983.

169. Share L, Claybaugh JR: Regulation of body fluids, *Ann Rev Physiol* 34:235-260, 1972.

170. Shirataki K, Chihara K, Shibata Y et al: Pituitary apoplexy manifested during a bromocriptine test in a patient with a growth hormone- and prolactin-producing pituitary ade-

noma, *Neurosurgery* 23:395-398, 1988.

171. Shome B, Parlow AF: Human pituitary prolactin (hPRL): the entire linear amino acid sequence, *J Clin Endocrinol Metab* 45:1112-1115, 1977.

172. Snyder PJ, Sterling FH: Hypersecretion of LH and FSH by a pituitary adenoma, *J Clin Endocrinol Metab* 42:544-550, 1976.

173. Sonksen PH, Ayres AB, Braimbridge M et al: Acromegaly caused by pulmonary carcinoid tumors, *Clin Endocrinol* 5:503-513, 1976.

174. Southwick JP, Katz J: Unusual airway difficulty in the acromegalic patient: indications for tracheostomy, *Anesthesiology* 51:72-73, 1979.

175. Spark RF, Baker R, Bienfang DC et al: Bromocriptine reduces pituitary tumor size and hypersecretion, *JAMA* 247:311-316, 1982.

176. Stanley TH, Philbin DM, Coggins CH: Fentanyl-oxygen anesthesia for coronary artery surgery, *Can Anaesth Soc J* 26:168-172, 1979.

177. Steer ML: Adenyl cyclase, *Ann Surg* 182:603-609, 1975.

178. Tashjian AH, Barowsky NJ, Jensen DK: Thyrotropin releasing hormone: direct evidence for stimulation of prolactin production by pituitary cells in cultures, *Biochem Biophys Res Commun* 43:516-523, 1971.

179. Taylor AL, Fishman LM: Corticotrophin-releasing hormone, *N Engl J Med* 319:213-222, 1988.

180. Teears RJ, Silverman EM: Clinicopathologic review of 88 cases of carcinoma metastatic to the pituitary gland, *Cancer* 36:216-220, 1975.

181. Tindall GT, Payne NS, Nixon DW: Transsphenoidal hypophysectomy for disseminated carcinoma of the prostate gland: results in 53 patients, *J Neurosurg* 50:275-282, 1979.

182. Tramu G, Beauvillain JC, Mazzuca M et al: Time dependent evaluation of pituitary prolactin adenomas under bromocriptine therapy. In Derome PJ, Jedynak CP, Peillon F, editors: *Pituitary adenomas: biology, physiopathology, and treatment,* Paris, 1980, Asclepios, p 343.

183. Trimble HG, Wood JR: Pulmonary hemorrhage: its control by the use of intravenous pituitrin, *Dis Chest* 18:345-351, 1950.

184. Turkalj LI, Braun P, Krupp P: Surveillance of bromocriptine in pregnancy, *JAMA* 247:1589-1591, 1982.

185. Uhl RR, Squires KC, Bruce DL et al: Effect of halothane anesthesia on the human cortical visual evoked response, *Anesthesiology* 53:273-276, 1980.

186. Van Thiel DH, Gavaler JS, Smith WS et al: Hypothalamic-pituitary-gonadal dysfunction in men using cimetidine, *N Engl J Med* 300:1012-1015, 1979.

187. Van Wyk JJ, Underwood LE: Relation between growth hormone and somatomedin, *Ann Rev Med* 26:427-441, 1975.

188. Venus B: Acromegalic patient: indications for fiberoptic bronchoscopy but not tracheostomy, *Anesthesiology* 52:100, 1980.

189. Veselis R, Korbon GA: A juvenile airway in an adult with suprasellar tumor, *Anesthesiology* 58:481-482, 1983.

190. Vigneri R, Goldfine ID: Pharmacologic therapy of patients with pituitary tumors secreting prolactin, growth hormone, and adrenocorticotropin, *Adv Intern Med* 25:69-89, 1980.

191. Wakai S, Fukushima T, Teramoto A et al: Pituitary apoplexy: its incidence and clinical significance, *J Neurosurg* 55:187-193, 1981.

192. Wayner MJ, editor: Thirst: proceedings of the first symposium held in May 1963, New York, 1964, Macmillan Publishing, p 570.

193. Weiss MH: Medical and surgical management of functional pituitary tumors, *Clin Neurosurg* 28:374-383, 1981.

194. Weiss MH, Teal J, Gott P et al: Natural history of microprolactinomas: six year follow up, *Neurosurgery* 12:180-183, 1983.

195. Weiss MH, Wycoff RR, Yadley R et al: Bromocriptine treatment of prolactin-secreting tumors: surgical implications, *Neurosurgery* 12:640-642, 1983.

196. Weitzman ED: Circadian rhythms and episodic hormone secretion in man, *Ann Rev Med* 27:225-243, 1976.

197. Wilkins RH: Hypothalamic dysfunction and intracranial arterial spasm, *Surg Neurol* 4:472-480, 1975.

198. Wilson WB, Kirsch WM, Neville H et al: Monitoring of visual function during parasellar surgery, *Surg Neurol* 5:323-329, 1976.

199. Wood JH: Neuroendocrinology of cerebrospinal fluid: peptides, steroids, and other hormones, *Neurosurgery* 11:293-305, 1982.

200. Woods WH, Holland RC, Powell EW: Connections of cerebral structures functioning in neurohypophyseal hormone release, *Brain Res* 12:26-46, 1969.

201. Yuen BH, Cannon W, Sy L et al: Regression of pituitary microadenoma during and following bromocriptine therapy: persistent defect in prolactin regulation before and throughout pregnancy, *Am J Obstet Gynecol* 142:634-639, 1982.

202. Zimmerman EA, Robinson AG: Hypothalamic neurons secreting vasopressin and neurophysin, *Kidney Int* 10:12-24, 1976.

30

Postoperative and Intensive Care

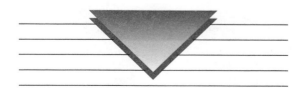

PATRICIA H. PETROZZA
DONALD S. PROUGH

GENERAL CARE
  Airway
  Mechanical ventilation
  Hemodynamic management: blood
    pressure control
  Perfusion assessment and management
  Hypoperfusion management
  Fluid management
  Management of disorders of sodium
    concentration
  Sedation and analgesia

Nutritional management
Infection
Transport of critically ill neurosurgical
  patients
IMMEDIATE POSTOPERATIVE CARE
  Carotid endarterectomy
  Craniotomy
  Vascular problems
  Laminectomy, spinal fixation, and spinal
    cord decompression
  Harrington rod placement and spinal

column stabilization
SPECIFIC CRITICAL CARE ISSUES
  Decreased level of consciousness
  Cerebral ischemia
  Acute intracranial hypertension
  Acute brain swelling
  Acute head injury
  Spinal cord injury
  Acute intracerebral hemorrhage
SUMMARY

After neurosurgical procedures or central nervous system (CNS) trauma, postoperative care and intensive care ensure that the outcome is as favorable as possible. The basic principles of management, such as airway maintenance, ventilatory assistance, and hemodynamic support, are identical to those used for other postoperative or critically ill patients; however, neurosurgical procedures also entail unique circumstances that require specific preparation and management. This chapter reviews the fundamentals of general supportive care, discusses aspects of the immediate postoperative care of specific neurosurgical procedures, and summarizes the approach to critical care issues that are unique to neurosurgery.

GENERAL CARE
Airway

Respiratory dysfunction after neurosurgical procedures encompasses three main categories: cranial nerve dysfunctions, airway reflex control abnormalities, and mechanical obstructions.[87] Many patients with slowly growing lesions are unaware of preoperative cranial nerve pareses.[109] Intraoperative damage either to cranial nerves or to cranial nerve nuclei may cause adverse postoperative sequelae. After procedures within the posterior fossa, tumor resections at the base of the skull, or carotid endarterectomy, cranial nerve injuries can compromise the airway. Careful presurgical examination, strict attention to the operative field, communication with the surgeon, and electromyographic (EMG) monitoring will often allow intraoperative recognition of those patients most prone to postoperative airway problems.

The integrity of the airway depends on proper function of cranial nerves V (trigeminal), VII (facial), IX (glossopharyngeal), X (vagus), and XII (hypoglossal). Swallowing dysfunctions related to injuries to nerves IX and X, as well as poor tongue function caused by compromise of cranial nerve XII, cause recurrent aspiration (Table 30-1). Injury to the vagus nerves is associated with bilateral vocal cord paralysis and the development of pulmonary edema as a complication of acute upper airway obstruction.[52] Cranial nerve injuries after carotid endarterectomy are surprisingly common, with unilateral vocal cord paralysis documented in as many as 6% to 7% of patients.[124] If cranial nerve dysfunction is anticipated in the immediate postoperative period, airway protection with a high-volume, low-pressure cuffed endotracheal tube should continue until recovery of swallowing and vocal cord function can be assessed. Slight residual neuromuscular blockade may also impair swallowing function.[91]

The control of respiration may be abnormal after intracranial surgery. Some postoperative patients never reinitiate breathing. Automatic control of respiration involves two pontine areas, the apneustic and pneumotactic centers, as well as pathways through the reticular formation of the medulla and the ventrolateral portions of the spinothalamic tract of the cervical cord. In the immediate postoperative period, apnea or highly irregular respiratory patterns may accompany brain stem compression, most often secondary to a rapidly expanding intracranial hematoma or to acute obstructive hydrocephalus. Delayed sequelae related to ischemia may present as ventilatory difficulty or deterioration of consciousness as late as 5 days postoperatively.[78] "Ondine's curse," a rare form of sleep-induced apnea, develops after bilateral percutaneous cervical cordotomy or, rarely, after intracranial procedures if edema, infarction, or hemorrhage has caused extensive damage at the pontomedullary junction. Although respiratory exchange is adequate in the waking state, patients cease to breathe during sleep, necessitating ventilatory support.

Among acromegalic patients, central sleep apnea occurs commonly. Disturbed ventilatory control, apparently unre-

lated to the also frequent problem of upper airway obstruction from enlarged anatomic structures, is usually self-limited.[74] Patients who have undergone bilateral carotid endarterectomy frequently manifest postoperative respiratory dysfunction related to bilateral cranial nerve injuries or to the loss of carotid body function. Without the usual compensatory circulatory or respiratory responses to hypoxia, the respiratory depressant effects of drugs such as narcotics may be exaggerated.[202]

After posterior fossa surgery, macroglossia secondary to venous obstruction, local trauma, or possibly neurogenic causes can cause airway obstruction.[135] Transoral surgical approaches to the rostral areas of the cervical spine necessitate the provision of a temporary airway postoperatively, with tracheostomy often electively performed. Selected patients may tolerate oral endotracheal intubation for approximately 48 hours to allow edema and swelling to subside. Plans for extubation of such patients must be made in concert with the surgical team.

Mechanical Ventilation

The first step in providing mechanical ventilatory support is to determine specifically whether a patient requires assistance with airway protection, carbon dioxide elimination, or oxygenation. Airway protection may be necessary because of preexisting or surgery-related cranial nerve damage or coma or because of residual anesthetics, narcotics, or neuromuscular blocking drugs. Even an alert patient with intact reflexes may require airway protection if vital capacity is inadequate (i.e., <12 ml/kg) to effect an adequate cough. Carbon dioxide elimination may be impaired by primary lung disease, weakness, depression of ventilatory drive, or residual anesthetic drugs or adjuvants. Impaired oxygenation requires mechanical support if oxygen supplementation (usually meaning a high-flow system with an Fio_2 ≤0.6) fails to increase oxyhemoglobin saturation to greater than 90%.

After specific requirements have been determined, a variety of modalities are available for airway support, ventilatory assistance (i.e., carbon dioxide removal), and oxygenation improvement.[179] If airway support is likely to be necessary for an extended period, a high–residual volume cuff on an endotracheal tube or tracheostomy tube may limit damage to the tracheal mucosa.

Ventilatory assistance may be provided with controlled mechanical ventilation (CMV), assist/controlled mechanical ventilation (AMV), intermittent mandatory ventilation (IMV), pressure support ventilation (PSV), or pressure control ventilation (PCV). CMV is appropriate for a patient who initiates no spontaneous breaths, regardless of the mechanism depressing ventilation. Typical settings, modified as necessary based on clinical presentation and arterial blood gases, include a tidal volume of 12 to 15 ml/kg and a ventilatory frequency of 8 to 10 breaths/min. AMV is suitable for patients who initiate spontaneous breaths but cannot maintain adequate minute ventilation without assis-

TABLE 30-1
Cranial Nerves and Swallowing Function

Cranial Nerve	Swallowing and Airway Function
V	Muscles of mastication
	Normal temporomandibular joint function
VII	Sensation to oral cavity
IX	Swallowing reflex trigger
	Pharyngeal phase of swallowing
X	Vocal cord movement, sensation
	Vocal cord pharyngeal coordination
	Cervical esophagus motion
XII	Tongue motion

tance. AMV supplies a full tidal volume (12 to 15 ml/kg) each time the patient initiates a breath. Therefore one of the main limitations of the technique is that some patients will maintain high ventilatory frequencies that result in significant hypocarbia or air trapping. IMV, often used as a primary ventilatory mode for the past 2 decades, provides a preset number of full tidal volumes per minute. These breaths may be delivered at fixed intervals or may be synchronized with spontaneous breaths. Between mechanical breaths the patient breathes from a parallel, continuous flow system or from a demand valve. PSV supplements spontaneous ventilation, as does IMV. However, PSV augments spontaneous breaths by pressurizing the circuit to a preset value until the patient terminates inspiration. The patient therefore determines tidal volume as well as frequency. In practice, clinicians commonly combine IMV and PSV. PCV, a newer modality that delivers a pressure-limited, time-cycled breath, partially overcomes the primary limitation of earlier pressure-cycled ventilators, which were more likely to deliver progressively less adequate tidal volumes as airway resistance increased or lung compliance decreased.

Mechanical ventilation can improve oxygenation through several techniques. One is simply to provide an assured Fio_2, without concern for the unavoidable dilution of inspired oxygen that occurs with conventional face mask delivery systems. Mechanical ventilation also improves oxygenation by providing tidal volumes that substantially exceed normal spontaneous tidal volumes (approximately 7 ml/kg). Positive end-expiratory pressure (PEEP) can be applied to increase functional residual capacity and reduce ventilation-perfusion mismatching. Another technique that has recently generated interest is inverse ratio ventilation, a modality that increases functional residual capacity, reduces ventilation-perfusion mismatching, and, if combined with PCV, does so at lower mean airway pressures than conventional CMV with PEEP.

Improved monitoring of oxygenation and carbon dioxide elimination should be valuable for neurosurgical and neurologic patients because of the greater vulnerability of the injured brain to hypoxemia and because of the risk of precipitating intracranial hypertension through hypoxemia or hypercapnia. Most patients who require ventilatory support should also have continuous noninvasive oxygen monitoring using pulse oximetry. Capnography may warn of increasing $Paco_2$, a risk in patients who have limited intracranial compliance, and may provide early evidence of accidental extubation. Decisions about direct arterial pressure monitoring should be based on the anticipated need for arterial blood gases as well as hemodynamic stability. Pulmonary artery catheterization can be very helpful in managing the occasional patient with severe hypoxemia requiring high levels (i.e., ≥ 15 cm H_2O) of PEEP. Calculation of the intrapulmonary shunt fraction may quantify the effects of changes in Fio_2, tidal volume, and PEEP. Thermodilution catheters permit detection of cardiac output (Q)

reduction, one of the major risks associated with application of PEEP.

Hemodynamic Management: Blood Pressure Control

After neurovascular or neurosurgical procedures, perioperative hypertension and tachycardia are associated with cerebral hemorrhage and myocardial ischemia.[11,188] As many as 80% of patients who undergo elective craniotomy may require treatment for postoperative hypertension, especially as anesthetic depth is reduced at the end of the procedure to afford a timely postoperative neurologic examination.[64] Common causes of postoperative hypertension, such as pain, bladder distention, or shivering, should be excluded, while remembering that extreme blood pressure elevation, accompanied by bradycardia and deteriorating consciousness, may signal intracranial catastrophe. The latter, termed the Cushing response, requires primary relief of brain stem ischemia rather than simple symptomatic management of the secondary hypertension.

Assuming that no correctable or ominous mechanism of hypertension is evident, a variety of antihypertensive agents can be selected, based on specific circumstances. These include the short-acting vasodilators sodium nitroprusside (SNP) and nitroglycerin; the ganglionic receptor antagonist trimethaphan; adrenergic receptor antagonists such as labetalol, a mixed beta- and alpha-receptor antagonist, and esmolol, a rapidly acting beta-receptor antagonist; hydralazine, a longer-acting vasodilator; and nifedipine, a calcium channel blocker.

Infusion of a vasodilator such as SNP or nitroglycerin may be useful in the immediate postoperative period. SNP, a predictably effective agent that rapidly reduces blood pressure, primarily through arteriolar dilation, is rapidly eliminated when the infusion is terminated. Because SNP-induced hypotension increases renin excretion, thus stimulating production of angiotensin I and the potent vasoconstrictor angiotensin II, rebound hypertension frequently occurs after cessation of the infusion. Slowly tapering SNP or adding beta-adrenergic receptor antagonists or angiotensin-converting enzyme (ACE) inhibitors will limit rebound hypertension until plasma renin levels return to normal.[199]

Intracranial pressure (ICP) and level of consciousness should be carefully monitored during SNP infusion in patients at risk for intracranial hypertension. Rapid administration of SNP is likely to cause an untoward increase in ICP when intracranial compliance is reduced.[32,82,125] In awake humans, SNP reduces mean arterial pressure, cerebral blood flow (CBF), and jugular venous bulb oxygen tension ($Pjvo_2$).[83] SNP may decrease CBF while increasing ICP, perhaps by increasing cerebral blood volume through dilation of cerebral capacitance vessels.[133] As blood pressure increases after termination of SNP, CBF may temporarily increase until SNP-induced cerebral vasodilation resolves.[133]

Several other considerations are important in the safe use of SNP. Tachyphylaxis to SNP can be complicated by loss of consciousness in critically ill patients.[146] Sensitivity to the hypotensive effects of SNP increases in elderly and hypovolemic patients. SNP inhibits platelet aggregation and impairs pulmonary hypoxic vasoconstriction. Frequent blood gas determinations are advisable to detect hypoxemia as well as metabolic acidosis, an indirect indicator of cyanide toxicity. Cyanide interferes with tissue oxygen utilization by interfering with cytochrome oxidase. If cyanide toxicity is suspected, the SNP infusion should immediately be discontinued. Sodium nitrite, 5 mg/kg, can be administered intravenously slowly, followed by sodium thiosulfate, 150 mg/kg, intravenously in cases of severe toxicity.[148]

Nitroglycerin, which also offers the advantage of a short plasma half-life (2 minutes), primarily dilates venous capacitance vessels, causing venous return, stroke volume, and cardiac output to diminish. Nitroglycerin, compared to SNP, promotes a more favorable distribution of coronary blood flow in patients with coronary artery disease.[2] Less predictably effective than SNP, especially in young patients, nitroglycerin occasionally may not achieve the desired level of blood pressure reduction. Nitroglycerin produces no toxic metabolites nor increases in plasma renin, thus averting rebound hypertension on discontinuation of the agent. During infusion of nitroglycerin, ICP may increase in patients with decreased intracranial compliance,[148] because cerebral capacitance vessels dilate and increase cerebral blood volume.[29]

Trimethaphan relaxes both resistance and capacitance vessels. The short half-life (1 to 2 minutes) reflects rapid inactivation by plasma cholinesterase with subsequent renal excretion. In patients who have decreased intracranial compliance, trimethaphan seldom increases ICP because ganglionic blockade generally spares the cerebral circulation.[211] Potential problems with trimethaphan include histamine release, bronchospasm, tachyphylaxis, and potentiation of succinylcholine-induced myoneural blockade. Ganglionic blockade also produces fixed, dilated pupils and may hinder accurate neurologic assessment.[148]

Labetalol, despite a relatively long duration of action (4.9 hours) is useful in managing postoperative hypertension, because the rapid onset of pressure reduction (≤ 5 minutes) permits easy titration.[129] Administered by either bolus or infusion (0.1% solution), labetalol decreases blood pressure promptly by decreasing cardiac output or systemic vascular resistance. However, dose requirements vary greatly among individuals, as do the relative effects on cardiac output and systemic vascular resistance. Myocardial oxygen consumption remains constant or decreases, because the $beta_1$ action prevents reflex tachycardia and the $alpha_1$-induced afterload reduction diminishes myocardial wall tension. One specific advantage of labetalol in neurosurgical patients is that it does not increase ICP, even when intracranial compliance is reduced.[205] The limitations of labetalol relate to its beta-blocking effects (i.e., bronchoconstriction and cardiac depression) and to its relatively pro-

longed half-life. Bradycardia secondary to labetalol administration may generate diagnostic confusion in the postanesthesia care unit (PACU) or intensive care unit (ICU). In addition, persistent beta blockade may blunt the usual adrenergic response to acute postoperative blood.

Esmolol is an intravenous, short-acting, cardioselective beta blocker with a rapid onset and elimination (half-life for beta = 9.2 minutes). Metabolized primarily by esterases and erythrocyte cytosol to an inactive metabolite, it is rapidly eliminated even in patients with hepatic or renal impairment. Esmolol has been successfully used to control hypertension after craniotomy and offers the advantage of relatively quick dissipation in the postoperative period.[64]

Hydralazine and nifedipine, other agents that may be useful in controlling perioperative hypertension, are somewhat more difficult to titrate and may cause intracranial hypertension.

Perfusion Assessment and Management

Two methods, conventional clinical assessment and invasive hemodynamic monitoring, are used to assess the adequacy of intravascular volume and perfusion. Clinical assessment begins with the recognition of settings in which deficits are likely, such as multiple trauma, aggressive diuresis, and prolonged fluid restriction. Tachycardia, supine hypotension, marked variation in pulse pressure induced by positive-pressure ventilation, oliguria, and a positive "tilt test" suggest the possibility of hypovolemia. Although supine hypotension implies a blood volume deficit exceeding 30%, arterial blood pressure within the normal range can represent relative hypotension in elderly or chronically hypertensive patients. Marked variations in pulse pressure, induced by positive-pressure ventilation, suggest hypovolemia.

Urinary output usually declines precipitously during moderate to severe hypovolemia. Therefore, in the absence of glycosuria or diuretic administration, a urinary output of 0.5 to 1.0 ml $\cdot$ kg^{-1} $\cdot$ hr^{-1} suggests adequate renal perfusion. Unfortunately, hypovolemic patients may be nonoliguric and normovolemic patients may be oliguric because of renal failure or stress-induced endocrine responses.[224] In the tilt test a positive response is defined as an increase in heart rate of 20 beats $\cdot$ min^{-1} or greater and a decrease in systolic blood pressure of 20 mm Hg or greater on assuming the upright position. However, classic studies[182] demonstrate that young, healthy subjects can withstand acute loss of 20% of blood volume while demonstrating only postural tachycardia and variable, usually mild, postural hypotension. In contrast, 20% to 30% of elderly patients may demonstrate orthostatic changes in blood pressure despite normal blood volume.[114] Noninvasively measured cardiac index and stroke volume index during orthostatic challenge appear to offer little advantage over conventional assessment.[216] Orthostatic changes in filling pressure, coupled with assessment of the response to fluid infusion, may represent a more sensitive test of the adequacy of circulating blood volume.[8]

Laboratory evidence that suggests hypovolemia or extracellular volume depletion includes increased blood urea nitrogen (BUN), increased serum creatinine (SCr), low urinary sodium (<10 mEq $\cdot$ L^{-1}), metabolic alkalosis, and metabolic acidosis. A ratio of BUN/SCr greater than 20 suggests dehydration. However, BUN, normally 8.0 to 20 mg $\cdot$ dl^{-1}, is increased by hypovolemia, high protein intake, gastrointestinal bleeding, or accelerated catabolism, whereas synthesis is decreased by hepatic dysfunction. In muscular or acutely catabolic patients, SCr, a product of muscle catabolism, may exceed the normal range (0.5 to 1.5 mg $\cdot$ dl^{-1}). SCr may be misleadingly low in elderly adults, females, and debilitated or malnourished patients. In prerenal oliguria, enhanced sodium reabsorption should reduce urinary sodium to less than 20 mEq $\cdot$ L^{-1}, and enhanced water reabsorption should increase urinary concentration (i.e., urinary osmolality >400; urine/plasma creatinine ratio $>40:1$). However, the sensitivity and specificity of measurements of urinary sodium, osmolality, and creatinine may be misleading in acute situations. Although hypovolemia does not generate metabolic alkalosis, mild-to-moderate extracellular volume depletion is a potent stimulus for the maintenance of metabolic alkalosis. Severe hypovolemia may result in systemic hypoperfusion and lactic acidosis.

In high-risk patients, invasive monitoring may be helpful. In patients undergoing extensive procedures, direct arterial pressure measurements are more accurate than indirect techniques and provide convenient access for obtaining arterial blood samples. Invasive measurement of cardiac output (Q) and pulmonary artery occlusion pressure (PAOP) may be useful in patients with known cardiac disease. However, Q can be normal despite severely reduced regional blood flow. Mixed venous oxygenation, a sensitive, specific indicator of poor systemic perfusion in experimental hemorrhagic shock,[168] nevertheless reflects average perfusion in multiple organs and cannot supplant monitors such as urinary output that reflect regional perfusion.

Hypoperfusion Management

Management of overt shock, manifested by lactic acidosis, frank hypotension, or acute oliguria, conventionally involves the use of a straightforward algorithm. The first intervention, in the absence of overt left-sided heart failure, is a series of fluid challenges. In patients who have decreased intracranial compliance, the challenges should consist of mildly hypertonic or isotonic fluids (i.e., 0.9% saline) rather than hypotonic fluids (i.e., lactated Ringer's solution). Colloid solutions are also an alternative. Fluid challenges will either improve shock, precipitate pulmonary edema, or produce no apparent change. Invasive hemodynamic monitoring is of greatest value in the latter two situations. Measurement of Q and PAOP and calculation of systemic vascular resistance and oxygen transport will usually guide rational decisions regarding the need for additional fluid vs. the indications for inotropic support or vasodilators.

In patients at high risk for hypoperfusion, such as patients who have suffered multiple trauma, unrecognized, subclinical, perioperative tissue hypoperfusion may explain postoperative complications, such as acute renal failure, hepatic failure, and sepsis.[23,183] In high-risk surgical patients who survive, average Q and systemic oxygen delivery (Do$_2$) are greater than in those who die.[23] In a single term, Do$_2$ combines Q and arterial oxygen content (Cao$_2$) according to the equation:

$$Do_2 = Q \times Cao_2 \times 10$$

where the factor 10 corrects Cao$_2$, usually measured in milliliters of O$_2$ $\cdot$ dl^{-1} to milliliters of O$_2$ $\cdot$ L^{-1}. One variable that is strongly associated with survival is a Do$_2$ greater than 600 ml O$_2$ $\cdot$ m^{-2} $\cdot$ min^{-1} (equivalent to a cardiac index of 3.0 L $\cdot$ m^{-2} $\cdot$ min^{-1}, a hemoglobin concentration of 14 g $\cdot$ dl^{-1}, and 98% oxyhemoglobin saturation).[183] In high-risk surgical patients treated to achieve a Do$_2$ of 600 ml O$_2$ $\cdot$ m^{-2} $\cdot$ min^{-1} as well as other hemodynamic goals, survival was improved and complications were reduced.[183] Pulmonary artery catheterization without specific management guidelines did not improve survival or morbidity. These data suggest that aggressive, goal-directed hemodynamic support in high-risk surgical patients reverses clinically inapparent hypoperfusion and thereby limits the incidence of mortality and morbidity. Similar goal-directed hemodynamic management also appears to improve outcome in septic patients.[203] Hemodynamic monitoring also may be useful in managing patients who undergo hypervolemic hemodilution as part of the management of vasospasm after subarachnoid hemorrhage.

Fluid Management
Maintenance

In healthy adults, sufficient water is required to balance gastrointestinal losses of 100 to 200 ml $\cdot$ day^{-1}, insensible (respiratory and cutaneous) losses of 500 to 1000 ml $\cdot$ day^{-1}, and urinary losses of 1000 ml $\cdot$ day^{-1}. Urinary output exceeding 1000 ml $\cdot$ day^{-1} may represent an appropriate physiologic response to ECV expansion or an inability to conserve salt or water. The daily adult requirement for sodium is 75 mEq. Patients with normal cardiac and renal reserve are capable of markedly increased excretion or extreme conservation (≤10 mEq excreted per day). Daily requirements for potassium, for which renal conservation is less efficient, slightly exceed 40 mEq. Physiologic diuresis typically induces an obligate potassium loss of at least 10 mEq $\cdot$ L^{-1} of urine.

To estimate maintenance water requirements using body weight, provide 4 mg $\cdot$ kg^{-1} $\cdot$ hr^{-1} for the first 10 kg, an additional 2 mg $\cdot$ kg^{-1} $\cdot$ hr^{-1} for the eleventh through twentieth kilograms, and 1 mg $\cdot$ kg^{-1} $\cdot$ hr^{-1} for each additional kilogram. Therefore the daily maintenance requirements for water, sodium, and potassium for a healthy, 70 kg adult consist of 2500 ml $\cdot$ day^{-1} of a solution containing Na$^+$ of 30 mEq $\cdot$ L^{-1} and K$^+$ of 15 to 20 mEq $\cdot$ L^{-1}. In practice, fluids containing free water should be used cautiously in neurosurgical patients because of the possibility of increasing cerebral edema.

Traditionally, glucose-containing intravenous fluids have been given perioperatively in an effort to prevent hypoglycemia and to limit protein catabolism. However, surgical and traumatic stress normally stimulates gluconeogenesis. Only infants and patients receiving insulin or drugs that interfere with glucose synthesis are at significant risk for hypoglycemia. In animals, hyperglycemia may aggravate global and focal neurologic ischemic injury.[103,119,157] In humans, although hyperglycemia is associated with worse outcomes in both ischemic[115] and traumatic[102] brain injury, it is likely that hyperglycemia is a secondary, hormonally mediated accompaniment of more severe injury.[117]

Fluid Resuscitation

Surgical patients require replacement of plasma volume and extracellular volume losses that result from wound or burn edema, ascites, and gastrointestinal secretions. Neurosurgical procedures and isolated head injury are associated with minimal loss of extracellular fluid, although associated injuries may necessitate aggressive fluid replacement. In general, surgical or traumatic losses in patients at risk for intracranial hypertension can be replaced using 0.9% saline. However, if cardiovascular or renal function is impaired, more precise replacement may require frequent assessment of serum sodium and potassium. Substantial or chronic loss of gastrointestinal fluids requires replacement of other electrolytes (i.e., potassium, magnesium, phosphate).

Replacement of fluid losses also must compensate for the sequestration of interstitial fluid that accompanies trauma, hemorrhage, and tissue manipulation. Patients studied during the first 10 days after resuscitation from massive trauma or sepsis actually demonstrate a slight percentage decrease in intracellular volume[24]; however, total body weight is increased in these patients as a consequence of a 55% increase in interstitial fluid volume. Based on estimates of fluid sequestration associated with extensive tissue manipulation, guidelines have been developed for replacement of third-space surgical losses. The simplest formula provides, in addition to maintenance fluids and replacement of estimated blood loss, $4 \ ml \cdot kg^{-1} \cdot hr^{-1}$ for procedures involving minimal trauma (e.g., uncomplicated neurosurgical procedures), $6 \ ml \cdot kg^{-1} \cdot hr^{-1}$ for those involving moderate trauma, and 8 to $15 \ ml \cdot kg^{-1} \cdot hr^{-1}$ for those involving severe trauma.[31]

The selection of a resuscitation fluid for patients who have decreased intracranial compliance requires an understanding of the relationship among intravenous fluids, brain water, and ICP. The blood-brain barrier, because of its relative impermeability to sodium, enhances the importance of changes in osmolality and proportionately reduces the importance of alterations in oncotic pressure.[201] Hypotonic solutions (including lactated Ringer's solution) increase brain water and ICP. Lactated Ringer's solution is more likely to increase brain water content than fluids such as 0.9% saline, 6.0% hydroxyethyl starch in 0.9% saline, or 5.0% albumin in 0.9% saline, all of which have higher osmolality.[151] Accordingly, rapid resuscitation with 6.0% hydroxyethyl starch in 0.9% saline increased ICP less than hemodynamically comparable resuscitation using hypotonic lactated Ringer's solution.[75] In experimental animals, resuscitation with hypertonic (3.0% to 7.5%) saline solutions was associated with lower ICP than resuscitation with isotonic or slightly hypotonic fluids.[155,214] Less hypertonic solutions ($Na^+ = 250 \ mEq/L$), infused at a rate sufficient to maintain stable cardiac output after resuscitation in dogs, were not appreciably superior to slightly hypotonic solutions.[214]

Management of Disorders of Sodium Concentration

Sodium, the primary cation and osmotically active solute in the extracellular compartment, is the principal determinant of total extracellular volume and contributes 90% to 95% of extracellular osmotic activity. Total body sodium consists primarily of extracellular sodium, because sodium is largely confined to the extracellular volume. Clinical disorders of sodium *concentration,* that is, hyponatremia and hypernatremia, usually reflect alterations of body water content and not the state of sodium balance.

Regulation of the quantity and concentration of sodium is accomplished by plasma volume receptors, endocrine regulation, and renal mechanisms. Increased plasma volume stretches the cardiac atria, triggering secretion of atrial natriuretic peptide (ANP). ANP increases renal sodium excretion, thereby decreasing plasma volume.[163,181,193] Aldosterone, the single most important hormonal regulator of renal sodium reabsorption, increases the exchange for sodium of potassium and hydrogen in the distal tubules and collecting ducts. Sodium concentration is regulated primarily by antidiuretic hormone (ADH). Increased secretion of ADH increases reabsorption of water in the renal collecting ducts and therefore dilutes plasma $[Na^+]$. A serum osmolality of 280 $mOsm \cdot kg^{-1}$ initiates ADH release; an osmolality of 294 $mOsm \cdot kg^{-1}$ (about a 2% increase in P_{Osm} above normal) results in maximally concentrated urine and may trigger thirst. ADH secretion can vary urinary volume from 0.4 to 20 $L \cdot day^{-1}$.

Hyponatremia

The signs and symptoms of hyponatremia ($[Na^+] \leq 135$ $mEq \cdot L^{-1}$) depend on both the rate and severity of the plasma $[Na^+]$ decrease. Plasma $[Na^+]$ less than 120 $mEq \cdot L^{-1}$ usually results in CNS symptoms such as disorientation, lethargy, coma, and possibly seizures (Table 30-2). The CNS manifestations of acute hyponatremia, more severe than those of chronic hyponatremia at identical levels of plasma $[Na^+]$, result from rapid transmembrane water equilibration across the blood-brain barrier, increasing both extracellular and intracellular brain water and brain edema. Compensation for brain edema occurs by loss

TABLE 30-2
Clinical Manifestations of Hyponatremia

Neurologic	Gastrointestinal	Muscular
Altered consciousness (lethargy, apathy)	Anorexia	Cramps
Coma	Nausea	Weakness
Seizures	Vomiting	Rhabdomyolysis
Cerebral edema		
Cheyne-Stokes respiration		
Hypothermia		
Pathologic reflexes		
Depressed deep tendon reflexes		

TABLE 30-3
Clinical Manifestations of Hypernatremia

Neurologic	Renal	Muscular
Thirst	Polyuria or oliguria	Increased muscle tone
Restlessness; irritability	Renal insufficiency	Hyperreflexia
Seizures; ataxia		
Intracranial hemorrhage		

of intracellular osmotically active solutes,[112] including potassium and organic osmolytes ("idiogenetic osmoles") such as taurine, phosphocreatine, glutamine, and glutamate.[195] Brain edema is minimal in chronic hyponatremia.[38,195]

Hyponatremia is classified as factitious or true. Factitious hyponatremia, which requires no treatment, occurs when hyperproteinemia or hyperlipidemia displaces water from plasma, thereby producing apparently low plasma [Na^+]. Factitious hyponatremia occurs if protein concentrations increase by two times normal or if hyperlipidemia is sufficiently severe to produce plasma lactescence. In such patients, *measured* serum osmolality will be normal. True hyponatremia may be associated with normal, high, or low serum osmolality. A discrepancy greater than 10 $mOsm \cdot kg^{-1}$ between the measured and calculated osmolality (calculated using the formula: $2 \times [Na^+]$ + glucose/18 + BUN/2.8) suggests either factitious hyponatremia or the presence of a nonsodium solute. BUN, included in the calculation of total osmolality, is excluded from the calculation of *effective* osmolality ($2 \times [Na^+]$ + glucose/18), because it distributes throughout *both* extracellular and intracellular volume. Hyponatremia with a normal or high serum osmolality results from the presence of a nonsodium solute, such as glucose or mannitol, which does not diffuse freely across cell membranes. The resulting osmotic gradient causes water to move from the intracellular volume to the extracellular volume, resulting in dilutional hyponatremia. For instance, plasma [Na^+] decreases approximately 1.6 mEq/L^{-1} for each 100 $mg \cdot dl^{-1}$ increase in plasma glucose concentration.

Hyponatremia with hypoosmolarity is associated with a high, low, or normal total body sodium and plasma volume. Hyponatremia with increased total body sodium is characteristic of edematous states such as congestive heart failure, cirrhosis, nephrosis, and renal failure. Hyponatremia with low total body sodium content (hypovolemia) occurs in association with nonrenal or renal losses of sodium (e.g., adrenal insufficiency). Volume receptors stimulate ADH secretion, sacrificing tonicity in an attempt to preserve intravascular volume.

Euvolemic hyponatremia is associated with a relatively normal total body sodium and extracellular volume. The syndrome of inappropriate ADH (SIADH) secretion often is associated with ectopic (neoplastic) ADH secretion or excessive hypothalamic-pituitary release of ADH (secondary to CNS pathologic conditions, pain, surgery, or endocrine abnormalities). Prospective studies suggest that at least 4.0% of surgical patients develop plasma [Na^+] <130 $mEq \cdot L^{-1}$.[10] Although neurologic manifestations are relatively uncommon, signs of hypervolemia may be present.[10] In extreme cases, administration of hypotonic fluids to women after surgery has resulted in severe neurologic symptoms and death secondary to transtentorial herniation.[61,112,192]

Hyponatremia associated with a normal or high serum osmolality (e.g., hyperglycemia) requires reduction of the elevated concentrations of the responsible solute (Fig. 30-1). SIADH management requires free water restriction sufficient to decrease total body water (TBW) by 0.5 to 1.0 $L \cdot day^{-1}$. The resultant reduction in glomerular filtration rate (GFR) enhances proximal tubular reabsorption of salt and water and stimulates aldosterone secretion. Demeclocycline and lithium antagonize the renal actions of ADH in refractory cases of SIADH.

Neurologic symptoms with profound hyponatremia ([Na^+] <115 to 120 $mEq \cdot L^{-1}$) require aggressive therapy. Three percent saline will increase total body sodium as well as TBW; nevertheless, plasma [Na^+] may only transiently increase, since extracellular volume expansion results in rapid urinary sodium excretion. Intravenous furosemide, combined with quantitative replacement of urinary sodium loss with 0.9% or 3.0% saline, can rapidly increase plasma [Na^+]. Hypertonic saline is most indicated in patients who have seizures or those who develop severe symptoms of water intoxication. In such cases, 3% saline, administered at a rate of 1 to 2 $ml \cdot kg^{-1} \cdot hr^{-1}$ to increase plasma [Na^+] by 1 to 2 $mEq \cdot L^{-1} \cdot hr^{-1}$,[164,194] should be monitored every 1 to 2 hours to avoid overcorrection. CNS signs and symptoms usually improve within 24 to 72 hours.

Excessively rapid correction of hyponatremia may result in permanent neurologic sequelae (i.e., central pontine myelinolysis or the osmotic demyelination syndrome),[39] cerebral hemorrhage, or congestive heart failure. The rapidity of correction appears to be a critical factor in osmotic demyelination. Most patients who develop fatal osmotic de-

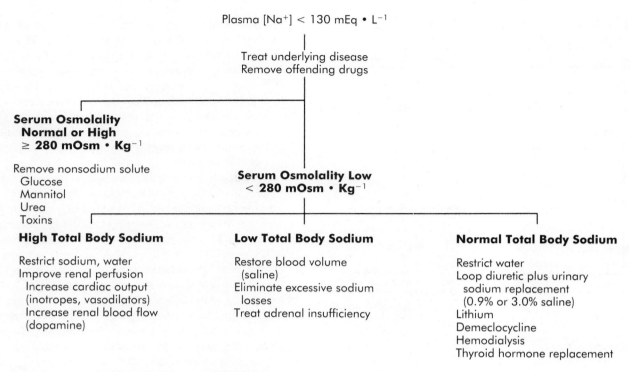

Plasma [Na$^+$] < 130 mEq · L^{-1}

Treat underlying disease
Remove offending drugs

**Serum Osmolality
Normal or High
≥ 280 mOsm · Kg^{-1}**

Remove nonsodium solute
  Glucose
  Mannitol
  Urea
  Toxins

**Serum Osmolality Low
< 280 mOsm · Kg^{-1}**

High Total Body Sodium

Restrict sodium, water
Improve renal perfusion
  Increase cardiac output
  (inotropes, vasodilators)
  Increase renal blood flow
  (dopamine)

Low Total Body Sodium

Restore blood volume
  (saline)
Eliminate excessive sodium
  losses
Treat adrenal insufficiency

Normal Total Body Sodium

Restrict water
Loop diuretic plus urinary
  sodium replacement
  (0.9% or 3.0% saline)
Lithium
Demeclocycline
Hemodialysis
Thyroid hormone replacement

FIG. 30-1   Hyponatremia is treated according to the underlying disease and etiology, serum osmolality, and clinical estimate of total body sodium.

myelination syndrome have undergone correction of plasma [Na$^+$] of more than 20 mEq · L^{-1} · day^{-1}.[17,39] Initially, plasma [Na$^+$] may be increased by 1 to 2 mEq · L^{-1} · hr^{-1}; however, plasma [Na$^+$] should not be increased more than 12 mEq · L^{-1} in 24 hours or 25 mEq · L^{-1} in 48 hours,[189] or to a concentration greater than 130 mEq · L^{-1}. Hypernatremia must be avoided.

Hypernatremia

Severe hypernatremia is associated with a high mortality. Most hypernatremic patients have severe associated illnesses[72] and may be hypovolemic from diabetes insipidus or osmotically induced loss of sodium and water. An increased volume of hypotonic urine is often the first clinical indicator of abnormal water balance.[22] The clinical consequences of hypernatremia are most serious at the extremes of age[73] and when hypernatremia develops abruptly. Brain tissue dehydration produces symptoms such as decreased mental status and seizures (Table 30-3)[73] and may stretch delicate cerebral vessels, leading to hemorrhagic complications.

Hypernatremia ([Na$^+$] >150 mEq · L^{-1}) indicates an absolute or relative water deficit (from the loss of free water or gain of sodium in excess of water) and is always associated with hypertonicity. Hypernatremia can exist in the setting of hypovolemia, euvolemia, or hypervolemia (Fig. 30-2).[22] As extracellular [Na$^+$] increases, intracellular water is shifted out of cells and cellular dehydration results.

The TBW deficit can be estimated from plasma [Na$^+$] using the equation:

$$\text{TBW deficit} = 0.6 \times (\text{body weight in kg}) - (140 \div \text{actual } [\text{Na}^+]) \times 0.6 \times (\text{body weight in kg})$$

Treatment of hypernatremia produced by water loss consists of water replacement as well as repletion of associated deficits of sodium and other electrolytes (Table 30-4). Hypernatremia must be corrected slowly because of the risk of neurologic sequelae such as seizures and cerebral edema.[22,73] The water deficit should be replaced over 24 to 48 hours, and the plasma [Na$^+$] should not be reduced by more than 1 to 2 mEq · L^{-1} · hr^{-1}. In the occasional patient who is both water depleted and sodium overloaded, sodium excretion can be accelerated using loop diuretics or dialysis, and volume can be replaced with hypotonic fluids.

After pituitary surgery, neurosurgical patients are at particular risk of developing transient or permanent diabetes insipidus,[175,207] usually presenting as one of three distinct patterns of polyuria. Fifty percent of patients demonstrate transient, acute ADH deficiency that resolves within 3 to 5 days, 33% exhibit permanent ADH deficiency, and a minority demonstrate a "triphasic" response, manifested by early diabetes insipidus, followed by return of urinary concentrating ability for 1 to 2 weeks and then recurrent and permanent diabetes insipidus.[160] Hypernatremia secondary to diabetes insipidus is managed according to whether its etiology is central or nephrogenic (Table 30-4). Central di-

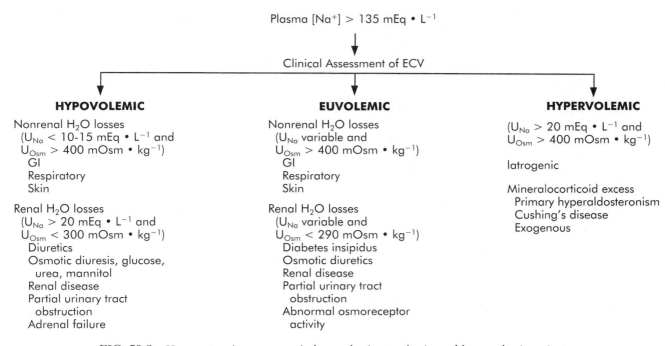

FIG. 30-2   Hypernatremia may occur in hypovolemic, euvolemic, and hypervolemic patients. Diagnostic categories are based on assessment of extracellular volume (ECV). U_{Na}, Urinary sodium; U_{Osm}, urinary osmolality.

TABLE 30-4
Hypernatremia: Treatment

Sodium Depletion (Hypovolemia)	Sodium Overload (Hypervolemia)	Normal Total Body Sodium (Euvolemia)
Correct hypovolemia with 0.9% saline	Enhance sodium removal (loop diuretics, dialysis)	Replace water deficit (hypotonic fluids)
Correct hypernatremia with hypotonic fluids	Replace water deficit (hypotonic fluids)	Central diabetes insipidus
		Aqueous vasopressin, 5-10 u sc, IM every 4-6 hr
		DDAVP,* 5-20 μg by nasal spray BID or 1-4 μg sc IV
		Chlorpropamide, 250-750 mg/day
		Clofibrate, 250-500 mg/6-8 hr
		Carbamazepine, 400-1000 mg/day
		Nephrogenic diabetes insipidus
		Restrict sodium and water intake
		Hydrochlorothiazide, 50-100 mg/day, orally

*1-Desamino-8-D-arginine vasopressin (Desmopressin).

abetes insipidus requires exogenous replacement of ADH with either Desmopressin (DDAVP) or aqueous vasopressin.[35,40,184,225] DDAVP may be given subcutaneously in a dose of 1 to 4 μg every 12 to 24 hours or intranasally in a dose five times larger. DDAVP lacks the vasoconstrictor effects of vasopressin and is less likely to produce abdominal cramping, probably owing to its enhanced V_2-receptor selectivity. Incomplete ADH deficits (partial diabetes insipidus) are effectively managed with chlorpropamide (250 to 750 mg/day^{-1}), clofibrate, or carbamazepine to stimulate ADH release and enhance the renal response to ADH.

Sedation and Analgesia

Neurosurgical patients have highly variable requirements for analgesia and sedation. Immediately after craniotomy, many patients experience little pain; unnecessary sedatives or narcotics may interfere with continued neurologic assessment. In contrast, patients with fractures of the vertebral column require substantial analgesia and sedation. Patients who have severe head injuries may receive sedative infusions to minimize cerebral metabolic demand and to counteract the effects of large amounts of circulating catecholamines.[30]

Several sedative and analgesic drugs have been or are currently administered by continuous infusion in the intensive care setting. Etomidate and althesin have largely been abandoned because of associated side effects. Midazolam, a water-soluble, nonanalgesic benzodiazepine with a rapid onset of action, induces sleep and angiolysis and decreases muscle tone. Midazolam reduces CBF and cerebral metabolism and does not affect or slightly decreases ICP. The usual loading dose is approximately 0.1 to 0.2 mg/kg administered over 30 minutes, followed by a continuous infusion of 0.05 mg/kg/hr adjusted to the patient's response. A qualitative scoring system assists with titration (Table 30-5). The elimination half-life of midazolam, normally 2 to 4 hours after a single dose, may be significantly prolonged in critically ill patients.[178] After discontinuation of a continuous infusion, mental status returns to baseline in approximately 90 minutes.[132] Case reports of prolonged sedation with midazolam are related to the drug's pharmacokinetics, which are markedly altered in critically ill patients secondary to multiple factors, including decreased hepatic perfusion and metabolic capacity, fluid shifts, altered protein binding, and the effects of concomitant medication.[5] Patients with multisystem organ dysfunction will have significant alterations in midazolam disposition.

Flumazenil, an imidazobenzodiazepine that acts as a benzodiazepine antagonist, has a very short half-life. When flumazenil is used to reverse the effects of sedative benzodiazepines, sedation or respiratory depression may recur. While specific information concerning pharmacokinetics in critically ill patients is limited, caution should be used in administering the drug, because rapid antagonism of sedation may result in hypertension and tachycardia.[36] Increases in ICP have been reported after the administration of flumazenil to patients with severe head injuries.

Propofol, an alkylphenol sedative drug formulated as a soybean and water emulsion, has reportedly produced satisfactory sedation in patients in ICUs. In patients with head injuries, propofol administered at an infusion rate of 2 to 4 mg · kg^{-1} · hr^{-1} provides satisfactory sedation without detrimental changes in cerebral perfusion pressure.[55] No adverse changes in serum lipid concentrations have been observed in ICU patients receiving propofol by continuous infusion for 3 days. Minor disturbances in blood coagulability have been reported in selected patients, however.[69]

Occasionally, patients with severe head injuries receive large doses of pentobarbital in an effort to decrease ICP. Careful monitoring of hemodynamics is essential, and drug levels may vary, owing to changes in plasma clearance related to enzyme induction.[53] The recent introduction of processed electroencephalographic monitoring into the ICU setting may allow more careful titration of sedative drugs in critically ill patients.[180]

Narcotics are an essential part of management of patients who have severe pain secondary to neurologic or associated nonneurologic injuries or procedures. Morphine, administered either by intermittent small boluses (2 to 4 mg IV) or by continuous infusion (2 to 3 mg · hr^{-1}), provides both analgesia and sedation. However, because of individual variations in pharmacokinetics and pharmacodynamics, sedation or respiratory depression may be excessive or prolonged.[208] A theoretic concern is the ability of morphine to cause a naloxone-reversible depression of the primary immune response.[4] Morphine also depresses the activity of the reticuloendothelial system and phagocytosis in other animal models.

Alfentanil, a synthetic opioid, possesses a limited duration of action, attributable to a short elimination half-life and a small volume of distribution. The hemodynamic effects of an alfentanil infusion are minimal, and recovery from respiratory depression is generally rapid. An initial infusion rate of 24 μg · kg^{-1} · hr^{-1} provides satisfactory analgesia for critically ill patients. Intermittent supplementation with midazolam (5 mg) can be used as necessary for sedation.[186] Plasma alfentanil levels vary during infusion, but sedation is adequate in those patients requiring mechanical ventilation. Although alfentanil produces no biochemical or hematologic alterations and no evidence of tolerance, it may cause increased cerebrospinal fluid (CSF) pressure in patients with brain tumors.[127] In the rare critically ill patient, alfentanil has been reported to have a prolonged elimination and duration of action.[41]

Nutritional Management

The most extensive studies of the nutritional needs of patients with acute neurosurgical disease have been performed in head-injured patients. Those with a Glasgow Coma Scale (GCS) score of 4 to 5 require nearly 70% more than predicted resting metabolic requirements.[159b] Heart rate, temperature, and the days elapsed after injury correlate significantly[195a] as do catecholamine levels[56] with measured energy expenditure. Because of intense catabolism after injury, protein-calorie malnutrition can develop within a few days, potentially leading to immunocompromise and infection, hypoalbuminemia, poor wound healing, and skin breakdown.[66a] Loss of amino acids from skeletal muscle produces muscle wasting and weight loss.[221a] Glucocorticoids, used for reduction of vasogenic edema in patients with brain tumors, increase nitrogen wasting in head-injured patients without increasing metabolic rate.[159a] Be-

TABLE 30-5
Scoring System for Assessment of Sedation in ICU Patients

Level	Response
1	Anxious, or agitated and restless, or both
2	Cooperative, oriented, and tranquil
3	Responds to commands only
4	Asleep but brisk response to glabellar tap or loud auditory stimulus
5	Asleep with sluggish response to glabellar tap or loud auditory stimulus
6	No response

Modified from Ramsay MA et al: Controlled sedation with alphaxalone-alphadolone, *Br Med J* 2:656, 1974.

cause of the extraordinary requirements for both calories and nitrogen in intensely catabolic patients, positive nitrogen balance may be difficult to achieve.[38a,38c] Aggressive enteral nutrition containing 22% protein may be sufficient in some patients to promote nitrogen equilibrium, however.[38b]

High circulating levels of catabolic hormones generate gluconeogenesis, reduce glucose tolerance, and may produce hyperglycemia despite increased insulin levels. Therefore, when feeding patients who have acute neurologic disease, hyperglycemia should be anticipated and blood glucose concentration controlled. Descriptive data implicate hyperglycemia in worse neurologic outcome after head trauma, cardiac arrest, and stroke.[103,116a,117,117a]

Although patients with severe head injury remain hypermetabolic for prolonged intervals, the appropriate level of nutritional support has yet to be defined,[98a] a problem similar for other critically ill patients with neurologic and neurosurgical disease. Undernutrition frequently is unrecognized.[66a] Although recent studies suggest caution,[98a] some investigators report improved mortality in patients who receive early parenteral nutrition, as opposed to early enteral nutrition, after head trauma.[151a,221b] Some patients with acute head injury tolerate enteral feeding poorly, with the greatest difficulty encountered in those patients with more severe injury and intracranial hypertension.[141a] The intolerance for enteral feeding may be related to delayed gastric emptying, reduced intestinal motility, or increased susceptibility to diarrhea.[141a] Nevertheless, many centers prefer enteral feeding, which does not require central venous catheterization and which may benefit gut integrity and immune competence. Hyperglycemia is less frequent with enteral compared to parenteral feeding; the incidence of regurgitation and aspiration can be reduced by head elevation and by ensuring that feeding tubes are placed within the duodenum. Early enteral nutrition may also improve the function of the immune system.[221b]

Many questions regarding nutrition of patients with neurologic and neurosurgical disease remain unanswered. Most clinicians tend to initiate either enteral or parenteral nutrition as soon as possible after acute head injury, generally preferring enteral nutrition if tolerated. An appropriate strategy is to provide sufficient calories and nitrogen to prevent catabolism without causing hyperglycemia.

Infection

Infection can be difficult to diagnose in postoperative and critically ill patients. Fever and leukocytosis, common findings in infection, are also common in patients with no evidence of infection. Stress responses, pontine injuries, or autonomic dysfunction accompanying bilateral frontal damage[182] may cause fever, but infectious causes must be excluded. Some types of therapy may increase the risk of infection. Glucocorticoids have long been associated with an increased rate of infection. Fifty-five percent of patients receiving barbiturates for uncontrolled intracranial hypertension developed infections.

Critically ill patients are at risk for pulmonary and nonpulmonary infections, because defense barriers must be violated in the course of care. Two fifths of head-injured patients develop pulmonary complications, with the peak incidence occurring 2 to 4 days after injury. In many patients with acute neurologic disease, pneumonia may develop as a consequence of secretion retention, atelectasis, and secondary infection. Compulsive turning therefore is essential for patients who cannot position themselves. Prevention of aspiration requires recognition of those at risk, gastric decompression, and, in patients who cannot protect their airways, endotracheal intubation. Overgrowth of pathogenic bacteria in the stomach may play a role in the genesis of pneumonia secondary to aspirated oropharyngeal material. Because stress ulceration and erosive gastritis are associated with high gastric acidity, treatment with antacids or H_2 blockers has been used to minimize the incidence of these complications. Aggressive antacid therapy or frequent administration of H_2 blockers may be necessary to control gastric pH; however, recent data demonstrate that gastric bacterial overgrowth is common if gastric pH is increased in an effort to prevent stress gastritis. Because of the increased risk of passive regurgitation of gastric contents with subsequent aspiration and infection, sucralfate may be preferable for ulcer prophylaxis.

Urinary tract infection may result from prolonged bladder catheterization. Maxillary sinusitis is surprisingly common among nasotracheally intubated head trauma patients,[87a] although the incidence may be no greater than in orally intubated patients.[36a] Otitis media occurs in one sixth of intubated head-injured patients.[36a] Ventriculitis and meningitis complicate penetrating trauma, surgical procedures that violate the dura, and indwelling intraventricular monitoring devices. Most clinicians believe that ventricular cannulae are acceptable in patients with head trauma for limited periods of time, if strict asepsis is maintained.[127a] The risk of intracranial infection appears to be less with subarachnoid bolts than with ventriculostomies.

Transport of Critically Ill Neurosurgical Patients

Many neurosurgical ICU patients require transport to other regions of the hospital for diagnostic studies. Computed tomographic (CT) scans of the head or abdomen are frequently requested on ICU patients.[88] However, transport of critically ill patients is associated with complications. As many as 70% of patients may demonstrate deterioration of gas exchange.[26] Hypotension, necessitating changes in drug infusions, is commonly associated with overzealous manual ventilation.[26] To avoid unnecessary complications, the decision to transport patients must be weighed carefully, considering the anticipated results of a planned diagnostic study and the likelihood that results will alter clinical management. Only 25% of 103 consecutive transports for diagnostic studies at a trauma unit led to a change in patient management.[113]

During transport of critically ill patients, the standards of intensive monitoring, nursing care, and respiratory care should be maintained. Suggested solutions include the design of a portable transport unit for patients to standardize care and the development of a separate transport team for critically ill patients, although the efficacy of this concept in intrahospital transport has not been evaluated.[113]

IMMEDIATE POSTOPERATIVE CARE
Carotid Endarterectomy

After carotid endarterectomy, the most important considerations relate to the occurrence of new neurologic deficits, hemorrhage, the hyperperfusion syndrome, hypertension, and hypotension. Although the overall incidence of serious postoperative complications is low, close observation is necessary to avoid unnecessary morbidity.

New neurologic deficits may develop because of occlusion of the operated carotid or perioperative embolic events. Recognition of a new deficit should prompt immediate diagnostic evaluation. Doppler ultrasound may demonstrate cessation of flow; angiography will confirm vascular occlusion. If occlusion is diagnosed, reexploration may be necessary, occasionally without diagnostic confirmation.

Hemorrhage after carotid endarterectomy may represent both a surgical and an anesthetic challenge. If hemorrhage is sufficiently severe to produce a large cervical hematoma, subsequent intubation may be difficult.[145] Anticipation of a difficult intubation may necessitate an induction sequence in which spontaneous ventilation is maintained until the larynx can be visualized and the airway secured.

The cerebral hyperperfusion syndrome is associated with postoperative hypertension, neurologic deficits, and increased CBF.[196] The pathogenesis appears to be sudden restoration of perfusion pressure in a vascular bed that has been chronically perfused at low pressure. Symptoms include headache and occasional seizures or intracerebral hemorrhage. Management consists of control of hypertension and treatment of associated complications such as seizures.

Hypertension and hypotension are common after carotid endarterectomy. Hypertension appears to be more common after general anesthesia, whereas hypotension is more common after regional anesthesia.[174] The etiology of blood pressure abnormalities is unclear, with hypertension attributed to circulating catecholamines and hypotension attributed to an abrupt increase in the perfusion pressure of the carotid sinus. Management of hypertension usually consists of administration of short-acting agents, such as sodium nitroprusside; hypertension typically resolves within a few days except in patients who had uncontrolled hypertension preoperatively. Management of hypotension can be accomplished with volume administration or the infusion of phenylephrine.[156] The use of an alpha agonist is appropriate, because most patients after carotid endarterectomy have adequate systemic perfusion and, in this population with a high incidence of coronary artery disease, the use of combined alpha and beta agonists has been associated with postoperative myocardial infarction.[159]

Craniotomy

A variety of minor and major challenges occur after craniotomy for tumor, hematoma drainage, aneurysm clipping, or other intracranial procedures. Decisions must be made regarding the timing of extubation, head elevation, maintenance of ventilation and oxygenation, control of pain, management of nausea and vomiting, treatment of hypovolemia, reversal of incidental or intentional hypothermia, termination of seizures, reduction of excessive blood pressure, diagnosis and drainage of intracranial hematomas, management of increased ICP, treatment of tension pneumocephalus, identification of peripheral nerve injuries, and recognition of upward transtentorial herniation.

After resection of a supratentorial tumor, most patients who have recovered sufficiently from anesthesia to follow commands can be safely extubated in the operating room. However, patients with compromised airway protection preoperatively should remain intubated postoperatively. After posterior fossa surgery, cranial nerve defects are common; therefore it is important to assess ability to handle secretions, because insidious aspiration is a frequent cause of postoperative morbidity.[109]

After movement from the operating table, most patients are positioned in a semirecumbent position with the head elevated 30 degrees to maximize cerebral venous drainage and are then transported to the PACU. Supplemental oxygen, direct arterial blood pressure monitoring, and pulse oximetry, if possible, should be continued during transport. The PACU staff should be informed about important details regarding preoperative status and intraoperative course, especially the patient's preexisting neurologic condition, nerve deficits, intraoperative administration of antiepileptics and diuretics, and parameters for hemodynamic management.

Patients who should be maintained in the supine rather than head-up position include those who have undergone drainage of a chronic subdural hematoma or repair of a CSF leak. After transsphenoidal surgery, patients have extensive nasal packing and must breathe through their mouths. Humidification of inspired gases improves postoperative comfort.

Ventilation should be assessed frequently in the immediate postoperative interval. Neuromuscular blockers should be fully reversed. Impaired swallowing ability may be related to residual neuromuscular blockade and not to cranial nerve dysfunction. A high percentage of newly admitted PACU patients demonstrate residual neuromuscular blockade.[16] After prolonged surgery, localized airway edema may respond to inhalational administration of racemic epinephrine (0.5 ml of a 2.0% solution added to 3.0 ml of saline for nebulization). In addition to ventilatory mechanics, attention should be paid to ventilatory rhythm. Unusual or irregular breathing patterns such as Cheyne-Stokes respiration may signal brain stem compression by edema or hematoma. Occasionally, if patients are not stimulated after narcotic-based anesthetic techniques, hypoventilation may occur.

In individual patients the need to maintain communication and repeatedly assess level of consciousness must be weighed against the need to relieve discomfort from pain or nausea. After a narcotic-based anesthetic technique, severe postoperative pain is unusual, but often small, carefully titrated doses of morphine (1 mg IV) can be administered without causing excessive sedation.

Postoperative nausea and vomiting in neurosurgical patients should be alleviated promptly, because these conditions may increase blood pressure and ICP. Refractory nausea should prompt consideration of the development of acute hydrocephalus or increased ICP secondary to brain edema or hematoma.[86] Droperidol, 0.625 to 2.5 mg intravenously, and promethazine, 12.5 to 25 mg intravenously or intramuscularly, both commonly employed to treat nausea and vomiting, are dopamine antagonists and may cause dystonic reactions or exacerbations of Parkinson's disease.

After craniotomy, patients may be relatively hypovolemic secondary to intraoperative use of diuretics or acute blood loss. As a first-line guide to the adequacy of blood volume, urinary output should be maintained at 0.5 ml/kg/hr through infusions of isotonic, non−glucose-containing solutions. Electrolytes should be measured early in the postoperative period to monitor changes in serum sodium and potassium, particularly if diuretics have been administered. If a suprasellar mass has been resected or the patient has experienced severe head injury, the onset of diabetes insipidus should be considered if urinary output exceeds 200 to 400 ml/hr and if specific gravity is less than 1.005.

Because mild hypothermia may protect the brain from ischemic injury, neurosurgical patients may be permitted to become somewhat hypothermic in the operating room and may arrive in the PACU in that state.[108] Mild degrees of hypothermia can prolong emergence from anesthesia, causing concern among the anesthetic and surgical staff. If the patient is allowed to shiver, oxygen consumption may increase as much as 400%, thereby risking hypertension and hypercarbia. Hypothermia should be corrected with warming lights or the application of a circulating warm air mattress. Infused fluids should be warmed.

Prevention of seizures in the postoperative period is critical. Seizures may precipitate serious complications, including secondary intracranial bleeding, hypoxia, and aspiration. If seizures occur despite preoperative administration of anticonvulsants, control should be obtained with small doses of benzodiazepines while ensuring an adequate airway. A recurrent intracranial mass should be suspected if a patient is not arousable within a short interval after termination of a seizure; a cranial CT scan is then indicated.

In neurosurgical patients, hypertension in the periopera-

tive and postoperative period may be a sign of developing intracranial hematomas.[96] Other causes of postoperative hypertension, including hypercarbia, pain, shivering, and bladder distention, also should be investigated. If there is no apparent primary cause of hypertension, aggressive efforts at control are warranted because of the risk that hypertension will precipitate intracranial hemorrhage or worsen cerebral edema. After supratentorial craniotomy for tumor, appropriate initial treatment consists of the administration of labetalol (5 to 10 mg increments IV) or small doses of esmolol. If hypertension persists and intracranial hypertension is unlikely, hydralazine (10 to 20 mg IV), nifedipine (10 to 20 mg sublingually), or, in rare cases, a continuous infusion of SNP may be required.

Although a variety of focal neurologic deficits may be present, a depressed level of consciousness is the most consistent clinical presentation of postoperative intracranial hematomas,[96] 15% of which present within 6 hours of surgery. Coagulopathy and hypertension are precipitating factors for hematomas after brain tumor surgery. In a survey of approximately 5000 intracranial procedures, most postoperative hematomas occurred in the operative site, whereas 17% occurred at remote sites.[96] Surgical positioning (supine or lateral vs. sitting) did not correlate with the occurrence of postoperative hematoma.[96] After surgery for drainage of traumatic intracranial mass lesions, pretraumatic alcohol intake and preoperative mannitol administration correlated with a higher incidence of postcraniotomy hematomas.[28] In some patients who have suffered head trauma, ICP fails to rise despite clinical deterioration, and detection of a postcranial hematoma may be delayed if the clinical examination is discounted.[28]

Even in the absence of intracranial hematomas, ICP commonly increases after elective intracranial surgery, with maximal pressure readings recorded approximately 16 hours postoperatively.[42] After brain tumor resection, the most common finding on a cranial CT scan of a patient with elevated ICP is brain edema.[42] Risk factors for postoperative intracranial hypertension include glioblastoma resection, repeat surgery, and protracted surgery (>6 hours). ICP monitoring performed in the supratentorial compartment may not accurately reflect pressures in the infratentorial compartment. During the first 12 hours postoperatively, monitored posterior fossa pressure was 50% greater than that of the supratentorial space.[162] Compliance also was markedly less in the posterior fossa compartment when compared to the supratentorial compartment (Fig. 30-3).[162] No untoward side effects were noted related to monitoring ICP in the posterior fossa with a Silastic catheter.[162] Some centers have also employed brain stem auditory evoked potentials to monitor posterior fossa dynamics in patients who are unresponsive after surgery.

Aggressive intraoperative cerebrospinal fluid drainage or diuretic administration can create a space between the dura and cranial vault, sometimes resulting in a tension pneumocephalus that is possibly exacerbated by nitrous oxide,

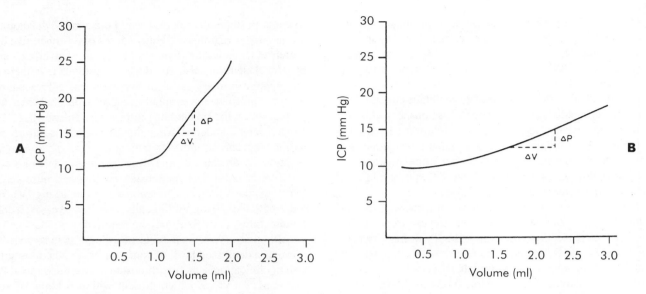

FIG. 30-3 Postoperative intracranial compliance curves. **A,** Infratentorial compartment. **B,** Supratentorial compartment. Compliance was less in the posterior fossa compartment when compared to the supratentorial compartment. *(From Rosenwasser RH, Kleiner LI, Krzeminski JP et al: Intracranial pressure monitoring in the posterior fossa: a preliminary report,* J Neurosurg *71:503, 1989.)*

as the cranial contents retract. In the PACU, focal neurologic signs or a generalized decrease in alertness may signal the presence of a symptomatic tension pneumocephalus. Prompt placement of a burr hole to release trapped gases frequently results in an improved level of consciousness.

Peripheral nerve injuries related to surgical positioning may be initially recognized in the PACU. Sciatic nerve injury and brachial plexus injury have been attributed to intraoperative positioning. Corneal abrasions, either related to damage to the fifth cranial nerve intraoperatively or to positioning, should be promptly suspected in patients who complain of eye pain.

A particularly worrisome complication that can occur after resection of a tumor at the cervical medullary junction is upward transtentorial herniation secondary to edema of the operative site.[191] Patients classically present with an abrupt decrease in the level of consciousness and with impaired ventilation. A high index of suspicion for this complication should be maintained in the patient who has undergone decompression at the cervical medullary junction.

Vascular Problems
Intracranial Aneurysm

Increasingly, patients with subarachnoid hemorrhage (SAH) secondary to a ruptured cerebral aneurysm undergo surgery to isolate the aneurysm shortly after admission to the hospital. So-called early surgery, which contrasts with the more traditional approach of waiting until the risk of postoperative vasospasm has decreased, permits more aggressive treatment of delayed cerebral ischemia secondary to cerebral vasospasm.

After uncomplicated aneurysm clipping, patients will most likely be extubated if the preoperative neurologic grade was favorable (Hunt and Hess grades I, II, and III). Intraoperative aneurysm rupture, acute hydrocephalus, brain swelling, or hemodynamic instability may prompt a decision to maintain intubation for a short interval postoperatively. In the PACU immediately after surgery, problems that may require attention include management of cardiac output and blood pressure, rewarming from moderate hypothermia, identification and control of electrolyte abnormalities, treatment of hypovolemia, prophylaxis against seizures, and recognition and evacuation of postoperative intracranial hematomas.

Hemodynamic management of patients who have experienced an SAH has generated considerable controversy. Before aneurysm obliteration, hypertension potentially can precipitate rerupture, although hypervolemic, normotensive hemodilution may reduce cerebral ischemic symptoms. Once an aneurysm has been clipped, many surgeons add moderate hypertension to hypervolemic hemodilution in patients who have symptomatic vasospasm. Prophylactic hypervolemic hemodilution, with or without hypertension, may be used in asymptomatic patients. Most clinicians monitor either central venous pressure (CVP) or use a pulmonary artery catheter to monitor cardiac output and PAOP in hemodiluted patients. Although results in some series are encouraging, randomized prospective studies evaluating prophylactic hypervolemic therapy are lacking.[99] Indeed, in patients with myocardial dysfunction, rapid expansion of volume may be detrimental, causing pulmonary edema and congestive heart failure.[144]

Although SAH is associated with electrocardiographic changes suggestive of myocardial ischemia, those abnormalities do not accurately predict myocardial function as assessed by echocardiography.[45] Myocardial dysfunction is more closely correlated with neurologic condition. In previously healthy individuals after SAH, CVP correlates poorly with PAOP and cardiac performance. A PAOP of 14 mm Hg was associated with maximum cardiac performance without the use of inotropes in one clinical series.[110]

Disturbances of CSF circulation occur in most patients after SAH. Although intracranial hypertension is related to the amount of intraventricular blood shown on CT scan, patients should be observed carefully in the PACU for decreases in level of consciousness. If an intraventricular drain is present, modest drainage of CSF may restore ICP to normal levels.[98]

A syndrome of salt wasting after SAH has been described. Hypovolemia, which may accompany relative hyponatremia in this group of patients, is frequently associated with the development of cerebral ischemia.[79] Marked increases in ANP precede natriuresis, and elevations of serum ADH levels are also reported.[215]

After craniotomy for aneurysm clipping, patients must be observed for seizures. Preoperative hypertension is a risk factor for epilepsy, and phenobarbital or phenytoin can be administered for prophylaxis.[143] Finally, careful monitoring of the level of consciousness and ICP in the PACU may alert the clinician to developing intracerebral hematomas, related to the operative site or to overzealous CSF drainage and tearing of the bridging dural veins.[9]

Arteriovenous Malformation

Most aspects of the care of patients who have undergone craniotomy for resection of aneurysms and arteriovenous malformations (AVMs) are similar. However, hemodynamic management after AVM resection emphasizes postoperative control of increases in mean arterial blood pressure. Patients who have undergone AVM resection are at risk for the development of the syndrome of normal pressure cerebral hyperperfusion (particularly if the AVM was large and contained feeding vessels perforating deep into the brain).[15] Of a large surgical series, 20% of patients developed evidence of cerebral edema and brain swelling approximately 48 to 72 hours after resection of large AVMs.[15] Experimental evidence indicates that areas of brain immediately bordering large AVMs may be chronically ischemic[14] but hyperreactive to increases in $Paco_2$.[222] After AVM resection, blood vessels that heretofore had been relatively hypoperfused become hyperperfused. Treatment may necessitate emergency reintubation, hyperventilation, administration of mannitol, and induction of barbiturate coma. In certain centers, extremely large AVMs are resected with the patient under barbiturate anesthesia sufficient to produce electroencephalographic burst suppression, and the patient is awakened slowly from anesthesia.[190]

In some patients after AVM resection, a hyperdynamic cardiovascular response, apparently centrally mediated, complicates management.[152] Marked increases in cardiac index, stroke index, left ventricular stroke work index, and heart rate have been observed for 24 hours or more postoperatively. Postoperative seizures after AVM resections are common, and prophylaxis must be continued in the perioperative period.

Vasospasm after Subarachnoid Hemorrhage

Seven percent of neurosurgical patients with aneurysms will die from vasospasm; others will suffer disabling neurologic morbidity.[84] Vasospasm causes delayed cerebral ischemic deficits in 20% to 30% of patients who survive SAH. Although 70% of patients develop radiographic evidence of vascular spasm, it is most often clinically asymptomatic.

Three to nine days after SAH, the patient with symptomatic vasospasm will characteristically become disoriented and drowsy over a period of hours. Focal deficits may follow. Vasospasm is presumed to be the etiology if repeat hemorrhage, mass lesion, intracranial hypertension, meningitis, or metabolic encephalopathy can be excluded through proper diagnostic studies.

Arteriography in patients who have vasospasm demonstrates luminal irregularities in large conducting vessels, although these are not the major site of precapillary resistance. CBF is not reduced until the angiographic diameter of the cerebral arteries is decreased by 50% or more compared to normal.[209] The intraparenchymal cerebral resistance vessels tend to dilate after the onset of spasm of the larger vessels, thus partially compensating for increased upstream resistance. ICP and cerebral blood volume may actually increase during vasospasm owing to dilation of cerebral capacitance vessels (veins) and accumulation of tissue edema resulting from cerebral ischemia.[100]

Recent positron emission tomography data indicate that in patients with focal deficits, CBF values are within the 10 to 20 ml/100 g/min range (50 ml/100 g/min being normal). In patients with regional CBF values less than 12 ml/100 g/min, clinical deficits are not reversible.[154] Global CBF is markedly reduced (10 to 30 ml/100 g/min) in patients who are stuporous because of severe diffuse vasospasm.[154]

The most common modality used clinically to confirm the presence of vasospasm is transcranial Doppler (TCD) ultrasonography,[1] which measures blood flow velocity in the large extracerebral arteries. In the basal cerebral, middle cerebral, and internal carotid arteries, blood flow velocity and blood vessel diameter relate inversely. Theoretically, TCD should be able to confirm the presence of vasospasm in more than 90% of patients with anterior circulation aneurysms who have involvement of the basal vessels.[187]

A *peak* flow velocity of 140 to 200 cm/sec is defined as moderate spasm, whereas peak flow velocities greater than 200 cm/sec are classified as severe (Fig. 30-4). Blood flow velocities, normal in the first 12 hours after ictus, tend to

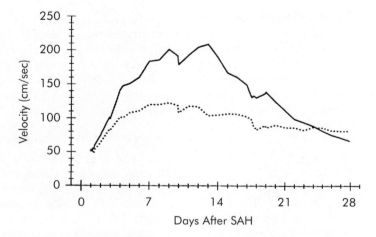

FIG. 30-4 Transcranial Doppler ultrasound data for five patients with permanent neurologic deficits from cerebral infarction. Curve shows the time course of severe symptomatic vasospasm. A peak flow velocity of 140 to 200 cm/sec in the middle cerebral artery is defined as moderate spasm, whereas velocities >200 cm/sec are classified as severe. *(Modified from Seiler RW, Grolimund P, Aaslid R et al: Cerebral vasospasm evaluated by transcranial ultrasound correlated with clinical grade and CT-visualized subarachnoid hemorrhage, J Neurosurg 64:594, 1986.)*

increase by the second postictal day, reach a plateau between the sixth and the ninth days, and remain elevated for 15 to 30 days depending on the amount of blood in the basal cisterns on CT scan.[177] In patients with severely elevated ICP, the diastolic component of large vessel flow is progressively lost; therefore TCD ultrasonography using only *mean* flow velocities may inaccurately evaluate the severity and time course of vasospasm and can produce false-negative results.[100]

Cerebrovascular reactivity is impaired in patients who have vasospasm. Pressure autoregulation is ineffective. In patients with symptomatic vasospasm the maximally dilated intraparenchymal resistance vessels are unable to dilate further in response to decreased perfusion pressure. Thus CBF decreases during induced hypotension.[210] Carbon dioxide reactivity persists but is abnormal. Hypocapnia, which enhances vasospasm both in patients with severe diffuse vasospasm (Hunt and Hess grades III and IV) and in those with better neurologic grade (Hunt and Hess grades I, II, and III),[210] may be detrimental in the presence of diffuse vasospasm. Interestingly, the response to hypercapnia in the group of patients with better neurologic grade is markedly diminished.

Cerebral infarction after the onset of vasospasm appears to correlate with the amount of blood seen on the patient's initial CT scan and with a history of hypertension.[19] Pathologically, vasospasm is associated with narrowed arteries and microscopic changes such as intraluminal platelet and white blood cell accumulation; intimal degeneration with swelling and proliferation; damage to the endothelium with subendothelial fibrosis; migration and necrosis of smooth muscle cells with medial infiltration of lymphocytes, plasma cells, and macrophages; and degeneration of perivascular nerves. These microscopic changes are observed within days of SAH.[99]

> **BOX 30-1**
> **ACTIONS OF OXYHEMOGLOBIN ASSOCIATED WITH CEREBRAL VASOSPASM**
>
> - Direct vasoconstriction
> - Release of prostaglandin (PGE$_2$)
> - Inhibition of endothelium-derived relaxant factor (EDRF)
> - Propagation of lipid peroxidation
> - Release of endothelin

Chemical factors may also play a synergistic role with the anatomic degeneration seen with vasospasm. Although many putative mediators have been proposed in the past 20 years, oxyhemoglobin currently appears to be the principal pathogenetic agent.[120] Oxyhemoglobin, released from lysis of subarachnoid red blood cells, is present in high concentrations in the CSF during vasospasm. Although oxyhemoglobin is a less potent vasoconstrictor than other agents, it promotes the release of vasoactive eicosanoids and endothelin from the arterial wall, inhibits endothelium-dependent relaxation, produces bilirubin and lipid peroxide, and causes damage to perivascular nerves (Box 30-1). As the blood clot undergoes lysis, oxyhemoglobin is liberated and converted to methemoglobin and superoxide anion. In the presence of iron the superoxide anion converts to the highly reactive hydroxy radical, which in turn reacts with fatty acids to cause destruction of membranes by lipid peroxidation.[121]

The observation that free radicals can cause injury by initiating a generalized inflammatory response prompted a small clinical trial of high-dose methylprednisolone administered to patients within 72 hours of SAH. Those patients receiving methylprednisolone (30 mg/kg IV every 6 hours for 3 days initially) were twice as likely to have an excellent outcome after SAH and half as likely to die as patients receiving placebo.[37] The incidence of severe, delayed cerebral ischemia also was reduced in the treated patients when compared to control patients. None of the small group of steroid-treated patients developed serious side effects attributable to steroid treatment. However, these results must be confirmed in a large clinical trial.

Other treatment modalities include fibrinolysis, angioplasty, calcium entry blockers, and hypervolemic hypertension. Fibrinolysis of the subarachnoid hematoma markedly reduces the effects of vasospasm. A continuous infusion of intracisternal recombinant tissue plasminogen activator has been used to promote clearance of blood from the subarachnoid space.[223] Although development of an intracranial hematoma is a risk, postoperative treatment with tissue plasminogen activator in serial doses is well tolerated and appears to be effective in reducing the severity of delayed cerebral vasospasm.[223]

When patients initially become symptomatic from vasospasm, angioplasty increases the caliber of spastic vessels, produces rapid clinical improvement, and significantly reduces flow velocities on TCD in selected patients. The effects of dilation of vasospastic arteries appear stable.[221]

Intracellular calcium, known to mediate tension development in vascular smooth muscle, enters the cell through leakage, receptor-mediated channels, and voltage-mediated channels.[59] A subtype of voltage-mediated channel, the L-type calcium channel, which is abundant in cardiac, cerebral, and skeletal vascular smooth muscle, is blocked by dihydropyridine drugs such as nimodipine and nicardipine. Nimodipine and nicardipine, which are highly lipid soluble, readily cross the blood-brain barrier. Clinical trials have demonstrated the efficacy of these drugs in preventing and treating delayed cerebral ischemia related to vasospasm.[65]

The initial report on the effectiveness of nimodipine was by Allen and co-workers,[7] who administered oral nimodipine, 0.7 mg/kg loading dose followed by 0.35 mg/kg every 4 hours, to a small group of patients in a randomized, double-blind prospective study. In these patients, who were Hunt and Hess grades I and II, nimodipine reduced the occurrence of severe neurologic deficits and mortality from vasospasm. Pickard et al.[150] found that oral nimodipine, 60 mg every 4 hours, reduced both the frequency of cerebral infarction and the percentage of patients with poor outcome in comparison to placebo treatment. In poor-grade aneurysm patients prospectively randomized to receive oral nimodipine therapy, 90 mg every 4 hours, outcome was improved 3 months after SAH and fewer patients developed delayed ischemic deficits from vasospasm, although angiographic evidence of vasospasm was unchanged.[149] In a randomized, double-blind, placebo-controlled study, nimodipine, 0.03 mg/kg/hr administered intravenously within 24 hours of the symptoms of delayed cerebral ischemia, was associated with reductions in mortality and severe morbid-

ity from vasospasm.[93] Nicardipine, which is available as an intravenous solution, is the therapeutic agent in an ongoing randomized clinical trial addressing prevention of vasospasm after SAH.[59]

As discussed previously, hypervolemic hemodilution has been advocated for prophylaxis and treatment of vasospasm in patients after SAH. Theoretic evidence supporting the need for volume expansion includes the observation that 10% to 33% of patients after SAH develop hyponatremia, associated with negative sodium balance and intravascular volume contraction.[141] Hyponatremic patients are more likely to develop vasospasm. In one series, prophylactic volume expansion was associated with outcomes as good as those achieved with calcium channel blocker prophylaxis.[131] Although no large clinical trials have used a controlled randomized design to compare volume expansion to other therapies for symptomatic vasospasm, many surgeons are convinced that patients demonstrate symptomatic improvement once blood volume has been expanded.

In general, clinical reports, with patients serving as their own controls, provide circumstantial evidence of the efficacy of hypervolemia and induced hypertension to treat vasospasm. One algorithm for producing hypervolemia and increasing cerebral perfusion pressure consists of pulmonary artery catheterization and infusion of fluid, either saline or colloid, to increase the PAOP to 15 ± 3 mm Hg. Associated therapeutic goals include a CVP of 10 ± 2 mm Hg, a systolic blood pressure of 180 ± 10 mm Hg (a mean arterial pressure of 130 ± 10 mm Hg), and adequate arterial oxygen content, defined as a hemoglobin of 11 g/dl and an oxyhemoglobin saturation of 95% (Box 30-2).[99] If volume expansion does not achieve these hemodynamic goals, vasopressors such as phenylephrine, 10 to 14 μg/min, or dopamine, 5 to 10 μg/kg/min, are added. With this protocol, most neurologic deficits attributed to vasospasm improve within 1 to 4 hours.[223] Although the use of pulmonary artery catheterization permits more precise quantification of systemic responses to hypervolemic therapy, central venous catheterization may provide adequate monitoring information in patients who have normal cardiovascular function.

Although hemodilution is popular in some clinical centers, its clinical efficacy is unproven. Hematocrit values in the range of 35% to 50% are consistent with normal cerebral oxygen delivery. At higher values an increase in oxygen capacity is offset by increased viscosity and decreased CBF. For hematocrit values below 35%, the decreased oxygen-carrying capacity is only partially offset by decreased viscosity and increased CBF.[9]

Occasionally, hypertensive hypervolemic therapy is required for up to 3 weeks until neurologic status remains stable as treatment is tapered. A suggested protocol for weaning therapy involves 48 hours of intensive volume expansion and then gradual discontinuation of therapy with careful monitoring of clinical neurologic signs.[99] Therapy may also be discontinued by decreasing mean arterial pressure in increments of 10 mm Hg every 4 to 6 hours until new neurologic symptoms appear, pretreatment blood pressure is achieved, or vasoactive drugs are stopped. Other investigators wean therapy when CBF increases and autoregulation or carbon dioxide responsiveness, determined by CBF measurements, becomes normal.[12] Recurrent evidence of ischemic symptoms necessitates a rapid return to previously effective hemodynamic goals.

Cardiac, hematologic, and pulmonary sequelae have been reported as consequences of volume expansion and induced hypertension. Recent evidence suggests that PAOP correlates with increases in cardiac index but not with CVP. In patients with no history of heart disease, a PAOP of 14 mm Hg is associated with maximum cardiac performance.[110]

Laminectomy, Spinal Fixation, and Spinal Cord Decompression
Laminectomy

In the early postoperative period after cervical laminectomy for disk disease, concerns relate to muscle spasms, to deficits caused by intraoperative positioning, and to hematoma formation in the surgical site. Spasms of the cervical musculature often cause considerable postoperative discomfort, which can usually be relieved by small doses of benzodiazepines in the PACU. Adequate monitoring of respiratory function is essential. After lumbar laminectomy, positioning injuries may become apparent in the PACU. Although a rare complication, a hematoma at the operative site may become apparent through a progressive decrease in neurologic function. Lumbar hematoma may be particularly suspected if the patient complains of difficulties with bowel and bladder function. Unexplained hypotension may result from previously unrecognized injury to the aorta or common iliac blood vessels.[48]

A rare complication after laminectomy relates to the relatively recent surgical practice of instilling narcotics such as morphine into the epidural space. Although this represents an extremely effective method of providing postoperative analgesia for many patients,[170] an unsuspected dural rent may allow rapid drug absorption and respiratory depression in the PACU.

Spinal Fixation

When patients with a recent cervical spinal cord injury undergo acute cervical spine fixation, they may present to the PACU still manifesting signs of the acute "spinal shock" phase of injury. Blood pressure support with dopamine and careful fluid administration may be required in the postoperative period. Because patients with high cervical cord injuries cannot thermoregulate normally, rewarming after exposure to the cold operating room environment may be necessary.

Patients with acute spinal cord injuries are prone to hypoxia and hypoventilation secondary to compromised respiratory mechanics. If preoperative respiratory mechanics have been marginal, it may be best to maintain intubation until postoperative function can be thoroughly assessed. In addition, certain fixation devices such as the halo fixator may complicate emergency reintubation should the endotracheal tube become dislodged. Borderline hypoxemia, unsuspected without oximetry monitoring, is associated with severe bradycardia in this group of patients.[106] Electrocardiographic monitoring may demonstrate persistent ST elevation related to sympathetic denervation.[107]

Patients with rheumatoid arthritis often undergo operations on the cervical area of the spine to prevent progressive neurologic deterioration. These patients often manifest cardiac and respiratory problems, related to their underlying connective tissue disease, that may require postoperative hemodynamic and respiratory support. In addition, bleeding from bone graft sites can cause significant hypotension. Paresthesias related to injury of the nerves around the iliac crest (frequently the site of bone graft donation) may be evident postoperatively.[167]

Occasionally, cervical cord decompression may be attempted through the transoral route. An artificial airway, either through prolonged orotracheal intubation or tracheostomy, must be provided while swelling and the acute operative effects of dissection in the oropharynx are allowed to recede.[77] Spinal column fixation in the cervical region is also attempted through an anterolateral approach, which employs a large retractor to separate the carotid vessels from the trachea and esophagus. Reported complications from this approach include hematomas that may be manifest in the immediate postoperative period as well as esophageal perforation. The latter complication may be recognized by spreading subcutaneous emphysema.[206]

Lumbar spinal fixation is often accomplished through a posterolateral interbody fusion procedure that involves complete eradication of the disk space and subsequent insertion of bone graft between the vertebral bodies. Postoperatively, patients may be hypovolemic from intraoperative blood loss or, very rarely, from a retroperitoneal hematoma. Injury to the bowel or major vascular intraabdominal structures is possible. Patients who have had lumbar spinal fusion may benefit from patient-controlled analgesia postoperatively. Nausea in this group of patients and those who have undergone spinal stabilization procedures should be treated promptly and effectively.

Spinal Cord Decompression

Spinal cord decompression and stabilization in the acutely traumatized patient may combine a transthoracic approach to the thoracic spine and a transabdominal approach to the lumbar spine. The transthoracic approach risks intraoperative or postoperative pneumothorax. Severe postoperative pain necessitates careful attention to postoperative analgesia. Often, extensive fluid resuscitation is required in the immediate postoperative period because of relatively large "third space" edema accumulation.

Spinal cord decompression for metastatic tumors is an emergent procedure. Because of preoperative debilitation, malignant bony destruction, and extensive intraoperative blood loss,[136] these patients may manifest hypovolemia, respiratory insufficiency, and electrolyte abnormalities such as hypomagnesemia or hypercalcemia.

A particularly severe complication of decompression laminectomy for spondylitic cervical myeloradiculopathy has recently been reported in four patients. Each patient had undergone cervical decompression without problems, but on initially being raised into the sitting position within 72 hours after surgery, developed extreme hypotension, necessitating resuscitative measures. When blood pressure was restored, three of the four patients experienced residual central cervical cord syndrome apparently related to the severe hypotension. Particular caution is advised in early mobilization of elderly patients, such as those described, who have a history of hypertension and signs of arteriosclerosis.[44]

Harrington Rod Placement and Spinal Column Stabilization

In adolescents and young adults with scoliosis, Harrington rod placement is performed to prevent progression of the deformity and disability. In older patients, Harrington rod placement is used to stabilize the spine. Because of the extent of the procedure and because of preoperative respiratory compromise by the chest deformity, postoperative respiratory complications, including pneumothorax, pneumonia, and atelectasis, occur frequently.[101] In patients with severe scoliosis accompanied by neuromuscular disease, postoperative ventilation is often anticipated. Other problems seen shortly after Harrington rod placement include fat embolism, wound hematoma, and paralytic ileus, as well as severe postoperative pain. Patient-controlled analgesia is effective in most patients, including the very young, after Harrington rod placement. Neurologic complications related both to positioning and to nerve root entrapment secondary to the Harrington rod apparatus or herniated disks secondary to the instrumentation have also been reported.[137] Nerve root compression problems related to Harrington rods may not be detected by intraoperative somatosensory evoked potential monitoring.[176]

SPECIFIC CRITICAL CARE ISSUES
Decreased Level of Consciousness

Impaired consciousness is nonspecific; however, recognition of changing consciousness may signal a variety of treatable conditions, including progression of intracranial hypertension, developing vasospasm in patients after subarachnoid hemorrhage, delayed posttraumatic intracranial hematomas, or systemic complications of intracranial pathologic conditions, such as hyponatremia, hypoxemia, or hypercarbia. Focal neurologic findings often suggest a specific lesion; that is, unilateral weakness or reflex changes developing after carotid endarterectomy suggest the possibility of ipsilateral carotid occlusion.

Frequent, accurately recorded neurologic examinations are an essential aspect of neurologic monitoring. Ideally, any neurologic examination will include a meaningful, easily interpreted description of the patient's ability to interact with the environment. Neurologic examination quantifies two key characteristics: changes in consciousness and focal brain dysfunction. The state of consciousness and the trend in neurologic function are the most important indications of the severity of neurologic disease and the most important predictors of survival. Comparable levels of consciousness imply different prognoses in patients who are improving vs. those who are deteriorating.

The Glasgow Coma Scale (GCS), originally developed as a prognostic tool and as a way to compare series of patients in different institutions,[197] has become popular as a brief estimate, with minimal interobserver variability, of level of consciousness in critically ill patients. The GCS score has been used successfully to stratify general ICU patients and predict mortality,[13] although discrimination in the intermediate ranges (GCS scores of 7 to 11) is poor. The scale, which includes observations regarding eye opening, motor response in the "best" limb, and verbal responses, is less useful in intubated patients who cannot make verbal responses. The GCS does not provide information regarding pupillary responses and brainstem functions. A first approximation of the likely etiology of deteriorating neurologic status includes level of consciousness, best motor response, pupillary response, corneal responses, ocular muscle function, and respiratory function.

Assessment of consciousness is by two means, verbal response and response to pain. The former includes spontaneous speech: oriented, confused, inappropriate, or incomprehensible. Response to pain is essential in assessing patients who make no verbal responses. Because consciousness waxes and wanes, the pain stimulus must be severe enough to elicit a response.

Motor responses are lost in the following sequence: obeying commands, localization of pain, withdrawal to pain, flexion to pain, and extension to pain. The likelihood of severe morbidity and mortality increases substantially in patients who have abnormal posturing.

Brainstem function (i.e., pupillary light responses)

should also be tested in all comatose patients to assist in establishing prognosis.[98,100,101] In paralyzed, intubated patients, the pupillary reaction provides the only clinical neurologic assessment. In the course of transtentorial herniation, the superficial location of the parasympathetic fibers on the third nerve results in early compression, resulting in ipsilateral pupillary dilation. Bilateral dilated pupils constitute a grave prognostic sign. Pupillary examination may be difficult in the presence of an associated orbital hematoma or erroneous with direct ocular or optic trauma. Corneal reflexes, important for protection of the eyes, are lost early after traumatic brain injury and have little prognostic significance.

Both the oculovestibular and the oculocephalic reflexes require the integrity of the third, fourth, and sixth cranial nerves, the medial longitudinal fasciculus, the eighth nerve afferents, and an intact brainstem. The oculocephalic reflex requires movement of the neck and is hence inappropriate in the presence of a cervical spine injury. The normal oculocephalic response, tested by abruptly rocking the head from right to left, is maintenance of the direction of gaze despite a shift in head position. If a normal oculocephalic (doll's eyes) response cannot or should not be elicited, the normal oculovestibular (ice-water caloric) response of a comatose patient to irrigation of the external ear canal with 10 to 20 ml of ice-cold water should be tonic gaze deviation of both eyes to the ipsilateral side.[102] The oculovestibular response requires a patent external auditory canal. Initial stimulation with measured cold saline should be performed with the patient's head in a neutral position if cervical spine injury is a consideration; however, neck flexion of 30 degrees may be required if the reflex is impaired. Impaired oculocephalic and oculovestibular reflexes are grave prognostic signs.

Neurologic examination may also suggest the possibility of intracranial hypertension in patients at risk. A patient able to follow simple commands, even if stuporous or lethargic, rarely has a raised ICP, whereas approximately 40% to 50% of head-injured patients with altered consciousness have intracranial hypertension. The symptoms and signs of raised ICP are not, however, uniformly reliable. In unconscious, head-injured patients, the probability of increased ICP is lower if the patient withdraws to painful stimuli or moans or grimaces. A frankly raised ICP is likely to be encountered with GCS scores of 4 to 6 in head-injured patients. Severe increases in ICP may present as the Cushing triad of hypertension, bradycardia, and respiratory irregularity; but the absence of the Cushing triad does not rule out intracranial hypertension. Pupillary dilation may herald transtentorial herniation but is a late manifestation of central herniation. Herniation, which could be a result of vascular insufficiency or direct compression and infarction of the brainstem, is a major catastrophe almost synonymous with imminent, extensive, and fatal brain damage. The presence of apnea is also a grave prognostic sign.

Cerebral Ischemia
Pharmacologic Management

After stroke the therapeutic window for pharmacologic or other interventions is narrow, probably less than 6 to 12 hours before injury is complete.[21] However, carotid cross-clamping during carotid endarterectomy and temporary occlusion of arteries during aneurysm clipping are surgical situations in which prompt intervention, whether initiated before, during, or after ischemia, might reduce morbidity and mortality. In addition to injury occurring during ischemia, experimental work suggests the likely occurrence of reperfusion injury, damage that occurs after restoration of flow in neural tissue or in the cerebral vasculature (Fig. 30-5). Reperfusion injury is a potential source of morbidity after pharmacologic or surgical recanalization for acute stroke, after temporary arterial occlusion during carotid endarterectomy or intracranial vascular surgery, and after restoration of cerebral perfusion after cardiac arrest. The therapeutic implications of progressive injury during reperfusion are obvious. Therapeutic interventions, even if initiated after restoration of perfusion, could perhaps decrease neurologic morbidity if the mechanisms underlying progressive injury can be identified and interrupted. Drugs that offer promise in ameliorating the effects of acute cerebral ischemia include calcium entry blockers, pentoxifylline, thrombolytic agents, antagonists of the excitotoxins (glutamate and aspartate), and gangliosides.

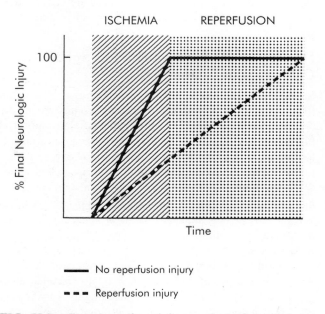

FIG. 30-5 Experimental work has emphasized the likely occurrence of reperfusion injury in the cerebral circulation. Reperfusion injury is damage that occurs in neural tissue or in the cerebral vasculature after cerebral blood flow (CBF) is restored. A central part of the reperfusion injury hypothesis is that ischemic injury is not maximal at the time that ischemia resolves.

Meta-analysis of five double-blind, placebo-controlled studies of the treatment of stroke with nimodipine, a calcium entry blocker that differentially dilates the cerebral vasculature, indicates that nimodipine improves mortality and outcome.[63] Efficacy is particularly evident if nimodipine administration occurs within 12 hours of the onset of stroke or if the patient is more than 65 years of age. Adverse reactions, primarily hypotension, are relatively mild. Nimodipine is administered orally in a total daily dose of 120 mg, most often as four divided doses.

Nicardipine, a more water-soluble calcium entry blocker that can be administered intravenously, has also been associated with encouraging results in a limited number of patients suffering from acute cerebral ischemia. Despite a significant incidence of hypotension, occasionally requiring discontinuation of therapy, patients starting therapy less than 6 hours after the onset of ischemic symptoms show neurologic improvement at 3-month follow-up.[161]

Pentoxifylline, a methylxanthine that reduces blood viscosity and improves distal circulatory flow in lower extremity claudication, increases CBF in low-flow areas in patients with chronic cerebrovascular disease.[140] If administered during the first few days after acute stroke, it produces clinical improvement that has not been sustained.[94] It may be efficacious as an adjunct to other modalities in acute stroke.

Cerebrovascular recanalization may improve CBF after acute thromboembolic events. Tissue plasminogen activator, recently available in sufficient quantities for clinical trials, is a relatively thromboselective agent that promotes thrombolysis when administered by intravenous infusion. A prospective, open-label, multicenter study of recombinant tissue plasminogen activator in acute thromboembolic and thrombotic stroke is now underway. Although preliminary results indicate that partial arterial recanalization occurs in all dosage groups, hemorrhagic transformation of the ischemic deficit is a common finding, occurring in 27% of patients studied at 24 hours after treatment.[47] Despite this fact, most patients demonstrated minimal change in clinical status after hemorrhagic infarction and followed a generally benign course.

Antagonists of the excitatory neurotransmitter glutamate may play an important role in mediating ischemic neuronal damage. Oral dextromethorphan, an n-methyl-D-aspartate antagonist, has neuroprotective properties in animal models of ischemia.[6] Preliminary studies indicate that this drug, when administered in a dose of 30 mg orally four times daily to patients at risk for brain ischemia, demonstrates little toxicity.[20] This preliminary study may allow the design of larger studies using the agent for therapy after stroke.

The monosialoganglioside GM_1 reduces excitatory amino acid–related neurotoxicity by limiting excitatory amino acid receptor stimulation and promoting neuronal regeneration.[33] If patients receive GM_1 daily (100 mg IV for 15 days) after a stroke, significant neurologic improvement

can be demonstrated with no increase in mortality.[66] Larger prospective studies are planned.

Hemodilution

Cerebral perfusion also can be improved by reducing blood viscosity with hemodilution. Hypervolemic hemodilution with dextran produces small, statistically insignificant increases in CBF in animals with normal cerebral vasculature.[219] However, in brain tissue distal to an experimental middle cerebral artery occlusion, dextran significantly improves CBF.[218,220] If cerebral oxygen delivery (CDo_2, the product of CBF and Cao_2) increases, tissue with borderline viability may be preserved. Hemodilution has been extensively studied in patients with stroke. In patients with acute stroke, normovolemic hemodilution increases CBF and improves EEG activity.[217]

However, widespread clinical application has been impeded by concern regarding two physiologic risks. First, hypervolemia may produce cardiac failure or myocardial ischemia in patients who have coexisting cerebrovascular and coronary occlusive disease. Second, although flow may be slightly improved by moderate hemodilution, the reduction in oxygen-carrying capacity may prevent any improvement in local oxygen delivery. The Scandinavian Stroke Study Group, which randomized 373 patients to receive either conventional therapy or normovolemic hemodilution after stroke, demonstrated an increased incidence of cardiovascular complications and an increased early mortality among hemodiluted patients.[169] The Italian Acute Stroke Study Group randomized 1267 patients to receive conventional therapy or normovolemic hemodilution and found no difference in outcome.[92] However, both studies were constrained by the cardiovascular risk of volume expansion. In contrast, the Hemodilution in Stroke Study Group used invasive cardiovascular monitoring to guide hypervolemic hemodilution with pentastarch and increase cardiac output in patients with acute ischemic stroke.[81] Although overall mortality and neurologic outcome were not superior in the hemodilution group, neurologic outcome was apparently improved in patients who were entered into the trial within 12 hours of the onset of stroke and in those who had an increase of cardiac output greater than or equal to 10% of baseline.

Acute Intracranial Hypertension

Control of increased ICP depends on effective control of cerebral tissue volume, cerebral blood volume, and CSF volume. The therapy of intracranial hypertension must either decrease the volume of the component that caused the original problem (e.g., tumor or hematoma removal) or decrease the volume of one of the other components (Fig. 30-6). On an emergent basis, intracranial hypertension is most quickly treated by reducing cerebral blood volume, often by intentionally using acute hyperventilation to decrease CBF.

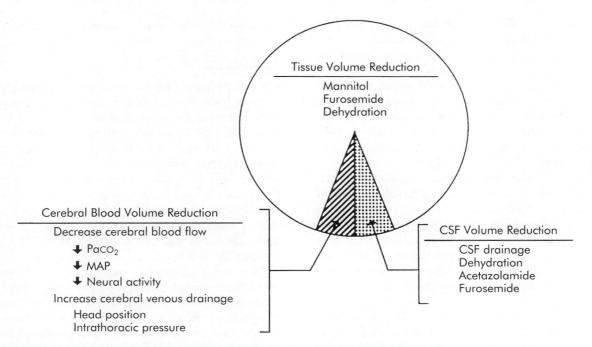

FIG. 30-6   Strategies for reducing intracranial pressure (ICP) based on the intracranial compartments: tissue volume, cerebrospinal fluid (CSF) volume, or cerebral blood volume. *MAP,* Mean arterial pressure. The therapy of intracranial hypertension must either decrease the volume of the component that caused the original increase in ICP or decrease the volume of one of the other components.

Reduction of Cerebral Tissue Volume

Brain tissue volume, often increased as a consequence of cerebral edema, can be reduced medically or surgically. Three types of cerebral edema have been described experimentally,[58] although in individual patients more than one type of edema may be present. Interstitial edema occurs with hydrocephalus. Vasogenic edema, which accompanies intracranial tumors, is associated with opening of the blood-brain barrier to protein. The most clearly established use of glucocorticoids in neurologic intensive care is to treat the vasogenic edema associated with brain tumors and brain abscesses.[158] Cytotoxic edema, which accompanies hypoxic or traumatic injury, is characterized by cellular swelling and is not responsive to glucocorticoids.[58] Therefore glucocorticoids appear to be ineffective in closed head injury[46,166] and in focal and global cerebral ischemia.[85,105]

Although chronic fluid restriction does not effectively reduce brain tissue volume, diuretics are commonly used to reduce acute intracranial hypertension associated with cerebral edema. Mannitol and other osmotic diuretics reduce brain volume primarily by osmotically removing water from uninjured brain in which the blood-brain barrier is intact. Mannitol and other osmotic diuretics also reduce blood viscosity and may improve microcirculatory flow.[85,138] This effect, in conjunction with the reduction in ICP produced by osmotic diuretics, limits the extent of infarction in animal models of focal ischemia.[85,115] Mannitol reduces ICP for 3 to 4 hours. An intravenous bolus of 1.0 to 1.5 g/kg

provides brain decompression in anticipation of surgical mass removal, that is, tumor removal or hematoma drainage. Smaller doses (0.25 to 0.5 g/kg) have been used effectively to maintain lower ICP in patients with closed head trauma. Mannitol is less effective in patients with severe, diffuse brain injury because the integrity of the blood-brain barrier is compromised. Furosemide, 20 to 40 mg intravenously, reduces ICP acutely in animal models and in patients.[43,158] Although the initial effect is to reduce brain water, furosemide also inhibits the elaboration of CSF, thereby reducing another of the three components of intracranial volume.

Reduction of Cerebral Blood Volume

Cerebral blood volume may be reduced by reducing CBF or facilitating cerebral venous drainage. Endotracheal intubation and mechanical ventilation maintain adequate gas exchange, thereby limiting the likelihood of inadvertent increases in CBF resulting from hypoxemia or hypercarbia. Adequate sedation and analgesia, by limiting the effects of brain stimulation on the cerebral metabolic rate for oxygen ($CMRo_2$) and CBF, are useful in the control of ICP. Patients with multiple injuries, including closed head trauma, may require potent narcotic analgesic agents in sufficient doses to control pain if intracranial hypertension is to be managed effectively. In such narcotized patients, control of ventilation is essential. Passive hyperventilation is commonly used to reduce CBF and cerebral blood volume, both as a sustained therapeutic measure and as an acute response to sudden increases in ICP; however, limited attention has been paid to the maintenance of adequate CBF during therapeutic hyperventilation. Mechanical hyperventilation frequently reduces the internal jugular venous oxygen saturation (Sjvo$_2$) below acceptable average levels.[142] Further studies are required to determine if monitoring of Sjvo$_2$, in conjunction with monitoring of ICP, can be used to improve outcome in patients with intracranial hypertension who require mechanical ventilation.

Blood pressure control represents a particularly difficult problem in patients with intracranial hypertension. Autoregulation is attenuated or abolished in areas of injured brain. Consequently, decreased systemic blood pressure may reduce CBF and worsen cerebral ischemia. Increased blood pressure may, in some patients, increase CBF and cerebral blood volume, thereby increasing ICP. Pharmacologic reduction of systemic blood pressure may have adverse effects on intracranial hemodynamics. SNP has been associated both with cerebral ischemia from rapid blood pressure reduction[76] and with intracranial hypertension. Nitroglycerin, like SNP, may increase ICP. When SNP or nitroglycerin is used to reduce blood pressure in patients with intracranial lesions, the net effect on ICP is the result of reduced cerebral blood volume in injured areas that do not autoregulate and increased cerebral blood volume in intact regions where the drug therapy itself inhibits autoregulation. Other antihypertensive drugs also influence CBF. The calcium entry blocker nifedipine maintains or increases CBF and may increase ICP.[18] Labetalol, a combination beta- and alpha-antagonist, causes little change in CBF in hypertensive patients.[147]

Reduction of Cerebrospinal Fluid Volume

CSF volume can be reduced mechanically through systemic dehydration or by pharmacologic intervention. CSF can be withdrawn through intraventricular catheters, which are placed more commonly in patients who have intraventricular hemorrhage and less commonly in other situations involving intracranial hypertension. Dehydration decreases the production of CSF. Drugs such as furosemide; acetazolamide, 250 mg orally or intravenously; and digoxin also reduce CSF production, although they are uncommonly used in acute situations.

Acute Brain Swelling

Bilateral, diffuse cerebral swelling typically occurs after head trauma in young children.[21] In contrast to increased brain water accumulation associated with cerebral edema, cerebral swelling represents vascular congestion. On computed tomography the cardinal diagnostic feature is symmetric compression of the lateral ventricles and cisterns and normal or increased white matter density. A lucid interval in children is more likely to result from generalized cerebral swelling or cerebral hyperemia rather than from an increasing intracranial mass. Management is best performed

with acute hyperventilation, which reduces inappropriately increased CBF. Mannitol, which may transiently increase CBF, is of less value than in states in which CBF is likely to be reduced. Hemispheric cerebral swelling, which usually represents both vascular congestion and edema, is commonly observed in association with ipsilateral subdural hematomas and epidural hematomas, in which groups it implies a mortality of nearly 90%.[116]

Acute Head Injury

The clinical concept governing the postoperative management of patients with closed head injury is that the ultimate risk of morbidity and mortality results from the cumulative effects of both the primary mechanical injury and the secondary injuries produced by associated physiologic derangements. Secondary insults, including hypoxemia, hypercapnia, hypotension, hypercapnia, and intracranial hypertension, complicate the course of 48% of comatose, head-injured patients (Table 30-6).[134] After trauma the brain is exquisitely sensitive to hypotension or hypoxia.[89,90] In experimental animals subjected to head injury, autoregulation was impaired; that is, hemorrhagic hypotension reduced CBF more than in uninjured animals,[111] and compensatory increases in CBF also failed to occur in response to hemodilution after hemorrhage.[50] The histopathologic evidence of cerebral ischemia frequently seen in fatal closed head injury illustrates the potential importance of recognizing and limiting secondary injury.[3] Therefore the focus of postoperative management of head-injured patients who require neurosurgical procedures, such as drainage of intracranial hematomas, elevation of depressed skull fractures, excision of contused brain tissue, or decompressive craniectomy, is on control of arterial blood gases, blood pressure, and intracranial pressure.

Before planning postoperative care of patients with head trauma, the clinician should anticipate the expected level of consciousness at the conclusion of surgery. Patients who preoperatively had decreased consciousness will usually be

TABLE 30-6

Influence of Remediable Causes of Secondary Injury on Outcome After Head Injury

Secondary Insult	Definition*	Poor Outcome (%)†
Hypoxemia	Pao$_2$ <60 mm Hg	59
Hypotension	SBP <90 mm Hg	65
Anemia	Hct <30%	62
Hypercarbia	Paco$_2$ >45 mm Hg	78
Intracranial hypertension	ICP >20, reducible	45
	ICP >20, not reducible	95

*SBP, Systolic blood pressure; Hct, hematocrit; ICP, intracranial pressure.
†Severe disability, persistent vegetative state, or death.
Modified from Miller JD et al: Further experience in the management of severe head injury, *J Neurosurg* 54:289, 1981.

in a similar condition postoperatively. In such patients, postoperative care, including intubation and mechanical ventilation, will be indistinguishable from that provided to head-injured patients who do not require surgery. Notable exceptions consist of acutely comatose patients who undergo emergent drainage of intracranial hematomas, after which acute improvement in cerebral perfusion will occasionally result in rapid awakening. Such patients can often be extubated soon after surgery.

Management of arterial blood gases in head-injured patients is based on several factors. First, maintenance of an artificial airway markedly reduces the probability that hypoxemia or hypercapnia will result from airway compromise, aspiration, or secretion retention. Second, acute head injury is associated with several potentially life-threatening respiratory problems, including transient apnea, aspiration of vomitus, and central neurogenic pulmonary edema.[118] Third, hyperventilation can be used as a means of reducing CBF and therefore ICP.

Hypoxemia is surprisingly common in patients who suffer closed head trauma. Ventilation-perfusion mismatching is evident even in patients who lack physical or radiographic evidence of pulmonary compromise.[173] Central neurogenic pulmonary edema,[123] an occasional accompaniment of severe injury, necessitates both prompt correction of intracranial hypertension and ventilatory support with positive end-expiratory pressure.

The physiologic rationale for routine hyperventilation recently has been questioned. Severely head-injured patients usually demonstrate a depressed $CMRo_2$, less markedly decreased CBF, and highly variable carbon dioxide reactivity. In some patients the reduced CBF appears to occur secondary to the reduction in $CMRo_2$ (i.e., CBF and $CMRo_2$ are coupled); in others, CBF may be less depressed than $CMRo_2$[142] (Fig. 30-7). Patients with coupled but reduced CBF and $CMRo_2$ may be vulnerable to excessive vasoconstriction during acute hyperventilation. Nearly 20% of patients develop a wide cerebral arteriovenous oxygen content difference ($AVDo_2$) during hyperventilation, suggesting that hyperventilation therapy perhaps should be accompanied by an estimate of the adequacy of cerebral perfusion.[142] Muizelaar et al.[139] have recently reported that routine hyperventilation may even be associated with worse neurologic outcome in head-injured patients.

Although elevated blood pressure is commonly observed in head-injured patients, hypotension actually may be more harmful than hypertension. Typically, head-injured patients are hypertensive and tachycardic and have increased cardiac output. In some patients, severely increased ICP precipitates reflex hypertension; in such cases, therapeutic reduction of ICP may interrupt the reflex response. Because of the vulnerability of the acutely injured brain to hypotension, prompt reversal of hypovolemic shock accompanying acute head injury is essential. Experimental and clinical data demonstrate that CBF after head trauma frequently depends on cerebral perfusion pressure rather than being in-

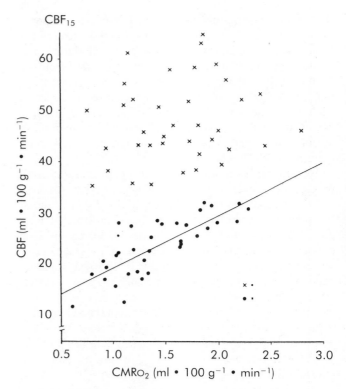

FIG. 30-7 Flow-metabolism coupling in patients who have acute head injury. The *solid circles* and the *regression line* demonstrate normal coupling of cerebral blood flow (CBF) and the cerebral metabolic rate for oxygen ($CMRo_2$), albeit at values lower than normal (CBF = 50 ml · 100 g^{-1} · min^{-1} and $CMRo_2$ = 3.5 ml · 100 g^{-1} · min^{-1}). The *xs* represent values of CBF that exceed metabolic need, i.e., uncoupled values. *(From Obrist WD, Langfitt TW, Jaggi JL et al: Cerebral blood flow and metabolism in comatose patients with acute head injury: relationship to intracranial hypertension,* J Neurosurg *61:241, 1984.)*

dependent of it (Fig. 30-8). Most patients with mass lesions demonstrate defective autoregulation; conversely, autoregulation remains intact in many patients without intracranial mass lesions.[27] In head-injured patients in whom autoregulation is intact, mannitol reduces ICP and does not change CBF; if autoregulation is defective, ICP changes little and CBF increases.[138] Despite impaired autoregulation, CBF may not increase to normal levels even at high levels of CPP.

Much of the current clinical strategy for the management of acute closed head injury is directed toward ICP reduction, since the control of intracranial hypertension appears to improve outcome.[165] Intracranial hypertension is a particularly important cause of secondary neural injury, because it is possible to monitor and reduce ICP effectively in most patients. As many as 30% of patients who develop increased ICP after head injury have a delayed rise, occurring 3 to 10 days after injury.[204] However, very aggressive control of ICP does not reverse the effects of the primary

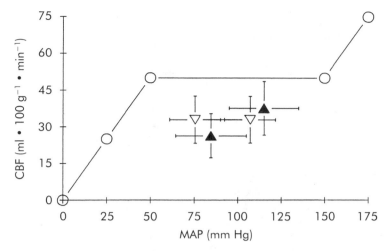

FIG. 30-8 In comparison to the normal autoregulatory curve, adult patients following closed head injury have reduced flow and, in some cases *(closed triangles)*, impaired autoregulation. Other patients have reduced flow and preserved autoregulation *(open triangles)*. *(From Muizelaar JP, Lutz III HA, Becker DP: Effect of mannitol on ICP and CBF and correlation with pressure autoregulation in severely head-injured patients,* J Neurosurg 61:700, 1984.)

injury. An overall approach to the management of intracranial hypertension was presented earlier in this chapter.

Therapeutic reduction of both CBF and $CMRo_2$, which can be accomplished with barbiturates, appears to be a physiologically sound strategy for the reduction of ICP without adversely affecting brain oxygenation. Marshall and associates[126] reported good results in a pilot study in which sodium pentobarbital, 3 to 5 mg/kg followed by an infusion of 100 to 200 mg every 30 to 60 minutes, was given to patients with severe closed head injury. Nevertheless, the overall response to barbiturate therapy after closed head trauma has been disappointing,[213] perhaps reflecting the variability in CBF responsiveness to barbiturates in this heterogeneous population, as well as variability in the extent of primary injury. Recently, Eisenberg et al.[54] have defined a limited role for barbiturates in closed head injury associated with refractory intracranial hypertension.

Spinal Cord Injury

Postoperative management of the patient with an acute spinal cord injury should attempt to limit the morbidity and mortality of common complications that occur in the first postinjury month, which includes the time during which patients are most likely to require surgery for acute spinal column stabilization. These complications include cardiovascular instability, inadequate pulmonary mechanics, and a variety of medical complications that contribute to morbidity. Pneumonia, pulmonary embolism, and sepsis are the most common factors contributing to death in spinal cord–injured patients.[49]

Cardiovascular Management

Acute spinal cord injury above T5 produces sympathectomy, which slightly decreases systemic vascular resistance and markedly dilates the venous capacitance vessels (spinal shock). If the lesion is cephalad to T4, loss of the input to the cardiac accelerator fibers reduces or eliminates compensatory tachycardia. Bradycardia secondary to unopposed vagal tone, particularly in association with hypoxemia, may precipitate cardiac arrest.[60] Sympathetic denervation also reduces myocardial compensation for sudden increases in preload and afterload.[122] As spinal shock resolves, usually within 2 to 3 weeks after injury, patients with spinal cord injuries cephalad to the level of splanchnic sympathetic innervation (T4 to T6) may manifest autonomic hyperreflexia,[172] a risk that is maximal approximately 4 weeks after injury. Of patients with lesions above T7, 66% to 85% manifest hyperreflexia at some time,[172] most commonly in response to distention of a hollow viscus.[171,212] In this disorder, loss of neurogenic control distal to the lesion results in profound vasoconstriction in response to noxious stimuli below the level of the lesion. Subsequent reflex activity of the carotid and aortic baroreceptors produces vasodilation above the level of the lesion, ventricular dysrhythmias, bradycardia, and occasionally heart block.

Postoperative cardiovascular management is directed at maintenance of intravascular volume, inotropic support as needed, avoidance of excessive fluid administration, and careful avoidance or prompt treatment of bradycardia. Spinal shock, which may continue for as long as 6 weeks after injury, requires intravascular volume maintenance and, in some cases, vasoactive drugs such as dopamine. Treatment of hypotension may also improve perfusion of the spinal cord. Although it is unclear whether autoregulation of spinal cord blood flow is impaired after spinal cord injury, it is likely that the traumatized spinal cord, like the traumatized brain, is extremely vulnerable to hypotension. During the spinal shock phase, sudden upright positioning may result in acute hypotension.[130] Bradycardia accompanied by hypotension may necessitate intermittent or prophylactic treatment with atropine, especially during vagotonic maneuvers such as tracheal suctioning. Management of autonomic hyperreflexia is first directed toward eliminating the causative stimuli and then using direct-acting vasodilators, such as SNP, and antiarrhythmic drugs.

Pulmonary Management

A T1 lesion eliminates the contributions of the intercostal muscles to both inspiration and expiration and of the abdominal obliques to expiration. Inspiratory reserve volume, total lung capacity, expiratory reserve volume, and forced vital capacity (FVC) are thereby reduced (Table 30-7).[58] Within the first few days after acute spinal cord injury, FVC typically decreases further and then begins to recover.[104] Diaphragmatic function gradually and progressively deteriorates for up to 5 days after injury, often accelerated by other pulmonary complications such as pulmonary edema or aspiration of vomitus. Despite partial respiratory paralysis, most patients who are able to generate a normal or nearly normal tidal volume remain normocarbic. However, hypoxemia occurs when FVC is less than $15 \text{ ml} \cdot \text{kg}^{-1}$ because of inability to cough and sigh. Acute onset of aspiration, atelectasis, or pneumonia may result in sudden respiratory compromise. Pulmonary edema occurs in up to 50% of patients with cervical spinal cord injuries, possibly because of massive sympathetic discharge immediately after high spinal cord injury.[198]

In general, spinal cord–injured patients require ventilatory assistance when FVC is less than $15 \text{ ml} \cdot \text{kg}^{-1}$, or a peak negative inspiratory pressure of $-25 \text{ cm H}_2\text{O}$ cannot be generated. The same measurements are used to guide weaning from mechanical ventilation (Table 30-8).[172] To reduce the risk of nosocomial pulmonary infections, close attention to pulmonary toilet, including chest physiotherapy, positioning, and tracheal suctioning, is essential,[128] especially in patients with borderline pulmonary mechanics.

In the acute phase of management an arterial catheter may be useful for blood pressure monitoring and management of blood gases. If persistent hypotension or pulmonary edema is present, pulmonary artery catheterization may clarify the need for additional intravascular volume replacement vs. the need for inotropic support.[122] However, because of the risk of infection after spinal cord injury, invasive monitoring should be used judiciously. Pulmonary monitoring is the same as that used for other critically ill patients and consists of pulse oximetry, capnography, and, as necessary, arterial catheterization to obtain arterial blood gases. Pulse oximetry may avert catastrophe in those patients who become bradycardic in response to hypoxemia.

Airway Management

The occasional patient who requires postoperative reintubation represents a technical and pharmacologic challenge. Despite the simultaneous risks of inadequate pulmonary function and aggravation of spinal cord damage, there are no universally accepted approaches to airway management in patients with acute spinal cord injury. The method chosen is determined by the severity of respiratory and hemodynamic compromise, the clinician's skills, the availability of equipment, and the diagnostic information about the cervical spine.[71,80] Cervical spine immobilization can be accomplished using Gardner-Wells tongs or manual in-line axial traction (MIAT),[71] a method used safely in more than 3000 patients.[70]

The method of choice for reintubation, even in nonemergent circumstances, may be orotracheal intubation, in conjunction with MIAT, after denitrogenation, supplemented by a small dose of a sedative/hypnotic and a neuromuscular blocker. If a patient is hypoxic, hypercapnic, or actively vomiting, direct visualization and orotracheal intubation are clearly preferable. If time permits, nasotracheal intubation may be performed either blindly or using fiberoptic guid-

TABLE 30-7

Pulmonary and Respiratory Muscle Function in Quadriplegic Patients with Mid to Lower Cervical Spinal Cord Injury

Variable*	C4 to C7 Injury†
Vital capacity	52 ± 11
FEV$_1$/FVC %	85 ± 3
Inspiratory capacity	71 ± 16
Expiratory reserve volume	21 ± 12
Total lung capacity	70 ± 4
Functional residual capacity	86 ± 14
Residual volume	141 ± 20
Maximum voluntary ventilation	49 ± 10
PI$_{max}$ cm H$_2$O	64 ± 12
PE$_{max}$ cm H$_2$O	41 ± 22

*FEV_1, Forced expiratory volume in 1 second; FVC, forced vital capacity; PI_{max}, maximum inspiratory pressure; PE_{max}, maximum expiratory pressure.
†Values expressed as percentage of predicted normal unless otherwise specified.
Modified from Findley LJ et al: The lungs and neuromuscular and chest wall diseases. In Murray JF, Nadel JA: *Textbook of respiratory medicine*, Philadelphia: 1988, Saunders.

TABLE 30-8

Weaning Criteria for Removal from Mechanical Ventilation

Weaning Criterion	Acceptable Value
Maximum peak negative inspiratory pressure	$>-20 \text{ cm H}_2\text{O}$
Maximum expiratory force	$>+20 \text{ cm H}_2\text{O}$
Vital capacity	$>1000 \text{ ml}$
Expiratory value	$>10 \text{ L/sec}$ (level dependent)
Pao$_2$/Fio$_2$	>250
Vd/Vt	>0.55
Lung thorax compliance	$>30 \text{ ml/cm H}_2\text{O}$

Modified from Schreibman DL et al: The trauma victim with an acute spinal cord injury, *Prob Anesth* 4:459, 1990.

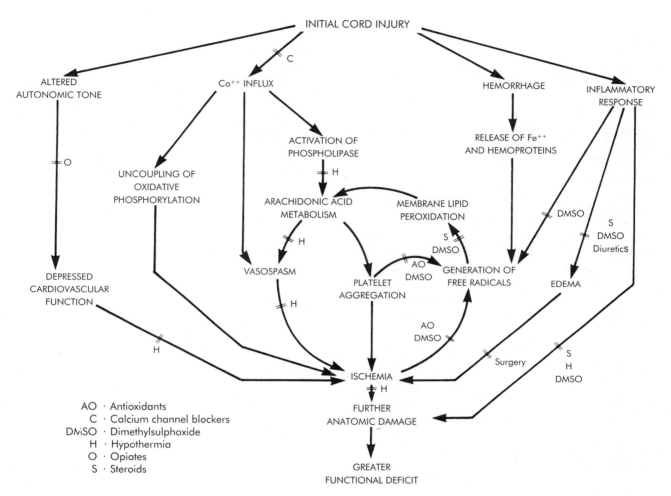

FIG. 30-9 Schematic illustration of proposed mechanisms of secondary spinal cord injury. Because of the progressive hemorrhagic infarction of the spinal cord that follows acute trauma, the pathophysiology of secondary, progressive injury has been extensively investigated. The processes interact, ultimately producing a greater deficit than could be attributed to the primary injury alone. Potential sites at which these interactive pathways could be interrupted are illustrated. *(From Janssen L, Hansebout RR: Pathogenesis of spinal cord injury and newer treatments: a review, Spine 14:23, 1991.)*

ance, except in the presence of basilar skull fracture, midface instability, or nasoseptal injury. Fiberoptic bronchoscopy requires specific training in the technique and an oropharynx relatively free of blood or foreign material.

If neuromuscular blocking agents must be used after the first 24 to 48 hours after spinal cord injury, it is necessary to recall that succinylcholine-induced hyperkalemia can be life threatening.[200] Studies in primates suggest that the critical interval begins 4 days after injury with peak increases ($\sim$5.5 mEq $\cdot$ L^{-1}) occurring at 14 days.[95] Spinal cord–injured patients appear to remain vulnerable to the hyperkalemic response to succinylcholine for more than 6 months after injury. A nondepolarizing agent such as vecuronium is preferable if more than 48 hours have elapsed.

Spinal Cord Preservation

Because of the progressive hemorrhagic infarction of the spinal cord that follows acute trauma, the pathophysiology of secondary, progressive injury has been extensively investigated (Fig. 30-9). Of the great variety of interventions that have been attempted after acute spinal cord injury, two (glucocorticoids and GM$_1$ gangliosides) have recently proven partially efficacious in clinical trials. A randomized, controlled clinical trial compared placebo, naloxone, and methylprednisolone given as a bolus of 30 mg $\cdot$ kg^{-1}, followed by a 23-hr infusion at a rate of 5.4 mg $\cdot$ kg^{-1} $\cdot$ hr^{-1}.[25] The single day of treatment was based on the rationale that short-term administration of glucocorticoids would be associated with fewer wound complications and infections but would still provide maximal effects during the most critical interval. Those subjects who received methylprednisolone within 8 hours of injury showed a significantly greater improvement in motor function and sensation to pinprick and touch than those who received placebo, naloxone, or methylprednisolone more than 8 hours after injury.[25] Although the differences were small, even slight improvement in motor function may substantially improve rehabilitation and quality of life of spinal cord–injured patients.

In a prospective, randomized, placebo-controlled, double-blind trial, GM$_1$ ganglioside (monosialotetrahexosylganglioside), a compound that enhances neurologic recovery after experimental spinal cord injury,[68] substantially enhanced improvement, assessed using the Frankel scale and the American Spinal Injury Association (ASIA) motor scores, after 1 year of follow-up.[62] The improvement appeared to be attributable to restoration of useful motor function in initially paralyzed muscles rather than to improving strength in paretic muscles.

Medical Complications

Common medical problems early after spinal cord injury include pulmonary embolism, gastric atony, urinary retention, and electrolyte abnormalities. Prevention of venous thrombosis and pulmonary embolism, a major cause of morbidity and mortality after spinal cord injury,[130] is an im-

portant part of the management of these patients. Low–molecular weight heparin is safer and more effective than conventional heparin in the prevention of thromboembolism in spinal cord–injured patients who have complete motor paralysis.[72] Gastric atony usually accompanies spinal shock. Because intestinal motility may be reduced for several weeks after injury, nasogastric intubation is mandatory. Prophylaxis against stress gastritis can be accomplished using antacids, H$_2$ blockers, or sucralfate. All patients with complete spinal cord injury and many patients with incomplete cord injury syndromes require urinary bladder drainage to relieve acute distention. Hypercalcemia, secondary to calcium release from immobility, usually develops within 2 weeks after spinal cord injury. Extensive bone demineralization increases vulnerability to fractures with minimal trauma, even that associated with transfer and positioning. Hyponatremia, a mild, common complication after spinal cord injury, occasionally results in severe water intoxication.[185] In part, this reflects a tendency of these patients toward high fluid intake plus impaired free water excretion.

Acute Intracerebral Hemorrhage

Nearly 60,000 patients per year suffer nontraumatic intracerebral hemorrhage not related to intracranial aneurysms. In patients who become comatose after intracerebral hemorrhage, mortality exceeds 50%.[67] Usually related to chronic systemic hypertension, primary intracerebral hemorrhage most commonly occurs in penetrating vessels in the basal ganglia, subcortical white matter, thalamus, cerebellum, and pons. The onset of primary brain hemorrhage is typically abrupt and rapidly progressive. Although the clinical picture may suggest the cause of neurologic deterioration, CT scanning provides the definitive diagnosis.[67] The indications for surgical evacuation of intracerebral hematomas vary with the location and size of the lesion. Cerebellar hematomas exceeding 2 to 3 cm in diameter and large lobar hematomas frequently require emergency evacuation to prevent brainstem compression or herniation. Surgical evacuation of hemorrhages from the brain stem, thalamus, and putamen remains controversial.

Nonsurgical or postsurgical treatment of primary intracerebral hemorrhage consists of intubation if coma is profound, seizure prophylaxis with phenytoin, control of blood pressure, and reduction of ICP (if necessary) with mannitol.[51,67] Endotracheal intubation should be performed with care to prevent reflex hypertension. Systolic blood pressure should be reduced to less than 150 to 160 mm Hg, ideally by using beta-adrenergic receptor antagonist drugs that reduce the impact of arterial pulsations on the damaged arterial wall. Labetalol, a combination alpha- and beta-receptor antagonist, appears to be particularly useful. The pure vasodilators nitroglycerin and SNP may increase ICP. Glucocorticoids are of no benefit.[153] ICP monitoring and control of intracranial hypertension may be useful in patients who present with or develop an altered sensorium.

▼

SUMMARY

Neurosurgical patients require careful attention to cardiorespiratory support, management of fluids and electrolytes, nutrition, and infection. In this respect they are identical to other high-risk postoperative and critically ill patients. However, equally close attention to the specific postoperative requirements of operations on the brain and spinal column and to key issues relating to support of patients with acute dysfunction of the central nervous system increases the likelihood of a satisfactory neurologic outcome.

References

1. Aaslid R, Huber P, Nornes H: A transcranial Doppler method in the evaluation of cerebrovascular spasm, *Neuroradiology* 28:11, 1986.
2. Abrams J: Nitrates, *Med Clin North Am* 72:1, 1988.
3. Adams JH, Graham DI, Gennarelli TA: Contemporary neuropathological considerations regarding brain damage in head injury. In Becker DP, Povlishock JT, editors: *Central nervous system trauma status report*, Bethesda, Md, 1985, National Institutes of Health.
4. Aitkenhead AR: Analgesia and sedation in intensive care, *Br J Anaesth* 63:196, 1989.
5. Aitkenhead AR, Pepperman ML, Willatts SM et al: Comparison of propofol and midazolam for sedation in critically ill patients, *Lancet* 2:704, 1989.
6. Albers GW: Potential therapeutic uses of N-methyl-D-aspartate antagonists in cerebral ischemia, *Clin Neuropharmacol* 13:177, 1990.
7. Allen GS, Ahn HS, Preziosi TJ et al: Cerebral arterial spasm: a controlled trial of nimodipine in patients with subarachnoid hemorrhage, *N Engl J Med* 308:619, 1983.
8. Amoroso P, Greenwood RN: Posture and central venous pressure measurement in circulatory volume depletion, *Lancet* 2:258, 1989.
9. Archer DP, Shaw DA, Leblanc RL et al: Haemodynamic considerations in the management of patients with subarachnoid haemorrhage, *Can J Anaesth* 38:454, 1991.
10. Arieff AI: Hyponatremia, convulsions, respiratory arrest, and permanent brain damage after elective surgery in healthy women, *N Engl J Med* 314:1529, 1986.
11. Asiddao CB, Donegan JH, Whitesell RC et al: Factors associated with perioperative complications during carotid endarterectomy, *Anesth Analg* 61:631, 1982.
12. Awad IA, Carter LP, Spetzler RF et al: Clinical vasospasm after subarachnoid hemorrhage: response to hypervolemic hemodilution and arterial hypertension, *Stroke* 18:365, 1987.
13. Bastos PG, Sun X, Wagner DP et al: Glasgow Coma Scale score in the evaluation of outcome in the intensive care unit: findings from the Acute Physiology and Chronic Health Evaluation III study, *Crit Care Med* 21:1459, 1993.
14. Batjer HH, Devous MD Sr, Meyer YJ et al: Cerebrovascular hemodynamics in arteriovenous malformation complicated by normal perfusion pressure breakthrough, *Neurosurgery* 22:503, 1988.
15. Batjer HH, Devous Sr MD, Seibert GB et al: Intracranial arteriovenous malformation: relationship between clinical factors and surgical complications, *Neurosurgery* 24:75, 1989.
16. Beemer GH, Rozental P: Postoperative neuromuscular function, *Anaesth Intensive Care* 14:41, 1986.
17. Berl T: Treating hyponatremia: what is all the controversy about? *Ann Intern Med* 113:417, 1990.
18. Bertel O, Conen D, Radu EW et al: Nifedipine in hypertensive emergencies, *Br Med J* 286:19, 1983.
19. Biller J, Godersky JC, Adams Jr HP: Management of aneurysmal subarachnoid hemorrhage, *Stroke* 19:1300, 1988.
20. Biller J, Love BB: Medical management of acute cerebral ischemia in the elderly, *Clin Geriatr Med* 7:455, 1991.
21. Biller J, Love BB: Nihilism and stroke therapy, *Stroke* 22:1105, 1991.
22. Black PL, Zervas NT, Candia GL: Incidence and management of complications of transsphenoidal operation for pituitary adenomas, *Neurosurgery* 20:920, 1987.
23. Bland RD, Shoemaker WC: Probability of survival as a prognostic and severity of illness score in critically ill surgical patients, *Crit Care Med* 13:91, 1985.
24. Böck JC, Barker BC, Clinton AG et al: Post-traumatic changes in, and effect of colloid osmotic pressure on the distribution of body water, *Ann Surg* 210:395, 1989.
25. Bracken MB, Shepard MJ, Collins WF et al: A randomized, controlled trial of methylprednisolone or naloxone in the treatment of acute spinal-cord injury, *N Engl J Med* 322:1405, 1990.
26. Braman SS, Dunn SM, Amico CA et al: Complications of intrahospital transport in critically ill patients, *Ann Intern Med* 107:469, 1987.
27. Bruce DA, Langfitt TW, Miller JD et al: Regional cerebral blood flow, intracranial pressure, and brain metabolism in comatose patients, *J Neurosurg* 38:131, 1973.
28. Bullock R, Hannemann CO, Murray L et al: Recurrent hematomas following craniotomy for traumatic intracranial mass, *J Neurosurg* 72:9, 1990.
29. Burt DER, Verniquet AJW, Homi J: The response of canine intracranial pressure to systemic hypotension induced with nitroglycerine, *Br J Anaesth* 54:665, 1982.
30. Butterworth JB, DeWitt DS: Severe head trauma: pathophysiology and management, *Crit Care Clin* 5:807, 1989.
31. Campbell IT, Baxter JN et al: IV fluids during surgery, *Br J Anaesth* 65:726, 1990.

32. Candia GJ, Heros RC, Lavyne MH et al: Effect of intravenous sodium nitroprusside on cerebral blood flow and intracranial pressure, *Neurosurgery* 3:50, 1978.

33. Carolei A, Fieschi C, Bruno R et al: Monosialoganglioside GM1 in cerebral ischemia, *Cerebrovasc Brain Metab Rev* 3:134, 1991.

34. Cernacek P, Maher E, Crawhall JC et al: Renal dose response and pharmacokinetics of atrial natriuretic factor in dogs, *Am J Physiol* 255:R929, 1988.

35. Chanson P, Jedynak CP, Dabrowski G et al: Ultra-low doses of vasopressin in the management of diabetes insipidus, *Crit Care Med* 15:44, 1987.

36. Chiolero RL, Ravussin P, Anderes JP et al: The effects of midazolam reversal by RO 15-1788 on cerebral perfusion pressure in patients with severe head injury, *Intensive Care Med* 14:196, 1988.

36a. Christensen L, Schaffer S, Ross SE: Otitis media in adult trauma patients: incidence and clinical significance, *J Trauma* 31:1543-1545, 1991.

37. Chyatte D, Fode NC, Nichols DA et al: Preliminary report: effects of high dose methylprednisolone on delayed cerebral ischemia in patients at high risk for vasospasm after aneurysmal subarachnoid hemorrhage, *Neurosurgery* 21:157, 1987.

38. Chung HM, Kluge R, Schrier RW et al: Postoperative hyponatremia: a prospective study, *Arch Intern Med* 146:333, 1986.

38a. Clifton GL, Robertson CS, Choi SC: Assessment of nutritional requirements of head-injured patients, *J Neurosurg* 64:895-901, 1986.

38b. Clifton GL, Robertson CS, Contant CF: Enteral hyperalimentation in head injury, *J Neurosurg* 62:186-193, 1985.

38c. Clifton GL, Robertson CS, Grossman RG et al: The metabolic response to severe head injury, *J Neurosurg* 60:687-696, 1984.

39. Cluitmans FH, Meinders AE: Management of severe hyponatremia: rapid or slow correction? *Am J Med* 88:161, 1990.

40. Cobb WE, Spare S, Reichlin S: Neurogenic diabetes insipidus: management with dDAVP (1-desamino-8-D-arginine vasopressin), *Ann Intern Med* 88:183, 1978.

41. Cohen AT, Kelly DR: Assessment of alfentanil by intravenous infusion as long-term sedation in intensive care, *Anaesthesia* 42:545, 1987.

42. Constantini S, Cotev S, Rappaport ZH et al: Intracranial pressure monitoring after elective intracranial surgery: a retrospective study of 514 consecutive patients, *J Neurosurg* 69:540, 1988.

43. Cottrell JE, Robustelli A, Post K et al: Furosemide- and mannitol-induced changes in intracranial pressure and serum osmolality and electrolytes, *Anesthesiology* 47:28, 1977.

44. Cybulski GR, D'Angelo CM: Neurological deterioration after laminectomy for spondylotic cervical myeloradiculopathy: the putative role of spinal cord ischaemia, *J Neurol Neurosurg Psychiatr* 51:717, 1988.

45. Davies KR, Gelb AW, Manninen PH et al: Cardiac function in aneurysmal subarachnoid haemorrhage: a study of electrocardiographic and echocardiographic abnormalities, *Br J Anaesth* 67:58, 1991.

46. Dearden NM, Gibson JS, McDowall DG et al: Effect of high-dose dexamethasone on outcome from severe head injury, *J Neurosurg* 64:81, 1986.

47. del Zoppo GJ: An open, multicenter trial of recombinant tissue plasminogen activator in acute stroke: a progress report, *Stroke* 21:IV174, 1990.

48. Desaussure RL: Vascular injury coincident to disc surgery, *J Neurosurg* 16:222, 1959.

49. DeVivo M, Kartus PL, Stover SL et al: Cause of death for patients with spinal cord injuries, *Arch Intern Med* 149:1761, 1989.

50. DeWitt DS, Prough DS, Taylor CL et al: Regional cerebrovascular responses to progressive hypotension after traumatic brain injury in cats, *Am J Physiol* 32: 1276, 1992.

51. Diringer MN: Intracerebral hemorrhage: pathophysiology and management, *Crit Care Med* 21:1591, 1993.

52. Dohi S, Okubo N, Kondo Y: Pulmonary oedema after airway obstruction due to bilateral vocal cord paralysis, *Can J Anaesth* 38(4):492, 1991.

53. Durbin Jr CG: Neuromuscular blocking agents and sedative drugs: clinical uses and toxic effects in the critical care unit, *Crit Care Clin* 7:489, 1991.

54. Eisenberg HM, Frankowski RF, Contant CF et al: High-dose barbiturate control of elevated intracranial pressure in patients with severe head injury, *J Neurosurg* 69:15, 1988.

55. Farling PA, Johnston JR, Coppel DL: Propofol infusion for sedation of patients with head injury in intensive care: a preliminary report, *Anaesthesia* 44:222, 1989.

56. Feldman Z, Contant CF, Pahwa R et al: The relationship between hormonal mediators and systemic hypermetabolism after severe head injury, *J Trauma* 34:806, 1993.

57. Findley LJ, Rochester DF: The lungs and neuromuscular and chest wall diseases. In Murray JF, Nadel JA: *Textbook of respiratory medicine,* Philadelphia, 1988, Saunders.

58. Fishman RA: Brain edema, *N Engl J Med* 293:706, 1975.

59. Flamm ES: The potential use of nicardipine in cerebrovascular disease, *Am Heart J* 117:236, 1989.

60. Frankel HL, Mathias CJ, Spalding JMK: Mechanisms of reflex cardiac arrest in tetraplegic patients, *Lancet* 2:1183, 1975.

61. Fraser CL, Arieff AI: Fatal central diabetes mellitus and insipidus resulting from untreated hyponatremia: a new syndrome, *Ann Intern Med* 112:113, 1990.

62. Geisler FH, Dorsey FC, Coleman WP: Recovery of motor function after spinal-cord injury—a randomized, placebo-controlled trial with GM-1 ganglioside, *N Engl J Med* 324:1829, 1991.

63. Gelmers HJ, Hennerici M: Effect of nimodipine on acute ischemic stroke: pooled results from five randomized trials, *Stroke* 21:IV81, 1990.

64. Gibson BE, Black S, Maass L et al: Esmolol for the control of hypertension after neurologic surgery, *Clin Pharmacol Ther* 44:650, 1988.

65. Gilsbach JM: Nimodipine in the prevention of ischaemic deficits after aneurysmal subarachnoid haemorrhage: an analysis of recent clinical studies, *Acta Neurochir Suppl* 45:41, 1988.

66. Giraldi C, Masi MC, Manetti M et al: A pilot study with monosialoganglioside GM1 on acute cerebral ischemia, *Acta Neurol* 12:214, 1990.

66a. Godbole KB, Berbiglia VA, Goddard L: A head-injured patient: caloric needs, clinical progress and nursing care priorities, *J Neurosci Nurs* 23:290-294, 1991.

67. Godersky JC, Biller J: Diagnosis and treatment of spontaneous intracerebral hemorrhage, *Compr Ther* 13:22, 1987.

68. Gorio A, Di Guillo AM, Young W et al: GM₁ effects on chemical traumatic and peripheral nerve induce lesions to the spinal cord. In Goldberger ME, Gorio A, Murray M, editors: *Development and plasticity of the mammalian spinal cord,* vol 3, Padua, Italy, 1986, Liviana Press.

69. Gottardis M, Khünl-Brady KS, Koller W et al: Effect of prolonged sedation with propofol on serum triglyceride and cholesterol concentrations, *Br J Anaesth* 62:393, 1989.

70. Grande CM, Barton CR, Stene JK: Appropriate techniques for airway management of emergency patients with suspected spinal cord injury, *Anesth Analg* 67:710, 1988 (letter).

71. Grande CM, Stene JK, Bernhard WN: Airway management: considerations in the trauma patient, *Crit Care Clin* 6:37, 1990.

72. Green D, Lee MY, Lim AC et al: Prevention of thromboembolism after spinal cord injury using low-molecular-weight heparin, *Ann Intern Med* 113:571, 1990.

73. Griffin KA, Bidani AK: How to manage disorders of sodium and water balance: five-step approach to evaluating appropriateness of renal response, *J Crit Illness* 5:1054, 1990.

74. Grunstein RR, Ho KY, Sullivan CE: Sleep apnea in acromegaly, *Ann Intern Med* 115:527, 1991.

75. Gunnar W, Jonasson O, Merlotti G et al: Head injury and hemorrhagic shock: studies of the blood brain barrier and intracranial pressure after resuscitation with normal saline solution, 3% saline solution, and dextran-40, *Surgery* 103:398, 1988.

76. Haas DC, Streeten DHP, Kim RC et al: Death from cerebral hypoperfusion during nitroprusside treatment of acute angiotensin-dependent hypertension, *Am J Med* 75:1071, 1983.

77. Hadley MN, Spetzler RF, Sonntag VKH: The transoral approach to the superior cervical spine: a review of 53 cases of extradural cervicomedullary compression, *J Neurosurg* 71:16, 1989.

78. Hanakita J, Kondo A: Serious complications of microvascular decompression operations for trigeminal neuralgia and hemifacial spasm, *Neurosurgery* 22:348, 1988.

79. Hasan D, Wijdicks EFM, Vermeulen M: Hyponatremia is associated with cerebral ischemia in patients with aneurysmal subarachnoid hemorrhage, *Ann Neurol* 27:106, 1990.

80. Hastings RH, Marks JD: Airway management for trauma patients with potential cervical spine injuries, *Anesth Analg* 73:471, 1991.

81. The Hemodilution in Stroke Study Group: Hypervolemic hemodilution treatment of acute stroke: results of a randomized multicenter trial using pentastarch, *Stroke* 20:317, 1989.

82. Henriksen L, Paulson OB: The effects of sodium nitroprusside on cerebral blood flow and cerebral venous blood gases. II. Observations in awake man during successive blood pressure reduction, *Eur J Clin Invest* 12:389, 1982.

83. Henriksen L, Paulson OB, Lauritzen M: The effects of sodium nitroprusside on cerebral blood flow and cerebral venous blood gases. I. Observations in awake man during and following moderate blood pressure reduction, *Eur J Clin Invest* 12:383, 1982.

84. Hijdra A, van Gijn J, Nagelkerke NJD et al: Prediction of delayed cerebral ischemia, rebleeding, and outcome after aneurysmal subarachnoid hemorrhage, *Stroke* 19:1250, 1988.

85. Hoff JT: Cerebral protection, *J Neurosurg* 65:579, 1986.

86. Horowitz NH, Rizzoli HV: *Postoperative complications of intracranial neurological surgery,* Baltimore, 1982, Williams & Wilkins.

87. Howard R, Mahoney A, Thurlow AC: Respiratory obstruction after posterior fossa surgery, *Anaesthesia* 45:222, 1990.

87a. Humphrey MA, Simpson GT, Grindlinger GA: Clinical characteristics of nosocomial sinusitis, *Ann Otol Rhinol Laryngol* 96:687-690, 1987.

88. Indeck M, Peterson S, Smith J et al: Risk, cost, and benefit of transporting ICU patients for special studies, *J Trauma* 28:1020, 1988.

89. Ishige N, Pitts LH, Berry I et al: The effects of hypovolemic hypotension on high-energy phosphate metabolism of traumatized brain in rats, *J Neurosurg* 68:129, 1988.

90. Ishige N, Pitts LH, Pogliani L et al: Effect of hypoxia on traumatic brain injury in rats. II. Changes in high energy phosphate metabolism, *Neurosurgery* 20:854, 1987.

91. Isono S, Ide T, Kochi T et al: Effects of partial paralysis on the swallowing reflex in conscious humans, *Anesthesiology* 75:980, 1991.

92. Italian Acute Stroke Study Group: Haemodilution in acute stroke: results of the Italian Haemodilution Trial, *Lancet* 1:318, 1988.

93. Jan M, Buchheit F, Tremoulet M: Therapeutic trial of intravenous nimodipine in patients with established cerebral vasospasm after rupture of intracranial aneurysms, *Neurosurgery* 23:154, 1988.

94. Janaki S: Pentoxifylline in strokes: a clinical study, *J Int Med Res* 8:56, 1980.

95. John DA, Tobey RE, Homer LD et al: Onset of succinylcholine-induced hyperkalemia following denervation, *Anesthesiology* 45:294, 1976.

96. Kalfas IH, Little JR: Postoperative hemorrhage: a survey of 4992 intracranial procedures, *Neurosurgery* 23:343, 1988.

97. Kassell NF, Peerless SJ, Durward QJ et al: Treatment of ischemic deficits from vasospasm with intravascular volume expansion and induced arterial hypertension, *Neurosurgery* 11:337, 1982.

98. Kasuya H, Shimizu T, Kagawa M: The effect of continuous drainage of cerebrospinal fluid in patients with subarachnoid hemorrhage: a retrospective analysis of 108 patients, *Neurosurgery* 28:56, 1991.

98a. Kaufman HH, Bretudiere J-P, Rowlands BJ et al: General metabolism in head injury, *Neurosurgery* 20:254-265, 1987.

99. Kirsch JR, Diringer MN, Borel CO et al: Cerebral aneurysms: mechanisms of injury and critical care interventions, *Crit Care Clin* 5:755, 1989.

100. Klingelhöfer J, Dander D, Holzgraefe M et al: Cerebral vasospasm evaluated by transcranial Doppler ultrasonography at different intracranial pressures, *J Neurosurg* 75:752, 1991.

101. Kostuik J: Adult scoliosis. In Bridwell KH, Dewald RL, editors: *Spinal surgery,* Philadelphia, 1991, Lippincott.

102. Lam AM, Winn HR, Cullen BF et al: Hyperglycemia and neurological outcome in patients with head injury, *J Neurosurg* 75:545, 1991.

103. Lanier WL, Stangland KJ, Scheithauer BW et al: The effects of dex-

trose infusion and head position on neurologic outcome after complete cerebral ischemia in primates: examination of a model, *Anesthesiology* 66:39, 1987.

104. Ledsome JR, Sharp JM: Pulmonary function in acute cervical cord injury, *Am Rev Respir Dis* 124:41, 1981.

105. Lee MC, Mastri AR, Waltz AG et al: Ineffectiveness of dexamethasone for treatment of experimental cerebral infarction, *Stroke* 5:216, 1974.

106. Lehmann KG, Lane JG, Piepmeier JM et al: Cardiovascular abnormalities accompanying acute spinal cord injury in humans: incidence, time course and severity, *J Am Coll Cardiol* 10:46, 1987.

107. Lehmann KG, Shandling AH, Yusi AU et al: Altered ventricular repolarization in central sympathetic dysfunction associated with spinal cord injury, *Am J Cardiol* 63:1498, 1989.

108. Leonov Y, Sterz F, Safar P et al: Mild cerebral hypothermia during and after cardiac arrest improves neurologic outcome in dogs, *J Cereb Blood Flow Metab* 10:57, 1990.

109. Levine TM: Swallowing disorders following skull base surgery, *Otolaryngol Clin North Am* 21:751, 1988.

110. Levy ML, Giannotta SL: Cardiac performance indices during hypervolemic therapy for cerebral vasospasm, *J Neurosurg* 75:27, 1991.

111. Lewelt W, Jenkins LW, Miller JD: Autoregulation of cerebral blood flow after experimental fluid percussion injury of the brain, *J Neurosurg* 53:500, 1980.

112. Lien YH, Shapiro JI, Chan L: Effects of hypernatremia on organic brain osmoles, *J Clin Invest* 85:1427, 1990.

113. Link J, Krause H, Wagner W et al: Intrahospital transport of critically ill patients, *Crit Care Med* 18:1427, 1990.

114. Lipsitz LA: Orthostatic hypotension in the elderly, *N Engl J Med* 321:952, 1989 (review).

115. Little JR: Modification of acute focal ischemia by treatment with mannitol and high-dose dexamethasone, *J Neurosurg* 49:517, 1978.

116. Lobato RD, Sarabia R, Cordobes F et al: Posttraumaic cerebral hemispheric swelling: analysis of 55 cases studied with computerized tomography, *J Neurosurg* 68:417, 1988.

116a. Longstreth WT, Inui TS: High blood glucose level on hospital admission and poor neurological recovery after cardiac arrest, *Ann Neurol* 15:59-63, 1984.

117. Longstreth WT Jr, Diehr P, Cobb LA et al: Neurologic outcome and blood glucose levels during out-of-hospital cardiopulmonary resuscitation, *Neurology* 36:1186, 1986.

117a. Longstreth WT Jr, Diehr P, Inui TS: Prediction of awakening after out-of-hospital cardiac arrest, *N Engl J Med* 308:1378-1382, 1983.

118. Luce JM: Medical management of head injury, *Chest* 89:864, 1986.

119. Lundy EF, Kuhn JE, Kwon JM et al: Infusion of five percent dextrose increases mortality and morbidity following six minutes of cardiac arrest in resuscitated dogs, *J Crit Care* 2:4, 1987.

120. Macdonald RL, Weir BKA: A review of hemoglobin and the pathogenesis of cerebral vasospasm, *Stroke* 22:971, 1991.

121. Macdonald RL, Weir BKA, Runzer TD et al: Etiology of cerebral vasospasm in primates, *J Neurosurg* 75:415, 1991.

122. Mackenzie CF, Shin B, Krishnaprasad D et al: Assessment of cardiac and respiratory function during surgery on patients with acute quadriplegia, *J Neurosurg* 62:843, 1985.

123. Malik AB: Mechanisms of neurogenic pulmonary edema, *Circ Res* 57:1, 1985.

124. Maniglia AJ, Han DP: Cranial nerve injuries following carotid endarterectomy: an analysis of 336 procedures, *Head Neck* 13:121, 1991.

125. Marsh ML, Aidinis SJ, Naughton KVH et al: The technique of nitroprusside administration modifies the intracranial pressure response, *Anesthesiology* 51:538, 1979.

126. Marshall LF, Smith RW, Shapiro HM: The outcome with aggressive treatment in severe head injuries. II. Acute and chronic barbiturate administration in the management of head injury, *J Neurosurg* 50:26, 1979.

127. Marx W, Shah N, Long C et al: Sufentanil, alfentanil, and fentanyl: impact on cerebrospinal fluid pressure in patients with brain tumors, *J Neurosurg Anesth* 11:3, 1989.

127a. Mayhall CB, Archer NH, Lamb VA et al: Ventriculostomy-related infections: a prospective epidemiologic study, *N Engl J Med* 310:553-559, 1984.

128. McMichan JC, Michel L, Westbrook PR: Pulmonary dysfunction following traumatic quadriplegia, *JAMA* 243:528, 1980.

129. McNulty S, Sharifi-Azad S, Farole A: Induced hypotension with labetalol for orthognathic surgery, *J Oral Maxillofac Surg* 45:309, 1987.

130. McVicar JP, Luce JM: Management of spinal cord injury in the critical care setting, *Crit Care Clin* 2:747, 1986.

131. Medlock MD, Dulebohn SC, Elwood PW: Prophylactic hypervolemia without calcium channel blockers in early aneurysm surgery, *Neurosurgery* 30:12, 1992.

132. Michalk S, Moncorge C, Fichelle A et al: Midazolam infusion for basal sedation in intensive care: absence of accumulation, *Intensive Care Med* 15:37, 1988.

133. Michenfelder JD, Milde JH: The interaction of sodium nitroprusside, hypotension, and isoflurane in determining cerebral vasculature effects, *Anesthesiology* 69:870, 1988.

134. Miller JD, Butterworth JF, Gudeman SK et al: Further experience in the management of severe head injury, *J Neurosurg* 54:289, 1981.

135. Moore JK, Chaudhri S, Moore AP et al: Macroglossia and posterior fossa disease, *Anaesthesia* 43:382, 1988.

136. More J, Sundaresan N: Complications of spine surgery in cancer patients. In Tarlov EC, editor: *Complications of spinal surgery: neurosurgical topics*, Park Ridge, Ill, 1991, American Association of Neurological Surgeons.

137. Mueller WM, Larson SJ: Complications of spinal instrumentation. In Tarlov EC, editor: *Complications of spinal surgery: neurosurgical topics*, Park Ridge, Ill, 1991, American Association of Neurological Surgeons.

138. Muizelaar JP, Lutz III HA, Becker DP: Effect of mannitol on ICP and CBF and correlation with pressure autoregulation in severely head-injured patients, *J Neurosurg* 61:700, 1984.

139. Muizelaar JP, Marmarou A, Ward JD et al: Adverse effects of prolonged hyperventilation in patients with severe head injury: a randomized clinical trial, *J Neurosurg* 75:731, 1991.

140. Müller R, Lehrach FR: Haemorrheology and cerebrovascular disease:

multifunctional approach with pentoxifylline, *Curr Med Res Opin* 7:253, 1981.

141. Nelson RJ, Roberts J, Rubin C et al: Association of hypovolemia after subarachnoid hemorrhage with computed tomographic scan evidence of raised intracranial pressure, *Neurosurgery* 29:178, 1991.

141a. Norton JA, Ott LG, McClain C et al: Intolerance to enternal feeding in the brain-injured patient, *J Neurosurg* 68:62-66, 1988.

142. Obrist WD, Langfitt TW, Jaggi JL et al: Cerebral blood flow and metabolism in comatose patients with acute head injury: relationship to intracranial hypertension, *J Neurosurg* 61:241, 1984.

143. Öhman J, Servo A, Heiskanen O: Risk factors for cerebral infarction in good-grade patients after aneurysmal subarachnoid hemorrhage and surgery: a prospective study, *J Neurosurg* 74:14, 1991.

144. Origitano TC, Wascher TM, Reichman OH et al: Sustained increased cerebral blood flow with prophylactic hypertensive hypervolemic hemodilution ("triple-H" therapy) after subarachnoid hemorrhage, *Neurosurgery* 27:729, 1990.

145. O'Sullivan JC, Wells DG, Wells GR: Difficult airway management with neck swelling after carotid endarterectomy, *Anaesth Intensive Care* 14:460, 1986.

146. Patel CB, Laboy V, Venus B et al: Use of sodium nitroprusside in postcoronary bypass surgery: a plea for conservatism, *Chest* 89:663, 1986.

147. Pearson RM, Griffith DNW, Woollard M et al: Comparison of effects on cerebral blood flow of rapid reduction in systemic arterial pressure by diazoxide and labetalol in hypertensive patients: preliminary findings, *Br J Clin Pharmacol* 8:195S, 1979.

148. Petrozza PH: Induced hypotension, *Int Anesthesiol Clin* 28:223, 1990.

149. Petruk KC, West M, Mohr G et al: Nimodipine treatment in poor-grade aneurysm patients: results of a multicenter double-blind placebo-controlled trial, *J Neurosurg* 68:505, 1988.

150. Pickard JD, Murray GD, Illingworth R et al: Effect of oral nimodipine on cerebral infarction and outcome after subarachnoid haemorrhage: British aneurysm nimodipine trial, *Br Med J* 298:636, 1989.

151. Poole Jr GV, Prough DS, Johnson JC et al: Effects of resuscitation from hemorrhagic shock on cerebral hemodynamics in the presence of an intracranial mass, *J Trauma* 27:18, 1987.

152. Porembka D, Ebrahim Z, Bloomfield E et al: The postoperative hyperdynamic cardiovascular response following intracranial excision of arterial venous malformation (AVM), *Anesthesiology* 75:A215, 1991 (abstract).

153. Poungvarin N, Bhoopat W, Viruyavejakui A et al: Effects of dexamethasone in primary supratentorial intracerebral hemorrhage, *N Engl J Med* 20:1229, 1987.

154. Powers WJ, Grubb RL Jr, Baker RP et al: Regional cerebral blood flow and metabolism in reversible ischemia due to vasospasm: determination by positron emission tomography, *J Neurosurg* 62:539, 1985.

155. Prough DS, Johnson JC, Stump DA et al: Effects of hypertonic saline versus lactated Ringer's solution on cerebral oxygen transport during resuscitation from hemorrhagic shock, *J Neurosurg* 64:627, 1986.

156. Prough DS, Scuderi PE, McWhorter JM et al: Hemodynamic status following regional and general anesthesia for carotid endarterectomy, *J Neurosurg Anesth* 1:35, 1989.

157. Pulsinelli WA, Kraig RP, Plum F: Hyperglycemia, cerebral acidosis, and ischemic brain damage. In Plum F, Pulsinelli W, editors: *Cerebrovascular diseases,* New York, 1985, Raven Press.

157a. Rapp RP, Young B, Twyman D et al: The favorable effect of early parenteral feeding on survival in head-injured patients, *J Neurosurg* 58:906-912, 1983.

158. Reulen HJ: Vasogenic brain oedema: new aspects in its formation, resolution and therapy, *Br J Anaesth* 48:741, 1976.

159. Riles TS, Kopelman I, Imparato AM: Myocardial infarction following carotid endarterectomy: a review of 683 operations, *Surgery* 85:249, 1979.

159a. Robertson CS, Clifton GL, Goodman JC: Steroid administration and nitrogen excretion in the head-injured patient, *J Neurosurg* 63:714-718, 1985.

159b. Robertson CS, Clifton GL, Grossman RG: Oxygen utilization and cardiovascular function in head-injured patients, *Neurosurgery* 15:307-314, 1984.

160. Robinson AG: DDAVP in the treatment of central diabetes insipidus, *N Engl J Med* 294:507, 1976.

161. Rosenbaum D, Zabramski J, Frey J et al: Early treatment of ischemic stroke with a calcium antagonist, *Stroke* 22:437, 1991.

162. Rosenwasser RH, Kleiner LI, Krzeminski JP et al: Intracranial pressure monitoring in the posterior fossa: a preliminary report, *J Neurosurg* 71:503, 1989.

163. Roy LF, Ogilvie RI, Larochelle P et al: Cardiac and vascular effects of atrial natriuretic factor and sodium nitroprusside in healthy men, *Circulation* 79:383, 1989.

164. Sarnaik AP, Meert K, Hackbarth R et al: Management of hyponatremic seizures in children with hypertonic saline: a safe and effective strategy, *Crit Care Med* 19:758, 1991.

165. Saul TG, Ducker TB: Effect of intracranial pressure monitoring and aggressive treatment on mortality in severe head injury, *J Neurosurg* 56:498, 1982.

166. Saul TG, Ducker TB, Saloman M et al: Steroids in severe head injury: a prospective randomized clinical trial, *J Neurosurg* 54:596, 1981.

167. Saunders RL: Complications of corpectomy. In Tarlov EC, editor: *Complications of spinal surgery: neurosurgical topics,* Park Ridge, Ill, 1991, American Association of Neurological Surgeons.

168. Scalea TM, Holman M, Fuortes M et al: Central venous blood oxygen saturation: an early, accurate measurement of volume during hemorrhage, *J Trauma* 28:725, 1988.

169. Scandinavian Stroke Study Group: Multicenter trial of hemodilution in acute ischemic stroke. I. Results in the total patient population, *Stroke* 18:691, 1987.

170. Schmidek HH, Cutler SG: Epidural morphine for control of pain after spinal surgery: a preliminary report, *Neurosurgery* 13:37, 1983.

171. Schonwald G, Fish KJ, Perkash I: Cardiovascular complications during anesthesia in chronic spinal cord injured patients, *Anesthesiology* 55:550, 1981.

172. Schreibman DL, Mackenzie CF: The trauma victim with an acute spinal cord injury, *Prob Anesth* 4:459, 1990.

173. Schumacker PT, Rhodes GR, Newell JC et al: Ventilation-perfusion imbalance after head trauma, *Am Rev Respir Dis* 119:33, 1979.

174. Scuderi PE, Prough DS, Davis Jr CH et al: The effects of regional and general anesthesia on blood pressure control after carotid endarterectomy, *J Neurosurg Anesth* 1:41, 1989.

175. Seckl JR, Dunger DB, Lightman SL: Neurohypophyseal peptide function during early postoperative diabetes insipidus, *Brain* 110:737, 1987.

176. Segal R, Pollack I, Segal E et al: Herniated L4-L5 disc after placement of Harrington instrumentation for a fracture of the thoracolumbar spine, *Neurosurgery* 29:135, 1991.

177. Seiler RW, Grolimund P, Aaslid R et al: Cerebral vasospasm evaluated by transcranial ultrasound correlated with clinical grade and CT-visualized subarachnoid hemorrhage, *J Neurosurg* 64:594, 1986.

178. Shafer A, Doze VA, White PF: Pharmacokinetic variability of midazolam infusions in critically ill patients, *Crit Care Med* 18:1039, 1990.

179. Shapiro BA: New ventilator technology: impact on patient care, In Carlson RW, Reines HD: *Critical care: state of the art,* vol 13, Anaheim, Calif, 1992, Society of Critical Care Medicine.

180. Shearer ES, O'Sullivan EP, Hunter JM: An assessment of the Cerebrotrac 2500 for continuous monitoring of cerebral function in the intensive care unit, *Anaesthesia* 46:750, 1991.

181. Shenker Y: Atrial natriuretic hormone effect on renal function and aldosterone secretion in sodium depletion, *Am J Physiol* 255:R867, 1988.

182. Shenkin HA, Cheney RH, Govons SR et al: On the diagnosis of hemorrhage in man: a study of volunteers bled large amounts, *Am J Med Sci* 208:421, 1944.

183. Shoemaker WC, Appel PL, Kram HB et al: Prospective trial of supranormal values of survivors as therapeutic goals in high-risk surgical patients, *Chest* 94:1176, 1988.

184. Shucart WA, Jackson I: Management of diabetes insipidus in neurosurgical patients, *J Neurosurg* 44:65, 1976.

185. Sica DA, Culpepper RM: Case report: severe hyponatremia in spinal cord injury, *Am J Med Sci* 298;331, 1989.

186. Sinclair ME, Sear JW, Summerfield RJ et al: Alfentanil infusions on the intensive therapy unit, *Intensive Care Med* 14:55, 1988.

187. Sloan MA, Haley Jr EC, Kassell HF et al: Sensitivity and specificity of transcranial Doppler ultrasonography in the diagnosis of vasospasm following subarachnoid hemorrhage, *Neurology* 39:1514, 1989.

188. Slogoff S, Keats AS: Does perioperative myocardial ischemia lead to postoperative myocardial infarction? *Anesthesiology* 62:107, 1985.

189. Snyder NA, Feigal DW, Arieff AI: Hypernatremia in elderly patients: a heterogeneous, morbid, and iatrogenic entity, *Ann Intern Med* 107:309, 1987.

190. Spetzler RF, Martin NA, Carter LP et al: Surgical management of large AVMs by staged embolization and operative excision, *J Neurosurg* 67:17, 1987.

191. Spiegelmann R, Hadani M, Ram Z et al: Upward transtentorial herniation: a complication of postoperative edema at the cervicomedullary junction, *Neurosurgery* 24:284, 1989.

192. Sterns RH: Severe symptomatic hyponatremia: treatment and outcome. A study of 64 cases, *Ann Intern Med* 107:656, 1987.

193. Sterns RH: Endocrine crises: the management of hyponatremic emergencies, *Crit Care Clin* 7:127, 1991.

194. Sterns RH, Riggs JE, Schochet Jr SS: Osmotic demyelination syndrome following correction of hyponatremia, *N Engl J Med* 314:1535, 1986.

195. Sterns RH, Thomas DJ, Herndon RM: Brain dehydration and neurologic deterioration after rapid correction of hyponatremia, *Kidney Int* 35:69, 1989.

195a. Sunderland PM, Heilbrun MP: Estimating energy expenditure in traumatic brain injury: comparison of indirect calorimetry with predictive formulas, *Neurosurgery* 31:246-253, 1992.

196. Sundt TM, Sharbrough FW, Piepgras DG et al: Correlation of cerebral blood flow and electroencephalographic changes during carotid endarterectomy, *Mayo Clin Proc* 56:533, 1981.

197. Teasdale G, Jennet B: Assessment of coma and impaired consciousness, *Lancet* 2:81, 1974.

198. Theodore J, Robin ED: Speculations on neurogenic pulmonary edema (NPE), *Am Rev Respir Dis* 113:405, 1976.

199. Thomsen LJ, Riisager S, Jensen KA et al: Cerebral blood flow and metabolism during hypotension induced with sodium nitroprusside and captopril, *Can J Anaesth* 36:392, 1989.

200. Tobey RE: Paraplegia, succinylcholine and cardiac arrest, *Anesthesiology* 32:359, 1970.

201. Tommasino C, Moore S, Todd MM: Cerebral effects of isovolemic hemodilution with crystalloid or colloid solutions, *Crit Care Med* 16:862, 1988.

202. Toung TJK, Sieber FE, Grayson RF et al: Chemoreceptor injury as probable cause of respiratory depression after a simultaneous, bilateral carotid endarterectomy, *Crit Care Med* 18:1290, 1990.

203. Tuchschmidt J, Fried J, Astiz M et al: Elevation of cardiac output and oxygen delivery improves outcome in septic shock, *Chest* 102:216, 1992.

204. Unterberg A, Kiening K, Schmiedek P et al: Long-term observations of intracranial pressure after severe head injury: the phenomenon of secondary rise of intracranial pressure, *Neurosurgery* 32:17, 1993.

205. Van Aken H, Puchstein C, Schweppe ML et al: Effect of labetolol on intracranial pressure in dogs with and without intracranial hypertension, *Acta Anaesthesiol Scand* 26:615, 1982.

206. van Berge Henegouwen DP, Roukema JA, de Nie JC et al: Esophageal perforation during surgery on the cervical spine, *Neurosurgery* 29:766, 1991.

207. Verbalis JG, Robinson AG, Moses AM: Postoperative and post-traumatic diabetes insipidus. In Czernichow P, Robinson AG, editors: *Diabetes insipidus in man: frontiers of hormone research,* vol 13, Basel, 1984, Karger.

208. Veselis RA: Sedation and pain management for the critically ill, *Crit Care Clin* 4:167, 1988.

209. Voldby B, Enevoldsen EM, Jensen FT: Regional CBF, intraventricular pressure, and cerebral metabolism in patients with ruptured intracranial aneurysms, *J Neurosurg* 62:48, 1985.

210. Voldby B, Enevoldsen EM, Jensen FT: Cerebrovascular reactivity in patients with ruptured intracranial aneurysms, *J Neurosurg* 62:59, 1985.

211. Wang HH, Liu LMP, Katz RL: A comparison of cardiovascular effects of sodium nitroprusside and trimethaphan, *Anesthesiology* 46:40, 1977.

212. Wanner MB, Rageth CJ, Zach GA: Pregnancy and autonomic hyperreflexia in patients with spinal cord lesions, *Paraplegia* 25:482, 1987.

213. Ward JD, Becker DP, Miller DJ: Failure of prophylactic barbiturate coma in the treatment of severe head injury, *J Neurosurg* 62:383, 1985.

214. Whitley JM, Prough DS, Brockschmidt JK et al: Cerebral hemodynamic effects of fluid resuscitation in the presence of an experimental intracranial mass, *Surgery* 110:514, 1991.

215. Wijdicks EFM, Ropper AH, Hunnicutt EJ et al: Atrial natriuretic factor and salt wasting after aneurysmal subarachnoid hemorrhage, *Stroke* 22:1519, 1991.

216. Wong DH, O'Connor D, Tremper KK et al: Changes in cardiac output after acute blood loss and position change in man, *Crit Care Med* 17:979, 1989.

217. Wood JH, Polyzoidis KS, Epstein CM, et al: Quantitative EEG alterations after isovolemic-hemodilutional augmentation of cerebral perfusion in stroke patients, *Neurology* 34:764, 1984.

218. Wood JH, Simeone FA, Fink EA et al: Hypervolemic hemodilution in experimental focal cerebral ischemia: elevation of cardiac output, regional cortical blood flow, and ICP after intravascular volume expansion with low molecular weight dextran, *J Neurosurg* 59:500, 1983.

219. Wood JH, Simeone FA, Kron RE et al: Experimental hypervolemic hemodilution: physiological correlations of cortical blood flow, cardiac output, and intracranial pressure with fresh blood viscosity and plasma volume, *Neurosurgery* 14:709, 1984.

220. Wood JH, Snyder LL, Simeone FA: Failure of intravascular volume expansion without hemodilution to elevate cortical blood flow in region of experimental focal ischemia, *J Neurosurg* 56:80, 1982.

221. Yamamoto Y, Smith RR, Bernanke DH: Mechanism of action of balloon angioplasty in cerebral vasospasm, *Neurosurgery* 30:1, 1992.

221a. Young B, Ott L, Phillips R et al: Metabolic management of the patient with head injury, *Neurosurg Clin N Am* 2:301-320, 1991.

221b. Young B, Ott L, Twyman D et al: The effect of nutritional support on outcome from head injury, *J Neurosurg* 67:668-676, 1987.

222. Young WL, Solomon RA, Prohovnik I et al: [133]Xe blood flow monitoring during arteriovenous malformation resection: a case of intraoperative hyperperfusion with subsequent brain swelling, *Neurosurgery* 22:765, 1988.

223. Zabramski JM, Spetzler RF, Lee KS et al: Phase I trial of tissue plasminogen activator for the prevention of vasospasm in patients with aneurysmal subarachnoid hemorrhage, *J Neurosurg* 75:189, 1991.

224. Zaloga GP, Hughes SS: Oliguria in patients with normal renal function, *Anesthesiology* 72:598, 1990.

225. Zornow MH, Todd MM, Moore SS: The acute cerebral effects of changes in plasma osmolality and oncotic pressure, *Anesthesiology* 67:936, 1987.

31

Management of Severe Head Injury

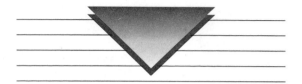

Shankar P. Gopinath
Claudia S. Robertson

EPIDEMIOLOGY OF HEAD INJURY

Trauma caused by accidents, homicide, and suicide accounts for 140,000 deaths in the United States each year. Trauma is the leading cause of death under the age of 45 years and constitutes nearly two thirds of the deaths in people aged 15 to 34 years. Head injury is responsible for nearly a third of all trauma deaths.[59]

In the United States, 470,000 people per year suffer traumatic brain injury. Approximately 15% of these people die before reaching the hospital. Nearly 40,000, or 10%, of the remaining patients have a severe brain injury.[70] Head injury occurs most commonly in young adults between the ages of 15 and 44 years. The average age in most series is approximately 30 years. Men are affected with head injuries more than twice as often as women. Approximately 49% of brain injury hospitalizations are due to automobile or motorcycle accidents, another 28% are caused by falls, and about 22% are due to guns and other causes. Although no accurate figures are available on the extent of disability produced by traumatic brain injury, virtually all severely brain-injured people sustain some degree of long-term disability.[70]

The loss to society from head injury is not just in lost lives but also in the resources required for hospitalization of head-injured patients and for rehabilitation and chronic care of disabled survivors. In addition, because most head-injured patients are teenagers and young adults, productivity is lost. These statistics illustrate the magnitude of the head injuries in the United States, but the problem is not confined to the United States and is rapidly becoming a ma-

661

jor public health concern in other developed and developing countries.

Two large data banks of severely head-injured patients have been collected and reported. The International Data Bank (IDB) consisted of 1000 comatose patients from three centers in Scotland, the Netherlands, and the United States when reported in 1979.[56] The Traumatic Coma Data Bank (TCDB), reported initially in 1991, consists of 1030 comatose patients from four centers in the United States.[31] Analysis of these data and data from individual head injury centers has been invaluable in developing approaches for systematically studying head injury and in understanding the factors that determine long-term recovery after a severe head injury.

CLASSIFICATION OF HEAD INJURY

Head injury has been classified in several ways based on mechanism, severity, pathology, and computed tomographic (CT) scan findings.

Mechanism of Injury

Head injuries can be divided into two general categories based on the mode of injury.[139] Nonmissile or closed head injuries are usually associated with motor vehicle accidents, falls, and assaults, and missile or penetrating injuries are most commonly due to gunshot wounds. Of all severe head injuries in the Traumatic Coma Data Bank (TCDB), 82% were closed head injuries, and the remaining 18% were due to gunshot wounds.[31] This differentiation is important primarily because the emphasis of surgical management and the outcome of missile injuries are somewhat different from nonmissile injuries.

Severity of Injury

Classification of head trauma by the severity of injury is useful because information about initial management and about prognosis is obtained. The neurologic examination performed in the emergency room after cardiopulmonary resuscitation is used to determine the severity of injury. Examinations obtained while patients are hypotensive or hypoxic are unreliable. The neurologic examination may dramatically improve with successful treatment of hypovolemic shock. In addition, alcohol or drug intoxication can suppress the neurologic examination. One study showed an improved Glasgow Coma Scale (GCS) score during the first 6 hours after injury in patients intoxicated with alcohol.[51] The emergency room examination is used to guide the initial management, but the neurologic examination at 6 hours after injury, when any drug effects have disappeared, is recommended for determining prognosis.[56]

The Glasgow Coma Scale (GCS), described by Teasdale and Jennett,[139] is used to quantitate the neurologic examination. The GCS is based on three parameters: eye opening, speech, and motor function (Table 31-1). Patients who open their eyes spontaneously, obey commands, and are

TABLE 31-1
Glasgow Coma Scale

Parameter	Score
Eye Opening	
Spontaneous	4
To speech	3
To pain	2
None	1
Best Motor Response	
Obeys	6
Localizes	5
Withdraws	4
Abnormal flexion	3
Extensor response	2
None	1
Verbal Response	
Oriented	5
Confused conversation	4
Inappropriate words	3
Incomprehensible sounds	2
None	1

oriented score the maximum of 15 points, and those who have no neurologic function score 3 points. Patients with a postresuscitation GCS score of 8 or less have suffered a *severe* head injury, and patients with a GCS score of 9 to 12 and 13 to 15 have a *moderate* and *mild* injury, respectively.[111]

The category of severe head injury generally implies that the patient is in coma. Jennett and Teasdale[55] defined coma strictly as the inability to obey commands, utter words, or open the eyes. Although no single GCS score within the range of 3 to 15 forms an absolute cut-off point for coma by this strict definition, a GCS of 8 or less has generally been considered synonymous with coma. Nine tenths of all patients with a sum score of 8 or less and none of those with a score of 9 or more are in coma, by Jennett and Teasdale's definition. Others have used the criteria of not following commands or a score on the motor section of the GCS of 5 or less to indicate coma.[5]

The GCS, in addition to its simplicity and low interobserver variability,[140] has good predictive properties.[132] The mortality rate of patients with both closed and penetrating injuries is closely related to their postresuscitation GCS score in the emergency room and to the classification of mild, moderate, or severe head injury. In closed head injuries, a consistent correlation has been found between the GCS sum score and subsequent recovery. Two large series of patients admitted to hospitals in the United States have described the relationship of GCS and outcome across the entire spectrum of head injury. Klauber et al.[66] described 1311 patients admitted to 10 hospitals in San Diego County during 1978. Most (1134) of the patients had an initial GCS score of 8 to 15 and a mortality rate of 0.3%. The mortality rate with a GCS score 6 to 7, 4 to 5, and 3 increased to 24%, 49%, and 83%, respectively. Rimel et al.[112,113] described 1248 patients hospitalized at the University of Virginia with head injury. Most (55%) had a GCS score of 13 to 15, 24% had a GCS score of 9 to 12, and 21% had a GCS score of 8 or less. The mortality rate was 3%, and the frequency of a good recovery was 78% for patients admitted with a GCS score of 9 to 12.[113] There were no deaths, and virtually all patients admitted with a GCS score of 13 to 15 had a good recovery.[112]

In penetrating head injuries, outcome also closely correlates with the admission GCS score. In the patient with a GCS score of 3, the mortality rate has been shown to be 100% regardless of therapy,[12,16] but in the patient with a GCS score of 9 to 15, the mortality rate is only 12% and significant recovery can be expected with operation.[95] We have studied 450 patients admitted to Ben Taub General Hospital during a 9-year period with gunshot wounds to the head.[97] Unlike closed head injuries, the distribution of GCS scores with gunshot wounds was bimodal, with the majority of patients being at the very low or the high end of the GCS spectrum. After resuscitation in the emergency room, 48% had a GCS score of 3 to 5, 12% had a GCS score of 5 to 7, 8% had a GCS score of 8 to 12, and 23% had a GCS score of 13 to 15. The outcome was closely related to the admission GCS score. Patients with a GCS score of 3 to 4 invariably died. The frequency of a good outcome was 13% with GCS score of 5 to 7, 32% with GCS score of 8 to 12, and 91% with GCS score of 13 to 15.

The GCS relays information primarily about the level of consciousness, while pupillary response to light and the oculocephalic/vestibular reflexes give complementary information about brainstem function. For patients with severe head injury (GCS ≤ 8), abnormalities of these reflexes have additional predictive power. In the IDB series,[56] the outcome was vegetative or dead in 39% of patients with reactive pupils and 91% in patients with bilaterally unreactive pupils. The outcome was vegetative or dead in 33% of patients with intact oculocephalic/vestibular reflexes, compared with 62% with impaired reflexes, and 90% with absent reflexes. In the TCDB series,[79] the outcome was vegetative or dead in only 9% of patients with bilaterally reactive pupils, 50% of patients with unilaterally unreactive pupils, and 74% of patients with bilaterally unreactive pupils.

Pathology of Injury

Autopsy studies of patients who have died of their head injury and the development of improved neuroimaging techniques for patients who survive have allowed a better understanding of the pathology of human head injury. Head injuries can be classified into two general categories by morphologic characteristics: skull fractures and intracranial lesions.

Skull Fractures

Skull fractures may or may not be associated with underlying brain injury. The incidence of an associated vault or basal skull fracture increases with the severity of the injury, from 3% in patients with mild head injury to 65% in patients with severe head injury.[55] It occurs in 80% of patients with fatal head injuries.[57] The cranial vault is fractured three times as often as the skull base, 62% compared with 20%.[55] The identification of skull fractures is important in the management of head injury because of the association with intracranial hematomas, cerebrospinal fluid fistula, and infection.

Probably the most important use of the plain skull x-ray in the emergency room is to identify patients with a mild head injury who are at a greater risk of having an intracranial hematoma because of the presence of a skull fracture. In a large series of over 180,000 patients presenting to an emergency room with head injury, there was a 1 in 4 chance of an intracranial hematoma in patients with impaired consciousness and a skull fracture. In patients who were oriented, there was a 1 in 32 chance of an intracranial hematoma with a skull fracture, compared with a 1 in 6000 chance in patients without any skull fracture.[82] Therefore a fracture increases the risk of intracranial hematoma by 400 times in a conscious patient and by 20 times in a comatose patient.

Most depressed fractures and all open or compound skull fractures with dural laceration require early surgical repair. A skull fracture is considered significantly depressed if the outer table of the skull lies below the inner table of the surrounding bone. Sometimes the depression is not evident on plain x-rays, but it is usually clearly seen on a CT scan.

A fracture associated with a scalp laceration or one that is in communication with paranasal sinuses or the middle ear is, by definition, an open fracture. CSF rhinorrhea and otorrhea are definite signs of a dural tear and predispose the acutely head-injured patient to the development of posttraumatic meningitis. CSF rhinorrhea is usually associated with an anterior basal skull fracture. In nearly 80% of cases, the CSF leak stops within a week. Transcranial or transsphenoidal surgery is considered after CT cisternography if the CSF leak persists beyond 2 weeks. CSF otorrhea is usually associated with transverse fractures of the petrous bone, and, in the majority of cases, the CSF leak stops spontaneously within a week. In rare cases, lumbar CSF drainage or surgery may be required.

In a study of posttraumatic bacterial meningitis, the incidence of meningitis was found to be 18% and 9% when associated with otorrhea and rhinorrhea, respectively, compared with 0.38% in the absence of a cerebrospinal fluid leak.[71] Tenney found a higher risk of infection with rhinorrhea than with otorrhea.[144] The efficacy of prophylactic antibiotics in patients with traumatic CSF fistula is controversial. Antibiotics are recommended only when symptons or signs of meningitis develop.

Intracranial Lesions

Although intracranial lesions are generally classified as focal or diffuse, the two may coexist. In the TCDB series,

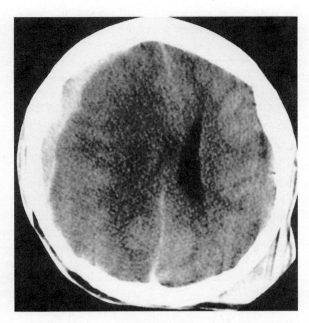

FIG. 31-1   CT scan demonstrating a subdural hematoma.

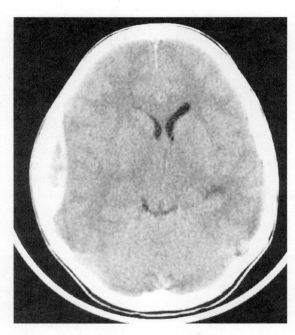

FIG. 31-2   CT scan demonstrating an epidural hematoma.

56% of patients with severe closed head injury had a diffuse injury, and 42% had a focal mass lesion. The mortality rate was generally higher with a focal lesion, 39% compared with 24% with a diffuse injury.[31]

The subdural hematoma is the most common focal intracranial lesion, occurring in 24% of patients with severe closed head injuries in the TCDB.[31] The hematoma is between the dura and the brain, usually resulting from a torn bridging vein between the cortex and the draining sinuses. An acute subdural hematoma identified within 72 hours after trauma usually appears on a CT scan as a high-density, homogenous crescent-shaped mass paralleling the calvarium (Fig. 31-1). However, if the patient is anemic, up to 10% of acute subdural hematomas may be isodense with brain because of the low hemoglobin content.[131] The mortality rate in patients with subdural hematomas was 50% in the TCDB series.[79] Two subtypes of acute subdural hematoma have been recognized: "pure" subdural hematoma and subdural hematoma associated with brain contusions.[142] In the latter type, because of the association with underlying severe cerebral injury, the outcome is worse than in the pure subdural hematoma group. Several studies report a decrease in the mortality or morbidity of patients who underwent an early evacuation of subdural hematoma.[5,34,124]

Epidural hematomas, or collections of blood between the skull and the dura, are less common. Epidural hematomas occurred in 6% of patients with severe closed head injuries in the TCDB series.[31] Although patients with subdural hematomas are usually immediately comatose, only a third of patients with an epidural hematoma are unconscious from the time of injury, one third have a lucid interval, and one third are never unconscious.[52] An epidural hematoma is almost always associated with a skull fracture (91% in adults and 75% in children).[55] The blood comes from torn dural vessels, usually arterial, from the fractured skull bone, or occasionally from torn venous sinuses. On CT scan (Fig. 31-2), an epidural hematoma is characterized by a biconvex, uniformly hyperdense lesion. Associated brain lesions are less common than with subdural hematomas. Epidural hematomas may also develop in a delayed fashion or on the contralateral side after evacuation of an initial epidural hematoma. The outcome of the patient with an epidural hematoma depends on the neurologic status at the time of surgery. The mortality rate varies from 0% for patients who are not in coma, to 9% for obtunded patients, to 20% for patients in deep coma.

Intracerebral blood can take the form of a hematoma or a contusion. Intracerebral hematomas are more common, occurring as the primary lesion in 10% of the severe closed head injuries in the TCDB series.[31] Occasionally, it may be difficult to differentiate a traumatic intracerebral hematoma from a spontaneous hemorrhage; however, the presence of associated contusion, fracture, or air fluid level in the sinus helps in identifying the hematoma as traumatic. In contrast to spontaneous hemorrhage, traumatic intracerebral hematomas are irregular and poorly marginated (Fig. 31-3). A zone of surrounding hypodensity denotes contusion or edema.

Most intracerebral hematomas are visualized as hyperdense mass lesions. They are usually located in frontal and temporal lobes and can be detected on a CT scan immediately after the trauma. However, delayed intracerebral he-

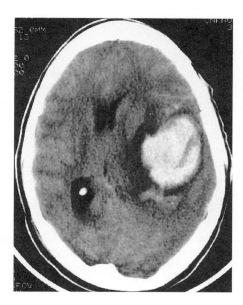

FIG. 31-3   CT scan demonstrating an intracerebral hematoma.

matomas may also be manifest during the hospital course. A delayed hematoma is one that is seen on a repeat CT scan within 24 to 48 hours of the injury or operation but is not present on the initial CT scan. Commonly, a delayed hematoma is associated with clinical deterioration. In one series, 19% of patients with a severe head injury who neurologically deteriorated after admission to the hospital had a large delayed intracerebral hematoma.[17]

Hemorrhagic contusions were present as the primary lesion in 3% of severe closed head injuries in the TCDB series.[31] Single contusions are located either below the region of the impact or opposite the region of impact. Contusions appear as heterogenous areas of brain necrosis, hemorrhage, and infarct representing mixed-density lesions on CT scan.[153] Multiple focal contusions have a "salt and pepper" appearance on CT scan.

Diffuse brain injuries have no mass lesions requiring surgery. Traumatic loss of consciousness of less than 6 hours is considered a concussion and is usually associated with amnesia for the events related to the injury. Traumatic coma of greater than 6 hours is defined as diffuse axonal injury (DAI). DAI is a frequent injury, occurring in nearly 60% of comatose head injuries. DAI is associated with microscopic damage scattered throughout the brain. Three severities of DAI are recognized: (1) mild DAI—coma of 6 to 24 hours duration, (2) moderate DAI—coma of more than 24 hours without decerebrate posturing, and (3) severe DAI—coma of more than 24 hours with decerebrate posturing or flaccidity. Severe DAI has a 50% mortality.[34]

CT Scan

A new classification of head injury based on information obtained in the initial CT scan was described from the TCDB data.[78] The scheme uses the status of mesencephalic cisterns, the amount of midline shift, and the presence or absence of surgical masses. Diffuse injuries were defined in all patients with no mixed or high-density lesions greater than 25 ml. The category of diffuse injuries was divided into four subgroups: Diffuse injury I included all head injuries with no visible pathology, diffuse injury II included all diffuse injuries with cisterns present and less than 5 mm shift, diffuse injury III included all diffuse injuries with compressed or absent cisterns but less than 5 mm shift, and diffuse injury IV included all diffuse injuries with more than 5 mm midline shift. The category of mass lesions, which included all patients with mixed or high-density lesions greater than 25 ml, was divided into those with the mass surgically evacuated (including operated subdural, epidural, and intracerebral hematomas) and those with nonevacuated mass lesions.

This classification scheme provided a better assessment of the risk of intracranial hypertension and of a fatal outcome. Patients with diffuse injury I had the lowest mortality rate of 10%, while the diffuse injury II, III, and IV groups had mortality rates of 14%, 34%, and 56%, respectively. The mortality rate of evacuated hematomas was 39%.

PRIMARY VS. SECONDARY INSULTS TO THE BRAIN

Neurologic injury from trauma is due to both primary and secondary brain insults.[87] The primary brain injury represents the biomechanical effect of energy dissipation onto the skull and brain substance occurring immediately with the impact. These early effects of the impact include direct neuronal and axonal disruption, vascular injury, direct brain laceration, and diffuse shearing injuries.[3] The primary injury is—at one end of the spectrum—a concussion or transient, reversible loss of consciousness and—at the other end of the spectrum—sudden death caused by physical disruption of the brainstem. The primary brain injury can, in turn initiate a more complex biochemical cascade resulting in secondary brain injury. This secondary damage can be considered as a complication of the original injury and includes intracranial hematoma, brain damage secondary to raised intracranial pressure, brain swelling, herniation of the brain, and hypoxic brain damage.[1] Several substances, such as proteolytic enzymes, biogenic amines (serotonin and histamine), neurotransmitters (glutamate), unsaturated fatty acids (arachidonic acid and its metabolites), free radicals, and the kallikrein-kinin system, have been implicated as mediators in the production of various reversible and irreversible pathophysiologic mechanisms causing secondary brain damage. These mechanisms might include production of vasogenic edema by altering the blood-brain barrier, secondary ischemia, and an increase of intracranial pressure (ICP) caused by induction of circulatory disturbances, cytotoxic edema, and cell necrosis. In addition, the cerebral

▼

BOX 31-1
Causes of Secondary Brain Injury

Systemic	Intracranial
Arterial hypotension	Epidural/subdural hematoma
Hypoxemia	Contusion/intracerebral hematoma
Hypercapnia	Raised intracranial pressure
Anemia	Cerebral edema
Hypoglycemia	Cerebral vasospasm
Hyponatremia and osmotic imbalance	Intracranial infection
Hyperthermia	Cerebral hyperemia
Sepsis	Posttraumatic epilepsy
Coagulopathy	
Hypertension	

circulation plays a significant role in secondary brain damage, which may result from microcirculatory disorders causing either delayed brain edema or secondary cerebral ischemia (Box 31-1).[58]

Prehospital Management of Head Injury

The most important goals of prehospital management are to maintain the airway and to support blood pressure to preserve cerebral perfusion pressure. Prehospital hypoxia and hypotension are common in severely head-injured patients. In a series of 100 patients with severe head injury presenting to the Medical College of Virginia, 13% were hypotensive, 12% were anemic, 30% were hypoxic, and 4% were hypercarbic on arrival in the emergency room.[87] Of 363 patients in coma admitted to a British hospital between 1959 and 1968, 8.5% were hypoxic, 15.1% were hypotensive, and 3.3% were both hypoxic and hypotensive.[107] In a head-injured patient, a systolic blood pressure of less than 90 mm Hg on admission to the hospital has been reported to double the mortality rate from 34% to 65%.[89,98] The incidence of a poor outcome ranges from 59% to 71% in patients who were hypoxic compared with 27% to 34% in patients who were never hypoxic. The combined effects of hypotension and hypoxia result in 100% mortality.[35,68] These observations from epidemiologic studies have been reproduced in the laboratory, where hypoxia or hypotension markedly worsen the outcome from experimental head injury.[48,49,50]

In addition, it is important to take the severely injured patient directly to a hospital that has neurosurgical support. If a surgical lesion is present, time to evacuation of the hematoma is an important determinant of outcome.[81,119] Optimal results with intracranial hematomas require surgical evacuation within 2 to 4 hours of the injury. This is only possible if patients are taken directly to a neurosurgical cen-

ter.[135] In instances where patients have been transferred secondarily to neurosurgical services, worse outcomes have been occasionally noticed.[9,134]

Approximately 2% to 5% of all patients with severe head injury have an associated spinal cord injury.[76] Stabilization of the neck until x-rays can demonstrate absence of a cervical spine fracture is important for all severely head-injured patients.

Emergency Room Management of Head Injury
Mild Head Injury

The majority (80%) of head-injured patients seen in the emergency room are classified as mild head injury, and most of these recover without incident although they may have neuropsychologic sequelae.[66,112] Approximately 3% of patients with an initial GCS score of 13 to 15, however, will deteriorate and require neurosurgical intervention.[24] The challenge of this group of patients is to identify the subgroup of patients at high risk of deterioration. Guidelines suggested by a multicenter study of 7035 head-injured patients at 31 hospitals[80] include:

- For low-risk patients, those who have minimal initial signs and symptons such as headache, dizziness, or scalp lacerations, discharge the patient to a reliable environment for observation.
- For moderate-risk patients, those who have initial signs such as vomiting, alcohol, or drug intoxication, posttraumatic amnesia, or clinical signs of a basilar or depressed skull fracture, a CT scan should be considered, and the patient should be closely monitored for 12 to 24 hours.
- For high-risk patients, those who have a depressed or decreasing level of consciousness, focal neurologic signs, or penetrating injuries, an emergency CT scan should be obtained.

Moderate Head Injury

There is a tendency to underestimate the severity of the injury in the group of patients with an initial GCS score of 9 to 12 because they are able to follow simple commands in the emergency room. However, these patients can deteriorate rapidly.[118] In addition, it has been shown that, although the mortality rate is 3%, morbidity is very high, with roughly 50% having a moderate disability at 3 months after injury.[113] Patients with a GCS score of 9 to 12 should have an emergent CT scan and be admitted for observation even though their initial CT scan is normal. The goals of monitoring are the same as for severe head injuries, except the neurologic status is monitored by serial neurologic examinations. ICP monitoring is reserved for those patients who clinically deteriorate, or possibly patients who, because of treatment of systemic injuries, cannot be followed with serial neurologic examinations.

Severe Head Injury
Resuscitation

The first goal of resuscitation of a severely head injured patient is cardiopulmonary stabilization. All patients are intubated to protect their airway from aspiration and to allow controlled ventilation. Hypotension is rapidly treated with volume replacement. In adults, hypotension is rarely caused by head injury alone, and another injury site should be sought.[47] Blood loss from another injury, an associated spinal cord injury, cardiac contusion or tamponade, and tension pneumothorax are other causes of hypotension to be considered. Standard resuscitation fluids include crystalloids, colloids, and blood products. Most studies show no advantages of colloid over crystalloid resuscitation in experimental head injury.[151,155] Crystalloids should not include glucose to minimize hyperglycemia. Experimental studies have suggested that hypertonic saline may replace volume loss with less increase in intracranial pressure than with colloids or crystalloids.[43]

ICP should be assumed to be elevated in patients with severe head injury before definitive treatment. Miller et al.,[86] in a series of 160 patients in whom ICP was measured in the emergency room after cardiopulmonary resuscitation, found that 98% of patients with a mass lesion had an elevated ICP, and 74% of patients with a diffuse injury had an elevated ICP. ICP is controlled temporarily with controlled ventilation ($Pao_2 > 100$ mm Hg, $Paco_2$ 30 to 35 mm Hg) to prevent hypoxia and hypercarbia, and with sedation and paralysis until definitive treatment of surgical lesions and an ICP monitor can be placed. Mannitol, 1 g/kg IV, is given, especially if the patient has signs of herniation or is neurologically deteriorating.

Diagnostic Evaluation

History. Even though obtaining a detailed history is often not possible in patients with severe head injury, the approximate time and mechanism of injury at the scene of the accident may be obtained from the paramedics. The time of intubation and the patient's vital signs and neurologic deficits at the scene of accident and during transportation, especially the presence of apnea and hypotension, will help in subsequent evaluations. In addition, progressive deterioration of the level of sensorium before the patient reaches the hospital suggests an expanding intracranial mass lesion, and the patient who was unconcious from the time of injury is more likely to have diffuse axonal injury.

Neurologic Examination. The main goal of the initial neurologic examination in patients with severe head injury is to document the degree of dysfunction of the cortex and various levels of brainstem and to identify evidence of any unilateral neurologic abnormality that would suggest a mass lesion. The neurologic examination should include, in addition to vital signs, the GCS score to assess functional capacity of cerebral cortex, the pupillary examination and the corneal reflex to assess brainstem function, and the oculocephalic and oculovestibular reflex to assess eye movement.

In addition to the neurologic examination, a general examination should be done with specific attention directed at identifying pneumothorax/hemothorax, visceral injuries of the abdomen, pelvic injuries, spinal injuries, and injuries involving extremities. Symptoms caused by systemic injuries may be delayed or obscured in the unconscious patient, and every effort must be made to rule out other injuries that might result in secondary insults to the brain by causing hypotension or hypoxia.

Radiologic Examination. Before the advent of CT scanning, the common radiologic procedures in the management of head-injured patients included skull x-ray, cerebral angiography, ventriculography, and radionuclide brain scanning. The radiologic procedure of choice at present in an acute trauma patient is the unenhanced CT scan. Contrast-injected studies are only required when an isodense subdural hematoma is suspected either from clinical history or from radiologic evidence of ventricular shift or sulcal effacement on the unenhanced scan.

Studies in minor head injury suggest that MR may be more sensitive than CT scan, identifying lesions in symptomatic patients even when the CT scan is normal. However, there is not yet sufficient experience with the use of MRI to recommend its use in the acute evaluation of the severely head-injured patient. In addition, the equipment necessary to monitor and support the critically ill head-injured patient may not always be usable in the MR scanner.

Cerebral angiography provides a specific diagnosis only in extracerebral lesions or in cases of vascular injury. At present, angiography is performed in head-injured patients only when CT scanning is not available, when an isodense subdural hematoma is suspected on CT, or when a vascular injury is considered.

Several investigators have studied the size of CT lesions, hematomas, contusion, size of the third ventricle, relation of basal cisterns, and other signs of brain swelling, as predictors of the frequency of intracranial hypertension and outcome. Toutant compared outcome in 218 patients in the pilot TCDB series with the status of the basal cisterns on the initial CT scan.[145] Mortality rate was 77%, 29%, and 22% with absent, compressed, and normal basal cisterns, respectively. This association was significant even after adjusting for GCS score. Van Dongen also found a relationship between the status of basal cisterns and outcome in 116 head-injured patients.[146] Mortality rate was 7%, 35%, 38%, and 93% in patients with normal scans, abnormal scan plus normal cisterns, abnormal scan plus compressed cisterns, and abnormal scan plus absent cisterns, respectively. Klauber et al. found the best predictors of intracranial hypertension after the first hospital day to be an increased ICP on day 1, the presence of hypotension, and the presence of abnormal ventricles (absent, small, or enlarged) on the initial CT scan.[67] Based on CT findings of presence or absence of contusion, hematoma, brain edema, or brain swelling alone or in combination, Richard et al. found the mortality rate to be higher (46%) with contusions in combination with brain swelling, while contusions in combination with brain edema and swelling had a mortality of 30%.[110]

SURGICAL MANAGEMENT OF HEAD INJURY
Closed Head Injuries

In general, all intracranial mass lesions are considered operable if there is a midline shift of 5 mm or more. In the majority of patients with contusions who also have compressed basal cisterns, surgery is needed. Patients with temporal lobe hematoma/contusions are at a greater risk of developing tentorial herniation than those with frontal/parietal lesions,[4] and, therefore, surgery must be considered in the light of clinical findings.

Most epidural hematomas require surgery, and mortality and morbidity of surgical evacuation is low if the patient is operated upon early. Although the type of craniotomy depends on the location of the epidural hematoma, generally the flap must allow for adequate exploration to locate the source of bleeding. If the patient's neurologic condition is deteriorating rapidly, the initial burr hole should be placed directly in relation to the site of the hematoma to allow rapid evacuation of the clot because release of even a small amount of blood clot will relieve the pressure on the brainstem. After this initial step, the craniotomy can be completed. The important step, after evacuation of the hematoma and securing of the bleeding points, is to tack up the dura to prevent reaccumulation of blood. An ICP monitor should be placed in patients who are unconscious.

Most acute subdural hematomas also require surgery. The rapidity of surgical evacuation[124] and the degree of associated brain damage are major determinants of outcome.

The principle of surgical management for acute subdural hematoma, which often is associated with underlying brain contusion, is based on two factors: (1) to relieve brainstem compression by removal of the subdural clot and contused brain and (2) to prevent the adverse effect of blood products on brain function. A large craniotomy trauma flap is preferred because it offers the advantages of exposing both subfrontal and subtemporal regions, permitting identification of the source of bleeding, especially near the midline, and allows effective clearing of the subdural space. Because postoperative brain swelling is common after evacuation of a subdural hematoma, an ICP monitor should be placed in patients with impaired consciousness.

The decision to operate on an intracerebral hematoma is based on the patient's general condition, associated brain injuries, site and size of the hematoma, the ICP, and the magnitude of the mass effect.[11] The indications for operative management of intracerebral hematoma are controversial. Generally accepted indications for surgery include (1) a hematoma associated with mass effect or in the anterior temporal lobe or in the cerebellum, (2) progressive neurologic deterioration, or (3) refractory intracranial hypertension. As a general principle, during the surgery, removal of contused brain should be continued until a margin of healthy brain is reached because contused brain, being irreversibly damaged, acts as a mass lesion and might cause further local brain swelling.

Sudden massive brain swelling may occur in a patient as the dura is opened or minutes after the clot or contusion has been removed; it is seen in up to one fifth of the patients with acute subdural hematoma.[73] It is thought to be due to defective cerebral autoregulation with reactive hyperemia and vascular engorgement,[6] but an important cause to recognize is a new acute hemorrhage. Intraoperative ultrasound is useful in distinguishing these possibilities.[101] One also must rule out systemic causes, such as venous engorgement, hypercapnia, hypoxia, pneumothorax, and hypertension. Treatment includes rapid and thorough resection of the hematoma/contusion, and reduction in brain volume by hyperventilation, mannitol, infusion of barbiturates such as thiopental or pentobarbital, or induced hypotension.

Penetrating Head Injuries

Penetrating head injury can be due to perforating stab wounds or to gunshot wounds. Civilian gunshot wounds are primarily from lower velocity missiles. An object protruding from the skull should not be removed until the patient is in the operating room and the craniotomy has been completed because profuse hemorrhage may follow removal. Extensive scalp laceration and profuse bleeding can be sufficient to produce hypovolemic shock. The clinical presentation can vary from a minimally depressed level of consciousness to a fully unconscious state. The operative principle of a penetrating injury includes evacuation of the hematoma through a small craniotomy, resection of necrotic brain tissue, removal of accessible bone and missile fragments, and repair and closure of the dura.[46,62] In case of uncontrolled bleeding from a venous sinus, ligation of the sinus may be required.[136]

INTENSIVE CARE MONITORING

The outcome from severe head injury to a large extent depends on anticipation, recognition, and early treatment of the preventable secondary brain damage. Intensive care monitoring offers the opportunity to identify early and therefore treat early the secondary posttraumatic insults that may impair ultimate recovery. Several studies have suggested that with aggressive monitoring and treatment, the mortality rate after severe head injury can be decreased.[5,9,86,122]

The ICU management of both surgically treated and nonsurgical patients is similar. Monitoring can be divided into two broad categories—monitoring of the brain and monitoring of the body although both systems interact with each other.

Neurologic Monitoring

To assess the neurologic status of the patient, one should include evaluation of mental status, cranial nerve, pupillary, and motor functions in the periodic neurologic examination. This will help in determining the progressive recovery, deterioration, or static nature during therapy. A 24-hour record of the patient should be available on one sheet, such as was described by Clifton and Grossman,[18] and should include information regarding vital signs and laboratory values,

Intracranial Pressure Monitoring

Normally, resting ICP is 0 to 15 mm Hg. Transient elevations of ICP occur normally with straining, coughing, or the Trendelenburg position. A sustained ICP greater than 20 mm Hg is clearly abnormal. An ICP between 20 and 40 mm Hg is considered moderate intracranial hypertension. An ICP greater than 40 mm Hg represents severe, usually life-threatening, intracranial hypertension.[74]

Intracranial Hypertension After Severe Head Injury

Intracranial hypertension develops in 50% of patients in coma caused by severe head injury. It is a misconception that ICP will always be low after operative evacuation of a large intracranial hematoma. Intracranial hypertension occurs in 50% to 70% of patients after evacuation of an intracranial hematoma.[86,87] This postoperative intracranial hypertension may be due to a postoperative hematoma, either at the site of the operation or at a new site, progressive swelling of focal contusion, diffuse brain swelling, and other systemic complications. The incidence of intracranial hypertension is greater after evacuation of an intracerebral

hematoma, 71% compared with 39% after evacuation of a subdural or epidural hematoma.[86] In patients with no mass lesions, an elevated ICP has been observed to occur during the hospital course in 30%[86] to 80%[10] of patients.

The association between the severity of intracranial hypertension and a poor outcome after severe head injury is well recognized. In one series, 77% of patients with an ICP below 15 mm Hg had a favorable outcome, compared with only 43% in patients with an ICP above 15 mm Hg.[77] Miller[88] reported that mortality rate increased from 18% to 92% and the frequency of good outcomes decreased from 74% to 3% in patients with normal ICP compared with patients who had intracranial hypertension that could not be reduced below 20 mm Hg. Similarly, Saul and Ducker reported a 69% mortality rate in patients with an ICP greater than 25 mm Hg, compared with a mortality rate of 15% if ICP remained less than 25 mm Hg.[122]

The relationship between an elevated ICP and a poor outcome is not simply a reflection of the severity of the initial neurologic injury. Severe intracranial hypertension can result in secondary injury to the brain through ischemia, produced by reducing cerebral perfusion pressure, and it can also distort and compress the brainstem. Although no randomized clinical trial has addressed this question, several clinical series have suggested that reduction of the ICP to less than 20 mm Hg does reduce mortality after severe head injury.[5,9,86,122]

Measurement of Intracranial Pressure in the ICU

To treat intracranial hypertension effectively, one must actually measure ICP. There are no reliable clinical indicators of intracranial hypertension in patients with severe head injury. Clinical symptoms of raised ICP, such as headache, nausea, and vomiting, are impossible to elicit in comatose patients. Papilledema is uncommon after head injury, even in patients with intracranial hypertension.[125] Although 54% of patients had an increased ICP, only 3.5% had papilledema on funduscopic examination. Other neurologic signs, including pupillary dilation and decerebrate posturing, can occur in the absence of intracranial hypertension. CT scan signs of brain swelling, such as midline shift and compressed basal cisterns, are predictive of raised ICP, but intracranial hypertension can occur without these findings.[65]

Monitoring of ICP can result in serious complications, however, and is indicated only in those patients at significant risk of developing intracranial hypertension (Fig. 31-4). Patients who are particularly at risk for developing elevated ICP include those with GCS scores of 8 or less after resuscitation and an abnormal CT scan, and those with GCS scores of 8 or less and a normal CT but adverse features such as age over 40 years, systolic BP of 90 mm Hg or less, or motor posturing.[96] Patients with a GCS score greater than 8 might be considered for ICP monitoring if they require treatment that would not allow serial neuro-

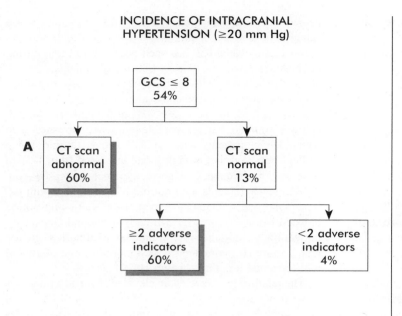

INCIDENCE OF INTRACRANIAL
HYPERTENSION (≥20 mm Hg)

A

GCS ≤ 8
54%

CT scan
abnormal
60%

CT scan
normal
13%

≥2 adverse
indicators
60%

<2 adverse
indicators
4%

INDICATIONS FOR ICP MONITORING

1. Greater than 50% chance of having an
   increased ICP:
   GCS ≥ 8 and abnormal CT scan
                    or
   GCS ≥ 8 and normal CT scan,
        but any two of the following
        adverse indicators:
        (a) Age > 40 years
        (b) Decerebrate
        (c) Hypotension
2. Inability to monitor serial
   neurologic examinations because
   of anesthesia for systemic
   injuries or pharmacologic
   paralysis for respiratory
   management
3. Need for a treatment that
   might increase ICP, such as
   high levels of PEEP for
   acute respiratory failure

B

FIG. 31-4 **A,** Incidence of intracranial hypertension in subgroups of comatose patients. **B,** Indications for ICP monitoring in head-injured patients. (**A,** *data from Narayan RK, Kishore RPS, Becker DP et al:* J Neurosurg *56:650, 1982*).

logic examinations,[141] such as prolonged anesthesia for surgery of multiple injuries or prolonged pharmacologic paralysis for ventilatory management, or if they require a treatment that might raise ICP, such as PEEP. A severe coagulopathy is the only major contraindication to ICP monitoring.

Although several new types of monitors have recently been marketed, the ventriculostomy catheter remains the preferred device for monitoring ICP and the standard against which all of the newer monitors are compared. The ventriculostomy catheter is positioned with its tip in the frontal horn of the lateral ventricle and is coupled by fluid-filled tubing to an external pressure transducer that can be reset to zero and recalibrated against an external standard. The ventriculostomy catheter provides the most reliable measurement of ICP throughout the normal and pathologic ranges. In addition, the ventriculostomy ICP monitor allows treatment of an elevated ICP by intermittent drainage of cerebrospinal fluid. However, the risk of ventriculitis and of intracranial hemorrhage is highest with the ventriculostomy,[96] and proper placement of the catheter tip in the lateral ventricle can be difficult in patients with small, compressed ventricles.

When the ventricle cannot be cannulated, alternative devices are used. The subarachnoid bolt was previously the most common alternative device. The bolt is placed subdurally through a twist drill hole and provides fluid coupling from the surface of the brain to an external transducer.

The main advantage of the bolt is that it does not require cannulation of the ventricle and therefore can be used in patients with small, compressed ventricles. The major disadvantage is the occurrence of falsely low ICP values caused by herniation of brain into the hollow bolt when the ICP is elevated. Fluid-coupled catheters can also be placed in the subdural or epidural spaces. Like the subarachnoid bolt, these catheters tend to become obstructed and to provide spuriously low ICP values when the ICP is elevated.

A number of nonfluid-coupled devices have become available for ICP monitoring and have replaced the subarachnoid bolt in most institutions. The Ladd fiberoptic device and the Camino fiberoptic catheter-tip transducers are the most widely available. The Ladd device is an epidural monitor. The Camino catheter can be inserted in the subdural space or directly into brain tissue. The main advantage of these monitors is the ease of insertion, especially in patients with compressed ventricles. They provide more reliable measures of ICP than fluid-coupled catheters in the subdural space because they have no lumen to become obstructed. The transducers, however, cannot be reset to zero after they are inserted into the skull, and they exhibit small amounts of drift over time.

For surgical patients the ICP monitor should be inserted during surgery. Those who do not require surgery are immediately transferred to the ICU after the initial CT scan, and an ICP monitor is then inserted. A pressure tracing should display the pulsatile nature of the ICP. A dampened tracing may not be a reliable measure of ICP. Monitoring should be continued as long as ICP remains elevated, during active management of ICP, or for 3 days in the absence of significant ICP elevation.

The two major complications of ICP monitoring are ventriculitis and hemorrhage. Infection may be confined to the skin wound, but in 1% to 10% of cases, ventriculitis occurs. Most studies have found a higher rate of infection in the ventriculostomy-monitored patients than in those monitored with subarachnoid bolts or subdural catheters.[96,99] In most studies, the rate of infection is directly related to the duration of monitoring, with very few infections in patients monitored for less than 3 days. The practice of replacing the ventriculostomy catheter after 5 days, if continued monitoring is required, has been recommended on the basis of these studies. Another study, however, demonstrated that most ventriculostomy-related infections occurred in the first week and were thus presumably due to contamination at the time of insertion of the catheter.[60] The authors of this study concluded that it was best not to replace uninfected ventriculostomy catheters routinely. No controlled studies have investigated this issue or the ability of prophylactic antibiotics to reduce the incidence of ventriculostomy-related infections.

The second major complication of ICP monitoring is intracerebral hemorrhage. Although the risk of hemorrhage has been shown to be consistently low (1% to 2%), it is an important complication to recognize and treat.[96] Ventriculostomy catheters are associated with a slightly higher risk of hemorrhage than subarachnoid or subdural devices. Patients with coagulopathies are at a greater risk of developing this complication.

Cerebral Perfusion Monitoring

Normal cerebral blood flow (CBF) is 0.54 plus or minus .12 ml/g/min in adults,[64] and 1.06 plus or minus .03 ml/g/min in children.[63] Normal cerebral metabolic rate of oxygen ($CMRo_2$) is 1.5 μmol/g/min. After a severe head injury, $CMRo_2$ is consistently reduced by approximately 50%. The severity of the suppression of $CMRo_2$ is directly related to the level of coma.[100] Although CBF is normally tightly coupled to metabolic rate, after a severe head injury, CBF can vary widely and independently of $CMRo_2$. CBF can also vary as a result of $Paco_2$. Most authors adjust CBF to a common $Paco_2$, such as 34 mm Hg, and compare with normal values for that $Paco_2$. By this convention, CBF is reduced in 45%, normal in 35%, and elevated in 20% of head-injured adults.[100] An elevated CBF occurs in as many as 30% of head-injured children.[93]

Cerebral Ischemia After Severe Head Injury

Ischemic brain damage has been found on neuropathologic examination in at least 88% of head-injured patients with fatal injuries.[41,42] Infarction can be identified on CT scan in approximately 15% of patients with severe head in-

jury.[116] The ischemia can be global or regional and can be due to intracranial or systemic causes.

Intracranial hypertension can cause global ischemia or local ischemia due to compression of intracranial vessels.[2] Global ischemia usually results from severe intracranial hypertension where cerebral perfusion pressure is reduced to less than 40 mm Hg. Refractory intracranial hypertension of this severity occurs in approximately 10% to 15% of all comatose head-injured patients and is associated with a mortality greater than 90%.[9] With less severe intracranial hypertension, circulation may be compromised in certain susceptible areas. Compression of the posterior cerebral arteries against the tentorium causes ischemia of the occipital lobes, resulting in the classic pathologic finding of intracranial hypertension, called "medial occipital necrosis." This type of infarction has been found at autopsy in 33% of patients who died of head injury.[41] The CT scan appearance is that of lucent areas in the occipital lobes, which can be unilateral or bilateral.

Normally the brain regulates CBF in a normal range despite variations in mean arterial pressure from 50 to 130 mm Hg. The ability of the brain to autoregulate CBF is commonly impaired after severe head injury.[72,148] Hypotension of a degree for which the brain would normally compensate without neurologic consequences can reduce CBF to critical levels and result in ischemic injury after head trauma. The watershed areas of the brain, typically between the anterior and middle cerebral artery distributions, are the most susceptible to ischemia caused by hypotension. This type of boundary zone infarction has been found at autopsy in 22% of patients who die of their injuries.

Infarctions in the distribution of arterial territories (other than posterior cerebral artery) occur in 9% of patients who die of head injury.[41] The most likely causes of these infarctions include arterial vasospasm, compression of vessels by mass lesions, and injury of major intracranial vessels. Angiographic evidence of vasospasm has been reported to occur in 19% of patients with moderate-to-severe head injury.[32,137,149] The incidence of ischemic injury caused by vasospasm is more difficult to estimate because the neurologic signs of ischemia are superimposed on the neurologic deficits of the traumatic injury. In a group of patients with fatal head injuries selected because they had both angiographic and neuropathologic examinations, the incidence of arterial spasm on the preoperative angiogram was 41%. The factors most strongly correlating with the subsequent development of arterial territory infarctions were the presence of intracranial hematomas and vasospasm. These studies suggested that mechanical factors generated by distortion and displacement of an intracranial hematoma can reduce regional cerebral blood flow to critical levels, especially when vasospasm is present.[75]

Injuries of the major intracranial arteries range from intimal dissection with thrombosis to complete transection. The incidence of this type of ischemic injury is not known

TABLE 31-2
Relationship Between CBF and Outcome in 202 Patients (p = .029; Chi-Square Test)

Three Month Glasgow Outcome Scale	Reduced CBF Number (% of Group)	Normal CBF Number (% of Group)	Elevated CBF Number (% of Group)
Good recovery/moderate disability	7 (15.9%)	30 (41.1%)	36 (42.4%)
Severe disability/vegetative	19 (43.2%)	26 (35.6%)	28 (33.0%)
Dead	18 (40.9%)	17 (23.3%)	21 (24.7%)
Total number	44 (100%)	73 (100%)	85 (100%)

but is probably lower than the other causes of arterial distribution infarctions. A review of 31 cases of intracranial carotid artery injury reported in the literature through 1987 demonstrated a generally poor outcome with 16 of 31 (51%) dying and 7 of 31(23%) surviving with a major neurologic deficit.[90]

Many studies reporting CBF measurements in head-injured patients have been published, but the lack of practical technologies for measuring CBF in the ICU and two unanswered questions have prevented measurements of CBF from widespread clinical use. The first question—how low does CBF have to be reduced to result in injury after head injury—is still unanswered while the second question—when does the ischemia occur—is beginning to be elucidated.

An extremely low CBF (<0.2 ml/g/min) has almost always been associated with a poor neurologic otucome. Overgaard et al.[103] showed, using intracarotid xenon CBF measurements, that rCBF values less than 0.2 ml/g/min occurred in 61% of patients who died or who were severely disabled or vegetative but in only 10% of patients with a good outcome. Overgaard and Tweed[104] reported that patients who died or remained vegetative often had very low rCBF in arterial boundary zones, and, as a group, had lower global CBF values than patients who recovered.

Other studies have suggested that a moderately reduced CBF is also more commonly associated with an unfavorable outcome. Tabbador et al.[138] found CBF and CMR_{O_2} to be lower in patients who died of their head injury. We reported an association between reduced CBF during the first 5 days after injury and a higher mortality and a poorer neurologic recovery in a group of survivors of 102 head-injured patients.[117] We have measured CBF in 202 patients with head injury and classified them as having a normal, reduced, or elevated CBF compared with normal values at Pa_{CO_2} of 34 mm Hg. The mortality rate increased from 19% in patients with a normal or elevated CBF to 41% in patients with a reduced CBF (Table 31-2). Although there is an association between a reduced CBF and a negative outcome, it is not clear whether moderately reduced CBF values are in themselves injurious or whether a reduced CBF predisposes to transient ischemia.

The epidemiologic studies of emergency room hypoxia and hypotension suggest that a large portion of the ischemic damage occurs before hospitalization. The early stud-

ies by Overgaard[103] and more recent studies by Bouma[8] and Muizelaar[92] suggest that most of the remaining sustained periods of very low CBF values occur within the first few hours after injury. Muizelaar found that in the first 24 hours after injury, patients with a good neurologic outcome had a higher CBF than those with a poor neurologic outcome.[92] After 24 hours, there was no relationship between CBF and outcome. Bouma found that within 6 hours of injury, the mean CBF was lower than at any time thereafter and was critically low in 33% of the cases.[8]

Transient ischemia, however, can occur throughout the early hospital course and from a variety of both intracranial and systemic causes. We reported finding transient periods of jugular venous desaturation (<50% saturation for at least 15 minutes) in 20 (44%) out of 45 patients when jugular venous oxygen saturation (Sj_{VO_2}) was monitored continuously during the first 5 days after injury.[128] We have monitored Sj_{VO_2} in 95 patients with severe head injury[106] and identified 66 episodes of transient jugular desaturation in 39 (41%) of the patients. The causes of the desaturation were intracranial on 27 occasions, systemic on 34 occasions, and both intracranial and systemic on 5 occasions (Table 31-3). The mortality rate was significantly related to the presence and the number of these episodes of desaturation (Table 31-4).

Measurement of Cerebral Perfusion in the ICU

Cerebral Perfusion Pressure. The simplest measure of cerebral perfusion is the cerebral perfusion pressure (CPP), which is calculated by subtracting the ICP from the

TABLE 31-3
Causes of Jugular Venous Desaturation in 39 of 95 Patients Monitored

Cause	Number of Episodes
Intracranial	
Intracranial hypertension	26
Vasospasm	1
Systemic	
Hypotension	8
Hypoxia	6
Hypocarbia	19
Anemia	1
Combination of intracranial and systemic	5

TABLE 31-4
Relationship of Transient Jugular Venous Desaturation and Outcome (p = .001; Chi-Square Test)

Three-Month Glasgow Outcome Scale	Episodes of Desaturation			
	None	One	Two or More	Total
Good recovery/moderate disability	23 (77%)	5 (17%)	2 (7%)	30
Severe disability/vegetative	23 (70%)	7 (21%)	3 (9%)	33
Dead	10 (31%)	10 (31%)	12 (38%)	32

mean arterial blood pressure. The normal lower limit of autoregulation for CPP is 50 mm Hg. In severely head-injured patients, the ability to autoregulate may be impaired, and cerebral blood flow may decrease with CPP values less than 50 mm Hg. CPP can be reduced through either decreases in blood pressure or increases in ICP. For equivalent levels of CPP, cerebral perfusion is impaired more by reductions in blood pressure than by increases in ICP.[85] Recent studies have suggested that outcome is improved if CPP is maintained above 70 to 80 mm Hg.[13,120] As a monitor for cerebral perfusion, CPP is widely available and convenient but limited in that only ischemia caused by increased ICP or by decreased blood pressure is assessed.

Cerebral Blood Flow. Recently, newer technologies have made measurement of CBF more feasible in the ICU. Measurement of global CBF by the classic Kety-Schmidt technique using nitrous oxide as the diffusible indicator can be performed at the bedside with a minimum of expense and equipment. Instruments for measuring regional CBF using the inhaled xenon technique are commercially available. However, both of these measurements of CBF are intermittent and require the patient to be hemodynamically stable during the 15 minutes required for the measurements. Therefore transient reductions in CBF or reductions of CBF in the acutely unstable patient are difficult to document with these technologies.

Two methods for continuously measuring local CBF are now commercially available, the thermal diffusion method and the laser Doppler method. Both methods are invasive, requiring the probe to be placed on the surface of the brain at surgery. Both methods measure CBF in only a small volume of brain, which may or may not be representative of the whole brain. However, the continuous nature of the measurements gives a dynamic picture of brain perfusion. Although there is extensive documentation of the reliability of these methodologies in the laboratory, there is currently limited experience in the ICU. However, for patients undergoing a craniotomy, these may become practical methods for monitoring CBF postoperatively.

Cerebral Oxygenation. Jugular venous oxygen saturation ($Sjvo_2$) has been used to monitor for cerebral hypoxia/ischemia.[23,33,128] The advantage is that jugular venous oxygen saturation will be reduced whenever oxygen availability is reduced relative to cerebral metabolic requirements, regardless of the cause. Jugular venous oxygen-

saturation can be measured intermittently or continuously with a fiberoptic oxygen-saturation catheter. The indications for $Sjvo_2$ monitoring are generally the same as for ICP monitoring. The contraindications include cervical neck fracture and severe coagulopathy. Goetting and Preston recently showed that a catheter can be safely placed in the jugular bulb of the head-injured patient without any rise in the ICP.[37]

Systemic Physiologic Monitoring

Head-injured patients should have close monitoring of systemic parameters, including ECG, heart rate, blood pressure, temperature, fluid intake and output. An arterial catheter is usually indicated to continuously monitor blood pressure and to provide easy access for blood sampling. Severely head-injured patients should be routinely monitored with pulse oximetry and capnography to avoid unrecognized hypoxemia or changes in arterial pco_2. Hypoxia and hypocapnia were among the most common systemic causes of jugular venous desaturation in our series (see Table 31-3). A central venous catheter and, in certain circumstances, a Swan-Ganz catheter may be needed to judge volume status. A Foley catheter is necessary for accurate measurement of urine output.

MEDICAL MANAGEMENT OF HEAD INJURY
Treatment of Intracranial Hypertension

Surgical lesions should always be ruled out by CT scan whenever severe intracranial hypertension develops unexpectedly, when intracranial hypertension is accompanied by a clinical neurologic deterioration, or when intracranial hypertension is refractory to medical management. Medical treatment of intracranial hypertension can be divided into two broad categories: general measures to prevent systemic factors that may exacerbate or cause intracranial hypertension and specific measures aimed at returning elevated ICP to acceptable levels.

General Measures

In all patients with severe head injury, simple measures can be taken to minimize systemic factors that can cause or aggravate intracranial hypertension. Commonly recommended practices include elevating the head of the bed 15 to 30 degrees, sedation, controlled ventilation, seizure prophylaxis, and treatment of systemic hypertension and fever when present.

Head Elevation. Elevation of the head of the bed and keeping the head in a neutral position to minimize compression of venous return from the brain has been standard neurosurgery practice for management of intracranial pressure in the past. However, the ideal head position for patient with head injury has been disputed in recent years. Rosner et al. have advocated keeping the patient's head flat, as part of an overall treatment program intended to maximize CPP.[120,121] Other studies have shown a reduction in ICP without a reduction in either CPP or CBF in most patients with elevation of the head to 30 degrees.[26,30] We have examined the effects of head position on ICP and cerebral hemodynamics in 22 patients with severe head injury.[30] Elevation of the head to 30 degrees reduced ICP and BP without changing CPP or CBF in most patients (Fig. 31-5). Therefore we usually keep the patient's head elevated to 30 degrees.

Treatment of Systemic Hypertension. Systemic hypertension associated with head injury is common and is characterized by a systolic blood pressure increase that is greater than diastolic increase. It is associated with a hyperdynamic state including tachycardia and increased cardiac output. Systemic hypertension is associated with sympathetic hyperactivity.[114] It is unwise to reduce systemic blood pressure in patients with hypertension associated with

untreated intracranial mass lesions, because cerebral perfusion is being maintained by the higher blood pressure. However, treatment of systemic hypertension (systolic blood pressure >160 mm Hg) during the postoperative course after a head injury is recommended by many neurosurgeons. Because autoregulation is frequently impaired after severe head injury, systemic hypertension may increase CBF and ICP[28] and may exacerbate cerebral edema.[25] However, others have emphasized the importance of maintaining CPP, even at the expense of a higher ICP.[13,121]

Often systemic hypertension will resolve with sedation. If antihypertensive drugs are required, vasodilating antihypertensive drugs, including hydralazine and nitroprusside, consistently increase ICP.[22,102] Sympathomimetic-blocking antihypertensive drugs, such as beta-blocking drugs (propanolol or labetalol) or centrally acting alpha receptor agonists (clonidine or alpha-methyldopa) are preferred because they reduce blood pressure without affecting the ICP.[114] We have compared the effects of labetalol and hydralazine in hypertensive head-injured patients.[38] Although both drugs reduced blood pressure by approximately 20 mm Hg, the ICP increased from 16 plus or minus 1 to 24 plus or minus 1 mm Hg with hydralazine but did not significantly change with labetalol. As shown in Table 31-5, the increase in ICP with hydralazine was accompanied by an increase in CBF and a decrease in CVR and AVDo$_2$. In addition, the systemic cardiovascular abnormalities re-

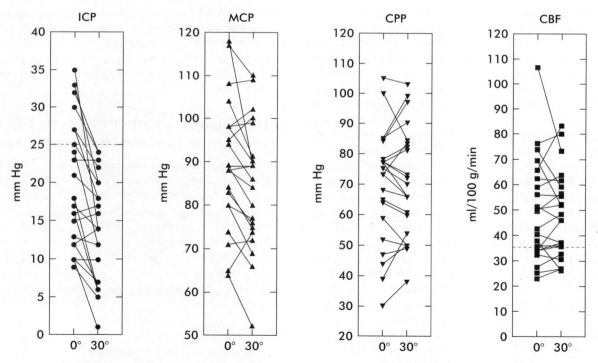

FIG. 31-5   Graph showing cerebral and systemic physiologic parameters at head elevations of 0 degrees and 30 degrees in 22 patients with severe head injury. *ICP*, intracranial pressure; *MCP*, mean carotid pressure; *CPP*, cerebral perfusion pressure; *CBF*, cerebral blood flow. *(From Feldman Z, Kanter MJ, Robertson CS et al: J Neurosurg 76:207, 1992).*

TABLE 31-5
Comparison of Hydralazine and Labetalol as Antihypertensive Drugs in Head-Injured Patients

	Hydralazine		Labetalol	
	Before	After	Before	After
ICP (mm Hg)	16 ± 1	24 ± 3*	16 ± 2	18 ± 3
CBF (ml/g/min)	0.51 ± 0.11	0.68 ± .0.12*	0.54 ± 0.07	0.45 ± 0.05
CVR (mm Hg/ml/g/min)	2.9 ± 0.6	1.8 ± 0.5*	2.6 ± 0.4	2.6 ± 0.4
AVDo$_2$ (μmol/ml)	1.8 ± 0.3	1.4 ± 0.1*	1.9 ± 0.4	2.3 ± 0.3
CMRo$_2$ (μmol/g/min)	0.88 ± 0.12	0.92 ± 0.12	0.90 ± 0.12	0.94 ± 0.14

*Change with hydralazine was significantly different from the change seen with labetalol (p < .05).

solved with labetalol but were exaggerated with hydralazine.

Controlled Ventilation. Hypoxia and hypercarbia can dramatically raise ICP. Patients with severe head injury can have periodic episodes of hypoventilation that precipitate episodes of intracranial hypertension. Controlled ventilation helps prevent these episodes of hypoventilation and intracranial hypertension.

Treatment of Fever. Fever is common during the recovery from a head injury. Fever is a potent cerebral vasodilator and can raise ICP. In addition, fever can raise cerebral metabolic requirements. Recent studies have suggested that rectal temperature may underestimate temperature in the brain, especially during a fever spike.[133] Temperatures greater than 38° F should be treated with antipyretics and/or cooling blankets. Infectious causes of fever should be investigated with appropriate cultures and treated with antibiotics.

Prevention of Seizures. The risk of posttraumatic seizure is 15% with severe head injury.[53] The use of anticonvulsants to prevent seizures is controversial. Young et al. found no difference in the incidence of seizures with prophylactically administered phenytoin.[152] Tempkin et al. recently reported results from a double-blind study in which 404 severely head-injured patients randomly received phenytoin or placebo for 1 year.[143] Phenytoin reduced the incidence of seizures during the first week but not thereafter. We give all severely head-injured patients in the emergency room phenytoin, 15 ml/kg IV at a rate that does not exceed 25 mg/min, followed by a daily maintenance dose adjusted to keep plasma levels in the therapeutic range. If no early seizures occur, we usually taper and discontinue the phenytoin after 1 week.

Specific Measures

For patients with sustained ICP greater than 20 mm Hg, despite the general measures described previously, specific measures are added in a stepwise fashion until the ICP is controlled (Fig. 31-6).

Pharmacologic Paralysis. ICP raised by purposeless agitation or coughing should be prevented by narcotics and nondepolarizing muscle relaxants that do not alter cerebrovascular resistance. We normally use morphine 5 to 10 mg

IV each hour for sedation and pancuronium bromide (Pavulon) 6 mg IV followed by 1 to 2 mg each hour as a muscle relaxant. Although the neurologic examination cannot be closely monitored while the patient is paralyzed, the muscle relaxants can be withheld once a day, usually before morning rounds, to obtain a brief neurologic examination.

Hyperventilation. Induced hyperventilation constricts cerebral blood vessels, reducing global CBF and cerebral blood volume. The effect of changes in Paco$_2$ on cerebral vessels is mediated by the change in pH induced in the extracellular fluid.[69] CO$_2$ reactivity is preserved in most patients with severe head injury, and therefore hyperventilation can rapidly lower ICP through the reduction in cerebral blood volume. The effects of hyperventilation on ICP are immediate, but the duration of the effect is controversial because the pH of the brain, at least in normal individuals, soon equilibrates to the lower Paco$_2$ level.

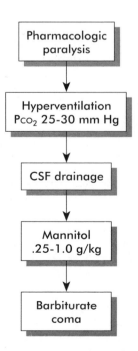

FIG. 31-6   Stepwise treatment of intracranial hypertension.

Hyperventilation reduces the ICP at the expense of cerebral perfusion. Whether hyperventilation can actually result in cerebral ischemia in head-injured patients is controversial. Hyperventilation (to $Paco_2$ of 20 mm Hg) has been shown to have a detrimental effect on outcome in one randomized trial.[94] The authors of this study recommended using hyperventilation only in patients with intracranial hypertension rather than as a routine in all head-injured patients. Cold recently reported in a study of 27 comatose patients that hyperventilation increased the frequency of finding rCBF values less than 0.2 ml/g/min from 5% to 16%.[20] A low rCBF before hyperventilation predisposed to this increased frequency.

We have examined the relationship of hyperventilation and global cerebral blood flow in a series of 171 head-injured patients during the first 10 days after injury.[44] Of 1212 CBF measurements in these patients, 132 (11%) were less than 0.25 ml/g/min. Of the 132 low CBF values, 71 (54%) were appropriately reduced relative to the lower $CMRo_2$, while 61 (46%) were associated with increased oxygen extraction and/or increased cerebral lactate production, suggesting a relative inadequacy of perfusion. The incidence of an inadequate CBF steadily increased as the $Paco_2$ decreased, and was 2%, 4%, 8%, and 23% when the $Paco_2$ was greater than 30, 25 to 30, 20 to 25, and less than 20 mm Hg, respectively. The incidence of an inadequate CBF was twice as high during the first 24 hours than on any other day (8% compared with 4%). The incidence was highest in the patients with a reduced CBF (11%) compared with patients with normal or elevated CBF (2%). We reserve induced hyperventilation for those patients who actually develop intracranial hypertension and do not lower $Paco_2$ to less than 25 mm Hg unless $Sjvo_2$ is monitored to make certain that ischemia is not being produced.

In patients who have been chronically hyperventilated, abruptly returning the $Paco_2$ to normal can result in a dramatic increase in ICP. Muizelaar showed, in an experimental study, that this phenomenon occurred after 24 hours of hyperventilation and was associated with vasodilation of cerebral vessels as the CSF pH equilibrates at the new lower $Paco_2$ level.[91] Hyperventilation should be withdrawn over several days to avoid this increase in ICP.

CSF Drainage. Although removal of 1 ml of CSF normally does not change ICP by more than 1 to 2 mm Hg, in patients with an elevated ICP, drainage of 1 to 2 ml of CSF through the ventriculostomy catheter can temporarily lower ICP. However, as the brain becomes more swollen, the ventricles collapse, less CSF is available for drainage, and the effectiveness of this modality is reduced.

Dehydration and Osmotherapy. Before a method for measuring ICP became available, dehydration therapy was common in the management of head-injured patients. However, we have found that normovolemia does not result in an increased rate of intracranial hypertension and eliminates severe electrolyte abnormalities and renal failure.[115] Fluid overload, however, should be avoided. Fluid restriction may be necessary in cases of hyponatremia caused by inappropriate antidiuretic hormone secretion.

The osmotic diuretic mannitol is given as an intravenous infusion of 0.25 to 1 g/kg and will maximally reduce the ICP within 10 minutes. The reduction in ICP usually persists for 3 to 4 hours. Serum osmolarity appears to be optimal when raised to 300 to 320 mOsm and should be kept below 320 mOsm to avoid side effects of therapy such as hypovolemia, hyperosmolarity, and renal failure. Loop diuretics, such as furosemide, decrease the CSF production and increase serum osmolarity by increasing the free-water clearance by the kidney. Given along with mannitol, furosemide (0.7 mg/kg) results in a greater (62% vs. 57%) and more sustained (5 hours vs 2 hours) decrease in ICP than mannitol alone.[105]

Barbiturate Coma. Barbiturate coma is another treatment modality that has been used to lower ICP in head-injured patients.[77,109] Barbiturates are protective during periods of cerebral hypoxia.[130] Although routine use of barbiturates in unselected patients has not been consistently effective in reducing morbidity or mortality after severe head injury,[123,147] a recent randomized multicenter trial demonstrated that instituting barbiturate coma in patients with refractory intracranial hypertension resulted in a twofold greater chance of controlling the ICP.[27]

Because of the hypotensive complications associated with barbiturates and because the neurologic examination is unavailable during treatment, barbiturate coma is usually reserved for patients with intracranial hypertension resistant to other modalities. Pentobarbital is given in both loading and maintenance doses. The loading dose is 10 mg/kg, given over 30 minutes, followed by 5 mg/kg each hour for three doses. This typically provides a therapeutic level after the fourth dose. The maintenance dose is 1 to 2 mg/kg/hr adjusted so that either the serum level is in the therapeutic range of 30 to 50 μg/ml or the EEG has a burst suppression pattern. Winer et al. recently reported that plasma and CSF pentobarbital levels do not accurately reflect the physiologic effects of pentobarbital and recommended monitoring the EEG instead of pentobarbital levels.[150] Pulmonary wedge pressure and cardiac output are monitored in all patients. Hypotension caused by pentobarbital is treated first with volume replacement and then with dopamine if necessary. The mechanism of ICP reduction by barbiturates is not entirely clear but is usually considered to be hemodynamic because of the immediate effect on ICP. Studies by Messeter et al. have suggested that the reduction in ICP with barbiturates is closely tied to the retention of CO_2 reactivity by the brain.[84,98]

We have examined the effects of pentobarbital on cerebral hemodynamics in 29 patients with refractory intracranial hypertension[61] (Fig. 31-7). ICP and BP were decreased by 11 and 15 mm Hg respectively after the loading dose of pentobarbital. Dopamine was required to treat systemic hypotension in 20 (69%) of the 29 patients. CPP was improved in only 11 (38%) of the patients and was decreased

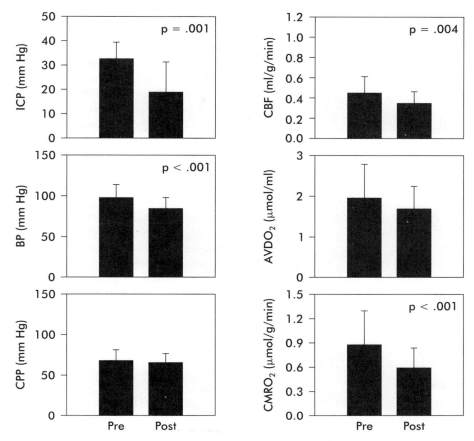

FIG. 31-7 Physiologic effects of loading dose of pentobarbital in 29 patients with refractory intracranial hypertension.

or unchanged in 18 (62%) patients. For the whole group, CPP averaged 65 plus or minus 15 mm Hg pretreatment and 62 plus or minus 13 mm Hg after the loading dose of pentobarbital. CBF and CMRo$_2$ were also significantly decreased after the loading dose of pentobarbital, by 25% and 34%, respectively. CVR, arterial Paco$_2$, AVDo$_2$, arteriovenous content difference of lactate, and cerebral metabolic rate for lactate were not consistently changed by pentobarbital when the whole group was considered.

Other Agents. Corticosteroids have been used in previous years to reduce the edema associated with head injury. Several randomized, double-blinded clinical trials have failed to demonstrate a beneficial effect of steroids.[21] Although most neurosurgeons have discontinued the routine use of steroids in head-injured patients because of these studies, the recent successful trial of methylprednisolone in spinal cord injury may renew interest in the use of steroids in head injury.

The role of subtemporal decompression is also being reexamined. Recent reports, such as the one by Gower et al.,[40] in which mortality rate for refractory intracranial hypertension was reduced from 82% to 40% with the addition of subtemporal decompression, have renewed interest in the procedure.

Treatment of Cerebral Hypoxia/Ischemia

The algorithm that we use for diagnosing and treating cerebral hypoxia/ischemia is shown in Fig. 31-8. Jugular venous desaturation is first confirmed by measuring So$_2$ in a blood sample drawn through the jugular venous oxygen saturation catheter. If an Sjvo$_2$ less than 50% is verified, treatable systemic causes for the desaturation are sought. Hypoxia and excessive hyperventilation are sought with an arterial blood gas. Anemia is sought by measuring hemoglobin concentration. Systemic hypotension is eliminated. Finally, intracranial hypertension and occasionally cerebral vasospasm are intracranial causes to consider if systemic causes are not found. The treatment is then specifically directed at the cause of the desaturation.

OUTCOME FROM SEVERE HEAD INJURY

Three indices have been used in measuring outcome in severely head-injured patients. The functional status of pa-

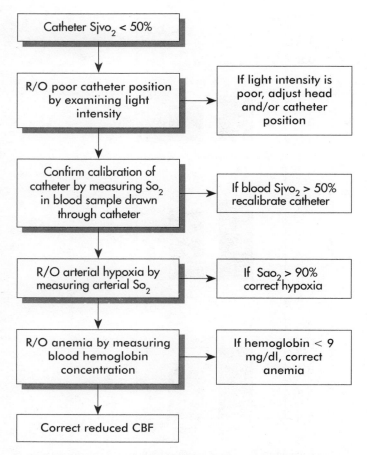

FIG. 31-8 Algorithm for diagnosing the cause of jugular venous desaturation. *(From Sheinberg M, Kanter JM, Robertson CS et al: J Neurosurg 76:212, 1992.)*

tients with severe head injury often continues to improve for months after the injury. Assessments before 6 months may significantly underestimate functional recovery.

Assessing Outcome
Glasgow Outcome Scale

In 1975, Jennett and Bond described a five-point scale, called the Glasgow Outcome Scale (GOS), for quantitating neurologic recovery afer head injury.[54] A good recovery means that the patient has returned to the preinjury level of function. A moderate disability describes a patient who has some neurologic impairment but is able to care for himself/herself. A severely disabled patient has some evidence of higher mental function but depends on others. A patient is vegetative who has no evidence of higher mental function. The fifth outcome category is death.

Disability Rating Scale

Although GOS has been used widely to categorize outcome in many patients, it is relatively insensitive to small changes in functional status that may occur in a patient over time

because of its five limited categories. An alternative method, called the Disability Rating Scale (DRS), was proposed by Rappaport et al.[108] It is a 30-point scale that ranges from 0 (full recovery without any functional impairment) to 30 (death). Based on a total score, the DRS distinguishes 10 levels of clinical disability. Sensitivity, especially at the high end, is greater with the DRS than with the GOS, but the DRS has been used less extensively.[39]

Neuropsychologic Tests

Neuropsychologic deficits long have been known to constitute the primary disability in long-term survivors of severe head injury, but this aspect has been given little attention because severe cognitive deficits often preclude effective testing, following the head-injured patient on a long-term basis is difficult, and these time-consuming tests cannot be done without a dedicated neuropsychologist. The important domains of neuropsychologic function for which measurement is recommended include (1) attention (digit symbol substitution), (2) memory (selective reminding), (3) language (controlled oral word association), (4) mental processing (trail making B), and (5) motor speed and coordination (grooved peg board).[19]

Predicting Outcome

Several models for predicting outcome from severe head injury have been developed from the large sets of data that have been collected at head-injury research centers. One of the easiest to apply clinically is illustrated in Fig. 31-9.[14] Such a model can be very useful for providing family members with information about chances for functional recovery. However, other models, such as the Leed's Prognostic Score, have been proposed to identify patients who will invariably die so that early withdrawal of medical treatment can be considered.[36] We have found these models to be less than 100% accurate. Caution must be exercised when the experience of one center is applied directly to another because of variations in demographic factors, mechanism, and severity of injury; delay between injury and treatment; management techniques; and other support systems. One cannot rely on these models to clarify the complicated emotional, moral, legal, and financial issues that surround the early termination of care in seriously head-injured patients.[29]

HEAD INJURY IN CHILDREN

Researchers have calculated that nearly 200/100,000 children annually sustain head injuries and that approximately 10/100,000 children die from head trauma.[127] The two common causes of head trauma in children, especially below the age of 4, are falls and automobile accidents. Although the statistics regarding child abuse as a cause of head injury are scarce, a significant proportion of head trauma is probably due to child battering, especially in the urban population. The presence of multiple fractures, bilateral frac-

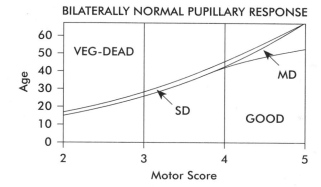

BILATERALLY NORMAL PUPILLARY RESPONSE

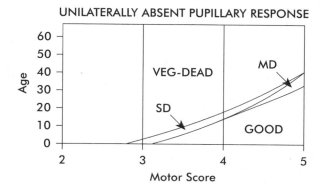

UNILATERALLY ABSENT PUPILLARY RESPONSE

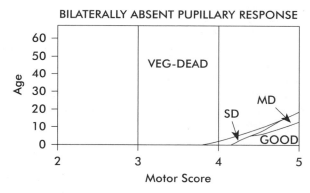

BILATERALLY ABSENT PUPILLARY RESPONSE

FIG. 31-9 Predicting outcome in severe head injury. The abbreviations are defined in the text. *(From Choi SC, Narayan RK, Anderson RL et al: J Neurosurg 69:381, 1988.)*

TABLE 31-7
Modification of the Glasgow Coma Scale for Children

Response	Score	Age
Eye Response		
Spontaneously	4	
To speech	3	
To pain	2	
None	1	
Best Motor Response in Upper Limbs (Score Highest Appropriate For Age)		
Obeys commands	6	>2 years
Localizes to pain	5	6 months—2 years
Normal flexion to pain	4	>6 months
Spastic flexion to pain	3	<6 months
Extension to pain	2	
None	1	
Best Verbal Response (Score Highest Appropriate For Age)		
Oriented to place	5	>5 years
Words	4	>12 months
Vocal sounds	3	>6 months
Cries	2	<6 months
None	1	

From Simpson D, Reilly P: *Lancet* 2:450, 1982.

uation of the level of the sensorium according to GCS, a modified GCS for children has been proposed (Table 31-6).[129] The best response appropriate for the age is recorded.

Although systemic arterial hypotension rarely results from brain injury alone, the exception occurs in infants, where intracranial or subgaleal bleeding may be sufficient to produce shock. Assessment of hypotension still should include thoracic or intraabdominal injuries and fracture of the extremities. Therapy should be expeditiously instituted because young children are not as able to tolerate blood loss compared with adults.

In children who are conscious with no history of unconsciousness or seizures, only a plain film x-ray of the skull may be necessary. However, the presence of skull fractures is four times higher in children more than 4 years of age and requires hospitalization because of a higher incidence of brain injury (8%).[45] ICP monitoring is strongly recommended, especially because the clinical presence of intracranial hematoma is less clearly recognized in the younger age groups. The incidence of increased ICP is seen in more than 50% of children with GCS lower than 8. In one series, the incidence of elevated ICP was documented in 86% of children with a GCS lower than 8.[126]

CT scan is the standard diagnostic procedure in children who have altered sensorium and who have had loss of consciousness/seizures; however, in infants, diagnostic ultrasonography may be a useful alternative in the evaluation of trauma. Extracranial hematomas can be of three types: subcutaneous hematoma, subgaleal hematoma, and cephalhematoma.[15] In none of these situations is aspiration indicated.

tures, and fractures crossing sutures may point toward the diagnosis of abuse.[83]

Several factors may influence the effect of trauma in pediatric age groups: (1) the relative immaturity of the nervous system in terms of myelinization, dendritic arborization, proliferation of glial cells, and integrity of blood-brain barrier and (2) characteristics of skull such as thinner, more pliable nature, unfused sutures, and the relative smoothness of the floor of the skull.

In the management of head injury of children, one must note the levels of the sensorium as well as seizures, both of which signify trauma significant enough to produce dysfunction of the nervous system. To reduce difficulty in eval-

Epidural hematoma is usually less common in children, especially infants, than in adults, probably because of the firm adherence of the dura to the calvarium. However, after it is discovered, surgery to remove the epidural hematoma is preferred although nonoperative management has been reported in neurologically intact patients. Although a lucid interval is usually seen in nearly half of patients with epidural hematoma (48%), children may remain conscious (12%), be comatose (23%), or may be drowsy and confused (20%) during the entire course.[15]

Acute subdural hematoma is the most common posttraumatic hematoma in children. A subdural hematoma in the newborn can be due to trauma occurring during delivery, particularly breech delivery. In the older infant and child, it occurs in about 25% of trauma cases, an incidence similar to adults. Pallor, irritability, and a tense fontanelle suggest an intracranial clot in a child. A comatose state may not be noted. If the lesion is more than 5 mm in thickness, it is surgically evacuated by a craniotomy. Intracerebral hematomas were noted in 3% of pediatric head injuries.[154] Evacuation is indicated only if there is progressive clinical deterioration.

Diffuse brain swelling has been reported to occur commonly in children, with an incidence of 29% to 44% of patients with severe head injury. It causes delayed neurologic deterioration.[7,10] It is characterized by a decrease in CSF spaces, compressed or obliterated mesencephalic cisterns, and small ventricles in the absence of other intracranial pathology. A recent report, although concurring that diffuse brain swelling commonly occurs in children compared with adults (2 to 1), noted a mortality rate of 53%, which was nearly three times that of children without diffuse brain swelling (16%).[2] However, secondary events such as hypoxia and hypotension are commonly associated with diffuse brain swelling and might play an important role.

The primary effort in the treatment of diffuse brain injury is to control elevated ICP, which can be secondary to several factors such as hyperemia, increased CBF, increased brain water, and probably reduced CSF absorption. On occasion, hyperventilation to extreme levels may have to be employed to control ICP, especially where increased CBF is the probable response to injury. At the same time, normal hemoglobin and arterial blood pressure should be maintained to prevent hypoxia. The other drugs that are used to reduce ICP include mannitol, glycerol, and sodium pentobarbital. However, a CT scan should be repeated when the patient does not respond to therapy because delayed hematomas or ventricular dilation could be the cause of elevated ICP. The objective of management is to have a normal CPP while controlling ICP.

Outcome from head injury depends on the severity of the injury, presence of focal lesion, duration of coma, and ICP course. A chronic vegetative state is rare in children (1% to 2%).[7,10] If the duration of coma is less than 3 months, the chance of a favorable outcome approaches 90%.[10] In general, outcome for children is clearly superior to that for adults, despite the comparable neural dysfunction as measured by GCS and brainstem signs. A mortality rate of 25% to 30% and good outcome of about 60% probably represent the expected outcome when one considers all the factors.

SUMMARY

The ultimate goal in the management of patients with severe head injury is to reduce the mortality rate and to prove the functional status of those who survive. In order to achieve this, prevention of secondary insults to the already injured brain and aggressive management at three different levels is required: prehospital transportation, emergency room, and operating room/intensive care unit.

Rapid transfer to a center where a neurosurgical service is available, maintenance of an adequate airway to prevent hypoxia, and prevention of hypotension are basic steps for pre-hospital transfer. In the emergency room, hemodynamic stability should be achieved in addition to the mechanical ventilation before transferring the patient for a CT of the head. Finally, all effort should be made to evacuate intracranial hematoma as quickly as possible. While in the operating room or in ICU, precaution should be taken to avoid obstruction to the cerebral venous outflow.

Transient episodes of hypotension, hypoxia, hypocarbia, and ischemia individually or in combination can occur while the patient is in ICU or while the patient is being transported to and from the ICU for diagnostic purposes. However, with the available new monitoring techniques, one should be able to recognize the secondary insults early enough to treat them or to prevent potential secondary insults to the brain.

References

1. Adams JH, Gennarelli TA, Graham DI: Brain damage in non-missile head injury: observation in man and subhuman primate. In Smith WT, Cavanaugh JB, editors: *Recent advances in neuropathology,* London 1982, Churchill-Livingstone, pp 165-190.

2. Adams JH, Graham DI: The relationship between ventricular fluid pressure and the neuropathology of raised intracranial pressure, *Neuropathol Appl Neurobiol* 2:323-332, 1976.

3. Adams JH, Mitchell D, Graham DI et al: Diffuse brain damage of immediate impact type — its relationship to "primary brainstem damage" in head injury, *Brain* 89:235-268, 1977.

4. Andrews BT, Chiles III BW, Oslen WL et al: The effect of intracerebral hematoma location on the risk of brain stem compression and on clinical outcome, *J Neurosurg* 69:518-522, 1988.

5. Becker DP, Miller JD, Ward JD et al: The outcome from severe head injury with early diagnosis and intensive management, *J Neurosurg* 47:491-502, 1977.
6. Becker DP: Acute subdural hematomas. In Vigouroux RP, editor: *Neurotraumatology,* Vienna, 1986, Springer-Verlag, pp 51-100.
7. Berger MS, Pitts LH, Lovely M et al: Outcome from severe head injury in children and adolescents, *J Neurosurg* 62:194-199, 1985.
8. Bouma GJ, Muizelaar PJ, Choi SC et al: Cerebral circulation and metabolism after severe traumatic brain injury: the elusive role of ischemia, *J Neurosurg* 75:685-693, 1991.
9. Bowers SA, Marshall LF: Outcome in 200 consecutive cases of severe head injury treated in San Diego County: a prospective analysis, *Neurosurgery* 6:237-242, 1980.
10. Bruce DA, Raphaely RC, Goldberg AI et al: The pathophysiology, treatment and outcome following severe head injury in children, *Child Brain* 5:174-191, 1979.
11. Bullock R, Golek J, Blake G: Traumatic intracranial hematoma: which patients should undergo surgical evacuation? CT scan features and ICP monitoring as a basis for decision-making, *Surg Neurol* 32:181-187, 1989.
12. Cavaliere R, Cavenago L, Siccardi D et al: Gunshot wounds of the brain in civilians, *Acta Neurochir (Wien)* 94:133-136, 1988.
13. Changaris DG, McGraw CP, Richardson JD et al: Correlation of cerebral perfusion pressure and Glasgow Coma Scale to outcome, *J Trauma* 27:1007-1013, 1987.
14. Choi SC, Narayan RK, Anderson RL et al: Enhanced specificity of prognosis in severe head injury, *J Neurosurg* 69:381-385, 1988.
15. Choux M: Extracerebral hematoma in children. In Vigouroux RP, editor: *Advances in neurotraumatology. Extracerebral collection,* Vienna, 1986, Springer-Verlag, pp 173-208.
16. Clark WC, Muhlbauer MS, Watridge CB et al: Analysis of 76 civilian gunshot wounds, *J Neurosurg* 65:9-14, 1986.
17. Clifton GL, Grossman RG, Makela ME et al: Neurological course and correlated computerized tomography findings after severe closed head injury, *J Neurosurg* 52:611-624, 1980.
18. Clifton GL, Grossman RG: Technical note: flowsheet for the neurosurgical intensive care units, *Neurosurgery* 11:280-283, 1982.
19. Clifton GL, Hayes RL, Levin HS et al: Outcome measures for clinical trials involving traumatic brain injured patients: report of a conference, *Neurosurgery* 31:975-978, 1992.
20. Cold GE: Does acute hyperventilation provoke cerebral oligaemia on comatose patients after acute head injury? *Acta Neurochir* 96:100-106, 1989.
21. Cooper PR, Moody S, Clark WK et al: Dexamethasone and severe head injury: a prospective double-blind study, *J Neurosurg* 51:307-316, 1979.
22. Cottrell JE, Patel K, Turndorf H et al: Intracranial pressure changes induced by sodium nitroprusside in patients with intracranial mass lesions, *J Neurosurg* 48:329-331, 1978.
23. Cruz J: Continuous versus serial global cerebral hemometabolic monitoring: applications in acute brain trauma, *Acta Neurochir* (suppl 42):33-39, 1988.
24. Dacey RG Hr, Alves WM, Rimel RW et al: Neurosurgical complications after apparently minor head injury: assessment of risk in a series of 610 patients, *J Neurosurg* 65:203-210, 1986.
25. Durward QJ, Del Maestro RF, Amacher AL et al: The influence of systemic arterial pressure and intracranial pressure on the development of cerebral vasogenic edema, *J Neurosurg* 59:803-809, 1983.
26. Durward QJ, Amacher AL, Del Maestro RF et al: Cerebral and cardiovascular responses to changes in head elevation in patients with intracranial hypertension, *J Neurosurg* 59:938-944, 1983.
27. Eisenberg HM, Frankowski RF, Contant CF et al: High-dose barbiturate control of elevated intracranial pressure in patients with severe head injury, *Neurosurgery* 69:15-23, 1988.
28. Enevoldsen EM, Jensen JT: Autoregulation and CO_2 responses of cerebral blood flow in patients with acute severe head injury, *J Neurosurg* 48:689-703, 1978.
29. Feldman Z, Contant CF, Robertson CS et al: Evaluation of the Leeds Prognostic Score for severe head injury, *Lancet* 337:1451-1453, 1991.
30. Feldman Z, Kanter MJ, Robertson CS et al: Effect of head elevation on intracranial pressure, cerebral perfusion pressure, and cerebral blood flow in head-injured patients, *J Neurosurg* 76:207-211, 1992.
31. Foulkes M, Eisenberg HM, Jane JA et al: The Traumatic Coma Data Bank: design, methods, and baseline characteristics, *J Neurosurg* 75(suppl):S8-13, 1991.
32. Friendenfelt H, Sunstrom R: Local and general spasm in the internal carotid system following trauma, *Acta Radiol (Diagn)* 1:278-283, 1963.
33. Garlick R, Bihari D: The use of intermittent and continuous recordings of jugular venous bulb oxygen saturation in the unconscious patient, *Scan J Clin Lab Invest* 47(suppl 188):47-52, 1987.
34. Gennarelli TA, Spielman GM, Langfitt TW et al: Influence of the type of intracranial lesion on outcome from severe head injury: a multicenter study using a new classification system, *J Neurosurg* 56:26-32, 1982.
35. Gentleman D, Jennett B: Hazards of inter-hospital transfer of comatose head injured patients, *Lancet* 2:853-855, 1981.
36. Gibson MR, Stephenson GC: Aggressive management of severe closed head trauma: time for reappraisal, *Lancet* 2:369-371, 1989.
37. Goetting MG, Preston G: Jugular bulb catheterization does not increase intracranial pressure, *Intensive Care Med* 17:195-198, 1991.
38. Gokaslan ZL, Villareal C, Robertson CS et al: Treating hypertension in neurosurgical patients. Forty-First Annual Meeting of the Congress of Neurological Surgeons, Orlando, Oct, 1991, Abstract #12.
39. Gouvier D, Blanton PD, LaPorte KK et al: Reliability and validity of the disability rating scale, and the level of cognitive functioning scale in monitoring recovery from severe head injury, *Arch Phys Med Rehabil* 68:94-97, 1987.
40. Gower DJ, Lee KS, McWhorter JM: Role of subtemporal decompression in severe closed head injury, *Neurosurgery* 23:417-422, 1988.
41. Graham DI, Adams JH, Doyle D: Ischaemic brain damage in fatal non-missile brain injuries, *J Neurol Sci* 39:213-234, 1978.
42. Graham DI, Ford I, Adams JH et al: Ischaemic brain damage is still com-

mon in fatal non-missile head injury, *J Neurol Neurosurg Psych* 52:346-359, 1989.

43. Grunner WP, Merlotti GJ, Barrett J et al: Resuscitation from hemorrhagic shock: alteration of the intracranial pressure after normal saline, 3% saline, and dextran-40, *Ann Surg* 204:686-692, 1986.

44. Hayes C, Robertson CS, Narayan RK et al: The effect of hyperventilation of cerebral blood flow in head injured patients. Sixtieth Annual Meeting of the American Association of Neurological Surgeons, San Francisco, April 1992, Abstract #1271.

45. Harhood-Nash, DC, Hendrick EB, Hudson AR: The significance of skull fractures in children—a study of 1187 patients, *Radiology* 101:151-155, 1977.

46. Hubschman O, Shapiro K, Baden M et al: Craniocerebral gunshot injuries in civilian practice. Prognostic criteria and surgical management: experiences with 82 cases, *J Trauma* 19:6-12, 1979.

47. Illingworth G, Jennett B: The shocked head injury, *Lancet* 2:511-514, 1965.

48. Ishige N, Pitts LH, Hashimoto T et al: The effects of hypoxia on traumatic brain injury in rats: part 1. Changes in neurological function, electroencephalograms, and histopathology, *Neurosurgery* 20:848-853, 1987.

49. Ishige N, Pitts LH, Posliani L et al: Effect of hypoxia on traumatic brain injury in rats: part 2. Changes in high energy phosphate metabolism, *Neurosurgery* 20:854-858, 1987.

50. Ishige N, Pitts LH, Berry I et al: The effects of hypovolemic hypotension of high-energy phosphate metabolism in traumatized brain in rats, *J Neurosurg* 68:129-136, 1988.

51. Jagger G, Fife D, Vernberg K et al: Effect of alcohol intoxication on the diagnosis and apparent severity of brain injury, *Neurosurgery* 15:303-306, 1984.

52. Jamieson KG, Yelland JDN: Extradural hematoma: report of 167 cases, *J Neurosurg* 29:13-23, 1968.

53. Jennett B: *Epilepsy after nonmissile head injuries*, ed 2, London, 1975, Heineman, pp 1-179.

54. Jennett B, Bond MR: Assessment of outcome after severe brain damage, *Lancet* 1:480-484, 1975.

55. Jennett B, Teasdale G, Galbraith S et al: Severe head injuries in three countries, *J Neurol Neurosurg Psych* 40:291-298, 1977.

56. Jennett B, Teasdale G, Braakman R et al: Prognosis of patients with severe head injury, *Neurosurgery* 4:283-289, 1979.

57. Jennett B: Significance of skull x-rays in the management of recent head injury, *Clin Radiol* 31:463-469, 1980.

58. Jennett B, Carlin J: Preventable mortality and morbidity after head injury, *Injury* 10:154-159, 1978.

59. Kalsbeek WD, McLaurin RL, Harris BSH et al: The National Head and Spinal Cord Injury Survey: major findings, *J Neurosurg* 53(suppl 5):19-31, 1980.

60. Kanter RK, Weiner LB: Ventriculostomy-related infections, *N Engl J Med* 311:987, 1984.

61. Kanter MJ, Gokaslan ZL, Robertson CS et al: Changes in cerebral physiology following barbiturate therapy in head injured patients with intractable intracranial hypertension, *J Neurosurg* 74:348A, 1991.

62. Kauffman HH, Makela ME, Lee F et al: Gunshot wounds to the head: a perspective, *Neurosurgery* 18:689-695, 1986.

63. Kennedy C, Sokoloff L: An adaptation of the nitrous oxide method to the study of cerebral circulation in children: normal values for cerebral blood flow and cerebral metabolic rate in childhood, *J Clin Invest* 36:1130-1137, 1957.

64. Kety SS, Schmidt CF: The nitrous oxide method for the quantitative determination of cerebral blood flow in man: theory, procedure and normal values, *J Clin Invest* 27:476-483, 1948.

65. Kishore PRS, Lipper MH, Becker DP et al: The significance of CT in head injury: correlation with intracranial pressure, *AJNR* 2:307-311, 1981.

66. Klauber MR, Marshall LF, Barrett-Conner E et al: Prospective study of patients hospitalized with head injury in San Diego County 1978, *Neurosurgery* 9:236-241, 1981.

67. Klauber MR, Toutant SM, Marshall LF: A model for predicting delayed intracranial hypertension following severe head injury, *J Neurosurg* 51:695-699, 1984.

68. Kohi YM, Mendelow AD, Teasdale GM et al: Extracranial insults and outcome in patients with acute head injury—relationship to the Glasgow Coma Scale, *Injury* 16:25-29, 1984.

69. Kontos HA, Raper AJ, Patterson JL Jr: Analysis of vasoactivity of local pH, pco_2, and bicarbonate on pial vessels, *Stroke* 8:358-360, 1977.

70. Kraus JF, Black A, Hessol N et al: The incidence of acute brain injury and serious impairment in a defined population, *Am J Epidemiol* 119:186-210, 1984.

71. Lau YL, Kenna AP: Post-traumatic meningitis in children, *Injury* 17:407-409, 1986.

72. Lewelt W, Jenkins LW, Miller JD: Autoregulation of cerebral blood flow after experimental fluid percussion injury, *J Neurosurg* 53:500-511, 1980.

73. Lobato RD, Sarabia R, Cordobes F et al: Post-traumatic hemispheric swelling: analysis of 55 cases studied with computerized tomography, *J Neurosurg* 68:417-423, 1988.

74. Lundberg N, Troupp H, Lorin H: Continuous recording of the ventricular fluid pressure in patients with severe acute traumatic brain damage. A preliminary report, *J Neurosurg* 22:581-590, 1965.

75. MacPherson P, Graham DI: Correlation between angiographic findings and the ischemia of head injury, *J Neurol Neurosurg Psychiatry* 41:122-127, 1978.

76. Maloney AF, Whatmore WJ: Clinical and pathological observation in fatal head injuries: a 5-year survey of 173 cases, *Br J Surg* 56:23-31, 1969.

77. Marshall LF, Smith RW, Shapiro HM: The outcome with aggressive treatment in severe head injury. I. The significance of intracranial pressure monitoring, *J Neurosurg* 50:20-25, 1979.

78. Marshall LF, Marshall SB, Klauber MR et al: A new classification of head injury based on computerized tomography, *J Neurosurg* 75(suppl):S14-20, 1991.

79. Marshall LF, Gautille T, Klauber MR et al: The outcome of severe closed head injury, *J Neurosurg* 75(suppl):S28-36, 1991.

80. Masters SJ, McClean PM, Arcarese JS et al: Skull x-ray examinations after head trauma: recommendations by a multidisciplinary panel and valida-

tion study, *N Engl J Med* 316:84-91, 1987.

81. Mendelow AD, Karmi NZ, Paul KS et al: Extradural hematoma: effect of delayed treatment, *Br Med J* 1:1240-1242, 1979.

82. Mendelow AD, Teasdale G, Jennett B et al: Risks of intracranial hematoma in head injured adults, *Br Med J* 287:1173-1176, 1983.

83. Meserry CJ, Towbin R, McLaurin RL et al: Radiographic characteristics of skull fractures in child abuse versus accidental injury, *AJNR* 8:455-457, 1987.

84. Messeter K, Nordstrom CH, Sundbarg G et al: Cerebral hemodynamics in patients with acute severe head trauma, *J Neurosurg* 64:231-237, 1986.

85. Miller JD, Stanek A, Langfitt TW: Concepts of cerebral perfusion pressure and vascular compression during intracranial hypertension, *Prog Brain Res* 35:411-432, 1971.

86. Miller JD, Becker DP, Ward JD et al: Significance of intracranial hypertension in severe head injury, *J Neurosurg* 47:501-516, 1977.

87. Miller JD, Sweet RC, Narayan R et al: Early insults to the injured brain, *JAMA* 240:439-442, 1978.

88. Miller JD, Butterworth JF, Gudeman SK et al: Further experience with the management of severe head injury, *J Neurosurg* 54:289-299, 1981.

89. Miller JD: Head injury and brain ischaemia—implications for therapy, *Br J Anaesth* 57:120-129, 1985.

90. Morgan MK, Besser M, Johnston I et al: Intracranial carotid artery injury in closed head trauma, *J Neurosurg* 6:192-197, 1987.

91. Muizelaar JP, van der Poel HG, Li ZC et al: Pial artery diameter and CO_2 reactivity during prolonged hyperventilation in the rabbit, *J Neurosurg* 69:923-927, 1988.

92. Muizelaar JP: Cerebral blood flow, cerebral blood volume, and cerebral metabolism after severe head injury. In Becker DP, Gudeman SK, editors: *Textbook of head injury,* Philadelphia, 1989, WB Saunders, pp 221-240.

93. Muizelaar JP, Marmarou A, DeSalles AAF et al: Cerebral blood flow and metabolism in severely head-injured children. Part 1: relationship with GCS score, outcome, ICP, and PVI, *J Neurosurg* 71:72-76, 1989.

94. Muizelaar JP, Marmarou A, Ward JD et al: Adverse effects of prolonged hyperventilation in patients with severe head injury: a randomized clinical trial, *J Neurosurg* 75:731-739, 1991.

95. Nagib MA, Rockswold GL, Sherman RS et al: Civilian gunshot wounds to the brain: prognosis and management, *Neurosurgery* 18:533-537, 1986.

96. Narayan RK, Kishore PRS, Becker DP et al: Intracranial pressure: to monitor or not to monitor: a review of our experience with severe head injury, *J Neurosurg* 56:650-659, 1982.

97. Neufield P, Pitts L, Kaktis JV: The influence of shock on mortality after head trauma, *Crit Care Med* 8:254, 1980.

98. Nordstrom CH, Messeter K, Sundbarg G et al: Cerebral blood flow, vasoreactivity, and oxygen consumption during barbiturate therapy in severe traumatic brain lesions, *J Neurosurg* 68:424-431, 1988.

99. North B, Reilly P: Comparison among three methods of intracranial pressure recording, *Neurosurgery* 18:730-732, 1986.

100. Obrist WD, Langfitt TW, Jaggi JL et al: Cerebral blood flow and metabolism in comatose patients with acute severe head injury: relationship to intracranial hypertension, *J Neurosurg* 61:241-253, 1984.

101. Ostrup R, Bejar R, Marshall L: Real-time ultrasonography: a useful tool in the evaluation of the craniectomized brain injured patient, *Neurosurgery* 12:225-227, 1983.

102. Overgaard J, Skinhoj E: A paradoxical cerebral hemodynamic effect of hydralazine, *Stroke* 6:402-404, 1975.

103. Overgaard J, Modsdal C, Tweed WA: Cerebral circulation after head injury. Part 3: does reduced regional cerebral blood flow determine recovery of brain function after blunt head injury? *J Neurosurg* 55:63-74, 1981.

104. Overgaard J, Tweed WA: Cerebral circulation after head injury. Part 4: functional anatomy and boundary-zone flow deprivation in the first week of traumatic coma, *J Neurosurg* 59:439-446, 1983.

105. Pollay M, Fullenwider C, Roberts A et al: Effect of mannitol and furosemide on blood-brain osmotic gradient and intracranial pressure, *J Neurosurg* 59:945-950, 1983.

106. Prakash GS, Robertson CS, Narayan RK et al: Transient jugular venous desaturation and outcome from severe head injury, *J Neurosurg* 76:398A, 1992.

107. Price DJE, Murray A: Influence of hypoxia and hypotension on recovery from head injury, *Injury* 3:218-224, 1972.

108. Rappaport M, Hall KM, Hopkins K et al: Disability Rating Scale for severe head trauma: coma to community, *Arch Phys Med Rehabil* 63:118-123, 1982.

109. Rea GL, Rockswold GL: Barbiturate therapy in uncontrolled intracranial hypertension, *Neurosurgery* 12:401-404, 1983.

110. Richard KE, Wirtelerz R, Frowein RA: Traumatic brain edema: frequency and prognosis, *Adv Neurosurg* 17:81-86, 1989.

111. Rimel JW, Jane JA, Edlich RF: An injury severity scale for comprehensive management of central nervous system trauma, *J Am Coll Emerg Phys* 8:64-67, 1979.

112. Rimel RW, Giordani R, Barth JT et al: Disability caused by minor head injury, *Neurosurgery* 9:221-228, 1981.

113. Rimel RW, Giordani B, Barth FP et al: Moderate head injury: completing the clinical spectrum of brain trauma, *Neurosurgery* 11:344-351, 1982.

114. Robertson CS, Clifton GL, Taylor AA et al: Treatment of hypertension associated with head injury, *J Neurosurg* 59:445-460, 1983

115. Robertson CS, Clifton GL, Grossman RG: Oxygen utilization and cardiovascular function in head-injured patients, *Neurosurgery* 15:307-314, 1984.

116. Robertson CS, Grossman RG, Goodman JC et al: The predictive value of cerebral anaerobic metabolism with cerebral infarction after head injury, *J Neurosurg* 67:361-368, 1987.

117. Robertson CS, Contant CF, Gokaslan ZL et al: Cerebral blood flow, $AVDo_2$, and outcome in head injured patients, *J Neurol Neurosurg Psych* 55:594-603, 1992.

118. Rockswold GL, Leonard PR, Nagib MG: Analysis of management in thiry-three closed head patients who "talked and deteriorated," *Neurosurgery* 21:51-55, 1987.

119. Rose J, Valtonen S, Jennett B: Avoidable factors contributing to

death after head injury, *Br J Med* 2:615-618, 1977.

120. Rosner MJ, Coley IB: Cerebral perfusion pressure, intracranial pressure, and head elevation, *J Neurosurg* 65:636-641, 1986.

121. Rosner MJ: Cerebral perfusion pressure: link between intracranial pressure and systemic circulation. In Wood JH, editor: *Cerebral blood flow, physiologic and clinical aspects*. New York, 1987, McGraw-Hill, pp 425-448.

122. Saul TG, Ducker TB: Effect of intracranial pressure monitoring and aggressive treatment on mortality in severe head injury, *J Neurosurg* 56:498-503, 1982.

123. Schwartz ML,Tator CH, Rowed DW et al: The University of Toronto Head Injury Treatment study: a prospective, randomized comparison of pentobarbital and mannitol, *Can J Neurol Sci* 11:434-440, 1984.

124. Seelig JM, Becker DP, Miller JD et al: Traumatic acute subdural hematoma: major mortality reduction in comatose patients treated within four hours, *N Engl J Med* 304:1511-1518, 1981.

125. Selhorst JB, Gudeman SK, Butterworth JF et al: Papilledema after acute head injury, *Neurosurgery* 16:357-363, 1985.

126. Shapiro K, Marmarou A: A clinical application of the pressure volume index in treatment of pediatric head injuries, *J Neurosurg* 56:819-825, 1982.

127. Shapiro K: *Pediatric head trauma*, New York, 1983, Futura Publishing, pp 1-10.

128. Sheinberg M, Kanter MJ, Robertson CS et al: Continuous monitoring of jugular venous oxygen saturation in head-injured patients, *J Neurosurg* 76:212-217, 1992.

129. Simpson D, Reilly P: Pediatric coma scale, *Lancet* 2:450, 1982.

130. Smith AL: Barbiturate protection in cerebral hypoxia, *Anesthesiology* 47:285-290, 1977.

131. Smith WP, Batnitzky S, Rengachary SS: Acute isodense subdural hematomas: a problem in anemic patients, *AJR* 136:543-546, 1981.

132. Starmark JE, Holmgren E, Stalhammar D: Current reporting of responsiveness in acute cerebral disorders: a survey of the neurosurgical literature, *J Neurosurg* 69:692-698, 1988.

133. Sternau LL, Thompson C, Ganges A et al: Human brain temperature following severe head injury, *J Neurotrauma* 9:70, 1992.

134. Stone JL, Rifai MHS, Sugar O et al: Subdural hematomas. I. Acute subdural hematomas: progress in definition, clinical pathology, and therapy, *Surg Neurol* 19:216-231, 1983.

135. Stone JL, Lone RJ, Jonasson O et al: Acute subdural hematoma: direct admission to a trauma center yields improved results, *J Trauma* 26:445-449, 1986.

136. Suddaby L, Weir B, Forsyth C: The management of 0.22 caliber gunshot wounds of the brain: a review of 49 cases, *Can J Neurol Sci* 14:268-272, 1987.

137. Suwanweh C, Suwanweh N: Intracranial arterial narrowing and spasm in acute head injury, *J Neurosurg* 26:314-323, 1972.

138. Tabbador K, Bhushan C, Pevsher PH et al: Prognostic value of cerebral blood flow (CBF) and cerebral metabolic rate of oxygen ($CMRo_2$) in acute head trauma, *J Trauma* 12:1053-1055, 1972.

139. Teasdale G, Jennett B: Assessment of coma and impaired consciousness, *Lancet* 2:81-84, 1974.

140. Teasdale G, Knill-Jones R, Van der Sande J: Observer variability in assessing impaired consciousness and coma, *J Neurol Neurosurg Psych* 41:603-610, 1978.

141. Teasdale G, Galbraith S, Jennett B: Operate or observe? ICP and the management of the "silent" traumatic intracranial hematoma. In Shulman K, editor: *Intracranial pressure IV*, Berlin, 1980, Springer-Verlag, pp 35-38.

142. Teasdale GM, Galbraith S: Acute traumatic intracranial hematomas. In H. Krayenbuhl, editor: *Progress in neurological surgery*, vol 10, Basel, Switzerland, 1981, S Karger, pp 252-290.

143. Tempkin NR, Dikmen SS, Wilensky AJ et al: A randomized, double-blind study of phenytoin for the prevention of post-traumatic seizures, *N Engl J Med* 323:497-502, 1990.

144. Tenny JH: Bacterial infection of the central nervous system in neurosurgery, *Neurol Clin* 4:91-114, 1986.

145. Toutant SM, Klauber MR, Marshall LF et al: Absent or compressed basal cisterns on first CT scan: ominous predictors of outcome in severe head injury, *J Neurosurg* 61:691-694, 1984.

146. Van Dongen KJ, Braakman R, Gelpke GJ: The prognostic value of computerized tomography in comatose head-injured patients, *J Neurosurg* 59:951-957, 1983.

147. Ward JD, Becker DP, Miller JD et al: Failure of prophylactic barbiturate coma in the treatment of severe head injury, *J Neurosurg* 62:383-388, 1985.

148. Wei EP, Dietrich WD, Povlishock JT et al: Functional, morphological, and metabolic abnormalities of the cerebral microcirculation after concussive brain injury in cats, *Circ Res* 46:37-47, 1980.

149. Wilkins RH, Odom GL: Intracranial arterial spasm associated with craniocerebral trauma, *J Neurosurg* 32:626-633, 1970.

150. Winer JW, Rosenwasser RH, Jimenez F: Electroencephalographic activity and serum and cerebrospinal fluid pentobarbital levels in determining the therapeutic endpoint during barbiturate coma, *Neurosurgery* 29:739-742, 1991.

151. Wisner D, Busche F, Sturm J et al: Traumatic shock and head injury: effects of fluid resuscitation on the brain, *J Surg Res* 46:49-59, 1989.

152. Young B, Rapp RP, Norton NA et al: Failure of prophylactically administered phenytoin to prevent early post-traumatic seizures. *J Neurosurg* 58:231-235, 1983.

153. Zimmerman RA, Bilaniuk LT, Dolinskas C et al: Computed tomography of acute intracerebral hemorrhagic contusion, *J Comput Assist Tomogr* 1:271-279, 1977.

154. Zimmerman RA, Bilaniuk LT: Computed tomography in pediatric head trauma *J Neuroradiology* 8:257-271, 1981.

155. Zornow MH, Scheller MS, Todd MM et al: Acute cerebral effects of isotonic crystalloid and colloid solutions following cryogenic brain injury in the rabbit, *Anesthesiology* 69:180-184, 1988.

32

Multisystem Sequelae of Severe Head Injury

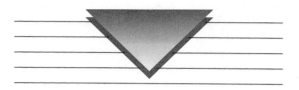

M. Jane Matjasko

CARDIOPULMONARY SEQUELAE OF
ACUTE HEAD INJURY
Initial pulmonary findings
Shock and the adult respiratory distress
syndrome (ARDS)
Neurogenic pulmonary edema (NPE)
Fat embolism
Electrocardiographic changes
Diaphragmatic paralysis

HEMATOLOGIC SEQUELAE
Trauma and coagulation
Disseminated intravascular coagulation
ENDOCRINOLOGIC SEQUELAE
Anterior pituitary insufficiency
Posterior pituitary dysfunction
METABOLIC SEQUELAE
Cerebrospinal fluid metabolic changes

Water and electrolyte balance
Glucose metabolism
Nonketotic hyperosmolar hyperglycemic
coma
GASTROINTESTINAL SEQUELAE
SKELETAL SEQUELAE
Maxillofacial injuries
SUMMARY

The nonneurosurgical, direct, indirect, and multisystem sequelae of head trauma are diverse. This chapter compiles the recognized sequelae of acute head injury and serves as a bibliographic source for those managing such patients on a day-to-day basis. This chapter is not meant to be an exhaustive manual of diagnosis and therapeutics but rather provides approaches to and controversies in pathophysiology, diagnosis, and management.

The commonly recognized nonneurosurgical sequelae of acute head injury are listed in Box 32-1. Appropriate management of these disorders as well as attention to aggressive comprehensive care protocols can significantly reduce mortality after head injury.

CARDIOPULMONARY SEQUELAE OF ACUTE HEAD INJURY

Outcome in head-injured patients can be directly related to inattention to the principles of airway management. This is true at the scene of the accident and during diagnostic studies, particularly CT scanning or magnetic resonance imaging. Expert airway care after severe head injury can help stabilize a patient for adequate neurodiagnostic studies and, at the same time, allow necessary airway protection, hyperventilation, and resuscitation to proceed simultaneously and without delay.

Initial Pulmonary Findings

At the time of concussion, acute elevations in ICP may temporarily or permanently affect the respiratory center, leading to apnea.[99] Perhaps this mechanism accounts for a certain percentage of immediately fatal head injuries. The unconscious state predisposes to upper airway obstruction, hypoxemia, and respiratory acidosis. At the time of injury, laryngeal and pharyngeal reflexes may be acutely depressed,[99] allowing silent or overt aspiration of blood, mucus, foreign body, or gastric contents, and the development of atelectasis, pulmonary edema, and secondary bronchopneumonia.

▼

BOX 32-1
MULTISYSTEM SEQUELAE OF ACUTE HEAD INJURY

Cardiopulmonary

Abnormal breathing patterns
Airway obstruction
Hypoxemia
Shock
Adult respiratory distress syndrome (ARDS)
Neurogenic pulmonary edema (NPE)
Fat embolism
Electrocardiographic changes
Diaphragmatic paralysis

Hematologic

Trauma and coagulation
Disseminated intravascular coagulation (DIC)

Endocrinologic

Anterior pituitary insufficiency
Posterior pituitary dysfunction
   Diabetes insipidus (DI)
   Syndrome of inappropriate antidiuretic hormone secretion (SIADH)

Metabolic

Metabolic response to head injury
Cerebrospinal fluid metabolic changes
Nonketotic hyperosmolar hyperglycemic coma (NHHC)

Gastrointestinal

Skeletal

Maxillofacial injuries

Abnormal breathing patterns were recorded at some time in 60% of 227 patients with head injury, intracranial tumor, or subarachnoid hemorrhage.[277] Periodic, irregular, and rapid breathing occurred equally commonly in all groups. Tachypnea (>25 breaths per minute) and hyperventilation ($Paco_2 < 30$ mm Hg) were associated with a poorer prognosis when they were combined; however, the breathing patterns observed did not correlate anatomically with the site of the lesion.

In the absence of airway obstruction, 30% to 50% of acutely head-injured patients demonstrate hypoxemia and spontaneous hyperventilation.* Isolated head-injured patients demonstrate an increased perfusion of hypoventilated alveoli in the presence of a normal chest roentgenogram and pulmonary capillary wedge pressure whether they are mechanically ventilated or breathe spontaneously.[330] These data imply that bronchoconstriction is present and that compensatory hypoxic pulmonary vasoconstriction is absent. Elevated cerebrospinal fluid (CSF) lactic acid or severe dysfunction of the medial pontine structures may be the stimulus for such a picture.[198,243] Supplemental oxygen often corrects the hypoxemia without terminating the hyperventilation. Severe refractory hypoxemia indicates a poor prognosis.[199,272] Brain-injured patients may have low CSF pH and bicarbonate levels and high lactic acid levels that correlate with the severity of injury[198,244]; hyperventilation will return CSF pH to normal.[69,334] Minute ventilation may be twice normal, particularly if carbon dioxide production is above normal, as in the decerebrate patient. The increased dead-space-to-tidal-volume ratio (as high as 0.6) in the absence of shock and the large intrapulmonary shunt

suggest an ill-defined effect of acute intracranial hypertension on ventilation-perfusion relationships.[136,184,233]

Shock and the Adult Respiratory Distress Syndrome (ARDS)

Thoracic and/or abdominal injuries leading to hypotension and shock occur in approximately 39% of head-injured patients.[30,88,324] Clearly, shock increases morbidity and mortality in these patients; resuscitation must be rapid and vigorous. High minute ventilation volumes may be needed to compensate for the increased dead space associated with head injury[136,184] and the pulmonary hypoperfusion of the shock state.[118,134] Swift volume replacement with blood and appropriate crystalloid and/or colloid is necessary to restore adequate organ perfusion, maximize oxygen-carrying capacity and cardiac output, and minimize alveolar dead space.[134,281] Cervical spine injury occurs in 5% to 10% of head-injured patients, and 20% to 25% of head-injured patients have associated spine injuries. Spinal shock (hypotension and bradycardia) may be present on admission or develop after careless manipulation of the neck during resuscitation. Cardiogenic shock can compound hemorrhagic shock because of the effects of the protracted low-flow state on myocardial muscle function.

Hemodynamic measurements in patients with isolated severe head trauma (Glasgow Coma Scale score less than 7, brain contusion or intracranial hematoma) obtained within 12 hours of injury demonstrate a maximum shunt of 11% to 16% and a low cardiac index that increased over 48 hours to normal in survivors. Initial pulmonary vascular resistance was high in both nonsurvivors and survivors but returned to normal by 48 hours in survivors. There was little correlation between ICP increases and hemodynamic

---

*References 1, 136, 199, 215, 258, 306, 344.

variables.[298] Other studies report conflicting results (variable cardiac index, high pulmonary artery pressure); the clinical picture obviously varies in these patients and may be related to vascular volume status, mannitol, and radiographic contrast dye administration.[50,329]

Serial serum creatine kinase levels in patients with severe closed head injury demonstrate an elevation in the myocardial isoenzyme (CK-MB) in 28 of 30 patients. The mean CK-MB levels remain elevated for at least 3 days after injury; however, the associated ECG abnormalities (prolonged QT, nonspecific ST-T wave changes) and clinical course are not consistent with myocardial infarction. CK-MB levels after myocardial infarction return to normal within 24 to 36 hours unless repeated infarcts or infarct extension occurs. The observed prolonged elevation of CK-MB in the head-injured patient implies ongoing myocardial cell injury, perhaps as a result of sustained sympathetic hyperactivity.[160] Myofibrillar degeneration[390] and subendocardial hemorrhage[197] have been observed histologically in patients dying after cerebrovascular accidents.

Neurogenic shock is rare.[185] In adults, a fatal degree of cerebral compression usually develops before there is vasomotor center collapse. In young children with an expansive skull and relatively small blood volume, a significant proportion of the blood volume may accumulate intracranially and lead to hypotension. Also in young children, small scalp lacerations can lead to a significant reduction in blood volume. In Clark's[74] study of 721 head-injured patients, 49 had shock attributable to the head injury; these patients were neurologically moribund, and 46 did not survive.

Approximately 20% of head-injured patients develop acute respiratory failure,[215] that is, progressive hypoxemia resistant to oxygen therapy[12,233,258] and continuous positive airway pressure. The respiratory failure is associated with measured reductions in functional residual capacity[215,258,306] and pulmonary compliance,[32,52,215] pulmonary hypertension,[405] and the typical radiologic findings indicative of "shock lung." Coincident shock and thoracic trauma predispose to respiratory failure. This can significantly impair cerebral perfusion and oxygenation, leading to a greater compromise of the injured brain and perhaps extension of ischemia and edema to noninjured cerebral tissue.

Pathologically, the lungs are stiff and heavy with varying degrees of hemorrhagic edema throughout the airways, alveoli, and interstitium.[12,387] Platelet aggregation and microthrombosis of pulmonary capillaries may initiate the release of vasoactive substances (serotonin, histamine),[37] leading to increases in pulmonary vascular resistance (perhaps primarily venular).[4,268,361] Metabolic and respiratory acidosis, endogenous catecholamines, prostaglandins,[174] and alveolar hypoxia all may lead to increased pulmonary vascular resistance.[4,20,387] Damage to the capillary and epithelial cells permits movement of fluid, cells, and protein into the interstitium. When the transport capacity of the pulmonary lymphatics is exceeded, edema develops in the loose connective tissues surrounding the respiratory bronchiole and its accompanying arteriole, venule, and lymphatics.[354,355] Peribronchiolar edema leads to an increase in small airway resistance; alveolar interstitial edema reduces lung compliance. Later, alveolar edema occurs. Inspired gases tend to be diverted to more compliant alveoli, leading to an increased intrapulmonary shunt. Functional residual capacity and compliance fall. Atelectasis, hyaline membrane formation, and diffuse fibrosis develop with virtual cessation of gas-exchange capability. As long as nitrogen is present in alveolar gas, alveoli with low ventilation-perfusion ratios tend to stay open. When the inspired oxygen tension is raised, the structurally important nitrogen tension decreases. With continued uptake of oxygen from a partially obstructed but totally perfused alveolus, the intraalveolar oxygen tension falls toward mixed venous levels and the alveolus tends to collapse.[100,240,396] Early treatment (i.e., intubation, mechanical ventilation with end-expiratory pressure, and careful fluid management), can abort or minimize the full-blown symptom complex. In many trauma centers, death from respiratory insufficiency has been reduced by expectant and early management.

Priorities in the management of hemorrhagic shock in the head-injured patient are airway control and volume replacement. Blood glucose and lactate levels are commonly increased in patients with severe head injury,[101] presumably related to central mechanisms and surgical stress. The increased glucose levels are potentially dangerous because hyperglycemia has been shown to exacerbate the severity of brain injury during ischemic conditions.[212] A retrospective study of severe head-injury patients (Glasgow Coma Scale score of 8 or less) shows that there is a correlation between severity of head injury and elevated serum glucose levels and that those with a poorer outcome have much higher serum glucose than those with good outcome.[211] In fact, a glucose level greater than 200 mg/dl was associated with a poor outcome. Abundant glucose substrate allows anaerobic metabolism to continue, and lactate and hydrogen ions accumulate. The resulting intracellular acidosis causes the hypoxic cascade—calcium entry into cells, lipolysis, release of free fatty acids and glutamate, and eventual cell membrane destruction. Attention to the presence of hyperglycemia and treatment with insulin or inhibition of glycolysis through an increase in the availability of ketone bodies via peripheral hyperalimentation may influence outcome by decreasing lactic acid production. Even moderate reductions in serum glucose may be therapeutic.[219,310]

Smooth intubation and airway control are indicated. The efficacy of prolonged hyperventilation has been questioned. Recent studies suggest that loss of bicarbonate buffers from the CSF during prolonged hyperventilation results in increased sensitivity of the cerebral vessels to $Paco_2$.[270] Sustained hyperventilation in an experimental fluid percussion model of head injury caused greater brain lactate production and greater depletion of oxidative stores than in control animals or those treated with tromethamine (THAM), a buffering agent that crosses the blood-brain barrier and causes some osmotic diuresis. THAM-treated animals had reduced lactate production and reduced brain water content.[402] In a randomized clinical trial in head-injured patients, prophylactic use of sustained hyperventilation for a period of 5 days retarded recovery from severe head injury, with outcome being significantly worse at 3 and 6 months but not at 12 months. THAM administration (0.3 M solution at a dose calculated to raise pH to 7.6 using the formula THAM [ml] = body weight [kg] × base deficit) by constant infusion at 1 ml/kg/hr over 5 days seemed to counteract the deleterious effects of prolonged hyperventilation, and its use may be beneficial when ICP control is difficult to attain. THAM may protect against the deleterious effects of hyperventilation by reducing brain edema and lactate levels.[269]

During the acute phase of head injury, adult comatose patients have reduced cerebral oxygen metabolism ($CMRo_2$), while CBF may be increased, decreased, or normal. Because cerebral $AVDo_2$ equals $CMRo_2/CBF$, $AVDo_2$ has been investigated as a clinically measurable parameter to assess the adequacy of CBF during many clinical conditions, including head injury. A normal $AVDo_2$ (5 to 7.5 vol %) suggests that $CMRo_2$ and CBF are normally coupled. A decreased $AVDo_2$ (less than 5 vol %) indicates that CBF is excessive for brain metabolic requirements (hyperemia); an elevated $AVDo_2$ (greater than 7.5 vol %) suggests cerebral ischemia caused by decreased CBF. A high $AVDo_2$ suggests that raising CBF by increasing $Paco_2$ or giving mannitol may be effective in improving outcome, whereas continuing hyperventilation in this setting may compromise CBF further and result in brain energy failure. $AVDo_2$ therefore may guide therapy. An increase in blood pH shifts the oxyhemoglobin dissociation curve to the left; therefore, for a given $AVDo_2$, the venous O_2 content will fall (the Bohr effect). Experimental results suggest that a low jugular venous oxygen content may indicate inadequate global CBF in the presence of increased ICP.[311,365] Much more clinical experience is required before this becomes fully accepted. Monitoring of $AVDo_2$ might prove to be valuable to guide therapy in comatose head-injured patients in whom cerebral ischemia may not be evident from the neurologic examination or ICP monitoring.[90,364]

Several recent studies support hypertonic fluid administration rather than fluid restriction as the optimal therapy in animals with cerebral (cryogenic) injury or hypovolemic shock.[238,336] A 24-hour infusion of hypertonic sodium lactate (500 mOsm/L) compared with hypotonic Ringer's lactate (270 mOsm/L) in pigs subjected to a cryogenic brain injury demonstrated a significantly lower ICP, higher CBF and oxygen delivery and, of course, a higher serum osmolality. Brain water content in the area of the lesion was similar in both groups, but in the uninjured hemisphere, it was lower in the hypertonic group. Hypertonic maintenance fluid improves intracranial compliance by reducing water content in the uninjured brain. The improved CBF in the hypertonic group may be due to dehydration of the cere-

brovascular endothelium and erythrocytes. Oxygen delivery to injured brain may be improved. In contrast, administration of hypotonic fluids may contribute to secondary injury after head trauma.[336] How much fluid and how long it should be administered are unclear at this time. Experimental microdialysis via cortically implanted catheters in head-injury patients has shown a rapid correlation between changes in metabolic products such as lactate, pyruvate, lactate:pyruvate ratio, glutamate, aspartate, and taurine and the severity of injury, the response to treatment, and the degree of cellular energy perturbation (i.e., ischemia). Despite the fact that the catheter dialysis method only samples a small area of cortex, it correlated remarkably rapidly with the existing clinical situation. The possibility of being able to directly and continuously assess the cerebral energy state to guide therapy is intriguing.[293]

Inspired oxygen tension must be adjusted serially, depending on the patient's response to therapy and recognizing that inspired tensions above 0.40 (Pao_2 250 mm Hg) can adversely affect pulmonary gas exchange in normal as well as traumatized patients.[240,396] In addition to microatelectasis, high inspired oxygen tensions may have ill-defined effects on pulmonary vasculature, leading to ventilation-perfusion mismatching and increased right-to-left shunting.

Positive end-expiratory pressure (PEEP) may restore functional residual capacity,[243,300] and PEEP-produced improvement in ventilation-perfusion relationships may allow reductions in inspired oxygen concentration.[258] PEEP-induced increases in mean alveolar pressure[115] are transmitted to the pleural cavity, heart, and great vessels in direct relation to the lung compliance; that is, as PEEP increases, the level at which cardiac output is depressed varies inversely with the lung compliance.[167,243] Alveolar pressure applied to the pulmonary capillary or the disease process itself may increase pulmonary vascular resistance,[300] and raising alveolar Po_2 may be instrumental in reversing hypoxic pulmonary vasoconstriction. Theoretically, increases in transpulmonary pressure may be transmitted principally to normal alveoli and thus reduce perfusion in these areas, leading to a worsening of the shunt.[13,193,257] High levels of PEEP may reduce cardiac output below levels sufficient for oxygen consumption; greater peripheral venous desaturation occurs because of this reduction in oxygen availability, and alveolar-to-arterial oxygen tension gradients can increase substantially in the presence of an unchanging venous admixture. In some patients, improvement in shunting can be more than offset by a fall in cardiac output with a consequent reduction in oxygen availability to the tissues (available oxygen = oxygen content × cardiac output). The cause of PEEP-induced reductions in cardiac output may be related to a reduction in venous return[363]; when PEEP is at low levels (less than 10 cm H_2O), the reduction in output can be reversed by blood volume expansion. In patients requiring higher levels of PEEP, a further decrease in cardiac output can occur and may be caused by acute right ventricular loading, resulting in a leftward shift of the interventricular septum,[188] or by increases in left ventricular afterload, reflected by an increase in left ventricular transmural pressure (left ventricular end diastolic pressure minus pleural pressure); PEEP may reduce left ventricular preload and left ventricular pressure while increasing intrapleural pressure.[64,362] Therefore mechanical ventilation with positive end-expiratory pressure may reduce shunting by increasing functional residual capacity and reducing hypoxic pulmonary vasoconstriction; it may also increase shunting by shifting pulmonary blood flow to nonventilated regions of the lung and by reducing cardiac output. Ideal management of these patients is best accomplished when serial cardiac output, oxygen consumption, oxygen availability, pulmonary vascular resistance, and blood gas measurements are available.[108,300,363]

Highly variable effects of PEEP on ICP and neurologic status have been noted in animals and humans. Aidinis et al.[3] demonstrated in cats with intracranial mass lesions that PEEP can initiate changes in ICP and systemic blood pressure. Reductions in cerebral perfusion pressure (CPP) were particularly damaging (electroencephalographic abnormalities, sudden increase in pupillary diameter) in animals with impaired autoregulation. Animals with oleic-acid–induced pulmonary damage had less severe reductions in CPP with PEEP application.

Application and removal of PEEP may be particularly dangerous. PEEP removal may precipitate a sudden increase in left ventricular preload, blood pressure, and cerebral perfusion pressure and lead to increased cerebral edema in patients with low intracranial compliance and loss of autoregulation.

PEEP application and removal and other clinical situations in which intrathoracic pressure is raised (intubation, coughing, suctioning, chest physiotherapy, Valsalva maneuver) may adversely affect CPP and ICP.[218,222] Intravenous barbiturates and lidocaine can prevent or treat acute intraoperative increases in ICP.[33,338] In a study of comatose, brain-injured patients, intravenous succinylcholine (1 mg/kg) was most effective in attenuating the ICP response to coughing during tracheal suctioning as compared with intravenous fentanyl (1 μg/kg), thiopental (3 mg/kg), and lidocaine (1.5 mg/kg). Intratracheal lidocaine (1.5 mg/kg) alone provoked coughing. Mean arterial pressure (MAP) was elevated and CPP was not significantly changed in all drug groups.[398] Muscle relaxants alone do not prevent increases in MAP; central nervous system depressants alone do not abolish the cough reflex and the accompanying increases in intrathoracic venous pressure. Acute reductions in CPP are possible if cerebral autoregulation is impaired or absent. CPP control may best be achieved in the individual patient by a combination of short-acting muscle relaxants, intravenous thiopental, lidocaine, or esmolol (a short-acting beta antagonist). The influence of muscle relaxants on ICP has been studied extensively. Succinylcholine should be used with caution in patients with intracra-

nial hypertension. "Precurarization" or a short-acting nondepolarizing muscle relaxant is suggested.[162,213,256,357]

Variable effects of PEEP have been reported in severely head-injured patients. McAslan et al.[239] exposed eight supine patients to increases in PEEP from 5 to 20 cm H_2O; no change in ventricular fluid pressure was observed until PEEP exceeded 15 cm H_2O. CPP remained above normal in all but one patient, whose blood pressure fell at 20 cm H_2O PEEP. No specific deteriorations in neurologic status were noted. Frost[137] exposed 10 patients (30-degree head-up tilt) to varying PEEP levels and observed no changes in ICP despite increases in central venous pressure and pulmonary wedge pressure. PEEP of 35 cm H_2O applied for 10 minutes, however, did lead to pressure waves indicating reduced intracranial compliance. Apuzzo et al.[9] applied 10 cm H_2O of PEEP to 25 severely head-injured patients (head position not stated). In 12 of 13 patients with increased elastance (decreased compliance), PEEP caused increases in ICP that were at times greater than double the baseline level; of these 12 patients, 6 had CPP below 60 mm Hg. In 12 of 12 patients with normal elastance, no change in ICP occurred with PEEP. Increases in ICP and reductions in CPP with PEEP application and removal may be "buffered" in patients who have reduced static pulmonary compliance (tidal volume [ml]/end-inspiratory pressure [cm H_2O]).[53] Caution must be exercised in the individual patient. PEEP should not be withheld when it is essential for improvement of functional residual capacity and venous admixture. The lowest effective PEEP level should be applied with simultaneous observance of its effect on ICP, cardiac output, MAP, CPP, and oxygen availability. This is important if high-dose barbiturate therapy is being used. Significant circulatory depression frequently occurs in this setting; continuous CPP measurement is mandatory.

Most head-injured patients are nursed in a slight head-up position (30 degrees) based on the clinical observation that this maneuver can reduce ICP by hydrostatic reductions in cerebral venous outflow pressure and ventricular fluid pressure. Most patients adjust to this postural change by a compensatory rise in peripheral vascular resistance and thus maintain blood pressure and CPP. Patients with a concomitant spinal cord injury or those who are moribund with elevated ICP and intracranial vasomotor paralysis may not be able to tolerate even transient small reductions in CPP without decompensation.

Frequent arterial blood gases, cardiac output, pulmonary arterial and wedge pressures, ongoing neurologic assessment, and ICP measurements are all necessary for intelligent management of this complex changing situation.

Weaning from mechanical ventilation must be individualized, based on the severity of respiratory involvement and associated injuries; however, the usual criteria apply—vital capacity of at least 10 ml/kg, maximum inspiratory force of at least −20 to −30 cm H_2O,[119,177,297] dead-space-to-tidal-volume ratio less than 0.6,[347] $A-aDo_2$ less than 300 to 350 mm Hg,[123] cardiovascular stability, and a normal metabolic state.[217]

Neurogenic Pulmonary Edema (NPE)

After a variety of central nervous system insults, fulminant pulmonary edema characterized by marked pulmonary vascular congestion, intraalveolar hemorrhage, and protein-rich edema fluid may develop. The syndrome most often occurs in the absence of underlying cardiopulmonary disease; traditional therapy for pulmonary edema of cardiac origin is ineffective, and the outcome is frequently fatal.[371] It is important to exclude other potential disease processes that could cause hypoxemia, such as aspiration pneumonitis, pneumonia, and congestive heart failure.

The association between central nervous system injury and pulmonary disease dates to 1874 when Nothnagel[279] reported the death of a rabbit from pulmonary congestion after probing of the brain at unspecified points. In 1918, Moutier[267] noted the frequent occurrence of fatal, acute pulmonary edema associated with battle injuries, namely gunshot wounds to the head. Pulmonary edema developed within 1 hour of injury and was associated with hypertension and bradycardia; deaths were attributed to overactivity of the suprarenal glands. To date, neurogenic pulmonary edema has been reported after a variety of conditions: head trauma,[55,79,111,114,341] intracranial hemorrhage,[72,375] tumors,[55,153,221,375] strokes,[55] seizures,[39,156,182] Guillain-Barré syndrome,[170] meningitis,[55] poliomyelitis,[23] venous air embolism,[66] intrathecal hypertonic saline,[372] and insulin shock treatment of schizophrenia.[276] Pulmonary edema has been produced in a variety of experimental animals, including primates, after an increase in ICP by means of gun impact,[29] wooden block blow,[228] inflation of an epidural balloon,* or infusion of saline,[49,112,169,178,314] blood,[56] or fibrin[56,322,323] into the intracranial space. Electrolytic lesions of the hypothalamus,[230,307] low cervical spinal cord transection,[48] and bilateral cervical vagotomy[121,122] have also led to neurogenic pulmonary edema.

The influence of raised ICP on circulatory dynamics was described by Harvey Cushing[91] in his classic study published in 1901. Dogs exposed to local and general cerebral compression developed an increase in ICP and a concomitant increase in systemic blood pressure, which tended to "find a level slightly above that of the pressure exerted against the medulla." This elevation in pressure apparently serves to spare medullary function. The systemic hypertension was not attenuated by cervical vagotomy but was totally abolished by cervical cord transection or topical cocainization of the medulla, implying a sympathetic-nervous-system–mediated mechanism. Cushing also exposed the small intestine and directly observed splanchnic vasoconstriction coincident with the systemic hypertension. Rhythmic variations in blood pressure (Traube-Hering waves) occurred during the intracranial hypertension; the

crests of the waves were higher and the valleys lower than the ICP. By direct observation through a cranial window, the crests of the blood pressure waves were associated with hyperemia of the cortical vessels and Cheyne-Stokes respiration. The valleys were accompanied by anemia of the cortical surface vessels and concomitant respiratory arrest. Although no animal developed pulmonary edema despite ICP greater than 200 mm Hg, respiratory rate and volume were affected. He concluded that an increase in ICP to levels greater than blood pressure led to medullary ischemia and vasomotor center stimulation, prompting a rise in blood pressure slightly above the pressure exerted against the medulla. This increase in blood pressure led to medullary reflow and vasomotor center inhibition, prompting a fall in blood pressure below ICP and initiation of the cycle again.[92]

Over the next 70 years, many investigators postulated humoral or neural mechanisms to account for the left ventricular failure and/or increased pulmonary capillary permeability of neurogenic pulmonary edema. Any pathophysiologic mechanism must account for the specific characteristic features of this syndrome, which include[369,370]:

1. Rapid onset
2. Relationship to hypothalamic lesions
3. Prevention or attenuation by alpha blockers and central nervous system depressants
4. Specific sequence of hemodynamic changes
5. High-protein-content edema fluid
6. Resemblance to epinephrine-induced pulmonary edema

The rapid onset suggests a massive neural discharge from the injured brain secondary to intracranial hypertension. In Vietnam, patients with penetrating head injuries without associated injuries to other organ systems showed a high incidence of pulmonary edema. Among patients who died within a few minutes after head injury, 17 of 20 had associated pulmonary edema. If cervical cord transection or massive hemorrhage accompanied the head injury, pulmonary edema did not occur.[341] Because of the rapid onset, conventional forms of heart failure are unlikely.

Specific hypothalamic electrolytic lesions in rats can produce pulmonary edema. Maire and Paton[230] postulate the existence of a hypothalamic "edemagenic center" whose impulses arise from postchiasmatic hypothalamic structures. This edemagenic center is normally inhibited by structures in the preoptic area; destructive preoptic lesions release this inhibition and lead to pulmonary edema. Vagotomy and cervical cord transection prevent edema after such lesions. Reynolds[307] offers an alternative interpretation: Electrolytic lesions cause pulmonary edema on the basis of irritation of the sympathetic pathways in the hypothalamus and subsequent massive neural discharge. It is probable that the hypothalamus would be vulnerable to dysfunction by a variety of proximal or distal brain insults. Perhaps the massive neural discharge of neurogenic pulmonary edema is centrally mediated with an important hypotha-

---

*References 34, 35, 57, 58, 112, 113.

lamic component. However, Chen et al.[68] have reported that the hypothalamus is not essential for the development of pulmonary edema because midbrain lesions producing decerebration in animals did not affect either the cardiovascular or pulmonary changes induced by cerebral compression.

Pretreatment of head-injured experimental animals with central nervous system depressants (phenobarbital, ether, chloral hydrate) and alpha adrenergic receptor antagonists prevented or attenuated the severity of pulmonary edema compared with untreated controls after the same head trauma.[29,44,228] Adrenalectomy offered no protection. Studies by Brown[49] suggest that neurogenic pulmonary edema is mediated largely through the sympathetic nervous system, specifically the alpha adrenergic system, and that the sympathetic nervous system response is centrally mediated because it is attenuated by central nervous system depressants. Dogs pretreated with dibenzyline do not exhibit massive increases in systemic blood pressure or peripheral resistance after acute intracranial hypertension.[49] Elevated blood catecholamine levels occur during intracranial hypertension; peak levels are reached when systemic hypertension is greatest.[316]

A specific sequence of hemodynamic changes has been observed in susceptible animals after head injury.* Animals show massive increases in systemic arterial, pulmonary arterial, pulmonary venous, and superior vena caval pressures accompanied by a dramatic increase in total peripheral resistance 20% of the time. As a result of the increase in peripheral resistance, blood shifts from the peripheral to the pulmonary vascular bed as documented by pressure and blood volume changes (increased size of left atrium, pulmonary venous engorgement). Within 15 minutes the lungs become cyanotic and edematous. In contrast, 80% of animals tend to have decreasing systemic, pulmonary arterial, and pulmonary venous pressures over the next few minutes and no pulmonary edema.[112]

After an initial phase of increased pulmonary vascular pressure, pulmonary edema persists while this pressure returns to normal. Pulmonary wedge pressure measurements in patients with NPE are rare, but they have been observed to be normal in these patients when pulmonary edema was well established. This observation suggests that pulmonary capillary membrane disruption has occurred.[165]

The electron microscope picture of vascular wall rupture with leakage of red blood cells and amorphous material into the perivascular and intraalveolar spaces and the clinical finding of high protein content in the edema fluid suggest that capillary membrane disruption is an important feature of neurogenic pulmonary edema.[68,181,325] Even though the hemodynamic abnormalities that produce the capillary structural damage subside quickly, altered pulmonary capillary permeability may persist, requiring extreme caution in respiratory and fluid management.

---

*References 49, 112, 113, 231, 322, 323.

The profound vasoconstriction that follows intravenous epinephrine[224,228,400] precipitates pulmonary edema, which can be prevented by pretreatment with alpha adrenergic antagonists. These studies indicate that the immediate cause of neurogenic pulmonary edema is a sudden increase in pulmonary capillary pressure and eventual capillary membrane disruption. Left atrial and left ventricular end-diastolic pressures rise as a result of increased afterload and decreased left ventricular compliance. Therefore changes in cardiac function are brief, based on an increase in cardiac work, and not related to intrinsic cardiac failure.[370]

The current working hypothesis relative to the pathophysiology of this condition is illustrated in Fig. 32-1. More recent experimental data suggest that neither systemic nor pulmonary hypertension is essential to the development of neurogenic pulmonary edema in cats subjected to sustained increases in ICP. Perhaps the massive sympathetic discharge caused by intracranial hypertension affects the pulmonary vascular bed directly.[140,179]

Experimental animals with intracranial hypertension[178] and humans with severe head injury uniformly exhibit increases in lung water, which appears to be common but clinically unrecognized (no neurogenic pulmonary edema, no or only moderate hypoxemia). Perhaps increased lung water is the earliest evidence of the pulmonary effects of head trauma, which in its extreme manifestation is neurogenic pulmonary edema.

Therapy consists of immediate pharmacologic or surgical relief of intracranial hypertension, continuous positive pressure ventilation, supplemental oxygen therapy, careful fluid management, and perhaps sodium nitroprusside, which may be useful because of its ability to directly dilate peripheral and pulmonary vessels.[80] Perhaps nifedipine should be administered in a controlled trial for the same reason.[27,81]

Vigorous inspiratory effort against a closed glottis or totally obstructed airway can generate severe negative intraalveolar pressures and lead to pulmonary edema. This mechanism may be operative in head-injured patients who are unconscious with upper airway obstruction.[286]

Various forms of noncardiac pulmonary edema—high altitude,[180,183,343] opiate-induced,[110,285] smoke inhalation, and pulmonary edema after decompression—have been explained on the basis of hypoxic pulmonary vasoconstriction leading to pulmonary hypertension,[150,196,292,356] arterial wall rupture, and leakage of protein-rich fluid into the interstitium and alveoli. An alternative theory is that damaged arterial walls attract fibrin and platelets, which form thrombi that may then shower the capillary and venous bed with microemboli, producing pulmonary capillary hypertension, capillary rupture, and edema formation.[208,342,397] Activated intravascular clotting or fibrinolysis may have an important role in high-altitude pulmonary edema.[154,174] Nifedipine, diamox (acetazolamide), and dexamethasone have been reported to be effective in preventing high-altitude pulmonary edema and treating it after it has occurred.[27] These

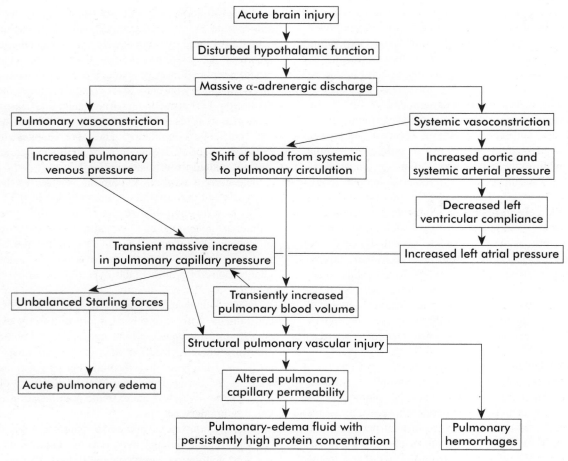

FIG. 32-1   Working hypothesis relative to the pathophysiology of neurogenic pulmonary edema (NPE).

forms of therapy have not been used in NPE to date but may be reasonable to try because the outcome with standard therapy is uniformly poor.

There are striking similarities in the pathologic and clinical picture of shock lung and neurogenic pulmonary edema. Moss[264-266] has subjected dogs to hypoxic cerebral perfusion (Pao_2 35 ± 5 mm Hg) without systemic ischemia, acidemia, hypercarbia, or hypotension. Within 2 hours the animals developed impaired pulmonary function pathologically similar to shock lung. He postulates that many respiratory distress syndromes have a common cerebral etiology; the initiating trauma interferes with hypothalamic cellular metabolism, which leads to autonomically mediated increased pulmonary venular resistance. This results in increased capillary pressures and vascular congestion, interstitial and intraalveolar edema and hemorrhage, and right-to-left shunting. Lung denervation can prevent these changes.[361] The transudate of plasma and resulting hyaline membrane formation inactivates surfactant and predispose to atelectasis. Systemic hypoxia, such as acute mountain sickness or high-altitude hypoxemia, should also produce

this syndrome. This is an attractive unifying theory to explain posttraumatic pulmonary insufficiency and adult respiratory distress syndrome, as well as the varied forms of noncardiac pulmonary edema, including neurogenic pulmonary edema.

Fat Embolism

Fat embolism may be associated with fractures of any bone containing marrow. Nearly all patients who die shortly after sustaining fractures have fat emboli in the lungs postmortem,[335] but only 1% to 2% of patients with fractures develop clinical features compatible with fat embolism.[315] Mortality has been reduced in recent years because of appropriate respiratory management.[106]

Clinical symptoms usually develop 24 to 48 hours after trauma; most frequent are changes in mental status from restlessness to coma. Accompanying findings are pyrexia, tachycardia, tachypnea, cyanosis, seizures, paralysis, and an evanescent petechial rash associated with thrombocytopenia best seen on the anterior axillary folds, neck, abdominal wall, and conjunctiva.[120] Ross reported on a group of

45 patients, 37 of whom had this classic petechial rash with or without other signs.[315] Failure to recover consciousness after general anesthesia may lead to suspicion of this diagnosis, particularly in the absence of head injury. Droplets lodging in the pulmonary circulation may lead to hypoxemia; they may be seen in sputum and, if they traverse the pulmonary capillary, they may be seen in retinal vessels and urine. It has been suggested that biochemical changes in the plasma during shock disrupt the lipid suspension system, allowing fatty acids and free fat to appear.[138] Free fat in the pulmonary capillary may cause a release of lipase, produced in the pulmonary parenchyma, with resultant breakdown of fat to free fatty acids.[11] Toxic free fatty acids may produce epithelial damage, platelet aggregation, inactivation of lung surfactant, increased capillary permeability, decreased lung compliance, and hypoxemia as a result of increased right-to-left shunting.[51,291] The associated anemia and thrombocytopenia in fat embolism have been explained on the basis of disseminated intravascular coagulation.[203] Differential diagnosis must include posttraumatic pulmonary insufficiency, shock, venous thromboembolism, and aspiration pneumonitis. Secondary deterioration in a head-injured patient may result from fat embolism.

The chest x-ray may show the characteristic "snowstorm" appearance of diffuse, fluffy, hazy infiltration. Other laboratory findings may be anemia, thrombocytopenia, and hypocalcemia caused by the interaction of fatty acids and calcium. No laboratory test is pathognomonic. Treatment must primarily be directed to correction of hypoxemia. Pharmacologic steroid therapy and heparinization may be of value.[14,106,203]

Electrocardiographic Changes

The first report of abnormal electrocardiographic changes associated with acute CNS disease appeared in 1947.[54] Jacobson and Danufsky[187] produced dysrhythmias in mice after experimental head injury; atropine pretreatment prevented these dysrhythmias, implying that vagal stimulation was responsible. Bradycardia, shortened QT interval, elevated ST segments, nodal rhythm, and increased T wave amplitude have been reported after experimental concussion in monkeys. Cardiac arrest may also occur.[244] Atrial fibrillation after head injury with and without intracranial hypertension also has been reported.[234] The pathogenesis of varied electrocardiographic abnormalities after head injury,[175,244,317] subarachnoid hemorrhage,* and cerebrovascular accidents[124] is obscure. Central autonomic stimulation at cortical, hypothalamic, or brainstem levels or interruption or spasm of deep perforating vessels to the hypothalamus could account for these observations.[176,389] Several reports point to the left-sided dominance of sympathetic innervation of the heart.† In some studies there seems to be

no correlation between intracranial hypertension or electrolyte imbalance and ECG changes in patients with subarachnoid hemorrhage, meningitis, or space-occupying lesions,[176] yet others report a correlation.[296]

Because many patients with isolated severe head injury have elevated serum CK-MB levels, and subendocardial hemorrhage has been detected at autopsy, it is possible that significant myocardial involvement may necessitate therapy[197,273] and in some cases preclude consideration of these patients as potential donors for cardiac transplantation. Echocardiographic evaluation may be valuable in assessing functional myocardial damage.[296]

Diaphragmatic Paralysis

Transient diaphragmatic paralysis after head trauma has been reported infrequently.[301] In stroke and hemiplegic patients contralateral diaphragmatic paralysis has been observed.[201] When the brain injury is diffuse, a possible cause of transient phrenic nerve dysfunction may be hyperextension of the neck, resulting in stretching, edema, or hemorrhage in the nerve without complete avulsion. Recovery occurred in 1 to 6 months in the cases reported by Prasad and Athreya.[301] Diaphragmatic paralysis may aggravate the respiratory problems of the head-injured patient and be responsible for difficulty in weaning because of inadequate lung expansion and poor coughing ability.

HEMATOLOGIC SEQUELAE
Trauma and Coagulation

The severely traumatized patient displays a multitude of clotting abnormalities.[16,166] Among 42 patients with a wide variety of traumatic injuries reported by Innes and Sevitt,[186] hypercoagulable and fibrinolytic states existed within the first few hours after trauma, probably as a result of release of tissue thromboplastin, presumably for hemostatic purposes. The duration of exaggerated fibrinolysis correlated with the severity of the injury. Hypocoagulability in these patients was probably related to clotting factor deficiencies (II, VII, platelets). Frequently these patients demonstrate an abrupt rebound antifibrinolysis, perhaps again a hemostatic mechanism. Adrenergic hyperactivity after trauma may trigger hypercoagulability.[59,60,335]

Good correlation exists between the severity of trauma and a decrease in platelets, prothrombin (factor II), proaccelerin (factor V), and plasminogen and an increase in fibrin degradation products. When intravascular coagulation is present, increased clinical morbidity in the form of respiratory and other organ failure usually develops.[359] It is recognized that multiple transfusions, shock, sepsis, and unknown factors may influence coagulation.[82,105] Head trauma has been shown to impair platelet aggregation in vitro and in vivo,[26,282,380,393] as have many drugs, including aspirin, phenylbutazone, chlorpromazine, penicillin, general anesthetics, and furosemide.

*References 7, 139, 176, 232, 247, 358, 373, 392.
†References 139, 152, 175, 273, 287, 317.

Disseminated Intravascular Coagulation

Disseminated intravascular coagulation (DIC) is a physiologic response to a variety of underlying stimuli that provoke a generalized activation of the hemostatic mechanism leading to the intravascular consumption of clotting factors with subsequent thrombosis and/or bleeding diathesis. This syndrome reflects the interplay of two basic processes. The first is a complex sequence of events leading to the evolution of thrombin; the second is a series of protective mechanisms employed by the body to defend itself against the disseminated clotting that would occur in the presence of unchecked thrombin activity. Therefore thrombin formation and fibrinolysis occur, leading to the clinical picture of simultaneous thrombosis and hemorrhage.[105] Etiologically, disseminated intravascular coagulation can be the result of three processes: (1) endothelial cell injury, which activates Hageman factor and the intrinsic clotting system; (2) tissue injury, which activates the extrinsic clotting system; and (3) red cell or platelet injury, with the release of coagulant phospholipids.[82] These processes lead to the formation of thrombin, which, in turn, cleaves fibrinogen, activates factor XIII (fibrin stabilizing factor), aggregates platelets, releases platelet constituents, and triggers secondary fibrinolysis. The fibrinolytic agent plasmin splits fibrinogen, producing fibrin degradation or split products that themselves have anticoagulant properties. Analysis of a series of 90 patients revealed that diagnostic criteria for disseminated intravascular coagulation require the presence of at least three abnormal screening tests (prolonged prothrombin time, decreased fibrinogen, decreased platelets). If only two of the three are abnormal, a test for fibrinolysis (thrombin time, euglobulin clot lysis, or fibrinogen degradation products) should be abnormal to establish the diagnosis.[82]

In the head-injured patient, several clotting abnormalities may be present, and disseminated intravascular coagulation has been reported after mild and severe cerebral trauma[109,148,242,383] and anoxic brain damage.[6] Reduced platelet aggregation associated with elevated cytoplasmic adenosine 3', 5' monophosphate (cyclic AMP) has been reported after head injury.[377,380] Several investigators have prospectively examined coagulation profiles in head-injured patients. In general, coagulation abnormalities or evidence of DIC was more likely in the presence of brain tissue destruction.[148,380,382]

In a series of 87 consecutive pediatric head injuries, 32% had evidence of disseminated intravascular coagulation and 71% had one or more abnormal clotting studies. Patients with penetrating injuries and mass lesions had a higher frequency of disseminated intravascular coagulation and a higher mortality than those with diffuse injury. Coagulation disorders returned to normal quickly in survivors; many patients died after the clotting studies had returned to normal, implying that the abnormal clotting was the result of massive brain tissue destruction.[255]

Delayed or recurrent posttraumatic intracranial hematomas are related to the presence of clotting abnormalities and disseminated intravascular coagulation. Intracerebral hematomas may occur at ventriculostomy sites in patients with disseminated intravascular coagulation; such clotting abnormalities should be corrected before catheter insertion.[200,302,359]

The pathogenesis of disseminated intravascular coagulation in head injury is uncertain. The severity of coagulation abnormalities correlates with the severity of head injury and associated multiple injuries. Shock, sepsis, extensive surgery,[82,105,166] and fat embolism[202] all have been associated with the development of disseminated intravascular coagulation and may be concurrent factors in the head-injured patient. Brain tumors are also known to predispose to disseminated intravascular coagulation.[235,379] The brain as a whole is rich in tissue thromboplastin and contains 50 units per gram of tissue. The lung is the only organ with higher thromboplastin levels than brain, up to 200 units per gram.[15] Takashima et al.[366] and Tovi[374] have shown that high levels of fibrinolytic activity are present in the brain, primarily in the highly vascular connective tissue of the choroid plexus and meninges. Fibrinolytic activity is low in brain tissue itself, and the amount of either substance liberated into the general circulation after head trauma is unknown. Hemorrhagic cerebral tissue was present within the sagittal sinus in a patient with fulminant disseminated intravascular coagulation associated with a skull fracture and severe head injury. Prothrombin time and partial thromboplastin time were greater than 800 seconds.[73]

The demonstration of increased myelin basic protein, a nervous-system-specific protein, in the serum of patients with severe head injury,[371] brain tissue emboli in pulmonary vessels after head injury,[365] and the high incidence of pulmonary microthrombi in rats subjected to minor head injury[376] support the direct relationship between head injury, brain tissue destruction, and disseminated intravascular coagulation.

Central nervous system mechanisms exist for the regulation of plasma levels of blood clotting factors. Gunn and Hampton[159] have reported that direct hypothalamic stimulation can lead to a decrease in factor VIII levels. Stimulation of permanent electrodes in subcortical areas of 12 dogs demonstrated that factor VIII levels were decreased by stimulation of ventral and lateral hypothalamic areas with the medial forebrain bundle overlying the optic tract, the ventral hippocampus, the nucleus supramammilaris, and the segmental fields of Forel. Factor VIII levels were increased by stimulation of the mesencephalic pontine reticular formation, central gray, lateral hypothalamic area, habenula, and habenular interpeduncular tract. There is a relationship between peripheral autonomic function and blood coagulation. Stress,[61] splanchnic nerve stimulation,[60] and epinephrine[60] administration may lead to hypercoagulability.

The mortality in disseminated intravascular coagulation associated with head injury is very high and may be caused by intractable cerebral edema, intracerebral or intraventricular hemorrhage, multiple organ failure as a result of microthrombosis, or uncontrollable hemorrhage. It is essential that appropriate coagulation studies be done early in the course of management of the head-injured patient. Therapy is directed primarily toward the underlying disease process. In the potentially salvageable patient, correction of hemostatic defects after head injury may occur spontaneously within hours, or it may require administration of cryoprecipitate (fibrinogen, factor VIII), fresh frozen plasma (factor V), platelet concentrates, and fresh red cells. Such therapy is of doubtful validity in the deeply comatose patient with evidence of irreversible brain damage. Heparin therapy may produce dramatic effects within a few hours, raising fibrinogen levels to normal, shortening thrombin times, raising the plasminogen levels, and allowing resynthesis of consumed clotting factors. However, heparin therapy may predispose the head-injured patient to intracranial hemorrhage and is therefore not recommended. Caution also should be exercised in the use of aspirin and steroids in the immediate posttrauma period because of deleterious effects on platelet function[26,282,393] and possible precipitation or aggravation of gastrointestinal bleeding.[145]

ENDOCRINOLOGIC SEQUELAE
Anterior Pituitary Insufficiency

Anterior pituitary insufficiency after head trauma is reported approximately one dozen times in the literature and is certainly a rare clinical condition.[5,147,290,394] At autopsy, however, recognizable pituitary or hypothalamic damage after head trauma is common.[116] Crompton[89] reported a 42% incidence of anterior hypothalamic ischemia or hemorrhage in a series of 106 patients who died soon after closed head injury. Multiple endocrine abnormalities, including unexplained elevations in growth hormone (GH), leutinizing hormone (LH), and follicle-stimulating hormone (FSH), are reported after mild, moderate, and severe head injury in the absence of diabetes insipidus.[205]

Patients with posttraumatic diabetes insipidus may have impaired anterior pituitary reserve for 1 or more hormones evident within one month after injury and often without clinical signs. The most common abnormality is GH deficiency, followed in order of frequency by adrenocorticotrophic hormone (ACTH), FSH, and LH. The severity of the anterior pituitary abnormalities did not appear to correlate with the severity of diabetes insipidus; however, the majority of patients had injuries to the temporal region. There are no reports of the duration and permanence of the observed anterior pituitary dysfunction.[25]

The pathogenesis of posttraumatic anterior pituitary insufficiency is not certain. Anterior lobe necrosis, similar in extent and location to the infarcted area after section of the pituitary stalk in animals and humans, has been observed in several autopsy series.[65,94] Pituitary infarction may be caused by traumatic rupture of the stalk or interruption of the vascular supply at the time of head injury. Because interruption of the long hypophyseal portal veins may cause

central anterior pituitary necrosis, Crompton[89] theorized that hypothalamic and stalk lesions were caused by shearing of small portal vessels at the time of impact. Hypopituitarism may be secondary to vascular collapse in the head-injured patient with associated hemorrhagic shock[339] or to traumatic hemorrhage into the pituitary gland.[312] It is more likely to occur in the patient with a skull fracture, especially of the middle fossa, and is frequently accompanied by transient or permanent diabetes insipidus[116]; normal ADH function can be maintained after pituitary stalk section because ADH can be released from fibers ending in the median eminence.[229,337]

Dzur and Winternitz[116] reported anterior pituitary insufficiency in a patient who sustained massive facial trauma and exhibited transient diabetes insipidus. Decreased ACTH, growth hormone, and gonadotropin and elevated prolactin levels were observed. These findings are consistent with a lesion separating the hypothalamus functionally from the anterior lobe of the pituitary and the loss of the hypothalamic inhibition leading to excessive prolactin secretion. Low or normal prolactin levels would be seen in conditions affecting the pituitary cells themselves because they are responsible for prolactin synthesis and release independent of the prolactin-inhibiting factor. Stimulation tests with synthetic thyrotropin-releasing factor (TRF) may show subnormal thyroid-stimulating hormone (TSH) and supranormal prolactin release by the anterior pituitary compatible with pituitary rather than hypothalamic dysfunction. In the presence of hypothalamic dysfunction, TRF would be expected to promote a significant release of TSH from the pituitary.[133,290]

Anterior pituitary insufficiency should be considered in patients with basal or temporal skull fractures and/or posttraumatic diabetes insipidus. Late developments are secondary amenorrhea, galactorrhea, regression of secondary sexual characteristics, poor recovery, posttraumatic psychosis, or persistent general malaise.[116] Appropriate replacement therapy is indicated when specific deficiencies are proved through endocrinologic testing. Precocious puberty is a rare sequela of head injury; however, discrete hypothalamic lesions visible with magnetic resonance scanning have been shown to be associated with a decrease in serum melatonin, an antigonadotropic amine. Anterior hypothalamic lesions have been linked to delayed puberty or hypogonadism.[237,332]

Posterior Pituitary Dysfunction
Diabetes Insipidus

Diabetes insipidus is a relatively common phenomenon after craniofacial trauma and basilar skull fracture[157] and can be permanent or transient, disappearing in a few days or weeks. McLaurin[245] reports that 6% of all cases of diabetes insipidus are caused by trauma. Hypoxic brain damage after cardiopulmonary arrest[318] and drug overdose[144] can cause diabetes insipidus. Hemorrhagic shock can predispose to necrosis of the posterior pituitary.[227,313] Diabetes insipidus has occurred after fat embolization to the posterior pituitary.[164,319]

Antidiuretic hormone, vasopressin, is an octapeptide synthesized in the supraoptic nuclei of the anterior hypothalamus and transported along the neurophyseal pathway attached to a large carrier protein, neurophysine, to be stored in the posterior lobe of the pituitary. It is released in response to many stimuli, the most important being increased plasma osmolality, hypovolemia, pain, emotional stress, drugs (nicotine, barbiturates, morphine, carbamazepine [Tegretol], tricyclic antidepressants, chlorpropamide, vincristine), hormonal mediators (thyroxin, angiotensin, glucocorticoids), cholinergic and beta-adrenergic stimulation, and positive airway pressure.* Head injury and acute intracranial hypertension can stimulate ADH production and release.[67,141] ADH secretion is inhibited by increased plasma volume, reduced plasma osmolality, alpha adrenergic stimulation, and several drugs such as ethanol, atropine, phenytoin, reserpine, and chlorpromazine.[126,207,260]

In the kidney, ADH attaches to the contraluminal side of the renal medullary tubular cell by means of a specific vasopressin receptor. It then activates renal medullary adenyl cyclase, which in turn stimulates production of cyclic AMP. Cyclic AMP activates a protein kinase on the luminal side of the cell, causing phosphorylation of membrane protein, leading to increased permeability of the cell to water, facilitating its transport into the intercellular spaces, into the renal medullary circulation, and back into the general circulation.[171,260,284] Adrenocortical insufficiency in humans is associated with a subnormal diuretic response to hydration and plasma hypoosmolality and sustained elevation of plasma ADH. Steroid replacement therapy lowers plasma ADH to normal and permits the normal diuretic response to hydration. Glucocorticoids may inhibit the secretory activity of the supraoptic neurons.[337]

Clinical manifestations of ADH deficiency include polyuria (greater than 2 to 3 L/day), polydipsia, hypernatremia, high serum osmolality (320 to 330 mOsm/kg), dilute urine, and a urine-to-serum osmolality ratio of less than one, implying a negative water balance. The differential diagnosis of polyuria after trauma or surgery in the area of the pituitary and hypothalamus may be difficult because there are a variety of causes. Solute diuresis may be the result of osmotic or loop diuretics, high urea levels, hypoglycemia, or the inability to retain sodium as a result of mineralocorticoid deficiency. During solute diuresis, urine specific gravity is between 1.009 and 1.035, urine osmolality is usually 250 to 320 mOsm/kg, serum sodium is normal or increased, and thirst is usually a prominent feature.[340]

The most commonly used diagnostic test of ADH deficiency is cautious fluid restriction with measurement of urine volume and osmolality.[260,261] A normal subject exposed to water deprivation can reduce urine flow to less than

0.5 ml/min and increase urine osmolality to greater than 800 mOsm/kg. Diagnosis can be confirmed by measurement of ADH levels in plasma and urine in relation to plasma osmolality. Response of the renal tubule can be tested by the administration of aqueous vasopressin intramuscularly or intravenously.[260,263,340]

Simultaneous measurement of urine and plasma osmolalities may be a useful rapid method of diagnosing diabetes insipidus, especially in a recently traumatized patient in whom water deprivation may be ill-advised. When plasma osmolality markedly exceeds urine osmolality, the diagnosis of diabetes insipidus is probable. Mild fluid restriction may then be done; if plasma osmolality still exceeds urine osmolality, the diagnosis is certain. This approach to screening may not be accurate in the presence of adrenal insufficiency, uremia, hyperglycemia, alcohol intoxication, or other conditions in which osmotically active substances are present in blood or urine (e.g., contrast material). High-dose steroid therapy (e.g., 16 mg dexamethasone) may also confuse the results. If polyuria is present, a therapeutic trial with synthetic vasopressin is indicated.[280]

Frequently, posttraumatic diabetes insipidus is transient; long-term therapy occasionally is necessary. Daily measurements of weight and careful records of intake and output, serum BUN, electrolytes, urine specific gravity, and osmolality are essential in the management of diabetes insipidus. For therapy, the patient's hourly urine output together with the usual estimate for insensible loss is replaced with solutions containing water and few or no electrolytes. The administration of sodium-containing solutions is perhaps the commonest error in the management of diabetes insipidus. Saline solutions deliver a continuing solute load to the kidneys and raise serum sodium rapidly because pure water is being lost.

If the patient is awake, alert, and able to take oral fluids, fluid balance can sometimes be maintained satisfactorily. If urinary output exceeds 250 ml/hr for 2 consecutive hours or 6 to 7 L/day, or the patient is unable to maintain fluid balance, exogenous vasopressin is indicated; aqueous vasopressin (5 to 10 IU intramuscularly or intravenously q 4 to 6 hours) or vasopressin tannate-in-oil (5 IU intramuscularly every 24 to 72 hours) may be used. Additional choices include lysine vasopressin nasal spray and DDAVP (1-deamino-8-D-arginine vasopressin). Lysine vasopressin nasal spray is a synthetic preparation that has a short duration of action and is associated with a high incidence of rhinitis. It is supplied in 5 ml bottles containing 50 IU/ml and can be administered by nasal instillation three to four times a day. Each spray delivers 2 IU. DDAVP is a long-acting synthetic analogue with no vasopressor action. It is supplied in 2.5 ml bottles with 100 µg/ml; the usual dose is 10 to 20 µg intranasally every 12 to 24 hours. Water intoxication (lethargy, confusion, seizures, and coma) can occur if excess vasopressin is administered.[28,340]

Nonhormonal treatment methods include chlorpropamide and thiazide diuretics. Chlorpropamide, an oral hypo-

---

*References 8, 260, 262, 271, 328, 350.

glycemic agent, is effective in reducing polyuria in hypothalamic but not nephrogenic diabetes insipidus. The drug is given in doses ranging from 50 to 250 mg/day. Chlorpropamide appears to act by potentiating the antidiuretic effect of low levels of endogenous ADH and is therefore most effective in mild cases.[71,254,388] Thiazide diuretics contract the extracellular fluid volume secondary to sodium loss and therefore reduce urine volume and raise urine osmolality by an indirect effect. The antidiuresis is enhanced by low sodium intake and diminished by a high sodium intake. Supplemental potassium is usually required.[117]

Syndrome of Inappropriate Antidiuretic Hormone Secretion

Schwartz[331] has described hyponatremia and renal salt-wasting unrelated to renal or adrenal disease in a variety of clinical conditions. The typical features of the syndrome of inappropriate antidiuretic hormone secretion (SIADH) are hyponatremia with corresponding hypoosmolality of the serum and extracellular fluid, continued renal excretion of sodium, absence of clinical evidence of volume depletion (normal skin turgor and blood pressure), urine osmolality greater than serum osmolality, and normal renal and adrenal function. The excessive water retention and renal sodium loss result in hypoosmolality of the extracellular fluid and lead to the picture of water intoxication. Symptoms include anorexia, nausea, vomiting, irritability, personality changes, and neurologic abnormalities (loss of reflexes, muscular weakness, bulbar or pseudobulbar palsy, positive Babinski sign, stupor, convulsions). The renal salt-wasting mechanism is obscure but is probably related to suppression of proximal tubular reabsorption of sodium in response to the expansion of extracellular fluid volume.[28] Aldosterone levels in patients with SIADH are in the normal range.[210] Many central nervous system conditions, including meningitis,[194] encephalitis,[320] head injury,[31,63,126,210,308] brain abscess, tumor,[63,132] Guillain-Barré syndrome,[85] acute intermittent porphyria,[28,275] and subarachnoid hemorrhage[191] have been associated with inappropriate ADH secretion, previously known as "cerebral salt-wasting."

Anesthesia and surgery can also cause elevations in blood ADH levels secondary to pain, stress, and various drugs.[104,259] In neurosurgical patients, all the cardinal features of SIADH can be produced by excess fluid administration to patients with increased ADH secondary to the stress of major trauma[42] or by the overvigorous administration of vasopressin in the therapy of diabetes insipidus.[216,331]

Continuous positive pressure ventilation (PEEP 10 cm H_2O) leads to water and sodium retention. The water retention (ADH release, increased urinary ADH) is related to a fall in cardiac output (decrease in right ventricular preload or reduced left ventricular filling caused by leftward displacement of the interventricular septum[188]) and is associated with a reduction in urinary output, renal blood flow, and glomerular filtration rate. This suggests that PEEP causes renal vasoconstriction and subsequent renin-angiotensin and aldosterone release, resulting in sodium retention.[8]

Other hyponatremic syndromes may be differentiated primarily on clinical grounds. True sodium-depletion hyponatremia is accompanied by evidence of a contracted blood volume (low blood pressure, decreased skin turgor, elevated hematocrit). In dilutional hyponatremia, edema is a prominent feature and there may be evidence of congestive heart failure or hepatic disease.[161] Urinary sodium is low (below 10 mmole/L) in both salt depletion and dilutional hyponatremia.

In a prospective study of 15 patients with facial bone fractures and associated cerebral injury, three had unequivocal SIADH. Inappropriate ADH secretion after head trauma probably results from overproduction or release of ADH in response to irritation of the hypothalamic-pituitary axis; limbic structures may facilitate or fail to inhibit ADH release.[31] Increased ADH secretion may be enhanced by stimulation of the intrathoracic volume receptors when patients are nursed in the head-up position. The head-up position may exacerbate SIADH if it is present; fluid restriction, common in the head-injured patient, may prevent the full-blown syndrome.[19]

In another series, SIADH developed in 84 (4.6%) of 1808 patients with head injury.[107] Excluding patients with mild head injury (842 patients), 8.2% of those with moderate or severe head trauma developed SIADH, which, when severe (serum sodium less than 125 mmole/L), caused marked neurologic deterioration.

The syndrome of inappropriate ADH secretion usually begins 3 to 15 days after trauma and with appropriate therapy lasts no more than 10 to 15 days. Treatment includes, most importantly, water restriction (600 to 800 ml 5% dextrose in 0.45% saline per 24 hours), with or without hypertonic saline; diuresis usually occurs in 36 to 48 hours. Patients in coma or with seizures may require hypertonic saline and diuretic therapy to promote water loss.[98] Rarely will it be necessary to institute specific therapy to inhibit ADH release (e.g., demeclocycline,[103,131] phenytoin[126,367]). Rapid correction of chronic hyponatremia has been associated with fatal central pontine and extrapontine myelinosis; on the other hand, severe acute hyponatremia can cause fatal cerebral edema and tentorial herniation. Despite the concern regarding rapid correction, a recent review suggests that rapid or slow treatment of acute or chronic hyponatremia with furosemide and isotonic or hypertonic saline is safe.[76]

In patients whose serum sodium is less than 110 mEq/L, 5% saline containing 855 mEq/L of sodium, or 3% saline containing 513 mEq/L can be used. Caution must be exercised in patients with heart disease, hypertension, or intracranial bleeding, and in the elderly. Phenytoin may be needed for control of seizures, and it has the desirable side effect of inhibiting ADH release in some patients with

SIADH, although routine oral or intramuscular administration has no significant clinical effect.[126]

It is conceivable that the hyponatremia after head injury is iatrogenic; that is, caused by excess fluid administration when ADH is increased because of the general stress reaction after major injury. Bouzarth and Shenkin[42] recommend 1000 ml of 2.5% glucose in 0.45% saline intravenously per 24 hours or 1 L of oral fluids, if tolerated. With this regime, sodium homeostasis was maintained in a group of 70 head-injured patients.

Fichman et al.[127] measured elevated ADH levels in 25 nonedematous patients on long-term thiazide therapy. These patients resembled those with inappropriate ADH syndrome, except that the low serum sodium was usually accompanied by hypokalemia and alkalosis. The potassium depletion of long-term diuretic therapy facilitates entry of sodium into cells, producing further extracellular fluid volume contraction; this may increase a volume-receptor–mediated release of vasopressin, with resultant water retention and hyponatremia.

Hyponatremia can occur after prolonged mannitol diuresis if sodium losses are not replaced, but in these patients total osmolality is increased and circulatory volume is reduced.

Although glucocorticoid therapy reduces ADH secretion and promotes renal free water clearance,[2,97] dexamethasone has no significant effect on salt and water balance in SIADH.[125]

METABOLIC SEQUELAE
Cerebrospinal Fluid Metabolic Changes

Cerebrospinal fluid (CSF) acid-base status more closely reflects brain interstitial fluid acid-base status than does either arterial or venous blood values.[246] Brain injury results in CSF lactic acidosis with low pH and bicarbonate concentration and systemic respiratory alkalosis.[198,246] The severity of CSF metabolic acidosis is related to the severity of the head injury and seems to depend on the amount of lactic acid produced by the injured and hypoxic brain tissue.[244] Persistently elevated CSF lactate would suggest continued cerebral ischemia and hypoxia.[246] Marked intracranial hypertension, causing a reduction in cerebral blood flow, is accompanied by long-lasting but reversible cerebral tissue lactic acidosis. The acidosis may explain the reactive hyperemia commonly seen in experimental models when blood flow is restored after a period of intracranial hypertension.[214]

A low CSF pH promotes spontaneous hyperventilation; lowering CSF carbon dioxide restores the normal 20:1 ratio of bicarbonate to carbon dioxide and returns CSF pH toward normal levels.[69]

Serotonin levels in CSF rise after head trauma; the higher the levels, the more severe the trauma.[383] CSF cyclic AMP levels were lowest in patients in the deepest grades of coma after head injury or spontaneous intracranial hemorrhage.[321]

Other reports indicate that acute brain injury can cause a temporary increase in brain and spinal fluid cyclic AMP.[385,395] The subnormal levels in comatose patients may reflect a depletion of brain cyclic AMP uniquely associated with prolonged coma after trauma or intracranial hemorrhage.[321]

CSF levels of brain-specific creatine kinase (CK-BB) isoenzyme correlate directly with the degree of head trauma as measured by the Glasgow Coma Scale. The highest isoenzyme values in the CSF are observed on admission or within 12 to 24 hours; the level is irregularly detectable for the next 24 to 72 hours. Secondary late increases in CK-BB were correlated with clinical evidence of secondary injury (hematoma, infarction, hypoxia, or pathologically increased ICP); its reappearance was associated with a 90% fatality rate. In general, the combination of a low Glasgow Coma Scale score and a high CK-BB level (greater than 200 U/L) was invariably fatal.[22]

Water and Electrolyte Balance

Head injury in the absence of exogenous steroids induces marked hypermetabolism and hypercatabolism. Head injury with brainstem involvement may elicit the greatest response.[403] Neurologic recovery occurs more rapidly in patients with better early nutritional support.[404] The majority of head-injured patients have no clinically detectable abnormalities of water and electrolyte balance. Sodium retention is a normal response to bodily injury. After head injury, sodium retention is related to the severity of injury, lasts 2 to 4 days, and appears to be related to aldosterone secretion and to hypothalamic stimulation with subsequent ACTH release. There is no relationship between the severity of sodium retention and the location of brain damage. Major trauma may lead to a mild degree of ADH-mediated water retention lasting 2 or 3 days. Prolonged retention is rare but does occur if inappropriate ADH secretion ensues. Despite sodium retention, head-injured patients may be mildly hyponatremic because of the concomitant water retention.[246] Negative water balance may be the result of diabetes insipidus. Fluid restriction, abnormal thirst mechanisms, high-protein hyperalimentation or tube feedings,[142] and prolonged osmotic diuresis reduce circulating volume and stimulate aldosterone-mediated salt retention. The hypertonicity promotes vasopressin-mediated water retention.[335]

Glucose Metabolism

Glucose intolerance is a common phenomenon after trauma.[204,244,335] High catecholamine levels diminish insulin release.[204,244] ACTH, serum cortisol, and growth hormone levels may be elevated after trauma.[206,246] Exogenously administered steroids are diabetogenic.[40] Serum immunoreactive insulin levels may be elevated but to levels lower than expected in relation to blood sugar elevations. Catecholamines and growth hormone oppose insulin release and cellular activity.[246] Steroids promote glyconeogenesis, increasing hepatic glucose production; they also may stimulate pancreatic beta cell function with ensuing exhaustion and degranulation of these cells, and peripheral glucose utilization is impaired through an unknown mechanism.[220] Severe diabetes develops in only a few patients receiving steroids, and in only patients with reduced insulin reserve (as in the adult-onset diabetic) is the diabetogenic action of steroids extreme.[10] Latent diabetes mellitus may be precipitated by trauma and may be detrimental to the patient's recovery if unrecognized.[246]

Nonketotic Hyperosmolar Hyperglycemic Coma

Nonketotic hyperosmolar hyperglycemic coma (NHHC) has been observed as a complication of many primary illnesses both in diabetic and nondiabetic patients.[10,241] Over a 3-year period, Park et al.[289] report a 10% incidence of this condition in seriously ill patients who died while in a neurosurgical intensive care unit. The patients had various neurosurgical conditions (transsphenoidal hypophysectomy for metastatic breast cancer, intracerebral hemorrhage, ischemic infarction, closed and penetrating head injury, brain tumor), and many had no previous history of diabetes mellitus. Diagnostic criteria for NHHC are listed in Box 32-2.

Blood sugars may range from 400 to 2700 mg/100 ml, sodium from 119 to 188 mEq/L, and plasma osmolality from 268 to 465 mOsm/kg; there may be severe potassium depletion and dehydration as a result of the osmotic diuresis. These patients may also exhibit leukocytosis, hemoconcentration, and azotemia with a BUN-to-creatinine ratio of 30:1 implying a prerenal extracellular fluid deficit; acute renal failure may also develop.[241] This condition has a 40% to 70% mortality rate. The average age of patients is 57 years. Two thirds of the patients have no previous history of diabetes mellitus; 50% have some precipitating event such as infection, dehydration caused by increased losses or inadequate replacement, or ingestion of drugs known to aggravate glucose homeostasis (thiazides,[46] steroids,[43,353] phenytoin,[146,294] and glycerol[333]). Many patients are febrile, in shock, and in coma; they may or may not have focal neurologic signs.[225] Coma and subsequent death are usually attributed to total body sodium depletion or to cellular dehydration, particularly in the brain,[303] although this may not be apparent at autopsy.[299] Patients with a normal level of consciousness have a considerably higher survival rate, less severe associated illness, and smaller requirements for insulin and fluid replacement.[241] Because serum glucose levels are not paralleled by high levels of glucose in brain and spinal fluid, an osmotic shift of free water into the intravascular space may occur, leading to severe intracellular dehydration of the brain and resultant coma.[75,303] In Park's series, autopsies on many of the patients did not show evidence of cerebral edema, transtentorial herniation, or brainstem damage, which implies that the central nervous system lesions present were compatible with survival except for the presence of NHHC. The causes of death in these patients were renal failure, dysrhythmias, cerebrovascular accidents, and systemic thromboembolic complications.[241,289]

In the neurosurgical patient, many factors predisposing to NHHC are present: steroids,[43,353] prolonged mannitol therapy,[21,143] hyperosmolar tube feedings,[142] phenytoin,[146,294] and limited water replacement. Whether hypothalamic damage predisposes to this condition is unknown. Nondiabetic severely head-injured patients who develop nonketotic hyperglycemia commonly have associated diabetes insipidus (not related to glucose loading), elevated ICP, and a uniformly fatal outcome.[252]

The pathogenesis of NHHC is not clear, particularly in those patients without a history of diabetes mellitus and who require no insulin therapy after resolution of NHHC. The absence of ketosis may reflect the antiketogenic effects of severe hyperglycemia or the effect of insulin on fat and carbohydrate metabolism. At very low plasma insulin concentrations (reported in patients with NHHC and maturity-onset diabetes mellitus), insulin has no effect on glucose uptake by cells, yet it still can inhibit release of free fatty acids from adipose tissue.[220,241]

Steroids have long been recognized for their diabetogenic potential secondary to increased hepatic glucose production, exhaustion of pancreatic beta cells, and decreased peripheral glucose utilization.[220] The diabetogenic action of steroids is extreme only when there is a reduced insulin reserve, as in the maturity-onset diabetic or in a patient with NHHC.[40,173] Hyperosmolar tube feedings may precipitate hypernatremia and hyperglycemia secondary to extracellular water deficits from osmotic diuresis or diarrhea. Thirst mechanisms are absent in the comatose patient, and there may be inattention to the state of hydration. Mannitol therapy in patients with acute renal failure or hepatic disease can lead to hyperosmolar states associated with increased or decreased serum sodium concentrations. Toxic serum phenytoin levels result in delayed and subnormal insulin response to a glucose load; hyperglycemia after phenytoin therapy has been observed in the critically ill diabetic and nondiabetic patient. Phenytoin has been shown to decrease tissue uptake of glucose and increase glycogenolysis in the liver.[146]

Before therapy, appropriate laboratory data must be obtained. Serum sodium may be high, low, or normal, de-

▼

BOX 32-2

DIAGNOSTIC CRITERIA FOR NONKETOTIC HYPEROSMOLAR HYPERGLYCEMIC COMA (NHHC)

Hyperglycemia	Plasma osmolality > 330 mOsm/kg
Glucosuria	Dehydration
Absence of ketosis	Central nervous system dysfunction

pending on the state of hydration. Urine sodium may be in the range of 10 to 50 mEq/L. Serum potassium is usually low because of the combined effects of the release of aldosterone stimulated by low extracellular fluid volume and the continued delivery of sodium to the distal tubule sodium-potassium exchange site as a result of the glucose diuresis. If lactic acidosis is also present, hydrogen ion may enter cells in exchange for potassium and result in elevated serum potassium in spite of total body depletion. When blood glucose rises above the renal threshold, glucose will appear in the urine and prevent maximal urine concentration even in the presence of ADH. Serum osmolality must be high to make the diagnosis of NHHC. Serum osmolality measured in an osmometer (freezing point depression) may be elevated because of the osmotic contribution of urea, which is free to move across the semipermeable cell membrane and therefore does not exert effective osmotic pressure in vivo. Effective osmolality can be calculated using the formula:

$$\text{Plasma osmolality} = 2(Na^+) + \text{glucose}/18$$

In an azotemic patient, this will be significantly lower than the osmolality measured in an osmometer, the difference representing the osmotic contribution of urea.

Hypovolemia and hypertonicity are the immediate threats to life. Hypotonic saline may not improve sodium and water deficits fast enough, therefore normal saline is used, unless a patient is hypertensive or edematous, until blood pressure and urine output are stabilized. If a patient is in hypovolemic shock, isotonic sodium chloride or plasma may be necessary regardless of the osmolality. Large amounts of insulin in such a patient may precipitate hypotension, shock, and subsequent renal failure because the drop in blood sugar may remove a significant percentage of the already inadequate plasma water.[128,368] Diuretics may be necessary if oliguria persists after sodium repletion. If plasma osmolality is normal or low in a hyperglycemic hyponatremic patient, there is excess water present; removal of the osmotic contribution of glucose by administering insulin or hypotonic saline may precipitate water intoxication.

Serial laboratory data are essential. After sodium deficits are replaced and blood pressure and urine output are stable, water deficits can be replaced with 0.45% saline. The volume of hypotonic fluid varies in individual patients but is usually greater than 5 L in the first 12 hours and averages 500 to 1300 ml/hr until plasma osmolality reaches 325 mOsm/L. Severe potassium losses may also have occurred as a result of the osmotic diuresis.

Hyperglycemia usually dramatically responds to relatively small doses of insulin. Large doses of insulin, with rapid lowering of serum glucose, may increase mortality by decreasing plasma volume before there has been adequate fluid and salt replacement, by producing cerebral edema or hypoglycemia. McCurdy recommends not exceeding 25 units of insulin per hour until sodium deficits have been replaced. When the effective plasma osmolality approaches 325 mOsm/L, decreased glucosuria permits renal mechanisms for salt and water homeostasis to finally restore osmolality and plasma volume to normal levels.[241]

Intermittent furosemide therapy for cerebral edema may obviate severe hyperosmolar stresses, particularly in the elderly, the adult-onset diabetic, or the patient with compromised renal function.[86]

GASTROINTESTINAL SEQUELAE

The relationship between intracranial disease and gastrointestinal bleeding has been known for over 100 years. Since Cushing's[93] paper on the coincidence of peptic ulceration and intracranial pathology, Cushing ulcer has been the term usually applied to all gastroduodenal ulcers coexisting with brain disease. In patients dying from intracranial disorders, the incidence of gastroduodenal ulceration and hemorrhage postmortem is twice that of those dying from all other causes (12.5% vs 6%). Esophageal ulceration seems to be more common in the neurologic population, but duodenal ulceration is more common in the nonneurologic population. The frequency of gastric lesions in both groups is approximately the same. There is no correlation between the type of neurosurgical disorder (diffuse or discrete) or intracranial hypertension and frequency of gastroduodenal hemorrhage or ulceration.[195]

In 433 patients with head injury of differing severity, the overall incidence of clinically detectable gastrointestinal bleeding (blood in gastric juice, melena detected at endoscopy) was 17%. There was a correlation between the severity of injury and the frequency of gastrointestinal bleeding. In comatose and decerebrate patients, the incidence was 30%. In severely injured patients receiving glucocorticoid therapy, the incidence was higher than in the less severely injured receiving steroid therapy. The presence of shock did not seem to predispose to bleeding.[192]

Cushing[93] thought that a diencephalic parasympathetic center stimulated vagal nuclei, inducing vagal hyperactivity and subsequent acid hypersecretion. French et al.[135] were able to produce prompt and excessive elevation of gastric acid secretion by direct anterior hypothalamic stimulation. Anterior hypothalamic ablative lesions frequently resulted in gastric mucosal and submucosal hemorrhages. Presumably the sympathetic center in the posterior hypothalamus was then unopposed and the hemorrhagic changes resulted from this imbalance. Prior sympathectomy protected animals from the hemorrhagic changes. Posterior hypothalamic lesions increased vagal tone, and pure gastric erosions occurred that could be prevented by vagotomy.

Watts and Clark[386] have reported gastric hyperacidity in patients comatose from head injury. Bleeding occurred in five of seven hypersecretors who were decerebrate with signs and symptoms of lower diencephalon or upper brainstem injury. Hyperacidity has not been demonstrated in patients with postburn (Curling) or postsurgical ulcers.[151]

Gastric mucosal barrier disruption may also play a role

in the pathogenesis of these ulcers.[348] As a group, patients with neurosurgical disease have normal gastric mucosal permeability. However, general surgical and neurosurgical patients who develop upper gastrointestinal bleeding have a significantly increased permeability and a higher incidence of sepsis, hypotension, respiratory failure, renal insufficiency, and jaundice than either of the groups with normal permeability.[151,346] Aspirin and ethanol increase gastric mucosal permeability.[249] Ethanol, in combination with aspirin and acid, is especially harmful and frequently produces mucosal bleeding.[95] Steroids do not alter gastric mucosal permeability but may increase the effect of other agents that do.[17,70]

The exact role of steroids in the production of gastroduodenal ulcerations is controversial. ACTH and cortisone[249] reduce the rate of renewal of surface epithelial cells and mucous secretion[250] in the canine gastric antrum. Gray et al.[155] have shown that human gastric acid and pepsin secretion increase after the administration of ACTH and cortisone and the physical stress of surgery. In Davis' series it was noted that neurosurgical patients with a previous history of gastrointestinal symptomatology experienced a reactivation of symptoms and frequently disastrous episodes of hematemesis after surgery.[96] Steroid ulcers are primarily antral and can effectively be prevented by antacid therapy.[149,309] Several prospective studies have failed to define the relationship between the frequency of peptic ulceration and steroid treatment.[83,84,253] In a prospective series of head-injured patients receiving steroids but not antacids, 79% had some evidence of gastrointestinal hemorrhage (as diagnosed by endoscopy); 37% of cases required 2 to 12 units of blood; and 16% required operative treatment. During the first 6 days after injury, no correlation between gastric hyperacidity, erosion, or hemorrhage and the presence of an intracranial mass, level of ICP, neurologic examination parameters, shock, hypoxemia, or sepsis could be demonstrated.[158]

Stress ulcer has been loosely used to refer to upper gastrointestinal lesions after major medical illnesses, surgery, trauma, severe burns, frostbite, neurosurgical procedures, or steroid therapy. Goodman has shown, in humans and in pigs, that ulcers after shock and sepsis are different clinically and pathologically from postburn, postneurosurgical, and steroid ulcers.[149] Evidence suggests that stress ulcers are not caused by circulating endogenous steroids. Ulcers after steroid therapy have a longer time course (4 to 10 days or longer) and tend to occur in the gastric antrum or duodenum, as opposed to the fundus.[145,309] In addition, Goodman and Osborne[149] were able to produce the typical fundal stress ulcer in adrenalectomized pigs. Long-term high-dose cortisone acetate therapy does not alter gastric antral or duodenal resistance to digestion by an acid pepsin stream.[391]

Hemorrhagic shock is a specific and sufficient stress for the production of superficial, linear erosions of the gastric fundus,[38,168,209] primarily on the crests of the rugal folds.

Most patients with these lesions eventually die from severe and persistent hemorrhage superimposed on their already grave clinical conditions. These lesions may be secondary to mucosal ischemia.[384] Hemorrhagic shock leads to elevated catecholamine levels. It is not clear whether hypovolemia alone or in combination with increased sympathetic tone is responsible for the observed severe reductions in mucosal blood flow. Klemperer[209] and Baronofsky[24] were able to produce arteriolar vasospasm and gastric ulceration after epinephrine administration. Vasoconstriction and resultant ischemia are regularly followed by mucosal hemorrhage and ulceration. It is possible that ulceration could result from hypercoagulable, hyperviscous, or hypoxic[288] states associated with various disease processes. The hypovolemia, hemoconcentration, high peripheral resistance, and reduced cardiac output in the immediate postburn period seem to predispose to decreased organ flow and may lead to gastric mucosal ischemia.[129,283,305]

The neurogenic ulcer tends to perforate as a result of esophagogastric malacia, whereas acute postshock ulcers rarely perforate.[93,149,352] Postburn ulcers are located primarily at the depths of the rugal folds of the gastric fundus and the duodenum.[149] They are round and deep, with well-defined margins, and may show bacterial colonies at their base.[283,305] Stress ulcers appear in the corpus of the stomach and involve the antrum and duodenum only in the most severe cases. These superficial lesions are common after multiple trauma and may develop in a few hours; the incidence of bleeding from stress ulcers is low, particularly with antacid prophylaxis.[251,304]

Goodman and Osborne suggest a reclassification of stress ulcers as follows: (1) ulcers after head trauma and intracranial operations are neurogenic ulcers; (2) postburn ulcers are Curling ulcers; (3) ulcers after long-term steroid therapy are steroid ulcers; and (4) posttraumatic and postsurgical ulcers associated with shock and sepsis are stress ulcers.[149]

Other sources of gastric irritation may be present in head-injured patients. Ethanol ingestion can produce hemorrhagic gastritis. Aspirin and phenylbutazone[236] cause shedding of gastric surface mucosal cells without a concomitant increase in the rate of cell renewal. They reduce antral mucous secretion, as do ACTH and cortisone.[102,248-250] Ethanol and aspirin increase gastric mucosal permeability.[350] Aspirin and phenylbutazone depress platelet aggregation[351,393,406] and may oppose prostaglandin regulation of gastric acid secretion.[378] Positive end-expiratory pressure and passive hyperventilation may lead to increased splanchnic vascular resistance and subsequent gastric mucosal ischemia.[190]

Signs and symptoms of gastrointestinal ulceration and/or perforation may include abdominal distention, ileus, anemia, hypotension, hematemesis, melena, and pain; the last symptom depends of course on the level of consciousness of the patient. Steroid-induced bleeding into the gastrointestinal tract may be painless. Antacid therapy administered orally or via nasogastric tube may be of value in preventing and treating postneurosurgical and steroid ulcers.[145] Anticholinergic drugs reduce acid secretion in comatose patients.[278] Maintaining gastric pH above 5 may be effective in reducing the need for surgical control of bleeding; however, double-blind series are lacking. Bleeding is usually self-limiting and requires nasogastric suction (perhaps cold saline lavage), fluid replacement, and transfusion if anemia is severe. When operative treatment is necessary for protracted hemorrhage, partial gastrectomy and vagotomy may be more effective operative treatment than vagotomy and pyloroplasty.[305,345]

Histamine appears to be the major, if not the only, stimulator of parietal cell hydrogen ion secretion.[78] The final common pathway is an H_2 receptor at the base of the parietal cell.[36,47] H_2 receptor blockers inhibit all forms of gastric secretion.[226] Both cimetidine and intensive antacid regimens reduce the incidence of gastric hemorrhage in the critically ill[163,304] and may be particularly indicated in patients with a peptic ulcer disease history.

H_2 receptor–blocking drugs can produce agranulocytosis.[87] Cimetidine treatment has been shown to stimulate prolactin secretion in humans but has no effect on thyrotropin, growth hormone, or thyroxine levels. Perhaps histamine has an important function in the regulation of prolactin secretion in humans.[62] Of interest is the effect of H_2 blockers on cerebrovascular reactivity. Cimetidine has been shown to inhibit the hypoxia-induced increase in cerebral blood flow in dogs subjected to FIo_2 0.10. Ranitidine did not prevent the increase at normal doses, but increased doses blunted the response.[8,77]

SKELETAL SEQUELAE

Cervical spine injury will be addressed comprehensively in Chapter 33; maxillofacial injuries are the focus in this section.

Maxillofacial Injuries

Blunt cervical trauma can lead to carotid artery injury. Compression or stretching of the vessel may lead to thrombosis, transient ischemic attacks, Horner syndrome, or lateral neck hematoma and airway obstruction.[189] Hyperextension of the neck combined with flexion or rotation can stretch the cervical portion of the carotid artery over the bony prominences of the cervical spine, usually the transverse process of C3. An intimal tear with dissection, throm-

bosis, and distal embolization may occur. The delayed onset of a neurologic deficit after trauma with a normal CT scan should prompt angiographic examination of the cervical portion of the carotid and vertebral vessels.[326,360] The vertebral artery is also vulnerable to hyperextension and rotational neck injuries[130] or mechanical compression at any fracture dislocation at and above the sixth cervical vertebra, particularly at the atlantoaxial level.[327] Basilar artery occlusion can result from clival fractures,[223] and thrombus propagation, internal dissection, or distal embolization can result from an endothelial injury to the vertebral artery.[274]

Horner syndrome may develop after neck trauma as a result of pressure or direct injury to the sympathetic supply to the face. Unilateral pupillary constriction that results may lead to confusion and overtreatment of a suspected intracranial mass. A combination of relative miosis, slight ptosis (narrowing of the palpebral fissure), slight enophthalmus, increase in temperature and sweating on the affected side of the face, and preservation of normal reflexes to light and convergence should lead to the diagnosis.[399]

Subcutaneous emphysema may result from frontal or ethmoid sinus fractures and has to be distinguished from that caused by thoracic, tracheal, or esophageal injury. Cribriform plate fractures may allow a nasogastric tube to enter the intracranial space.[401] In such circumstances, these tubes must be placed under direct vision through the mouth. Position of the tube must be verified radiographically before application of suction or injection of air or irrigating fluids.[41] Gastrostomy may be indicated.

▼

SUMMARY

Head injury cannot be considered an isolated, single-system injury. Head-injured patients frequently sustain other organ trauma. Equally important are the multisystem effects of trauma to any part of the body and the unique effects of head trauma on the hypothalamic-pituitary axis, which influences such diverse pansystemic functions as blood coagulation, pulmonary venular tone, gastric acid secretion, renal water conservation, and glucose metabolism. Management of most head injuries is nonsurgical, and quality functional survival obviously depends on attention to these multisystem derangements.

References

1. Abrams JS, Deane RS, Davis JH: Pulmonary function in patients with multiple trauma and associated severe head injury, *J Trauma* 16:543-549, 1976.

2. Ahmed ABJ, George BC, Gonzalez-Auvert C et al: Increased plasma arginine vasopressin in clinical adrenocortical insufficiency and its inhibition by glucosteroids, *J Clin Invest* 46:111-123, 1967.

3. Aidinis SJ, Lafferty J, Shapiro HM: Intracranial responses to PEEP, *Anesthesiology* 45:275-286, 1976.

4. Allardyce B, Hamit HF, Matsumoto T et al: Pulmonary vascular changes in hypovolemic shock: radiography of the pulmonary microcirculation and the possible role of platelet embolism in increasing vascular resistance, *J Trauma* 9:403-411, 1969.

5. Altman R, Pruzanski W: Posttraumatic hypopituitarism, *Ann Intern Med* 55:149-154, 1961.

6. Anderson JM, Brown JK: Brain ischemia and disseminated intravascular coagulation, *Lancet* 1:373-374, 1972.

7. Andreoli A, diPasquale G, Pinelli G et al: Subarachnoid hemorrhage: frequency and severity of cardiac arrhythmias. A survey of 70 cases studied in the acute phase, *Stroke* 18:558-564, 1987.

8. Annat G, Viale JP, Xuan BB et al: Effect of PEEP ventilation on renal function, plasma renin, aldosterone, neurophysins and urinary ADH, and prostaglandins, *Anesthesiology* 58:136-141, 1983.

9. Apuzzo MLJ, Weiss MH, Petersons V et al: Effect of positive end expiratory pressure ventilation on intracranial pressure in man, *J Neurosurg* 46:227-232, 1977.

10. Arieff AL, Carroll HJ: Nonketotic hyperosmolar coma with hyperglycemia: clinical features, pathophysiology, renal function, acid-base balance, plasma-cerebrospinal fluid equilibria and the effects of therapy in 37 cases, *Medicine* 51:73-94, 1972.

11. Armstrong HJ, Kuenzig MC, Peltier LF: Lung lipase levels in normal rats and rats with experimentally produced fat embolism, *Proc Soc Exp Biol Med* 124: 959-961, 1967.

12. Ashbaugh DG, Bigelow DB, Petty TL et al: Acute respiratory distress in adults, *Lancet* 2:319-323, 1967.

13. Ashbaugh DG, Petty TL: Positive end-expiratory pressure: physiology, indications and contraindications, *J Thorac Cardiovasc Surg* 65:165-170, 1973.

14. Ashbaugh DG, Petty TL: The use of corticosteroids in the treatment of respiratory failure associated with massive fat embolism, *Surg Gynecol Obstet* 123:493-500, 1966.

15. Astrup T: Assay and content of tissue thromboplastin in different organs, *Thromb Diath Haemorrh* 14:401-416, 1965.

16. Attar S, Boyd D, Layne E et al: Alterations in coagulation and fibrinolytic mechanisms in acute trauma, *J Trauma* 9:939-965, 1969.

17. Aubrey DA, Burns GP: Topically administered prednisolone and the antral phase of gastric secretion, *Arch Surg* 105:448-453, 1972.

18. Audibert G, Sauvier C, Hartemann D et al: Effects of H_2-receptor blockers on response of cerebral blood flow to normocapneic hypoxia, *Anesth Analg* 72:532-537, 1991.

19. Auger RG, Zehr JE, Siekert RG et al: Position effect on antidiuretic hormone, *Arch Neurol* 23:513-517, 1970.

20. Aviado DM: Adenosine diphosphate and vasoactive substances, *J Trauma* 8:880-890, 1968.

21. Aviram A, Pfau A, Czaczkes JW et al: Hyperosmolality with hyponatremia, caused by inappropriate administration of mannitol, *Am J Med* 42:648-650, 1967.

22. Bakay RAE, Ward AA: Enzymatic changes in serum and cerebrospinal fluid in neurological injury, *J Neurosurg* 58:27-37, 1983.

23. Baker AB: Poliomyelitis 16: a study of pulmonary edema, *Neurology* 7:743-751, 1957.

24. Baronofsky I, Wangensteen OH: Erosion or ulcer (gastric and/or duodenal) experimentally produced through the agency of chronic arterial spasm invoked by the intramuscular implantation of epinephrine or pitressin in beeswax, *Bull Am Coll Surg* 30:59-60, 1945.

25. Barrecca T, Perria C, Samnia A et al: Evaluation of anterior pituitary function in patients with posttraumatic diabetes insipidus, *J Clin Endocrinol Metab* 51:1279-1282, 1980.

26. Barrer MJ, Ellison N: Platelet function, *Anesthesiology* 46:202-211, 1977.

27. Bartsch P, Magglorini M, Ritter M et al: Prevention of high-altitude pulmonary edema by nifedipine, *N Engl J Med* 325:1284-1289, 1991.

28. Bartter FC, Schwartz WB: The syndrome of inappropriate secretion of antidiuretic hormone, *Am J Med* 42:790-806, 1967.

29. Bean JW, Beckman DL: Centrogenic pulmonary pathology in mechanical head injury, *J Appl Physiol* 27:807-812, 1969.

30. Beck GP, Neill LW: Anesthesia for associated trauma in patients with head injuries, *Anesth Analg* 42:687-695, 1963.

31. Becker RM, Daniel RK: Increased antidiuretic hormone production after trauma to the craniofacial complex, *J Trauma* 13:112-115, 1973.

32. Beckman DL, Bean JW, Baslock DR: Neurogenic influence in pulmonary compliance, *J Trauma* 14:111-115, 1974.

33. Bedford RF, Persing JA, Pobereskin LH et al: Lidocaine or thiopental for rapid control of intracranial hypertension? *Anesth Analg* 59:435-437, 1980.

34. Berman IR, Ducker TB: Pulmonary, somatic, and splanchnic circulatory responses to increased intracranial pressure, *Ann Surg* 169:210-216, 1969.

35. Berman IR, Ducker TB: Changes in pulmonary, somatic, and splanchnic perfusion with increased intracranial pressure, *Surg Gynecol Obstet* 128:8-14, 1969.

36. Black JW, Duncan WAM, Durant CJ et al: Definition and antagonism of histamine H_2-receptors, *Nature* 236:385-390, 1972.

37. Blaisdell FW, Lim RC, Stallone RJ: The mechanism of pulmonary damage following traumatic shock, *Surg Gynecol Obstet* 130:15-22, 1970.

38. Boles RS, Riggs HE, Griffiths JO: The role of the circulation in the production of peptic ulcer, *Am J Dig Dis* 6:632-636, 1939.

39. Bonbrest HC: Pulmonary edema following an epileptic seizure, *Am Rev Resp Dis* 91:97-100, 1965.

40. Bookman JJ, Drachman SR, Schaefer LE et al: Steroid diabetes in man: the development of diabetes during treatment with cortisone and corticotropin, *Diabetes* 2:100-111, 1953.

41. Borovich B, Braun J, Yosefovich T et al: Intracranial penetration of nasogastric tube, *Neurosurgery* 8:245-247, 1981.

42. Bouzarth WF, Shenkin HA: Is "cerebral hyponatremia" iatrogenic? *Lancet* 1:1061-1062, 1982.

43. Boyer MH: Hyperosmolar anacidotic coma in association with glucocorticoid therapy, *JAMA* 202:1007-1009, 1967.

44. Brashear RE, Ross JC: Hemodynamic effects of elevated cerebrospinal fluid pressure: alterations with adrenergic blockade, *J Clin Invest* 49:1324-1333, 1970.

45. Braunstein PW: Medical aspects of automotive crash injury research, *JAMA* 163:249-255, 1957.

46. Brenner WI, Lansky Z, Engelman RM et al: Hyperosmolar coma in surgical patients: an iatrogenic disease of increasing incidence, *Ann Surg* 178:651-654, 1973.

47. Brimblecombe RW, Duncan WAM, Durant CJ: Cimetidine— a nonthiourea H_2-receptor antagonist, *J Intern Med Res* 3:86-92, 1975.

48. Brisman R, Kovach RM, Johnson DO et al: Pulmonary edema in acute transection of the cervical spinal cord, *Surg Gynecol Obstet* 139:363-366, 1974.

49. Brown FK: Cardiovascular effects of acutely raised intracranial pressure, *Am J Physiol* 185:510-514, 1956.

50. Brown RS, Mohr PA, Carey JS et al: Cardiovascular changes after cerebral injury and increased intracranial pressure, *Surg Gynecol Obstet* 125:1205-1211, 1967.

51. Bruecke P, Burke JF, Lam KW et al: The pathophysiology of pulmonary fat embolism, *J Thorac Cardiovasc Surg* 61:949-955, 1971.

52. Brueggemann MW, Loudon RG, McLaurin RL: Pulmonary compliance changes after experimental head injury, *J Trauma* 16:16-20, 1976.

53. Burchiel KJ, Steege TD, Wyler AR: Intracranial pressure changes in brain-injured patients requiring positive end-expiratory pressure ventilation, *Neurosurgery* 8:443-449, 1981.

54. Byer E, Ashman R, Toth LA: Electrocardiogram with large, upright T waves and long QT intervals, *Am Heart J* 33:796-806, 1947.

55. Cameron GR: Pulmonary oedema, *Br Med J* 1:965-972, 1948.

56. Cameron GR, De SN: Experimental pulmonary edema of nervous origin, *J Pathol Bacteriol* 61:375-387, 1949.

57. Campbell GS, Haddy FJ, Adams WL et al: Circulatory changes and pulmonary lesions in dogs following increased intracranial pressure and the effect of atropine upon such changes, *Am J Physiol* 158:96-102, 1949.

58. Campbell GS, Visscher MB: Pulmonary lesions in guinea pigs with increased intracranial pressure and the effect of bilateral cervical vagotomy, *Am J Physiol* 157:130-134, 1949.

59. Reference deleted in proofs.

60. Cannon WB, Gray H: Factors affecting the coagulation time of blood. II. The hastening or retarding of coagulation by adrenalin injections, *Am J Physiol* 34:232-242, 1914.

61. Cannon WB, Mendenhall WL: Factors affecting the coagulation time of blood. IV. The hastening of coagulation in pain and emotional excitement, *Am J Physiol* 34:251-261, 1914.

62. Carlson HE, Ippoliti AF: Cimetidine, an H_2-antihistamine, stimulates prolactin secretion in man. *J Clin Endocrinol Metab* 45:367-370, 1977.

63. Carter NW, Rector FC, Seldin DW: Hyponatremia in cerebral disease resulting from inappropriate secretion of antidiuretic hormone, *N Engl J Med* 264:67-72, 1961.

64. Cassidy SS, Eschenbacher WL, Robertson CH et al: Cardiovascular effects of positive pressure ventilation in normal subjects, *J Appl Physiol* 47:453-461, 1979.

65. Ceballos R: Pituitary changes in head trauma (analysis of 102 consecutive cases of head injury), *Ala J Med Sci* 3:185-198, 1966.

66. Chandler WF, Dimcheff DG, Taren JA: Acute pulmonary edema following venous air embolism during a neurosurgical procedure, *J Neurosurg* 40:400-404, 1974.

67. Chang LR, Chen CF, Chai CY: The effect of head injury on antidiuretic hormone synthesis or release in rats, *Arch Int Physiol Biochem* 80:679-684, 1972.

68. Chen HI, Sun SC, Chai CY: Pulmonary edema and hemorrhage resulting from cerebral compression, *Am J Physiol* 224:223-229, 1973.

69. Christensen MS: Acid-base changes in cerebrospinal fluid and blood, and blood volume changes following prolonged hyperventilation in man, *Br J Anaesth* 46:348-357, 1974.

70. Chung RSK, Field M, Silen W: Effects of methylprednisolone on hydrogen ion absorption in the canine stomach, *J Clin Invest* 62:262-270, 1978.

71. Cinotti GA, Stirati G, Ruggiero F: Abnormal water retention and symptomatic hyponatremia in idiopathic diabetes insipidus during chlorpropamide therapy, *Postgrad Med* 48:107-112, 1972.

72. Ciongoli AK, Poser CM: Pulmonary edema secondary to subarachnoid hemorrhage, *Neurology* 22:867-870, 1972.

73. Clark JA, Finelli RE, Netsky MG: Disseminated intravascular coagulation following cranial trauma, *J Neurosurg* s2:266-269, 1980.

74. Clark K: The incidence and mechanisms of shock in head injury, *South Med J* 55:513-517, 1962.

75. Clements R, Prockop L, Winegrad A: Acute cerebral edema during treatment of hyperglycemia, *Lancet* 2:384-386, 1968.

76. Cluitmans FHM, Meinders AE: Management of severe hyponatremia: rapid or slow correction? *Am J Med* 88:161-166, 1990.

77. Clozel HP, Amend P, Sauvier C et al: Cimetidine inhibits the hypoxia-induced increase in cerebral blood flow in dogs, *Crit Care Med* 13:976-981, 1985.

78. Code CF: Reflections on histamine, gastric secretion and the H_2-receptor, *N Engl J Med* 296:1459-1462, 1977.

79. Cohen HB, Gambill AF, Eggers GWN: Acute pulmonary edema following head injury: two case reports, *Anesth Analg* 56:136-139, 1977.

80. Cohn JN, Franciosa JA: Vasodilator therapy of cardiac failure, *N Engl J Med* 297:254-258, 1977.

81. Colice GL: Neurogenic pulmonary edema, *Clin Chest Med* 6:473-489, 1985.

82. Colman RW, Robboy SJ, Minna JD: Disseminated intravascular coagula-

tion (DIC): an approach, *Am J Med* 52:679-684, 1972.

83. Conn HO, Blitzer BL: Nonassociation of adrenocorticosteroid therapy and peptic ulcer, *N Engl J Med* 294:473-479, 1976.
84. Cooper PR, Moody S, Clark WK et al: Dexamethasone and severe head injury, *J Neurosurg* 51:307-316, 1979.
85. Cooper WC, Green IJ, Wang S: Cerebral salt wasting associated with the Guillain-Barré syndrome, *Arch Intern Med* 116:113-119, 1965.
86. Cottrell JE, Robustelli A, Post K et al: Furosemide- and mannitol-induced changes in intracranial pressure and serum osmolality and electrolytes, *Anesthesiology* 47:28-30, 1977.
87. Craven ER, Whittington JM: Agranulocytosis four months after cimetidine therapy (letter), *Lancet* 2:294-295, 1977.
88. Crighton HC, Giesecke AH: One year's experience in the anesthetic management of trauma, *Anesth Analg* 45:835-842, 1966.
89. Crompton MR: Hypothalamic lesions following closed head injury, *Brain* 94:165-172, 1971.
90. Cruz J, Allen SJ, Miner ME: Hypoxic insults in acute brain injury, *Crit Care Med* 13:284, 1985.
91. Cushing H: Concerning a definite regulatory mechanism of the vasomotor centre which controls blood pressure during cerebral compression, *Johns Hopkins Hosp Bull* 12:290-292, 1901.
92. Cushing H: Some experimental and clinical observations concerning states of increased intracranial tension, *Am J Med Sci* 124:375-400, 1902.
93. Cushing H: Peptic ulcers and the interbrain, *Surg Gynecol Obstet* 55:1-34, 1932.
94. Daniel PM, Prichard MML, Treip CS: Traumatic infarction of the anterior lobe of the pituitary gland, *Lancet* 2:927-930, 1959.
95. Davenport HW: Gastric mucosal hemorrhage in dogs: effects of acid, aspirin, and alcohol, *Gastroenterology* 56:439-449, 1969.
96. Davis RA, Wetzel N, Davis L: Acute upper alimentary tract ulceration and hemorrhage following neurosurgical operations, *Surg Gynecol Obstet* 100:51-58, 1955.

97. Davis BB, Bloom ME, Field JB et al: Hyponatremia in pituitary insufficiency, *Metabolism* 18:821-832, 1969.
98. Decaux G, Waterlot Y, Genette F et al: Treatment of the syndrome of inappropriate secretion of anti-diuretic hormone with furosemide, *N Engl J Med* 304:329-330, 1981.
99. Denny-Brown D, Russel WR: Experimental cerebral concussion, *Brain* 64:93-164, 1941.
100. Dèry R, Pelletier J, Jacques A et al: Alveolar collapse induced by denitrogenation, *Can Anaesth Soc* 12:531-544, 1965.
101. De Salles AAF, Muizelaar JP, Young HF: Hyperglycemia, cerebrospinal fluid lactic acidoses, and cerebral blood flow in severely head injured patients, *Neurosurgery* 21:45-50, 1987.
102. Desbaillets L, Menguy R: Inhibition of gastric mucous secretion by ACTH: an experimental study, *Am J Dig Dis* 12:582-588, 1967.
103. DeTroyer A, Demanet JC: Correction of antidiuresis by demeclocycline, *N Engl J Med* 293:915-918, 1975.
104. Deutsch S, Goldberg M, Dripps RD: Postoperative hyponatremia with the inappropriate release of anti-diuretic hormone, *Anesthesiology* 27:250-256, 1966.
105. Deykin D: The clinical challenge of disseminated intravascular coagulation, *N Engl J Med* 283:636-644, 1970.
106. Dines DE, Linscheid RL, Didier EP: Fat embolism syndrome, *Mayo Clin Proc* 47:237-240, 1972.
107. Doczi T, Tarjanyi J, Huszka E et al: Syndrome of inappropriate secretion of antidiuretic hormone (SIADH) after head injury, *Neurosurgery* 10:685-688, 1982.
108. Downs JB, Klein EF, Modell JH: The effect of incremental PEEP on Pao_2 in patients with respiratory failure, *Anesth Analg* 52:210-215, 1973.
109. Drayer BP, Poser CM: Disseminated intravascular coagulation and head trauma: two case studies, *JAMA* 231:174-175, 1975.
110. Duberstein JL, Kaufman DM: A clinical study of an epidemic of heroin intoxication and heroin-induced pulmonary edema, *Am J Med* 51:704-714, 1971.
111. Ducker TB: Increased intracranial

pressure and pulmonary edema, I. Clinical study of 11 patients, *J Neurosurg* 28:112-117, 1968.
112. Ducker TB, Simmons RL: Increased intracranial pressure and pulmonary edema. II. The hemodynamic response of dogs and monkeys to increased intracranial pressure, *J Neurosurg* 28:118-123, 1968.
113. Ducker TB, Simmons RL, Anderson RW: Increased intracranial pressure and pulmonary edema. III. The effect of increased intracranial pressure on the cardiovascular hemodynamics of chimpanzees, *J Neurosurg* 29:475-483, 1968.
114. Ducker TB, Simmons RL, Martin AM: Pulmonary edema as a complication of intracranial disease, *Am J Dis Child* 118:638-641, 1969.
115. Dueck R, Wagner PD, West JB: Effects of positive end-expiratory pressure on gas exchange in dogs with normal and edematous lungs, *Anesthesiology* 47:359-366, 1977.
116. Dzur J, Winternitz WW: Posttraumatic hypopituitarism: anterior pituitary insufficiency secondary to head trauma, *South Med J* 69:1377-1379, 1976.
117. Earley LE, Orloff J: The mechanism of antidiuresis associated with the administration of hydrochlorthiazide to patients with vasopressin-resistant diabetes insipidus, *J Clin Invest* 41:1988-1997, 1962.
118. Eckenhoff JE, Enderby GEH, Larson A et al: Pulmonary gas exchange during deliberate hypotension, *Br J Anaesth* 35:750-758, 1963.
119. El-Naggar M: Weaning, *Mid East J Anaesth* 3:401-406, 1972.
120. Evarts CM: The fat embolism syndrome: a review, *Surg Clin North Am* 50:493-507, 1970.
121. Farber S: Studies on pulmonary edema. II. The pathogenesis of neuropathic pulmonary edema, *J Exp Med* 66:405-411, 1937.
122. Farber S: Neuropathic pulmonary edema, *Arch Pathol* 30:180-197, 1940.
123. Feeley TW, Hedley-Whyte J: Weaning from controlled ventilation and supplemental oxygen, *N Engl J Med* 292:903-906, 1975.
124. Fentz V, Gormsen J: Electrocardiographic patterns in patients with cerebrovascular accidents, *Circulation* 25:22-28, 1962.
125. Fichman MP, Bethune JE: The role

of adreno-corticoids in the inappropriate antidiuretic hormone syndrome, *Ann Intern Med* 68:806-820, 1968.

126. Fichman MP, Kleeman CR, Bethune JE: Inhibition of antidiuretic hormone secretion by diphenylhydantoin, *Arch Neurol* 22:45-53, 1970.

127. Fichman MP, Vorherr H, Kleeman CR et al: Diuretic-induced hyponatremia, *Ann Intern Med* 75:853-863, 1971.

128. Fitzgerald MG, O'Sullivan DJ, and Malins JM: Fatal diabetic ketosis, *Br Med J* 1:247-250, 1961.

129. Fletcher DG, Harkins HN: Acute peptic ulcer as a complication of major surgery, stress, or trauma, *Surgery* 36:212-226, 1954.

130. Ford FR, Clark D: Thrombosis of the basilar artery with softenings in the cerebellum and brain stem due to manipulation of the neck, *Johns Hopkins Med J* 98:3742, 1956.

131. Forrest JN, Cox M, Hong C et al: Superiority of demeclocycline over lithium in the treatment of chronic syndrome of inappropriate secretion of antidiuretic hormone, *N Engl J Med* 298:173-177, 1978.

132. Fox JL, Falik JL, and Shalhoub RJ: Neurosurgical hyponatremia: the role of inappropriate antidiuresis, *J Neurosurg* 34:506-514, 1971.

133. Frantz AG: Prolactin, *N Engl J Med* 298:201-207, 1978.

134. Freeman J, Nunn JF: Ventilation-perfusion relationships after haemorrhage, *Clin Sci* 24:135-147,1963.

135. French JD, Porter RW, von Amerongen FK et al: Gastrointestinal hemorrhage and ulceration associated with intracranial lesions, *Surgery* 32:395-407, 1952.

136. Froman C: Alterations of respiratory function in patients with severe head injuries, *Br J Anaesth* 40:354-360, 1968.

137. Frost EAM: Effects of positive end-expiratory pressure on intracranial pressure and compliance in brain-injured patients, *J Neurosurg* 47:195-200, 1977.

138. Fuchsig P, Brucke P, Blumel G et al: A new clinical and experimental concept on fat embolism, *N Engl J Med* 276:1192-1193, 1967.

139. Galloon S, Rees GAD, Briscoe C.E et al: Prospective study of electrocardiographic changes associated with subarachnoid hemorrhage, *Br J Anaesth* 44: 511-515, 1972.

140. Garcia-Uria J, Hoff JT, Miranda S et al: Experimental neurogenic pulmonary edema. II. The role of cardiopulmonary pressure change, *J Neurosurg* 54:632-636, 1981.

141. Gaufin L, Skowsky WR, Goodman SJ: Release of antidiuretic hormone during mass-induced elevation of intracranial pressure, *J Neurosurg* 46:627-637, 1977.

142. Gault MH, Dixon ME, Doyle M et al: Hypernatremia, azotemia, and dehydration due to high-protein tube feeding, *Ann Intern Med* 68:778-791, 1968.

143. Gipstein RM, Boyle JD: Hypernatremia complicating prolonged mannitol diuresis, *N Engl J Med* 272:1116-1117, 1965.

144. Glauser FL: Diabetes insipidus in hypoxemic encephalopathy, *JAMA* 235:932-933, 1976.

145. Glenn F, Grafe WR: Surgical complications of adrenal steroid therapy, *Ann Surg* 165:1023-1034, 1967.

146. Goldberg EM, Sanbar SS: Hyperglycemic, nonketotic coma following administration of Dilantin (diphenylhydantoin), *Diabetes* 18:101-106, 1969.

147. Goldman KP, Jacobs A: Anterior and posterior pituitary failure after head injury, *Br Med J* 2:1924-1926, 1960.

148. Goodnight SH, Kenoyer G, Rapaport SI et al: Defibrination after brain tissue destruction; a serious complication of head injury, *N Engl J Med* 290:1043-1047, 1974.

149. Goodman AA, Osborne MP: An experimental model and clinical definition of stress ulceration, *Surg Gynecol Obstet* 134:563-571, 1972.

150. Gopinathan K, Saraja D, Spears JR et al: Hemodynamic studies in heroin- induced acute pulmonary edema, *Circulation* (suppl 3), vol 41 and 42, pp III-44, 1970.

151. Gordon MJ, Skillman JJ, Zervas NT et al: Divergent nature of gastric mucosal permeability and gastric acid secretion in sick patients with general surgical and neurosurgical disease, *Ann Surg* 178:285-294,1973.

152. Grad A, Kiauta T, Osredkar J: Effects of elevated plasma norepinephrine on electrocardiographic changes in subarachnoid hemorrhage, *Stroke* 22:746-749, 1991.

153. Graf CJ, Rossi NP: Pulmonary edema and the central nervous system: a clinico-pathological study, *Surg Neurol* 4:319-325, 1975.

154. Gray GW, Bryan AC, Freedman MH et al: Effect of altitude exposure on platelets, *J Appl Physiol* 39:648-652, 1975.

155. Gray SJ, Ramsey C, Reifenstein RW et al: The significance of hormonal factors in the pathogenesis of peptic ulcer, *Gastroenterology* 25:156-172, 1953.

156. Greene R, Platt R, Matz R: Postictal pulmonary edema, *NY State J Med* 75:1257-1261, 1975.

157. Griffin JM, Hartley JH, Crow RW et al: Diabetes insipidus caused by craniofacial trauma, *J Trauma* 16:979-984, 1976.

158. Gudeman SK, Wheeler CB, Miller JD et al: Gastric secretory and mucosal injury response to severe head trauma, *Neurosurgery* 12:175-179, 1983.

159. Gunn CG, Hampton JW: CNS influence on plasma levels of factor VIII activity, *Am J Physiol* 212:124-130, 1967.

160. Hackenberry LE, Miner ME, Rea GL et al: Biochemical evidence of myocardial injury after severe head trauma, *Crit Care Med* 10:641-644, 1982.

161. Haden HT, Knox GW: Cerebral hyponatremia with inappropriate antidiuretic hormone syndrome, *Am J Med Sci* 249:381-390, 1965.

162. Haigh JD, Nemoto EM, DeWolf AM et al: Comparison of the effects of succinylcholine and atracurium on intracranial pressure in monkeys with intracranial hypertension, *Can Anaesth Soc J* 33:421-426, 1986.

163. Halloran LG, Zfass AM, Gayle WE et al: Prevention of acute gastrointestinal complications after severe head injury: a controlled trial of cimetidine prophylaxis, *Am J Surg* 139:44-48, 1980.

164. Hansen OH: Fat embolism and post-traumatic diabetes insipidus, *Acta Chir Scand* 136:161-165, 1970.

165. Harari A, Rapin M, Regnier B et al: Normal pulmonary-capillary pressures in the late phase of neurogenic pulmonary edema, *Lancet* 1:494, 1976.

166. Hardaway RM: Disseminated intravascular coagulation in experimental and clinical shock, *Am J Cardiol* 20:161-173, 1967.

167. Harken AH, Brennan MF, Smith B et al: The hemodynamic response to positive end-expiratory ventilation in hypovolemic patients, *Surgery* 76:786-793, 1974.

168. Harjola PT, Sivula A: Gastric ulceration following experimentally induced hypoxia and hemorrhagic shock: in vivo study of pathogenesis in rabbits, *Ann Surg* 163:2128, 1966.

169. Harrison W, Liebow AA: The effects of increased intracranial pressure on the pulmonary circulation in relation to pulmonary edema, *Circulation* 5:824-832, 1952.

170. Haymaker W, Kernohan JW: The Landry-Guillain-Barré syndrome, *Medicine* 28:59-141, 1949.

171. Hays RM: Antidiuretic hormone, *N Engl J Med* 295:659-665, 1976.

172. Hedley-Whyte J, Burgess GE, Freeley TW et al: *Applied physiology of respiratory care*, Boston, 1976, Little Brown & Co, p 57.

173. Henry DP, Bressler R: Serum insulin levels in nonketotic hyperosmotic diabetes mellitus, *Am J Med Sci* 256:150-154, 1968.

174. Henton E, Ross AM, Takeda VA et al: Alterations in blood coagulation at high altitude, *Adv Cardiol* 5:32-40, 1970.

175. Hersch C: Electrocardiographic changes in head injuries, *Circulation* 23:853-860, 1961.

176. Hersch C: Electrocardiographic changes in subarachnoid hemorrhage, meningitis, and intracranial space-occupying lesions, *Br Heart J* 26:785-793, 1964.

177. Hodgkin JE, Bowser MA, and Burton GG: Respirator weaning, *Crit Care Med* 2:96-102, 1974.

178. Hoff JT, Nishumura M: Experimental neurogenic pulmonary edema in cats, *J Neurosurg* 48:383-389, 1978.

179. Hoff JT, Nishimura M, Garcia-Uria J et al: Experimental neurogenic pulmonary edema. I. The role of systemic hypertension, *J Neurosurg* 54:627-631, 1981.

180. Houston CS: Acute pulmonary edema of high altitude, *N Engl J Med* 263:478-480, 1960.

181. Hücker H, Frenzel H, Kremer B et al: Time sequence and site of fluid accumulation in experimental neurogenic pulmonary edema, *Res Exp Med* 168:219-227, 1976.

182. Huff RW, Fred HL: Postictal pulmonary edema, *Arch Intern Med* 117:824-828, 1966.

183. Hultgren HN, Spickard WB, Hellriegel K et al: High altitude pulmonary edema, *Medicine* 40:289-313, 1961.

184. Huang CT, Cook AW, and Lyons HA: Severe craniocerebral trauma and respiratory abnormalities, *Arch Neurol* 9:545-554, 1963.

185. Illingworth G, Jennett WB: The shocked head injury, *Lancet* 2:511-514, 1965.

186. Innes D, Sevin S: Coagulation and fibrinolysis in injured patients, *J Clin Pathol* 17:1-13, 1964.

187. Jacobson SA, Danufsky P: Marked electrocardiographic changes produced by experimental head trauma, *J Neuropathol Exp Neurol* 13:462-466, 1954.

188. Jardin F, Farcot JC, Boisante L et al: Influence of positive end-expiratory pressure on left ventricular performance, *N Engl J Med* 304:387-392, 1981.

189. Jernigan WR, Gardner WC: Carotid artery injuries due to closed cervical trauma, *J Trauma* 11:429-435, 1971.

190. Johnson EE: Splanchnic hemodynamic response to passive hyperventilation, *J Appl Physiol* 38:156-162, 1975.

191. Joynt RJ, Afifi A, Harbison J: Hyponatremia in subarachnoid hemorrhage, *Arch Neurol* 13:633-638, 1965.

192. Kamada T, Fusamoto H, Kawano S et al: Gastrointestinal bleeding following head injury: a clinical study of 433 cases, *J Trauma* 17:44-47, 1977.

193. Kanarek DJ, Shannon DC: Adverse effect of positive end-expiratory pressure on pulmonary perfusion and arterial oxygenation, *Am Rev Resp Dis* 112:457-459, 1975.

194. Kaplan SL, Feigin RD: The syndrome of inappropriate secretion of antidiuretic hormone in children with bacterial meningitis, *J Pediatr* 92:758-761, 1978.

195. Karch SB: Upper gastrointestinal bleeding as a complication of intracranial disease, *J Neurosurg* 37:27-29, 1972.

196. Karliner JS: Noncardiogenic forms of pulmonary edema, *Circulation* 46:212-215, 1972.

197. Kaste M, Hernesniemi J, Somer H et al: Creatine kinese isoenzymes in acute brain injury, *J Neurosurg* 55:511-515, 1981.

198. Katsurada K, Sugimoto T, Onji Y: Significance of cerebrospinal fluid bicarbonate ions in the management of patients with cerebral injury, *J Trauma* 9:799-805, 1969.

199. Katsurada K, Yamada R, Sugimoto T: Respiratory insufficiency in patients with severe head injury, *Surgery* 73:191-199, 1973.

200. Kaufman HH, Moake JL, Olson JD et al: Delayed and recurrent intracranial hematomas related to disseminated intravascular clotting and fibrinolysis in head injury, *Neurosurgery* 7:445-449, 1980.

201. Keltz H, Kaplan S, Stone DJ: Effect of quadriplegia and hemidiaphragmatic paralysis on thoracoabdominal pressure during respiration, *Am J Phys Med* 48:109-115, 1969.

202. Reference deleted in proofs.

203. Kieth RG, Mahoney LJ, Garvey MB: Disseminated intravascular coagulation: an important feature of the fat embolism syndrome, *Can Med Assoc J* 105:74-76, 1971.

204. King LR, Knowles HC, McLaurin RL et al: Glucose tolerance and plasma insulin in cranial trauma, *Ann Surg* 173:337-343, 1971.

205. King LR, Knowles HC, McLaurin RL et al: Pituitary hormone response to head injury, *Neurosurgery* 9:229-235, 1981.

206. King LR, McLaurin RL, Lewis HP et al: Plasma cortisol levels after head injury, *Ann Surg* 172:975-984, 1970.

207. Kleeman CR, Rubini ME, Lamdin E et al: Studies on alcohol diuresis. II. The evaluation of ethyl alcohol as an inhibitor of the neurohypophysis, *J Clin Invest* 34:448-455, 1955.

208. Kleiner JP, Nelson WP: High altitude pulmonary edema: a rare disease? *JAMA* 234:491-499, 1975.

209. Klemperer P, Penner A, Bernhein AL: The gastro-intestinal manifestations of shock, *Am J Dig Dis* 7:410-414, 1940.

210. Knochel JP, Osborn JR, Cooper EB: Excretion of aldosterone in inappriate secretion of antidiuretic hormone following head trauma, *Metabolism* 14:715-725, 1965.

211. Lam AM, Winn HR, Cullen BF et al:

Hyperglycemia and neurological outcome in patients with head injury, *J Neurosurg* 75:545-551, 1991.

212. Lanier WL, Strangland KJ, Scheithauer BW et al: The effects of dextrose infusion and head position on neurologic outcome after complete cerebral ischemia in primates: examination of a model, *Anesthesiology* 66:39-48, 1987.

213. Lanier WL, Iaizzo PA, Milde JH: Cerebral function and muscle afferent activity following intravenous succinylcholine in dogs anesthetized with halothane: the effects of pretreatment with a defasciculating dose of pancuronium, *Anesthesiology* 71:87-95, 1989.

214. Lassen NA: The luxury-perfusion syndrome and its possible relation to acute metabolic acidosis localized within the brain, *Lancet* 2:1113-1115, 1966.

215. Laver MB, Lowenstein E: Lung function following trauma in man, *Clin Neurosurg* 19:133-174, 1972.

216. Leaf A, Bartter FC, Santos RF et al: Evidence in man that urinary electrolyte loss induced by pitressin is a function of water retention, *J Clin Invest* 32:868-878, 1953.

217. Lecky JH, Ominsky AJ: Postoperative respiratory management, *Chest* 62(suppl):50S-57S, 1972.

218. Leech P, Barker J, Fitch W: Changes in intracranial pressure and systemic arterial pressure during the termination of anaesthesia, *Br J Anaesth* 46:315-316, 1974.

219. Le May DR, Gehua L, Zelenock GB et al: Insulin administration protects neurologic function in cerebral ischemia in rats, *Stroke* 19:1411-1419, 1988.

220. Levine R, Mahler RR: Production, secretion, and availability of insulin, *Ann Rev Med* 15:413-432, 1964.

221. Lipinska D, Kurzaj E: Neurogenic pulmonary oedema in the course of increased intracranial pressure, *J Neurosurg Sci* 18:239-243, 1974.

222. Lofgren J: Airway pressure—neurosurgical aspects, *Anesthesiology* 45:269-272, 1976.

223. Loop JW, White LE, Shaw CM: Traumatic occlusion of the basilar artery within a clivus fracture, *Radiology* 83:36-40, 1964.

224. Luisada AA: Mechanism of neurogenic pulmonary edema, *Am J Cardiol* 20:66-68, 1967.

225. Maccario M: Neurological dysfunction associated with nonketotic hyperglycemia, *Arch Neurol* 19:525-534, 1968.

226. MacDonald AS, Steele BJ, Bottomley MG: Treatment of stress-induced upper gastrointestinal haemorrhage with metiamide, *Lancet* 1:68-70, 1976.

227. Machiedo G, Bolanowski PJP, Bauer J et al: Diabetes insipidus secondary to penetrating thoracic trauma, *Ann Surg* 181:31-34, 1975.

228. Mackay EM: Experimental pulmonary edema. IV. Pulmonary edema accompanying trauma to the brain, *Proc Soc Exper Biol Med* 74:695-697, 1950.

229. Magoun HW, Ranson SW: Retrograde degeneration of the supraoptic nuclei after section of the infundibular stalk in the monkey, *Anat Rec* 75:107-123, 1939.

230. Maire FW, Patton HD: Neural structures involved in the genesis of preoptic pulmonary edema, gastric erosions and behavior changes, *Am J Physiol* 184:345-350, 1956.

231. Malik AB: Pulmonary vascular response to increase in intracranial pressure: role of sympathetic mechanisms, *J Appl Physiol* 42:335-343, 1977.

232. Marion DW, Segal R, Thompson ME: Subarachnoid hemorrhage and the heart, *Neurosurgery* 18:101-106, 1986.

233. Markello R, Schuder R, Border J: Arterial-alveolar N_2 differences documenting ventilation-perfusion mismatching following trauma, *J Trauma* 14:423-426, 1974.

234. Marks J: Central nervous system influence in the genesis of atrial fibrillation, *Ohio State Med J* 52:1054-1055, 1956.

235. Matjasko MJ, Ducker TB: Disseminated intravascular coagulation associated with removal of a primary brain tumor, *J Neurosurg* 47:476-480, 1977.

236. Max M, Menguy R: Influence of adrenocorticotropin, cortisone, aspirin, and phenylbutazone on the rate of exfoliation and the rate of renewal of gastric mucosal cells, *Gastroenterology* 58:329-336, 1976.

237. Maxwell M, Karaostas D, Ellenbo-

gen RG et al: Precocious puberty following head injury, *J Neurosurg* 73:123-129, 1990.

238. Mazzoni MC, Borgström P, Arfors KE et al: Dynamic fluid redistribution in hypersmotic resuscitation of hypovolemic hemorrhage, *Am J Physiol* 255:H629-H637, 1988.

239. McAslan TC, Turney S, Paul R et al: The effect of stepwise increase in airway pressure on ventricular fluid pressure in humans with severe head injury. Presented at Annual American Society of Anesthesiologists Meeting, San Francisco, Oct., 1976.

240. McAslan TC, Matjasko-Chiu J, Turney SZ et al: Influence of inhalation of 100% oxygen on intrapulmonary shunt in severely traumatized patients, *J Trauma* 13:811-821, 1973.

241. McCurdy DK: Hyperosmolar hyperglycemic nonketotic diabetic coma, *Med Clin North Am* 54:683-699, 1970.

242. McGauley JL, Miller CA, Penner JA: Diagnosis and treatment of diffuse intravascular coagulation following cerebral trauma; case report, *J Neurosurg* 43:374-376, 1975.

243. McIntyre RW, Laws AK, Ramachandran PR: Positive expiratory pressure plateau; improved gas exchange during mechanical ventilation, *Can Anaesth Soc J* 16:477-486, 1969.

244. Reference deleted in proofs.

245. McLaurin RL, King LR: Recognition and treatment of metabolic disorders after head injuries, *Clin Neurosurg* 19:281-300, 1972.

246. McLaurin RL, King LR: Metabolic effects of head injury, *Handbook Clin Neurol* 23:109-131, 1975.

247. Melin J, Fogelholm R: Electrocardiographic findings in subarachnoid hemorrhage, *Acta Med Scand* 213:5-8, 1983.

248. Menguy R, Desbaillets L: Influence of phenylbutazone on gastric secretion of mucus, *Proc Soc Exp Biol Med* 125:1108-1111, 1967.

249. Menguy R, Masters YF: Effect of cortisone on mucoprotein secretion by gastric antrum of dogs: pathogenesis of steroid ulcer, *Surgery* 54:19-28, 1963.

250. Menguy R, Masters YF: Effects of aspirin on gastric mucous secretion, *Surg Gynecol Obstet* 120:92-98, 1965.

251. Menguy R: The prophylaxis of stress

ulceration *N Engl J Med* 302:461-462, 1980.

252. Merguerian PA, Perel A, Wald U et al: Persistent nonketotic hyperglycemia as a grave prognostic sign in head injured patients, *Crit Care Med* 9:838-840, 1981.

253. Messer J, Reitman D, Sachs HS et al: Association of adrenocorticosteroid therapy and peptic ulcer disease, *N Engl J Med* 309:21-24, 1983.

254. Miller M, Moses AM: Mechanism of chlorpropamide action in diabetes insipidus, *J Clin Endocrinol Metab* 30:488-496, 1970.

255. Miner ME, Kaufman HH, Graham SH et al: Disseminated intravascular coagulation fibrinolytic syndrome following head injury in children: frequency and prognostic implications, *J Pediatr* 100:687-691, 1982.

256. Minton MD, Stirt JA, Bedford RF et al: Intracranial pressure after atracurium in neurosurgical patients, *Anesth Analg* 64:1113-1116, 1985.

257. Modell JH: Ventilation/perfusion changes during mechanical ventilation, *Dis Chest* 55:447-451, 1969.

258. Monaco V, Burdge R, Newell J et al: Pulmonary venous admixture in injured patients, *J Trauma* 12:15-23, 1972.

259. Moran WH, Miltenberger FW, Shuayb WA et al: The relationship of antidiuretic hormone to surgical stress, *Surgery* 56:99-108, 1964.

260. Moses AM: Diabetes insipidus and ADH regulation, *Hosp Prac* 12:37-44, 1977.

261. Moses AM, Miller M: Urine and plasma osmolality in differentiation of polyuric states, *Postgrad Med* 52:187-190, 1972.

262. Moses AM, Miller M: Drug-induced dilutional hyponatremia, *N Engl J Med* 291:1234-1239, 1974.

263. Moses AM, Miller M, Streeten DHP: Pathophysiologic and pharmacologic alterations in the release and action of ADH, *Metabolism* 25:697-721, 1976.

264. Moss G: The role of the central nervous system in shock: the centroneurogenic etiology of the respiratory distress syndrome, *Crit Care Med* 2:181-185, 1974.

265. Moss G, Staunton C, Stein AA: Cerebral etiology of the shock lung syndrome, *J Trauma* 12:885-890, 1972.

266. Moss G, Stein AA: Cerebral etiology of the acute respiratory distress syndrome: diphenylhydantoin prophylaxis, *J Trauma* 15:39-41, 1975.

267. Moutier F: Hypertension et mort par oedema pulmonaire aigu, *Presse Medicale (Paris)* 26:108-109, 1918.

268. Murakami T, Wax SD, Webb WR: Pulmonary microcirculation in hemorrhagic shock, *Surg Forum* 21:25-27, 1970.

269. Muizelaar JP, Marmarou A, Ward JD et al: Adverse effects of prolonged hyperventilation in patients with severe head injury: a randomized clinical trial, *J Neurosurg* 75:731-739, 1991.

270. Muizelaar JP, van der Pael HG, Li ZC et al: Pial arteriolar vessel diameter and CO_2 reactivity during prolonged hyperventilation in the rabbit, *J Neurosurg* 69:923-927, 1988.

271. Murdaugh HV, Sieker HO, Manfredi F: Effect of altered intrathoracic pressure on renal hemodynamics, electrolyte excretion and water clearance, *J Clin Invest* 38:834-842, 1959.

272. Naeraa N: Blood-gas analyses in unconscious neurosurgical patients on admission to hospital, *Acta Anaesthesiol Scand* 7:191-199, 1963.

273. Neil-Dwyer G, Cruickshank JM, Stratton C: Beta blockers, plasma total creatine kinase and creatine kinase myocardial isoenzyme and the prognosis of subarachnoid hemorrhage, *Surg Neurol* 25:163-168, 1986.

274. Nezami AH, Bremer AM: Basilar artery occlusion in multiple trauma: case report, *Neurosurgery* 7:267-270, 1980.

275. Nielsen B, Thorn A: Transient excess urinary excretion of antidiuretic material in acute intermittent porphyria with hyponatremia and hypomagnesemia, *Am J Med* 38: 345-358, 1965.

276. Nielsen JM, Ingham SD, Von Hagen KO: Pulmonary edema and embolism as complications of insulin shock in the treatment of schizophrenia, *JAMA* 111:2455-2458, 1938.

277. North JB, Jennett S: Abnormal breathing patterns associated with acute brain damage, *Arch Neurol* 31:338-344, 1974.

278. Norton L, Greer J, Eiseman B: Gastric secretory response to head injury, *Arch Surg* 101:200-204, 1970.

279. Nothnagel H (quoted by Benassi G): Traumatismes cranio-encephaliques et oedema pulmonaire, *Paris Med* 103:525-532, 1937.

280. Notman DD, Mortek MA, Moses AM: Permanent diabetes insipidus following head trauma: observations on ten patients and an approach to diagnosis, *J Trauma* 20:599-602, 1980.

281. Nunn JF, Freeman J: Problems of oxygenation and oxygen transport during hemorrhage, *Anaesthesia* 19:206-216, 1964.

282. O'Brien JR: Effects of salicylates on human platelets, *Lancet* 1:779-783, 1968.

283. O'Neill JA, Pruitt BA, Moncrief JA et al: Studies related to the pathogenesis of Curling's ulcer, *J Trauma* 7:275-287, 1967.

284. Orloff J, Handler JS: The cellular mode of action of antidiuretic hormone, *Am J Med* 36:686-697, 1964.

285. Osler W: Oedema of left lung-morphia poisoning, *Montreal Gen Hosp Rev* 1:291, 1880.

286. Oswalt CE, Gates GA, Holmstrom FMG: Pulmonary edema as a complication of acute airway obstruction, *JAMA* 238:1833-1835, 1977.

287. Otteni JC, Potlecher T, Bronner G et al: Prolongation of the Q-T interval and sudden cardiac arrest following right radical neck dissection, *Anesthesiology* 59:358-361, 1983.

288. Palmer ED, Sherman JL: Hypoxia of abnormal physiologic origin as the final common pathway in gastroduodenal ulcer genesis, *Arch Intern Med* 101:1106-1117, 1958.

289. Park BE, Meacham WF, Netsky MG: Nonketotic hyperglycemic hyperosmolar coma: report of neurosurgical cases with a review of mechanisms and treatment, *J Neurosurg* 44:409-417, 1976.

290. Paxson CL, Brown DR: Post-traumatic anterior hypopituitarism, *Pediatrics* 57:893-896, 1976.

291. Peltier LF: A few remarks on fat embolism, *J Trauma* 8:812-820, 1968.

292. Penaloza D, Sime F: Circulatory dynamics during high altitude pulmonary edema, *Am J Cardiol* 23:369-378, 1969.

293. Persson L, Hillered L: Chemical monitoring of neurosurgical intensive care patients using intracerebral microdialysis, *J Neurosurg* 76:72-80, 1992.

294. Peters BH, Samaan NA: Hyperglycemia with relative hypoinsulinemia in diphenylhydantoin toxicity, *N Engl J Med* 281:91-92, 1969.

295. Plum F, Swanson AG: Central neurogenic hyperventilation in man, *Arch Neurol Psychiatry* 81:535-549, l959.

296. Pollick C, Cujec B, Parker S et al: Left ventricular wall motion abnormalities in subarachnoid hemorrhage: an echocardiographic study, *J Am Coll Cardiol* 12:600-605, 1988.

297. Pontoppidan H, Laver MB, Geffin B: Acute respiratory failure in the surgical patient, *Adv Surg* 4:163-254, 1970.

298. Popp AJ, Gottlieb ME, Paloski WH et al: Cardiopulmonary hemodynamics in patients with serious head injury, *J Surg Res* 32:416-421, 1982.

299. Poser CM: Hyperglycemic nonketotic coma: role of sodium in the pathogenesis of the neurologic manifestations, *Dis Nerv Sys* 33:725-729, 1972.

300. Powers SR, Mannal R, Neclerio M et al: Physiologic consequences of positive end-expiratory pressure (PEEP) ventilation, *Ann Surg* 178:265-272, 1973.

301. Prasad S, Athreya BH: Transient paralysis of the phrenic nerve associated with head injury, *JAMA* 236:2532-2533, 1976.

302. Pretorius ME, Kaufman HH: Rapid onset of delayed traumatic intracerebral haematoma with diffuse intravascular coagulation and fibrinolysis, *Acta Neurochir* 65:103-109, 1982.

303. Prockop L: Hyperglycemia, polyol accumulation and increased intracranial pressure, *Arch Neurol* 25:126-140, 1971.

304. Priebe HJ, Skillman JJ, Long PC et al: Antacid versus cimetidine in preventing acute gastrointestinal bleeding: a randomized trial in 75 critically ill patients, *N Engl J Med* 302:426-430, 1980.

305. Pruitt BA, Foley FD, Moncrief JA: Curling's ulcer: a clinical-pathology study of 323 cases, *Ann Surg* 172:523-539, 1970.

306. Ramachandran PR, Fairley HB: Changes in functional residual capacity during respiratory failure, *Can Anaesth Soc J* 17:359-369, 1970.

307. Reynolds RW: Pulmonary edema as a consequence of hypothalamic lesions in rats, *Science* 141:930-932, 1963.

308. Richards DE, White RJ, Yashon D: Inappropriate release of ADH in subdural hematoma, *J Trauma* 11:758-762, 1971.

309. Robert A, Nezamis JE: Ulcerogenic property of steroids, *Soc Exp Biol Med Proc* 99:443-447, 1958.

310. Robertson CS, Goodman JC, Narayan RK et al: The effect of glucose administration on carbohydrate metabolism after head injury, *J Neurosurg* 74:43-50, 1991.

311. Robertson CS, Narayan RK, Gokaslan ZL et al: Cerebral anteriovenous oxygen difference as an estimate of cerebral blood flow in comatose patients, *J Neurosurg* 70:222-230, 1989.

312. Robertson JD, Kirkpatrick HFW: Simmond's disease (hypopituitarism) in a man due to traumatic hemorrhage into the pituitary gland, *Lancet* 1:1048-1051, 1951.

313. Robinson RO, Pagliero KM: Polyuria after cardiac surgery, *Br Med J* 3:265-266, 1970.

314. Rodbard S, Reyes M, Mininni G et al: Neurohumoral transmission of the pressor response to intracranial compression, *Am J Physiol* 176:341-346, 1954.

315. Ross APJ: The fat embolism syndrome: with special reference to the importance of hypoxia in the syndrome, *Ann R Coll Surg Engl* 46:159-171, 1970.

316. Rossi NP, Graf CJ: Physiological and pathological effects of neurologic disturbances and increased intracranial pressure on the lung: a review, *Surg Neurol* 5:366-372, 1976.

317. Rotem M, Constantini S, Shir Y et al: Life-threatening Torsades de Pointes arrhythmias associated with head injury, *Neurosurgery* 23:89-92, 1988.

318. Rothschild M, Shenkman L: Diabetes insipidus following cardiorespiratory arrest, *JAMA* 238:620-621, 1977.

319. Rottenberg DA, Bennett WM, Wolpow ER: Transient diabetes insipidus complicating systemic fat embolization, *J Trauma* 12:731-733, 1972.

320. Rovit RL, Sigler MH: Hyponatremia with herpes simplex encephalitis: possible relationship of limbic lesions and ADH secretion, *Arch Neurol* 10:595-603, 1964.

321. Rudman D, Fleischer A, Kutner MH: Concentration of 3'5' cyclic adenosine monophosphate in ventricular cerebrospinal fluid of patients with prolonged coma after head trauma or intracranial hemorrhage, *N Engl J Med* 295:635-638, 1976.

322. Sarnoff SJ, Sarnoff LC: Neurohemodynamics of pulmonary edema. II. The role of sympathetic pathways in the elevation of pulmonary and system vascular pressures following the intracisternal injection of fibrin, *Circulation* 6:51-62, 1952.

323. Sarnoff SJ, Sarnoff LC: Neurohemodynamics of pulmonary edema. I. Autonomic influence on pulmonary vascular pressures and the acute pulmonary edema state, *Dis Chest* 22:685-698, 1952.

324. Saul TG, Ducker TB: Management of severe head injuries, *Md State Med J* 30:45-48, 1981.

325. Schäfer U, Hücker H, Meinen K: Early morphological alterations of the rat lung with increased intracranial pressure. II. A scanning electron microscopic study using different fixation procedures, *Res Exp Med* 165:1-8, 1975.

326. Scherman BM, Tucker WS: Bilateral traumatic thrombosis of the internal carotid arteries in the neck: a case report with review of the literature, *Neurosurgery* 10:751-753, 1982.

327. Schneider RC, Crosby EC: Vascular insufficiency of brain stem and spinal cord in spinal trauma, *Neurology* 9:643-656, 1959.

328. Schrier RW, Berl T: Nonosmolar factors affecting water excretion, *N Engl J Med* 292:141-145, 1975.

329. Schulte AM, Esch J, Murday H et al: Haemodynamic changes in patients with severe head injury, *Acta Neurochir* 54:243-250, 1980.

330. Schumaker PT, Rhodes GR, Newell JC et al: Ventilation-perfusion imbalance after head trauma, *Am Rev Respir Dis* 119:33-43, 1979.

331. Schwartz WB, Bennett W, Curelop S et al: A syndrome of renal sodium loss and hyponatremia probably resulting from inappropriate secretion of antidiuretic hormone, *Am J Med* 23:529-542, 1957.

332. Scoble JE, Havard CWH: Anosmia and isolated ACTH deficiency following a road traffic accident, *J Neurosurg* 73:453-454, 1990.

333. Sears ES: Nonketotic hyperosmolar hyperglycemia during glycerol therapy for cerebral edema, *Neurology* 26:8994, 1976.

334. Severinghaus JW, Mitchell RA, Ri-

chardson BW et al: Respiratory control at high altitude suggesting active transport regulation of CSF pH, *J Appl Physiol* 18:1155-1166, 1963.

335. Sevitt S: The boundaries between physiology, pathology, and irreversibility after injury, *Lancet* 2:1203-1210, 1966.

336. Shackford SR, Zhuang J, Schmoker J: Intravenous fluid tonicity: effect on intracranial pressure, cerebral blood flow, and cerebral oxygen delivery in focal brain injury, *J Neurosurg* 76:91-98, 1992.

337. Sharkey PC, Perry JH, Ehni G: Diabetes insipidus following section of hypophyseal stalk, *J Neurosurg* 18:445-460, 1961.

338. Shapiro HM, Galindo A, Wyte SR et al: Rapid intraoperative reduction of intracranial pressure with thiopental, *Br J Anaesth* 45:1057-1062, 1973.

339. Sheehan HL: Post-partum necrosis of the anterior pituitary, *J Pathol Bacteriol* 45:189-214, 1937.

340. Shucart WA, Jackson I: Management of diabetes insipidus in neurosurgical patients, *J Neurosurg* 44:65-71, 1976.

341. Simmons RL, Martin AM, Heisterkamp CA et al: Respiratory insufficiency in combat casualties. II. Pulmonary edema following head injury, *Ann Surg* 170:39-44, 1969.

342. Singh I: High altitude pulmonary edema, *Am Heart J* 70:435-439, 1965.

343. Singh I, Khanna PK, Srivastava MC et al: Acute mountain sickness, *N Engl J Med* 280:175-184, 1969.

344. Sinha RP, Ducker TB, Perot P: Arterial oxygenation: findings and its significance in central nervous system trauma patients, *JAMA* 224:1258-1260, 1973.

345. Skillman JJ, Bushnell LS, Goldman H et al: Respiratory failure, hypotension, sepsis, and jaundice, *Am J Surg* 117:523-530, 1969.

346. Skillman JJ, Gould SA, Chung RSK et al: The gastric mucosal barrier: clinical and experimental studies in critically ill and normal man, and in the rabbit, *Ann Surg* 172:564-584, 1970.

347. Skillman JJ, Malhotra IV, Pallotta JA et al: Determinants of weaning from controlled ventilation, *Surg Forum* :198-200, 1971.

348. Skillman JJ, Silen W: Acute gastroduodenal "stress" ulceration: bar-

rier disruption of varied pathogenesis? *Gastroenterology* 59:478-482, 1970.

349. Smith BM, Skillman JJ, Edwards BG et al: Permeability of the human gastric mucosa; alteration by acetylsalicylic acid and ethanol, *N Engl J Med* 285:716-721, 1971.

350. Smith HW: Salt and water volume receptors, *Am J Med* 23:623-652, 1957.

351. Smith JB, Willis AL: Aspirin selectively inhibits prostaglandin production in human platelets, *Nature (New Biol)* 231:235-237, 1971.

352. Spencer JA, Morlock CG, Sayre GP: Lesions in upper portion of the gastrointestinal tract associated with intracranial neoplasms, *Gastroenterology* 37:20-27, 1959.

353. Spenney JG, Eure CA, Kreisberg RA: Hyperglycemic, hyperosmolar, nonketoacidotic diabetes; a complication of steroid and immunosuppressive therapy, *Diabetes* 18:107-110, 1969.

354. Staub NC: The pathophysiology of pulmonary edema, *Human Pathol* 1:419-432, 1970.

355. Staub NC: Pathogenesis of pulmonary edema, *Am Rev Respir Dis* 109:358-372, 1974.

356. Steinberg AD, Karliner JS: The clinical spectrum of heroin pulmonary edema, *Arch Intern Med* 122:122-127, 1968.

357. Stirt JA, Grosslight KR, Bedford RF et al: "Defasciculation" with metocurine prevents succinylcholine-induced increases in intracranial pressure, *Anesthesiology* 67:50-53, 1987.

358. Stober T, Anstatt T, Sen S et al: Cardiac arrhythmias in subarachnoid haemorrhage, *Acta Neurochir* 93:37-44, 1988.

359. String T, Robinson AJ, Blaisdell FW: Massive trauma: effect of intravascular coagulation on prognosis, *Arch Surg* 102:406-410, 1971.

360. Stringer WL, Kelly DL: Traumatic dissection of the extracranial internal carotid artery, *Neurosurgery* 6:123-130, 1980.

361. Sugg WL, Craver WD, Webb WR et al: Pressure changes in the dog lung secondary to hemorrhagic shock: protective effect of pulmonary reimplantation, *Ann Surg* 169:592-598, 1969.

362. Summer W, Bromberger-Barnea B,

Shoukas A et al: The effects of respiration on left ventricular function, *Circulation* 53(suppl):11-13, 1976.

363. Suter PM, Fairley HB, Isenberg MD: Optimum end-expiratory airway pressure in patients with acute pulmonary failure, *N Engl J Med* 292:284-289, 1975.

364. Sutton LN, McLaughlin AC, Dante S et al: Cerebral venous oxygen content as a measure of brain energy metabolism with increased intracranial pressure and hyperventilation, *J Neurosurg* 73:927-932, 1990.

365. Tackett LR: Brain tissue pulmonary emboli, *Arch Pathol* 78:292-294, 1964.

366. Takashima S, Koga M, Tanaka K: Fibrinolytic activity of human brain and cerebrospinal fluid, *Br J Exp Pathol* 50:533-539, 1969.

367. Tanay A, Yust I, Peresecenschi G et al: Long term treatment of the syndrome of inappropriate antidiuretic hormone secretion with phenytoin, *Ann Intern Med* 90:50-52, 1979.

368. Taubin H, Matz R: Cerebral edema, diabetes insipidus, and sudden death during the treatment of diabetic ketoacidosis, *Diabetes* 17:108-109, 1968.

369. Theodore J, Robin ED: Pathogenesis of neurogenic pulmonary oedema, *Lancet* 2:749-751, 1975.

370. Theodore J, Robin ED: Speculations on neurogenic pulmonary edema (NPE), *Am Rev Respir Dis* 113:405-411, 1976.

371. Thomas DGT, Palfreyman JW, Ratcliffe JG: Serum myelin-basic-protein assay in diagnosis and prognosis of patients with head injury, *Lancet* 1:113-115, 1978.

372. Thompson GE: Pulmonary edema complicating intrathecal hypertonic saline injection for intractable pain, *Anesthesiology* 35:425-427, 1971.

373. Tobias SL, Bookatz BJ, Diamond TH: Myocardial damage and electrocardiographic changes in acute cerebrovascular hemorrhage: a report of three cases and review, *Heart Lung* 16:521-526, 1987.

374. Tovi D: Fibrinolytic activity of human brain; a histochemical study, *Acta Neurol Scand* 49:152-162, 1973.

375. Urabe M, Segawa Y, Tsubokawa T et al: Pathogenesis of the acute pulmonary edema occurring after brain

operation and brain trauma, *Jpn Heart J* 2:147-169, 1961.

376. Van der Sande JJ, Emeis JJ, Lindeman J: Intravascular coagulation: a common phenomenon in minor experimental head injury, *J Neurosurg* 54:21-25, 1981.

377. Van Woerkom TCAM, Huijbers WAR, Teelken AW et al: Biochemical and ultrastructural aspects of the inhibited phagocytosis by neutrophil granulocytes in acute brain-damaged patients, *J Neurol Sci* 31:223-235, 1977.

378. Vane JR: Prostaglandins and the aspirin-like drugs, *Hosp Prac* 7:61-71, 1972.

379. Vardi Y, Streifler M, Schujman E et al: Diffuse intravascular clotting associated with a primary brain tumour, *J Neurol Neurosurg Psychiatr* 37:987-990, 1974.

380. Vecht CJ: Additional studies on platelet function. In Minderhoud JM, Braakman R, editors: *Haemostasis in acute neurologic disorders (monographs on clinical neurology and neurosurgery),* vol 2, Assen, The Netherlands, 1975, Van Gorcum, pp 113-124.

381. Vecht CJ, Smit Sibinga CT: Head injury and defibrination, *Lancet* 2:905, 1974.

382. Vecht CJ, Smit Sibinga CT, Minderhoud JM: Disseminated intravascular coagulation and head injury, *J Neurol Neurosurg Psychiatry* 38:567-571, 1975.

383. Vecht CJ, Van Woerkom TCAM, Teelken AW et al: Homovanillic acid and 5-hydroxyindoleacetic acid cerebrospinal fluid levels, *Arch Neurol* 32:792-797, 1975.

384. Virchow R: Historisches, kritisches und positives zur lehre der unterleibsaffektionen, *Arch Pathol Anat* 5:281-375, 1853.

385. Watanabe H, Passonneau JV: Cyclic adenosine monophosphate in cerebral cortex: alterations following trauma, *Arch Neurol* 32:181-184, 1975.

386. Watts CC, Clark K: Gastric acidity in the comatose patient, *J Neurosurg* 30:107-109, 1969.

387. Webb WR: Pulmonary complications of nonthoracic trauma: summary of the National Research Council Conference, *J Trauma* 9:700-711, 1969.

388. Webster B, Bain J: Antidiuretic effect and complications of chlorpropamide therapy in diabetes insipidus, *J Clin Endocrinol Metab* 30:215-227, 1970.

389. Weinberg SJ, Fuster JM: Electrocardiographic changes produced by localized hypothalamic stimulations, *Ann Intern Med* 53:332-341, 1960.

390. Weidler DJ: Myocardial damage and cardiac arrhythmias after intracranial hemorrhage: a critical review, *Stroke* 5:759-764, 1974.

391. Weinshelbaum EI, Ferguson DJ: The effect of cortisone on mucosal resistance to ulceration, *Gastroenterology* 44:52-56, 1963.

392. Weintraub BM, McHenry LC: Cardiac abnormalities in subarachnoid hemorrhage: a resume, *Stroke* 5:384-392, 1974.

393. Weiss HJ, Aledort LM, Kochwa S: The effect of salicylates on the hemostatic properties of platelets in man, *J Clin Invest* 47:2169-2180, 1968.

394. Weiss SR, Jacobi JD, Fishman LM et al: Hypopituitarism following head trauma, *Am J Obstet Gynecol* 127:678-679, 1977.

395. Welch KMA, Meyer JS, Chee ANC: Evidence for disordered cyclic AMP metabolism in patients with cerebral infarction, *Eur Neurol* 13:144-154, 1975.

396. West JB: Continuous distributions of ventilation-perfusion ratios in normal subjects breathing air and 100% O_2, *J Clin Invest* 54:54-68, 1974.

397. Whayne TF, Severinghaus JW: Experimental hypoxic pulmonary edema in the rat, *J Appl Physiol* 25:729-732, 1968.

398. White PF, Sclobohm RM, Pitts LH et al: A randomized study of drugs for preventing increases in intracranial pressure during endotracheal suctioning, *Anesthesiology* 57:242-244, 1982.

399. White PR: Horner's syndrome and its significance in the management of head and neck trauma, *Br J Oral Surg* 14:165-170, 1976.

400. Worthen M, Placik B, Argano B et al: On the mechanism of epinephrine-induced pulmonary edema, *Jpn Heart J* 10:133-141, 1969.

401. Wyler AR, Reynolds AF: An intracranial complication of nasogastric intubation; case report, *J Neurosurg* 47:297-298, 1977.

402. Yoshida K, Marmarou A: Effects of tromethamine and hyperventilation on brain injury in the cat, *J Neurosurg* 74:87-96, 1991.

403. Young B, Ott L, Norton J et al: Metabolic and nutritional sequelae in the non-steroid treated head injury patient, *Neurosurgery* 17:784-791, 1985.

404. Young B, Ott L, Twyman D et al: The effect of nutritional support on outcomes from severe head injury, *J Neurosurg* 67:668-676, 1987.

405. Zapol WM, Snider MT: Pulmonary hypertension in severe acute respiratory failure, *N Engl J Med* 296:476-480, 1977.

406. Zucker MB, Peterson J: Effect of acetylsalicylic acid, other nonsteroidal anti-inflammatory agents, and dipyridamole on human blood platelets, *J Lab Clin Med* 76:66-75, 1970.

33

Spinal Cord Injury

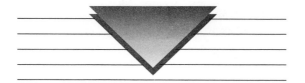

MAURICE S. ALBIN

INTRODUCTION AND DEMOGRAPHICS

In the not-too-distant past, the fate of a patient with a complete spinal cord injury (SCI) involved a chronic bedridden state with recurrent pulmonary infections, elimination incontinence, extensive infected decubiti, underlying osteomyelitis, eventual renal failure, and death. The success in dealing with the manifold problems of SCI during the past 5 decades has been due, in large part, to the pioneering efforts of the late Sir Lionel Guttman at the Stoke-Mandeville Spinal Cord Injury Centre in Great Britain, who made systematic studies of the basic physiologic problems and needs of the patient with SCI and developed the basic therapeutic concepts used today.[132] Although the life expectancy of a person with paraplegia who survives the first year after injury and receives adequate therapy is near normal, the health care insurance crisis and the fragmentation of health services in the United States have a negative impact on the ability of such an individual to receive an adequate contin-

uum of care. SCI is a catastrophic event that acutely impacts on the patient and the familial support group. It creates huge economic costs as well as significant morbidity and mortality.

In 1982 the National Head and Spinal Cord Injury Survey indicated that, each year, there are roughly 10,000 acute spinal cord injuries that result in paraplegia and quadriplegia.[25] About 4000 of these patients die before reaching a hospital, and 1000 die during hospitalization.[63,165,238] Thus the acute death rate for SCI is about 50%. In the United States, approximately 4000 new traumatic quadriplegia cases are added to the national pool each year, and it is estimated that in 1980 there were about 200,000 persons in the United States with complete or partial paralysis resulting from trauma.[202] The overall incidence of SCI appears to be about 28 to 50 per million population.[202]

Epidemiologic data from many countries appear to indicate that the etiologic factors of SCI are (in order of decreasing incidence) vehicular accidents,[250] falls, and sports injuries, particularly from diving.[32,127,238] There appears to be a much higher incidence of SCI in males and most patients range from 15 to 35 years of age. Not surprisingly, younger and middle-aged persons are the victims of occupational injuries, whereas older persons are more likely to suffer SCI after falls at home. Within this group of older patients (>50 years), there appears to be a high percentage of cervical SCI unaccompanied by bone injury.[116,196,211] Sadly, a major cause of SCI in the metropolitan areas in the United States is due to penetrating injuries caused by handguns. Green et al. noted that "if you live in a metropolitan area in the United States and you are black and under 40, you have a one in twelve chance of dying of a handgun-inflicted wound."[124]

The overall mortality rate of those with SCI appears to be about 10% the first year although some centers report a mortality rate reaching 40% in those with quadriplegia.[124,144] First-year hospital costs for patients with acute cervical cord injury now range from $50,000 to $150,000, with lifetime costs of greater than $1 million per individual.[3,202,203] If we add to this the loss to the Gross National Product, SCI presents a staggering multibillion-dollar annual health care problem. The direct medical cost of these injuries to the federal government exceeds $4 billion per year, and lost earnings are thought to be more than $3,400,000,000 (in 1987 dollars) annually.[203]

With the motor vehicle accident being the most common cause of SCI, it has been noted that during 1986 in the United States as many as 5000 individuals died of SCI at the scene of the accident.[124] Interestingly, the decreased incidence in overall mortality and paralysis after establishment of the 55 mph speed limit has been changing recently since the federal government has allowed states to raise the speed limits on the interstate highways outside metropolitan areas to 65 mph. Along the same lines, the use of seat belts has been shown to decrease the incidence of SCI in the United States, Australia, and Japan.[124] Nevertheless, the tragic consequences of imbibing alcohol in the home or workplace or while driving has contributed significantly to the incidence of SCI. It has been estimated that in nearly half of the motor vehicle accidents occurring in the United States, alcohol intake has been implicated. As a corollary, Goldbaum et al. evaluated the rate of failure to use seat belts from 1981 to 1983 and found that the drunk driver was less likely to use seat belts.[119]

The key to dealing with the problem of SCI lies in developing an all-encompassing, integrated systems approach, including prevention, emergency medical services, emergency room management, acute inpatient care, rehabilitation, and a follow-up care program. This systems approach emphasizes educational programs to prevent SCI, techniques for minimizing lesion exacerbation during initial care, placement of the patient in a milieu of professional health care workers familiar with the problem of SCI, and provision for physical, social, mental, and vocational reha-

bilitation. Such an approach is extremely cost effective. Unfortunately, our health care insurance system has fragmented care and has made adequate funding for these patients difficult. In essence—with rare exceptions—we now treat the majority of these patients with a "non-system," unless an individual patient is fortunate enough to have the economic wherewithal to afford treatment costs. Further discussion of these issues is beyond the scope of this chapter, but it is important to realize the socioeconomic conditions underlying the attempts to handle this type of an injury.

In this chapter, we deal principally with the patient with acute cervical SCI because this individual requires the maximal use of resources and presents the most difficult management problems. We also place other aspects of SCI in perspective and delineate some of the mechanisms involved in the development of autonomic dysreflexia. Finally, we weave within this therapeutic carpet the important multidisciplinary threads concerning orthopedic, urologic, rehabilitative, neurosurgical, and nursing considerations.

BIOMECHANICS

To understand the forces acting on the spine and reflected onto the spinal cord, one must have knowledge of the biomechanical factors that occur during impact.[58,232] External loading of the spine can produce flexion, extension, compression, tension, rotation, and shear stress; these forces can result in SCI. The complexity of spinal deformation often involves various combinations of these biomechanical stresses, making it extremely difficult to classify the injuries. Spinal injuries may also be associated with impacts that transmit inertial force to the vertebral column. The cervical vertebral column is particularly susceptible to injuries, such as those caused by sudden and rapid acceleration or deceleration. Injuries to the upper cervical spine may involve fractures at the atlas, with associated fractures of the anterior, posterior, or lateral arches; the odontoid process; and the axis. An impact of sufficient force to the head—which produces an axial load on the vertex of the skull—drives the occipital condyles down into the atlas, causing fractures of the anterior and posterior arches.

Fracture of the arches of the atlas is most likely to occur at the grooves where the vertebral arteries lie. The exploding fragments are driven outward, tending to widen the spinal column at the cervicomedullary junction, leaving the spinal cord uninjured in some cases.[241] In a heavy direct impact to the vertex in which the skull or cervical vertebral column does not sustain fracture, force can be transmitted directly down the spinal axis through the brainstem and into the cervical spinal cord at the C2 level. Injuries of this nature result in immediate respiratory paralysis and death resulting from microhemorrhages in the upper spinal cord.[121,241,243]

During impact loading to the head or inertial loading to

the neck (e.g., as a result of whiplash [extension] motion), internal stresses and strains in the ligaments and muscles may exceed their limits, resulting in hemorrhage and rupture of ligaments, with dislocation or fracture of the cervical vertebrae or both. Ligament trauma has also been observed when column strain resulting from tension exceeds 50%.[111,240] Fractures of the anterior arch of the atlas may also be associated with flexion injuries. An impact producing cervical flexion has been shown to cause transverse ligament rupture with anterior movement of the atlas. A flexion-producing force of 2200 (N) (495 lb) appears necessary before rupture of the transverse ligament occurs.[107]

From a biomechanical standpoint, the cervical spine appears to be relatively strong with compression and flexion but weak during torsion. When the head and jaw are swung laterally, unilateral dislocation often occurs between two cervical facets.[231] Dislocations of the C1 and C2 vertebrae may involve fractures of the odontoid process and/or tears or stretching of the supporting ligaments without fracture but with disruption of the normal anatomic alignments. Fractures of the odontoid process can be caused by impact to the face, side, or back of the head. Extension loading of the cervical spine with 4410 N (991 lb) has been shown to disrupt the longitudinal ligament and cause transverse fracture of the odontoid process in fresh cadaver experiments.[238] In studies where lateral and flexion loading of the cervical column were carried out, transverse fracture of the odontoid process was observed at 2500 N (562 lb).[238] At this force, substantial disruption of the anterior and posterior longitudinal ligaments also occurred. The odontoid process may also impinge onto the base of the medulla after atlantoaxial dislocation, resulting in substantial compression of the pyramidal tracts.[225,242,247]

Fracture dislocations between C2 and C3 were first described by Wood-Jones as the injury resulting from judicial hanging.[289] In motor vehicle accidents, similar injuries were reported to occur when the face or chin impacted the steering wheel or dashboard. There is hyperextension of the neck, producing shear stresses on the C2 to C3 vertebral unit. The laminar arches of the C2 vertebral body avulse with some degree of dislocation between C2 and C3.[241] Mertz and Patrick suggested that the C2 to C3 unit can withstand an applied shear force of approximately 8900 N.[197,198] In judicial hanging, C2 arches fracture, and the medulla and spinal cord are placed into traction by the downward pull of the body. Subsequent dislocation between C2 and C3 severs the vertebral arteries and compresses the cervicomedullary junction.[242] Hyperextension of the neck secondary to motor vehicle accidents also results in fracture of the neural arches. However, because the body remains supported during the impact sequence, the avulsed arches act to decompress the cervicomedullary junction and usually mild or no neurologic deficits occur.[243]

In experiments in which a cadaver's neck was hyperextended to the point of the anterior longitudinal ligament's failure, bone fracture and separation of the C2 to C3 intervertebral disk occurred. In relation to football injuries, the bending moment or stresses on the cervical spine can be limited by contact of the rear of the helmet to the shoulder pads or neck at midcervical level. It was estimated that high-cut helmets would allow 13 degrees more extension, making it easier for higher strains to develop in the cervical spine between C2 and C5.[62]

Lower cervical spine injuries between C5 and C7 are the most common of the cervical vertebral column injuries.[206,249,290] Hyperextension injuries, which account for most of the lower neck injuries, squeeze the spinal cord between the posterior aspect of the vertebral body and the ligamentum flavum and lamina.[21,117] The resulting spinal cord dysfunction is usually severe, with permanent paralysis or paresis. Individuals who have degenerative spine disease are at particular risk for hyperextension injuries. The degenerative disease process destabilizes the column sufficiently so that even moderate degrees of hyperextension may produce spinal cord injury. Injuries that are associated with normal-appearing spinal radiography are most probably hyperextension injuries.[282]

Hyperflexion injuries often involve trauma to the posterior ligamentous structures, and, as such, account for much of the chronic neckache that is associated with this injury. Injury to the nerve roots and spinal cord is rare. Hyperflexion, however, in combination with rotation is often associated with either unilateral or bilateral facet dislocation, which may also result in facet locking. Intraspinous ligaments are disrupted, along with the facet capsules and the posterior and anterior longitudinal ligaments.[282] Unilateral facet subluxation often involves entrapments and compression of the nerve root and is most frequently associated with moderate cord injury. Bilateral facet dislocation, on the other hand, often produces extensive damage to the spinal cord.[282]

Hyperflexion, in association with compression, generally produces compression injuries to the vertebral bodies. Flexion loadings between 1500 and 4500 N (337 to 1012 lb) were observed to produce cervical vertebral column failure. Massive axial forces applied to the neck during flexion result in a crush fracture at the vertebral body, followed by posterior displacement into the spinal canal. The extent of cord myelopathy appears to be related to the level of flexion at the time of impact.[282]

Laterally applied forces to the cervical column result in fracture injuries to the articular, transverse, and uncinate processes; the vertebral body; and the oncovertebral joints. Subsequent injury to proximal nerve roots and vertebral artery usually occurs. However, extensive damage to the spinal cord is unusual.[282] Dislocation of the cervical column at C6, resulting from direct impact with shear forces of 845 N (190 lb), was demonstrated by Sances et als.[238]

The greater mobility of the thoracolumbar vertebral column contributes significantly to the frequency of spinal injuries in that region. Mechanical stability of the upper thoracic column is strengthened by the rib cage and sternum.

Injury to the thoracolumbar spinal column can result in wedge fracture at the vertebral body, with destruction of the laminae pedicles and facets. Protrusion of the vertebral body into the spinal cord occurs when the injury is severe.[74] Axial compression of sufficient magnitude can cause vertebral burst fractures and bony protrusion into the spinal canal.[154,238] Burst fractures of the thoracic vertebra in seated cadavers were reported to occur at 1554 to 2705 N (350 to 608 lb). The force required for producing these fractures was also shown to vary inversely with the initial degree of vertebral column flexion.[238] The addition of torque results in fracture-dislocations of the thoracic vertebral column. Failure of the vertebral column unit can occur either through the disk or the vertebral body. In general, higher forces are required to fracture and dislocate the thoracic vertebral column between T1 and T9. Injuries to the thoracolumbar vertebral column are also associated with general injury to thoracic organs.[154] Lumbar fractures have been reported to occur infrequently and are the result of flexion and compression.[201,238] Because these injuries involve only the cauda equina, neurologic recovery is potentially high.

In addition to the mechanical properties of the spinal vertebrae, variations in loading characteristics and the strength of muscles and ligaments are vital to the development of spinal injury criteria. Clearly, deformation of the vertebral column and bony fracture depend on the location and magnitude of the loading components—namely, tension, compression, shear, and torsion. The loading characteristics for spinal injuries are more complicated than those for analyzing the head injury.

ANATOMY

Spinal anatomy may be divided arbitrarily into three broad biomechanical categories. The first includes the vertebral bony column and its attendant ligaments and muscles (the vertebral unit); the second is the spinal cord and its associated nerve roots and membrane investments, including the dura (the cord unit); and the third consists of the spinal cord vasculature (the spinal vascular unit). These categories are not strictly accurate because all tissues that compose the spinal system are intimately related. However, the categories are clinically useful in relating biomechanical distortion of the vertebral and spinal vascular units to function of the cord unit.

Vertebral Unit

The spinal column consists of 33 vertebrae: 7 cervical, 12 thoracic, 5 lumbar, 5 fused sacral, and 1 coccygeal that results from the fusion of four separate bodies. The stability and mobility afforded the human body is the mechanical responsibility of this unit. All of the individual bony elements composing the spine articulate by virtue of intravertebral disks and by posterolateral joints, with the exception of the first two cervical and the sacral vertebrae. The very strong annulus fibrosis of the disk provides stability to the synarthroses between the vertebral bodies. The diarthrodial apophyseal joints are stabilized by their capsule as well as the intrasupraspinous ligaments and ligamentum flava. The ligamentous structures—as a result of their intrinsic tensile strength and elasticity, as well as the engineering design used in their points of origin and termination—provide an almost ideal structural unit for stability and mobility. The articular processes are flat and small in the cervical region, whereas those in the upper thoracic region are directed upward and backward. In the lumbar region, the articular surfaces are large, and they point inward and outward. In all cases, the upper facets of the lower vertebrae articulate with the lower facets of the superior vertebrae. Further stability is afforded the thoracic spine through rigidity of the thoracic cage.

Spinal Cord Unit

The spinal cord is a cylindric extension of the brainstem, suspended by means of a series of nerve roots and ligaments in a fluid-filled cavity confined by a relatively inelastic fibrous membrane (the dura). The true spinal dura is an uninterrupted extension of the inner layer of the cranial dura, firmly attached circumferentially at the foramen magnum. It is frequently in close apposition with the posterior surfaces of the first and second cervical vertebrae and more loosely associated with the posterolongitudinal ligament in both the lumbar and cervical regions. At the second sacral level, the dural investment is penetrated by the filum terminale, a direct extension of the pia mater that is in direct continuity with the inferior tapering spinal cord. The filum terminale and its covering of narrowed dura continue as a multilayered structure to blend, finally, with the periosteum of the dorsal surface of the coccyx as the coccygeal ligament.

The interface between the spinal dura and the vertebral column is a true space—known as the *epidural space*—that contains numerous venous plexuses, fat, and ligaments of the vertebral unit. Also through this space passes the entering and exiting nervous elements of the cord as well as significant numbers of vascular structures supplying the cord substance.

Within the dural sac, two additional membranes surround the spinal cord, and, collectively with the dura, they are known as the *spinal meninges*. One of these membranes, the *pia mater,* is intimately applied to the external surface of the cord. A loosely arranged structure, referred to as the *arachnoid,* is interposed between the dura proper and the pia and constitutes the third element of the spinal meninges. The spinal dura and the leptomeninges, by virtue of their intimate relationship to the existing nerve roots, virtually cuff these structures as they terminate their association at the intervertebral foramen.

The ligamentous suspensory elements of the cord itself are known as *dentate ligaments*. Of these processes, 21 are attached to the inner surface of the dura and the lateral surface of the cord. The first dentate ligament is just cephalad to the first cervical roots, and the lowest ligament is found between the last thoracic or just above the first lumbar roots. While the significance of their supportive function to cord remains controversial, these tough small triangular ligaments securely anchor the cord to the dural surface.

The paired spinal roots present a constant reminder of the segmental arrangement present in the substance of the spinal cord. They are divided anatomically into the anterior (motor) and posterior (sensory) roots and are blended together to form the spinal nerves exiting through their cuff of spinal dura at the intervertebral foramen. Aside from their obvious neurophysiologic function, they are also considered by some to provide mechanical fixation for the cord, especially at the cervical level in certain pathologic states.

Vascular Unit

Anatomically, the substance of the spinal cord is supplied by branches from a number of major vessels, including the vertebral and posterocerebellar arteries. Regional perfusion is provided by branches from the thoracic and abdominal aorta as well as from the deep cervical, intercostal, lumbar, and lateral sacral arteries. Lateral spinal arteries, originating from all of these parent vessels, eventually terminate in the anterior and posterior radicular arteries. The anterior radicular artery entering at each side of the cord with each anterior root (only six to eight of these vessels are of significant caliber) joins with the anterior spinal artery, which descends on the ventral surface of the cord after its formation from branches of both vertebral arteries. Within the cranium, small branches of the vertebral or posteroinferior cerebellar arteries continue caudally over the dorsal surface of the cord, usually as two small trunks known as the *posterior spinal arteries*. Only five to eight of the posterior radicular arteries are of sufficient size to provide meaningful perfusion to the cord. The largest of the radicular arteries, both anterior and posterior branches, usually enters the cord circulation in the upper lumbar region. While the venous drainage of the spinal cord may be variable, its anatomic pattern is similar to that of the arteries.

Rheology

Recent work concerning autoregulation of spinal cord blood flow by Hickey et al.[149] demonstrates clearly the close parallelism between spinal cord and cerebral blood flow and emphasizes the need to consider spinal cord perfusion pressure along the same lines as cerebral perfusion pressure. Hickey's group found that spinal cord blood flow autoregulated between mean arterial blood pressures of 60 and 120 mm Hg. Below the lower and above the upper limit, flow becomes pressure dependent. Thus spinal cord ischemia may be exacerbated in situations of sustained spinal cord perfusion pressure below the lower limits of autoregulation. This is also important in light of our knowledge of the vascular dynamics of spinal cord blood flow, which indicates that blood flows from the opposite ends of the spinal cord via the cervical cord vessels and the paired posterior and

anterior spinal arteries.[82] Thus the "watershed areas" can be found at equidistant points from the radicular artery bifurcations. It appears that the lower cervical area, because it is farthest from collateral pathways, would be the most vulnerable to ischemia. These rheologic considerations have been shown to have clinical relevance in humans. Turnbull et al.[273] studied autopsy material demonstrating the presence of only one anterior radicular artery supplying the cervical cord. Fried et al.[113] collected three human spinal cords showing a paucity of radicular arteries. Manners performed a postmortem review of 215 spinal cords and showed only one anterior radicular artery in the cervical cord.[185] Confirmation of the clinical response to the cervical "watershed" can be seen in Jellinger's analysis[153] of the distribution of chronic ischemic cord lesions in 60 cases of advanced arteriosclerosis. He noted the preferential area of ischemia was located between C5 and T2. In Manners' postmortem review mentioned previously, there were 25 spinal cord infarctions in geriatric cases in which the selective site for small softening was at the C5 to C8 levels, with the greatest number of infarcts being at the C6 segment. The rhesus monkey study of Fried et al. demonstrated that the area most vulnerable to ischemia is at C6 because the blood flow splits into compartments flowing up and down the anterior spinal artery.[113] Thus the lower cervical area is farthest from the collateral pathways (via the vertebral and intercostal arteries). These facts underline the dangers in allowing arterial hypotension to continue below the lower limits of autoregulation for any sustained period. There are also hazards in manipulating the head and neck during positioning for surgical procedures because neck manipulation may compromise blood flow to these vulnerable areas.

Physiopathology

The past three decades have changed much of the thinking related to acute spinal cord injury.[54] Formerly it was thought that acute spinal trauma was irreversible and hopeless, and, therefore, efforts were focused on improving the functional ability of the patient with this type of lesion by bettering the rehabilitative process. Albin et al.,[11-14,16] as well as White et al.,[283-285] gave impetus to a new understanding of the physiopathology of spinal cord injury by reviving and modifying the impact injury animal model first developed by Allen[20] and studied by Freeman and Wright in 1953.[112] Albin et al. and White demonstrated (1) that the acute cord lesion progressively develops time-dependent characteristics, involving primarily gray matter vascularity; (2) that up to a point (4 hr), it is possible to arrest this destructive process by localized spinal cord hypothermia, and (3) that it is possible to use somatosensory cortically evoked responses (SCER) to test the completeness of the lesion.[16,122,285] These findings have been verified in elegant histologic studies by Dohrman et al.,[84-86] Wagner et al.,[276,277] Goodkin and Campbell,[120] and Assenmacher and

Ducker.[28] Changes in oxygen tensions have been indicated by Kelly et al.[159] and Ducker et al.,[95] whereas Donaghy and Numoto,[90] Perot;[220] Rowed et al.,[236] and Grundy and Friedman[130] have shown the sensitivity of the SCER as a diagnostic and prognostic tool. Lewin et al.[176] and Eidelberg et al.[98] implicated changes in Na^+ and K^+ in the injured spinal cord secondary to tissue edema and necrosis, whereas Kakari et al.[157] thought the release of lysosomal enzymes was important in the development of the lesion. An important development in the understanding of this pathologic process involving spinal cord injury was made by Osterholm and Mathews,[214,216,217] who described an increase in norepinephrine in the gray matter of the contused spinal cord and noted that blocking norepinephrine synthesis by alpha methyltyrosine could prevent lesion expansion. Although this finding was not corroborated by others, these investigators can be credited with opening the area of spinal cord injury to neurochemical evaluation.[55,56,77,207]

In terms of the dynamics of experimental impact injury, trauma can bring with it mechanical destruction of neuronal elements, hemorrhage, or both; a decreased vascular perfusion; and lowering tissue Po_2, edema, and necrosis.[84,85] The critical nature of the time dependence has been shown by Albin et al.[9] Inhibition of axoplasmic transport (using tritiated leucine) can be seen 2 hours after injury, with a marked block occurring 4 hours after trauma and complete inhibition at 6 hours. It is important to realize that Drummond and Moore[92] noted in animals that neurologic dysfunction increased in the presence of dextrose administration after temporary spinal cord ischemia.

Unfortunately, experimental responses to new therapies are difficult to evaluate because of the large variety of methods used to produce the injury.[161] They range from the weight-drop technique (developed by Allen,[20] tested by Freeman and Wright,[112] and reintroduced by Albin et al.[11,13] in the 1960s) to open compressive techniques. Typically, most investigators use the Allen technique of weight drop. However, it is open to criticism related to the laminectomy, which (1) exposes the cord to infection and other cellular changes; (2) removes the anatomic energy-attenuating structures (e.g., hair, skin, bone, and muscle mass) so that a relatively small amount of force can produce major damage; (3) lacks correlation with pathologic changes found in humans; (4) does not allow the study of the biomechanical factors concerning the vertebral body, posterior elements, and ligaments; and (5) is variable in lesion development because of differences in design of weight-dropping systems. To obviate the limitations of the Allen model, our research group has developed an experimental closed impact injury technique, which uses a missile impacting on an impounder resting between the T9 to T10 interspace.[57] The impounder is seated in an electronic collar that records the force exerted on impact. It was found that 0.8×10^7 dynes/kg of force (or greater) caused irreversible paraplegia and created lesions that indicated complete histologic damage in the spinal cord of the animals used. It is felt that this new closed impact injury model for studying acute impact injury to the spinal cord is superior to the presently-used Allen technique because it shows more relevancy to injury in the human and is more suitable for drug evaluation and biochemical studies. We believe that it is imperative that standardization of a spinal cord injury model occur so that investigators will be able to make critical comparisons of a relevant nature and have a benchmark bereft of experimental variables.

THERAPY

Therapeutic modalities evaluated in the experimental animal have involved localized selective hypothermia as described by Albin et al.,[11-14,16] White et al.,[283,285] Ducker et al.,[95] Kelly et al.,[159] Hansebout et al.,[137] and Kuchner and Hansebout.[166] In 1961, Albin et al.[12] described perfusion cooling of the subarachnoid space after laminectomies at T9 and T10 in which intrinsic spinal cord temperatures of 10° C or lower could be reached and maintained. The choice of 10° C as a target temperature was made because the somatosensory evoked potentials passing through the cord were abolished at this temperature, indicating a substantial decrease in metabolic activity.[13] Subsequently, paraplegia was produced (in dogs and monkeys) using the weight-drop technique developed by Allen,[20] studied by Freeman and Wright,[112] and reintroduced by Albin et al.[11] With the same force as used in the control group, perfusion cooling after attaining a cord temperature of 10° C, was carried out for 3 hours after a 4-hour delay following injury. Although there was evidence of histologic damage in the hypothermic group, motor function returned in these animals, while the control group remained paraplegic. Unfortunately, in the enthusiasm generated by the publication of this paper, uncontrolled clinical studies were carried out that demonstrated limited efficacy. In these five clinical studies, inadequate cooling was carried out with spinal cord temperatures not being measured, localized hypothermia initiated many hours or days after the recommended optimal 4-hour postinjury period, and perfusion cooling carried out for only short periods.[2,49,163,194,246] Tator and Deecke[262] did not find spinal cord hypothermia effective against balloon compression injury and thought that normothermic perfusion was helpful. On the other hand, Thienprasit et al.[267] found localized cord cooling useful against balloon compression injury, whereas Albin and White[10] found normothermic perfusion valueless against the impact injury preparation.

Hyperosmotic agents have been shown by Joyner and Freeman[156] (urea) and by Richardson and Nakamura[230] (mannitol) in experimental animals to have a beneficial effect. Hyperbaric oxygenation (three atmospheres) has also been used by Hartzog et al.[139] on baboons with impact injury and resulted in improvement when compared with controls. Other experimental therapies reported include the use of vasopressors to maintain adequate spinal cord perfusion pressure, epsilon aminocaproic acid by Naftchi et al.[207] for cell membrane stabilization, and dimethyl sulfoxide by de la Torre et al.[76] to reduce edema and to scavenge free radicals. Naloxone has been reported to be useful in experimental spinal cord injury with striking preservation of sensory function and SEP at 24 hr after injury. This finding by Faden[99-101] has stimulated an enormous amount of investigative effort because it was hypothesized that the release of endogenous opioids after central nervous system injury contributes to the developing injury by affecting flow through the microcirculation. Thus the posttraumatic ischemia that is characteristic of impact injury to the spinal cord is partially potentiated by these endogenous opioids and attenuated by the narcotic-antagonist naloxone. However, controlled, randomized multicenter clinical studies using naloxone in patients with spinal cord injury indicated that this drug had no ameliorating effect on SCI.

Similarly, other opiate receptor antagonists—such as naltrexone, betafunaltrexamine, and naloxonazine—have been evaluated in the experimental animal.[99] Interestingly, Wallace and Tator[278] recently reported that naloxone did not improve spinal cord blood flow or cardiac output after SCI produced by a 50-g force clip injury. Black et al.[37,38] also reported the failure of naloxone (at high or megadoses) to improve recovery, using a dynamic loading impact injury similar to that employed by Faden. Thyrotropin-releasing hormone (TRH) has also been employed against SCI (the impact injury model) because of its capability to antagonize endorphins.[99] Faden[103] has compared TRH, naloxone, and dexamethasone in experimental impact injury to the spinal cord and noted that both TRH and naloxone significantly improved neurologic outcome, while the corticosteroid had no benefit.

On the other hand, the glucocorticoids were noted by Ducker et al.[94,95] and Black and Markowitz[39] to be efficacious in experimentally injured animals. Osterholm and Mathews[215-217] and Osterholm[214] reasoned that steroids depress postinjury catecholamine metabolism and accumulation. However, the norepinephrine depression by steroids was less striking than the depression observed during localized hypothermia of the spinal cord. Eidelberg et al.[97] did not find significant differences between the steroid and control group when a more severe experimental injury was used. The use of high-dose corticosteroids for acute SCI characterized much of the experimental therapeutic thinking in the 1980s.[106] From rationales similar to those promoting use of methylprednisolone in septic shock, it was thought that cell membranes could be stabilized by inhibiting the release of lysosomes and by inhibiting complement activation.[26,45-47,102,136] Similarly, the action of high-dose corticosteroids was also thought to involve the scavenging of oxygen-free radicals, thus attenuating the cascade that resulted in neuronal breakdown and the release of eicosanoids.[24,45,78] Clinical trials with methylprednisolone (MP) were carried out under the National Acute Spinal Cord Injury Study (NASCIS) umbrella. In the first study (NAS-

CIS I), low-dose MP (100 mg IV loading, followed by 100 mg daily for 10 days) was compared against a high-dose regimen of MP (1 g IV loading, followed by 1 g daily for 10 days).[42] No difference between the groups was found in the six-point scale for motor power and the three-point scale for sensation. Believing that the NASCIS I MP dose was too small and responding to the experimental evidence showing that naloxone enhanced spinal cord blood flow in the area of injury, NASCIS II was initiated.[44,100] This prospective study randomized treatment to one of three treatment groups—placebo, naloxone (5.4 mg/kg IV loading dose, followed 45 min later by 4 mg/kg/h for 23 hours), and MP (30 mg/kg IV loading dose, followed 45 min later by 5.4 mg/kg/h for 23 hours). Motor and sensory functions were evaluated by neurologic examination on admission, 6 weeks and 6 months after injury. It is important to point out that outcome evaluation was made on the basis of neurologic evaluation and not on functional ability. There were 154 patients in the naloxone group, 162 patients in the MP group, and 171 patients in the control group. Patients treated with naloxone or those given MP more than 8 hours after injury showed no difference in neurologic outcome, when compared with the placebo group. Those patients receiving MP within 8 hours after injury had significant improvement in motor responses at 6 months, when compared with placebo. There was similar mortality and morbidity in all three groups. It must be emphasized that while there were positive changes in the neurologic examination, this study has not demonstrated that improved function occurred as a result of MP therapy. In the discussion concerning the improvement seen with MP, Bracken et al.[44] speculated that the major effect of this therapy is to inhibit cell membrane perturbation by inhibiting lipoperoxidation and the resulting arachidonic acid cascade. In a follow-up to the NASCIS II trial, the patients were again evaluated at 1 year. This evaluation confirmed the results noted at the 6-month evaluation.[43] Patients treated with either steroid or naloxone after 8 hours actually did worse than did the placebo-treated controls. MP patients treated within 8 hours of injury showed statistically significant improvements in both motor and sensory scores.

It has been noted that the anesthetic ketamine hydrochloride (KH) reduces neuronal excitation mediated by the aspartate N-methyl-D-aspartate (NMDA) subclass of the postsynaptic excitatory amino acid (EAA) receptor.[71,186] This NMDA antagonistic effect of KH has been shown to reduce ischemic hippocampal neuronal injury and to block NMDA receptor–mediated late neuronal loss in cortical cell cultures.[70,187] Robertson et al.[233] reported that KH increased the duration of spinal cord ischemia (produced by aortic occlusion) needed to cause hindlimb paralysis in the rabbit. Rigamonti et al.[231] produced spinal cord ischemia with paraplegia in the rat through the intrathecal injection of the endogenous opiate peptide dynorphin A. Dynorphin-treated animals remained paralyzed and showed extensive pathology throughout the lumbosacral cord. Rats injected with dynorphin plus KH demonstrated protection of the lumbar enlargement and lower lumbar segment. The animals treated with KH plus dynorphin were able to bear weight.

Recent work has indicated the exacerbation of neurologic deficits after spinal cord ischemia when the animal was pretreated with dextrose, resulting in hyperglycemia.[106,169,173,174,179] This is similar to the finding that an increased blood glucose level before cerebral ischemia is associated with poorer neurologic outcome in humans.[288] The pathogenesis of this poorer outcome may be that the increased glucose results in a higher intracellular lactic acid accumulation during the ischemic period.

Secondary physiopathologic responses after dynamic spinal cord injury include reflux of prostaglandins, oxygen-free radicals, arachidonic acid metabolites, vasogenic amines, and reperfusion phenomenon involving calcium, oxygen, and glucose. All these biochemical factors have antagonists that are being evaluated for treatment of intestinal, myocardial, and cerebral ischemia. Some of the compounds that have been tested under experimental and clinical conditions are superoxide dismutase, catalase, prostacyclins, dimethylsulfoxide (DMSO), calcium channel blockers, allopurinol, and antioxidants, such as vitamin E.[65,76,190]

The relationship of driving while intoxicated to spinal cord and head trauma is obvious to all. What has not been appreciated is that Flamm et al.[105] reported exacerbation of experimental spinal cord and intracranial lesions with ethanol intoxication resulting—to a great extent—from an increase in oxygen-free radicals and subsequent lipoperoxidation with cellular damage. Albin and Bunegin[6] reported a marked increase in intracranial lesion volume after pressure-induced focal ischemia under conditions of prior ethanol loading (200 mg per dl). These intracranial lesions could be markedly attenuated by treatment with DMSO, a compound that has free-radical scavenging properties.[6]

The application of the therapies just mentioned is difficult to evaluate in humans, unless a standardized, randomized study with rigid selection criteria is effected. The primary difficulty involves rapidly getting the patient to a hospital center equipped to initiate therapy. Clinically, spinal cord cooling has been used with inconsistent results in humans, as reported by Acosta-Rua,[2] Koons et al.,[163] White et al.,[283] Meachem et al.,[195] and Bricolo et al.[49] Our own experience has been hampered by difficulties in delivering and evaluating the patient in order to begin cooling within the 4-hr period.[4] Recent information has noted that moderate hypothermia (a decrease of 2° to 3° below normothermia) is neuroprotective against cerebral ischemia and that moderate hypothermia has an effect in decreasing the concentration of leucotrienes during cerebral ischemia, hence attenuating the development of the neurodestructive cascade.[59,79]

EFFECTS OF ANESTHETIC AGENTS AND ADJUVANTS ON THE SPINAL CORD

Recent work concerning autoregulation of spinal cord blood flow (SCBF) by Hickey et al.[149] demonstrated succinctly the close parallelism between spinal cord and cerebral blood flow and emphasized the need to consider spinal cord perfusion pressure along the same lines as cerebral perfusion pressure. Hickey's group found that SCBF autoregulated between mean arterial blood pressures of 60 to 120 mm Hg. Below the lower and above the upper limit, flow becomes pressure dependent. Thus spinal cord ischemia may be exacerbated if the spinal cord perfusion pressure is sustained below the lower limits of autoregulation.

There is a paucity of information concerning the effects of anesthetic agents on autoregulation of SCBF. After pentobarbital was administered to rats, Hickey et al.[149] noted that autoregulation of spinal cord and cerebral blood flow occurred between the range of 60 to 120 mm Hg. They also noted that autoregulation was abolished after ketamine was administered (40.0 mg/kg) and described autoregulation of SCBF after halothane administration ranging between 70 and 110 mm Hg in the rat[147,148] (Figs. 33-1 and 33-2). While spinal cord research has centered on the physiopathologic, therapeutic, and regenerative processes related to spinal cord injury, there is a lack of experimental data concerning the effects of anesthetics per se on traumatic and/or ischemic SCI. Cole et al.[73] demonstrated the protective effects of fentanyl/N_2O, spinal lidocaine, and halothane in the setting of experimental acute SCI due to expansion of an epidural balloon in rats. The balloon catheter was inflated for varying periods, and the duration of balloon inflation required to produce hindlimb paralysis was determined for each group. Cole et al. were able to demonstrate an improved tolerance for epidural spinal cord compression in all three anesthetic groups, as compared with awake controls. The times required to produce a neurologic deficit (hindlimb paralysis) for spinal lidocaine, halothane, and fentanyl/N_2O were 19.6, 19.8, and 37.9 minutes, respectively, compared with 10 minutes in controls. Seven days after the injury, the incidence of sustained neurologic injury in the anesthetic exposure group was lower than in controls. No specific conclusions were drawn about the precise properties affording this apparent protection.

Conversely, Koike et al.,[162] reported that a neurologic deficit developed more rapidly in ketamine- and halothane-anesthetized rabbits than in control animals in an experimental ischemic SCI model. Because rabbits have poorly developed collateral flow to the lower spinal cord, occlusion of the infrarenal aorta in these animals resulted in an ischemic injury to the lower cord. The rabbits received intraperitoneal injections of ketamine, fentanyl, naloxone, or saline during the period of occlusion. Another group was maintained with halothane. The time to total neurologic deficit in 50% of animals (ED_{50}) was determined for each

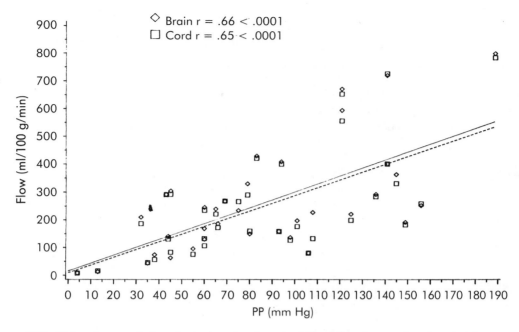

FIG. 33-1 Autoregulation of spinal cord and cerebral blood flow in rats after the administration of ketamine hydrochloride. Autoregulation is abolished, as noted by the regression equation. The horizontal axis *(PP)* represents cerebral and spinal cord perfusion pressures, and the vertical axis is blood flow expressed as ml per 100 g of brain or spinal cord tissue per minute. *(From Hickey R, Albin MS, Bunegin L:* Anesthesia Rev *15:78-79, 1988).*

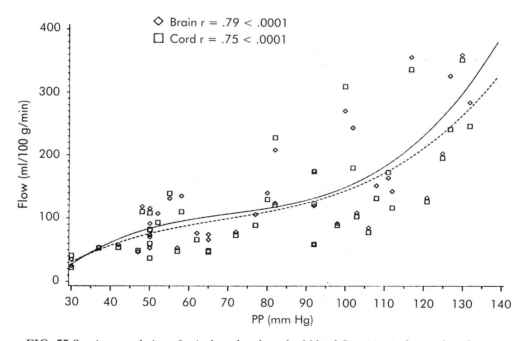

FIG. 33-2 Autoregulation of spinal cord and cerebral blood flow in rats during the administration of halothane. Autoregulation is modified as noted by the regression equations. The axes are the same as Fig. 33-1. *(From Hickey R, Albin MS, Bunegin L:* Anesthesia Rev *15:78-79, 1988.)*

group. The ED_{50} in control animals was 35.1 min, compared with 37.5 min in the naloxone group and 51.3 min in the fentanyl group. Those animals receiving ketamine and halothane demonstrated a decrease in the ED_{50} to 22.5 and 23.3 minutes, respectively. Despite the failure of fentanyl to demonstrate a change in the ED_{50}, the ability of naloxone to extend the period of ischemia suggested to the authors that anesthetic doses of narcotics may also shorten the time to neurologic injury. They concluded that "anesthesia" may be detrimental for patients with spinal pathology or recent stroke. More recently, Salzman et al.[237] have shown that rats receiving weight-drop SCI during halothane-induced anesthesia had better neurologic scores at all levels of injury, when compared with animals receiving pentobarbital. They also demonstrated that hypotension and hypoventilation did not contribute to the worsened outcome with pentobarbital. In addition, hypothermia was not associated with the improved outcome observed with halothane.

While these are the only studies that have been specifically designed to assess the effect of anesthetics on SCI, alterations in outcome have been demonstrated with other anesthetic agents. Barbiturates have been shown to be protective in models of focal ischemic cerebral injury, and a similar effect has been shown in ischemic SCI.* The protective benefits of barbiturates were also noted in experimental SCI using the weight-drop technique.[66]

One of the limitations in comparing data between studies of experimental SCI is the lack of standardization between methods used to create the injury. To date, the methods have included the use of weight-drop techniques (on both exposed and closed spinal cords),[16,89] acute compression of the spinal cord by clips[131,213] and balloons,[73,267] ischemia created by temporary vessel occlusion,† and compression caused by the implantation of tumor cells[251,274] and expandable synthetic materials.[27,33,128,263]

With experimental impact injury, the trauma occasions mechanical destruction of neuronal elements, hemorrhage, decreased cord perfusion, tissue hypoxia, edema, and necrosis. It also requires that a laminectomy be performed, which increases the risk of infection and other cellular changes and removes the anatomic energy-attenuating structures (e.g., hair, skin, bone, and muscle mass), so that a relatively small amount of force produces major damage.

There are some models of SCI that do have close ties to potential SCI in humans. Aortic occlusion models described in the rabbit, dog, and rat may be analogous to the situation in which spinal cord ischemia and injury develop during clamping and repair of thoracoabdominal aneurysms.[170,177,191] Other investigators have modeled the problem of spinal cord compression secondary to neoplasm by creating an experimental model of epidural cord compression using implanted tumor cells[251] or expandable synthetic materials.[27,33,128]

Grissom et al.[128] evaluated the effects of isoflurane, fentanyl/N_2O, and ketamine on a model of chronic spinal cord injury that used a hydrophilic expansible mass. They found that neurologic outcome was adversely affected by ketamine, whereas the other anesthetics demonstrated little change from controls.

CLINICAL CONSIDERATIONS WITH ACUTE SPINAL CORD INJURY

The protean nature of acute cervical SCI is manifested by changes in cardiopulmonary responses, fluid and electrolyte disorders, temperature control dysfunction, and abnormal responses to drugs.

Respiratory

The major early cause of death in patients with acute SCI is respiratory failure, which is usually secondary to paralysis of respiratory muscles.[253] The degree of respiratory insufficiency depends on the level of spinal cord injury. The spinal cord respiratory center, which is the origin of the phrenic nerve, is composed of the C4 segment of the cervical spinal cord with small contributions from the C3 and C5 segments. If the SCI occurs below the C4 level and the C4 nerve root is functioning under cervical control, voluntary control of breathing is expected, with a vital capacity (VC) of 20% to 25% of normal.[258] When the traumatic lesion is above the C4 level, voluntary diaphragmatic respiration mediated by the phrenic nerve is not possible. Injury to the upper part of the cervical cord involves nuclei of the lower cranial nerves. Such a lesion causes impairment of peripheral facial sensation and paralysis of the sternocleidomastoid and trapezius muscles. Most spinal cord injuries extend several segments superiorly and interiorly from the main traumatic area; therefore the damage may extend into the brain stem and affect motor control of the pharynx and sensation of the face.[218,258] Functional levels of SCI paralysis were classified by Stauffer and Bell.[258] The upper cervical lesions were divided into two groups. Pentaplegia is characterized by involvement of the lower cranial nerves and accessory muscles, with injury level at the brainstem to C1, and motor and sensory loss of the neck, arms, legs, and diaphragm. The patient with respiratory quadriplegia has a typical C2 and C3 functional level lesion in which all cranial and the upper two or three cervical nerves remain intact and thereby retains full sensation of the head and upper neck remains intact, as well as control of the sternocleidomastoid and accessory muscles of the neck. Such a patient has paralysis of the diaphragm and all four extremities and obviously requires ventilatory support. Cervical lesions at C6 or below spare diaphragmatic innervation but affect intercostal muscles to various degrees. Diaphragmatic respiration might be further restricted in patients with

---

*References 18, 66, 68, 150, 200, 210, 222, 233.
†References 66, 68, 89, 131, 162, 210, 213.

TABLE 33-1
Ventilatory Changes After Cervical Spinal Cord Injury

Innervation	Level	Ventilation
Accessory muscles spared Diaphragm paralyzed	C2	Ventilatory assistance
Total	C3	Ventilatory assistance
Partial	C4-C6	Greatly affected
Intercostal muscles paralyzed		Diaphragmatic

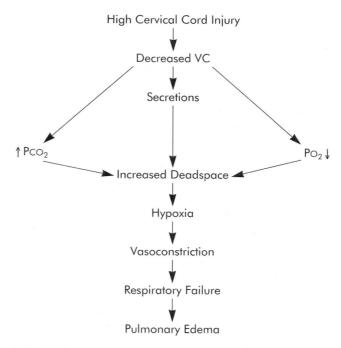

FIG. 33-3 Respiratory responses to high cervical spinal cord injury. *VC*, vital capacity.

quadriplegia by abdominal distention, usually resulting from acute gastric dilation. Paralysis of intercostal muscles alone decreases alveolar ventilation, causing paradoxical respiration—the inward motion of the upper thorax during upper intercostal contraction in inspiration, which prevents the patient from coughing effectively.[178,226] Such patients are unable to lift their ribs for enlarging the volume of their chest and are deprived of that volume of gas normally contributed by intercostal activity. In normal individuals, expansion of the rib cage accounts for 60% of the tidal volume.[34] Table 33-1 shows ventilatory changes after cervical cord injury.

Body positioning markedly affects alveolar ventilation in the patient with quadriplegia.[114] Gravity has an adverse effect on the mechanism of respiration in the upright position. The flaccid abdominal muscles protrude, abdominal contents move toward the pelvis, and the diaphragm lowers. Inspiration then results from a shorter descent of the diaphragm. With expiration, no abdominal rebound occurs to return the diaphragm to its resting position. The absence of elasticity of the abdominal muscles compromises pulmonary ventilation in the upright position.[193,194] Ventilation is markedly improved in the supine position, with descent of the diaphragm accompanied by compression of the abdominal contents and forward position of the flaccid abdominal wall.[193] At the end of inspiration in the supine position, the elastic recoil of the abdominal wall—combined with movement of the abdominal contents—moves the diaphragm cephalad, decreasing the end-expiratory volume and allowing for greater excursion of the diaphragm on the next inspiration. These facts become important to remember when placing the patient with quadriplegia in the head-up position before induction of anesthesia and during endotracheal intubation.

The expiratory reserve volume is low in those with quadriplegia, and maximal expiratory pressure is significantly reduced.[64] Inability to cough effectively leads to retention of secretions, atelectasis, and hypoxia. Possible aspiration of stomach contents presents additional respiratory problems and may occur at the time of or soon after the accident when the patient may regurgitate secondarily to hypoxia.[69] Fig. 33-3 summarizes the consequences of high cervical cord injury on respiration.

Pulmonary function has been studied extensively in SCI patients.* In 1955, Cameron et al.[60] showed that VC in patients with tetraplegia is less than normal and is affected by the posture of the patient (i.e., greater when the patient was tilted head down and least when tilted feet down). This was attributed to postural effects and paralysis of the abdominal muscles. In 1958, Hemingway et al.[145] confirmed Cameron's findings that patients with tetraplegia had reduced VC (two thirds of the predicted normal) and found in addition that maximal breathing capacity was reduced. Silver[252] in 1963 and Bergofsky[34] in 1964 independently showed that work of breathing in patients with tetraplegia is markedly increased. McKinley et al.[193] studied eight subjects with traumatic transection of the cervical cord in quadriplegia for an average of 27 months after injury. They found that VC ranged from 36% to 91% of that predicted and that there was no evidence of obstructive changes. Arterial blood gas levels and dynamic pulmonary compliance were normal. The thoracic component of ventilation was calculated to be 22% to 90% of total ventilation. Correlation between the level of SCI and results of bedside spirometry were described by Ohry et al.[212] As was expected, forced vital capacity (FVC) and forced expiratory volume in 1 second (FEV_1) were lowest for those with cervical lesions and highest for those with lumbar lesions.[212] Studying the flow volume curves of 20 patients with quadriplegia, Forner et al.[109] found that in the supine and Trende-

---

*References 34, 60, 108, 109, 152, 171, 193, 194, 212, 253.

lenburg positions the mean values of FVC were significantly higher than in the sitting position. This study showed the correlation between spirometry results and body positioning. Fugl-Meyer and Grimby,[114] while performing pulmonary function studies in patients with quadriplegia, showed a decrease in total lung capacity (TLC), a decrease in VC to 66% of that predicted, a decrease in the expiratory reserve volume (ERV) to 33% of that predicted, and an increase in residual volume (RV) to 107%; however, the functional residual capacities (FRC) were normal. In 1980, Forner[108] studied the mechanics of breathing and lung volumes in patients with quadriplegia and found the relation FEV_1/FVC to be normal, indicating the absence of airway obstruction. Also, VC and ERV—as well as peak expiratory flow and maximal expiratory flows at 25%, 50%, and 75% of VC—were found to be reduced. Respiratory assessment by pulmonary function testing was presented by McMichan et al.[194] in 1980. The usefulness of intermittent spirometric examination in the management of patients with SCI was demonstrated. The majority of observations, however, have been made on patients after the acute stage of injury, usually between 2 months and 5 years after injury. Ledsome and Sharp[171] measured pulmonary function in the patient as soon as possible after injury to the cervical region of the spinal cord. Initial measurements were recorded at 3 days of spinal cord injury on admission to the hospital and thereafter at 3 weeks, 5 weeks, 3 months, and 5 months. During the first week, the measurements of FVC, FEV_1, and maximal mid-expiratory flow rate (FEF of 25% to 75%) were reduced to about 30% of predicted values. Significant improvement occurred in the fifth week after injury. The average FEV_1/FVC percentage was normal, indicating that significant airway obstruction was not usually a problem.

Holmstrom and Babinski[151] carried out bedside spirometry for early pulmonary assessment in patients with acute SCI. During a 2-year period, 17 patients with various degrees of neuromuscular paralysis after acute trauma to the spinal cord were studied. There were 12 patients with cervical lesions and 5 with thoracic. In 9 patients, associated injury to the chest or abdomen complicated their hospital course. Bedside spirometry, using a Stead-Wells respirometer, was performed within 24 hours after trauma with all patients supine and horizontal. Additional measurements were done at intervals during their hospital stay. Two patients with C2 to C3 injuries had minimal neurologic deficits; the decrease in FVC resulted from immobilization and traction. The group with lower cervical lesions showed an initial decrease in FVC to about 22% of that predicted, with further deterioration for the fourth day, and gradual improvement through the second and third weeks. No other group of patients showed such a decrease. This early deterioration in respiratory status probably represents a transient upward spread of the cord lesion, affecting the additional phrenic nerve elements and to some degree the accessory muscles. FVC returned to the first-day values within a week and improved to 30% of that predicted in 3 weeks. Improvement occurs when spinal shock subsides and muscle spasticity increases. The decrease in FVC in patients with thoracic injury was related to the degree of intercostal involvement, as well as associated injuries to the chest. These studies also demonstrated that, based on a FEV_1/FVC ratio, there is no obstructive element seen at any cord injury level. Pulmonary function test studies, when initiated early and used periodically, facilitate the management of patients with acute SCI. Comparison of changes in FVC and apparent lesion level assist in determining the need for intubation or tracheostomy, the need for and duration of mechanical ventilation, and the likelihood of pulmonary complications. Pulmonary function tests should be a mandatory part of the preoperative evaluation of such a patient.

Additional pathologic events in the acute period of SCI that can further impair alveolar ventilation are extension of the lesion, pulmonary embolism, and pulmonary edema.[226,287] The initial level of the lesion may ascend or descend to involve other portions of the spinal cord. Deterioration in a patient's condition may be caused by the upward spread of spinal cord edema and hemorrhage. Such extensions of the cone of hemorrhage or edema in the spinal cord can involve the anterolateral portion of the cord in the C2 to C4 area. This usually occurs without any prior changes in objective respiratory findings.[205,264] An awake patient shows adequate alveolar ventilation but while asleep can develop apnea. Experience with percutaneous cordotomies has shown that the greatest danger of sleep apnea is during the first 5 nights after the insult to the spinal cord.[205,264]

Two main pathologic disturbances of the general circulation during the acute stage of SCI can affect respiration. Pulmonary embolism is often the cause of death within the first month after the acute injury. The incidence of pulmonary embolism in patients dying in the early stages of SCI was found by Wolman[287] to be 15.2%—5 fatalities in a series of 33 acute cases. Pulmonary embolism was found to occur only in the acute stage and was never a cause of death after the first month.[287] The incidence of pulmonary edema in the patient with acute SCI is rather high.[199,224,287] It is related to the acute insult to the central nervous system and, in many cases, to overtransfusion. In 44 cases of acute injury to the cervical spine presented by Wolman,[287] 30 patients died within 11 days of the accident. Of these 30 cases, 23 died of acute respiratory failure—accompanied by severe pulmonary edema in 20 and massive pulmonary collapse in 3.[287] Meyer et al.[199] presented hemodynamic studies of 9 battle casualties who suffered acute quadriplegia. Four of the 9 patients developed severe pulmonary edema 11 to 34 hr after wounding. Although chest trauma and other factors may have contributed to the development of pulmonary edema, the most likely cause was fluid overload during resuscitation.[199] An interesting observation was the increase in total peripheral resistance (TPR) in these patients after injury. In one case, TPR increased by 40% in 25 hr and in the other, by approximately 230% in 95 hr. This sudden increase in autonomic neural activity could trigger an acute volume overload of the vascular system and precipitate acute pulmonary edema. Poe et al.[224] described a case of acute pulmonary edema diagnosed within 10 to 12 hr after acute injury to the cervical spine. There was no concomitant head injury or other respiratory complications, and the authors considered neurogenic pulmonary edema (NPE) to be the causative factor (NPE will be discussed in greater detail later). It is important to emphasize that fluid overload or "iatrogenic" pulmonary edema probably occurs more frequently than is reported in the literature. Because of the hypotension brought on by the spinal shock, overly vigorous fluid therapy to bring the mean arterial pressure to normal levels by those unfamiliar with or forgetting the dynamics of acute SCI can result in pulmonary edema. It is often forgotten that because the patient with SCI is usually younger than 30 years of age, the autoregulation of spinal cord and cerebral blood flow generally remains within normal limits, indicating that these individuals may tolerate a decreased perfusion pressure.

Cardiovascular-Neurogenic

When first evaluated, the patient with complete acute cervical SCI demonstrates the stigmata of spinal shock—namely, hypotension, bradycardia, and increased venous capacitance. To this one can add a decrease in myocardial contractility and poikilothermia. In controlled animal experiments, trauma to the spinal cord at about the T10 vertebral level produces a brief immediate vasopressor response, characterized by arterial hypertension,[228] an increase in pulse pressure, bradycardia, and cardiac arrhythmias.[15,129] After this brief hypertensive phase (2 to 6 min), prolonged hypotension results, with continued bradycardia, decreased systemic vascular resistance, and decreased myocardial contractility. The physiologic consequences of this second phase are similar to that of the onset of spinal shock found in humans. Thus acute transection of the spinal cord may initiate a transitory sympathetic-mediated response, followed by a reaction consistent with denervation of the sympathetic outflow.[268] In experimental animals, Albin et al.[8] demonstrated that acute transection of the spinal cord at C4 initiates immediate transitory sympathetic mediated responses. They observed a marked increase in mean arterial blood pressure, followed by significant hypotension; increases in pulmonary capillary wedge pressure, extravascular lung water, intracranial pressure (ICP), brain water, and blood-brain barrier permeability; and a decrease in cerebral blood flow (CBF). Pretreatment with an alpha-adrenergic blocking agent, phentolamine, followed by transection blocked the rise in arterial blood pressure but did not affect the increase in ICP, brain water, blood-brain barrier permeability, and extravascular lung water, or the

TABLE 33-2
Summary of Findings after Experimental Spinal Cord Transection at the Vertebral C2 Level, Without and With Pretreatment of 2-mg Intravenous Phentolamine

Variable	Transection Alone	Phentolamine + Transection
Mean arterial pressure	↑	No Change
Intracranial pressure	↑	↑
Blood-brain barrier	↑	↑
Brain water	↑	↑
Cerebral blood flow*	↓	↓

*Microsphere technique.

decrease in CBF (Table 33-2). The changes found by Albin et al. appear to have significant correlates in the human situation. The development of pulmonary edema secondary to neurologic dysfunction was initially reported after head injuries; it has also been noted after trauma to the spinal cord, strokes, ICP, and central nervous system disease, including seizures, tumors, and intracranial hemorrhage.* A large body of experimental data exists, and the association of pulmonary edema with primary central nervous system pathology has been termed *neurogenic pulmonary edema,* a term originally coined by Sarnoff and Sarnoff[239] in 1952. Neurogenic pulmonary edema (NPE) appears to be characterized by the following: (1) the absence of a cardiopulmonary pathologic condition such as a primary process of the lung or heart or both, (2) an extraordinary rapid onset occurring within seconds to minutes after injury, (3) the presence of critical anatomic areas, that, when lesioned or stimulated, will cause pulmonary edema (hypothalamus or medulla oblongata or both), (4) inhibition of pulmonary edema by alpha-adrenergic blockers, anesthetics, or central nervous system depressants, (5) similarity to the fulminating onset of pulmonary edema found after epinephrine infusion at high doses, (6) the high protein content of the pulmonary edema exudate, and (7) an initial transitory increase in pulmonary and systemic vascular resistance, followed by pulmonary edema, while the pulmonary and systemic vascular resistance return to normal.[265] This points to a centrogenic pathogenesis involving intense sympathetic hyperactivity possibly secondary to stimulation of hypothalamic, medullary, or brainstem areas in the brain caused by trauma, compression, stimulation, or increases in ICP.†

The production of neurogenic pulmonary edema by induced intracranial hypertension, as pioneered by Campbell et al.[61] and developed by Ducker and Simmons,[93,96] has provided a useful model for evaluating many of the pathophysiologic features of this entity. Malik[184] and Van der

*References 36, 104, 146, 204, 224, 281, 287.
†References 31, 40, 51, 67, 83, 93, 96, 115, 123, 183, 184, 229.

Zee et al.[275] investigated the pulmonary vascular response to increased ICP and the lung fluid exchange during increased ICP. They were interested in evaluating the role of sympathetic mechanisms, and, in addition to cardiopulmonary dynamics, they also measured lung lymph flow and protein concentration during an increase in ICP to near-mean arterial blood pressure levels. They also pretreated one series of sheep with an alpha-blocker, phenoxybenzamine, and created a series of both pretreated and posttreated animals with increased ICP by use of another alpha-blocker, phentolamine (2.0 mg/kg).[184,275] In the untreated sheep, the increased ICP resulted in a significant increase in mean arterial blood pressure, systemic vascular resistance, lymph flow, lymph protein concentration, lymph-plasma protein concentration ratio, and lymph clearance and a decrease in plasma protein concentration. In the group with phentolamine pretreatment, the ICP elevation did not produce the marked alteration in lymph flow and lymph-protein concentration ratios. The researchers also found no increase in mean arterial blood pressure, systemic vascular resistance, pulmonary artery pressure, or pulmonary blood flow. They pointed out that only modest increases in left atrial pressure occurred as a result of increased ICP, even when the mean ICP was raised above mean arterial blood pressure. It was noted by Guyton and Lindsay[133] that left atrial pressure must be elevated and maintained at or above 25 mm Hg for 2 to 3 hours to produce pulmonary edema. It was postulated that increased ICP caused an increase in lung vascular permeability, and the increase was independent of hemodynamic mechanisms.[184,275] Thus it was concluded that the increase in vascular permeability to protein during increased ICP was due to sympathetic stimulation. Phentolamine, on the other hand, prevented the increase in permeability and increases in lung lymph flow. Bowers et al.[41] and Brigham et al.[50] also noted increased lung vascular permeability after induced intracranial hypertension in sheep, as evidenced by the increased flow of protein-rich lymph under the conditions of near-normal pulmonary vascular pressures. They speculated that the increased vascular permeability could be affected by vasoactive substances, such as histamine (normally present in the lung), with release occurring from neural stimuli.[41,50] Another explanation was that a direct neuronal pathway was involved that may increase the pulmonary vascular permeability.

Interestingly, Nathan and Reis[209] reported that bilateral electrolytic lesions of the anterior hypothalamus produced within a period of 2 hr arterial hypertension, tachycardia, hyperthermia, and increased motor activity, leading to pulmonary edema and death in unrestrained rats. The same course occurred with paralyzed, anesthetized, and ventilated rats. Phentolamine at the concentration of 1 mg/kg reversed the mean arterial blood pressure rise and the elevated peripheral resistance and brought the decreased cardiac output to normal levels.[207] Bilateral adrenalectomy, adrenal demodulation, or adrenal denervation before lesion placement prevented the increased mean arterial blood pressure

and pulmonary edema, as well as changes in peripheral resistance, cardiac output, and body temperature. The researchers concluded that a cardiovascular mechanism involved the release of catecholamines from the adrenal medulla and that pulmonary edema resulted from myocardial failure caused by ventricular overload. It was thought that the pathway passing through the anterior hypothalamus may exert control over the adrenal medulla that is independent of the vasomotor neurons.

Albin et al.[8] envisioned a resonating circuit with pivotal loci in the brain and spinal cord that modulated and integrated the functional and neurohumoral responses between the brain, lungs, and cardiovascular system and which controlled the level of activity involving blood-brain barrier permeability and CBF. The moment the spinal cord segment of this loop is disrupted by transection, the loop is opened and dysfunction occurs until the circuit is reestablished at a different functional level (spinal shock). In both groups with transection only and phentolamine plus transection, the changes in CBF could not be due to deficient perfusion because the cerebral perfusion pressure was at or above a mean of 100 mm Hg during the time the CBF was studied. Although physiologic responses involving both acute and complete transection of the cervical spinal cord and the development of the Cushing reflex (through increased ICP) may have some similarities, the initiation of these responses is markedly different.[35,36] The reaction to transection is extraordinarily rapid in terms of its effects on ICP, blood-brain barrier permeability, brain water, and CBF, and evanescent in the cardiovascular responses that occur. The rise in extravascular lung water appears to be a later response, and similar to ICP, blood-brain barrier permeability, brain water, and CBF, it is not markedly attenuated by pretreatment with the alpha-blocker phentolamine.

If one can transpose this information to humans, it emphasizes the exquisite physiologic vulnerability of the patient with acute transection of the cervical spinal cord during the first few hours after transection. In the 1960s, Albin et al.[11,16] and White et al.[283] emphasized the rapidity of the intrinsic physiopathologic response to transection of the spinal cord and the concurrent need for rapid movement of this type of patient to a center where evaluation and therapy could be initiated. With both the brain and lungs at risk, the development of an associated head injury with hypoxia, hypercarbia, hypovolemia, or all three could have—and probably does have—devastating effects.

As a corollary, Albin and Bunegin[7] measured the ICP wave generated by closed impact injury with a paraplegia-producing force (1.0×10^7 dynes/kg) to the lower thoracic spine. They found that the CSF pressure within the cranium after impact had a mean amplitude of 30 mm Hg over a period of 8 msec, with the peak pressure occurring approximately 3.8 msec after impact. This may have relevance to the patient with a cervical cord injury who also suffers craniocerebral trauma (vehicular or diving accident).

Human studies have also documented cardiovascular disturbances after acute SCI. The initial hypertensive response documented in animals has not been detected in humans, but this is probably due to the time delay from injury to examination.[19] Lehmann et al.[172] studied the frequency and time course of cardiovascular abnormalities in 71 patients with acute SCI. They divided the patients into three groups: severe cervical (complete loss of motor function—31 patients), milder cervical (partial loss of motor function—17 patients), and thoracolumbar (23 patients). They found that persistent bradycardia (mean daily heart rate of <60 beats per minute for 1 day during the 14-day study period) occurred in all 31 patients with severe cervical cord injury, but it was less common in those with milder cervical injury (35%) or thoracolumbar injury (13%). Hypotension (systolic blood pressure of <90 mm Hg on at least two consecutive measurements) and primary cardiac arrest occurred only in the severe cervical injury group, with frequencies of 68% and 16% of patients, respectively. Supraventricular arrhythmias occurred in the severe cervical (19%) and milder cervical (6%) injury groups. It was also found in this study that the frequency of bradyarrythmias peaked on day 4 after injury and then gradually declined, with complete resolution by 2 to 6 weeks after SCI.

Winslow et al.,[286] in a study of 374 patients with SCI, noted that the prevalence of bradycardia in patients with quadriplegia caused by a complete cervical SCI was 26%. Bradycardia was not noted in patients with incomplete or no paralysis from cervical SCI or in patients sustaining thoracic or lumbar SCI. They also noted that the bradycardia was self-limited to 3 to 5 weeks after SCI and did not require permanent pacemaker therapy. Winslow et al.[286] and other authors[1,110,189] have noted a frequent occurrence of bradycardia with suctioning or changes in body position. Vagal stimulation that cannot be compensated for by an integrated sympathetic response is felt to be the mechanism underlying the bradycardia associated with these events.[286] Hypoxemia also plays a role during tracheal suctioning.[1,110,189,286] Bradycardic episodes are treated with vagolytic therapy (atropine, propantheline bromide) and, if associated with tracheal suctioning, increased ventilation and oxygenation. The hemodynamic status of the patient with acute SCI can be further depressed during anesthesia because of anesthetic and narcotic analgesic drugs that have myocardial depressant and vasodilating effects.[80] Hypoxia or hypercarbia may result from respiratory failure, airway obstruction, or excessive airway pressures during anesthesia and interference with venous return. Normally, the reflex response to elevated mean intrathoracic pressure compensates for the decreased venous return by increasing the peripheral vascular tone and maintaining the pressure gradient between the intrathoracic vein and peripheral circulation. This compensatory response is lost in patients with SCI.[189] Respiratory alkalosis produced by hyperventilation should be avoided because it may further depress the myocardium.[266] A patient with SCI can have an associated injury and might also be in hemorrhagic shock. Hypovolemia resulting from blood loss in such patients is poorly tolerated. A sudden change in position during the administration of an anesthetic can lead to orthostatic hypotension.[218] Patients with high cervical spinal cord lesions in whom nasopharyngeal or tracheal suctioning is carried out are at risk for reflex bradycardia and cardiac arrest; this is more likely to occur when the patient is hypoxic. The bradycardia appears to be due to the vagovagal reflex also; hypotension caused by spinal shock and the effect of anesthetic agents may reduce the spinal cord perfusion pressure below the lower levels of autoregulation.

Fluid and Electrolyte Balance

In the patient with acute SCI, fluid and electrolyte balance can be affected by respiratory acidosis resulting from alveolar hypoventilation, metabolic alkalosis resulting from vomiting or gastric suction, and hypocholemia resulting from vomiting, gastric suction, or fluid loss into dilated gut.[69] The antidiuretic hormone system remains intact because of impulses arising from atria and carotid arteries. These do not travel via the spinal cord but outside of it; hence the ability to release the antidiuretic hormone is preserved.[69]

Temperature Control

Transection of the spinal cord above C7 destroys the sweating centers. Some patients become poikilothermic; because their body temperature depends on the temperature of the environment, they are often prone to develop hyperthermia. Cheshire and Coats[69] reported that during a heat wave, a patient with acute quadriplegia developed hyperthermia because of his inability to lower body temperature by sweating. Such patients also are prone to excessive heat loss during surgical procedures and become hypothermic, possibly prolonging recovery from anesthesics. With this in mind, it becomes important to monitor the patient's temperature—both in and out of the operating room—and to ensure that the patient remains normothermic.

Autonomic Dysreflexia

After spinal cord transection, sensory and motor functions below the level of injury are abolished and the reflex functions in the isolated spinal cord are held in abeyance (spinal shock). In addition to the cardiovascular effects, structures and functions below the level of the lesion are affected, including bladder, bowel, erection and ejaculation, autonomic control of blood vessels, and skeletal muscles. This is manifested by contracted bladder and rectal sphincters, with atonic detrusor and smooth muscles. Thus the urinary bladder fills and the sphincter opens when the intraluminal pressure overrides the sphincter pressure (overflow incontinence). Paralytic ileus develops because of loss of peristalsis, as well as the passive distention of the bowel.

The genital reflexes are also depressed or abolished. In general, spinal shock can last up to 6 weeks, but it must be pointed out that incomplete lesions can result in few or none of the characteristics that signify this syndrome.

As the period of spinal shock subsides, reflex activity starts returning, becoming stronger with time and recruiting additional muscle masses. The Babinski sign can now be elicited with fanning of the other toes. Withdrawal movements of the foot, leg, and thigh occur, triggered by tactile stimulation of the foot. This is then followed by the return of the Achilles and patellar reflexes, reflex defecation, and voiding of urine by active contraction of the detrusor muscle. At this point the withdrawal reflexes become greatly exaggerated, and piloerection, sweating, and an automatic bladder are also present. This type of "mass reflex" can be provoked by external stimulation or by an internal stimulus, such as a full bladder. Above the level of the spinal cord lesion, profuse flushing, diaphoresis in the head and neck, chest pain, headache, hypertension, and reflex bradycardia can occur—signaling the development of autonomic dysreflexia (AD).[81] Kendrick et al.[160] found AD in some form if the lesion was above the T7 spinal dermatome (splanchnic outflow); it appears that 85% of those with quadriplegia develop AD, accompanied by paroxysmal hypertension (PH). Head and Riddoch[143] have described PH, noting loss of consciousness and seizures; Kurnick[167] has described retinal and fatal subarachnoid hemorrhages. Bladder distention can provoke PH.[143,167] Kendrick describes 12 cases, with systolic blood pressure increases ranging from 80 to 120 mm Hg and diastolic blood pressure increases of 40 to 60 mm Hg.[160] Cardiac irregularities included sinus bradycardia, P wave changes, increased duration of P-R interval, ectopic beats, P waves independent of QRS complexes, and incomplete heart block—all indicating signs of vagal hyperactivity. The mechanism of the PH has become clearer because of better understanding of the roles of the neurotransmitters involved. Classical neurophysiology notes that in a complete cervical cord lesion, there is a functional separation between the thoracolumbar sympathetic outflow and the brain, allowing the spinal reflex activity to remain uninhibited from the higher centers. Naftchi et al.[208] have indicated that during bladder stimulation, intense vasoconstriction occurred in the upper and lower extremities in patients with quadriplegia. This generalized vasoconstriction below the level of the lesion correlated with arterial hypertension, increased serum beta-hydroxylase levels, and increased excretion of catecholamine metabolites.[72,75] Buttressing this idea is the work of Roussan et al.,[235] who found that calf blood flow decreases during autonomic dysreflexia and that, consequent to the expansion of the urinary bladder, there was a gradual facilitation of the spinal cord as a primary cause for reduced circulation in the calf musculature. They thought that the arterial hypertension was due to the sudden shifts of large blood volumes from skeletal muscle circulation to the capacitance vessels. Thus blood volume shifts into capacitance vessels may act as *positive feedback*, causing compensatory vasodilation, profuse flushing diaphoresis in head and neck, chest pain, and headache.[208] The neurotransmitter factors, norepinephrine (NE) and 5-hydroxytryptamine (5-HT), disappear below the level of transection and accumulate rostrally. This suggests that one of these biogenic amines may be an inhibitory neurotransmitter within the spinal cord because NE and 5-HT depress the activity of anterior horn cells and Renshaw cells.[221,280] Therefore it is thought that the loss of inhibitory neurotransmitters after cord transection may cause permanent facilitation of the cord below the level of the lesion.[23,182] It also appears that the prostaglandins may play a role during PH because they may be part of a compensatory mechanism that decreases adrenergic activity.[208] Prostaglandin E_2 has also been known to cause headaches, as well as flushing in the face, neck, and upper trunk.[158]

Administering an anesthetic to the patient with AD is a difficult challenge because the anesthesiologist must balance the need for adequate depth of anesthesia to prevent the onset of PH with the dangers of hemodynamic instability intrinsic to this condition that could be exacerbated by the anesthetic. It appears that the hypertensive response cannot be attenuated by withholding anesthesia, with sedation, or by using topical anesthesia.[168] Halothane/N_2O, isoflurane/N_2O, and spinal and epidural anesthesics have been used to prevent or attenuate PH.[17,80,91,234,244,272] Blockers—including hexamethonium, trimethaphan, sodium nitroprusside, labetalol, and esmolol—have also been used to control PH. Although spinal and epidural anesthesics have been used to prevent AD, the limiting factors relate to difficulties in determining the sensory level in the patient with quadriplegia, the possibility of severe hypotension caused by compromised vascular tone and dysreflexia, and difficulties in performing the spinal or epidural puncture. Nevertheless, Lambert et al.[168] reported that there was no difference between spinal and general anesthesics in terms of preventing PH in patients at risk. In terms of adequate analgesia and a workable surgical field, regional and general anesthesics have been used satisfactorily.*

Because one cannot predict the occurrence of PH in the patient with paraplegia or quadriplegia, one must conclude that either general, epidural, or spinal anesthesics should be employed in these patients. This is especially true in the pregnant patient with quadriplegia or the patient with SCI in labor.[192,279] The development and use of new adrenergic blockers and vessel wall dilators during the past two decades have allowed for easier and more predictable attenuation of PH without the need to invoke deep general anesthesia. Similarly, these pharmacologic agents may be used cautiously in a special care unit, where autonomic dysreflexia may be caused by a stimulus not related to surgery. Postoperatively, the patient should be closely monitored in

---

*References 17, 91, 219, 234, 244, 272, 279.

a recovery room or other special unit for PH because it can occur with a full bladder or distended rectum.

THERAPEUTIC CONSIDERATIONS
Initial Response

The need for transporting the patient with SCI as rapidly as possible to a specialized treatment unit because of the importance of time in the development of the injury has been emphasized in numerous studies[4,5,9,16] and in a model developed by Green et al.[124] That rapid evacuation can be efficacious in limiting the progression of neurologic damage is demonstrated by the experience of Gregg and Wilmot[125,126] in Eire, where a special "flying squad" consisting of a physician and a nurse is helicoptered to the scene of the accident, and the patient is retrieved by helicopter on a specially designed stretcher and transported with the team to the National Rehabilitation Centre in Dublin. Their high percentage of incomplete cervical cord lesions indicates the effectiveness of this approach. Coordination of ground and ambulance service is best exemplified by the Swiss Air Rescue Unit, which transports all patients with SCI to a Spinal Cord Center. The average time elapsed is 50 minutes instead of the 4 hours found with a conventional ambulance system.[134,135] It is obvious that rapid, safe transportation to a unit specializing in the care of patients with SCI is one of the keys to successful therapy. Protocols should be developed on a geographic basis to standardize evacuation and delivery of the patient to a specialized center. Similarly, standards for SCI centers should be delineated and coordinated with air and highway transportation.

Whether the patient with a cervical cord injury is first seen by a "flying squad" or an ambulance unit with a paramedical staff, the patient should be immobilized on a spine board with the head and neck placed in a neutral position. All comatose patients and/or patients with multiple trauma should be treated as if SCI has occurred. Evaluation of adequacy of ventilation must be made and assistance given where needed. Training of emergency medical technicians in ventilatory management of these patients, and recognition of neurologic symptoms is critical. Adequate equipment—including spine boards, collars, ventilating bags and masks, intravenous solutions, and volume expanders—should be considered part of normal operations. A centralized communication system with operational control handled by an emergency medical service assistance group allows for optimal triage and the opportunity to interpose specialist consultation when needed. If there is any hope of preventing the incomplete cervical cord lesion from becoming complete—let alone salvaging the patient with multiple trauma, including head and cord injury—then these modern systems of integrated communication and command must be established. The parochialism involved in mandating that local ambulance services transport patients to the nearest hospital (even though it has minimal facilities to take care of these acute problems) must give way to extri-

cation and transportation to the unit with optimal facilities for acute care—in this case, the SCI center.[124]

The essential purpose of the first response is to extricate, identify, and move the patient with a cord lesion to the appropriate medical institution without exacerbating existing neurologic damage, while maximally supporting the cardiovascular and pulmonary systems. Attempts at bony reduction should not be made at the scene of the accident (or anywhere) without adequate diagnostic studies.

A flow chart with documentation of movement—as well as frequent neurologic checks—should be begun because the patient may be taken to many different service areas of the hospital—emergency department, radiology, patient unit, or operating theater.

Neurologic Syndromes

Except for injury to the spine that does not produce neurologic dysfunction, the classification of neurologic injury patterns is based on the degree and distribution of neurologic dysfunction. In complete SCI, total paralysis and loss of sensation result from a complete interruption of the ascending and descending pathways below the level of the lesion. Functional levels of complete lesions have been classified by Stauffer and Bell.[258] High cervical lesions with damage to the brainstem to C1 result in pentaplegia, and patients with pentaplegia have paralysis of the lower cranial nerves and accessory muscles, as well as sensory and motor loss to the arms and legs. Patients with respiratory quadriplegia have functional levels at C2 to C3, leaving the face, neck, sternocleidomastoid, and accessory muscles intact. These patients require ventilatory support because diaphragmatic control is lost. Quadriplegia involves loss of the arms and legs (injury to C4 to C8), and paraplegia involves loss of the legs only (injury to T1 to S1). Perineal paraplegia involves loss of sacral roots S2 to S5, causing dysfunction of the bowel, bladder, and sexual function.

In an incomplete injury, there is preservation of some of the sensory and/or motor fibers below the lesion. Incomplete injuries can be delineated according to the anatomic damage sustained and include several symptom complexes. Anterior SCI syndrome is characterized by immediate motor paralysis of the upper and lower extremities, hypesthesia, and hypalgesia, but preservation of position sense, vibration sense, and light touch. Anterior compression of the spinal cord by a ruptured disk or dislocation of vertebrae affects the lateral corticospinal tract and spinothalamic tract but preserves the posterior columns.

Brown-Séquard syndrome is a lesion of the lateral half of the spinal cord and is manifested by ipsilateral paresis and contralateral loss of pain and temperature one or more levels below the lesion. This entity is commonly seen in stab wounds and occasionally with blunt trauma. Central cord syndrome occurs when there is more cellular destruction in the center of the cord than in the periphery, giving a disproportionate degree of motor paralysis in the upper extremities, as compared with the lower. This is accompanied by varying degrees of sensory loss. One finds central destruction of the spinal cord resulting from hemorrhage or necrosis, with sparing of the peripheral leg area in the lateral corticospinal tract.

Thoracic anterior spinal artery syndrome is characterized by fracture or dislocation in the lower thoracolumbar area, with sensory and motor loss that appears at a higher level than the lesion itself because of ischemia and edema after vascular compromise to the midthoracic cord. The cauda equina syndrome involves peripheral nerves, instead of the spinal cord directly. When complete, it is signaled by paralysis of the lower extremities, sensory loss, and bowel and bladder dysfunction. When incomplete, symptoms may include sciatica, numbness, patchy sensation, and bowel and bladder dysfunction with saddle anesthesia. Because peripheral nerves possess the ability to regenerate, when compared with the spinal cord, there appears to be a better prognosis for recovery with this syndrome.

One specialized form of incomplete lesion is the patient with sacral sparing. In these patients, the lesion appears to be complete, except for the presence of function in the sacral area, such as rectal tone, perianal sensation, or deep touch. The identification of this condition, as well as the differentiation of other incomplete lesions from complete lesions, is important because the prognosis is often better than for other complete lesions if aggressive early care is provided.[245]

Surgical Criteria

Immobilization at the scene of the accident is critical, and, for cervical spine injuries, a rigid cervical collar, sand bags, and spine board should be used to immobilize the head, neck, and body. After emergency room evaluation—including a complete physical examination, neurologic evaluation, and laboratory and neuroradiologic tests (including enhanced CT and/or MR scans and myelography, if indicated), patients with a complete cord lesion and no demonstrated pathology can be moved to a kinetic nursing bed. Alignment and stability may be maintained using halo traction in some of the spinal fractures. Candidates for emergent surgery are those with incomplete sensory-motor paralysis, where closed reduction has failed or where a fracture-dislocation has been reduced and the CT scan indicates bone or disk fragments in the canal or an extrinsic lesion that affects the cord. Maroon and Abla[188] note that the surgical approach is determined by which area of cord or spine is injured. Thus the objective of decompressive operative procedures is to avoid further injury to the cord and to relieve any developing pressure. If a fracture-dislocation persists, bone healing is likely to be retarded, and, if angulation results, a delayed neurologic loss can occur (Box 33-1)

Associated Injuries

Associated injuries are very common in patients with spinal cord trauma, and their incidence ranges from 25% to 65%.[53,72,257,271] In general, head injuries are the most common. Chest injury associated with a serious injury to the thoracic spine is also frequent. No part of the body is immune to trauma, and two or more associated injuries are not uncommon.[256] Attention to ventilatory problems; evaluation of "silent areas," such as the chest, head, and abdomen, and long bones; and placement of nasogastric and urinary catheters can all help determine the extent of suspected associated injury.

▼

BOX 33-1
CLASSIFICATION OF CERVICAL AND THORACOLUMBAR INJURIES

A. **Unstable Displaced Fracture with Partial Spinal Cord or Cauda Equina Lesion**
  1. Brust fracture
  2. Unilateral articular process dislocation
  3. Perched lesion of facet
  4. Minimal anterior or posterior vertebral body subluxation (5 mm)
  5. Disk rupture

B. **Unstable Displaced Fracture with Complete Cord or Cauda Equina Lesion**
  1. Articular process dislocation
  2. Burst fracture
  3. Fracture dislocation
  4. Shear fracture

C. **Unstable Displaced Fracture ± Spinal Cord or Cauda Equina Lesion**
  1. Compression fracture
  2. Burst fracture
  3. Fracture due to subluxation
  4. Subluxation 3 mm
  5. Disk rupture
  6. Laterolisthesis with fracture of posterior elements
  7. Anterolisthesis

D. **Stable ± Displaced Bone Fracture ± Spinal Cord or Cauda Equina Lesion**
  1. Linear fracture through body and lamina
  2. Compression fracture
  3. Fracture of pedicle and lamina
  4. Fracture of lamina
  5. Fracture of dens
  6. C1 fracture
  7. Fracture of articular facet
  8. Fracture of pars interarticularis
  9. Fracture of pedicle
  10. Naked facet
  11. Hangman's fracture

From Maroon JC, Abla AA: *Crit Care Clin* 3:655-677, 1987.

Airway Management

Inadequate alveolar ventilation with CO_2 retention is not uncommon in those with acute cervical cord injury. This compromise in respiratory function makes it difficult for the patient to cough and clear existing secretions, thereby further compromising oxygenation (see Fig. 33-3). In an elective, relatively nonemergent situation, the criteria for intubation and mechanical ventilation can be assessed easily using arterial blood gas measurements, evaluating the chest film, and carrying out easily performed pulmonary function tests. The intubation criteria, noted in Table 33-3, have been developed by Mackenzie and Ducker[180,181] and are quite useful. Endotracheal intubation will also secure the airway and help prevent aspiration of gastric contents. If the cervical spine is unstable, mechanical traction using Gardner-Wells tongs or halo traction is applied to provide stability and reduce external compression. When tracheal intubation must be performed before application of the traction device, longitudinal (axial) traction must be applied manually. A person stands at the head of the patient's bed, places his/her hands on the patient's mastoid process, and applies a traction force of 5 to 10 pounds in the cephalad direction while keeping the mastoid processes in line with the axis of the spine. This will counter any extension or flexion of the cervical spine during laryngoscopy and tracheal intubation. If it is known that the lower cervical spine is unstable, more effective traction may be applied by placing the hands at the midpoint of a line connecting the external auditory canal and the lateral angle of the eye.

Patients scheduled for decompressive surgery on the spinal column and who are not in respiratory failure are intubated in the operating room. These patients are placed in mechanical traction, which will not prevent extension or flexion of the cervical spine related to manipulation during laryngoscopy. A review of the literature on the optimal technique for endotracheal intubation reveals marked differences of opinion among those with experience in dealing with patients with acute SCI. The major consensus appears to indicate that the endoscopist should be experienced with this problem, the patient should be appropriately immobilized, and the intubation technique specifically tailored

to the neurologic and pathophysiologic conditions present. Thus patients with a potential for basilar skull injury should not be intubated using the nasal approach, and, although the patient with unstable cervical cord injury generally does poorly with neck flexion and may improve with neck extension, in patients with fractures of the odontoid process, extension maneuvers may prove to be hazardous. In nonemergent situations, a number of experienced practitioners recommend nasotracheal intubation using a topical anesthesic with the patient awake.* The availability of the fiberoptic bronchoscope/laryngoscope has facilitated atraumatic intubations. On the other hand, Kopaniky[164] believes that nasotracheal intubation has few indications because it requires a small diameter tube, can be traumatic, and determining the position of the tube necessitates capnography.

The patient with acute SCI who is unconscious, in shock, and has associated injuries—or who has cardiovascular and/or respiratory distress—requires immediate attention. These individuals may have a full stomach, or they may be intoxicated. For these reasons, heavy sedation and sustained efforts to use topical anesthesics may be dangerous. Mackenzie and Ducker[180] do not use topical anesthesics in these patients, and instead, intubation is carried out after the administration of succinylcholine and a sleep dose of thiopental. Suderman et al.[261] evaluated intubation methods against neurologic outcome in a retrospective study of 150 patients with cervical SCI after induction of general anesthesia in 83 of the patients; the remaining patients were intubated while they were awake. Of the patients, 71% had oral intubation and the remainder were intubated nasally. No changes in neurologic outcome were noted, whether the patients were intubated while awake or after receiving an anesthetic or whether oral or nasal intubation was used.

In the emergent difficult intubation of a patient with an unstable cervical fracture, cricothyrotomy or tracheostomy may have to be considered. One must also not forget the possible use of jet ventilation via the cricothyroid membrane. Once adequate ventilation has been effected with the jet ventilator, it is then possible to move the needle in the trachea so the needle points in the cephalad direction; disconnect the needle from the jet ventilation unit; insert a J-wire guide, so that it can exit via the oropharynx or nasopharynx; and then pass over it a stylet, followed with the endotracheal tube. A complete retrograde intubation kit is now available commercially from Cook, Inc., Bloomington, Indiana.

Preoperative Evaluation

The anesthesiologist must try to ensure that a complete workup is available, including an ECG; chest film; hematocrit level; blood chemistry, including glucose, creatinine, and electrolyte levels; arterial blood gas levels; and, when-

TABLE 33-3

Indications for Intubation and Mechanical Ventilation in Patients with Acute Quadriplegia

Intubation Criteria	Value Indicating Need for Intubation
Maximal expiratory force	$< +20$ cm H_2O
Maximal inspiratory force	< -20 cm H_2O
Vital capacity	< 15 ml/kg or < 1000 ml
Pao_2/FIo_2	< 250
Chest x-ray examination	Atelectasis or infiltrate

From MacKenzie CF, Ducker TB: Cervical cord injury. In Matjasko J, Katz J, editors: *Clinical controversies in neuroanesthesia and neurosurgery,* Orlando, 1986, Grune & Stratton.

*References 30, 118, 180, 181, 223, 257.

ever possible, respiratory assessment using bedside spirometry. It is important to ensure that a complete neurologic evaluation has been carried out to secure a baseline for comparison and to help pinpoint location of the lesion. The enhanced CT scan and MR have been important advances in delineating the nature and localization of vertebral and spinal cord pathology. If there is any suggestion in the history or physical examination that craniocerebral trauma might be present as an associated injury, then appropriate neuroradiologic diagnostic procedures should be performed. In general, preoperative medication is not used, especially with patients suspected of having head injuries. Such drugs as barbiturates, narcotics, and tranquilizers should be avoided because they might affect the neurologic evaluation and depress ventilation. In the event that the patient demonstrates a marked bradycardia, atropine should be given. Mackenzie and Ducker[180] recommend the use of atropine if the patient has a pulse rate less than 70 beats per minute (0.02 mg/kg IV). These same authors found atropine to be useful in the patient with quadriplegia who is hypotensive, bradycardic, and in cardiac failure with pulmonary edema.

Cardiovascular Stabilization

When persistent hypotension and bradycardia is accompanied by diminished mentation, urine output of less than 0.5 ml $\cdot$ kg^{-1} $\cdot$ hr^{-1}, developing metabolic acidosis, or an ascending temperature gradient in the lower extremities, therapeutic intervention is required. Systemic hypotension should be judiciously treated with volume expansion using the Swan-Ganz catheter as a guide. Unfortunately, peripheral vasoconstrictors have been heralded as a means to restore adequate ventricular function. Severe hypotension, causing reduced tissue perfusion, actually is due to declining cardiac output and not to decreases in systemic vascular resistance (SVR).[227] Thus alpha agonists—such as methoxamine, mephenteramine, and phenylephrine—should not be used under these conditions because they increase the tissue oxygen debt and lactic acidosis. Cardiac function can be improved by using centrally-acting positive inotropic drugs that directly affect cardiac output. Because hypotension at or below the lower limits of autoregulation of spinal cord blood flow may be deleterious to the recovery of function, it is critical to maintain an adequate perfusion pressure. Under these conditions, inotropic agents—such a atropine, isoproterenol, dopamine, or dobutamine—can be used after a fluid challenge.[180]

Patients with SCI exhibit a low circulating blood volume, at least in relation to their expanded vascular bed.[81] Initial judicious expansion of total blood volume would therefore seem appropriate before resorting to vasopressor agents. Mackenzie et al.[181] have established that a pulmonary artery occluded pressure (PAOP) of 18 mm Hg produces optimal left-ventricular function in the patient with acute quadriplegia.[180] It is obvious, therefore, that should

cardiovascular instability exist in a patient with SCI, the passage of a balloon-tipped flow-directed pulmonary artery catheter is highly desirable. These same authors correctly state that increasing SVR increases left-ventricular work and myocardial oxygen consumption, reversing the favorable cardiac effects of low peripheral vascular tone. The value of increasing circulating blood volume, as compared with the use of dopamine or gamma hydroxybutarate, to increase spinal cord blood flow (SCBF) was also reported in 1982 by Dolan and Tator.[88]

It is helpful to use repeated fluid challenges, until evidence of hypoperfusion has reversed or until the PAOP exceeds 18 mm Hg and does not fall to lower levels within 5 minutes of completion of the fluid challenge. Usually, perfusion is restored at pressures of 10 to 12 mm Hg, but fluid administration is also curtailed if evidence of increasing pulmonary interstitial edema develops. This is indicated by an increase in the work of breathing, increasing pulmonary shunt fraction, decreasing static compliance, and by chest x-ray film changes.

Only if fluid therapy fails are vasopressor agents used. We prefer dobutamine. Unlike dopamine, this drug does not increase pulmonary vascular resistance, which could exacerbate pulmonary capillary leak. Dobutamine has proved effective, provided that ventricular filling pressures are optimized.

Controversy exists as to whether crystalloid or colloid fluids should be used. Experience in all types of capillary leak syndromes (adult respiratory distress syndrome, near drowning) has shown a clear preference for colloids, provided that the serum osmolality level is less than 320 mOsm/L.[226] This has also been confirmed by other workers[141,142,248] and may result from the fact that with colloids the total fluid required to expand the circulating blood volume is less than with crystalloids, and, as a result, pulmonary microvascular hydrostatic capillary pressure is lower.[140]

Respiratory Support

It has been our repeated clinical observation that except in SCI above C4, very few patients exhibit acute respiratory difficulty. Provided that the patient retains some diaphragmatic function and can use the sternocleidomastoid, scalene, and trapezius muscles, and, in the absence of an acute pulmonary event (such as aspiration or pulmonary edema), respiratory deterioration develops gradually during the first 4 days after injury.[69,151] Recovery then progresses through the second or third week. Failure to recognize this course of events has led to many problems with respiratory management in the past and may have contributed significantly to mortality.

Early Management

In recent years the mortality associated with tetraplegia has fallen dramatically[124]; this is substantially the result of improvements in respiratory management because most early deaths have resulted from pulmonary complications. Provided there is some sparing of diaphragmatic action (lesion at C4 or below), there is little difference in mortality among patients with SCI.[95] Mortality improves even more for thoracic or lumbar injuries.

Damage to cord segments C3 to C5 involves the phrenic nerve nuclei and causes partial or complete bilateral hemidiaphragmatic paralysis. In addition, the intercostal muscles caudad to the lesion are paralyzed, and the combined effect is to limit lateral expansion of the rib cage. Use of the accessory muscles of respiration results in an increase in the anteroposterior dimension of the upper rib cage and pulls the diaphragm cephalad. As the diaphragm ascends, negative intraabdominal pressure is created, producing paradoxical respiration.[60]

Even where the phrenic nerve nuclei are intact, diaphragmatic activity is compromised because of the inability of the paralyzed intercostal muscles to stabilize the rib cage. Diaphragmatic activity thus results in a paradoxical inward motion of the upper and middle rib cage during inspiration and is further compromised by the diaphragm's inability to contract from the domed position that it assumes as a result of loss of opposing forces from the abdominal musculature.

As a result of this marked respiratory muscle dysfunction, those with cervical quadriplegia exhibit loss of functional residual capacity, diminished static pulmonary compliance, retention of secretions, increased V/Q mismatch, and poor ability to sigh and cough. Alveolar hypoventilation is more pronounced during sleep, presumably because of diminished CO_2 responsiveness.[34]

If intubation is performed, it is usually desirable to institute ventilatory support. If vital capacity after intubation is greater than 9 ml/kg, static pulmonary compliance is greater than 30 ml/cm of water pressure, and oxygenation index (arterial oxygen tension in mm Hg divided by fractional inspired oxygen concentration, Pao_2/FIo_2) is greater than 250, the patient can be allowed to breathe spontaneously. However, pulmonary function must be monitored closely because—as discussed earlier—deterioration is particularly likely to occur in the first 4 days after injury.

The spontaneously breathing patient essentially has acute restrictive lung disease, and further loss of volume will occur. If the patient is intubated, the epiglottic retard mechanism is lost, predisposing to further loss of functional residual capacity. The use of a limited respiratory work CPAP circuit is most effective in maintaining FRC, reducing V/Q mismatch, and limiting work of breathing. With this system, end-expiratory pressure minus end-inspiratory pressure (EEP − EIP) should be 3 cm of water or less. Forced vital capacity (FVC) and negative inspiratory force are measured on a daily basis to monitor respiratory progress.

If immediate intubation is not necessary, aggressive chest physiotherapy is required to maintain pulmonary function. This can take the form of incentive spirometry, aerosol therapy to a preset limit by pressure-driven nebulizer, percussion and vibration chest physiotherapy to treat any areas of infiltrate or atelectasis, limited postural drainage, frequent changes of position, warm mist humidification of oxygen-enriched air delivered through wide bore tubing, and avoidance of anticholinergics.

Retention of secretions may require blind nasal tracheal suctioning with a soft suction catheter, and, if a major lung segment appears to be collapsed because of a mucous plug, fiberoptic bronchoscopy may be indicated. During such maneuvers, care must be taken to avoid severe bradyarrhythmias resulting from abnormal tracheal reflexes.[189] These are said to be caused by an imbalance of opposing vagal and sympathetic reflex responses, but they are more often the result of unrecognized borderline hypoxemia exacerbated by a tracheal suctioning procedure.

Assistance with coughing can be provided with an abdominal push maneuver, and much can be done to re-educate and strengthen the diaphragm.[22,48] Use of an abdominal corset when the patient is upright enables the diaphragm to assume its normal resting position and improve its function.

Gastric stasis and intestinal atony accompany spinal shock in many cases. This can lead to abdominal distention and risk of aspiration. The passage of a nasogastric tube and control of gastric pH is desirable. However, the combination of antacids, hydrogen ion loss in gastric aspirate, the metabolic effect of diuretic therapy, and maintenance of ionic balance in total parenteral nutrition by addition of acetate can all lead to significant metabolic alkalosis. Once the base excess is greater than 9 or 10, there is a risk of respiratory compensation for the metabolic alkalosis with hypoventilation, further loss of lung volume, and increased V/Q mismatch. If this complication develops, the cause of the alkalosis must be eliminated. Acetazolamide (250 mg IV in two doses 12 hr apart) facilitates correction.

If, despite the previously described therapeutic interventions, respiratory function continues to deteriorate, intubation and ventilation should not be delayed. There is an emotional component to the tendency to withhold ventilator support if the patient has been breathing adequately for 24 to 48 hours. To excessively delay providing ventilator support leads to patient anxiety, dyspnea, exhaustion, and unnecessary retention of secretions, with loss of lung volume and further deterioration in static pulmonary compliance. These changes may allow a significant pulmonary infection to become established.

Once the decision is made to ventilate the patient, ventilator settings are used that provide close to full respiratory support, requiring only relatively modest respiratory work from the patient. It is desirable to use a ventilator that imposes minimal respiratory work when the patient takes a spontaneous breath. The ventilator is used in SIMV mode, and, the pressure support component is not added, unless lung volumes are very low or compliance is excessively compromised by pulmonary interstitial edema or infiltrates. A low level of PEEP ($+5$ cm H_2O) is added as soon as cardiovascular stability is attained.

Weaning

Weaning parameters of FVC, negative inspiratory force, and oxygenation index are checked daily. The satisfaction of these weaning parameters often occurs suddenly between the tenth and twenty-first day after injury. If, at this time, the lungs are clear and secretions are minimal, weaning and extubation can proceed quickly. Our general policy is to use a gradual weaning technique with progressive reduction in the SIMV rate, but we have found that once the patient with SCI meets weaning parameters (Table 33-4), a rapid interval weaning technique is very effective.

Because of possible laryngeal incompetence, it is wise to suspend enteral feeding in the periextubation period (e.g., from 4 hr before until 12 hr after extubation). The patient should be encouraged to take sips of water at an early stage and proceed to a normal diet as tolerated. Tracheostomy is seldom indicated, and patients can be kept intubated for up to 3 weeks without problems.

MONITORING

Because of the effects of acute cervical cord injury on the cardiopulmonary and CNS system, these patients require indepth monitoring (Box 33-2). Because fluid-electrolyte-volume management is critical, it is important to place arterial, pulmonary artery and urinary catheters before induction of anesthesia. In general, radial artery cannulation and Swan-Ganz catheter placement should be carried out as soon as possible after the patient's admission to the hospital. The depressed myocardium, loss of sympathetic reflexes, and a markedly expanded vascular space in patients with acute quadriplegia predispose them to the development of pulmonary edema because of overtransfusion. Large swings in left-ventricular filling pressure and pulmonary artery pressure (PAP) may occur without any changes in

CVP. Thus using a central line for CVP monitoring is of little value because any abrupt increase in CVP is a late change. Continuous monitoring of PAP and intermittent monitoring of pulmonary capillary wedge pressure allows for optimal management of cardiac function and intravascular volume. Somatosensory evoked potentials (SSEP) have been useful for evaluating the functional integrity of the spinal cord. The SSEP has been used intraoperatively to monitor posterior column function during stabilization and decompressive procedures on the spine and spinal cord. The problem with the SSEP is that it reflects the electrophysiologic status of the posterior column and not the anterior spinal cord where the motor pathways course. Thus one may have quadriplegia with disruption of the anterior spinal artery, but, because the posterior column may be intact, the SSEP can be normal.[130,175] It is possible that the motor evoked potential (MEP) might prove to be a useful tool for evaluating the function integrity of the spinal cord because it reflects function of the motor pathways.

ANESTHESIA

After the trachea has been intubated in the awake patient, movement onto the operating table occurs. An advantage of the fully awake patient is that the neurologic status can be determined during and after positioning. For posterior operative procedures on the spine, the patient must be moved into the prone position without causing any distraction or in any way stressing the unstable spine, so neither torque nor compression is applied to the already damaged spinal cord. Transfer of the patient from the stretcher or Stryker frame onto the operating table is done with manually applied traction. After completion of the maneuver into the prone position, care must be taken to ensure proper placement if a headrest is used to avoid pressure points and to make sure no direct pressure is placed on ocular globes.

TABLE 33-4
Weaning Criteria for Removal from Mechanical Ventilation

Weaning Criteria	Acceptable Value for Removal
Maximal inspiratory force	>-20 cm H_2O
Maximal expiratory force	$>+20$ cm H_2O
Vital capacity	>1000 ml
Expiratory flow	>10 L/sec (level dependent)
Pao_2/FIo_2	>250
Vd/Vt	$<.55$
Lung thorax compliance	>30 ml/cm H_2O

From MacKenzie CF, Ducker TB: Cervical cord injury. In Matjasko J, Katz J, editors: *Clinical controversies in neuroanesthesia and neurosurgery*, Orlando, 1986, Grune & Stratton.

BOX 33-2
VARIABLES TO BE MONITORED IN PATIENTS WITH
ACUTE CERVICAL SPINAL CORD INJURY

Arterial blood pressure, direct measurement
Central venous, Swan-Ganz catheter
Electrocardiogram
Minute, tidal volume, and airway pressure
Urinary output
Neuromuscular blockade (estimated with the use of a nerve stimulator)
Blood gas levels
Hematocrit level
Serum and/or urine osmolality levels
Electrolyte, glucose levels
Temperature

The endotracheal tube and its connectors should be so secured that a disconnect is not possible, and the tube is not kinked or under tension. A wire reinforced tracheal tube can be useful. While moving the patient into the prone position, one must provide lateral support using rolls, bolsters, or special supports to ensure adequate ventilation and to avoid high caval pressures. After positioning and neurologic evaluation, general anesthesia is gradually induced. Commonly-used induction drugs include thiopental, fentanyl, fentanyl-droperidol, sufentanil, and etomidate. The use of the newest anesthetic drug—propofol—in patients with SCI has not been defined, but one should be concerned with the hypotension that may result. Of importance is that the induction drug should only minimally affect myocardial contractility and not produce hypotension. Maintenance of anesthesia can occur with inhalational drugs—such as N_2O, halothane, and isoflurane—or with intravenous drugs. Mackenzie and Ducker[180] believe that the inhalation drugs have an advantage over intravenous drugs in terms of maintenance in that they can easily be reversed in the face of hypotension. They also noted no differences in cardiovascular and pulmonary function in a series of 22 patients anesthetized within 5 days of acute SCI, comparing those receiving halothane with those receiving the fentanyl/droperidol combination. Our own method is to induce anesthesia slowly—with a sleep dose of thiopental, etomidate, fentanyl, or sufentanyl—and to use the nondepolarizing muscle relaxant vecuronium bromide while monitoring the state of neuromuscular blockade with a nerve stimulator (Box 33-3).

At the termination of the anesthesia, the muscle relaxant is reversed (if necessary), and the patient is transferred with all monitoring lines in place to the ICU or special care unit. The patient usually remains intubated and often requires postoperative ventilatory care. Even though the ventilatory status may have been adequate before the induction of anesthesia, the residual effects of the anesthetic drugs—together with the neurologic deficit—certainly might influence alveolar ventilation. Ventilatory support also prevents the development of postoperative atelectasis. According to Pasteyer et al.[218] extubation should be considered in those patients with lesions below C5, who have adequate arterial blood gas levels, no associated head or chest injury, an absence of excessive respiratory secretions, and satisfactory respiratory parameters, including a tidal volume of greater than 400 ml and minute ventilation of higher than 8 L.

SUCCINYLCHOLINE

The hyperkalemic response to succinylcholine involving severe cardiovascular reactions in the patient with spinal cord and other types of CNS injury has been well documented.*

_____

*References 52, 254, 255, 259, 260, 269, 270.

BOX 33-3
A PLAN FOR ANESTHETIC MANAGEMENT OF THE PATIENT WITH ACUTE SCI

Preanesthesia Evaluation
Respiratory, cardiovascular, neurologic, renal, associated injury

Preanesthetic Medication
Atropine if needed

Application of Monitoring
ECG, intraarterial catheter, IV, Swan-Ganz catheter, urinary catheter

Awake Nasotracheal Intubation
Light sedation, topical anesthesic, nerve blocks if indicated, blind intubation or with fiberoptic laryngoscopy

Transfer and Positioning of the Patient
Tracheal tube and monitoring lines secured
Transfer with continuous manual traction

Induction of General Anesthesia
Barbiturate or etomidate, nondepolarizing muscle relaxant, narcotic

Maintenance of Anesthesia
Low concentration of isoflurane, narcotics
Hypotension — positioning or anesthetic agents, use of vasopressor inotropes
Blood loss — blood or fluid administration with monitoring: PAP, CVP, PCWP, BP, ECG, pulse oximeter
Additional monitoring — breath and heart sounds, temperature, urine output, sensory evoked potentials, motor evoked potentials

Emergence from Anesthesia
Intubated patient — requires ventilatory support
Extubated patient with low level of injury requires adequate respiration

_____

From Babinski MF: *Crit Care Clin* 3:619-636, 1987.

Stone et al.[259,260] reported cardiac arrest in a patient with C6 quadriplegia who was given succinylcholine 46 days after SCI, with serum K^+ increasing from 4.6 to 16 mEq/L by approximately 2 minutes after injection. Studies also noted hyperkalemia in animals by 28 days after cord transection.[260] After SCI, the mechanism of hyperkalemia involves the pharmacologic receptor area of the endplate's developing hypertrophy, increased sensitivity, and decreased reentry permeability to K^+.[29,52,138,269,270] This change in the cholinergic receptor can be noted as early as 3 days after injury.[155] Tobey[270] noted that pretreatment with a nondepolarizing relaxant will decrease the rise in K^+ but will not totally suppress it. The duration of succinylcholine hypersensitivity is not totally clear because Smith[254] reported cardiac arrest in a quadriplegic patient 6 months after injury and Quinby et al.[227] felt that 8 months appears to be the minimal time after injury that one should wait before using succinylcholine. Thus a window for avoiding the use of succinylcholine appears to range from 3 days to 8 months. Unless there is some overriding need to use succinylcholine, we generally avoid its use until a year after injury has passed. Our practice is to use a nondepolarizing drug, such as vecuronium bromide, because it has a minimal effect on the cardiovascular system.

SUMMARY

The protean nature of acute spinal cord injury necessitates an acute awareness of the impact of this type of trauma on nearly every organ system in the body. This is especially true for complete cervical spinal cord injury at or above the C4 vertebral level. The major concerns are with autoregulation of spinal cord blood flow and spinal cord perfusion pressure, ventilation, cardiovascular and cerebrovascular dynamics, fluid and electrolyte disturbances, temperature control, and associated injuries. Anesthetic management of spinal cord injury patients is based on these substrates as well as on an understanding of responses to anesthetic agents and adjuvants. Unfortunately, there is no definitive information as to the choice of an optimal anesthetic agent. Caution must be exercised in the use of succinylcholine because of hyperkalemia and in the use of parenteral solutions containing dextrose because they may exacerbate neurologic dysfunction. Endotracheal tube placement must be carried out with caution and with the head-neck area immobilized and stabilized maximally. Preoperative, intraoperative, and postoperative monitoring modalities can be critical in establishing the physiologic baseline and progress of the patient, and the use of the triple lumen catheter can be useful. Positive interactions between the anesthesiologist, neurosurgeon, and intensivist are critical for a high-level continuum of care.

References

1. Abd AG, Braun NMT: Management of life threatening bradycardia in spinal cord injury, *Chest* 95:701-702, 1989.
2. Acosta-Rua G: Treatment of traumatic paraplegic patients by localized cooling of the spinal cord, *J Iowa Med Soc* 60:326-328, 1970.
3. Albin MS: Epidemiology, physiopathology and experimental therapeutics of acute spinal cord injury, *Crit Care Clin* 3:441-452, 1987.
4. Albin MS: Resuscitation of the spinal cord, *Crit Care Med* 5:270-276, 1978.
5. Albin MS, Aronica MJ, Black WA Jr et al: Report, Spinal Cord Injury Task Force, Health Advisory Council, Department of Health, Commonwealth of Pennsylvania, *Penn Med* 81:28-54, 1978.
6. Albin MS, Bunegin L: An experimental study of craniocerebral trauma during ethanol intoxication, *Crit Care Med* 14:841-846, 1986.
7. Albin MS, Bunegin L: ICP and biomechanical responses after closed impact injury to the spinal cord. In Hoff JT, Betz AL, editors: *Intracranial pressure VI,* Heidelberg, 1989, Springer-Verlag.
8. Albin MS, Bunegin L, Wolf S: Brain and lungs at risk after cervical cord transection: intracranial pressure, brain water, blood-brain barrier permeability, cerebral blood flow and extravascular lung water changes, *Surg Neurol* 24:191-205, 1985.
9. Albin MS, Helsel P, Bunegin L et al: Axoplasmic transport patterns after experimental spinal cord crush injury, *Anat Rec* 190:603, 1978.
10. Albin MS, White RJ: Evaluation of normothermic spinal cord perfusion after impact injury, *Proceedings of the Society for Neuroscience Third Annual Meeting,* Nov 1973.
11. Albin MS, White RJ, Acosta-Rua G et al: Study of functional recovery produced by delayed localized cooling after spinal cord injury in primates, *J Neurosurg* 29:113-120, 1968.
12. Albin MS, White RJ, Donald DE et al: Hypothermia of the spinal cord by perfusion cooling of the subarachnoid space, *Surg Forum* 12:188-189, 1961.
13. Albin MS, White RJ, Locke GE et al: Localized spinal cord hypothermia: anesthetic effects and application to traumatic injury, *Anesth Analg* 46:8-16, 1967.
14. Albin MS, White RJ, Locke GE et al: Spinal cord hypothermia by localized perfusion cooling, *Nature* 210:1059-1060, 1966.
15. Albin MS, White RJ, Taslitz N: Initial cardiovascular responses following cervical cord transection, *Anat Rec* 157:347, 1967.
16. Albin MS, White RJ, Yashon D et al: Effect of localized cooling in spinal cord trauma, *J Trauma* 9:1000-1008, 1969.
17. Alderson JD, Thomas DG: The use of halothane anesthesia to control autonomic hyperreflexia during transurethral resection in spinal cord injury patients, *Paraplegia* 13:183-188, 1975.
18. Aldfield EH, Plunkett RJ, Nylander WA et al: Barbiturate protection in acute experimental spinal cord isch-

emia, *J Neurosurg* 56:511-516, 1982.

19. Alexander S, Kerr FWL: Blood pressure responses in acute compression of the spinal cord, *J Neurosurg* 21:485-491, 1964.

20. Allen AR: Surgery of experimental lesion of spinal cord equivalent to crush injury of fracture dislocation of spinal column: a preliminary report, *JAMA* 57:878-880, 1911.

21. Allen BL Jr, Ferguson RL, Lehmann TR et al: A mechanistic classification of closed indirect fractures and dislocations of the lower cervical spine, *Spine* 7:1-27, 1982.

22. Alvarez E, Peterson M, Lunsford BR: Respiratory treatment of the adult patient with spinal cord injury, *Phys Ther* 61:1737-1745, 1981.

23. Anden NE, Haggendal E, Magnusson T et al: Time course of the disappearance of noradrenaline and 5-hydroxytryptamine in spinal cord after transection, *Acta Physiol Scand* 62:115-118, 1964.

24. Anderson DK, Means ED: Lipid peroxidation in spinal cord, *Neurochem Path* 1:249-264, 1983.

25. Anderson DW, McLauren RL, editors: Report on the National Head and Spinal Cord Injury Survey, *J Neurosurg* 53:1-43, 1980.

26. Anderson DK, Means ED, Waters TR et al: Microvascular perfusion and metabolism in injured spinal cord after methylprednisolone treatment, *J Neurosurg* 56:106-113, 1982.

27. Arbit E, Galicich W, Galicich JH et al: An animal model of epidural compression of the spinal cord, *Neurosurgery* 24:860-863, 1989.

28. Assenmacher DR, Ducker TB: Experimental traumatic paraplegia: the vascular and pathologic changes seen in reversible and irreversible spinal cord lesions, *J Bone Joint Surg* 53:671-680, 1971.

29. Axelsson J, Thesleff S: A study of supersensitivity in mammalian skeletal muscle, *J Physiol* 149:178-181, 1957.

30. Babinski MF: Anesthetic management in the patient with acute spinal cord injury, *Crit Care Clin* 3:619-636, 1987.

31. Bean JW, Beckman DL. Centrogenic pulmonary pathology in mechanical head injury, *J Appl Physiol* 27:807-812, 1969.

32. Bedbrook GM: Spinal injuries with tetraplegia and paraplegia, *J Bone Joint Surg* 61B:267-284, 1979.

33. Bennett MH, McCallum JE: Experimental decompression of spinal cord, *Surg Neurol* 8:63-67, 1977.

34. Bergofsky EH: Mechanism for respiratory insufficiency after cervical cord injury, *Ann Intern Med* 61:435-447, 1964.

35. Bhargava KP, Kulsreshtha JK. Pharmacological analysis of the spinal compression vasomotor response, *Arch Int Pharmacodyn Ther* 127:67-84, 1960.

36. Bhargava KP, Kulsreshtha JK: The spinal compression vasomotor response as a pharmacological tool, *Arch Int Pharmacodyn Ther* 120:85-96, 1959.

37. Black P, Markowitz RS: Experimental spinal cord injury in monkeys: comparison of steroids and hypothermia, *Surg Forum* 22:409-411, 1971.

38. Black P, Markowtiz RS, Keller S et al: Naloxone and experimental spinal cord injury. I. High dose administration in a static load compression model, *Neurosurgery* 19:905-908, 1986.

39. Black P, Markowitz RS, Keller S et al: Naloxone and experimental spinal cord injury. II. Megadose treatment in a dynamic load model, *Neurosurgery* 19:909-913, 1986.

40. Blessing WW, West MJ, Chalmers J: Hypertension, bradycardia and pulmonary edema in the conscious rabbit after brainstem lesions coinciding with the AI group of catecholamine neurons, *Circ Res* 49:949-958, 1981.

41. Bowers RE, Ellis EF, Brigham KL et al: Effects of prostaglandin cyclic endoperoxides on the lung circulation of unanesthetized sheep, *J Clin Invest* 63:131-137, 1979.

42. Bracken MB, Collins WF, Freeman DF et al: Efficacy of methylprednisolone in acute spinal cord injury, *JAMA* 251:45-52, 1984.

43. Bracken MB, Collins WF, Freeman DF et al: Methylprednisolone or naloxone treatment after acute spinal cord injury: 1-year follow-up data, *J Neurosurg* 76:23-31, 1992.

44. Bracken MB, Shephard MJ, Collins WF et al: A randomized, controlled trial of methylprednisolone and naloxone in the treatment of acute spinal-cord injury, *N Engl J Med* 322:1405-1411, 1990.

45. Braughler JM, Hall ED: Correlation of methylprednisolone levels in cat spinal cord with its effects on Na^+,K^+, ATPase, lipid peroxidation, and alpha motor neuron function, *J Neurosurg* 56:838-844, 1982.

46. Braughler JM, Hall ED: Effects of multi-dose methylprednisolone sodium succinate administration on injured cat spinal cord neurofilament degradation and energy metabolism, *J Neurosurg* 61:290-295, 1984.

47. Braughler JM, Hall ED, Means ED et al: Evaluation of an intensive methylprednisolone sodium succinate dosing regime in experimental spinal cord injury, *J Neurosurg* 67:102-105, 1987.

48. Braun SR, Giovannoni R, O'Connor M: Improving the cough in patients with spinal cord injury, *Am J Phys Med* 63:1-10, 1984.

49. Bricolo A, Dalle-Oro G, DaPian R et al: Local cooling in spinal cord injury, *Surg Neurol* 6:101-105, 1976.

50. Brigham KL, Owen PJ: Increased sheep lung vascular permeability caused by histamine, *Circ Res* 37:647-657, 1975.

51. Brisman R, Kovach RM, Johnson DO et al: Pulmonary edema in acute transection of the cervical spinal cord, *Surg Gynecol Obstet* 139:363-366, 1974.

52. Brooke MM, Donovan WH, Stolov WC et al: Paraplegia: succinylcholine induced hyperkalemia in cardiac arrest, *Arch Phys Med Rehabil* 59:306-309, 1978.

53. Brookman R: Traumatic lesions of the spine. In Rosenberg RN, Grossman RG, editors: *The clinical neurosciences*, New York, 1983, Churchill Livingstone.

54. Bucy PC: Acute cervical spinal injury, *Surg Neurol* 20:427-429, 1983 (editorial).

55. Bunegin L, Albin MS, Jannetta PJ: Catecholamine responses to experimental spinal cord impact injury. I. Intrinsic spinal cord synthesis rates, *Exp Neurol* 53:274-280, 1976.

56. Bunegin L, Albin MS, Jannetta PJ: Catecholamine responses to experimental spinal cord impact injury. II. Fate of intravenous $_3$H-NE, *Exp Neurol* 53:281-284, 1976.

57. Bunegin L, Albin MS, Martinez J et al: A new closed impact injury model for experimental spinal cord injury, *Neurosci Abstracts* 12:388, 1986.

58. Bunegin L, Hung TK, Chang GL:

Biomechanics of spinal cord injury, *Crit Care Clin* 3:453-470, 1987.

59. Busto R, Globus MYT, Dietrich WD et al: Effect of mild hypothermia on ischemia-induced release of neurotransmitters and free fatty acids in rat brain, *Stroke* 20:904-910, 1989.

60. Cameron GS, Scott JW, Jousse AT et al: Diaphragmatic respiration in the quadriplegic patient and the effect of position on his vital capacity, *Ann Surg* 141:451-456, 1955.

61. Campbell GS, Hoddy FJ, Adams WL et al: Circulatory changes and pulmonary lesions in dogs following increased intracranial pressure and the effect of atropine upon such changes, *Am J Physiol* 158:96-102, 1949.

62. Carter DR, Frankel VH: Biomechanics of hyperextension injuries to the cervical spine in football, *Am J Sports Med* 8:302-309, 1980.

63. Carter RE: Etiology of traumatic spinal cord injury: statistics of more than 1100 cases, *Texas Med* 73:61-65, 1977.

64. Carter RE: Medical management of pulmonary complications of spinal cord injury. In Thompson RA, Green JR editors: *Advances in neurology,* New York, 1979, Raven Press.

65. Cerutti P: Prooxidant states and tumor production, *Science* 227:375-381, 1985.

66. Chang JL, Chang GL, Nemoto EM et al: Barbiturate protection in experimental spinal cord injury, *Anesthesiology* 63:A400, 1985.

67. Chen HI, Liao JF, Kuo L et al: Centrogenic pulmonary hemorrhagic edema induced by cerebral compression in rats. Mechanism of volume and pressure loading in the pulmonary circulation, *Circ Res* 47:366-373, 1980.

68. Cheng MK, Robertson C, Grossman RG et al: Neurological outcome correlated with spinal evoked potential in a spinal cord ischemia model, *J Neurosurg* 60:786-795, 1984.

69. Cheshire DJE, Coats DA: Respiratory and metabolic management in acute tetraplegia, *Paraplegia* 3:178-181, 1965.

70. Choi DW: Ketamine reduces NMDA receptor mediated neurotoxicity in cortical cultures. In Domino EF, editor: *Status of ketamine in anesthesiology,* Ann Arbor, 1990, NPP Books.

71. Choi DW, Maulucci-Gedde MA, Kriegstein AR: Glutamate neurotoxicity in cortical cell culture, *J Neurosci* 7:357-368, 1987.

72. Claus-Walker JL, Carter RE, Lipocomb HS et al: Analysis of daily rhythms of adrenal function in men with quadriplegia due to spinal cord section, *Paraplegia* 6:195-207, 1968.

73. Cole DJ, Shapiro HM, Drummond JC et al: Halothane, fentanyl/nitrous oxide, and spinal lidocaine protect against spinal cord injury in the rat, *Anesthesiology* 70:967-972, 1989.

74. Cook WA, Hardaker WT: Injuries to the thoracic and lumbar spine. In Wilkins RH, Rengachany SS, editors: *Neurosurgery,* New York, 1985, McGraw-Hill.

75. Dahlstrom A, Fuxe K: Evidence for the existence of monamine neurons in the central nervous system. II. Experimentally induced changes in the intraneuronal amine levels of bulbospinal neuron systems, *Acta Physiol Scan Suppl* 64:1-85, 1965.

76. De La Torre JC, Johnson CM, Goode DJ et al: Pharmacologic treatment and evaluation of permanent experimental spinal cord trauma, *Neurology* 25:508-514, 1975.

77. De La Torre JC, Johnson CM, Harris LH et al: Monoamine changes in experimental head and spinal cord tissue: failure to confirm previous observations, *Surg Neurol* 2:5-11, 1974.

78. Delattre JY, Arbit E, Rosenblum MK et al: High dose versus low dose dexamethasone in experimental epidural spinal cord compression, *Neurosurgery* 22:1005-1007, 1988.

79. Dempsey RJ, Combs DJ, Maley ME et al: Moderate hypothermia reduces postischemic edema development and leucotriene production, *Neurosurgery* 21:177-181, 1987.

80. Desmond J: Paraplegia: problems confronting the anaesthesiologist, *Can Anaesth Soc J* 17:435-450, 1970.

81. Desmond JW, Laws AK: Blood volume and capacitance vessel compliance in the quadriplegic patient, *Can Anaesth Soc J* 21:421-426, 1974.

82. Di Chiro G, Freed LC: Blood flow currents in spinal cord arteries, *Neurology* 21:1088-1096, 1971.

83. Doba N, Reis DS: Acute fulminating neurogenic hypertension produced by brainstem lesions in the rat, *Circ Res* 32:584-593, 1973.

84. Dohrmann GJ, Wagner FC, Bucy PC: The microvasculature in transitory traumatic paraplegia: an electron microscopic study in the monkey, *J Neurosurg* 35:263-271, 1971.

85. Dohrmann GJ, Wagner FC, Bucy PC: Transitory traumatic paraplegia: electron microscopy of the early alterations in myelinated nerve fibers, *J Neurosurg* 36:407-415, 1972.

86. Dohrmann GJ, Wick KM, Bucy PC: Blood flow pattern in the intrinsic vessels of the spinal cord following contusion: an experimental study, *Trans Am Neurol Assoc* 97:189-192, 1972.

87. Dohrmann GJ, Wick KM, Bucy PC: Spinal cord blood flow patterns in experimental traumatic paraplegia, *J Neurosurg* 38:52-58, 1973.

88. Dolan EJ, Tator CH: The effect of blood transfusion, dopamine, and gamma hydroxybutyrate on posttraumatic ischemia of the spinal cord, *J Neurosurg* 56:350-358, 1982.

89. Dolan EJ, Tator CH, Endrenji L: The value of decompression for acute experimental spinal cord compression injury, *J Neurosurg* 53:749-755, 1980.

90. Donaghy RMP, Numoto M: Prognostic significance of sensory evoked potential in spinal cord injury, *Proc Spinal Cord Inj Conf* 17:251-257, 1969.

91. Drinker AS, Helrich M: Halothane anesthesia in the paraplegic patient, *Anesthesiology* 24:399-400, 1963.

92. Drummond JC, Moore SS: The influence of dextrose administration on neurologic outcome after temporary spinal cord ischemia in the rabbit, *Anesthesiology* 70:64-70, 1989.

93. Ducker TB: Increased intracranial pressure and pulmonary edema. I. Clinical study of 11 patients, *J Neurosurg* 28:112-117, 1968.

94. Ducker TB, Hamit HF: Experimental treatments of acute spinal cord injury, *J Neurosurg* 30:693-697, 1969.

95. Ducker TB, Russo GL, Bellegarrique R et al: Complete sensorimotor paralysis after cord injury: mortality, recovery and therapeutic implications, *J Trauma* 19:837-840, 1979.

96. Ducker TB, Simmons RL: Increased intracranial pressure and pulmonary edema. II. The hemodynamic response of dogs and monkeys to increased intracranial pressure, *J Neurosurg* 28:118-122, 1968.

97. Eidelberg E, Staten E, Watkins LJ et al: Treatment of experimental spinal cord injury in ferrets, *Surg Neurol* 6:243-246, 1976.

98. Eidelberg E, Sullivan S, Brigham A: Immediate consequences of spinal cord injury: possible role of potassium in axonal conduction block, *Surg Neurol* 3:317-321, 1975.

99. Faden AI: Opiate antagonists and thyrotropin releasing hormone, *JAMA* 252:1452-1454, 1984.

100. Faden AI, Jacobs TP, Holaday JW: Endorphins in experimental spinal injury: therapeutic effects of naloxone, *Ann Neurol* 10:326-332, 1981.

101. Faden AI, Jacobs TP, Holaday JW: Opiate antagonist improves neurologic recovery after spinal injury, *Science* 211:493-494,1981.

102. Faden AI, Jacobs TP, Patrick DH et al: Megadose corticosteroid therapy following experimental traumatic spinal injury, *J Neurosurg* 60:712-717, 1984.

103. Faden AI, Jacobs TP, Smith MT et al: Comparison of thyrotropin-releasing hormone (TRH), naloxone and dexamethasone treatments in experimental spinal cord injury, *Neurology* 33:673-679, 1983.

104. Felman AH: Neurogenic pulmonary edema: observations in 6 patients, *AJR* 112:393-396, 1971.

105. Flamm ES, Demopoulos HB, Seligman ML et al: Ethanol potentiation of central nervous system trauma, *J Neurosurg* 46:328-335, 1977.

106. Foltz R, Robertson CS, Grossman RG et al: Protection against experimental spinal cord injury, *J Neurosurg* 64:633-642, 1986.

107. Ford RWJ: A reproducible spinal cord injury model in the cat, *J Neurosurg* 59:268-275, 1983.

108. Forner JV: Lung volumes and mechanics of breathing in tetraplegics, *Paraplegia* 18:258-266, 1980.

109. Forner JV, Llombert RL, Valledor MCV: The flow-volume loop in tetraplegics, *Paraplegia* 15:245-251, 1977.

110. Frankel HL, Mathias CJ, Spalding JMK: Mechanisms of reflex cardiac arrest in tetraplegic patients, *Lancet* 2:1183-1185,1975.

111. Frankel VH, Norden M: *Basic biomechanics of the skeletal system,* Philadelphia, 1980, Lea & Febiger.

112. Freeman LW, Wright TW: Experimental observations of concussion and contusion of the spinal cord, *Ann Surg* 137:433-443, 1953.

113. Fried LC, Doppman JL, Di Chiro G: Direction of blood flow in the primate brain, *J Neurosurg* 33:325-330, 1970.

114. Fugl-Meyer AR, Grimby G: Ventilatory function in tetraplegic patients, *Scand J Rehab Med* 3:151-160, 1971.

115. Gamble JE, Parton JD: Pulmonary edema and hemorrhage from preoptic lesions in rats, *J Physiol* 72:623-631, 1953.

116. Gehrig R, Michaels LS: Statistics of acute paraplegia and tetraplegia on a national scale, *Paraplegia* 6:93-95, 1968.

117. Gehwerles JA Jr, Clark WM, Schoaf RE et al: Cervical spine trauma: the common combined conditions, *Radiology* 130:77-86, 1979.

118. Gilbert J: Critical care management of the patient with acute spinal cord injury, *Crit Care Clin* 3:549-567, 1987.

119. Goldbaum GM, Remington PL, Powell KE et al: Failure to use seat belts in the United States: the 1981-1983 behavioral risk factor surveys, *JAMA* 255:2459-2462, 1986.

120. Goodkin R, Campbell JB: Sequential pathologic changes in spinal cord injury, a preliminary report, *Surg Forum* 20:430-432, 1969.

121. Gosch HH, Gooding E, Schneider RC: Distortion and displacement of the brain in experimental head injuries, *Surg Forum* 20:425-426, 1969.

122. Gossman M, White RJ, Taslitz N et al: Electrophysiological responses immediately after experimental injury to the spinal cord, *Anat Rec* 160:473, 1968.

123. Graf CJ, Rossi NP. Pulmonary edema and the central nervous system—a clinico-pathological study, *Surg Neurol* 4:319-325, 1975.

124. Green BA, Eismont FJ, O'Heir JT: Spinal cord injury—a systems approach: prevention, emergency medical services, and emergency room management, *Crit Care Clin* 3:471-493, 1987.

125. Gregg TM: Organization of a spinal injury unit within a rehabilitation centre, *Paraplegia* 5:163-166, 1967.

126. Gregg TM, Wilmot CB: The flying squad and the paraplegic unit (preliminary report), *Paraplegia* 2:15-16, 1964.

127. Griffiths ER: Spinal injuries from swimming and diving treated in the Spinal Department of Royal Perth Rehabilitation Hospital, 1956-1978, *Paraplegia* 18:109-117, 1980.

128. Grissom TE, Mitzel HC, Bunegin L et al: Neurologic outcome to anesthetics after chronic spinal cord injury (SCI) in rats, *J Neurosurg Anesthesiol* 2:216, 1990.

129. Groat RA, Peele TL: Blood pressure response to acutely increased pressure upon the spinal cord, *Am J Physiol* 44:578-587, 1945.

130. Grundy BL, Friedman W: Electrophysiological evaluation of the patient with acute spinal cord injury, *Crit Care Clin* 3:519-548, 1987.

131. Guha A, Tator CH, Endrenyi L et al: Decompression of the spinal cord improves recovery after acute experimental spinal cord compression injury, *Paraplegia* 25:324-339, 1987.

132. Guttman L: *Spinal cord injuries: comprehensive management and research,* Oxford, 1976, Blackwell.

133. Guyton AC, Lindsey AW: Effect of elevated left atrial pressure and decreased plasma protein concentration on the development of pulmonary edema, *Circ Res* 12:649-657, 1959.

134. Hachen HJ: Emergency transportation in the event of acute spinal cord lesion, *Paraplegia* 12:33-37, 1974.

135. Hachen HJ: Idealized care of the acutely injured spinal cord in Switzerland, *J Trauma* 17:931-936, 1977.

136. Hall ED, Wolf DL, Braughler JM: Effects of a single large dose of methylprednisolone sodium succinate on experimental posttraumatic spinal cord ischemia, *J Neurosurg* 61:124-130, 1984.

137. Hansebout RR, Kuchner EF, Romero-Sierra C: Effects of local hypothermia and of steroids upon recovery from experimental spinal cord compression injury, *Surg Neurol* 4:531-536, 1975.

138. Harris EJ, Nicholls JG: The effect of denervation on the rate of entry of potassium into the frog muscle, *J Physiol* 131:473-476, 1956.

139. Hartzog JT, Fisher RG, Snow C: Spinal cord trauma: effect of hyperbaric oxygen therapy, *Proceedings of the Seventeenth Spinal Cord Injury Conference,* 1969.

140. Haupt MT, Rackow EC: Colloid osmotic pressure and fluid resuscitation

with hetastarch, albumin, and saline solutions, *Crit Care Med* 10:159-162, 1982.

141. Haupt MT, Teerapong P, Green D et al: Increased pulmonary edema with crystalloid compared to colloid resuscitation of shock associated with increased vascular permeability, *Circ Shock* 12:213-224, 1984.

142. Hauser CJ, Shoemaker WC, Turpin I et al: Oxygen transport responses to colloids and crystalloids in critically ill surgical patients, *Surg Gynecol Obstet* 150:811-816, 1980.

143. Head H, Riddoch J: Autonomic bladder, excessive sweating, and some other reflex conditions in gross injuries of the spinal cord, *Brain* 40:188-263, 1917.

144. Heiden JS, Weiss MH, Rosenberg AW et al: Management of cervical spinal cord trauma in Southern California, *J Neurosurg* 43:732-736, 1975.

145. Hemingway A, Price WM: The autonomic nervous system and regulation of body temperature, *Anesthesiology* 29:693-701, 1968.

146. Hess L: Uber Lungenodem bei organischen Nervenerkrankungen, *Wien Med Wochenschr* 84:255-288, 1934.

147. Hickey R, Albin MS, Bunegin L: Alterations in spinal cord and cerebral autoregulation during halothane anesthesia, *Anesth Rev* 15:78-79, 1988.

148. Hickey R, Albin MS, Bunegin L: Ketamine abolishes central nervous system autoregulation, *Anesth Rev* 15:77-78, 1988.

149. Hickey R, Albin M, Bunegin L et al: Autoregulation of spinal cord and cerebral blood flow: is the cord a microcosm of the brain? *Stroke* 17:1183-1189, 1987.

150. Hoff JT, Smith HL, Hankinson HL: Barbiturate protection from cerebral infarction in primates, *Stroke* 6:28-33, 1975.

151. Holmstrom F, Babinski M: Spirometry in acute spinal cord injury, *Crit Care Med* 8:253, 1980.

152. James WS, Minh V, Minteer MA et al: Cervical accessory respiratory muscle function in a patient with a high cervical cord lesion, *Chest* 71:59-64, 1977.

153. Jellinger K: Spinal cord arteriosclerosis and progressive vascular myopathy, *J Neurol Neurosurg Psychiat* 30:195-206, 1967.

154. Jelsnia RK, Kirsch PT, Rice JF, et al: The radiographic description of thoracolumbar fractures, *Surg Neurol* 18:230-236, 1982.

155. John DA, Tobey RE, Homer LD et al: Onset of succinylcholine induced hyperkalemia following denervation, *Anesthesiology* 45:294-299, 1976.

156. Joyner J, Freeman LW: Urea and spinal cord trauma, *Neurology* 13:69-72, 1963.

157. Kakari S, DeCrescito V, Tomasula JJ et al: Long term studies of histochemical and cytochemical changes in the contused feline spinal cord, *J Neuropath Exp Neurol* 35:109, 1976.

158. Karim SM, Filskie GM: The use of prostaglandin E_2 for therapeutic abortion, *J Obst Gynec* 79:1-13, 1972.

159. Kelly DL Jr, Lasiter RL, Calogero JA et al: Effects of local hypothermia and tissue oxygen studies in experimental paraplegia, *J Neurosurg* 33:554-563, 1970.

160. Kendrick WW, Scott JW, Jouse AT et al: Reflex sweating and hypertension in traumatic transverse myelitis, *Treatment Serv Bull* 8:437-441, 1953.

161. Khan M, Griebel R: Acute spinal cord injury in the rat: comparison of three experimental techniques, *Can J Neurol Sci* 10:161-165, 1983.

162. Koike M, Roizen MF, Zivin J et al: Adverse effects of some anesthetics on spinal cord ischemic injury, *Anesthesiology* 57:A312, 1982.

163. Koons DD, Gildenberg PL, Dohn DF et al: Local hypothermia in the treatment of spinal cord injuries: report of seven cases, *Cleve Clin Q* 39:109-117, 1972.

164. Kopaniky DR: Pathophysiology and management of spinal cord trauma. In Frost EAM, editor: *Clinical anesthesia in Neurosurgery,* Boston, 1991, Buttersworth-Heinemann.

165. Kraus JF: Epidemiologic features of head and spinal cord injury. In Shoenberg BS, editor: *Advances in neurology,* vol 19, New York, 1978, Raven Press.

166. Kuchner EF, Hansebout RR: Combined steroid and hypothermia treatment of experimental spinal cord injury, *Surg Neurol* 6:371-376, 1976.

167. Kurnick NB: Autonomic hyperreflexia and its control in patients with spinal cord lesions, *Ana Intern Med* 44:678-689, 1956.

168. Lambert DH, Deane RS, Mazuzan JE: Anesthesia and the control of blood pressure in patients with spinal cord injury, *Anesth Analg* 61:344-348, 1982.

169. Lanier WL, Stangland KJ, Scheithauer BW et al: The effects of dextrose infusion and head position on neurologic outcome after complete cerebral ischemia in primates: examination of a model, *Anesthesiology* 66:39-48, 1987

170. Laschinger JC, Cunningham JN Jr, Cooper MM et al: Prevention of ischemic spinal cord injury following aortic cross-clamping: use of corticosteroids, *Ann Thor Surg* 38:500-507, 1984.

171. Ledsome JR, Sharp JM: Pulmonary function in acute cervical cord injury, *Am Rev Resp Dis* 124:41-44, 1981.

172. Lehman KG, Lane JG, Piepmeier JM et al: Cardiovascular abnormalities accompanying acute spinal cord injury in humans: incidence, time course and severity, *J Am Coll Cardiol* 10:46-52, 1987.

173. LeMay DR, Lu AC, Zelenock GB et al: Insulin administration protects from paraplegia in the rat aortic occlusion model, *J Surg Res* 44:352-358, 1988.

174. LeMay DR, Neal S, Zelenock GB et al: Paraplegia in the rat induced by aortic cross-clamping: model characterization and glucose exacerbation of neurological deficit, *J Vasc Surg* 6:383-390, 1989.

175. Levy WJ, Yok DH: Evoked potentials from the motor tract in humans, *Neurosurgery* 12:422-429, 1983.

176. Lewin MG, Hansebout RB, Papius HM: Chemical characteristics of traumatic spinal cord edema in cats, *J Neurosurg* 40:65-75, 1974.

177. Little JW, Harris RM, Sohlberg RC: Locomotor recovery following subtotal spinal cord lesions in a rat model, *Neurosci Lett* 87:189-194, 1988.

178. Luce JM, Culver BH: Respiratory muscle function in health and disease, *Chest* 81:82-90, 1982.

179. Lundy EF, Ball T, Mandell MA et al: Dextrose administration increases sensory/motor impairment and paraplegia after infrarenal aortic occlusion in the rabbit, *Surgery* 102:737-742, 1987.

180. MacKenzie CF, Ducker TB: Cervical cord injury. In Matjasko J, Katz J editors: *Clinical controversies in neuroanesthesia and neurosurgery,* Orlando, 1986, Grune & Stratton.

181. MacKenzie CF, Shin B, Krishna-pradad D et al: Assessment of cardiac and respiratory function during surgery on patients with acute quadriplegia, *J Neurosurg* 63:843-849, 1985.

182. Magnusson T, Rosengren E: Catecholamines of the spinal cord normally and after transection, *Experimentia* 19:229-230, 1963.

183. Maire FW, Patton MD: Neural structures involved in the genesis of preoptic pulmonary edema, gastric erosions and behavior changes, *Am J Physiol* 184:345-350, 1956.

184. Malik AB: Pulmonary vascular response to increase in intracranial pressure: role of sympathetic mechanisms, *J Appl Physiol* 42:335-343, 1977.

185. Manners T: Vascular lesions in the spinal cord in the aged, *Geriatrics* 21:151-160, 1966.

186. Marcaux FW, Goodrich JE, Dominick MA: Ketamine prevents ischemic neuronal injury, *Brain Res* 452:329-335, 1988.

187. Marcaux FW, Goodrich JE, Dominick MA: Ketamine anesthesia reduces ischemic hippocampal neuronal injury. In Domino EF, editor: *Status of ketamine in anesthesiology,* Ann Arbor, 1990, NPP Books.

188. Maroon JC, Abla AA: Classification of acute spinal cord injury, neurological classification and neurosurgical considerations, *Crit Care Clin* 3:655-677, 1987.

189. Mathias CJ: Bradycardia and cardiac arrest during tracheal suction—mechanisms in tetraplegic patients, *Eur J Inten Care Med* 2:147-156, 1976.

190. McCord JM: Oxygen-derived free radicals in postischemic tissue injury, *N Engl J Med* 312:159-163, 1986.

191. McCullough JL, Hollier LH, Nugent M: Paraplegia after thoracic aortic occlusion: influence of cerebrospinal fluid drainage, *J Vasc Surg* 7:153-160, 1988.

192. McGregor JA, Meevusen J: Autonomic hyperreflexia: a mortal danger for spinal cord–damaged women in labor, *Am J Obstet Gynecol* 151:330-333, 1985.

193. McKinley AC, Auchincloss JH, Gilbert R et al: Pulmonary function, ventilatory control, and respiratory complications in quadriplegic subjects, *Am Rev Resp Dis* 100:526-532, 1969.

194. McMichan JC, Michel L, Westbrook PR: Pulmonary dysfunction following traumatic quadriplegia: recognition, prevention and treatment, *JAMA* 243:528-531, 1980.

195. Meachem W, McPherson W: Local hypothermia in the treatment of acute injuries of the spinal cord, *South Med J* 66:95-97, 1973.

196. Meinecke FW: Frequency and distribution of associated injuries in traumatic paraplegia and tetraplegia, *Paraplegia* 5:196-209, 1968.

197. Mertz JH Jr, Patrick LM: Strength and response of the human neck, *Proc 19th Stapp Car Crash Conf Soc of Auto Engrs,* 1971.

198. Mertz JH Jr, Patrick LM: Investigations of the kinematics and kinetics of whiplash, *Proc 19th Stapp Car Crash Conf Soc of Auto Engrs,* 1971.

199. Meyer GA, Berman IR, Doty DB et al: Hemodynamic responses to acute quadriplegia with or without chest trauma, *J Neurosurg* 34:168-177, 1971.

200. Michenfelder JD, Milde JH: Influence of anesthetics on metabolic, functional and pathological responses to regional cerebral ischemia, *Stroke* 6:405-410, 1975.

201. Miller CA, Dewey RL, Hunt WE: Impact fracture of the lumbar vertebrae with dural tear, *J Neurosurg* 53:765-771, 1980.

202. *Morbidity and Mortality Weekly Report* (Centers for Disease Control) 37:285-286, 1988, US Department of Health, Education, and Welfare, Public Health Service Center for Disease Control, Atlanta, Georgia.

203. *Morbidity and Mortality Weekly Report* (Centers for Disease Control) 38:743-746, 1989, US Department of Health, Education, and Welfare, Public Health Service Center for Disease Control, Atlanta, Georgia.

204. Moss G, Staunton C, Stein AA: Cerebral etiology of the "shock lung syndrome," *J Trauma* 12:885-890, 1972.

205. Mullan S, Hosobuchi Y: Respiratory hazards of high cervical percutaneous cordotomy, *J Neurosurg* 28:291-297, 1968.

206. Murray GC, Persellin RH: Cervical fracture complicating ankylosing spondylitis: a report of eight cases and review of the literature, *Am J Med* 70:1033-1041, 1981.

207. Naftchi NE, Demeny M, Decrescito V et al: Biogenic amine concentrations in traumatized spinal cords of cats: effects of drug therapy, *J Neurosurg* 40:52-57, 1974.

208. Naftchi NE, Wooten GF, Lowman EW et al: Relationship between serum dopamine-beta-hydroxylase activity, catecholamine metabolism and hemodynamic changes during paroxysmal hypertension in paraplegia, *Circ Res* 35:850-861, 1974.

209. Nathan MA, Reis DJ: Fulminating arterial hypertension with pulmonary edema from release of adrenomedullary catecholamines after lesions of the anterior hypothalamics in the rat, *Circ Res* 37:226-235, 1975.

210. Nylander WA, Plunkett RJ, Hammon JW Jr, et al: Thiopental modification of ischemic spinal cord injury in the dog, *Ann Thorac Surg* 33:64-68, 1982.

211. Nyquist RH: Mortality in spinal cord injury: follow-up report, *Calif Med* 103:417-419, 1965.

212. Ohry A, Molho M, Rozin R: Alterations of pulmonary function in spinal cord injured patients, *Paraplegia* 13:101-108, 1975.

213. Olmarker K, Rydevik B, Holm S: Edema formation in spinal nerve roots induced by experimental, graded compression, *Spine* 14:569-573.

214. Osterholm JL: The pathophysiological response to spinal cord injury: the current status of related research, *J Neurosurg* 40:5-33, 1974.

215. Osterholm JL, Mathews GJ: Altered norepinephrine metabolism following experimental spinal cord injury. I: Relationship to hemorrhagic necrosis and post-wounding neurological deficits, *J Neurosurg* 36:386-393, 1972.

216. Osterholm JL, Mathews GJ: Altered norepinephrine metabolism following experimental spinal cord injury. II. Protection against traumatic spinal cord hemorrhagic necrosis by norepinephrine synthesis blockade with alpha methyl tyrosine, *J Neurosurg* 36:395-401, 1972.

217. Osterholm JL, Mathews GJ: Treatment of severe spinal cord injuries by biochemical norepinephrine manipulation, *Surg Forum* 22:415-417, 1971.

218. Pasteyer J, Sigmor MB, Honnart F: Anesthesìe et réanimation chirurgicale dans la chirurgie du rachis cer-

vical avec troûbles neurologiques, *Ann Anesth Franc* 15:1-8, 1974.

219. Patel C, Miller SM, Chalon J et al: Anesthesia and spinal cord lesions, *Bull NY Acad Med* 54:924-930, 1978.

220. Perot PL: The clinical use of somatosensory evoked potentials in spinal cord injury, *Clin Neurosurg* 20:367-381, 1973.

221. Phillis JW, Tebecis AK, York DH: Depression of spinal motoneurones by noradrenaline, 5-hydroxytryptamine and histamine, *Eur J Pharmacol* 4:471-475, 1968.

222. Pierce EC Jr, Lambertson CJ, Deutsch S: Cerebral circulation and metabolism during thiopental anesthesia and hyperventilation in man, *J Clin Invest* 41:1664-1671, 1962.

223. Pitts LH: The management of cervical and spinal cord trauma, *American Society of Anesthesiologists Refresher Course Lecture* 121, 1981.

224. Poe RH, Reisman JL, Rodenhouse TG: Pulmonary edema in cervical cord injury, *J Trauma* 18:71-73, 1978.

225. Pong D, Wilberger WE Jr: Traumatic atlanto-occipital dislocation with survival case report and review, *Neurosurgery* 7:503-508, 1980.

226. Pontoppidan H, Rie M: Pathogenesis and therapy of acute lung injury. In Prakash O, editor: *Applied physiology in clinical respiratory care*, Boston, 1982, Nijhof.

227. Quinby CW, Williams RN, Greifenstein FE: Anesthetic problems of the acute quadriplegic patient, *Anesth Analg* 52:333-340, 1973.

228. Rawe SE, Perot PL Jr: Pressor response resulting from experimental contusion injury to the spinal cord, *J Neurosurg* 50:58-63, 1979.

229. Reynolds RW. Pulmonary edema as a consequence of hypothalamic lesions in rats, *Science* 41:930-932, 1963.

230. Richardson HD, Nakamura S: An electron microscopic study of spinal cord edema and the effects of treatment with steroids, mannitol and hypothermia, *Proceedings of the Thirty-ninth Annual Meeting of the American Association of Neurological Surgery,* April 1971.

231. Rigamonti DD, Martinez-Arizola A, Long JB: Neuroprotective effects of ketamine in a rodent model of peptide induced spinal cord injury: ana-

tomical and physiological correlates. In Domino EF, editor: *Status of ketamine in anesthesiology,* Ann Arbor, 1990, NPP Books.

232. Roaf R: A study of the mechanics of spinal injury, *J Bone Joint Surg* 60B:95-106, 1978.

233. Robertson CS, Faltz R, Grossman RG et al: Protection against experimental ischemic spinal cord injury, *J Neurosurg* 64:633-642, 1986.

234. Rocco AG, Vandam LD: Problems in anesthesia for paraplegia, *Anesthesiology* 20:348-353, 1959.

235. Roussan MS, Abramson AS, Lippman HI et al: Somatic and autonomic responses to bladder filling in patients with complete transverse myelopathy, *Arch Phys Med Rehab* 47:450-456, 1966.

236. Rowed EW, McLean JAG, Tator CH: Somatosensory evoked potentials in acute spinal cord injury: prognostic value, *Surg Neurol* 9:203-210, 1978.

237. Salzman SK, Mendez AA, Sabato S et al: Anesthesia influences the outcome from experimental spinal cord injury, *Brain Res* 52:33-39, 1990.

238. Sances A Jr, Myklebust JB, Maiman DS et al: The biomechanics of spinal injuries, *Crit Rev Biomech Eng* 11:1-76, 1984.

239. Sarnoff SJ, Sarnoff LC: Neurohemodynamics of pulmonary edema. The role of sympathetic pathways in the elevation of pulmonary and systemic vascular pressure following the intracranial injection of fibrin, *Circulation* 6:51-61, 1952.

240. Scher AT: The high rugby tackle—an available cause of cervical spinal injury? *S Afr Med J* 53:1015-1018, 1978.

241. Schneider RC, Crosby EC: Craniocerebral, cervicomedullary and spinal injuries. In Schneider RC, Kahn EA, Crosby EC, et al, editors: *Correlative neurosurgery,* ed 3, Springfield, Ill, 1982, Charles C Thomas.

242. Schneider RC, Livingston KE, Cave AJE et al: Hangman's fracture of the cervical spine, *J Neurosurg* 22:141-154, 1965.

243. Schneider RC: High cervical injuries. In Wilkins RH, Rengachany SS editors: *Neurosurgery,* New York, 1985, McGraw-Hill.

244. Schonwald G, Fish KJ, Perkash I: Cardiovascular complications during anesthesia in chronic spinal cord in-

jured patients, *Anesthesiology* 55:550-558, 1981.

245. Schrader S, Sloan TB, Toleikis JR: Detection of sacral sparing in acute spinal cord injury, *Spine* 12:533-535, 1987.

246. Selker RG: Ice water irrigation of the spinal cord, *Surg Forum* 22:411-413, 1970.

247. Sheik HH: Fractures of the atlas and odontoid process, *Orthop Clin North Am* 9:973-984, 1978.

248. Shoemaker WC, Hauser CJ: Critique of crystalloid versus colloid therapy in shock and shock lung, *Crit Care Med* 7:117-124, 1979.

249. Shrosbree RD: Neurological sequelae of reduction of fracture dislocations of the cervical spine, *Paraplegia* 17:212-221, 1979.

250. Shrosbree RD: Spinal cord injuries as a result of motorcycle accidents, *Paraplegia* 16:102-112, 1979.

251. Siegal T, Siegal TZ, Sandbank U et al: Experimental neoplastic spinal cord compression: evoked potentials, edema, prostaglandins, and light and electron microscopy, *Spine* 12:440-448, 1987.

252. Silver JR: The oxygen cost of breath in tetraplegic patients, *Paraplegia* 1:204-208, 1963.

253. Silver JR, Moulton A: The physiological and pathological sequelae of paralysis of the intercostal and abdominal muscles in tetraplegic patients, *Paraplegia* 7:131-141, 1969.

254. Smith RB: Hyperkalemia following succinylcholine administration in neurological disorders. A review, *Can Anaesth Soc J* 18:199-201, 1971.

255. Snow JC, Kripke BJ, Sessions GP et al: Cardiovascular collapse following succinylcholine in a paraplegic patient, *Paraplegia* 11:109-204, 1973.

256. Soderstrom CA, McArdle DQ, Ducker TB et al: The diagnosis of intra-abdominal injury in patients with cervical cord trauma, *J Trauma* 23:1061-1065, 1983.

257. Sokol MD: Anesthetic management of patients with spinal cord injuries, *American Society of Anesthesiologists Refresher Course Lecture* 131, 1980.

258. Stauffer ES, Bell GD: Traumatic respiratory quadriplegia and pentaplegia, *Orthop Clin North Am* 9:1081-1089, 1978.

259. Stone WA, Beach TP, Hamelberg

W: Succinylcholine-danger in the spinal cord injured patient, *Anesthesiology* 32:168-169, 1970.

260. Stone WA, Beach TP, Hamelberg W: Succinylcholine-induced hyperkalemia in dogs with transected sciatic nerves or spinal cords, *Anesthesiology* 32:515-519, 1970.

261. Suderman VS, Crosby ET, Lui A: Elective oral tracheal intubation in cervical spine-injured patients, *Can J Anaesth* 38:785-789, 1991.

262. Tator CH, Deecke L: Value of normothermic perfusion, hypothermic perfusion, and durotomy in the treatment of experimental acute spinal cord trauma, *Neurosurgery* 39:52-64, 1973.

263. Taylor AR, Byrnes DP: Foramen magnum and high cervical cord compression, *Brain* 97:473-480, 1974.

264. Tenicela R, Rosomoff HL, Feist J et al: Pulmonary function following percutaneous cervical cordotomy, *Anesthesiology* 29:7-16, 1968.

265. Theodore J, Robin ED: Speculations in neurogenic pulmonary edema (NPE), *Am Rev Respir Dis* 113:405-411, 1976 (editorial).

266. Theye RA, Milde JH, Michenfelder JD: Effect of hypocapnia on cardiac output during anesthesia, *Anesthesiology* 27:778-782, 1966.

267. Thienprasit P, Bantli H, Bloedel JR et al: Effect of delayed local cooling on experimental spinal cord injury, *J Neurosurg* 42:150-154, 1975.

268. Tibbs PA, Young B, McAllister RG et al: Studies of experimental cervical spinal cord transection, I. Hemodynamic changes after acute cervical spinal cord transection, *J Neurosurg* 49:558-562, 1978.

269. Tobey RE: Paraplegia, succinylcho-line and cardiac arrest, *Anesthesiology* 32:359-364, 1970.

270. Tobey RE, Jacobsen PM, Kable CT et al: The serum potassium response to muscle relaxants in neural injury, *Anesthesiology* 37:332-337, 1972.

271. Tribe CR: Causes of death in early and late stages of paraplegia, *Paraplegia* 1:19-47, 1963.

272. Troll GF, Dohrman GJ: Anesthesia of the spinal cord injured patient: cardiovascular problems and their management, *Paraplegia* 13:162-171, 1975.

273. Turnbull IM, Breig A, Hassler O: Blood supply of the cervical cord in man: a microangiographic study, *J Neurosurg* 24:951-965, 1966.

274. Ushio Y, Posner R, Posner JB et al: Experimental spinal cord compression by epidural neoplasms, *Neurology* 27:422-429, 1977.

275. Van der Zee H, Malik AB, Lee BC et al: Lung fluid and protein exchange during intracranial hypertension and role of sympathetic mechanism, *J Appl Physiol* 48:273-280, 1980.

276. Wagner FC Jr, Dohrmann GJ, Bucy PC: Histopathology of transitory traumatic paraplegia in the monkey, *J Neurosurg* 35:272-276, 1971.

277. Wagner FC Jr, Taslitz N, White RJ et al: Vascular phenomena in the normal and traumatized spinal cord, *Anat Rec* 163:281, 1969.

278. Wallace MC, Tator CH: Failure of naloxone to improve spinal cord blood flow and cardiac output after spinal cord injury, *Neurosurgery* 18:428-432, 1986.

279. Watson DW, Downey GO: Epidural anesthesia for labor and delivery of twins of a paraplegic mother, *Anesthesiology* 52:259-261, 1980.

280. Weight FF, Salmoiraghi GC: Adrenergic responses of Renshaw cells, *J Pharmacol Exp Ther* 154:391-396, 1966.

281. Weisman SJ: Edema and congestion of the lungs resulting from intracranial hemorrhage, *Surgery* 6:722-729, 1939.

282. Weiss MH: Mid and lower cervical spine injuries. In Wilkins RH, Rengachany SS, editors: *Neurosurgery,* New York, 1985, McGraw-Hill.

283. White RJ: Current status of spinal cord cooling, *Clin Neurosurg* 20: 400-408, 1973.

284. White RJ, Albin MS: Spine and spinal cord injury. In Gurdijian ES, Lange WA, Patrick LM et al, editors: *Impact injury and crash protection,* Springfield, Ill, 1970, Charles C Thomas.

285. White RJ, Albin MS, Harris LS et al: Spinal cord injury: sequential morphology and hypothermic stabilization, *Surg Forum* 20:432-434, 1969.

286. Winslow EBJ, Lesch M, Talano JV et al: Spinal cord injuries associated with cardiopulmonary complications, *Spine* 11:809-812, 1986.

287. Wolman L: The disturbance of circulation in traumatic paraplegia in acute and late stages: a pathological study, *Paraplegia* 1:213-226, 1965.

288. Woo E, Chan YW, Yu YL et al: Admission glucose level in relation to mortality and morbidity outcome in 252 stroke patients, *Stroke* 19:185-191, 1988.

289. Wood-Jones F: The ideal lesion produced by judicial hanging, *Lancet* 1:53, 1913.

290. Young JS, Cheshire JE, Pierce JA et al: Cervical ankylosis with acute spinal cord injury, *Paraplegia* 15:133-146, 1977.

34

Ethical Considerations in the Care of Patients with Neurosurgical Disease

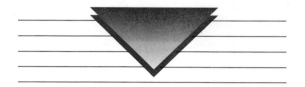

Jonathan D. Moreno
Connie Zuckerman

Research advances and heightened clinical capabilities have enabled those who care for patients with neurosurgical disease to make great strides toward the restoration of health and well being for such patients and in reducing their morbidity and mortality. Yet for every new technologic advance and clinical application, there have also arisen new questions for care givers, such as (1) the appropriate selection of patients for the application of new technologies, (2) the involvement of patients and families in balancing the risks of new treatments vs. their possible benefits, and (3) how to make decisions for patients who may not be able to participate in the decision-making process, yet for whom significant decisions must be made concerning the kind of care to be delivered.

Such questions demand that clinicians must sometimes look beyond their clinical training and subspecialty exper-

tise when they grapple with the genuine ethical dilemmas that are now an integral part of the clinical setting. Determining whether one's actions are "right" or "wrong" has become a troubling and sometimes arduous process for even the most enlightened of clinicians. Thus a system of "clinical ethics" has emerged over the last 30 years, which permits clinicians to apply philosophic reasoning and ethical analysis to the problems they encounter in the course of practice.

Heightened sensitivity to ethical concerns in the clinical setting has also been accompanied by increased awareness of, and concern for, the role of the legal system in clinical practice. As medical and surgical care has become ever more sophisticated and developments in the legal process have both educated and encouraged patients to assert themselves in the provider-patient relationship, physicians have naturally become more sensitive to the legal status of their actions. A clinical ethics framework that incorporates a perspective of legal concerns as it also tries to determine the appropriateness of an action may lay well beyond narrow legal definitions applicable in a particular situation. While it is incumbent on the clinician to be aware of the legal backdrop for clinical practice, it is also essential to recognize that many of the ethical dilemmas that confront the clinician move beyond mere legal technicalities and instead involve the clinician in an evaluation of concurrent and—at times—conflicting duties, rights, and values that are an inevitable part of the provider-patient relationship. In this chapter, we address the ethical issues that confront care givers of the neurosurgical patient population.

AN INTRODUCTION TO THE HISTORY AND THEORY OF MEDICAL ETHICS

This chapter begins with an overview of the historic development of medical ethics. The account concentrates mainly on the Western secular tradition that begins with followers of Hippocrates and emerges in a fundamentally altered form in the current framework of clinical ethics. We then describe the essential features of the current framework.

Origins of Contemporary Medical Ethics

Western medical ethics is normally thought to have originated with the Hippocratic cult (about 450 to 300 BC), a group of mystic physicians who are thought to have been heavily influenced by the Pythagorean thinkers. In addition to their accomplishments in mathematics, the Pythagoreans developed a moral philosophy that emphasized respect for life. This would account, for example, for the apparent strictures on abortion and euthanasia, which are features of a prominent version of the Hippocratic Oath. For different reasons, the Oath also prohibits surgery, which was not regarded as a proper part of physician activities. The attitudes held by the Hippocratic physicians apparently were not widely held among other physician cults of the ancient world.[10]

Perhaps the most striking feature of the Hippocratic Oath is its emphasis on what might be called "medical etiquette." This concept includes both the provision of professional courtesy and the maintainance of professional secrecy. Also associated with these standards is the expectation that physicians would use all their skills for the benefit of patients and that they would avoid harming them. Other Hippocratic documents, such as the Precepts, describe what would today be called "impression management techniques" to inspire in the patient feelings of confidence in the physician. The texts suggest a highly sophisticated appreciation for the placebo effect when no reliable curative measure was available, as was almost always the case, and part of the physician's job was to help the patient endure the affliction and to provide comfort and hope to the terminally ill.[21]

In the medieval world, Christianity contributed a spirit of self-sacrifice and self-abnegation to the ministrations of the physician. Rather than focusing on comportment and trading practices, the physician was thought to be only acting in concert with Jesus' healing ministry and was sometimes even seen as an extension of divine purpose. This shift in role conceptualization helps to account for the somewhat divided self-image of the modern profession, which values both guildlike physician self-determination and a degree of personal exertion on behalf of a patient that is more than normally required of human beings in relations with others.[22]

Conspicuous by its absence is the now ubiquitous notion of patient self-determination, which culminated in the doctrine of informed consent. To understand how this view became so prominent, one must first recall the technical breakthroughs in surgery and anesthesiology during the early and mid-nineteenth century and the development of the germ theory somewhat later. These developments increased both the ability of surgeons to intervene and the ability of physicians to diagnose. The therapeutic power and scientific basis of modern medicine that emerged by the turn of the century was accompanied, on the political front, by the consolidation of the authority of scientific medicine over its competitors, such as Thompsonianism, homeopathy, and osteopathy.[41]

One result of medicine's successes was, paradoxically, that its practitioners would be subject to gradually increasing scrutiny, precisely because of their remarkably enhanced power to predict and intervene. The latter part of the nineteenth and early part of the twentieth centuries saw a number of legal cases involving surgical patients whose consent to excision of tissues had not been obtained.[38] Under prevailing legal theories, these actions were at first considered torts, such as battery or unconsented-to-touching.[26] As the medical and judicial systems evolved, they were then gradually brought under a negligence theory.[26] This strengthened the growing expectation that informing the patient of the reason for the procedure and obtaining consent for it were proper parts of the doctor-patient relationship.[37] In theory, at least, obtaining the patient's informed consent became an essential aspect of the developing standard of care. However, honoring this legal requirement in clinical reality awaited the increased attention to ethical issues that emerged in the late 1960's.

Although our focus in this chapter is clinical ethics, no survey of the history of medical ethics can omit reaction to the abuses of human beings perpetrated by pseudoscientists and so-called physicians in Nazi Germany. The revelations at Nuremberg led to the promulgation of international standards for the protection of research subjects in Helsinki and Geneva.[14] Unfortunately, these efforts did not prevent blatantly unethical practices in the context of subsequent research by American investigators.[5] As a result, strict statutory protections were established to ensure the informed consent of research participants, including protocol review by institutional committees.[42,44] Public recognition of research abuses led to heightened scrutiny of the physician-patient relationship in the clinical setting and increased support for the concept of informed consent.

Technologic advances once again profoundly influenced the direction of medical ethics, beginning in the latter 1960s with the arrival of practical artificial respiratory equipment and, in the early 1970s, with the development of materials that facilitated artificial hydration and nutrition. These advances—combined with social and political changes, including the civil rights movements—culminated in the celebrated legal case of Karen Ann Quinlan in 1976.[36] In the *Quinlan* decision, the New Jersey Supreme Court established that the right to refuse medical treatment was fundamental and could be exercised on behalf of an incompetent patient by informed surrogates, knowledgeable about the patient's previous values and lifestyle.[36] The family was found to be in an excellent position to represent these wishes of their close relative.[36]

In summary, the history of Western medical ethics has featured a transition from the "beneficence" orientation (doing good for the patient) of premodern medicine to the view that it is ultimately the patient who must decide what his/her best interests are after going through a process of informed consent. Both morally and legally, patient self-determination has become the gold standard of modern biomedical ethics. In the next section, we review the prevailing philosophic principles and theories that are often used to further assess ethical problems in modern medicine.

Prevailing Theories and Principles

The term "medical ethics," as it is used in contemporary society, is somewhat ambiguous. It may refer to those rules of conduct that are established by the formal bodies of the medical profession in the course of regulating itself, such as the prohibition of the sexual exploitation of one's patients; or it may refer to novel ethical dilemmas that actually confront health care workers and have no obvious solution in terms of traditional values and ethical codes, such as the removal of life support systems from irreversibly comatose patients.

Two philosophic approaches dominate the literature. One is the deontologic approach, which is identified most closely with the philosopher Immanuel Kant.[23] Deontology is, literally, the study of duties that persons have toward one another. Thus deontologic ethics is often called "duty-based" ethics. The second dominant philosophic approach to medicine is utilitarianism, which is identified most closely with John Stuart Mill.[28] Utilitarianism is the view that actions or policies are to be morally evaluated according to the extent to which they promote happiness or well-being. There are, to be sure, other important intellectual traditions that have been applied to philosophic questions in medicine, but deontology and utilitarianism have been cited most often.

Both philosophic approaches are appealing in the medical context although for different reasons. Deontology is reminiscent of the familiar notion that doctors have certain special duties of care toward their patients, whereas utilitarianism is consistent with the preoccupation that most health care providers have with the outcomes or consequences of an intervention. Interestingly, neither approach on its face calls immediate attention to the idea of patient self-determination or autonomy although both are thought to be compatible with it.

The principle of autonomy is commonly regarded as the first principle of contemporary medical ethics.[4] But it is usually seen as conceptually balanced by the principle of beneficence or the obligation to do good for the patient.[4] Beneficence is closely associated with the traditional Hippocratic obligation to at least not harm the patient, or the principle of nonmaleficence.[4] Arguments that establish the moral basis of beneficence and nonmaleficence are also thought to be available in both deontologic and utilitarian moral philosophies.[4]

ISSUES OF CLINICAL DECISION MAKING
The Provider-Patient Relationship
Self-Determination

Strictly speaking, autonomy refers to the potential for the individual to be self-determining. Self-determination is, in this line of thinking, regarded as a good thing in itself and also as a means to an end. It is the expression of an individual's personality. Self-determination is thought to be the best means of identifying an individual's best interest, a determination that involves the incorporation of the values of that person into a decision. This concept suggests that each individual is in the best position to assess aspects of decision making in the context of his/her own value system. In the clinical setting, self-determination is exercised through the informed consent process, which allows the patient to ultimately determine the most individually appropriate health care choice, based on his/her own values and preferences.[35]

Because self-determination is regarded as good, certain individuals may be obligated to foster another's self-determination if they have certain types of relationships with that individual. An example of such a relationship is that of the parent, who has a unique opportunity to help the developing child realize his/her individuality by helping to prepare the child to make his/her own choices. Choices are not thought to be truly the result of self-determination until they are considered judgments that encompass the person's reflective deliberation. It is implicit that these judgments would then also be authentic and reliable representations of that person's character and values.

The promotion of a patient's self-determination is a major responsibility, and it is not hard to see how many conditions could prevent its realization in the clinical setting.[24] One of these is the sense of vulnerability that can accompany illness. Physicians and other health care providers are in a very powerful position, either to exploit this sense of vulnerability or to reduce it and instead promote a feeling that the patient has some measure of control over the situation. Ensuring the patient's control would be a first important step in promoting the patient's self-determination. A second important step would be to help the patient identify his/her own authentic preferences among the diagnostic or treatment options available.

Confidentiality

Confidentiality is one of the pillars of the Hippocratic tradition,[21] and it is a fundamental concept that still forms an essential aspect of the physician-patient relationship.[26] While maintaining its strong theoretic basis, however, it is a concept under continuous assault in the clinical setting, where the computerization of previously confidential information, team coverage of patient needs, and the demands of third-party insurers have all converged to threaten this fundamental aspect of the bond between patient and provider.[40]

At its core, the concept of confidentiality means that all information that the patient shares with the provider during the course of being treated should remain private and confidential; it should not be revealed to those outside of the patient-provider relationship. The trusting bond and fiduciary nature of the relationship should allow the patient to feel comfortable revealing to the provider all information necessary to ensure a comprehensive understanding of the patient's circumstances and a correct diagnosis of the patient's condition, thereby fostering an individually appropriate care giver response. In turn, as a means to encouraging the patient to be forthcoming, the provider ensures that no one else will come to know this highly personal and perhaps embarrassing information. Currently, there are permitted "intrusions" into this relationship—for example, multiple caregivers who learn of the patient's circumstances in acute care settings or insurance companies who learn of the patient's condition to determine whether reimbursement is warranted. Nonetheless, the notion that those who do not need to know these intimate details of the patient's condition will not know is still an essential factor in the bond that ties the patient to the provider.

The costs of not guaranteeing confidentiality or breaching it when previously assured are significant both for the individual patient and for society at large. Patients who believe they cannot trust their providers and are therefore less than candid in their descriptions are likely to suffer the consequences of an incomplete assessment or even a misdiagnosis of their condition. They lose out on what their physician may have to offer.[6] As well, providers who breach their duty to keep information confidential fail in their ultimate obligation to act beneficently toward their patients and to do them no harm.[6] Moreover, society as a whole is not served well when individuals in need of medical care feel inhibited or are unwilling to seek out that care.

Our legal system has recognized the fundamental requirement of confidentiality between patient and provider.[26]

Under most circumstances, information that passes between patient and provider during the course of care is "privileged," that is, it is inaccessible in a court of law; a judge or jury will be unable to learn of it.[26] This special exclusion of possibly relevant information further ensures that patients do not feel inhibited when conversing with providers. Despite the essential drive in our court systems to bring out all possibly pertinent information in an individual case, society has nonetheless recognized that our interests as a whole are better served when patients and providers can feel assured that their discussions are private and confidential.

Nonetheless, there are certain circumstances where other societal interests are believed to outweigh the interests served by confidentiality. For example, in the midst of certain public health epidemics, where the obligation to protect the health of society may conflict with the desire to maintain individual confidentiality, there is a societal consensus that it is morally and legally justifiable to breach individual confidentiality under certain limited conditions.[26] One example are laws requiring the reporting of certain diagnoses to health departments[26] and perhaps the tracing of contacts who may have been exposed to an individual's illness. Another example concerns the need to protect the public from harm. Under the state's "police power," physicians have the obligation to report certain medical conditions, such as gunshot wounds.[45] A third example occurs with respect to the state's obligation to protect its most vulnerable members, also known as the state's *parens patriae* power, so that health care providers are routinely obligated to breach confidentiality and report instances of known or suspected child abuse.[26] While the circumstances permitting the breach of confidentiality are limited, it is clear that they represent instances where other significant societal interests make such a breach justifiable and even desirable, despite the potential harm that may befall an individual patient.

The Informed Consent Process

As has already been stated, the informed consent process permits the expression of individual self-determination in the clinical setting. From a legal perspective, this means that providers are obligated to disclose to patients all information that will allow them to arrive at an informed decision about their choices, including such information as the patient's diagnosis and prognosis, a description of the proposed intervention and its risks and benefits to the patient, and the existence of alternative interventions, along with their risks and benefits.[3] In some jurisdictions, there is the requirement that information "material" to that individual patient be disclosed.[3,9,11,46] This requirement might obligate the provider to disclose certain details he/she might not normally discuss under routine circumstances. Overall, it is essential that the physician provide information to the patient, so that the patient can then consider the options and select that choice which promotes the patient's best interests as the patient assesses those interests.

Philosophically, autonomy and its promotion both undergird and exert greater demands than does the legal doctrine of informed consent.[35] Indeed, one seminal philosophic account of the informed consent process exhibits a far more fully fleshed-out conceptual scheme than is found in the law (Box 34-1).[4]

Competence

The possession of sufficient capacity to either consent to or refuse a proposed intervention is obviously a "threshold" requirement in the informed consent process.[35] That is, only those patients capable of making health care choices reflective of personal values have the ability to give informed consent and be considered self-determining. Patients with impaired or lost decisional capacity are generally considered unable to integrate factual information with personal preferences and are thus viewed as in need of assistance or even protection from harmful choices through either the use of a surrogate decision maker or some other method of deciding on care.[35] It is therefore essential to consider how "capacity to decide" is to be determined in the clinical setting.

Strictly speaking, the word *competence* denotes a legal concept.[3] This means that only a court of law can determine whether to suspend the legal presumption of competency, which generally attaches to all who reach the age of 18. The legal presumption of competency enables adults to involve themselves in all fundamental activities of citizenship, including the ability to vote, to contract with another, to write a will, and to get married. It is an empowering concept, covering a range of activities in which the individual is presumed capable of participating. A judicial declaration of incompetency is generally intended to apply globally—that is, to formally disempower the individual in most, if not all, major aspects of controlling his/her life.[3]

The routine assessment of competence in the clinical setting usually has little connection with the sort of global assessment that informs a judicial determination. Rather, competence in this setting is generally judged in the context of whether the patient is capable of either consenting to or refusing a particular proposed intervention.[8] The determination is usually made by an attending physician, sometimes with assistance of a professional from another discipline, such as a psychiatrist.[26]

Competence to decide about medical treatment may call on various abilities, depending on the demands of the task at hand.[8,16] Yet there are some general abilities required in the process of becoming involved in treatment decisions. These include the ability to understand or appreciate the nature of various alternatives and their consequences as well as the ability to communicate a preference.[35] In reaching a personal preference, one must also be capable of reasoning and deliberation, the latter term signaling that this is a decision process in which the decision maker's own values are gradually brought to bear on the question.[35] Accordingly, too, the competent decision maker's values will be more or less stable and consistent over time; they will be values that the decision maker recognizes as his/her own.

Information

The patient with decisional authority (or the properly identified surrogate decision maker) is entitled to all the information available about his/her condition that would be relevant to making a decision about treatment. This not only includes known or estimated risks and benefits of proposed therapies and their alternatives but also the implications of having no treatment at all.[27] The free flow of information to the patient—however sensitively it may need to be conveyed—is obviously vital for a valid consent process. As well, for the provider to suggest an individually appropriate treatment course for that patient, the patient must be encouraged to communicate openly with the provider.[35]

It has already been mentioned that full information is one of the legal pillars of informed consent, the other being the free and uncoerced consent itself.[35] Exceptions to such disclosure do exist—namely the "therapeutic privilege," which permits the physician to withhold information from the patient or to seek consent from an appropriate surrogate—if the provision of such information would be so detrimental that the result would be counter-therapeutic and would bring about harm to the patient.[3] In fact, concern is often expressed, particularly by physicians in fields in which terminal illness is common, about the "inhumanity" of telling the patient the unvarnished truth.[32] It is important, however, to distinguish between the inherently unwelcome nature of bad medical news vs. information that might actually induce negative physical consequences in the patient. The vast majority of patients who have been surveyed desire to have information given, even if it foretells their coming demise.[18] In fact, the real need for the therapeutic privilege is quite rare if it is employed for its actual intent, rather than for the purpose of affording the physician the opportunity to avoid an admittedly difficult discussion.

▼

BOX 34-1
The Elements of Informed Consent

1. Competence (a threshold requirement)

Information Requirements
2. Information
3. Understanding

Consent Requirements
4. Consent
5. Authorization
Our interpretation of these elements may not in all instances be identical with Beauchamp and Childress.

From Beauchamp T, Childress JF: *Principles of biomedical ethics,* ed 3, New York, 1989, Oxford University Press.

While it is appropriate that information be imparted in a sensitive manner, imparted it should be, nonetheless.

At such times it might be tempting to speak first with, for example, the patient's adult child, to enlist his/her support before an encounter with an older patient. For several reasons, this temptation should be avoided. First, certain classes of patients, such as those who are elderly, are too easily stereotyped as unable to manage emotionally powerful information, even though they may be quite functional in other areas of their lives and lacking any psychiatric history relevant to this issue. Second, the information is, after all, confidential information. Because it is of more concern to the patient than to anyone else, he/she has the right to hear it first. Third, the misguided attempt to enlist the adult child's help could backfire in several ways. The grown child may not be prepared for the loss of a parent, may not enjoy the patient's confidence, or may even have a personal agenda that is in conflict with or opposed to the best interests of the patient. There is no barrier to asking the patient whether it would be desirable for the physician to have a conversation with a particular relative, whether privately or with the patient, so that all three can cooperate in planning for the patient's future. In the final analysis, however, the confidentiality of the patient must be respected.

Understanding

A somewhat different objection to the idea of the patient rendering informed consent is the argument that some medical decisions are so complex that the lay patient cannot be expected to understand their components, thus calling into question the entire foundation of the informed consent concept. Clearly a medical school education should not be a prerequisite for a workable consent process; fortunately, that is not required. Some patients will benefit from a technical presentation of their situation, but that is not necessarily required for the consent process to be valid. Information should be conveyed to patients so that they will clearly understand how the proposed or available options will affect their lives; patients should be able to clearly articulate and understand the risks and benefits of choices as they concretely pertain to that individual lifestyle and preferences. Such an informing process is inevitably more satisfactory for both patient and provider when the informer knows the patient personally and understands the values that infuse the patient's life.[35] This is an admittedly difficult relationship to achieve, particularly for specialists who only briefly come to know the patient in the context of a specific acute situation. Nonetheless, a certain level of intimacy with the patient is essential to truly adhere to the principles that underlie the informed consent process and to help ensure that the patient truly understands the information of critical relevance to his/her personal decision.[3]

Clinically, there are certain factors inherent in both the patient's condition and the environment of care that may lessen or even prevent the patient from understanding the information conveyed, no matter how precisely or sensi-

tively it has been imparted. For example, a provider may be unsure whether a patient in an intensive care unit who has been sedated for pain relief can understand sufficiently to engage in informed consent. As well, the distracting machinery of the environment or the disrupted schedule to which patients must conform also work against full comprehension and understanding on the patient's part. It is incumbent on the provider to do all that is possible to lessen or even remove impediments that prevent the patient from fully participating in an informed consent process. Such actions might include temporarily moving a patient to more private or serene quarters to carry on a conversation, or perhaps lessening a dosage of pain medication so that, while less comfortable, the patient may nonetheless better comprehend and consider the choices that lay before him/her. As well, the physician should be satisfied that there is no metabolic basis (such as a toxic reaction to new medication) for the patient's lack of understanding.

Consent

Consent refers to the voluntary and uncoerced agreement of the patient. Consent is a more active process than mere assent or dissent. Ideally, it implies deliberation and perhaps also reflection based on one's own values. Obstacles to truly reflective consent in the hospital include such previously cited factors as the physical conditions commonly associated with treatment for acute illness and the disorientation imparted by impersonal hospital routines and protocols. For example, mechanical restraints may be used for legitimate or illegitimate purposes, but it is certain that they compromise the sense of control and voluntariness that enables a person to make well-considered choices.

Other sorts of constraints on the patient may be more subtle but no less undermining. Examples range from pressures associated with familial dynamics to concern with the financial consequences of one alternative as compared with another. In extreme circumstances the physician may be justified in assuming an active role as patient advocate in attempting to determine whether a stated choice is truly what the patient would want for himself/herself, or whether it is reflective of certain pressures inflicted on the patient.

Authorization

An action is authorized when the individual with the appropriate authority gives approval. In accordance with the previous discussion, this will be either the patient or some appropriately appointed representative of the patient. In certain circumstances—such as when an incompetent patient requires emergency care—the requirement for authorization is usually suspended because the immediate needs of the patient are felt to be so critical that time cannot be expended locating someone other than the patient to provide authorization.[26] In true emergency situations, when a patient's background is unknown (i.e., providers are not aware of any previously expressed wish on the patient's part to decline the type of care about to be provided) and care must be provided immediately to avoid irreparable harm to the patient, the requirement for authorization is generally waived.[26] In such cases, there is a legal presumption that (1) reasonable persons would consent to such necessary care, (2) there is no reason to believe this patient would refuse the proposed care, and (3) the time needed to locate an appropriate surrogate might otherwise jeopardize the patient's condition.[3] Such a suspension of consent is temporary, however, because if the patient should subsequently regain capacity, or an appropriate surrogate later becomes identified, then, of necessity, authorization would have to be obtained for any future interventions.

In a system preoccupied with documentation and record keeping, the signed consent form—presumably giving authorization—has tended to substitute for the consent process itself.[3] Of course, a form that purports to represent an actual event (that of informing the patient) but does not is neither ethically nor legally valid. Similarly, verbal consent without a form signed by the patient or surrogate may be valid although obviously documentation of one kind or another is usually advisable (though sometimes not possible).[2] Of overall importance, of course, is the dialogue that supports the documentation and that the consent form theoretically reflects.

Decision Making for Incapacitated Patients
The Importance of Prior Discussions

There is perhaps no more common remark about the medical profession in the modern world than that some of the physician's traditional "art" has succumbed to a preoccupation with applied science. Patients are often examined more in terms of their discrete diseases requiring investigation and intervention than as suffering individuals who face the dilemmas and perhaps deterioration brought on by medical crises. Whether this criticism is fair or even historically accurate, it is hard to dispute the concept that a great many of the dilemmas arising out of confusing treatment circumstances could be ameliorated if the wishes of the patient were expressed and discussed with the physician before the patient's loss of capacity.[31] Admittedly, given the fact that many people in our health care system do not have regular contact with a physician before the onset of serious illness, the opportunity for such ongoing discussions will not be available to everyone.[30] In addition, because few physicians are specially trained to undertake such intimate and personal discussions and because such discussions often require a significant amount of (unreimbursed) time, modern conditions for providing care are often not hospitable to fostering this kind of dialogue.[30]

Still, conversations with patients by either primary care physicians or specialists who have ongoing relationships with the patient provide excellent occasions for the practice of what is known as "preventive ethics." Properly conducted and documented, such conversations can provide critical guidance to—even if they do not determine—the nature of treatment for a patient who is no longer cogent.

The point of such information gathering is not merely to relieve the professional of legal liability. Rather, when physicians discuss preferences in advance, they are acting in a respectful manner that the vast majority of patients appreciate. These discussions permit the patient to maintain control and self-determination, despite any future loss of capacity, which may render the patient nonautonomous.[7]

Advance Directives and Proxy Appointments

Because patients' prospective treatment wishes often involve matters of withholding or withdrawing life-sustaining treatment and because of the potential for legal involvement when such treatment decisions are made, it is advisable that attempts be made to document these advance discussions. Such documentation is more likely to provide clarity in the midst of uncertainty or memory lapses and may also provide the type of legal evidence that may be necessary before life-sustaining care can be withheld or withdrawn.[31]

It is always wise that the medical record reflects the details of discussions between providers and patients, and specific mechanisms exist in most communities to highlight the nature of these advance planning discussions. Depending on the legal jurisdiction, patients and physicians have the opportunity to document such preferences via several methods. (Readers should consult their local medical society for the precise arrangements legally available in their own jurisdictions.) The two most commonly accepted methods for such advance planning documentation are the "Living Will"[31] and the "Durable Power of Attorney for Health Care," also known as the "Health Care Proxy."[31] Both mechanisms are used only if the patient loses the capacity to participate in the decision-making process. Both afford the patient and provider ample opportunity to specify particular wishes and preferences although the benefits of each method differ. Depending on patient circumstance, one method may be preferable to the other.

A living will is a document that patients execute before their loss of decisional capacity. The document serves to record for care givers and loved ones what the patient's preferences are about future treatment options, either in terms of treatment the patient would desire or treatment the patient would wish to be withheld or withdrawn.[27] Typically, such documents detail the types of interventions that patients wish to avoid as the end of their lives approaches. Many states have specified the precise form and content such documents must follow to be legally binding; other states are generally more concerned with the clarity and the substance contained in the document.[27]

In general, when executing a living will, patients should be as explicit as possible, using precise language that is not susceptible to differing interpretations or misunderstanding. For example, language discussing "heroic" or "extraordinary" care might have different meanings to different interpreters. If a patient is specifically concerned about such potentially intrusive interventions as mechanical ventilation or artificial nutrition and hydration, then it is wise for the patient to state such precisely.[27] It would also be advisable for patients to specify the precise physical circumstances under which they would want to trigger such withholding or withdrawal.[27] For example, they should make clear whether they desire that permanent loss of consciousness or unremitting pain be present before treatment is withheld or withdrawn. The average lay person would of necessity need the input of a medical provider, both in terms of deciphering what future options may face the patient and in determining the benefits and burdens of each option.

Even the most precise and specific living will may not cover every possible option that may confront the incapacitated patient; in addition, certain decisions may not be discernable from the contents of the document.[17] Written documents are also only helpful if they are available (as opposed to being locked away in a drawer) and actually enforced. Therefore many individuals choose to accompany or even replace their living wills with a durable power of attorney for health care or health care proxy.[2] Such a mechanism allows the patient (known as the principal) to legally empower another individual to make whatever treatment decisions the patient would have made had the patient had capacity.[30] Such a mechanism ensures that a vocal advocate will be legally available to assert the patient's prior wishes and also permits flexibility and interpretation should a situation arise that the patient had not previously addressed.[30]

Surrogate Decision Making: Who Decides and on What Basis?

Surrogates or agents specifically appointed by the patient in advance usually have the moral and legal authority to substitute for the patient if the patient becomes incapacitated.[30] Depending on the jurisdiction, legally binding mechanisms can be used before the loss of capacity. In some circumstances, court appointment of a surrogate may be necessary.[26] In some jurisdictions, the fact of biologic or spousal connection may be sufficient to both morally and legally empower the surrogate, regardless of a lack of a previously executed document or the lack of court involvement.[26]

Once an appropriate surrogate becomes identified, that person then has the responsibility to determine the best course of action for the now-incapacitated patient. Just as for the patient, so too would it be essential for the surrogate to go through an "informed consent" process with the patient's providers to ascertain all of the clinically relevant details necessary to understanding the patient's circumstances.[3] However, as has already been made clear, such decisions clearly extend beyond the realm of medicine and usually involve value judgments that the patient brings to the process. When a surrogate substitutes for the patient, the ideal method of decision determination is to consider and account for those values which defined the patient while capable, infused that patient's actions, and determined the patient's lifestyle.[30] What is ideally required is that the surrogate render a "substituted judgment" on the patient's be-

half, making the same sort of choice the patient would have had he/she had the capacity to participate.[30] Admittedly, this is no easy task, although the existence of a well-documented advance directive usually provides the surrogate with the type of information necessary to render such a judgment. In some circumstances, the surrogate may have to interpret or surmise what the patient would have wanted, based upon the surrogate's knowledge of the patient as a person and how he/she lived his/her life.[31] It should be noted that in some jurisdictions, such surrogate "interpretations" may not be legally acceptable, depending on the nature of the surrogate appointment and the clarity of the patient's previously expressed wishes.[30]

If such a substituted judgment is not possible, either because the surrogate has insufficient knowledge of the patient as a person or because whatever knowledge is available sheds little light on the current choice at hand, the surrogate would then be morally obligated to make that choice which promotes the patient's "best interests."[4] This judgment is meant to incorporate considerations of a more "objective" nature, such as patient prognosis, patient pain and suffering,[34] and the patient's present and projected quality of life, relative to the life the patient previously experienced, rather than a derogatory evaluation of personal worth in comparison with other members of society.[27] In most circumstances, particularly those involving decisions to withhold or withdraw life-sustaining treatment, surrogates work with providers to determine the patient's best interests in light of what can be done for the patient's current situation, the patient's underlying health and prognosis, and the burdens the patient may experience as a result of any measurable benefits to be achieved.[34] It is necessary to note again, however, that in certain jurisdictions the legality of such judgments may be challenged and that there is always a concern about bias or prejudice when discussions about "quality of life" emerge.[4]

Particularly when discussion of the patient's best interests focuses on what treatments might be "futile" and in no way beneficial to the patient, there is the potential for tremendous discord, because the precise meaning of the concept of "futility" may change, depending on the specific orientation of the decision maker.[19] For example, clinicians may view a course of treatment as "futile" if it does nothing to address the underlying condition that forms the subtext of the patient's current situation.[39] Yet others may regard "futility" as only apparent if no measurable benefit of any sort can be derived from a particular intervention.[31] In terms of the best interests standard, those cases embarking on the most controversial of courses and those in which such fundamental terms are in genuine dispute are the cases most likely to find their way to a judicial arena.[1,20]

The Never Legally Competent Patient: Decision Making for Minors

For some incapacitated patients, there is little, if any, possibility of making the kind of substituted judgment discussed previously. That has to do more with the nature of the patient, rather than any judgment flaws on the part of the surrogate. In this category, two types of patients require specific attention: children and those adults who never possessed decisional capacity.

Children. By law and in accord with typical maturation and emotional development, children are generally incapable of participating in treatment decision making or of rendering informed consent or refusal.[31] They lack the judgment and cognitive skills to weigh risks and benefits, and they are usually unable to consider short-term burden for long-term gain. Further, their choices of values and priorities are in constant transition and are easily influenced.

In most circumstances, those under the age of 18 are considered legally incompetent to make health care decisions on their own behalf (although well-defined exceptions do exist in most jurisdictions, which relate to the specific life circumstance of the child in question and often hinge on the precise nature of the treatment involved).[26] Parents are the natural surrogates for their children, because they are considered uniquely capable and privileged to both influence their child's development and maturity and to ascertain what activities suit their particular child's best interests.[26]

As surrogates, parents cannot call on their child's background or lifestyle to form a "substituted judgment." The natural course of surrogate decision making is one that relies on evaluation of the child's best interests, and in such determinations, the parents are generally afforded significant latitude to discern the nature and course of their child's care.[31] When parental decisions stand clearly in contrast with promoting their child's health and medical well-being, others may be empowered to challenge the choice made by the parents.[26] For these reasons, should parental conduct appear concretely neglectful—or even abusive—of a child's needs, grounds might then be found to disempower the parents and allow others to decide on the child's behalf. Principled choices of parents—which they could assert for themselves, such as prioritizing religious faith above risk of death—are considered unacceptable when applied to the children of such individuals.[26] Therefore parents who subscribe to the Jehovah's Witness faith may refuse life-saving blood transfusions for themselves, but not on their child's behalf. Parental empowerment does not include the ability to risk death for a child who has not yet attained the capacity to choose such a course for himself/herself.[26]

Children who are on the cusp of capacity (i.e., those approaching the murky line that separates adolescence from adulthood) may in certain circumstances be considered to possess sufficient judgment to participate in the decision-making process.[26] Even if their consent is technically not required, from a moral perspective, their concerns and desires should warrant serious attention and play a significant, if not determinative, part in the deliberation process.[31]

The Never Competent. Decision making for patients who never possessed capacity is similar to the process described for children; an appropriate surrogate must decide on behalf of the patient, based on an evaluation of what promotes the best interests of the patient.[35] Those who are congenitally retarded or severely impaired for other reasons never had the opportunity or ability to develop a system of values and preferences, which could be used to direct the course of care despite the lack of capacity. Thus "substituted judgment" cannot be rendered on their behalf, because they never possessed the original judgment.[35] Rather, the needs and course of care for those never competent must be determined based on an objective determination of their specific circumstances. This includes an examination of their diagnosis and prognosis and the benefits and burdens to be achieved by the various options in terms of pain, suffering, palliation, extension of life and other determinable measures, and perhaps a consideration of their "quality of life," again in comparison to that which they previously knew, rather than some comparison based on a more functional person's perspective.[19]

Critical Care and End-of-Life Decision Making: Special Concerns

The circumstances that surround critical care and end-of-life decision making are often made more controversial and problematic for both patients and providers because of uncertainty about the moral and legal permissibility of certain actions or decisions. This is particularly so when death is a likely or even intended consequence of a choice. In addition, many philosophically-based terms are sometimes interjected into discussions without universal clarity or certainty about their intended meanings. So, for example, words such as "ordinary" vs. "extraordinary," or "withholding" vs. "withdrawing" sometimes conjure up misguided notions about what is or is not acceptable in the course of delivering patient care.[34] The unnecessary inclusion of confusing terms often serves to cloud the underlying reasons and justifications for choices made either by or on behalf of a patient.

For patients who possess decisional capacity, the choice of whether to initiate, withhold, or withdraw care is one solely within the ambit of the patient's value system. This is so, even if the likely or intended consequence of the patient's choice is significant harm or even death.[34] Despite the discomfort many providers have with this concept, it is one in accord with the moral and legal frameworks supporting patient autonomy. Thus a patient can decline the option of life-prolonging surgery, can ask for the withholding of mechanical ventilation should respiratory distress occur, and can even ask for the withdrawal or cessation of such life-prolonging measures as dialysis, artificial nutrition, or hydration (in most jurisdictions), as long as the patient possesses the capacity and information to assess the benefits and burdens of such choices.[19] It should be noted, however, that in some jurisdictions, such choices may nonetheless require a legal process to carry out the request.[26] This may stem more from concern about injecting safeguards into such decision processes, rather than any move away from fundamental moral or common law support for such patient decisions. Moreover, in most jurisdictions, such patient requests would be accorded respect even if they were transmitted through an appropriately executed living will or appointed surrogate once the patient loses decisional capacity.

Questions of whether there is any moral or legal difference between withholding or withdrawing care, whether the care involved is of an "ordinary" vs. "extraordinary" nature, or whether it is acceptable to omit an action that may lead to the patient's death, but not to purposefully act in such a way that may bring about death, raise concerns about word origins and their current meaning and significance in the context of care. Many of these terms—while perhaps drawing some useful distinctions in their earlier, theologic origins or perhaps pointing to areas that warrant additional attention—in and of themselves do not determine the morality or legality of the choice carried out.[34] For example, a provider who makes the distinction that "extraordinary" care may be withheld or withdrawn, yet "ordinary" care must be initiated or continued, tells us little about the precise nature of the care or its effect on the patient at issue.[27]

While in simpler times it was perhaps easier to distinguish what was ordinary from what was not, the sophistication of the machinery or commonness of its application in today's sophisticated acute care environment creates situations where what is appropriate for one patient may not be acceptable or even beneficial to another similarly situated patient. In such determinations, what becomes important is not what the care is labeled, but rather how it affects that patient and fits into the patient's perspective in terms of benefits vs. burdens.[34] One patient may believe the receipt of artificial nutrition via a gastrostomy tube is desirable and acceptable, whereas another may view this as extraordinarily burdensome and inconsistent with his/her view of what best suits his/her interests. Such different meanings between patients only serves to underscore how physicians and patients may view decision choices very differently. Providers should not presume that patients consider a certain course of care in a way similar to the provider's perspective.[4]

Similarly, attempts to explain omissions or withholdings as being morally or legally permissible and actions or withdrawals as impermissible only serve to confuse and distort the reasons and justifications that will make such choices either permissible or not. Merely because a provider decides not to initiate a process does not necessarily relieve that provider of responsibility if the outcome was one intended or foreseen.[27] This is particularly so in the context of patient-provider relationships, where the provider owes duties to the patient and decisions not to act may be as influential and responsible for patient outcomes as any concrete activity that the provider undertakes. For example, a decision to withdraw artificial ventilation from a patient—which may or may not bring about the patient's death—is not necessarily any less permissible or unacceptable than the choice

to omit or withhold its use in the first place. While some may believe a distinction exists between an act that is believed to cause the death of the patient and one that merely holds back a possibility from an already dying patient, in fact—from a moral and legal point of view—arguments used to withhold treatment should be equally justifiable and binding as decisions to withdraw or cease.[19] Judicial decisions that have addressed this matter concur that no logical distinction exists.[19]

A decision not to initiate care can be viewed as just as "causative" in terms of patient outcome as any act of withdrawing, if the outcome was one that was foreseen and could have been avoided if a different choice was made. What is important in such circumstances is not so much whether one is acting or omitting or withholding or withdrawing, but rather why one is undertaking that course and whether it can be justified in terms of patient preference or the best interests of the patient as determined by an appropriate surrogate.[31] Moreover, many commentators have made clear that decisions not to initiate care because of fear that once started, a treatment cannot later be stopped may in fact work to harm certain patient populations.[27] Some patients might stand to benefit from a trial of therapy, although it may later be determined that the therapy no longer serves the patient's interests and should be withdrawn in the name of beneficence, nonmaleficence, or patient autonomy. Not to have tried an intervention for fear of not being able to stop lacks logic and defies the nature of providing medical care, which often means that certain risks are undertaken for certain potential benefits. One must always remember the provider's duty to relieve pain and suffering and not to cause harm to the patient.[27]

Nonetheless, certain actions on the part of providers and requests on the part of patients do trigger additional scrutiny and other societal interests that may take priority over a pure vision of patient autonomy or provider beneficence. For example, societal interests in the sanctity of life and concern for the prevention of suicide are generally used to deny support for patient requests of suicide assistance[19] or for provider services to purposefully administer a medication or other intervention for the purpose of causing the patient's death (what is sometimes known as "active euthanasia").[19] While much sympathy is generated for the plight of desperately ill patients seeking relief from their terminal conditions and often grand jury investigations of such matters fail to indict involved parties,[27] there currently still exists strict theoretic sanctions and prohibitions on provider involvement in such cases, despite the growing public discussion concerning this matter.

The debate centers around the precise role of the physician and the nature of physician-patient relations in an era of such sophisticated and often ambiguously successful care, when it is difficult to discern whether an intervention benefits or burdens a patient. Some argue that supporting physician involvement in the intended death of a patient destroys the essential role of the provider as healer and would create an air of uncertainty that would ultimately damage the trust that exists between patient and provider.[33] Others believe that one essential role of the modern physician is relief of suffering, and the possibility of such physician involvement might encourage otherwise desperate patients to try one more round of therapy or intervention, comforted by the knowledge that failure would not lead to unremitting pain or unendurable misery.[33] The debate has intensified[33] and is now the focus of increasing public policy attention,[19] with many states considering legislation in this area. The future may lead to a shift in societal consensus about how to prioritize values when fundamental questions about the meaning of life and death are at issue.

It should be made clear that all judicial decisions that have examined cases of the withholding or withdrawal of patient care have distinguished such circumstances from cases of active euthanasia or other forms of killing or suicide.[27] No physician who has participated in treatment decisions to withhold or withdraw care has ever been found criminally liable and responsible for the patient's death.[27] Cases of assisted suicide and euthanasia have been distinguished based on the nature of the patient's prognosis and clinical circumstances. Patients who refuse care or ask for its withdrawal and who will then die from their underlying conditions are not considered to be committing suicide, nor are providers who respect such decisions considered to be assisting suicide or killing the patient.

One final distinction deserves examination: the administration of pain relief with the knowledge, though perhaps not the intent, that such medication may ultimately shorten the patient's life or even cause the patient's death. Under the theologic doctrine of "double effect," such action is usually explained and justified by referring to the primary effect and intent of the action, that of relieving pain, while recognizing the possibility or even likelihood that another effect, that of the patient's shortened life or even death, is a possible result of the action.[4] The action is considered permissible because the intent was to relieve suffering, not cause death.

Theoretically, in current legal climates, the knowledge that an outcome is possible—though not necessarily intended—might still lead to liability on the part of the provider.[34] However, the authors know of no successful litigation against a provider for administering pain relief to a patient with significant need, even if the outcome of the relief also meant an earlier death for the patient. Justification for such actions are usually, in current climates, based on either patient choice to risk death to achieve pain relief (or a similar decision by an authorized surrogate) or on the widely recognized additional role of the provider to relieve pain when possible. Such provider actions are generally distinguished in legal forums from more common examples of "active euthanasia."[17] In fact, many commentators have suggested that it would be unusually cruel and harmful to a patient to respect their wish that care be withdrawn or withheld, yet not provide them with pain medication to ease their transition to death.[34]

Treatment Decisions Requiring Special Attention

DNR (Do Not Rescucitate) Orders

Decisions as to whether to attempt rescucitative measures in the event that a patient experiences a cardiac or pulmonary arrest should theoretically be no different from other patient treatment choices. Ideally, a provider would discuss the possible options and their risks and benefits with the patient in advance of any intervention, so that a decision to initiate cardiopulmonary resuscitation (CPR) would reflect patient desire that the provider intervene in such circumstances.

However, the reality and mythology that has developed around acute care decisions to rescucitate or to not rescucitate a patient has, for several reasons, brought this particular treatment situation into a different category. CPR protocols for the restoration of oxygenation and circulation have been remarkably successful, both in terms of their standardization (by the National Research Council in 1966) and their public acceptance: by 1977 more than 12 million people had been trained in CPR.[15] Second, because the use of CPR is often brought on by emergency circumstances, there may have been no prior discussion of patient preference and often no knowledge of the patient at all. Third, decisions not to resuscitate require consent not to intervene, which stands in contrast to the normal situation of consent to intervene in a particular circumstance. DNR orders require a conscious and perhaps courageous effort on the part of a team to recognize before a catastrophic event the inevitability of its occurrence and the likely outcome of intervention. Such forethought must happen in a climate that does little to foster discussion of death and does much to encourage the escalated use of sophisticated acute care technology merely because of its existence, rather than because of its likely benefit.

While in one state (New York), legislation exists to actually define the legal parameters of DNR orders,[29] in most jurisdictions the use of such orders must of necessity become one more familiar and comfortable process for those who frequently confront patients in the midst of an arrest. Just as with any other treatment decision, the ethically preferable process for making the DNR decision would be to undergo an informed consent process with the patient or, if incapacitated, with an appropriate surrogate. In the course of such discussion, it would be incumbent on the provider to disclose the likelihood and definition of "success" for a person in this particular patient's circumstances and would as well require a thorough discussion of all possible aspects of the intervention, including the possibility of connection to a ventilator or injury resulting from the aggressive nature of some resuscitative attempts.[34] While it is true that many patients unexpectedly have an arrest, other patients are likely to fall into a category of arrest "suspects"; their clinical condition would dictate that a discussion of DNR, among other possible treatment interventions, would be mandatory as early into their hospitalization as possible.[17] The goal is to solicit patient input and foster self-determination before the patient loses the capacity to participate in the decision-making process.

Ideally, advance discussions of DNR orders would come in the context of a more general discussion of future treatment options for a person in this patient's condition. However, that does not always happen, and it is possible that permission will be given to place a DNR order in the patient's chart, yet the patient or the surrogate will nonetheless insist on other types of aggressive care that may seem inconsistent with the decision to consent to a DNR order. Such inconsistency may be due to a lack of mutual agreement or understanding about the goals of the treatment process; it may also be the result of a reasoned decision on the part of the patient or surrogate that some interventions are worth certain risk, whereas others are not.[34] For example, a patient may be willing to undergo the toxic side effects of aggressive, experimental chemotherapy or the bruising recovery that may follow significant surgery, yet be unwilling to risk the possibility of winding up on a ventilator as a result of a resuscitation attempt. From the patient's or surrogate's perspective, such choices may not appear inconsistent, although providers would be wise to have the patient or surrogate vocally express reasons for the specific treatment choices made so as to ensure that there is full understanding and comprehension on the part of both the patient and the provider.

Of particular concern and difficulty are surgical candidates with preexisting DNR orders in place. Such patients typically have underlying chronic or terminal illnesses that provide the basis for the patient's previous decision to consent to a standing DNR order. However, there may be circumstances when such patients nonetheless become candidates for surgical intervention, perhaps for palliative purposes or for reasons unconnected to their underlaying disease process. In such cases, the decision as to whether the DNR order will remain in place during the surgical intervention should be thoroughly discussed by the patient, surrogate (if involved), surgeon, and anesthesiologist, if possible. Of critical importance for patients or their surrogates to realize is the distinct nature and characteristics of the cardiac arrest during the perioperative period. In particular, the fact that cardiac arrest during that period is often directly linked to either the surgical or anesthetic intervention, and that resuscitative interventions during such arrests have a very high success rate, must be made clear to a patient who seeks surgery for certain, specific objectives. In fact, for many providers, the concept of a DNR order during surgery seems incompatible with professional and moral obligations to a patient during the surgical procedure. The often direct linkage between the care giver's actions and the patient's arrest creates an inescapable obligation for many providers to intervene in the case of arrest.

An evolving approach to this difficult dilemma involves the protocol of "required reconsideration" whenever a patient with a DNR order in place becomes a candidate for surgery.[12,43] Such an approach demands active reconsideration of the DNR decision before the surgical intervention. Such discussion must necessarily involve the patient and the patient's surrogate, if appropriate, and should carefully review the distinct quality of perioperative arrest, as well as the goals of the patient for the surgical intervention. In most cases, an accommodation can be worked out whereby a temporary suspension of the DNR order is agreed on, with specific parameters set for its reinstitution, either dependent on the cause of the perioperative arrest or because of circumstances that arise after the patient's recovery from the surgical intervention. Such a protocol should reflect the patient's values and wishes to the extent possible. If an acceptable agreement cannot be worked out, the involved physicians may either have the option to proceed with the surgery, with a carefully delineated DNR order in place, or they may choose to decline to intervene, with the obligation to assist the patient in accessing other providers who may be willing to perform the surgery, despite the constraint of the existing DNR order.

Ultimately, when considering the applicability of a DNR order for a particular patient, one must remember that while the decision not to resuscitate might logically be accompanied by other choices about reducing the aggressiveness of care, this does not necessarily have to be so. A patient may logically, ethically, and legally desire intensive care intervention, yet be unwilling to be rescucitated should an arrest occur. Each type of intervention should be considered in its own distinct context, and the merits of any particular intervention should be judged on the patient's (or surrogate's) valuation of the risk/benefit ratio of the particular intervention.

Artificial Nutrition and Hydration

The use of artificial means to nourish and hydrate patients who are unable to take in food on their own has generated significant debate concerning definitions of "medical care" vs. "comfort care."[17] For many care givers, it raises the question of whether there are any limits to patient self-determination or provider obligations in the context of the physician-patient relationship. Many believe that it is permissible to withhold or withdraw "medical care" in accord with patient self-determination, whereas the provision of artificial nutrition and hydration represents the intrinsic "caring" nature of human interaction and therefore must always be provided as a fundamental demonstration of humanity and compassion.[25]

All courts of law that have addressed this question, including the United States Supreme Court, have equated the use of artificial nutrition and hydration with other medical technologies and have thus permitted its withholding or withdrawal in accord with the interests of patient self-determination.[13] Other groups have nonetheless made a clear distinction between such "high-tech" progenies as mechanical ventilation or dialysis and the provision of nutrients. In the political arena, some legislatures have even made exceptions to their living will or health care proxy legislation to make allowance for such a distinction[26] and, in some circumstances, to refuse to grant permission for patients or surrogates to have such care withheld or withdrawn.[26] Given the sometimes passionate nature of the debate, a compromise has been reached in many instances that recognizes both the right of individuals to determine the course of their care and the pluralistic nature of our society, particularly when providers feel unable to abide by such patient requests. This accommodation usually calls on either individual or institutional providers to disclose to patients and families, before the onset of a relationship, the perspective of the provider about this type of care.[31]

Dilemmas in Team Decision Making: The Role of the Anesthesiologist

In concluding this chapter, it is important to note that dilemmas in the clinical setting may emerge not only from interaction with patients and families, but also may arise in the relationships that are forged under a system of team coverage of patient care needs. Particularly for the neurosurgical patient—whose problems may span the disciplines of neurology, surgery, and anesthesiology, among others—the collection of providers who coalesce to meet the specific needs of an individual patient may generate interdisciplinary disputes, rivalry, or even antagonisms, which may subtly—or perhaps not so subtly—affect patient care. In this regard, we may briefly examine the role of the consultant anesthesiologist as just one example.

A cardinal rule of the Hippocratic tradition, which emphasized the appropriateness of calling in consultants, was that physicians were never to disagree with their colleagues in front of the patient.[21] In our own time, the notion of a "united front" before the laity has perhaps a greater command over medicine than in other professions, so that even when physicians are in substantial disagreement over the appropriate course, they rarely present their disagreement to the patient. Considering that the patient whose condition is serious enough to warrant consultation is often in an emotionally vulnerable position, this might not seem to be an unwise policy.

However, modern legal analysis and case law support the independent authority and responsibility of the anesthesiologist, separate and distinct from other members of the health care team. While the anesthesiologist may have little or no participation in the initial decision to intervene surgically, he/she does have separate responsibility to review the patient's condition and to obtain an independent informed consent directly from the patient or the patient's surrogate for the use of anesthesics. In effect, the anesthesiologist must review the feasibility of anesthetic intervention

for the particular patient and separately determine whether the surgery should proceed on the basis of this review. No longer are the actions or determinations of the anesthesiologist viewed as subordinate to those of the surgeon. The anesthesiologist has an independent duty to the patient, separate and apart from that of the surgeon or any other member of the care team. Such duty carries through the entire perioperative period, until such time as the anesthesiologist discharges the patient from his/her care.

▼

SUMMARY

Full and comprehensive care of the neurosurgical patient requires a thorough understanding of the ethical principles that guide the treatment decision-making process. Care givers must be sensitive to the right of patients to be self-determining and to participate in the treatment decision-making process to the extent possible. While decisional incapacity may render a patient unable to participate, the involvement of informed surrogates and the use of advance directives will help ensure that treatment decisions are in accord with patient wishes and values, even if the patient can no longer participate. It is essential to plan proactively for decisional incapacity through the use of advance planning mechanisms.

Particular problems may arise in connection with neurosurgical intervention, such as may occur when DNR orders are in place or the use of other life-sustaining measures create a dilemma. Clinicians must be cognizant of the autonomous rights of patients, yet patients and surrogates must also be informed of the unique and special characteristics of neurosurgical interventions, which may give rise to a reexamination of the reasons to withhold or withdraw life-sustaining treatments. Providers have a particular obligation to communicate such issues to patients. Anesthesiologists have separate and distinct obligations to the patient, including the obligations to interact directly with the patient, review the patient's readiness for anesthetic intervention, and monitor and oversee the patient's condition during the entire perioperative process in connection with the use of anesthesics.

Acknowledgements

The authors wish to thank Ho Jung Yoon for his research and editorial assistance with this manuscript.

References

1. Angell M: The case of Helga Wanglie—a new kind of right to die case, *N Engl J Med,* 325:511, 1991.

2. Annas G: *The rights of patients,* ed 2, Totowa, NJ, 1992, Humana Press, pp 92-93, 210-211.

3. Appelbaum P, Lidz C, Meisel A: *Informed consent: legal theory and clinical practice,* New York, 1987, Oxford University Press.

4. Beauchamp T, Childress J: *Principles of biomedical ethics,* ed 3, New York, 1989, Oxford University Press.

5. Beecher HK: Ethics and clinical research, *N Engl J Med* 274:1354-1360, 1966.

6. Brody BA, Englehardt HT: *Bioethics: readings and cases,* Englewood Cliffs, NJ, 1987, Prentice-Hall, pp 291-294.

7. Brody H: The physician/patient relationship. In Veatch R, editor: *Medical ethics,* Boston, 1989, Jones & Bartlett, pp 65-91.

8. Buchanan A, Brock DW: *Deciding for others: the ethics of surrogate decision making,* New York, 1989, Cambridge University Press, pp 17-84

9. *Canterbury v. Spence,* 464 F.2d 772 (D.C. Circ. 1972), *cert. denied,* 409 U.S. 1064 (1972).

10. Carrick P: *Medical ethics in antiquity,* Dordrecht, Holland, 1985, D Reidel Publishing.

11. *Cobbs v. Grant,* 8 Cal. 3d 229, 502 P.2d 1, 104 Cal. Rptr. 505 (1972).

12. Cohen CB, Cohen PJ: Do-not-resuscitate orders in the operating room, *N Engl J Med* 325:1879-82, 1991.

13. *Cruzan v. Director,* 110 U.S. 2841 (1990).

14. Declaration of Geneva, *World Med Assoc Bull,* 1:109-110 (1949).

15. Donegan JH: New concepts in cardiopulmonary resuscitation, *Anesth Analg* 60:100, 1981.

16. Drane J: The many faces of competency, *Hastings Cent Rep* 15:17-21, 1985.

17. Dubler NN, Nimmons D: *Ethics on call,* New York, 1992, Harmony Books, pp 173-175, 351-354, 357.

18. Harris L and Associates: Views of informed consent and desicion making: Parallel surveys of physicians and the public. In President's Commission for the Study of Ethical Problems in Medicine and Biomedical and Behavioral Research: *Making health care decisions, vol 2, appendices (empirical studies of informed consent)* Washington, DC, 1982, US Government Printing Office.

19. The Hastings Center: *Guidelines on the termination of life sustaining treatment and the care of the dying,* Bloomington, 1987, Indiana University Press.

20. *In re Helga Wanglie,* No. PX-91-283 (4th Judicial District Ct. Hennepin County, Minn., July 1, 1991).

21. Hippocrates: *Oeuvres completes d' Hippocrate,* translated by Littré, 10 vol, Paris, 1939-1961, Javal et Bourdeaux.

22. Jonsen A: Watching the doctor, *N Engl J Med* 308:1531-5, 1983.

23. Kant I: *Foundations of the metaphysics of morals,* translated by Beck LW, Indianapolis, Indiana, 1959, Bobbs-Merrill.

24. Katz J: Informed consent—a fairy tale? Law's vision, *U Pitt L Rev* 39:137-174, 1977.

25. Lynn J, Childress JF: Must patients always be given food and water? *Hastings Cent Rep* 13:17-21, 1983.

26. MacDonald M, Meyer K, Essig B: *Health care law,* New York, 1991, Matthew Bender & Co.

27. Meisel A: *The right to die,* New York, 1989, John Wiley & Sons.

28. Mill JS: *On liberty,* London, 1863, JW Parker.

29. New York State Public Health Law, Article 29-B (McKinney Suppl 1992).

30. The New York State Task Force on Life and the Law: *Life-sustaining treatment: making decisions and appointing a health care agent,* July 1, 1987, The New York State Task Force on Life and the Law.

31. The New York State Task Force on Life and the Law: *When others must choose: deciding for patients without capacity,* March 1992, The New York State Task Force on Life and the Law.

32. Novack DH, Plumer R, Smith RL: Changes in physicians' attitudes toward telling the cancer patient, *JAMA* 241:897, 1979.

33. Pelligrino E: Doctors must not kill, *J Clin Ethics* 3:98, 1992.

34. President's Commission for the Study of Ethical Problems in Medicine and Biomedical and Behavioral Research: *Deciding to forego life-sustaining treatment,* Washington, DC, 1983, US Government Printing Office.

35. President's Commission for the Study of Ethical Problems in Medicine and Biomedical and Behavioral Research: *Making health care decisions,* vol 1, Washington, DC, 1982, US Government Printing Office.

36. *In re Quinlan,* 70 N.J. 10, 355 A.2d 647, rev'g 137 N.J. Super. 227, 348 A.2d 801 (1975), *cert. denied,* 429 U.S. 922 (1976).

37. *Salgo v. Leland Stanford Jr. University Board of Trustees,* 154 Cal. App. 2d 560, 317 P.2d 170 (1st Dist.) (1957).

38. *Schloendorff v. Society of New York Hospital,* 211 N.Y. 125, 105 N.E. 92 (1914).

39. Schneiderman LJ, Jecker NS, Jonsen AR: Medical futility: its meaning and ethical implications, *Ann Intern Med* 112:949-954, 1990.

40. Siegler M: Confidentiality in medicine—a decrepit concept, *N Engl J Med* 307:1518-1521, 1982.

41. Starr P: *The social transformation of American medicine,* New York, 1982, Basic Books.

42. The National Commission for the Protection of Human Subjects of Biomedical and Behavioral Research: *The Belmont report: ethical principles and guidelines for the protection of human subjects of research,* DHEW Publication No. (OS) 78-0012, Appendix I, DHEW Publication No. (OS) 78-0013, Appendix II, DHEW Publication No. (OS) 78-0014, Washington, DC, 1978, US Goverment Printing Office.

43. Truog RD, Rockoff MA: DNR in the OR: further questions, *J Clin Anesth* 4:177-180, 1992.

44. United States Department of Health and Human Services: Protection of Human Subjects. *Title 45; Code of Federal Regulations,* Part 46: Revised as of March 8, 1983.

45. *Whalen v. Roe,* 429 U.S. 589 (1977).

46. *Wilkinson v. Vesey,* 110 R.I. 606, 295 A.2d 676 (1972).

Index

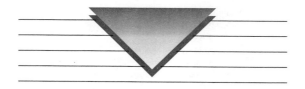